Operative
Obstetrics and Gynecology

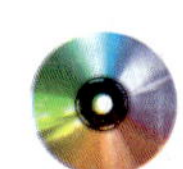

System requirement:

- Operating System – Windows XP or above
- Web Browser – Internet Explorer 8 or above, Google Chrome, Mozilla Firefox
- Essential plugins – Java & Flash player
  - Facing problems in viewing content – it may be your system does not have java enabled.
  - If Videos don't show up – it may be the system requires Flash player or need to manage flash setting. To learn more about flash setting click on the link in the help section.
  - You can test java and flash by using the links from the help section of the CD/DVD.

Accompanying CD/DVD ROM is playable only in Computer and not in DVD player.

CD/DVD has Autorun function – it may take few seconds to load on your computer. If it does not works for you then follow the steps below to access the contents manually:

- Click on my computer
- Select the CD/DVD drive and click open/explore – this will show list of files in the CD/DVD
- Find and double click file – "launch.html"

For more information about troubleshoot of Autorun click on: http://support.microsoft.com/kb/330135

Operative
Obstetrics and Gynecology

Second Edition

Editors

Narendra Malhotra MD FICOG FICMCH

Director, Malhotra Nursing and Maternity Home (P) Ltd
MD and Consultant, Global Rainbow Healthcare
Agra, Uttar Pradesh, India
Professor, Dubrovnik International University, Croatia
President, FOGSI 2008
Dean, ICMU 2008

Randhir Puri MD

WHO Fellow (Materno Fetal Medicine)
Gynecologist, Military Hospital
Belgaum, Karnataka, India

Jaideep Malhotra MD FICOG FICMCH

Director, Malhotra Nursing and Maternity Home (P) Ltd
MD and Consultant, Rainbow IVF
Agra, Uttar Pradesh, India
President, Elect ASPIRE 2010
Secretary, ICOG

Co-editors

Kavita N Singh

Professor, Jabalpur Medical College
Jabalpur, Madhya Pradesh, India

Parul Mittal

Consultant, Rainbow Hospital
Agra, Uttar Pradesh, India

Shobhna Mohandas

Consultant Gynecologist, Elite Mission Hospital
Thrissur, Kerala, India

Neharika Malhotra Bora

Assistant Professor, Bharati Vidyapeeth University
Pune, Maharashtra, India

Arun Nagrath

Professor, HOD and Dean
Rural Institute of Medical Sciences and Research
Safai, Etawah, Uttar Pradesh, India

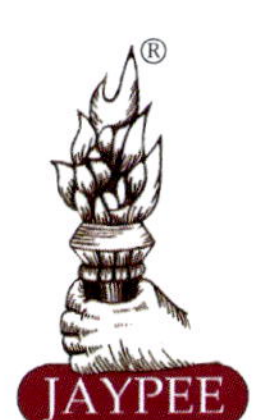

JAYPEE BROTHERS MEDICAL PUBLISHERS (P) LTD

New Delhi • London • Philadelphia • Panama

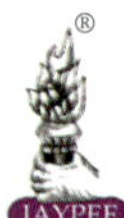

Jaypee Brothers Medical Publishers (P) Ltd

Headquarters

Jaypee Brothers Medical Publishers (P) Ltd
4838/24, Ansari Road, Daryaganj
New Delhi 110 002, India
Phone: +91-11-43574357
Fax: +91-11-43574314
Email: jaypee@jaypeebrothers.com

Overseas Offices

J.P. Medical Ltd
83 Victoria Street, London
SW1H 0HW (UK)
Phone: +44-2031708910
Fax: +02-03-0086180
Email: info@jpmedpub.com

Jaypee-Highlights Medical Publishers Inc.
City of Knowledge, Bld. 237, Clayton
Panama City, Panama
Phone: +1 507-301-0496
Fax: +1 507-301-0499
Email: cservice@jphmedical.com

Jaypee Medical Inc.
The Bourse
111 South Independence Mall East
Suite 835, Philadelphia, PA 19106, USA
Phone: +1 267-519-9789
Email: jpmed.us@gmail.com

Jaypee Brothers Medical Publishers (P) Ltd
17/1-B Babar Road, Block-B, Shaymali
Mohammadpur, Dhaka-1207
Bangladesh
Mobile: +08801912003485
Email: jaypeedhaka@gmail.com

Jaypee Brothers Medical Publishers (P) Ltd
Bhotahity, Kathmandu
Nepal
Phone: +977-9741283608
Email: kathmandu@jaypeebrothers.com

Website: www.jaypeebrothers.com
Website: www.jaypeedigital.com

Inquiries for bulk sales may be solicited at: jaypee@jaypeebrothers.com

Operative Obstetrics and Gynecology

First Edition: 2009
Reprint: 2012
Second Edition: **2014**

ISBN: 978-93-5152-161-7

Printed at Replika Press Pvt. Ltd.

Dedicated to

Teachers—for giving us wholeheartedly
Parents—for their affection and love
Family—for bearing with us for their valuable time and space
Last but not least
Our patients—for being edifice of our learning and their adulation

Contributors

Abha Majumdar
New Delhi, India
Chapter-43 (43.3)

Ajita Mandlekar
Mumbai, Maharashtra, India
Chapter-36 (36.1)

Alka Kriplani
New Delhi, India
Chapter-22

Alka Saraswat
Agra, Uttar Pradesh, India
Chapter-26

Anupam Gupta
Agra, Uttar Pradesh, India
Chapter-34

Anurag Gupta
Appendix-D

Aparna Hegde
Mumbai, Maharashtra, India
Chapter-3

Ariella J Setton
Chapter-42 (42.12)

Arun Tiwari
Agra, Uttar Pradesh, India
Chapter-52

Ashis Kumar Mukhopadhyay
Kolkata, West Bengal, India
Chapter-28

Ashwini Bhalerao-Gandhi
Mumbai, Maharashtra, India
Chapter-37 (37.7)

Atul Munshi
Ahmedabad, Gujarat, India
Chapters-40 (40.6), 41(41.3)

Avtar Singh
Punjab, India
Chapter-10

Barun Sarkar
Agra, Uttar Pradesh, India
Chapter-38 (38.4)

Bimal John
Kerala, India
Chapter-42 (42.4)

Bimal Mody
Mumbai, Maharashtra, India
Chapter-37 (37.7)

Ckumar
Chapter-12 (12.4)

Chandrawati
Lucknow, Uttar Pradesh, India
Chapter-39 (39.4)

CN Purandare
Mumbai, Maharashtra, India
Chapter-41(41.2)

Col Krishan Kapur
Delhi Cantt, New Delhi, India
Chapter-30

Paniel S Seiedman
Chapter-42 (42.12)

Deepika Deka
New Delhi, India
Chapters-31, 32

Devendra Gupta
Agra, Uttar Pradesh, India
Appendix-A

DK Tank
Mumbai, Maharashtra, India
Chapter-41 (41.9)

Duru Shah
Mumbai, Maharashtra, India
Chapter-42 (42.8)

Fessy Lauist
Chapter-42 (42.12)

Gautam N Allahbadia
Mumbai, Maharashtra, India
Chapters-2, 41 (41.7)

Geetha D Balsarkar
Mumbai, Maharashtra, India
Chapter-39 (39.6)

Gian Carlo Di Renzo
Germany
Chapter-41 (41.6)

Harshad Parasnis
Pune, Maharashtra, India
Chapter-41 (41.4)

Hemant Deshpande
Pune, Maharashtra, India
Chapter-25

Jaideep Malhotra
Agra, Uttar Pradesh, India
Chapter-39 (39.3), 50, 55

Jasleen
Patiala, Punjab, India
Chapter-38 (38.8)

Jayakrishnan K
Chapter-42 (42.12)

JD Tank
Mumbai, Maharashtra, India
Chapter-41 (41.9)

Kamal Gupta
Jalandhar, Punjab, India
Chapter-39 (39.7)

Kartik Bhagat
Mumbai, Maharashtra, India
Chapter-19

Kavita N Singh
Jabalpur, Madhya Pradesh, India
Chapters-13, 40 (40.2)

Kishore M Nadkarni
Vati, Gujarat, India
Chapters-51, 52

KK Gopinathan
Chapter-42 (42.12)

Kusum Gupta
Agra, Uttar Pradesh, India
Chapter-34

Lakhbir Dhaliwal
Chandigarh, India
Chapter-38 (38.6)

Lakhvinder Singh
Jalandhar, Punjab, India
Chapter-45

Madhu Nagpal
Amritsar, Punjab, India
Chapter-12 (12.3)

Madhuri A Patel
Mumbai, Maharashtra, India
Chapter-41 (41.2)

Mahendra N Parikh
Mumbai, Maharashtra, India
Chapter-1

Mala Arora
Mumbai, Maharashtra, India
Chapter-39 (39.5)

Mala Raj
Chapter-42 (42.1B)

Malini KV
Bengaluru, Karnataka, India
Chapter-37 (37.6)

Malvika Sabharwal
Delhi, India
Chapter-42 (42.2)

Manashi Ray
Chandigarh, India
Chapter-39 (39.8)

Mandakini Parihar
Mumbai, Maharashtra, India
Chapters-40 (40.5), 42 (42.9)

Maninder Ahuja
Faridabad, Haryana, India
Chapters-15, 16

MB Bellad
Karnataka, India
Chapter-40 (40.1)

Meenakshi Bharath
Bengaluru, Karnataka, India
Chapter-42 (42.9)

Michael Stark
Germany
Chapter-41(41.6)

Mitra Sexena
Rewari, Haryana, India
Chapter-21

Mohita
Agra, Uttar Pradesh, India
Chapter-24

Monesh Shah
Pune, Maharashtra, India
Chapter-50

Monica S Chauhan
Chapter-40 (40.2)

MS Agrawal
Agra, Uttar Pradesh, India
Chapter-27

MS Urala
Manipal, Karnataka, India
Chapter-38 (38.1)

Murad E Lala
Mumbai, Maharashtra, India
Chapter-37 (37.7)

Nandita Palshetkar
Mumbai, Maharashtra, India
Chapter-43 (43.2)

Narayan Jana
Kolkata, West Bengal, India
Chapter-28

Narendra Malhotra
Agra, Uttar Pradesh, India
Chapters-37 (37.2), 39 (39.3)

Neeta Singh
New Delhi, India
Chapters-23, 37 (37.3)

Nidhi Gupta
Agra, Uttar Pradesh, India
Chapters-10, 11, 23, 39 (39.7)
Appendix-D

Nikhil Datar
Mumbai, Maharashtra, India
Chapter-11

Nikhil Jani
Mumbai, Maharashtra, India
Chapter-42 (42.5)

Nikhil Purandare
Chapter-41 (41.8)

NS Sreedevi
Chapter-41 (41.10)

Nutan Agarwal
New Delhi, India
Chapter-31

Nutan Jain
Muzaffarnagar, Uttar Pradesh, India
Chapter-42 (42.6)

Pankaj Desai
Baroda, Gujarat, India
Chapter-25

Parimala Devi
Bengaluru, Karnataka, India
Chapter-40 (40.7)

Partha Guha Roy
Mumbai, Maharashtra, India
Chapter-29

Parul Mittal
Agra, Uttar Pradesh, India
Chapters-56, 56

PB Pai Dhungat
Mumbai, Maharashtra, India
Chapter-41 (41.7)

PG Paul
Bengaluru, Karnataka, India
Chapter-43 (43.4)

Phool Chandra
Patiala, Punjab, India
Chapter-38 (38.8)

PK Shah
Mumbai, Maharashtra, India
Chapter-3

PL Gautam
Punjab, India
Chapter-10

Prabha Malhotra
Agra, Uttar Pradesh, India
Chapter-37 (37.1)

Pranay Shah
Mumbai, Maharashtra, India
Chapters-42 (42.1, 3, 7, 10, 11), 43 (43.1)

Pratap Kumar
Karnataka, India
Chapter-42 (42.4)

Priti Kumar
Lucknow, Uttar Pradesh, India
Chapter-39 (39.4)

Rajalaxmi Walavalkar
Chapter-41 (41.8)

Rajni Sundar
Chapter-12 (12.4)

Rajyashri Sharma
Aligarh, Uttar Pradesh, India
Chapter-41 (41.1)

Randhir Puri
Belgaum, Karnataka, India
Chapters-5, 9, 14 (14.1), 33, 35, 37 (37.4, 5), 53

Reena Srivastava
Gorakhpur, Uttar Pradesh, India
Chapter-4

Reshma Rafi
Mumbai, Maharashtra, India
Chapter-49

Richa Saxena
New Delhi, India
Chapter-56

Rishma Pai
Mumbai, Maharashtra, India
Chapter-43 (43.2)

RN Goel
Appendix-C

Rooma Sinha
Hyderabad, Andhra Pradesh, India
Chapter-44

Sadhana Desai
Mumbai, Maharashtra, India
Chapter-29

Safala Shroff
Mumbai, Maharashtra, India
Chapter-42 (42.8)

Sandeep Agarwal
Agra, Uttar Pradesh, India
Chapter-48

Sandhya Gupta
Chapter-12 (12.1)

Sandro Gerli
Germany
Chapter-41 (41.6)

Sanjay Gupte
Pune, Maharashtra, India
Chapter-11
Appendix-B

Sanjay Sinha
Hyderabad, Andhra Pradesh, India
Chapter-44

Sarita Bhalerao
Mumbai, Maharashtra, India
Chapter-49

Saroj Singh
Agra, Uttar Pradesh, India
Chapter-24

Shailesh Kore
Mumbai, Maharashtra, India
Chapter-3

Shilpa Mangal
Mumbai, Maharashtra, India
Chapter-40 (40.5)

Shilpi Srivastava
Muzaffarnagar, Uttar Pradesh, India
Chapter-42 (42.6)

Shlomo B Cohen
Chapter-42 (42.12)

Shobhana Mohandai
Thrissur, Kerala, India
Chapter-42 (42.1B)

Shyam Desai
Mumbai, Maharashtra, India
Chapters-20, 42 (42.5)

S Inamdar
Appendix-E

SK Rath
Bikaneer, Rajasthan, India
Chapter-38 (38.7)

SN Daftary
Mumbai, Maharashtra, India
Chapter-18

Sonia Kamboj
Jalandhar, Punjab, India
Chapter-39 (39.2)

SPS Kochar
Pune, Maharashtra, India
Chapters-46, 47

S Singh
Agra, Uttar Pradesh, India
Chapter-38 (38.5)

SS Sheth
Mumbai, Maharashtra, India
Chapter-41 (41.5)

SS Trivedi
New Delhi, India
Chapter-38 (38.2)

Subhas Nargolkar
Pune, Maharashtra, India
Chapter-21

Suchitra Pandit
Mumbai, Maharashtra, India
Chapter-38 (38.3)

Sujal Munshi
Ahmedabad, Gujarat, India
Chapters-40 (40.6), 41 (41.3)

Sukhpreet Patel
Mumbai, Maharashtra, India
Chapter-42 (42.8)

Sukumar Barik
Howrah, West Bengal, India
Chapter-28

Sulbha Arora
Mumbai, Maharashtra, India
Chapter-2

Sumana G
Delhi, India
Chapter-22

Sumit Bansal
Agra, Uttar Pradesh, India
Chapter-27

Surveen Ghumman
Delhi, India
Chapter-39 (39.1)

Sushma Gupta
Agra, Uttar Pradesh, India
Chapter-54

Suvarna Khadilkar
Chapter-12 (12.2)

Swaraj Batra
Delhi, India
Chapter-38 (38.5)

Tamkeen Rabbani
Aligarh, Uttar Pradesh, India
Chapter-40 (40.3)

Tejshree Singh
New Delhi, India
Chapter-43 (43.3)

Tony Thomas
Kochin, Kerala, India
Chapter-43 (43.4)

Uday Thanawala
Mumbai, Maharashtra, India
Chapter-19

Umesh Gupta
Chapter-14 (14.2)

Usha R Krishna
Mumbai, Maharashtra, India
Chapter-36 (36.1, 2)

Usha Saraiya
Mumbai, Maharashtra, India
Chapter-49

Usha Sharma
Muzaffarnagar, Uttar Pradesh, India
Chapter-40 (40.4)

Vandana Walvekar
Mumbai, Maharashtra, India
Chapter-39 (39.6)

Veena Chandra
Champa, Chattisgarh, India
Chapters-6, 9, 14 (14.1), 35, 37 (37.4, 5)

Vinay Tiwari
Agra, Uttar Pradesh, India
Chapters-6, 7, 8

VL Lahiri
Agra, Uttar Pradesh, India
Chapter-39 (39.8)

Zehra Mohsin
Aligarh, Uttar Pradesh, India
Chapter-41 (41.1)

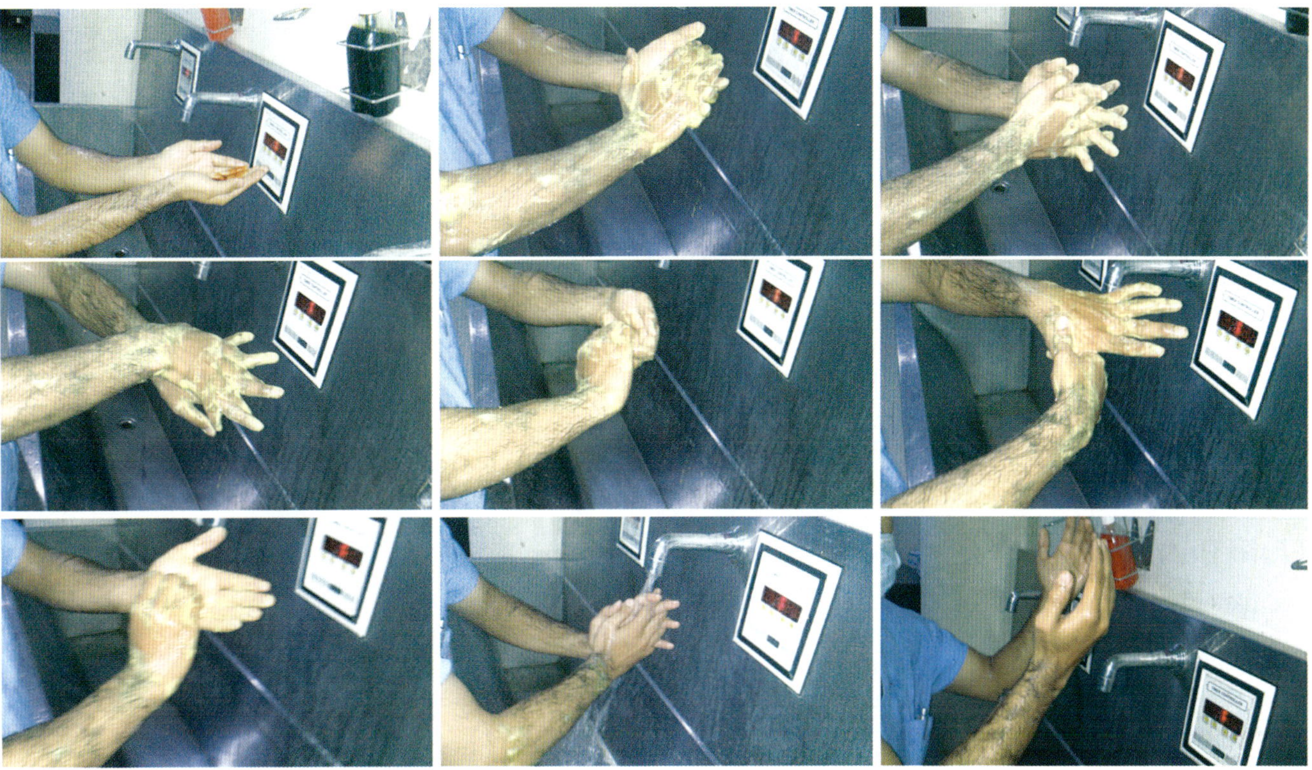

Fig. 3: Handwashing covering all surfaces from finger tip to elbow

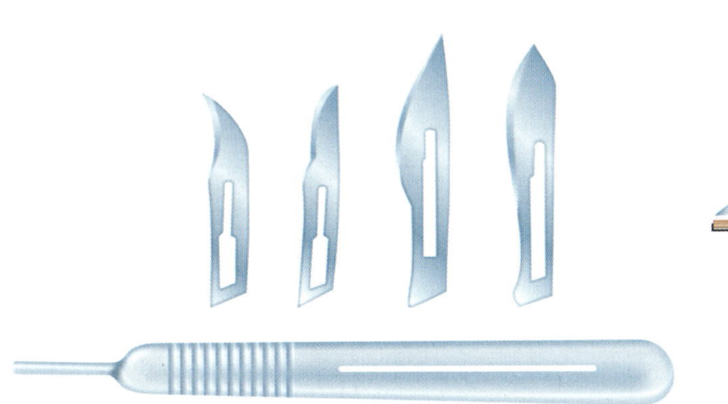

Fig. 4: Bard parker knife handle with different types of blades

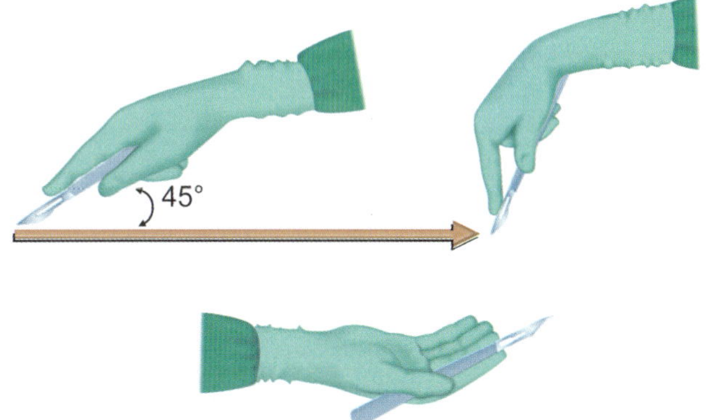

Fig. 5: Different knife holding positions

POSTOPERATIVE CARE

Environment

A postoperative patient should be provided with privacy for adequate rest, but at the same time, with all facilities for close observation by adequately skilled nursing staff round the clock.

Monitoring

Proper monitoring of the patient forms the bedrock of efficient postoperative management. It helps not only in preventing complications but also assists in early recovery. Monitoring would include evaluation of vital signs, catheter drainage including urinary catheters, nasogastric tubes and intraperitoneal drains, pulmonary and cardiovascular status, abdominal examination, and looking for vaginal bleeding.

Nutrition

In general patients undergoing elective gynecologic surgery have adequate nutritional stores and do not require nutritional support. However, all patients should have a nutritional assessment, especially those undergoing surgery for gynecologic cancer and other major gynecology procedures in which a prolonged postoperative recovery is expected. Weight loss, a serum albumin of less than 3.2 mg/dL (32 g/L) or a total lymphocyte count of less than 3,000 per μL may signify malnutrition and an increased perioperative risk. Dieticians should be available in ward. Also, associated medical problems like diabetes, renal diseases, etc. have to be considered so as to give the patient an ideal diet and proper recovery. Most patients following minor surgeries and hysterectomy would go on oral diet as soon as bowel peristalsis returns. However, in cases where oral intake is to be restricted for prolonged periods as in cases of surgeries for malignancies and those involving bowel, total parenteral nutrition may be required.

Fluid Replacement

For patients undergoing major abdominal and vaginal surgery, IV fluid replacement is required to replace blood and fluid loss and to allow for a period of decreased intake postoperatively. An average patient requires about 2.5–3 L of fluid per 24 hours. Proper management of electrolytes is also important in postoperative patients. Potassium loss may be increased by persistent vomiting and replacement should be made accordingly. In cases with high fluid loss, as in those with pelvic drains, long abdominal surgery, pyrexia etc., adequate replacement should be provided. Acute severe hyponatremia sometimes occurs following elective surgical procedures. It is usually due to the combination of appropriate postoperative stimulation of antidiuretic hormone secretion endogenously and injudicious administration of excess free water in the first few postoperative days. Totally sodium-free IV fluids (e.g. dextrose and water) should be given with great caution postoperatively, since occasionally the resulting hyponatremia can be associated with sudden death from a flaccid heart or with severe permanent brain damage.

Postoperative Analgesia

Satisfactory postoperative analgesia is easily achievable with currently available methods.

In cases of extended surgery, anesthetics and narcotics administered in epidural space are amongst the most potent analgesic agents available.

Nonsteroidal anti-inflammatory drugs (NSAIDs) are becoming increasing popular for postoperative treatment of pain. Long-acting preparations like diclofenac rectal suppositories provide very effective analgesia. Diclofenac skin patches are also available now.

Centrally acting opioid analgesics, like tramadol, work well in combination with NSAIDs to give pain relief.

Management of Drains

Drains are inserted in cases with risk of hemorrhage. In cases of abscess or drainage of hematoma, after lymphadenectomy drains may be kept for longer period, otherwise they can be safely removed after 24 hours, if loss is minimal (less than 30 mL per 24 hours) (Figs 6A and B).

Management of Urinary Catheters

Indwelling urinary catheters at the time of major pelvic surgery not only reduce the risk of bladder damage but are also important for the patients' comfort during recovery. Following uncomplicated surgeries, catheters should

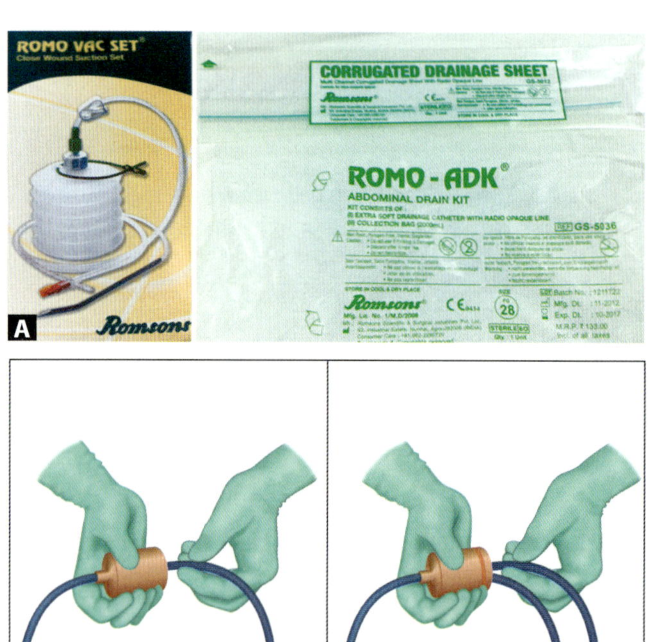

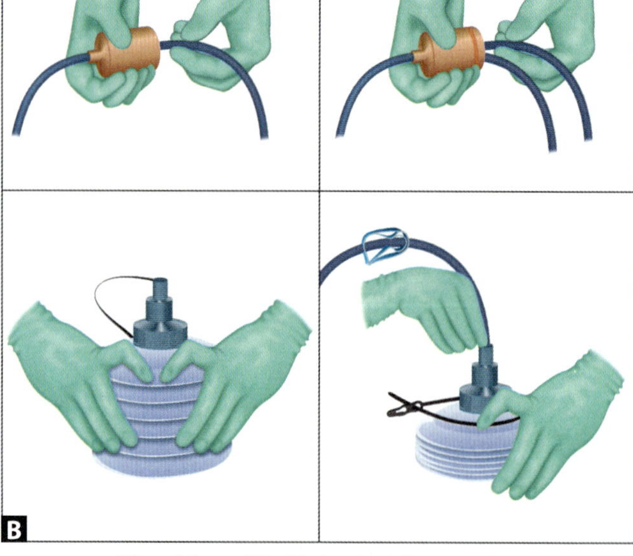

Figs 6A and B: Abdominal drainage kit

be removed as soon as patient is able to move. In cases where bladder has been injured during surgery, 7–10 days of in situ catheters is advised. Irrespective of the period of catheterization, care of the catheters is necessary to prevent infection and injury to lower genital tract. Simple measures, such as strapping the catheter to medial aspect of thigh, cleansing of vulva and catheter in proximity to vulva with antiseptic solutions helps in reducing chance of ascending infection.

Mobilization and Physiotherapy

Early mobilization is useful not only in reducing risk of thromboembolic disease and respiratory infection but also helps the patient to come back to normal activity as early as possible.

Physiotherapy plays a vital role in preventing complications and speeding recovery.

Wound Care

After wound closure a sterile dressing should be given which protects the suture line (Fig. 7). Suture removal for vertical wound should be delayed as vertical wounds may require 7–10 days to heal. A check dressing can be done on day 5 to look for edema, erythema, induration or discharge. If infection is suspected, wound swab is sent for culture and sensitivity, daily dressing and debridement is done. Appropriate antibiotic coverage should be given.

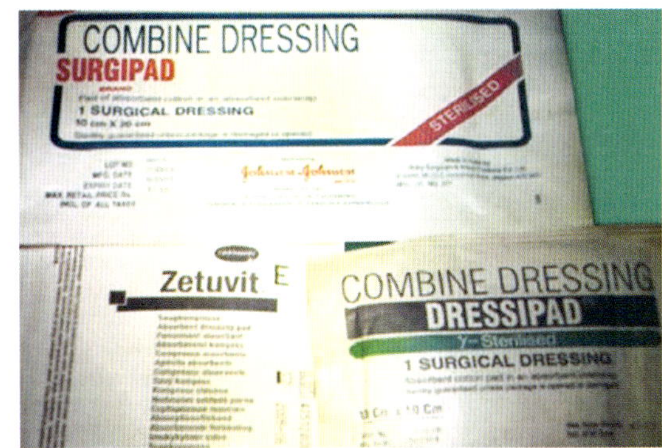

Fig. 7: Commonly used disposal dressing materials

Prevention of Bed Sores

Frequent change of posture, cleaning pressure areas such as sacral promontory, greater trochanter and heels with alcohol and keeping them dry with talc will prevent formation of bedsores. Care should be taken especially in patients requiring prolonged immobilization.

Psychological Care

Treatment of mind goes along with treatment of body. Providing a cheerful homely environment, giving time to hear patient's grievances and a few soothing words are of tremendous help in elevating patients' mood, which helps in early recovery.

BIBLIOGRAPHY

1. American College of Obstetricians and Gynecologists. Ethical dimensions of informed consent. Committee Opinion, No 108 Washington, DC: ACOG; 1992.
2. Brulicardi FC, Anderson DK, Billiar TR, et al. Swhwartz's Principles of Surgery, 7th edition. New York: McGraw-Hill Education; pp. 57-63.
3. Cain JM. Principles of patient care. In Berek JS (Ed). Novak's Gynecology, 13th edition. Lippincott Williams & Wilkins; 2002. pp. 21-30.
4. Eagle KA, Rihal CS, Mickel MC, et al. Cardiac risk in noncardiac surgery: influence of coronary disease and type of surgery in 3368 operations. Circulation. 1997;96:1882-7.
5. Goldman L, Caldera D, Nussbam SR, et al. Multifactoral index of cardiac risk in noncardiac surgical procedures. N Engl J Med. 1977;297:845-50.
6. Jewell ER, Persson AV. Preoperative evaluation of the high-risk patient. Surg Clin North Am. 1985;675:4.
7. Jonsen AR, Siegler M, Winslade WJ. Clinical Ethics. New York: McGraw Hill; 1992. pp. 5-61.
8. Karnath BM. Preoperative cardiac risk assessment. American Family Physician. 2002;95:21-6.
9. Norma V. Preoperative assessment of common diseases in the outpatient settings. Ambulatory anaesthesia. Anaesthesiology Clinical of North America 1996;14(4):631-8.
10. Rao MS. Morbid obesity-Anaesthesia management. Morbid obesity. 2003.
11. Sanford M. Markham, Rock JA. Preoperative care. In: Rock JA, Jones HW (Eds). Telinde's Operative Gynecology, 9th edition. Wolters Kluwer/Lippincott Williams & Wilkins; 2003. pp. 103-21.
12. Standards for the diagnosis and care of patients with chronic obstructive pulmonary disease. Am J Resp Crit Care Med. 1995;152(5):S77-121.
13. Townsend CM, Beauchamp RD, Evers BM, et al. In: Sabiston Textbook of Surgery: Biological Basis of Modern Surgical Practice, 15th edition. WB Saunders Company; pp. 1594-616.
14. Yamada D, Swietzer B, McHale MT. Preoperative assessment for gynecologic surgery. Contemporary OB/ GYN. 2005.

CHAPTER

4 Intravenous Fluids, Blood Products and Transfusion

Reena Srivastava

INTRODUCTION

Why do we need to learn and talk about intravenous fluids, blood products and transfusion separately in obstetrical conditions, especially during labor and surgeries? We all know that circulatory system undergoes a significant change in its structure and function during pregnancy and labor with more deviated adaptations during special conditions like pregnancy-induced hypertension (PIH) and intrauterine growth retardation (IUGR), diabetes, preterm labor, etc. So, requirement of intravenous fluid and transfusion have to be designed and matched with the changed physiological scenario of circulatory system during pregnancy and labor, otherwise instead of good we may do worse to the mother and fetus as well.

PHYSIOLOGICAL CHANGES AND ADAPTATION DURING PREGNANCY

Pregnancy is a state of hypervolemia. There is active retention of sodium, potassium, and water. But the increase is disproportionate, causing decreased sodium and potassium concentration and decreased osmolality. Total serum calcium is decreased, magnesium (extracellular) level is decreased, and phosphate is unchanged. Blood volume starts increasing from about 6th week to a maximum of 40–50% at 30–32 weeks. Plasma volume increases to a maximum of 50%, red blood cell (RBC) volume to the extent of 20–30% and total hemoglobin (Hb) is increased by 18–20%. The increase in plasma volume and RBC is disproportionate causing hemodilution. Near term, cardiac output is increased to 40%, stroke volume to 27%, and heart rate to 17% of the nonpregnant values. Blood pressure (BP) remains either unaffected or may show a midtrimester diastolic fall of 5–10 mm Hg. Venous pressure shows an increase of 100%; colloid oncotic pressure, a fall of 14%; systemic vascular resistance, a fall of 21%; and pulmonary vascular resistance, a fall of 34% near term.

These physiological changes undergo further change and adaptation in special conditions like PIH, heart disease, diabetes, etc., posing a further challenge to the obstetrician.

Fluid and Electrolytes in Normal Labor

With various physiological changes of pregnancy, the issues arising during labor have also to be addressed. During labor there is muscle exertion with increased demand of energy. The insensible loss through skin and lungs is more with significant hypotonic loss and the ability to excrete water is impaired. Forty percent of laboring women show positive ketonuria. If the labor is of normal duration these issues do not pose much threat, but same becomes more relevant in long and protracted labor.

How to maintain hydration during labor? What should be preferred—oral or intravenous route? Keeping the patient nil orally to avoid aspiration during anesthesia is not very valid now. Because if patient is kept nil orally the pH was found to be even less than 2.5 and increased gastric fluid volume, while if 150 mL of water is given 2 hours before surgery, gastric fluid volume is less than fasting. The study by Sleutel and Golden evaluated the risk of maternal mortality due to aspiration as 7 in 10 million births. Increased intravenous hydration showed less incidence of prolonged labor and less use of oxytocin than the group receiving limited fluids in labor. The recommendation is that oral fluid rich in carbohydrates should be given for quick energy and safe hydration, e.g. soups, fruit juices, electral powder solution because solid food specially rich in fat takes more time to digest, would not serve the quick requirement of energy during labor. When do we need parenteral infusion in labor?

Intravenous infusion in labor is required when laboring woman is disinclined to oral intake, there is repeated vomiting, dehydration of prolonged labor and special conditions. Selection of a proper intravenous fluid during labor is vital because the infusion used crosses the placenta readily and equilibrates with the fetal vascular compartment. Before recommending an intravenous fluid it is important to know normal water balance of the body (Fig. 1), composition, osmolality and metabolism of intravenous fluids for its final effect.

Various Intravenous Fluids

Crystalloid solutions (Figs 2A and B) do not stay in the extracellular compartment for long. Colloid solutions (Fig. 3) are large molecules, so are retained in the vascular system and are effective plasma volume expanders. The duration of effect is about 24–36 hours (Table 1).

Glucose solution metabolizes leaving back free water of zero osmolality to move to other compartments with high osmolality. So, it is not right fluid for hypovolemic shock. Infusion of more than 3,000 mL, 5% dextrose (D5) can cause maternal postpartum cerebral edema, hemolytic jaundice, and should be also dangerous for hypoxic fetus causing cerebral edema and acidosis.

Isotonic saline (0.9% NaCl) provides major extracellular electrolyte, maintains osmolality of extracellular fluid (ECF) and bring about increase in intravascular volume so is useful for hypovolemic conditions. But excess input may cause pulmonary edema in hypertensive, preeclampsia (toxemia) (PET), congestive heart failure (CHF), renal and liver diseases.

Dextrose saline provides energy as well as NaCl, maintains plasma volume, so given in hypovolemic shock with dehydration.

Ringer's lactate (RL) has an osmolality very close to plasma and almost similar to it in terms of electrolytes. It is very effective in severe hypovolemia and postoperative patients. It should not be given with blood transfusion as calcium binds with anticoagulant in blood.

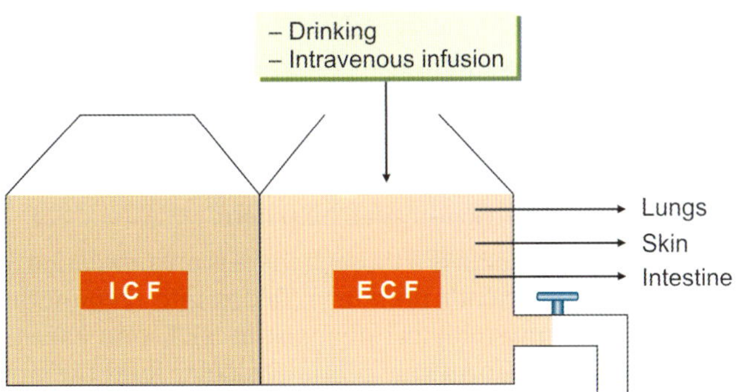

Fig. 1: Normal water balance

Isolyte G provides electrolytes lost by gastric juice and calories and corrects metabolic alkalosis.

Isolyte M is richest source of potassium so very useful in hypokalemia, supplies energy and corrects acidosis but to be strictly avoided in renal impairment.

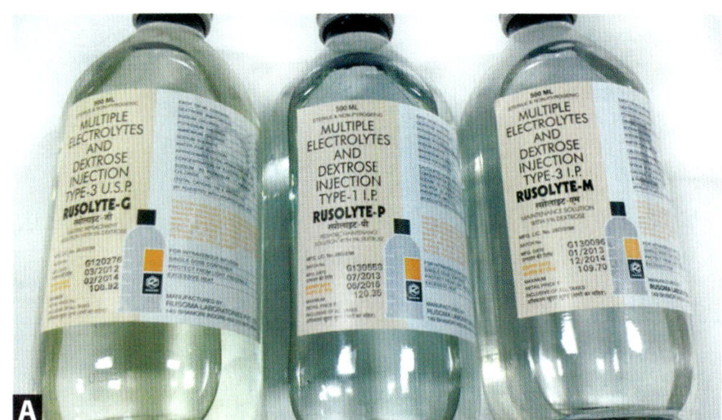

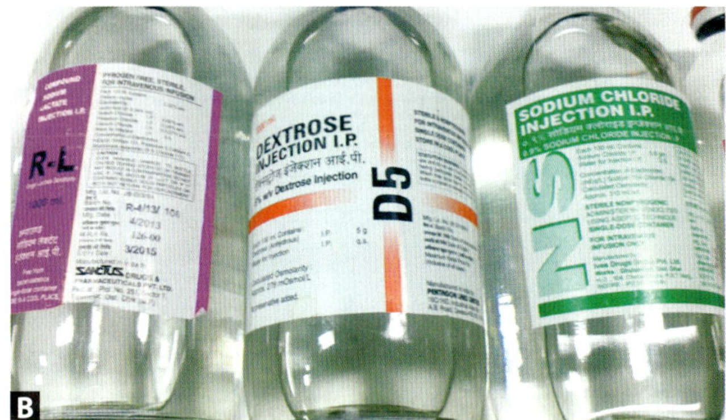

Figs 2A and B: Available bottled pyrogen free crystalloids fluids

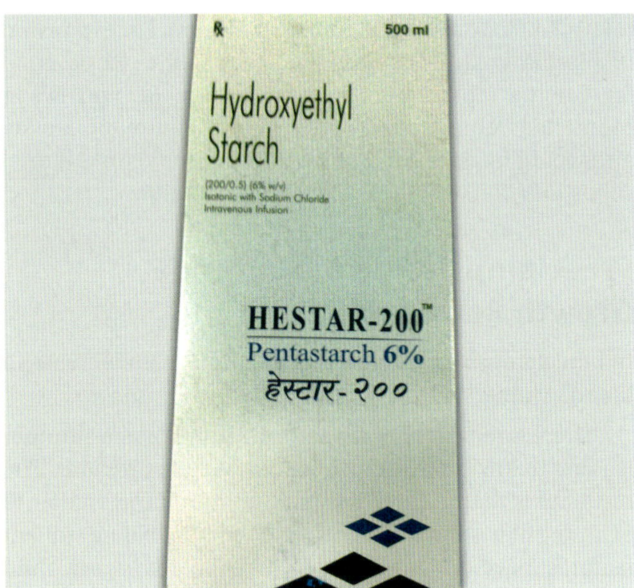

Fig. 3: Colloid fluids

Table 1: Composition and osmolality of crystalloids

	Dextrose	Na	K	Cl	Acetate	Lactate	NH_4Cl	Ca	Mg	HP_4	Citrate	mOsm/L
5% Dextrose	50	–	–	–	–	–	–	–	–	–	–	278
0.9% Saline	–	154	–	154	–	–	–	–	–	–	–	308
D-5%, 0.45% Saline	50	77	–	77	–	–	–	–	–	–	–	432
Dextrose saline	50	154	–	154	–	–	–	–	–	–	–	586
Ringer's lactate	–	130	04	109	–	28	–	03	–	–	–	274
Isolyte-G	50	63	17	150	–	–	70	–	–	–	–	580
Isolyte-P	50	25	20	22	23	–	–	–	–	03	03	368
Isolyte-E	50	140	10	103	47	–	–	05	03	–	08	595
Plasma osmolality												
Nonpregnant women	285 mOsm/kg											
Pregnant women	275 mOsm/kg											

Isolyte E is the only intravenous fluid, which helps in magnesium deficiency, provides energy water replacement, and corrects metabolic acidosis.

With the knowledge of various intravenous fluids, hemodynamics and circulatory changes during pregnancy and labor, we can now shape the recommendations in normal labor as well as labor in special conditions.

Normal Labor

The recommendations during normal labor is to allow the women to eat and drink in early labor and to switch on to oral intake of fluids only in active phase of labor. Intravenous fluids are usually not required in early phase of labor. In advanced labor, small amount of intravenous glucose can be given at a rate of not more than 6–15 g/hour (500 mL of 5% dextrose to run in 3–4 hours). For expansion of plasma volume choice is normal saline. RL is good for volume replacement in hemorrhage. RL and D5 in protracted labor could cause accumulation of lactate and would be harmful to the compromised fetus. Normal saline infusion would be safer in this situation.

Preeclampsia and Intrauterine Growth Retardation

In preeclampsia BP is elevated and there is no increase in blood volume.

There is renal leak of albumin and low plasma albumin leading to low intravascular colloid oncotic pressure. The resultant is that there is loss of fluid from intravascular to extravascular compartments and edema. Some salient features have to be considered while managing fluid therapy in PET, i.e.

- A reduced blood volume
- A low colloid oncotic pressure in the intravascular compartment
- More likely to suffer volume depletion in vomiting, hemorrhage and diuresis
- There might be damaged capillaries leading to extravasation of fluid
- There is sodium retention with an increase in total body sodium, but sodium restriction and use of diuretics can cause hyponatremia
- Sodium excretion is delayed to twice in the normal pregnant women
- Oliguria has to be taken into account. It may be associated with different subsets of pathophysiological changes.
  - If oliguria is secondary to hemorrhage there shall be low wedge pressure, moderately increased systemic vascular resistance, a low to normal cardiac output and hyperdynamic left ventricular function. Volume expansion will correct the situation
  - If oliguria is secondary to isolated renal arterial spasm there shall be persistent oliguria inspite of normal intravascular volume. These will have normal systemic vascular resistance. Diuretics will help in this situation
  - If oliguria is secondary to elevated systemic vascular resistance, there will be raised wedge pressure and low cardiac output. After load reduction and volume restriction shall help here.

Pulmonary edema is a threat if there is an imbalance of hydrostatic and oncotic pressures. Taking into account the various pathophysiological changes in PET, one cannot recommend a uniform rule of intravascular fluid therapy to all patients.

Recommendations for PET and IUGR

- Close monitoring of fluid intake and output and serum electrolytes
- Maintenance of crystalloid solutions (RL, normal saline) form is the mainstay of fluid therapy. They raise the cardiac output, lower vascular resistance and increase uterine blood flow. But the effect is short lasting and it is difficult to maintain central venous pressure (CVP) to 5–6 mm Hg as fluid extravasates to tissues
  - Hartmans solution (RL) 85 mL/hour
  - Any oral intake should be substracted from maintenance.
- A colloid infusion for volume expansion could be dangerous provoking pulmonary edema. A selective colloid expansion is useful in oliguria with low wedge pressure. If initial hematocrit is more than 35%, 500 mL of colloid can be given in 20 minutes then continue crystalloids with CVP measurement. Therefore, it has to be under care of intensive care management
- Oxytocin is advantageous because of its antidiuretic effect causing volume expansion but too energetic use can cause pulmonary edema, especially in oliguria
- Glucose infusion is not recommended because it can cause cerebral edema to these patients
- Use of diuretics can cause hyponatremia
- Only a 50% correction of sodium deficit is advocated as sodium excretion is delayed. Three percent of NaCl solution may be used
- A selective monitoring of CVP is required in cases of hemorrhage, oliguria, significant fall in platelet count, and liver tenderness
- Diuretics are recommended in pulmonary edema
- Cases of oliguria have to the managed according to CVP and urine output. Oliguria is defined as urine output less than 100 mL/4 hours. If CVP is less than 4 mm Hg, and there is no pulmonary edema, manage expectantly with fluid challenge. If CVP is greater than 8 mm Hg, careful assessment of pulmonary edema is required. If oliguria is persistent dopamine infusion (5 μg/kg/min) should be considered to enhance renal blood flow.

Induction and Augmentation of Labor

Oxytocin used for augmentation or induction of labor requires intravenous fluids as vehicle.

Oxytocin has an antidiuretic effect. When oxytocin infusion is prolonged and the infusion approaches 40 mIU/min, there is a dramatic drop in urinary output and may lead to water intoxication (retention of water and hyponatremia). Rapid intravenous infusion of oxytocin has been noted to cause severe maternal hypotension and electrocardiographic (ECG) changes of cardiac ischemia.

If a 5% glucose solution is used for oxytocin infusion, glucose gets metabolized leaving back free water causing hyponatremia. So glucose solution and oxytocin both would cause hyponatremia causing neonatal jaundice. The recommendation is to use normal saline as vehicle for oxytocin specially, if more than 500 mL of intravenous fluid is required. A concentrated solution and less drip rate would limit total fluid input.

Epidural and Spinal Analgesia

Epidural and spinal blockades cause chemical sympathectomy and can lead to hypotension. Infusion of 5% dextrose or dextrose saline did not decrease the incidence of hypotension. Rapid infusion of dextrose solutions can cause increased incidence of hyperinsulinemia in the fetus and pulmonary edema in mother. A preload of 500–1,000 mL of normal saline limits the fall of BP in response to sympathetic blockade. 500 mL of colloid is recommended for preload in cases of PET.

Fetal Distress

In conditions of fetal distress there is fetal hypoxia. In this situation if a 5% or 10% dextrose solution is given intravenous, there shall be anaerobic oxidation and lactate accumulation further deteriorating the fetal condition and increasing the chances of cerebral edema. So, glucose solution and Ringer lactate are best avoided. Parenteral fluid of choice in fetal distress is slow rate of normal saline which would expand the blood volume increasing uteroplacental flow.

Hypovolemia

Hemorrhage is one of the most common obstetric problems requiring immediate intervention. In acute situation, it is necessary to correct hypovolemia by parenteral fluids till arrangements for blood transfusion are being made. Now, the question is crystalloid or colloid. Colloids, such as polygeline or gelofusine are preferred as the first fluid for resuscitation because it is isooncotic, holds itself in the circulation, does not interfere with platelet function, grouping and cross matching, has long shelf life, and needs nominal storage requirements. But sometimes there are anaphylactic reactions. Among crystalloids, normal saline and RL are the solutions of choice for correcting hypovolemia immediately but these do not stay long in circulation. The recommendation is immediate use of colloid or crystalloid followed by blood transfusion to maintain Hb percentage, platelet and clotting factors replacement according to need.

Hypervolemia

Normally, hypervolemia does not occur unless very fast infusion is given. It is possible in oliguric renal failure usually associated with preeclampsia, abruptio placentae, disseminated intravascular coagulation (DIC), puerperal or postabortal sepsis, systemic lupus erythematosus, etc. It is also possible in cases of cardiac failure. In these cases, fluid intake should be restricted to 1,000–1,500 mL or per day output + 600 mL or urine output in per hour + 25 mL, sodium should be restricted.

Preterm Labor

Whilst intravenous hydration has theoretical potential, the available evidence suggests that its use is unlikely to be beneficial in the treatment of threatened preterm labor for the prevention of spontaneous preterm birth. If at all hydration is being considered first line intravenous fluid is saline. If ritodrine is being used for tocolysis one should be cautious for pulmonary edema.

Diabetes Mellitus

A strict control of maternal blood sugar level is required during labor, the reason being twofold, to prevent ketoacidosis in mother and hyperglycemia and distress in the neonate. During active phase of labor patient is kept nil orally, parenteral fluid 5% dextrose in saline is recommended. Insulin pump containing 40 units of actrapid insulin in 40 mL of normal saline should be connected by Y-tube. Glucose in a dose of 2.5 mg/kg/min and fluid in a dose of 75–150 mL/hour is usually required. Dose of insulin has to be titrated according to blood glucose charting. Blood glucose is controlled at 4.4–6.6 mmol/L (80–120 mg/dL). If oxytocin is required, it should be given in a different bottle. Ketoacidosis during labor requires a different regimen. First of all, normal saline 1–2 L should be infused in 30–60 minutes to correct dehydration and intravascular volume. Thereafter, the infusion is maintained at 200–250 mL/hour D5% to be given only after blood glucose level falls to below 200 mg/dL. Insulin is given as 0.1 IU/kg. Body weight (BW) as intravenous bolus is followed by 0.1 IU/kg BW per hour with the rest of the titration according to blood glucose level. Bicarbonates are given when the pH is below 7.1 and potassium (K) is added when serum K falls below 3.0 mEq/L. Because initially serum K is higher, with insulin therapy it comes down. So, these patients require intensive care monitoring.

To conclude, laboring women is allowed to eat and drink during passive phase of labor. Oral fluids are recommended in uncomplicated labor. Antacids and hydrogen (H_2) receptor blockers within 4 hours before surgery is effective against aspiration. Normal saline is the intravenous solution of choice during labor except when betamimetic therapy is on or patient is in renal or cardiac failure. All intravenous infusions have to be given slowly except hemorrhage and diabetic ketoacidosis. Total input should not exceed 3L/24 hours. Dextrose solution is best avoided in labor. Dextrose solution and RL may be harmful in fetal distress. For oxytocin therapy normal saline is recommended as a vehicle. The appropriate type and quality of intravenous fluids matching to various situations during labor have to be selected separately for a healthy maternal and neonatal outcome.

BLOOD COMPONENT TRANSFUSION OBSTETRIC INTENSIVE CARE PATIENT

Obstetric hemorrhage often requires transfusion of blood and blood products. In modern practice, it is more appropriate to use blood component therapy to treat specific derangements in the patient's blood instead of a blanket whole blood transfusion. If the blood component is taken from one donor it is termed as blood component and if from many donors it is known as blood products. Whole blood transfusion poses a significant risk of circulatory overload when many units are required.

Whole blood contains clotting factors, platelets, red cells and white cells.

- After one day of extravascular storage, platelets and granulocytes are lost, 2,3-diphosphoglycerate is depleted and oxygen carrying capacity of RBCs is significantly decreased
- After 1 week of extravascular storage, labile clotting factors (factor V and VII) are lost
- Later on increase in plasma level of K and ammonia occurs.

The blood products that are most commonly used in pregnancy are subdivided into cellular or plasma components.

CELLULAR COMPONENTS (TABLE 2)

Red Blood Cells

- One unit of RBC contains 250 mL of RBCs and 50 mL of plasma and has a hematocrit of 80%

Table 2: Characteristics of intravenous colloid fluids per 100 mL infusions

Type fluid	Effective plasma volume expansion	Duration of expansion
5% Albumin	70–130 mL	16 hours
25% Albumin	400–500 mL	16 hours
6% Hetastarch	100–130 mL	24 hours
10% Pentastarch	150 mL	8 hours
10% Dextran-40	100–150 mL	6 hours
6% Dextran-70	80 mL	12 hours

- Has a shelf life of 6 weeks when stored at 1–6°C
- Frozen RBCs can be stored for years at –70°C, but then freezing destroys WBCs
- Transfusion of one unit of RBCs would increase the Hb by 1 g/dL in a 70 kg person
- When WBCs have been removed from a unit of blood, the blood is considered *"leukocyte-poor"* and poses a decreased risk of febrile transfusion reactions.

Platelet Concentrates

- Can be collected from single or multiple donors
- One unit of platelets is equivalent to the number of platelets typically found in one unit of whole blood. This increases the number of platelets by approximately 7,500/mm^3 in a 70 kg person. The platelets will equilibrate within 10 min of transfusion
- Platelet concentrates contain serum bound RBCs to cause alloimmunization to red cell antigens. Therefore, there is a chance of rhesus (Rh) immunization in Rh negative female recipients
- Platelet concentrates are indicated in hemorrhage due to thrombocytopenia (quantitative) or thrombocytopathia (qualitative)
- Most cases (99%) of thrombocytopenia during pregnancy are related to hypertensive disorders, i.e. preeclampsia and eclampsia and gestational thrombocytopenic purpura. When evaluating the parturient with thrombocytopenia, there are two specific issues to consider. The first concern is whether the disorder is static or dynamic. The second issue is whether platelet function is normal or abnormal (thrombocytopathia). If it is dynamic and abnormal (e.g. in PET, immune thrombocytopenic purpura or gestational thrombocytopenic purpura) it is dangerous and needs serial estimations. If it is stable and normal in function, it is not so dangerous
- Thrombocytopenia in pregnancy is considered when the platelet count falls below 10,000/mm^3. Bleeding following major surgery rarely occurs when the platelet count is 50,000/mm^3 or above if platelet function is normal. When this count ranges between 20,000/mm^3 and 50,000/mm^3, bleeding during surgery can occur. Prophylactic platelet transfusion may be required with platelet counts 20,000/mm^3 or less even in nonbleeding case
- The cause of thrombocytopenia or thrombocytopathia must be determined. In the presence of immune thrombocytopenic purpura, where platelets are destroyed via an antibody mediated process, corticosteroids rather than platelets represent the best therapy
- Platelet transfusion is contraindicated in thrombotic thrombocytopenic purpura.

PLASMA COMPONENTS (TABLE 3)

Fresh Frozen Plasma

- Fresh frozen plasma (FFP) is plasma extracted from whole blood within 6 hours of collection and freezing. A unit of FFP contains 250 mL of fluid and 700 mg of fibrinogen

Table 3: Blood components

Component	Contents	Volume (mL)	Shelf life	Indications	Expected effect
Cellular components					
Platelets	Platelets, some plasma, RBCs, few WBCs	50	Up to 5 days	Bleeding due to thrombocytopenia	Increase total platelet count 7500/mm^3 per unit
Packed RBCs	Red cells, some plasma, few WBCs	300	42 days	Correct anemia	Increase hematocrit (Hct) 3% per unit Hb 1 g/unit
Leukocyte poor blood	RBCs, some plasma, few WBCs	250	21–24 days	Correct anemia, reduce febrile reactions	Increase Hct 3% per unit, Hb 1 g/unit
Plasma components					
Fresh frozen plasma	Fibrinogen, plasma clotting factors V, XI, XII	250	2 hours thawing, 12 months freezing	Treatment of coagulation disorders	Increase total fibrinogen 10–15 mg/dL per unit
Cryoprecipitate	Fibrinogen factors V, VIII, XIII von Willebrand's factor	40	4–6 hours thawing	Hemophilia A, von Willebrand's disease, fibrinogen deficiency	Increase total fibrinogen 10–15 mg/dL per unit

- One unit of FFP will increase the fibrinogen level by approximately 10-15 mg/dL. The dose of FFP is 15 mL/kg (target serum fibrinogen level is 100 mg/dL)
- Indicated in multiple clotting factor deficiency in bleeding patients arising from liver disease, vitamin K deficiency and DIC. It may be used in specific factor deficiencies, e.g. factors II, V, VII, IX, X and XI. It can be used in warfarin reversal where there is immediate requirement of correction of vitamin K dependent factors (II, VII, IX, and X).

Cryoprecipitate

- It is extracted from whole blood, which has been frozen and then allowed to thaw at refrigerator temperatures
- It is a cold insoluble fraction of FFP which precipitates under these conditions
- It is a single donor product so has a lower risk of infections
- It is rich in factor VIII (80-120 units), fibrinogen (200 mg), von Willebrand's factor and factor XIII
- Indications of use are von Willebrand's disease, factor VIII deficiency and fibrinogen deficiency.

Laboratory Tests Required in Coagulation Disorders

- Full blood count
- Platelet count
- Prothrombin time
- Activated partial thromboplastin time
- Thrombin time (TT): Particularly helpful in establishing presence or absence of DIC
- Fibrinogen: Normal concentration at term should be 4.0-6.0 g/L
- Fibrin degradation products (FDPs).

If laboratory tests are available, they may indicate the following and accordingly a selection of blood product for infusion can be done:

- Reduced coagulation factors (so all coagulation tests are prolonged)
- Low fibrinogen and FDPs
- Fragmented red cells on the blood film
- Reduced platelet count.

ALTERNATIVES AND TECHNIQUES TO AVOID TRANSFUSION

1. Colloid solution's estimated duration of effect is 24-36 hours
2. Autologous transfusion device
3. Acute normovolemic hemodilution.

Autologous Blood

- It is the collection and reinfusion of the patient's own RBCs. Donor and recipient are the same so it eliminates many transfusion related complications
- Until now, pregnant women were not allowed to donate blood. But a growing database suggests that it is safe for certain pregnant women to donate blood during pregnancy.
  - A predonation hemoglobin of 11g/dL or more
  - Autologous blood donation should be done no earlier than 6 weeks before their anticipated use because RBCs would destroy after that
  - One week should elapse between donations
  - More costly and does not totally eliminate the possibility of homologous transfusion.

Acute Normovolemic Hemodilution

- Patients at risk for intraoperative hemorrhage
- In preoperative period blood is collected from the patient into special storage bags containing an anticoagulant. Patient is given large amount of crystalloid in 3:1 ratio resulting in hemodilution. Blood lost intraoperatively is more dilute. When blood loss is controlled the blood is reinfused

Table 4: Complications of transfusion

Risk	Incidence (per unit of blood)
Delayed hemolytic reaction	1:2,500–1:600
Febrile, nonhemolytic reaction	1:100
Allergy	1:100–1:300
Anaphylaxis	1:2,000–1:50,000
Transfusion-related acute lung injury	Unknown; rare
Viral infections	
HIV	1:913,000
Hepatitis B virus	1:63,000–1:200,000
Hepatitis C virus	1:250,00–1:500,000
Prior infections	
Creutzfeldt-Jakob disease, Variant Creutzfeldt-Jakob disease	Theoretical risk only
Bacterial infection	<1:1 million
Fatal sepsis (e.g. *Yersinia enterocolitica*)	
Parasitic infections	1:400,000–1:4
Malaria	Million

- It is not indicated in fetal compromise, anemic status, coronary artery disease, pulmonary disease, and renal or hepatic insufficiency.

Complications of Transfusion

Complications related to transfusion are given in Table 4.

CONCLUSION

Obstetrics hemorrhage mostly requires transfusion of blood and blood products and it would be more appropriate to investigate and pin point the exact deficiency and transfuse the required component of blood instead of whole blood transfusion.

BIBLIOGRAPHY

1. American Society of Hospital Pharmacists. AHFS drug information. Bethesda ASHP. 1993. pp. 2039-41.
2. Arias F. Hypertension during pregnancy. In: Arias E (Ed). High Risk Pregnancy and Delivery. Toronto: Mosby; 1984.
3. Chesley LC. Sodium retention and pre-eclampsia. Am J Obstet Gynecol. 1966;95:127-32.
4. Clark SL, Greenspoon J, Aldahl D. Severe pre-eclampsia with persistent oliguria: Management of haemodynamic subsets. Am J Obstet Gynecol. 1986;154:490-4.
5. Consensus Conference. Fresh Frozen plasma: indications and risks. JAMA. 1985;253(4):551.
6. Consensus Conference. Perioperative red blood cell transfusion. JAMA. 1988;260(18):2700.
7. Consensus Conference. Platelet transfusion therapy. JAMA. 1987;257(13):1777.
8. Dumoulin J, Faulkes J. Ketonuria during labor. British J Obstet Gynecol. 1984;91:97-8.
9. Horne CH, Howie PW, Goudie RB. Serum alpha 2-macroglobulin, transferrin, albumin and IgG levels in pre-eclampsia. J Clin Pathol. 1970;23:514-8.
10. Kenepp NB, Shelly WC, Kumar S, et al. Fetal and neonatal hazards of maternal hydration with 5% dextrose before caesarean section. Lancet. 1982;1:1150-2.
11. Roberts, et al. Restricting oral intake leads to lower pH and there is paradoxical increase in gastric fluid during fasting.
12. Sleutel M, Golden SS. Fasting in labor Pelvic or requirement. J Obstet Gynecol Neonat Nurs. 1999;28:507-12.
13. Spencer SA, Mann NP, Smith ML, et al. The effects of intravenous therapy during labor on maternal and accord serum sodium levels. Br J Obstet Gynecol. 1981;88:480-3.
14. Studd JW, Blainey JD, Bailey DE. Serum protein changes in the pre-eclampsia eclapmsia syndrome. J Obstet Gynecol Br Wlth. 1970;77:796-801.
15. Transfusion alert: Indications for the use of red blood cells, platelets and fresh-frozen plasma. NIH Publication No. 89-2974 a, May 1989.

CHAPTER

5

Incisions and Sutures

Randhir Puri

Paré said,

"I dress the wounds, God heals them."

TYPES OF INCISIONS (FIG. 1)

Paramedian

Paramedian incisions are rarely used (Fig. 2). This incision provides little additional exposure beyond a midline incision. The blood and nerve supply to the abdominal wall enters from either side and may cross the midline poorly.

For this reason paramedian incisions have an increased risk of rendering part of the abdominal wall anesthetic and ischemic. The result is poor wound healing and increased risk of hernias.

Lower Midline

Lower midline incisions (Fig. 3) are used for complex appendicitis, sigmoid colonic, rectal, urological, and overlap obscuring the linea alba and making division of the muscle necessary in lower midline incisions.

In general, these incisions are well tolerated by patients but are often painful. The weight of the abdominal contents and an obese abdominal wall may put additional strain on

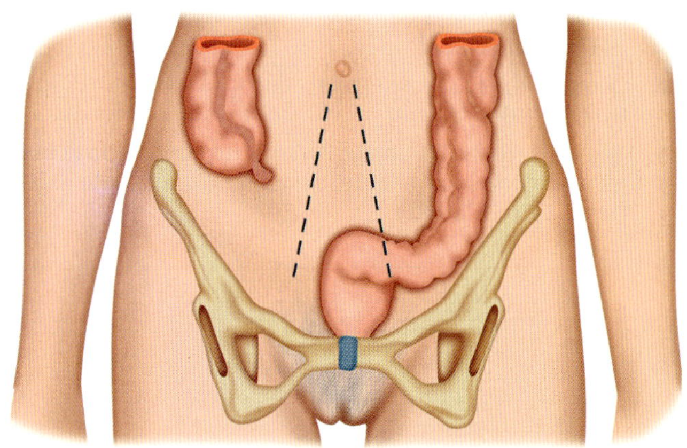

Fig. 2: Paramedian incision

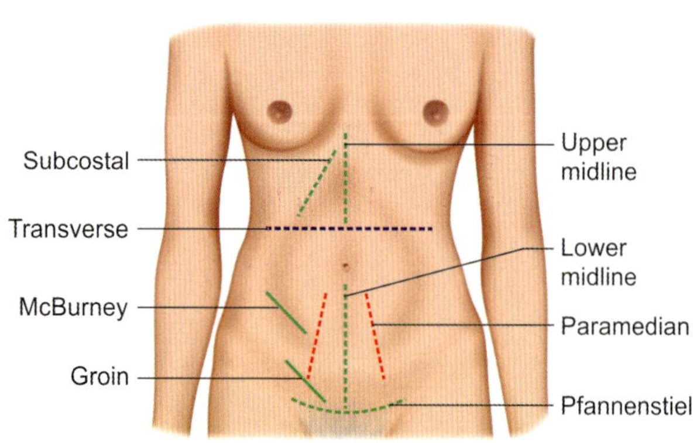

Fig. 1: Types of incisions

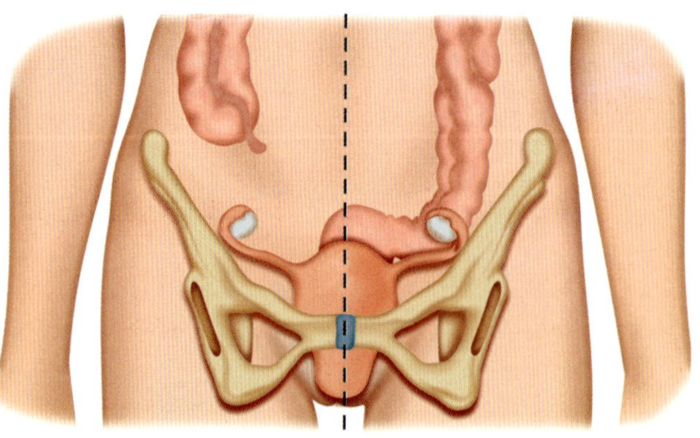

Fig. 3: Midline, vertical infraumbilical incision

such incisions, increasing the risk of hernia formation. For very obese patients, stretching of the abdominal wall can occur. Access to the pelvis is best achieved through an upper abdominal or periumbilical incision in these cases.

The principle advantage of the lower midline incision is that the incision can be extended superiorly for processes or operations that involve the upper abdominal viscera or require extra exposure. Similarly, the best exposure of the pelvis is gained by a lower midline incision to the pubis.

Groin Incision

Groin incisions may be oblique or within the skin lines and nearly transverse. Generally, they end medially at the level of the external ring, usually 1–2 finger breadths above the external ring. Laterally, these incisions usually extend for 10–12 cm, depending on the size of the patient, the size of the hernia and prior surgery. Staying out of the inguinal crease reduces the risk of infection. Such incisions are closed in layers. The oblique inguinal incision may be on the right or left side and is used for hernia repair. The superficial epigastric vein is usually encountered in the subcutaneous tissue. It is ligated and divided.

BASICS OF WOUND CLOSURE AND HEALING

There are many circumstances in which sutures are used to repair tissue and facilitate healing. The techniques that are used, the suture material used and the specific type of needle that is used will vary depending on whether one is closing a simple laceration on the foot, a complex laceration on the face, a gastrointestinal anastomosis, a vascular anastomosis or closing a median sternotomy.

TISSUE RESPONSE TO INJURY

There are three phases of healing

1. Hemostasis and inflammation.
2. Fibroplasia.
3. Wound maturation.

The recovery time for tissues incised is as follows:

- At 2 weeks the wound has achieved about 20% of its prewound strength
- By 5 weeks it is at about 50%
- By 10 weeks it is at about 80% of prewound strength
- Remodeling and maturation of the scar will continue for a year or more
- The principles of wound closure are dictated by the biology of healing.

Surgical Skill Methods Facilitating Healing

The goal of wound closure is to achieve healing with:

- No infection
- Normal function
- An excellent cosmetic result.

These goals are facilitated by handling tissues gently. As early as the 1500s, a barber-surgeon named Ambroise Paré demonstrated the importance of gentle handling of tissue:

- *Minimize bacterial contamination*: Bacterial contamination can be reduced by irrigating the wound with large amounts of sterile saline or Ringer's solution under moderate pressure. One method is to use a 50 cc syringe with a 16 or 18 gauge needle. Sterile saline can be aspirated and a pulsatile irrigating stream can be created by depressing the plunger with force. Small wounds with little contamination can be irrigated with 100–200 cc of saline but larger volumes should be used for larger or more contaminated wounds. Generally, antiseptics should not be used to irrigate wounds because they impair wound healing
- Remove foreign bodies and devitalize tissue
- Achieve hemostasis (blood is a culture medium)
- *Handle tissue gently*: Use fine-toothed forceps such as an Adson forceps; do not use smooth forceps, since these crush tissue because they require greater pressure to grasp
- *Approximate—don't strangulate:* The wound edges should just be approximated. Sutures that are too tight accentuate cross-hatching and cause ischemia of the wound edges, increasing the risk of infection.

Needles

Most sutures come as a single piece, with the suture material swaged onto the base of the needle. The needle should be grasped in the tip of the needle holder about two-third of the way back from the point (Figs 4A and B). Grasping further back at the swaged end tends to weaken the needle and its attachment to the suture, and you are likely to bend the needle.

There are many different needle types, but the chief distinction to be made here is the difference between taper or "smooth" needles in contrast to cutting needles. Taper needles do just what their name implies; they gradually taper to the point, and a cross-section anywhere along the shaft would reveal a round shaft as shown in the inset (Fig. 4B). Taper needles are used for tissue that is easy to penetrate such as bowel or blood vessels (Fig. 5A).

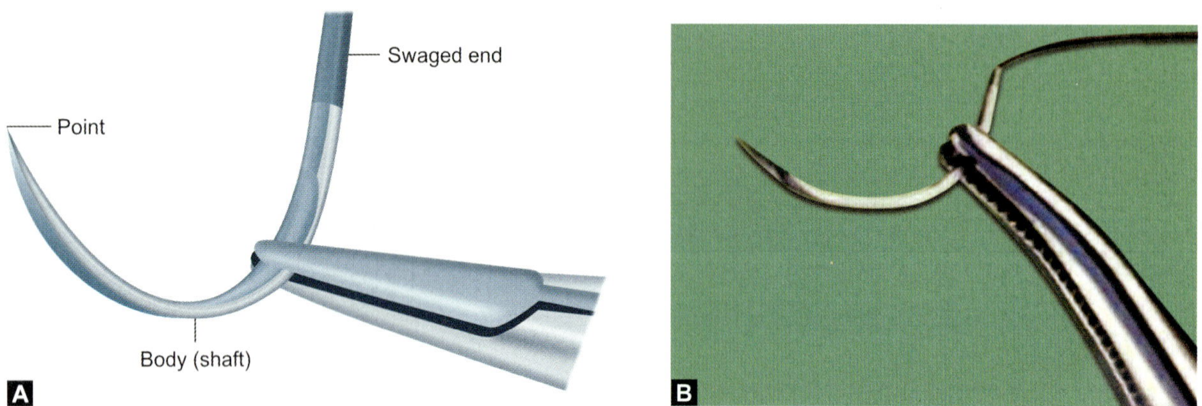

Figs 4A and B: (A) Anatomy of a needle; (B) Taper needle held at two-third distance from tip as shown

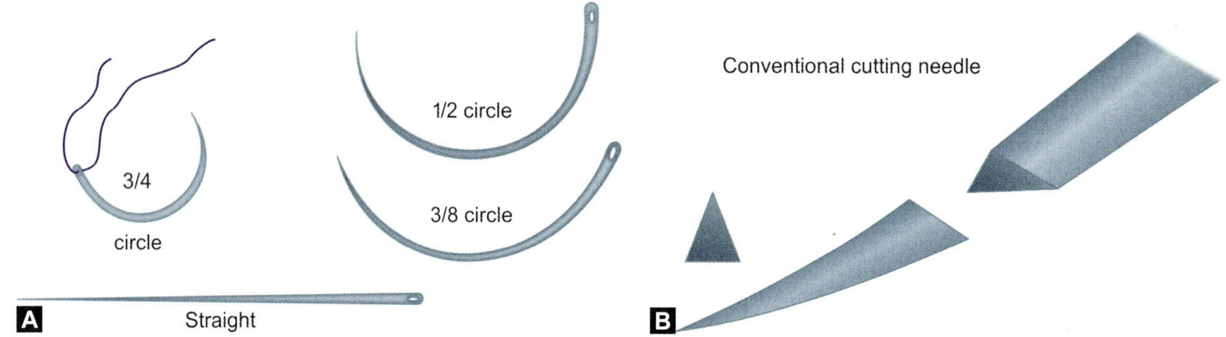

Figs 5A and B: (A) Types of needles; (B) Diagrammatic representation of cutting needle

In contrast, the tip of cutting needles (Fig. 5B) is triangular in shape, and the apex forms a cutting surface, which facilitates penetration of tough tissue such as skin. Cutting needles make it much easier to penetrate tough tissue. Penetrating skin with a taper needle is very difficult and causes excess trauma to the skin because of difficulty in penetration and the need to grasp the skin edge very tightly with forceps. Consequently, you should never use taper needles to suture skin.

The reverse cutting needle is similar to a conventional cutting needle, except that the cutting edge faces down instead of up. This may decrease the likelihood of sutures pulling through tissue in some cases.

SUTURES

Nonabsorbable sutures are made of materials that are not readily broken down by the body's enzymes or by hydrolysis. There are naturally occurring nonabsorbable materials (e.g. silk, cotton and steel) and synthetic non-absorbable materials (e.g. nylon, prolene and Mersilene (Figs 6 to 8).

In some cases, they are left in place indefinitely (e.g. when used to close the abdominal fascia), and in other cases they are removed after adequate healing has occurred (e.g. nylon sutures to close a superficial laceration).

Absorbable suture materials are those that are broken down. The original absorbable suture materials were plain and chromic "cat gut", which actually consisted of processed collagen derived from the submucosa of animal intestines. Plain gut is broken down enzymatically after about 7 days. Chromic gut is collagen treated with chromium salts to delay break down. Chromic gut, typically, loses its strength after 2–3 weeks and is completely digested after about 3 months. Now, there are many synthetic absorbable materials made from polymers (e.g. Vicryl and Monocryl). These materials are broken down nonenzymatically by hydrolysis; water penetrates the suture filaments and causes breakdown of the polymer chain. As a result, synthetic absorbables tend to evoke less tissue reaction than plain or chromic gut.

Vicryl retains 75% of its original tensile strength at 2 weeks and retains 50% at 3 weeks. Monocryl retains 60–70% of its strength at 1 week and 30–40% at 2 weeks. Polydioxanone suture (PDS) II is a soft, pliable monofilament material that retains about 50% of its strength at 4 weeks after implantation.

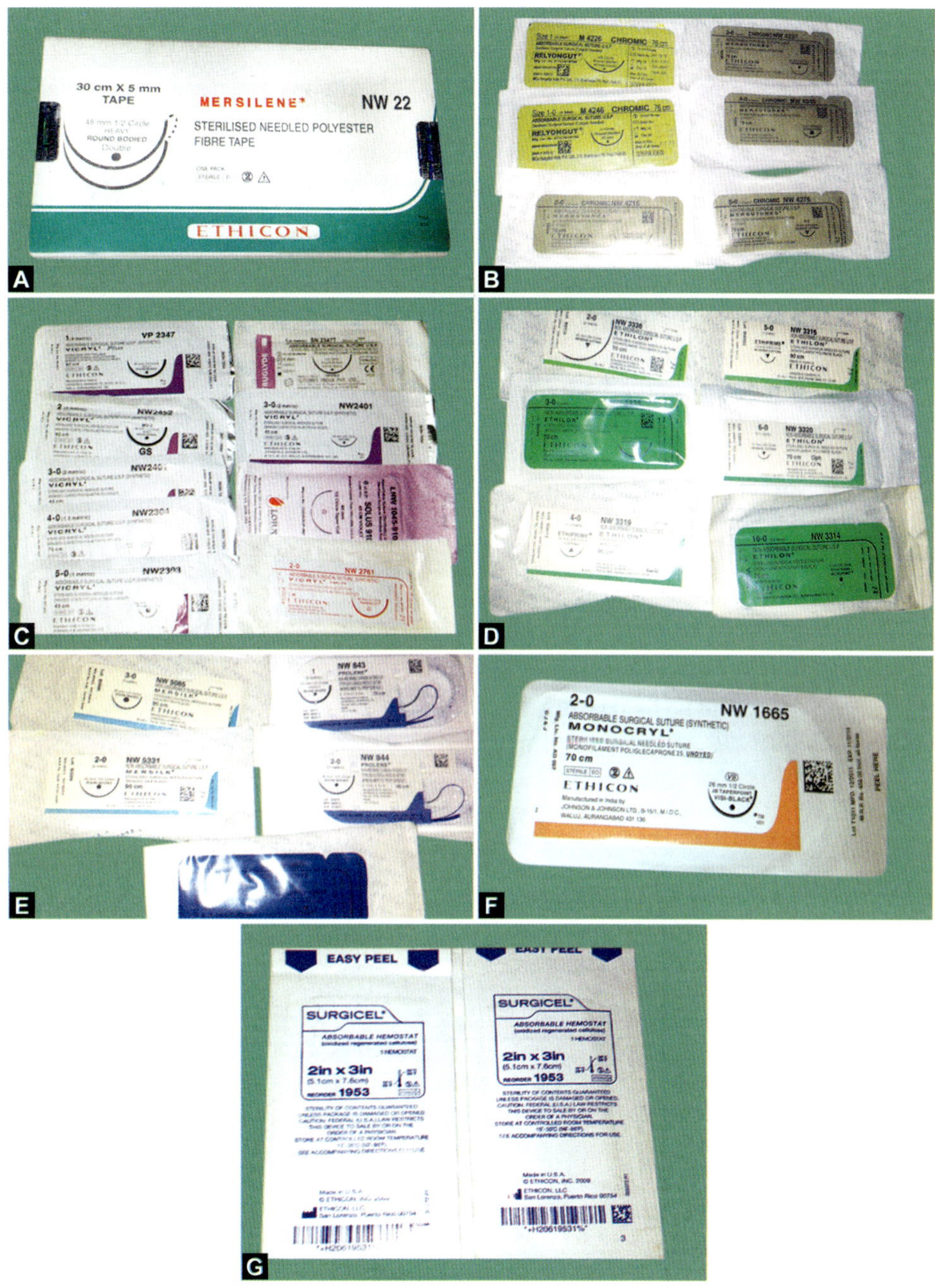

Figs 6A to G: Different types of sutures

Monofilament versus Multifilament

It should also be noted that some of these suture materials consist of a single smooth strand (monofilament) and others consists of multiple fibers woven together (multifilament). Characteristically, multifilament suture material (e.g. silk or Mersilene) tends to be easier to handle and tie, and knots in multifilament material are less likely to slip. On the other hand, monofilament materials (e.g. nylon or Prolene) are less traumatic, since they glide through tissues with less friction and they may be associated with lower rates of infection.

Since monofilament materials are more likely to slip, one generally ties knots with five or six "throws" when using monofilament materials (in contrast to three throws with silk or Mersilene). Despite the greater number of knots required, monofilament materials such as nylon are generally preferred for skin closure because they stimulate less tissue reaction, are less traumatic, may have less likelihood of infection and provide a better cosmetic result.

Among the absorbable suture materials, Vicryl is a multifilament material, but there is also a coated Vicryl that provides decreased drag through tissue. For this reason, coated Vicryl is used by some surgeons for the interior layer of bowel anastomoses. Monocryl is an absorbable monofilament material, but has excellent lability and provides easy handling and good knot security.

Scalpels

The most commonly used scalpel blades are the #10 and the #15 blade (Fig. 9). The #10 blade is better for long, straight incisions, and is held with the shaft of the scalpel in the palm of the hand with the index finger on top of the blade (Fig. 10A).

The smaller #15 blade is well suited for short, tortuous incisions; for this type of incision holding the scalpel as if it were a pencil may facilitate control (Fig. 10B).

Forceps

For skin closure, use a fine-toothed forceps, such as an Adson forceps (Fig. 11). The forceps should be held so one arm is an extension of thumb and the other is an extension of your index finger. The base of the forceps should rest on the dorsal surface of the web space between the thumb and index finger.

Use only forceps with teeth. Use the arm with a single tooth to gently elevate the skin edge. Avoid crushing the skin edges with the forceps. This further traumatizes the wound edge and impedes healing.

The forceps allow you to create counter traction and control the position of the skin edge to facilitate passage of the needle perpendicularly through the skin.

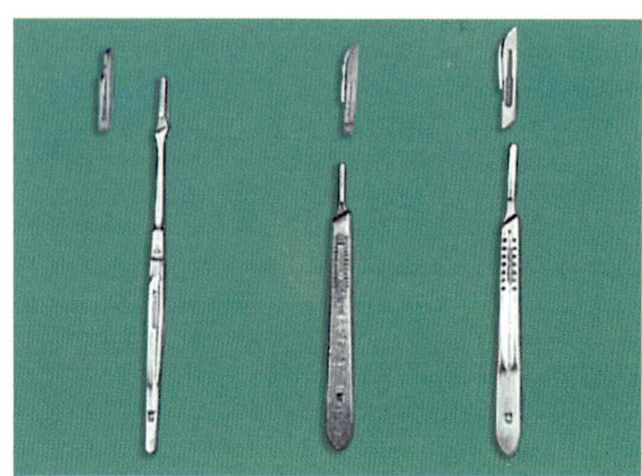

Fig. 9: Types of scalpels

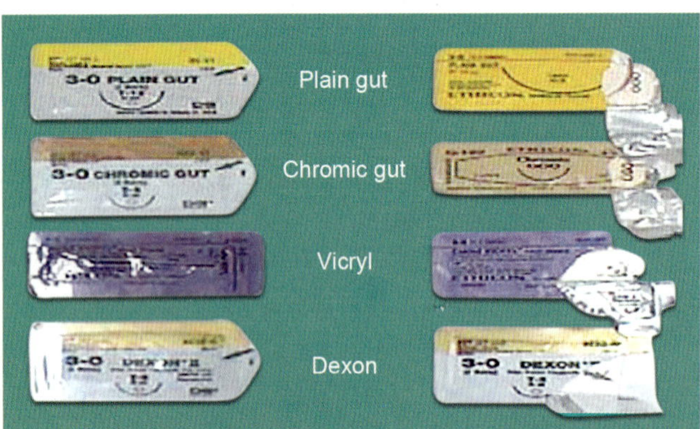

Fig. 7: Absorbable sutures

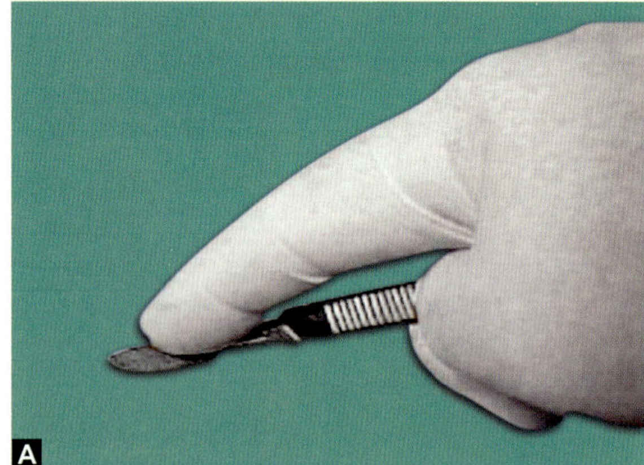

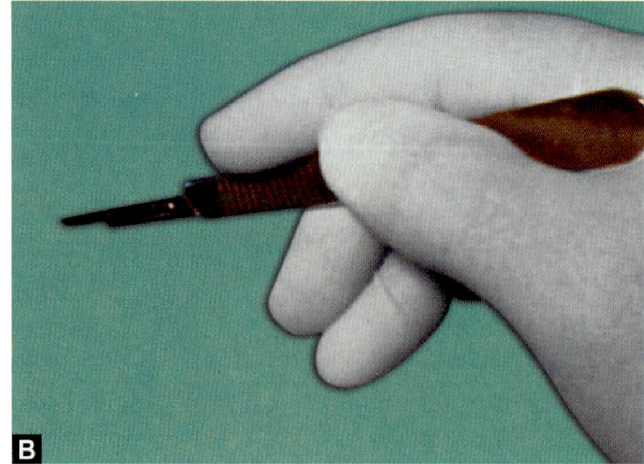

Figs 10A and B: Knife holding positions

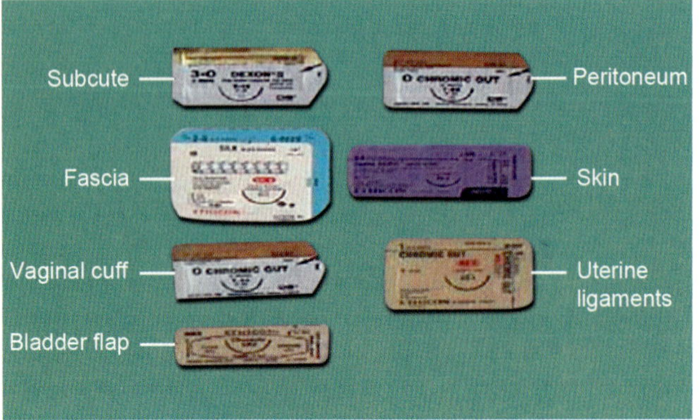

Fig. 8: Suture materials for abdominal hysterectomy

The forceps should also be used to grasp the needle when repositioning it in the needle holder. Needle should not be touched with fingers.

Skin Hooks

Instead of using forceps, the skin edges can also be controlled using skin hooks, which have the advantage that they do not crush the skin edge (Fig. 12).

Needle Holder

There are several techniques for holding the needle holder (Figs 13A and B). The most common method is to place the thumb and ring finger slightly into the instrument's rings. This allows you to pronate and supinate and to open and close the jaws of the needle holder. Avoid inserting the fingers far into the rings of the instrument, since this will tie up the fingers and impede the mobility. Some surgeons do not put their fingers into the rings at all and simply grasp the rings and body of the needle holder in the palm of their hand.

Remember to Create Right Angles

The ideal skin suture should form a rectangle, penetrating the epidermis and dermis perpendicular to the skin surface, then turning at a right angle to traverse the depth of the wound parallel to the skin surface, and then turning again to emerge from the opposite skin edge perpendicular to the skin surface (Figs 14A and B).

The distance between the skin edge and the emerging suture should be the same on both sides of the wound. When tied, a suture placed in this fashion will form a rectangle and will provide optimal approximation of the wound edges.

Getting the suture path to follow the rectangular course described above may seem counterintuitive, since the needle is curved. However, a rectangular path can be achieved by taking advantage of the needle's curvature and rotating the needle in such a way that the body of the needle stays perpendicular to the skin. Think of the skin as the tangent to the arc formed by the needle; in this case, the tangent is stationary and the arc rotates.

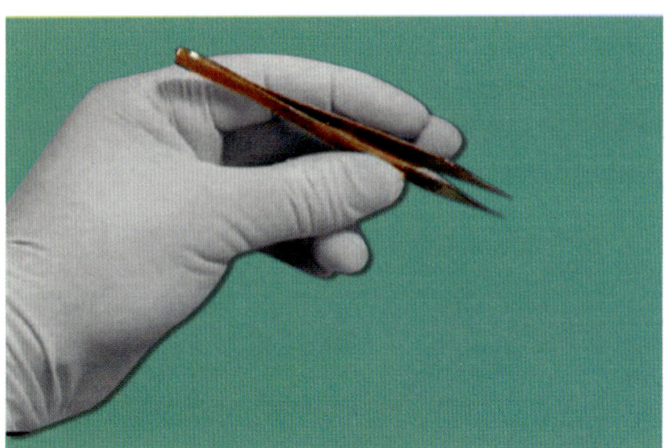

Fig. 11: Fine-toothed forceps

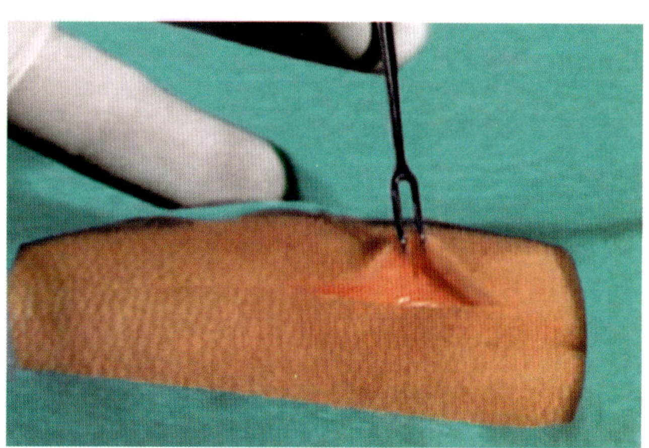

Fig. 12: Demonstration of skin hook usage

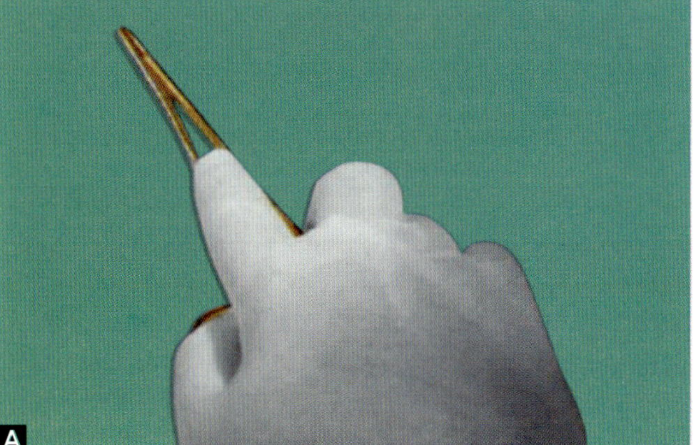

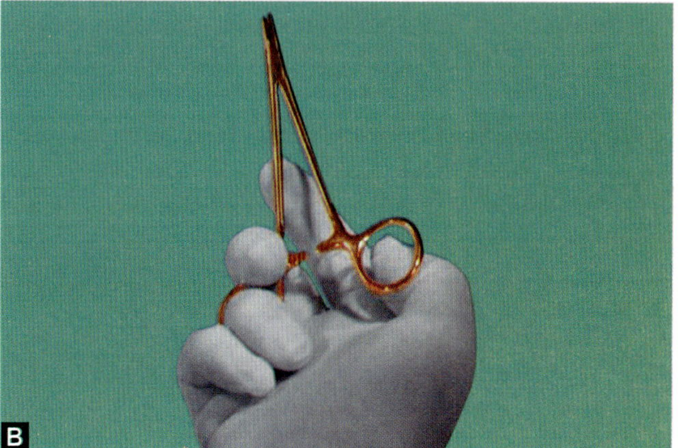

Figs 13A and B: Technique of holding the needle holder

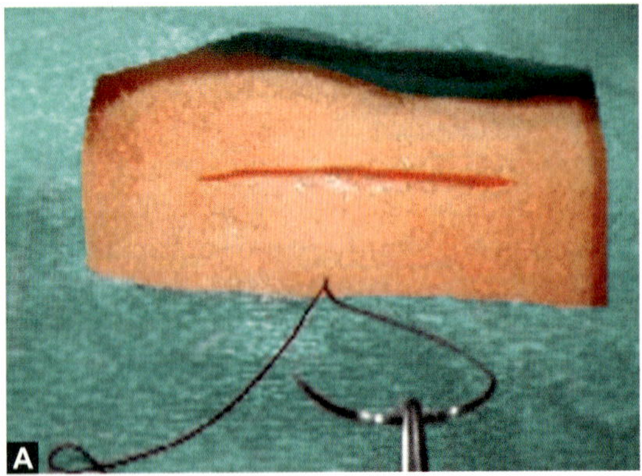

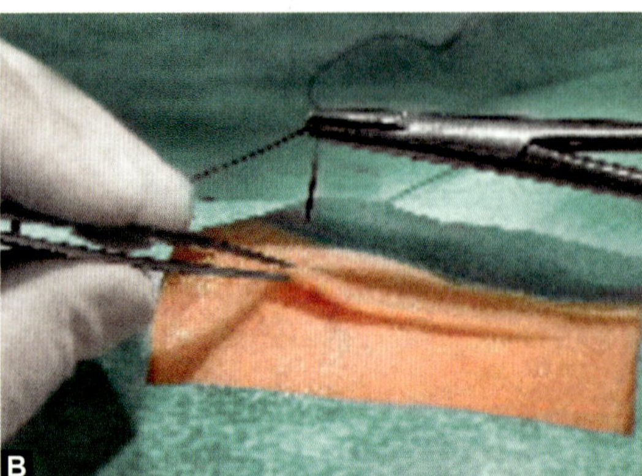

Figs 14A and B: Remember to create right angles

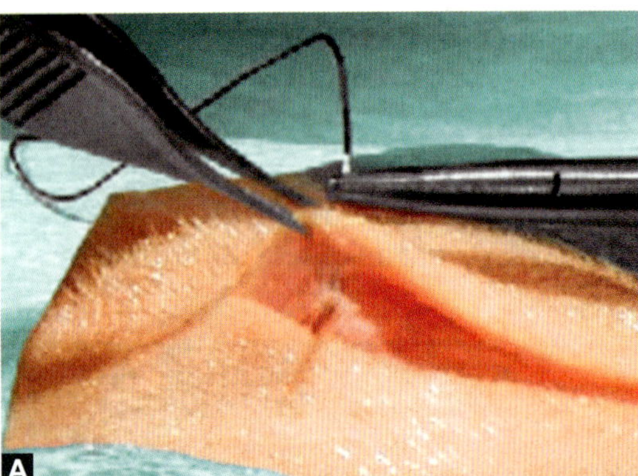

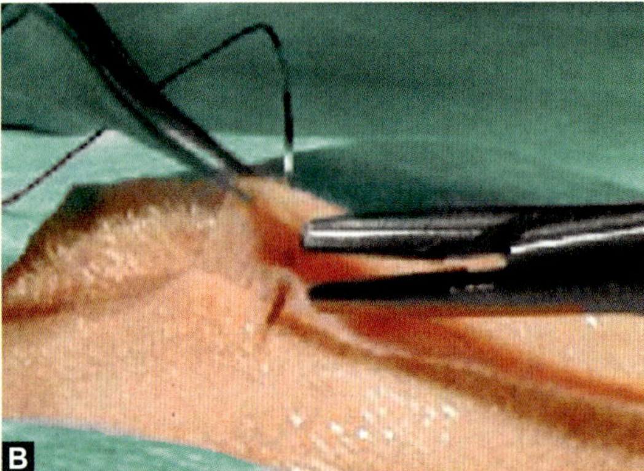

Figs 15A and B: Coordinated hand and instrument movements

Coordinated Use of the Forceps and Needle Holder

Efficient and atraumatic placement of sutures which follow the rectangular path described above requires coordinated use of the forceps and needle holder. One can best take advantage of the natural curvature of the needle by alternately pronating and supinating the hand with the needle holder (Figs 15A and B).

The tip of the needle holder should grasp the needle about two-third of the way back from the point. The needle holder and needle should be roughly perpendicular.

The far skin edge is elevated with the forceps in the left hand, while the right hand is pronated to "cock" the needle in preparation for taking the first "bite". The tip of the needle should penetrate the skin perpendicularly about 5–10 mm from the wound edge, and the needle should be rotated all the way through the epidermis and dermis by supinating the right hand to rotate the needle through its arc.

A KEY MANEUVER

The tip of the needle should now be seen protruding into the wound from the subcutaneous tissue. At this point, it is important to maintain the position of the skin edge using the forceps. A common error here is to release the forceps from the skin edge, but this allows the skin to retract, and the needle may move and retract beneath the skin edge (Fig. 16).

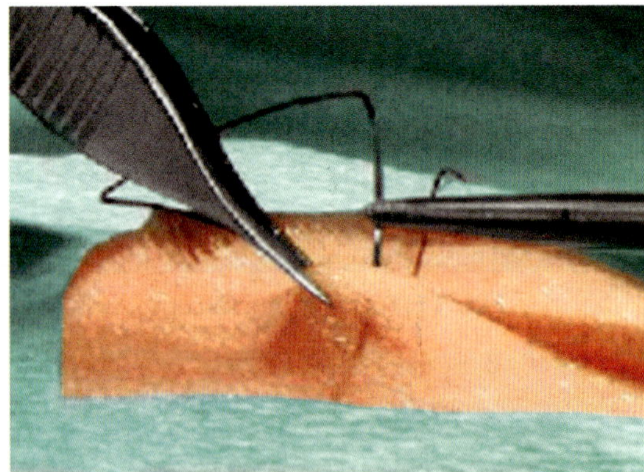

Fig. 16: Maintain steady position of skin by not releasing the skin forceps

The key is to maintain the position of the skin edge while releasing the needle from the needle holder. This will maintain the position of the needle tip. After the needle is released from the needle holder, the right hand should be fully pronated before regrasping the needle. The "bite" can then be completed by supinating the right hand in order to complete the rotation of the needle through the skin.

If it is necessary to reposition the needle in the needle holder before taking the second "bite", the needle should be grasped with the forceps, not with fingers.

The forceps then elevate the near skin edge in preparation for the second "bite". Once again, the right hand is cocked by pronating it and the needle is passed upward through the near skin edge by supinating the right wrist in order to keep the body of the needle perpendicular to the tissue it is passing through at all times. The needle should emerge about 4–5 mm from the wound edge (equidistant on both sides of the wound).

Scissors

Scissors are generally held with the thumb slightly in one ring and the ring finger in the other. The index finger stabilizes the instrument by resting on the shaft (Fig. 17).

Suture Removal

While cutting sutures, some recommend sliding the tips of the scissors down the strands to the point where they will be cut, but it probably makes more sense to simply move the tips of the scissors directed to the point where the cuts have to be made. For external nonabsorbable sutures, it is important to leave 4–5 mm "ears" to facilitate suture removal (Fig. 18).

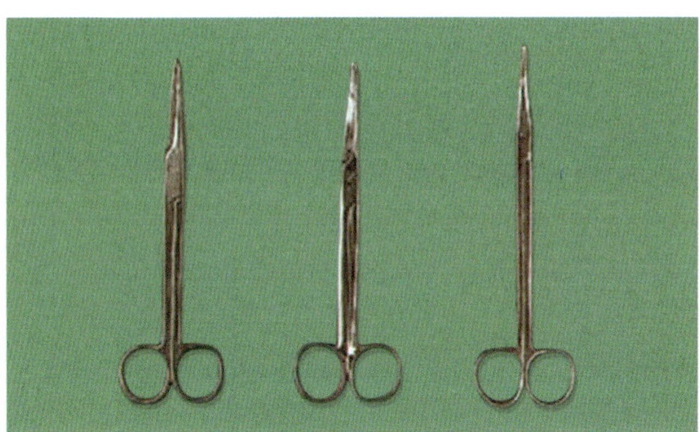

Fig.17: Various scissors

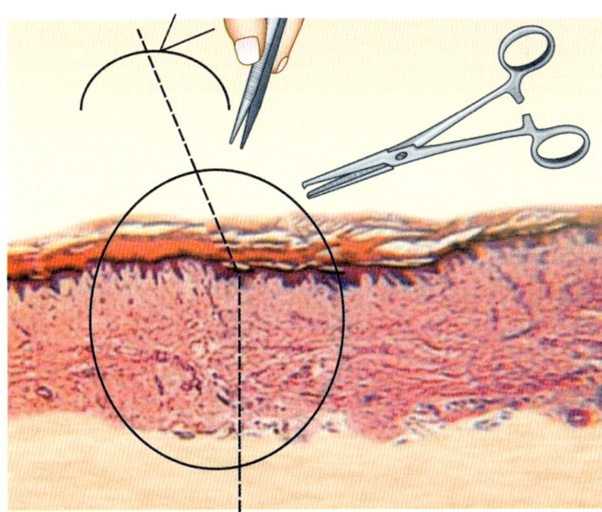

Fig. 18: Suture removal

When to Remove

Face: 3–4 days
Scalp: 5 days
Trunk: 7 days
Arm or leg: 7–10 days
Foot: 10–14 days

Steps of Suture Removal

Many patients are very apprehensive about suture removal, so the first step is to reassure the patient that the procedure is not painful. The skin should be cleansed. Hydrogen peroxide is a good choice for gently removing dried blood and exudate.

Then grasp one of the "ears" of the suture with a forceps to elevate the suture just enough to slip the tip of a small scissor under the suture in order to cut it. This should be done close to the skin edge in order to minimize the amount of contaminated suture that will be dragged through the stitch path. The suture is then gently removed by pulling with the forceps. It is frequently a good idea to reinforce the wound with tapes. These are narrow adhesive strips that are placed perpendicularly across the wound at intervals.

BASIC KNOT: ANATOMY AND METHODOLOGY

A square knot consists of two "throws" of the suture to form a loop and then throw (Figs 19 to 21). Here, the short

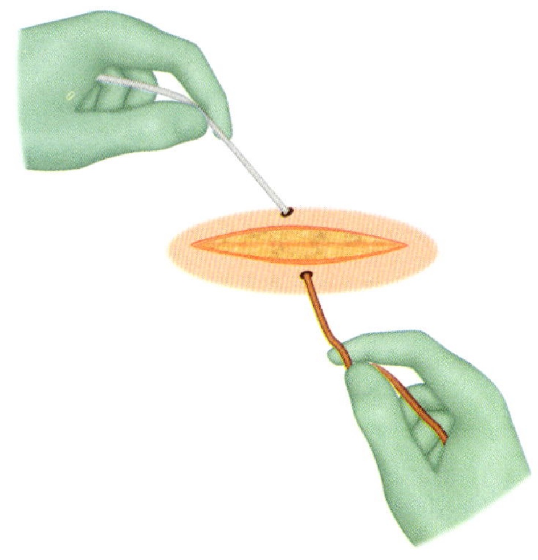

Fig. 19: During knot construction, the surgeon's hands should be on each side and parallel to the suture loop

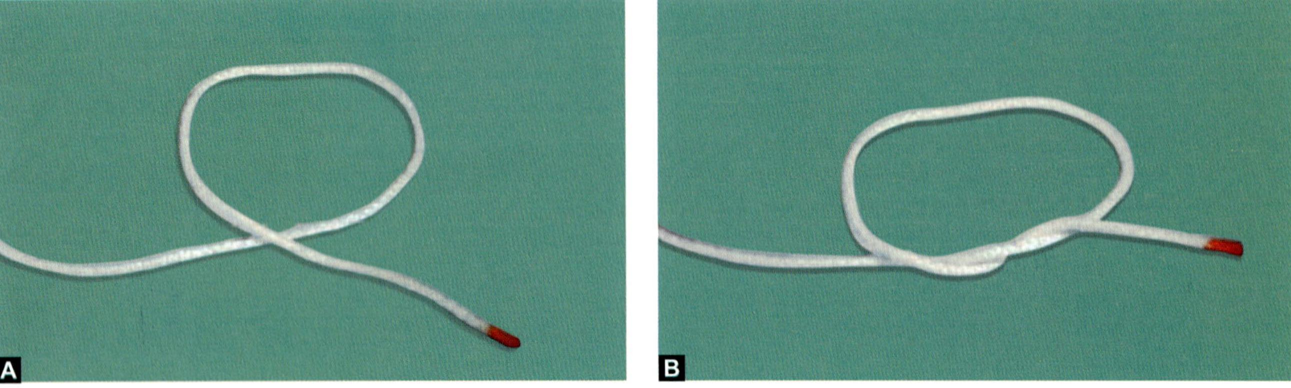

Figs 20A and B: The short end has been wrapped around the long end by passing it under the long end and up through

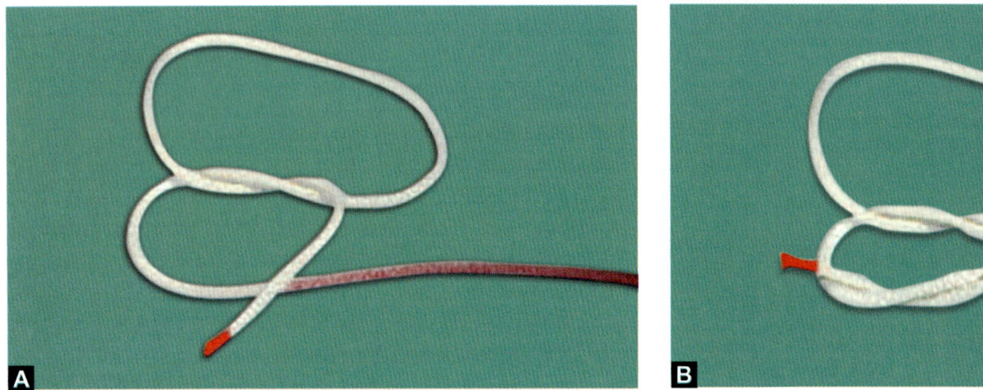

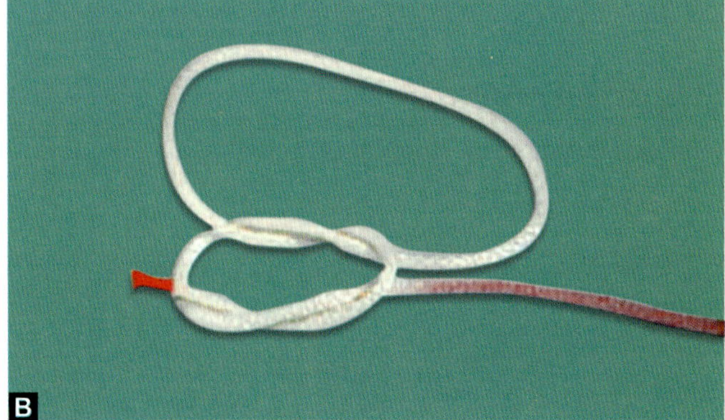

Figs 21A and B: The loop for the second throw is initiated by once again crossing the short end over the long strand from right to left

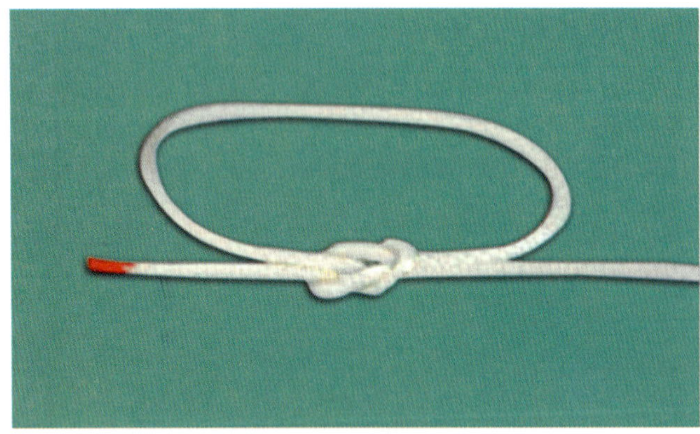

Fig. 21C: The knot has now been tightened and the result is a square knot

end has been crossed. Throws are constructed by crossing the ends, wrapping one end of the suture around the long end to form a loop.

COMMON TYING TECHNIQUES

Various tying techniques are used in the closure of skin wound (Figs 22 and 23). These can be broadly divided into:

- Continuous
- Interrupted.

For Satisfactory Wound Healing

- The wound edge is slightly everted to avoid wound depression
- The tissue is not constricted by suture
- The dead space is closed to reduce the risk of infection, hematoma and wound depression
- The wound edges are joined loosely since there is always some postoperative swelling.

After Care

- Earlier the sutures are removed, less is the likelihood of persistent puncture marks but the greater the risk of

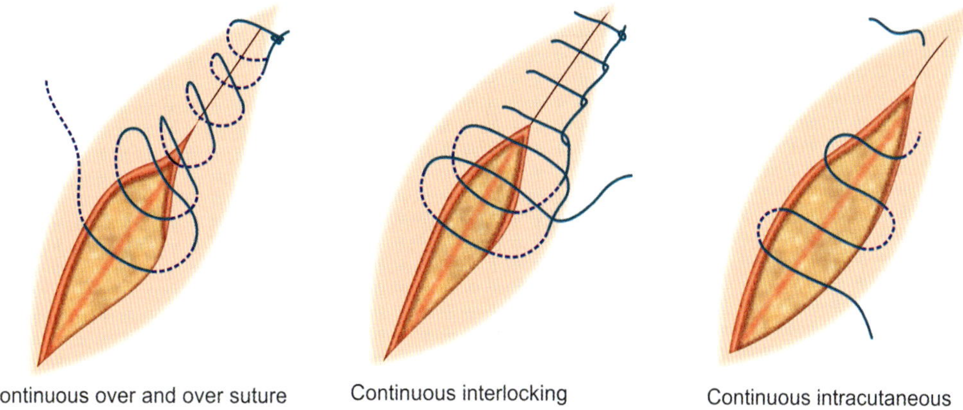

Fig. 22: Showing various suturing techniques

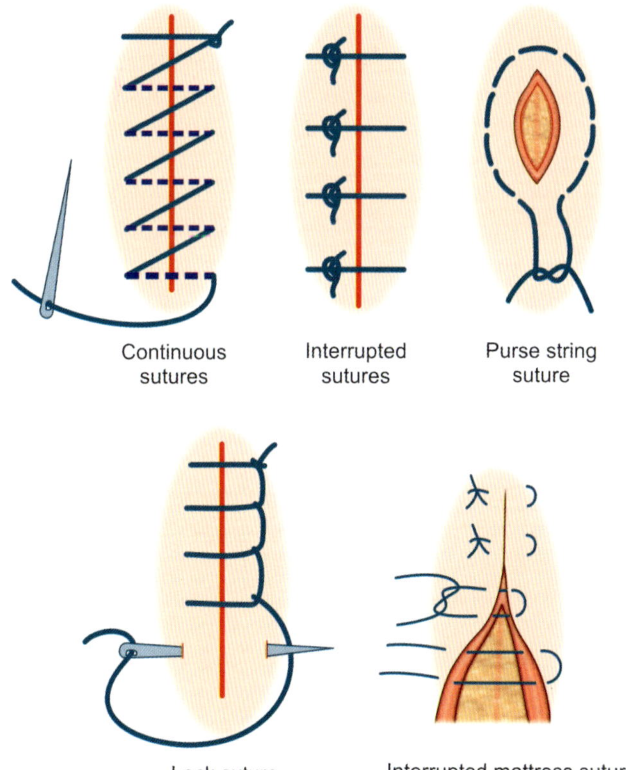

Fig. 23: The other types of suturing techniques

dehiscence. As an approximate guide, sutures on the face should be removed after 5 days. However, those sutures at the lid margin should be left for at least 10 days to avoid the risk of dehiscence.

Continuous Sutures

Continuous sutures have the advantage of evenly distributing the wound tension. However, if the suture or a knot breaks, wound dehiscence can easily occur. In this respect interrupted sutures give a better security.

The continuous intracutaneous is ideal for creating inconspicuous wound such as that in direct brow lift operation.

SMEAD-JONES/FAR-AND-NEAR

It is a double loop technique alternating far and near stitches, and possessing greater mechanical strength than continuous or simple interrupted sutures. It is commonly used for approximating fascial edges, especially for patients at risk for fascial disruption or infection.

CONCLUSION

Learning the basic surgical skills correctly at start of learning curve goes long way to inculcate best practice. These techniques are not difficult to master, surgical interns ab initio should put in sufficient mind and effort to learn the basic nunance of these skills.

CHAPTER

6

Perioperative Assessment and Drugs: Antibiotics, Analgesics, Others

Vinay Tiwari, Veena Chandra

PREOPERATIVE PREPARATION OF PATIENTS

Anesthesia, Outpatient Department, and Preoperative Consultation

One of the most striking changes, which have taken place in the recent times has been the short stay of the surgical patient in the hospital. Approximately 60% of surgical cases are ambulatory; another 20% are admitted to the hospital on the day of surgery; and, only about 20% are available in the hospital for preoperative anesthetic evaluation, a day before surgery. Patient's age and medical conditions, as well as surgical procedure and length, no longer determine the time of admission to hospital. What difference does the preoperative assessment make? Do the preoperative history and physical examination change anesthetic management or affect outcome? Although there is evidence to the contrary, preanesthetic evaluation is an important component of anesthetic care. Gibby et al. stated that in 20% of the patients, most of whom were American Society of Anesthesiologists (ASA) physical status I or II, the anesthetic care plan was modified by information obtained by the preanesthetic history or physical examination; to what degree the outcome is affected by the preoperative evaluation, is not yet clear.

Preoperative assessment of the patients begins in anesthesia outpatient departments (OPDs). It is advantageous to see patients at least a week before surgery, particularly in the presence of accompanying cardiovascular or lung diseases, which are likely to add to the risk of surgery or when special techniques of anesthesia, such as controlled hypotension, are to be used. Treatment of associated diseases can be instituted as an outpatient to ensure that the patient is as fit as possible before surgery. The patient is followed up by repeated attendances at the clinic; she is admitted to the hospital only when declared fit for surgery, thus, ensuring minimal stay in the hospital. The patient's general history is taken, physical examination and review of laboratory data are done, decisions regarding the need for further consultation and patient instructions regarding, which medications should be continued or discontinued or initiated before surgery, are taken.

In the preoperative interview, the stress is on her medical history, her current physical status, current medication and previous anesthetic exposure, if any. The patient's personal history of anesthesia-related problems [e.g. difficult airway, need for postoperative mechanical ventilation, unanticipated intensive care unit (ICU) admission, poorly controlled pain, persistent nausea and/or vomiting] and the patient's family history of anesthesia-related problems [e.g. malignant hyperthermia (MH), pseudocholinesterase deficiency] is obtained. Appropriate laboratory tests and cross-matching of blood, if required, are done. Autologous blood donation can be organized at this time. Also, patient's questions, if any, are answered.

The preanesthesia physical examination tends to focus primarily on the airway, heart, and lungs; it also seeks to identify disorders and abnormalities of other organ systems that may compromise or be exacerbated by intraoperative management and postoperative care.

Anesthesia-specific Disorders

A vital aspect of the anesthesiologist's preoperative assessment involves identifying the patients who are at risk because of the anesthetic agents that may be used during surgery. If a patient gives a personal or family history of requiring intubation for several hours after relatively minor surgery, then the potential for atypical or decreased pseudocholinesterase levels should be explored. These result in an inability to metabolize succinylcholine.

Several hours of paralysis may occur after administration of this short-acting muscle relaxant. It can be identified by a blood test.

There are disorders that may precipitate life-threatening systemic responses to commonly used anesthetic agents. MH is an inherited disorder of calcium flux and may be precipitated by use of succinylcholine and inhalation anesthetic agents. Patients of muscular dystrophy, neurofibromatosis and strabismus are more likely to have MH. MH is not diagnosed until a crisis develops. The key to safe management is preoperative identification and avoiding use of the known provoking agents. However, the strongest evidence of MH susceptibility is a history of an MH episode (with hypercarbia, hyperthermia, arrhythmias, acidosis, rigidity, increased creatinine kinase and/or myoglobinuria) in a patient or family member. Confirmation of the disease is with a muscle biopsy and positive caffeine–halothane contraction test.

Life-threatening responses to neuromuscular blocking drugs may occur in major tissue trauma, denervating injuries (e.g. stroke or major nerve injury) myopathies, muscle disorders (e.g. muscular dystrophy) and burn injury. Use of succinylcholine can result in life-threatening hyperkalemia. Not uncommonly, patients in the intensive care setting require reintubation for which succinylcholine is often used; this could precipitate MH or hyperkalemia.

Prolonged muscle paralysis may also be precipitated by anesthesia in the patient with myasthenia gravis, which results in exaggerated responses to nondepolarizing muscle relaxants, such as pancuronium, vecuronium, atracurium, and rocuronium. The key to successful management of patient with myasthenia gravis is determining if anticholinesterase drugs, given to treat the disease, can be discontinued the night before surgery. The stopping of anticholinesterase drugs facilitates intraoperative management because they may interfere with the use of neuromuscular blocking agents. However, withdrawal of anticholinesterase drugs should not be attempted in patients who are anticholinesterase-dependent and who develop severe muscle weakness.

Preanesthetic Assessment

After the usual history and general examination is completed in the outpatient anesthesia clinic, evaluation of the patient for anesthesia is done. Particular attention is paid to oral cavity, personal habits, such as smoking, alcohol intake and drug therapy for associated diseases. Of utmost importance is the evaluation of the cardiorespiratory systems and assessment of the airway.

Oral cavity is a potential source of infection. There may be loose teeth that might get dislodged during endotracheal intubation. A dental consultation may be necessary.

Smoking should be stopped 4–6 weeks before surgery to reduce postoperative pulmonary morbidity. Stopping smoking for 12–24 hours benefits the cardiovascular system (CVS) by withdrawing carbon monoxide and nicotine; stopping for a few days will benefit ciliary activity; stopping for 1–2 weeks will reduce sputum volume. Postoperative chest complications in abdominal operations are six times more frequent in smokers than in nonsmokers.

Obesity is the enemy of both surgeon and anesthesiologist. Defined as body weight in excess of 20% of predicted body weight, obesity is associated with higher incidence of diabetes, hypertension and cardiac disease. Obesity results in more rapid oxygen desaturation. Obese patients are at a greater risk of aspiration pneumonitis because of higher volume and lower pH of gastric contents. Pharmacokinetics of drugs is altered. Finally, regional anesthesia is more difficult to administer and often unsuccessful. Treated properly by a 1,000-calorie diet along with exercise, excellent results can be obtained, even in the little time at the anesthetist's disposal. Walking for 1 hour expends 300 calories. Failure to lose weight is no reason to accept an unnecessarily fat patient for anesthesia.

Occasionally, patients are terrified of anesthesia or may fear a particular anesthetic technique (face-mask, spinal anesthesia). A little time spent in discussion with these patients is invaluable and may in fact bring some patients into hospital who would otherwise default. It should rarely be necessary to force an unwelcome technique on a patient.

Medical History

This can be facilitated by asking the patients to complete a preoperative questionnaire. Important points to glean from the notes are:

- *Previous illnesses, operations and anesthetics*: Complications of previous anesthetic administrations may be avoided on this occasion
- *Drug therapy*, e.g. corticosteroids, insulin, antihypertensive drugs, calcium antagonists, tranquillizers, digitalis, monoamine oxidase inhibitors, tricyclic antidepressants, anticoagulants, barbiturates, diuretics, drug allergies and drug addiction
- *Symptoms referable to the respiratory system*: Respiratory reserve, cough, sputum, bronchospasm, ability to expel secretions, smoking habits, etc.
- *Cardiovascular system*: Exercise tolerance, hypertension, breathlessness, chest pain, previous myocardial infarction (MI), etc.
- *Tendency to postanesthetic vomiting*: This will affect the choice of anesthetic drugs
- *Alcohol intake*: Alcoholic patient may suffer from cirrhosis of the liver, cardiomyopathy, diminished

adrenocortical response to stress, electrolyte imbalance, hypoglycemia, bone marrow depression, neuropathy, and psychosis.

Medical Examination

- *Assessment of pulmonary function*: Stress is on clinical and monitored signs of respiratory disease, respiratory pattern and character, presence of added sounds on auscultation, localizing signs, mediastinal shift, finger clubbing, cyanosis, etc.
- Assessment of the CVS and an attempt at prediction of cardiac risk in noncardiac surgery is made. Serious heart disease can be asymptomatic. Acute MI can be present without obvious symptoms. The aim is to look for coronary artery disease (CAD), valvular lesions, arrhythmias and to assess the cardiac reserve
- *The airway and oral cavity*: Dentition, e.g. prominent front teeth, loose teeth, artificial dentures, crown caps at the front—their presence should be recorded. Assessment and grading of the airway for difficulty/ease of endotracheal intubation is made
- *Nutrition*: The state of nutrition, malnutrition or obesity is noted
- *Color*: Look for cyanosis, jaundice, pigmentation or pallor
- *Nervous system*: Examination of the nervous system including the spine particularly where spinal or epidural block is planned
- *Psychological state*: Whether the patient is calm, apprehensive, unstable, etc.
- *Veins*: The state of the veins is noted
- *Diseases*: The presence or absence of associated diseases is noted.

Simple additional tests, which can be carried out in the anesthetic outpatient clinic include:

- Exercise tolerance
- *The breath-holding test of Sabrasez*: While resting, patient takes a full inspiration and holds his breath. A time of 25 second or longer may be taken as normal. A time of 15 second or less indicates diminished cardiorespiratory reserve
- The forced expiratory volume and vital capacity can be readily measured by pocket-sized microspirometers
- The Wright peak flow meter can be used to measure peak expiratory flow rate
- Pulse oximetry will give an idea of the state of oxygenation of the patient.

Pulmonary Evaluation

Despite improvement in surgical and anesthetic techniques, lung complications remain a major problem. Seventy percent of patients with chronic obstructive pulmonary disease (COPD) develop postoperative atelectasis and pneumonia. Gold and Helvich reported 24% incidence of operative and postoperative complications in asthmatic patients. The incidence increases markedly after the age of 50 years because of changes in air flow rates, lung volumes, lung elasticity, and ventilation-perfusion mismatch, all of which result in less efficient respiratory function. Tissue hypoxia is more likely in this group because circulatory responses to hypoxia are diminished.

Any patient with a history of respiratory symptoms needs further evaluation. Specific questions about frequency and productivity of cough and volume of sputum are asked; quantitative assessment of degree of dyspnea at rest and the level of exercise that causes symptoms is made. Inspection of thorax for limitations of mobility, physical deformity, muscular weakness or atrophy is made. Auscultation of chest during quiet breathing and forced expiration is done to detect rales, rhonchi or wheezes, and differences in the intensity of breath sounds. Bronchospasm and increased airway sensitivity are detected by the presence of expiratory rhonchi. Fine inspiratory crepitations which do not clear after one or two deep breaths are caused by pulmonary congestion from left ventricular failure; coarse crepitations indicate excess bronchial secretions. Plural effusion is indicated by dull percussion node and absent or reduced breath sounds. A chest X-ray shows the condition of the lungs, pleura and the bony cage.

The patient is asked to blow out a lighted match stick held at a distance of 15 cm with the mouth wide open. The patients who can perform this test should maintain adequate ventilation after surgery. Auscultation over trachea during forced expiration is done; breath sounds audible for less than 5 seconds rule out obstruction; if heard for more than 6 seconds, it denotes airway obstruction.

Spirometry is the screening test of pulmonary function. From this tracing forced vital capacity (FVC), forced expiratory volume in 1 second (FEV_1), FEV_1/FVC ratio and many other values are obtained. Spirometer also generates a flow-volume curve which identifies small airways obstruction, usually not detected on chest auscultation but can cause hypoxemia during surgery.

Preoperative blood gas studies can also be performed, if needed. Increased arterial carbon dioxide (CO_2) tension indicates inadequate ventilation. Low arterial oxygen tension is due to ventilation-perfusion mismatch, diffusion defect, or shunting.

Indicators of potential postoperative respiratory complications are:

- COPD on chest X-ray
- Severe thoracic deformity on chest X-ray
- FVC less than 50% of predicted value
- FEV_1 less than 2 L or less than 50% of predicted value

- Partial pressure of oxygen (PaO_2) less than 65 mm Hg
- Partial pressure of carbon dioxide ($PaCO_2$) greater than 45 mm Hg.

Postoperative pulmonary complications (PPCs) occur in approximately 30–80% of patients, but fortunately they are not always serious. Risk factors for PPCs include smoking, chronic respiratory disease, emergency surgery, upper abdominal surgery, anesthetic time more than 180 minutes and age more than 70 years. Pain and abdominal distention are frequent causes of respiratory complications because of their limiting effects on ventilatory capacity.

Patients with obstructive lung diseases should be admitted to the hospital several days before surgery. Smoking is stopped. Bronchial infection is suspected if there is productive cough; appropriate antibiotics are started after culture and sensitivity. Bronchodilators and mucolytic agents are used in presence of bronchospasm. Adequate hydration is extremely important and patients should drink at least eight glasses of water daily. Physiotherapy of chest is very helpful in these patients; they breathe more efficiently and instructions on postural drainage and effective coughing will improve the ability to mobilize secretions.

Cardiac Evaluation

Cardiovascular disease is a significant cause of perioperative morbidity and mortality, which, if not treated, could lead to collapse or death. ASA has issued guidelines on clinical risk stratification and appropriate use of diagnostic testing (Tables 1 to 3).

Functional capacity of the heart is more important than the nature of the structural damage. The grading is done according to the patient's tolerance to effort, the presence or history of atrial fibrillation, and the existence of pulmonary congestion. Patients who could exercise to 85% of their peak maximal heart rate, even in the presence of a positive stress test, were at lower risk when compared with those who could not reach the desired heart rate. If a patient can walk a mile without becoming breathless, then the possibility of extensive CAD is small; alternatively, if the patient has dyspnea associated with chest pain during minimal exertion, then the possibility of CAD is higher.

Surgical procedure itself has a significant impact on perioperative risks; for minor surgical OPD procedures and day-care surgery not associated with significant stress, perioperative management is rarely altered by CVS status. On the other hand, vascular surgery represents high risk; intra-abdominal, thoracic, and orthopedic procedures are intermediate risk.

Coronary Artery Disease

Coronary artery disease continues to be a major cause of death; patients with preexisting cardiac disease are more likely to experience cardiac complications in the postoperative period than gynecological problems. Cadanelli and associates reported a 13.5% incidence of cardiac disease in 1,664 cases of gynecologic surgery;12% of these showed clinical or electrocardiographic (ECG) deterioration. The overall mortality was less than 1%; this low figure was possibly due to preoperative recognition and understanding of the disease process.

Clinical history will identify cardiorespiratory symptoms but patients with serious heart disease are not always symptomatic. Acute myocardial ischemia may be present without obvious symptoms. Classical symptoms of chest pain are well known and easily recognized but angina should also be suspected if pain or discomfort is felt anywhere between the waist and jaw on effort or due to emotion. Angina associated with breathlessness is indicative of left ventricular dysfunction. A recent history of MI is of particular importance as it increases the risk of perioperative MI (Table 2).

A diastolic murmur is unequivocal evidence of heart disease. A systolic murmur with no interval between

Table 1: Risks in surgical patients with cardiovascular disorders

S. No.	Disorder	Risk factors	Precautions
1	Arteriosclerotic heart disease	Unstable angina	Delay elective surgery for 6 months
		Recent MI	ECG and invasive monitoring
		Arrhythmias	Evaluation of LV function by echocardiography or thallium
		CHF	
2	Valvular heart disease	Endocarditis	Antibiotic prophylaxis
		CHF	Echocardiography
		Critical AS	Invasive monitoring
		Anticoagulants	

Abbreviations: MI, myocardial infarction; CHF, congestive; ECG, electrocardiogram; LV, left ventricular; AS, aortic stenosis

Table 2: Risk of perioperative myocardial infarction

Time since MI	Incidence of perioperative MI
<3 months	36%
3–6 months	16%
>6 months	6%

Table 3:. The degree of risk of cardiovascular disease can be assessed by using the Goldman index

Risk factor	Score
Third heart sound/gallop rhythm	11
MI within 6 months	10
>5 ventricular ectopics per min	7
Rhythm other than sinus	7
Age >70 years	5
Emergency surgery	5
Aortic stenosis	3
Abdominal or thoracic operation	3
Poor general condition	3

Note: A total of more than 13 gives a poor prognosis (11% life threatening complications); total of more than 26 has a mortality of 50% and only lifesaving operations should be considered. It is almost entirely based upon clinical findings.

the murmur and the second heart sound is likely to be associated with organic disease. Presence of a thrill, vascular bruits, gallop rhythm, abnormal venous pulsations and peripheral edema are equally important signs of cardiac or vascular disease. Preoperative congestive cardiac failure has been associated with increased incidence of perioperative cardiac morbidity.

Stabilization of ventricular function and finding the cause of pulmonary congestion is necessary because perioperative monitoring and treatment would depend on it. Congestive symptoms could be due to nonischemic cardiomyopathy or mitral or aortic valve disease. Patients with cardiac prostheses are likely to be on anticoagulant therapy, and this should not be stopped unless very necessary.

Routine laboratory investigations often fail to unmask the extent of cardiac disease. Resting abnormal ECG is helpful but a normal tracing associated with symptoms of progressive anginal pain is of no help. An exercise ECG is the least invasive and most cost effective method with reasonable sensitivity and specificity for identifying CAD. A significant number of patients are either unable to exercise or have contraindications to exercise; for them pharmacological stress testing (Thallium-201) has become popular. The ambulatory ECG (Holter) provides a means of continuously monitoring the ECG for significant ST segment changes during the perioperative period. Raby demonstrated that silent ischemia is a strong predictor of bad outcome.

Echocardiography accurately determines the size of various cardiac chambers, evaluates the ventricular wall motion, the size of different valve orifices and intracardiac thrombus or myxoma. Recently, stress echocardiography has received attention as a preoperative test. The appearance of new or worsened regional wall motion abnormalities is considered a positive test; these represent areas at risk for myocardial ischemia. Dobutamine echocardiography has been found to be the best predictive test; those patients who develop wall motion abnormalities at low heart rates are at greatest risk.

Noncardiac surgery should be deferred till a patient with CAD is stabilized by appropriate drug therapy or surgery; MI in the previous 6 months should be considered an unstable condition; surgery in this period is associated with high incidence of reinfarction and mortality.

Serum electrolytes are important in patients with arrhythmias. Chest X-ray in most cases is enough to show the size of cardiac shadow and the state of lung fields.

Valvular Heart Diseases

Mitral valve prolapse (MVP) is now the most common valvular lesion seen in women with a decline in the incidence of rheumatic fever. MVP exhibits vague symptoms of chest pain, fatigue and palpitation. Aortic stenosis increases the risk of surgery and is not always symptomatic. Valvular disease places the patient at risk according to their functional status. Risks are greatest in patients of ASA grades 3 and 4. Most of these patients are on digitalis, diuretic and a vasodilator. Surgery is delayed till heart failure is controlled and patient is clinically stable. They need invasive monitoring, echocardiography and antibiotic prophylaxis against endocarditis [ampicillin 2 g intravenous (IV) or intramuscular (IM) and gentamicin 1.5 mg/kg IM, given 1 hour before surgery, repeated 8 hours later. Vancomycin 1g IV slowly can be used in place of ampicillin].

Patients with valve prostheses may be on anticoagulants; warfarin sodium is discontinued for several days preoperatively till prothrombin time is about 15 seconds; surgery is performed and warfarin started as soon as it is deemed safe. IV heparin is used till the patients are back on warfarin.

Airway Assessment

Maintenance of an adequate airway at all times is one of the prime duties of an anesthesiologist. Endotracheal intubation must be smooth and quick; to achieve this end, preoperative airway evaluation is done; it requires no equipment, is entirely noninvasive and takes less than a minute to perform. The examination first focuses on the teeth; if the upper incisors are big or the maxillary teeth are anterior to mandibular teeth then there is difficulty in inserting the laryngoscope blade in the oral cavity. If the patient is able to protrude the mandible beyond the maxilla, this signifies good temporomandibular joint function and good mouth opening resulting in easy insertion of the laryngoscope. If the distance between the upper and lower incisors, on opening the mouth, is more than 3 cm, then laryngoscopy is easy. A large tongue or a narrow, highly arched palate reduces the oropharyngeal volume and make the laryngoscopy and visualization of the glottis difficult. If the distance between the thyroid cartilage and symphysis menti is more than 5 cm, intubation is easy. A short, thick neck and restricted movement of head and neck make intubation difficult. If endotracheal intubation is anticipated to be difficult, then the anesthesiologist has the time to plan and take suitable measures to overcome the problem.

Laboratory Investigations (Box 1)

Preoperative Laboratory Testing

They are aimed at discovering a medical condition that would adversely affect surgical outcome. The value of any preoperative test is directly proportional to the likelihood of discovering defects or disease. Previously, extensive laboratory tests were ordered; one advantage was that they provided baseline values for most potential disorders. However, disadvantages were many; the greater the number of preoperative tests performed, the greater the probability of finding a false-positive result. Moreover, such routine testing in healthy, asymptomatic and young patients is expensive, rarely alters perioperative management, often ignored, and may result in unnecessary delays. As age or symptoms increase, more diligent testing is justified. Laboratory testing should be based on information obtained during the preoperative assessment, such as the following:

- The presence of a disease condition determined from the preoperative history and physical examination
- If the patient belongs to a high-risk group based on epidemiology (e.g. ECG for male patient more than 45 years old)
- If a baseline value is beneficial because of likely intra- and postoperative changes
- If it affects the postoperative management.

The "basic" indication for testing is based on age; no testing required in a healthy patient less than 50 years old who is undergoing minor surgery. Additional testing may be required based on specific aspects of surgery and for various medical conditions to assess readiness for surgery as well as to provide important baseline information.

Box 1 Recommended laboratory testing

These tests may be required for administration of anesthesia and are not intended to limit those required by surgeons for issues specific to their surgical management.

Age less than 50 years, healthy

- No tests unless specified by surgeon for specific surgical issues.

Electrocardiogram

- Age 50 years or older
- Age greater than 40 years with risks factors (hyperlipidemia, hypertension diabetes, family history)
- Hypertension
- Irregular pulse
- Cardiac drugs (digoxin; antihypertensives)
- Current or past significant cardiac disease/circulatory disease
- Cardiothoracic procedure.

Chest X-ray

- Major respiratory condition with change of symptoms or acute episode in past 6 months
- Malignancy
- Cardiothoracic procedure.

Serum chemistry

- Renal disease
- Adrenal, thyroid, diabetes or other major metabolic disorders
- Digoxin, diuretic, angiotensin converting enzyme (ACE) inhibitors and steroid therapy
- Chemotherapy.

Urinalysis

- Genitourologic procedure.

Complete blood count

- Known/suspected anemia
- Condition causing preoperative blood loss
- History of bleeding/bruising disease
- Anticoagulant drugs
- Symptomatic cardiovascular or pulmonary disease
- Chronic diseases (rheumatoid, renal disease)
- Hematologic disorder (sickle cell disease; thalassemia)
- Vascular procedure
- Chemotherapy.

Clotting screen

- Liver disease
- Bleeding/bruising disease
- Anticoagulant therapy.

Liver function test

- Liver disease
- Excess alcohol consumption.

Testing should be performed within 30 days of surgery but results obtained from the medical record within 6 months of surgery are acceptable if the patient's medical history has not changed substantially. More recent testing, including repeat testing on the day of surgery, may be indicated if there is development of new or exacerbation of preexisting signs and symptoms or when test results may play a role in the selection of a specific anesthetic technique (e.g. regional anesthesia in the context of anticoagulation therapy).

Hemoglobin, hematocrit, total and differential blood counts, and complete urine analysis are a part of every preoperative workup. Symptoms suggestive of hepatic, renal or metabolic disease are thoroughly investigated by laboratory studies specific for the system concerned. For liver function: enzyme determinations, total protein with albumin-globulin ratio, prothrombin time and bilirubin levels are advised. Renal disease requires evaluation with an intravenous pyelogram (IVP), blood urea nitrogen, serum creatinine with complete urine analysis and urine culture.

Suspected metabolic diseases, such as thyroid dysfunction or diabetes are assessed by a thyroid panel or a fasting or 2-hour postprandial blood glucose level or both.

Patients with abnormal uterine bleeding should have blood coagulation studies, such as fibrinogen, platelet count, prothrombin time, bleeding and clotting time, as well as an endometrial biopsy or pelvic ultrasound.

All extensive surgery should be preceded by a baseline electrolyte panel as a basis for postoperative fluid and electrolyte replacement therapy. Serum sodium, potassium and calcium levels are important.

An IVP is obtained in the differential diagnosis of a pelvic mass, together with a barium enema if bowel involvement is suspected.

The need for routine ECGs is debated. Goldberger and O'Konski recommended ECGs for:

- Patients with a history and physical examination suggestive of cardiovascular disease
- Patients with systemic disease or other conditions that may be associated with unrecognized heart disease such as hypertension or diabetes
- Patients taking medications that might have cardiac toxicity
- Patients at risk for electrolyte disturbances
- Patients undergoing major surgical procedures
- Patients older than 40 years should have an ECG before surgery.

Chest X-ray examination with anteroposterior and lateral views is a routine hospital admission procedure. It may be useful as a baseline for postoperative care. It does carry a small risk of radiation damage; routine chest radiography of patients not being operated for chest or heart condition has been questioned.

Computerized tomography and magnetic resonance imaging can also be useful in differentiating uterine leiomyomas from adenomyosis. These imaging techniques should not be considered where the diagnosis is already confirmed but used only when necessary.

Ultrasonography can be a useful diagnostic tool for distinguishing uterine from adnexal disease and for measuring the growth of uterine myomas.

In certain cases it is desirable to refer the patient to other departments for advice (e.g. diabetes, hypertension, cardiac failure, infections, and respiratory failure).

Optimization of Patient Medications

Often patients are taking drugs for associated illness when they come for surgery. It is important for the anesthesiologist to know about these drugs because they can adversely affect the course of anesthesia. Medications typically continued till surgery includes cardiac, asthma, antiseizure, endocrine, steroid and gastrointestinal medications. Analgesics [except, possibly nonsteroidal anti-inflammatory drugs (NSAIDs) and aspirin containing drugs], antianxiety (except possibly monoamine oxidase inhibitors (MAOIs) and tricyclic antidepressants) and antihypertensive medications (except possibly angiotensin-converting enzyme inhibitors and angiotensin II receptor blocker) are also continued on the morning of surgery. An appreciation of subtle differences among medications is critical to perioperative management. For example, while it is common to continue H_2-blockers and proton pump antagonists to decrease the risk of acid aspiration, particulate antacids are withheld on the morning of surgery in light of their deleterious effects if aspirated.

Antibiotics

Large parenteral doses (e.g. mega-doses poured into wound or peritoneum) of the aminoglycosides, neomycin, streptomycin and dihydrostreptomycin and the lincomycins can cause a neuromuscular block, which is potentiated by the volatile agents or depolarizing muscle relaxants. Other antibiotics, that may cause a similar effect include kanamycin, tobramycin, polymyxin B, biomycin, bacitracin, and colistin. Use of depolarizing muscle relaxants does not obviate this danger because there has been a report of this syndrome when suxamethonium had been used as the relaxant, presumably due to the onset of dual block. This is not a common problem.

Psychotropic Drugs

Many psychotropic drugs potentiate the effects of anesthetics. Extrapyramidal effects (Parkinsonism, akathisia, dystonia and dyskinesia) can occur, especially with butyrophenones. Dystonia may respond dramatically to injection of antiparkinsonism drugs, such as benztropine, 1–2 mg IV.

Grand mal epilepsy can be precipitated by tricyclic antidepressants, lithium and major tranquillizers as well as by abrupt withdrawal of benzodiazepines. Major tranquillizers and tricyclic antidepressants have anticholinergic side effects. Tricyclic antidepressants block the reuptake of monoamines into adrenergic nerve terminals so that circulating catecholamines are increased. Adrenaline is best avoided. Sinus tachycardia and ventricular dysrhythmias can occur. Conversely, sudden withdrawal of tricyclic antidepressant therapy can lead to malaise, fatigue, muscle pains, vomiting, and diarrhea.

Lithium should be stopped 48–72 hours before a relaxant is given. It interacts with barbiturates to prolong recovery. Cardiac dysrhythmias are common. It potentiates the nondepolarizing relaxants. In emergency cases, suxamethonium and regional blocks should be considered.

Monoamine Oxidase Inhibitors

These drugs should be discontinued 2–3 weeks before elective surgery. The mode of action of this group of drugs is imperfectly understood. Reactions to pethidine, fentanyl and morphine have been reported in patients taking these drugs and deaths have occurred. Reactions include severe depression, coma, muscle twitching, hypotension, ataxia, ocular palsies, cerebral excitement and Cheyne-Stokes respiration. Relief has been obtained following administration of 25 mg of prednisolone hemisuccinate or chlorpromazine. Not all patients receiving treatment with MAOIs show adverse reactions. IV test doses of 5 mg, 10 mg, then 20 mg pethidine may be given, and the effect on blood pressure (BP) and pulse rate observed. Severe hypertensive effects and even death may occur when pressor drugs (e.g. the adrenaline in local analgesic solutions) are given to patients on MAOIs, but may be counteracted with phentolamine. For postoperative analgesia, a combination of chlorpromazine and codeine has been used without ill effect. Regional blocks and nonsteroidal anti-inflammatory drugs are also suitable.

Phenothiazine Derivatives

These cause peripheral vasodilatation and a fall in BP in some subjects, which may become severe during anesthesia. Narcotics are potentiated. Other side effects include liver dysfunction, antianalgesia and pseudoparkinsonism.

Levodopa

There is a slight risk of tachycardia and ventricular dysrhythmias, so it may be stopped on the day of operation only. Levodopa inhibits prolactin secretion and stimulates growth hormone production, which may make diabetic patients more liable to hyperglycemia. The danger of stopping levodopa for longer than the day of operation is the reappearance of severe parkinsonism, dysphagia and the risk of aspiration pneumonia. Butyrophenones antagonize the action of levodopa on dopaminergic receptors in the brain and should be used with caution.

Steroid Therapy

Any patient receiving steroids or who has received them within the last 12 months may have adrenal suppression and requires steroid cover during the perioperative period. For minor procedures hydrocortisone 100 mg is given along with premedication followed by 50 mg every 6 hours for 24 hours followed by the usual maintenance dose. For major surgery, hydrocortisone 100 mg along with premedication is given; during intraoperative and postoperative period 50–100 mg every 6 hours is given for 72 hours.

Antihyperglycemic Medications

Oral hypoglycemic agents are routinely withheld on the morning of surgery and these drugs may even be temporarily discontinued on the evening before surgery if the patient is prone to hypoglycemia before breakfast. Additionally, before major surgery, metformin may be withheld for 48 hours because of its potential to exacerbate lactic acidosis.

Antihypertensive Medications

Hypertension alone is not a major risk for surgery unless associated with renal or cardiac complications. It is a major anesthetic risk if systolic blood pressure (SBP) is greater than 180 mmHg or diastolic blood pressure (DBP) is greater than 110 mmHg. The objectives of evaluating hypertensive patients are to identify secondary causes, to assess target organ damage and to identify the cardiovascular risk factors. Drugs commonly used to treat mild to moderate hypertension include diuretics, calcium channel blockers, ACE inhibitors and beta blockers. The current trend is to continue the drugs in the perioperative period.

Hypertension has been associated with an increased perioperative risk ranging from benign BP fluctuations to pronounced hyper- and hypotension with myocardial ischemia and stroke. Hypertensive patients scheduled for surgery may present with left ventricular hypertrophy, CAD, poor exercise tolerance, chronic renal insufficiency and/or cerebrovascular disease. These patients often have persistent vasoconstriction, which is associated with increased afterload and hypovolemia. If end-organ damage is suspected, an ECG and serum creatinine measurement should be obtained preoperatively. Also, look for evidence of secondary hypertension, such as pheochromocytoma, hyperthyroidism, increased intracranial pressure, coarctation, hyperadrenalism, renal disease, renal artery stenosis, acromegaly, hypercalcemia, extreme anxiety, and pain.

Unless there is evidence of end-organ damage, patients with stage I (mild) and stage II (moderate) hypertension (SBP < 180 mmHg and DBP < 110 mmHg) do not appear to be at significantly increased risk for adverse cardiovascular outcomes during the perioperative period. However, moderate hypertension may predispose the patient to dangerously high pressures intraoperatively. The patient with BP greater than 160/100 mmHg would benefit from enhanced at-home therapy and may also require acute treatment on the morning of surgery.

The American College of Cardiology (ACC)/American Heart Association (AHA) guidelines recommendations are:

Blood pressure should be "controlled" before elective noncardiac surgery in patients with stage III (severe) hypertension (SBP >180 mmHg or DBP >110 mm Hg). The decision to delay surgery for stabilization of BP versus acutely correcting the hypertension, must take into account the potential benefits and the urgency of the surgical procedure. Except in cases of extreme stage III hypertension or severe end organ injury, it is characteristic to proceed with surgery by acutely controlling elevated BP if it is deemed important not to postpone surgery. If attempted, acute antihypertensive therapy should be titrated carefully so as not to precipitate hypotension, bradycardia and consequent organ ischemia. Optimal BP control must be maintained in the postoperative period to avoid rebound hypertension.

Patients are maintained on their antihypertensive medications, especially β-blockers, through the morning of surgery. Withdrawal of β-blockers can be associated with "rebound" hypertension and perioperative tachycardia. Diuretics are withheld on the morning of surgery to avoid excessive bladder filling during surgery, in the absence of a urinary catheter, unless these medications are vital to the management of congestive heart failure or continued treatment is necessary for fluid and electrolyte disturbances. Those receiving alpha-2 agonists like clonidine can have a hypertensive crisis if clonidine is withdrawn.

If patients develop hypertension during anesthesia, the most appropriate response is to deepen anesthesia and increase analgesia. If it persists beta-blockers are used; there is evidence that halothane is a safe agent in these circumstances; now calcium antagonists, ACE inhibitors, angiotensin II receptor blockers are the newer options available. Bradycardia, due to unopposed vagal action, is treated with atropine or glycopyrrolate.

Angiotensin-converting Enzyme Inhibitors

These are given orally, so may have to be withdrawn following abdominal surgery. They may be given on the day of operation and resumed as soon as oral intake is restarted. These drugs can result in significant intraoperative hypotension because of myocardial depression, hypovolemia, pronounced blood loss and vasodilatation that may be associated with general, spinal or epidural anesthesia. Patients on ACE inhibitors often respond inadequately to ephedrine and need more aggressive vasopressor therapy. Thus, it is recommended to withhold these drugs on the day of surgery, unless continuation is considered necessary to reduce afterload in a failing heart.

Calcium Channel Blockers

These should not be stopped prior to surgery without a very specific reason because an exacerbation of angina may occur.

Angina Prophylaxis Drugs

These drugs should be continued through the perioperative period. If the oral route is impossible, transdermal glyceryl trinitrate patch dressings placed on the lateral chest wall last about 24 hours. Reapplication should be at a fresh site.

Antithrombotic Medications

Many patients who have CAD, atrial fibrillation, cardiac valve prosthesis or a history of deep venous thrombosis, are on antithrombotic medications, which have important anesthetic implications. Vitamin E (in doses >400 units/day), fish oil and herbal supplements have antiplatelet and anticoagulant effects. In many situations, the antithrombotic effects are the "side effects" of agents administered for other purposes such as NSAIDs or aspirin used for analgesia.

A normal prothrombin time should be confirmed before surgery, particularly before a neuraxial block. These drugs should be stopped before surgery. NSAIDs are stopped 5–10 days, aspirin 10 days, and warfarin, vitamin E, fish oil and herbal supplements should be discontinued approximately 5 days before surgery. However, if discontinuation of these drugs prove to be harmful, then the risk/benefit evaluation of continuing or discontinuing these medications must be done. Often a suitable replacement (e.g. cyclooxygenase type 2 inhibitor instead of a NSAID) can be administered. If a patient cannot tolerate prolonged discontinuation of anticoagulation, then low molecular weight heparin can be administered because they have a relatively short half-life (4–6 h) with a quicker return to normal hemostasis.

Of greater concern, is the need to continue antithrombotic therapy before surgery. The disease process being treated, determines the choice of antithrombotic therapy and how these medications are to be adjusted during the perioperative period. The need to maintain aggressive antiplatelet therapy may necessitate delaying elective surgery for several weeks.

Successful regional anesthesia will reduce perioperative opioid requirements, may decrease blood loss and the incidence of deep vein thrombosis. However, administration of a regional anesthetic may cause bleeding when antiplatelet or anticoagulation medication is used. This does not necessarily rule out a neuraxial block but suggests the need for increased vigilance. The decision to continue or discontinue drug should be based on a consensus among the surgeon, physician and anesthesiologist. This decision should also take into consideration other medications and patient conditions that may affect bleeding.

Tocolytic Therapy

Tocolytics are often administered to inhibit premature labor or they may be used to manage acute fetal distress, while preparations are being made for delivery. It may be necessary to administer anesthesia in the presence of these agents. Tocolytics are sympathomimetic drugs with predominantly beta-2 but also some beta-1 activity. Heart rate and cardiac output increase; myocardial ischemia, pulmonary edema or even cardiac failure can occur after prolonged beta-mimetic therapy. Betamimetics stimulate release of antidiuretic hormone (ADH) and act directly on renal tubules to increase sodium reabsorption; therefore, these patients are at risk of fluid overload. They should be discontinued for 30 minutes before induction of general anesthesia (GA). Laryngoscopy and intubation may generate severe tachycardia and hypertension. Esmolol is useful drug to prevent these side effects. Avoid agents that cause tachycardia; halothane can cause arrhythmias, hence avoided. Hyperventilation is avoided because resulting hypocarbia enhances hypokalemia of beta-mimetic therapy. If regional anesthesia is chosen, it should be instituted cautiously. Prehydration is not necessary and can result in pulmonary edema. Vasopressors may elicit an exaggerated response. Magnesium sulfate is also widely used for tocolysis. It is also associated with pulmonary edema. The concerns regarding prehydration are similar to betamimetics. Magnesium potentiates both depolarizing and nondepolarizing muscle relaxants.

PREECLAMPTIC PATIENT

Severely preeclamptic patient should not be rushed unprepared into the operation theater (OT) for emergency cesarean (C) section in an effort to prevent convulsions. In the absence of fetal compromise, mother's BP must be stabilized, bringing the DBP to a range of 90–105 mmHg. Hydrazaline and labetalol are most commonly used for this purpose. Oral nifedipine has been found to be effective. If fetal distress necessitates an emergent C section, then IV nitroprusside may be used. Magnesium sulfate has been used for prophylaxis of eclampsia.

A lumbar epidural block provides safe, excellent analgesia for labor, improves uteroplacental perfusion, and may improve fetal condition; blockade to T8 level results in significantly reduced levels of circulating catecholamines. Safe administration of regional anesthesia in preeclamptic patients requires absence of significant coagulopathy, a DBP less than 110 mmHg and an adequate circulating blood volume. Coagulation abnormalities most often encountered are low platelets count, abnormal platelet function and prolonged thrombin time.

Circulating blood volume is often low and central venous pressure (CVP) of –1 to –4 cm of H_2O is common; correction of hypovolemia is necessary before a regional block, yet overhydration remains a danger in these patients who may develop pulmonary edema. CVP monitoring is usually instituted to assist in gauging adequacy of fluid therapy. IV fluids are given to raise the CVP to 3 to 4 cm of H_2O to prevent hypotension during regional anesthesia. The compliance and degree of compromise of the right and left ventricle in preeclampsia is often unequal. Urinary output may be unreliable as a guide to hydration, as it can be compromised by glomerular endotheliosis. Therefore, in cases of refractory oliguria or if signs of CHF are present, monitoring with pulmonary artery catheter may be more appropriate than a CVP line.

For C section, an epidural block may be safer than a spinal block because of the danger of sudden maternal hypotension; however, this can be countered by using a low dose local anesthetic alone or in combination with fentanyl for spinal. The level of an epidural block should be raised slowly; preeclamptic patients have an increased systemic vascular resistance (SVR) that can fall suddenly in the presence of sympathetic blockade. If hypotension does occur, ephedrine can be used in small doses of 5–10 mg, IV and hydration increased. Preeclamptic women may have exaggerated responses to exogenous or endogenous catecholamines. If GA is to be used for C section, it must be remembered that the patient may have received magnesium sulfate preoperatively; laryngeal edema may diminish the size of airway and create difficulty in intubation. Preeclamptic patients may have a marked hypertensive response to laryngoscopy and intubation. Antihypertensive drugs, such as esmolol and nitroprusside should be available; isoflurane is perhaps the volatile agent of choice in these patients.

FIT FOR SURGERY

This is a vague concept but usually implies that the patient, who is not unduly old, lives a normal life, is free from serious signs and symptoms of disease, is not receiving drug treatment for abnormalities, has reasonable exercise tolerance for his age, is not unduly overweight and appears emotionally stable. In the light of the more detailed ASA status analysis, the global concept of "fit" is outmoded. Physical status is close to, but not the same as "risk".

CANCELING CASES

The paramount concern is the safety of the patient. More and more of the decisions about the patient's fitness for surgery are being left to the anesthetist. This calls for skillful judgment. Occasionally, it may not be in the sick patient's interest that the surgery be cancelled and calculated risks may have to be taken with agreement of the patient or relatives. Operations may be cancelled in the following circumstances:

1. Because of inadequate preparation, e.g. blood test results or blood transfusion not available at the preoperative visit.
2. Because of risk arising from the poor condition of the patient.

The anesthetist should ask, "Is there any way in which this patient can be improved?", if so, the operation may be postponed. If not, the question becomes, "Is the risk of anesthesia justified by the probable benefits of the operation?", if the answer is "no", then, "Would a different type of anesthesia be suitable (e.g. regional analgesia or ketamine)?". If the answer to this is negative, it may either be due to shortcomings in the patient's health or shortage of facilities in the hospital, e.g. lack of intensive care, nursing shortage, etc. The anesthetist has a right to refuse a patient for anesthesia, either temporarily or permanently. He also has a right to postpone surgery (even for an "emergency" case) if he thinks that the patient's condition can be improved by delaying surgery.

Once the patient has been assessed, anesthetist must formulate a plan for the anesthetic management which involves ensuring that the patient is in the best condition possible. This will include correction of anemia, dehydration, control of heart failure, and optimization of lung function with physiotherapy, bronchodilators and antibiotics. Advice from physicians may be helpful in difficult cases. In emergency cases, it is vital to have replaced blood loss with appropriate fluids prior to induction of anesthesia.

SUMMARY

The preoperative preparation of patients should be based on a thorough clinical history and examination. Further investigations, if available, will confirm the clinical findings but should not be used as primary diagnostic methods. A plan of management should be formed before the start of every anesthetic and the anesthetist must be satisfied that the patient is in the best condition possible. The decision that the patient is "*fit for anesthesia*" is the sole responsibility of the anesthetist.

BIBLIOGRAPHY

1. Akhtar W, Reeves WC, Movahed A. Indications for anticoagulation in atrial fibrillation. Am Fam Physician. 1998;58:130-6.
2. American College of Physicians. Preoperative pulmonary function testing. Ann Intern Med. 1990;112:793-4.
3. American Society of Anesthesiologists task force on preanesthetic evaluation. Anesthesiology. 2002;96:485-96.
4. American Society of Anesthesiologists. (1963). Physical status classification system: new classification of physical status. Available from http://www.asahq.org/Home/For-Members/Clinical-Information/ASA-Physical-Status-Classification-System. [Accessed November, 2013].
5. American Society of Regional Anesthesia and Pain Medicine: Recommendations for Neuraxial Anesthesia and Anticoagulation. Reg Anesth. 1998;23(Suppl 2):129-94.
6. Arens JF. A practice parameters overview. Anesthesiology. 1993;78:229-30.
7. ASA Taskforce on preoperative fasting. Anaesthesiology. 1990; 90896-905.
8. Belli G, Ellis SG, Topol EJ: Stenting for ischemic heart disease. Prog Cardiovas Dis. 1997;40:159-82.
9. Berlauk JF, Abrams JH, Gilmour IJ, et al. Preoperative optimization of cardiovascular hemodynamics improves outcome in peripheral vascular surgery: A prospective, randomized clinical trial. Ann Surg. 1991;214:289-97; discussion 298-9.
10. Bertrand M, Godet G, Meersschaert K, et al. Should the angiotensin II antagonists be discontinued before surgery? Anesth Analg. 2001;92:26-30.
11. Bishop MU, Shoemaker WC, Appel PL, et al. Prospective randomized trial of survivor values of cardiac index: Oxygen delivery and oxygen consumption as resuscitation endpoints in severe trauma. Trauma. 1995;38:780-7.

12. Boyd O, Grounds RM, Bennett ED. A randomized clinical trial of the effect of deliberate perioperative increase of oxygen delivery on mortality in high-risk surgical patients. JAMA. 1993;270:2699707.
13. Boyd O, Grounds RM, Bennett ED. A randomized controlled trial of the effect of deliberate preoperative increase of oxygen delivery on mortality and morbidity in high-risk surgical patients. JAMA. 1993;270:2699-707.
14. Brabant SM, Bertrand M, Eyraud D, et al. The hemodynamic effects of anesthetic induction in vascular surgical patients chronically treated with angiotensin II receptor antagonists. Anesth Analg. 1999;89:1388-92.
15. Cadanelli GP, Cavatorta E, Verrilli D. Chirurgia gynecologia e cardiopatie. Quad Clin Obstet Gynecol. 1967;22:911.
16. Carlson RW, Weiland DE, Srivathsan K. Does a full-time, 24-hour intensivist improve care and efficiency? Crit Care Clin. 1996;12:525-51.
17. Chan WS. What is the optimal management of pregnant women with valvular heart disease in pregnancy? Haemostasis. 1999;29(Suppl):105-6.
18. Clozel JP, Ertel EA, Ertel SI. Discovery and main pharmacological properties of mibefradil (Ro 40-5967), the first selective T-type calcium channel blocker. J Hypertens .1997;15:S17-26.
19. Curran JE, Grounds RM. Ward versus intensive care management of high-risk surgical patients. Br J Surg. 1998;85:956-61.
20. Diener HC. Stroke prevention: Antiplatelet and antithrombotic therapy. Haemostasis. 2000;30(Suppl 3):14-26.
21. Eagle K, Berger P, Calkins H, et al. ACC/AHA guideline update for perioperative cardiovascular evaluation for noncardiac surgery—executive summary: a report of the American College of Cardiology/American Heart Association Task Force on practice guidelines. J Am Coll Cardiol. 2002;39:542-53.
22. Eagle K, Berger PB, Calkins H, et al. Guidelines for perioperative cardiovascular evaluation of non cardiac surgery. Circulation. 1996;93:1278-317.
23. Farmer W, Silverman DG. Herbal medicines: What the anesthesiologist needs to know. In: Hines RL (Ed). Seminars in Anesthesia: Pharmacology Update. Philadelphia: WB Saunders; 2001.
24. FitzGerald GA, Patrono C. Drug therapy: The coxibs, selective inhibitors of cyclooxygenase-2. N Engl J Med. 2001;345:433-42.
25. Flancbaum L, Ziegler DW, Choban PS. Preoperative intensive care unit admission and hemodynamic monitoring in patients scheduled for major elective noncardiac surgery: A retrospective review of 95 patients. J Cardiothorac Vasc Anesth. 1998;12:3-9.
26. Fleisher LA, Rosenbaum SH, Nelson AH. Preoperative dipyridamole thallium imaging and ambulatory electrocardiographic monitoring as a predictor of perioperative cardiac events and long-term outcome. Anaesthesiology 1995;83:906-17.
27. Fleisher LA. Preoperative evaluation of the patient with hypertension. . JAMA. 2002;287:2043–6.
28. Gallagher EG, White M, Ward S, et al. Prophylaxis against acid aspiration syndrome. Anesthesia. 1988;43:1011-4.
29. Garrison RN, Wilson MA, Matheson PJ, et al. Preoperative saline loading improves outcome after elective, noncardiac surgical procedures. Am Surg. 1996;62:223-31.
30. Gibby GL, Gravenstein JS, Layon AJ, et al. How often does the preoperative interview change anesthetic management? Anesthesiology. 1992;77:A1134.
31. Goel C, Anand LK, Gomber KK. Comparative evaluation of single dose intravenous pantoprazole and ranitidine on gastric pH and volume: A double blind study. J Anaesth Clin Pharmacol. 2006;22(2):145-9.
32. Gold MJ, Helvich M. A study of the complications related to anesthesia in asthmatic patients. Anesth Analg (Cleve). 1963;42:283.
33. Goldberger AL, O'Konski J. Utility of routine ECG before surgery and on general hospital admission. Ann Intern Med. 1986;105:552.
34. Goldman L, Caldera DL, Nussbaum SR, et al. Multifactorial index of cardiac risk. N Engl J Med. 1977;297:845-50.
35. Gribes AR. The high-risk surgical patient and the role of preoperative management. Neth J Med. 2000;57:98-105.
36. Gronert J. Cardiac arrest after succinylcholine: Mortality greater with rhabdomyolysis than receptor upregulation. Anesthesiology. 2001;94:523-9.
37. Hankey GJ.: Non-valvular atrial fibrillation and stroke prevention. National Blood Pressure Advisory Committee of the National Heart Foundation. Med J Aust. 2001;174:234-9.
38. Hart RG, Halperin JL. Atrial fibrillation and stroke: Concepts and controversies. Stroke. 2001;32: 803-8.
39. Horlocker TT, Wedel DJ, Benzon H, et al. Regional anesthesia in the anticoagulated patient: Defining the risks. Reg Anesth Pain Med. 2003;28:172-97.
40. Ingelmo P, Barone M, Fumagalli R.: Importance of monitoring in high risk surgical patients. Minerva Anesthesiology. 2002;68:226-30.
41. Ivanov R, Allen J, Calvin JE. The incidence of major morbidity in critically ill patients managed with pulmonary artery catheters: A meta-analysis. Crit Care Med. 2000;28:615-9.
42. Jakobsen CJ, Blom L, Brondjerg M, et al. Effect of metoprolol and diazepam on pre-operative anxiety. Anesthesia. 1990;45(1):40.
43. Jewell ER, Persson AV. Preoperative evaluation of the high-risk patient. Surg Clin North Am. 1985;65:3-19.
44. Kehlet H. Multimodal strategies to improve surgical outcome. Am J Surg. 2002;183:630-41.
45. Kern JW, Shoemaker WC. Meta-analysis of hemodynamic optimization in high-risk patients. Crit Care Med. 2002;30:1686-92.
46. Lee TH, Marcantonio ER, Mangione CM, et al. Derivation and prospective validation of a simple index for prediction of cardiac risk of major noncardiac surgery. Circulation. 1999;100:1043-9.
47. Mangano R. Preoperative cardiac assessment. Philadelphia: Lippincott; 1990.
48. Martin C, Dott C. High-risk surgical patients: Who are they and how should they be treated? Presse Med. 1996;25:1419-24.

49. Mc Phail N, Calvi JE, Shariatmadar A, et al. The use of preoperative exercise testing to predict cardiac complications. J Vasc Surg. 1998;7(1) :60-8.
50. National study by R Coll. Radiol Lancet. 1979;2:83.
51. Ornstein DL, Hong-Dice YG, Papini JR. Low-molecular-weight heparins for the prevention and treatment of venous thrombosis. Mil Med. 2001;166:593-601.
52. Palda VA, Detsky AS. Preoperative assessment and management of risk for coronary artery disease. Ann Intern Med. 1997;127:313-28.
53. Pederson T, Viby-Mogensen J, Ringsted C, et al. Anesthetic practice and post operative pulmonary complications. Acta Anaesthesiol. Scand. 1992:36;812-8.
54. Peverill RE. Warfarin or aspirin: Both or others? Med J Aust. 1999;171:321-6.
55. Poldermans D, Arnese M, Fioretti PM, et al. Improved cardiac risk stratification with dopamine-atropine stress echocardiography. J Am Coll Cardiol. 1995;26(3):648-53.
56. Prys-Roberts C, Foex P, Biro GP, et al. Studies of anaesthesia in relation to hypertension: Adrenergic beta-receptor blockade. Br J Anaesth. 1973;45:671-81.
57. Prys-Roberts C. Isolated systolic hypertension: pressure on the anesthetist? Anaesthesia. 2001;56 :505-10.
58. Psaty BM, Smith NL, Siscovick DS, et al. Health outcomes associated with antihypertensive therapies used as first-line agents: a systematic review and meta-analysis. JAMA. 1997;277(9):739-45.
59. Pulmonary Embolism (PEP) Trial. Prevention of pulmonary embolism and deep vein thrombosis with low dose aspirin. Lancet. 2000;355:1295302.
60. Raby KE, Goldman L, Creager MA, et al. Correlation between perioperative ischemia and major cardiac events. N Engl J Med. 1989;321:1296-300.
61. Richards MJ, Skues MA, Jarvis AP, et al. Total I.V. anaesthesia with propofol and alfentanil: dose requirements for propofol and the effect of premedication with clonidine. Br J Anaesth. 1990;65:157.
62. Ronco JJ, Fenwick JC, Tweeddale MG. Does increasing oxygen delivery improve outcome in the critically ill? No. Crit Care Clin. 1996;12:645-59.
63. Sabrasez. Bordeaux Med. J. 1902.
64. Savitz SL, Gupta G, Singh M, et al. Antithrombotic and thrombolytic therapy for ischemic stroke. Clin Geriatr Med. 2001;17:149-61.
65. Shapira Y, Vaturi M, Sagie A. Anticoagulant management of patients with mechanical prosthetic values undergoing non-cardiac surgery: Indications and unresolved issues. J Heart Valve Dis. 2001;10:380-7.
66. Shoemaker WC, Appel PL, Kram HB, et al. Perspective trial of supranormal values of survivors as therapeutic goals in high-risk surgical patients. Chest. 1998;94:1176-86.
67. Siegel D, Lopez J. Trends in antihypertensive drug use in the United States: Do the JNC V recommendations affect prescribing? JAMA. 1997;278(21):1745-8.
68. Silverman DG, Donati F. Factors affecting pseudocholinesterase and the pharmacokinetics and pharmacodynamics of succinylcholine. In: Silverman DG (Ed). Neuromuscular block in anesthesia and intensive care. Philadelphia: JB Lippincott; 1995.
69. Silverman DG, Donati F. Undesirable effects of succinylcholine. In: Silverman DG (Ed). Neuromuscular block in anesthesia and intensive care. Philadelphia: JB Lippincott; 1995.
70. Silverman DG, Halaszynski T, Sinatra R, et al. Rofecoxib does not compromise platelet aggregation during anesthesia and surgery: [Le rofecoxib n'altere pas l'agregation plaquettaire pendant l'anesthesie et la chirurgie]. Can J Anaesth. 2003;50:1004-8.
71. Silverman DG, Rosenberg H. Malignant hyperthermia: etiology, risks, and assessment of susceptibility. In: Silverman DG (Ed). Neuromuscular block in anesthesia and intensive care. Philadelphia: JB Lippincott; 1995.
72. Silverman DG, Rosenberg H. Malignant hyperthermia: signs, symptoms, and treatment. In: Silverman DG (Ed). Neuromuscular block in anesthesia and intensive care. Philadelphia: JB Lippincott; 1995.
73. Silverman DG, Rosenberg H. Other muscle disorders. In: Silverman DG (Ed). Neuromuscular block in anesthesia and intensive care. Philadelphia: JB Lippincott; 1995.
74. Silverman DG. Myasthenia gravis and the myasthenic syndrome. In: Silverman DG (Ed). Neuromuscular block in anesthesia and intensive care. Philadelphia: JB Lippincott; 1995.
75. Sinatra RS, Shen QJ, Halaszynski T, et al. Preoperative rofecoxib oral suspension as an analgesic adjunct after lower abdominal surgery: The effects on effort-dependent pain and pulmonary function. Anesth Analg. 2004;98:135-40.
76. Sinclair S, James S, Singer M. Intraoperative intravascular volume optimisation and length of hospital stay after repair of proximal femoral fracture: Randomised controlled trial. BMJ. 1997;315:909-12.
77. Steltzer H, Hiesmayr M. The relationship between oxygen delivery and uptake in the critically ill: Is there a critical or optimal value? A Meta-analysis. Anesthesia. 1994;49:229-36.
78. The sixth report of the joint national committee on prevention, detection, evaluation and treatment of high blood pressure. Arch Intern Med. 1997;157(21):2413-46.
79. Topol EJ. The future of antiplatelet therapy: Optimizing management in patients with acute coronary syndrome. Clin Cardio. 2000;23(Suppl 6):23-8.
80. Valentine RJ, Duke ML, Inman MH, et al. Effectiveness of pulmonary artery catheters in aortic surgery: A randomized trial. J Vasc Surg. 1998;27:203-11; discussion 211-2.
81. van Der Hiejden JF, Hutten BA, Buller HR, et al. Vitamin K antagonists or low-molecular-weight heparin for the long-term treatment of symptomatic venous thromboembolism. Cochrane Database Syst Rev. 2000;4.
82. Varon AJ, Hudson-Civetta JA, Civetta JM, et al. Preoperative intensive care consultations: Accurate and effective. Crit Care Med. 1993;21:234-9.
83. Velmahos GC, Demetriades D. Endpoints of resuscitation of critically injured patients: Normal or supranormal? Ann Surg. 2000;232:409-18.

Table 3: Systemic opioids

Drugs	Dose	Peak (hour)	Duration (hour)	Precautions
Morphine	10 mg IM	1–2	2.5–4	Impaired ventilation
	2.5 mg IV	0.3	1.5–2	Asthma, liver failure, increase in ICT
Pethidine	50–75 mg IM	0.5–1	3–4	Accumulation of metabolites can cause seizures; interact with MAO inhibitors
	20–50 mg IV		2–3	
Fentanyl	50–100 µg IM		1–2	Cumulative effect
	25–50 µg IV		0.5–1	
Remifentanil	1 µg/kg bolus			Very short acting potent drug
	Infusion at 0.1–2 µg/kg/min			
Pentazocine	40–60 mg IM	0.5–1		May cause psychomimetic effects
	20–40 mg IV			
Butorphanol	2 mg IM	0.5–1	4–6	Psychomimetic effects; maternal sedation
	1 mg IV		3–4	

Abbreviation: ICT, intracranial tension; MAO, monoamine oxidase

unsuitable for labor analgesia because of poor analgesic properties; they are used mainly for their anxiolytic effects.

Systemic Opioids

They provide effective analgesia but with undesirable side effects (Table 3). Opioids cross the placenta and depress the fetus; hence, used only in early labor. In the mother, they cause nausea, vomiting, drowsiness and disorientation. Morphine has a more potent depressant effect on the neonate, hence pethidine is more popular. Pethidine 10-25 mg intravenous (IV) or 25-50 mg intramuscular (IM) (maximum dose 100 mg) is used in early labor, where delivery is not expected for at least 4 hours. Promethazine 25-50 mg IM alone or combined with pethidine, reduces anxiety, nausea and opioid requirement without much effect on fetus.

Fentanyl (50-100 µg/h IV), sufentanil, alfentanil and remifentanil has also been used. Continuous infusion or patient controlled administration of opioids can provide useful analgesia when regional blocks are contraindicated.

Remifentanil

Remifentanil is an ultra-short acting opioid, which does not accumulate in the body even after prolonged administration. It is a potent, short-acting drug that has been approved for clinical use; it is metabolized by nonspecific esterases throughout the blood and muscles resulting in an extremely short duration of action. Its estimated half-life is 1.3 minutes and prolonged administration does not cause accumulation of this drug. Fetal exposure to the drug is minimized because of its rapid metabolism or redistribution. These properties make it an attractive alternative to systemic analgesics in parturients in whom regional anesthesia is contraindicated. A bolus dose of 0.25 µg/kg with a 2-minute lockout has been successfully used. Using patient-controlled analgesia system, IV remifentanil in a bolus dose of 0.4 µg/kg with a lockout time of 1 minute has shown good results. A continuous infusion of remifentanil at 0.05 µg/kg/min with a bolus of 25 µg and a lockout time of 5 minutes provides satisfactory labor analgesia. It has been used for 34 hours continuously with no adverse effects.

Although preliminary reports have been promising, it is still somewhat premature to advocate the use of remifentanil until larger studies have fully evaluated its safety and optimum administration technique and dosing.

Ketamine

Ketamine alone or in combination has been used to provide pain relief during labor. It is most useful when given just before delivery or as adjuvant to regional anesthesia.

Used as a continuous infusion after a bolus of 0.2 mg/kg intravenously, it is found to provide adequate analgesia for first stage of labor (Box 1).

Box 1 Ketamine analgesia

1. Preanesthetic evaluation; antacid prophylaxis
2. First stage labor: bolus of 10–12 mg followed by infusion at the rate of 0.5–1 mg/kg/min
3. Monitor sensorium
4. At crowning: 0.2–0.4 mg/kg (total dose 12.5–25 mg) Do not exceed 100 mg

Source: Gupta S, Kumar GS, Singhal H. Acute pain-labor analgesia. Indian J Anaesth. 2006;50(5):363-9.

During second stage of labor, 12.5-25 mg helps to provide good sedation and effective analgesia.

Higher doses of ketamine (>1 mg/kg) lead to emergent psychomimetic effects and respiratory depression in mother, low APGAR score and rigidity in the neonate.

Regional Analgesia Techniques

- Spinal
- Epidural
- Combined spinal-epidural analgesia.

They are the most popular methods of pain relief during labor, providing excellent pain relief yet awake and a cooperative patient during labor.

Opioids and local anesthetics alone can provide analgesia; combining both results in good analgesia reduced dose requirements with few maternal and fetal side effects.

Pain of first stage of labor is initially confined to T11–T12 dermatome but later on involves T10–L1 dermatomes. Pain during late first stage and second stage of labor involves the S2, S3 and S4 dermatomes.

Absolute Contraindications to Regional Anesthesia

- Infection over injection site
- Bleeding diathesis
- Anticoagulant therapy
- Marked hypovolemia
- Sensitivity to local anesthetics
- Patient refusal
- Raised intracranial pressure.

Relative Contraindications

- Preexisting neurological disease
- Disorders of spine
- Cardiac diseases.

Intrathecal (Spinal) Opioids

Preservative free opioids are given intrathecally as a single dose or intermittently or continuously via an intrathecal catheter. They are suitable for high risk patients with significant cardiovascular disease such as aortic stenosis, Fallot's tetralogy, Eisenmenger's syndrome, mothers in very advanced first stage labor and in need of instrumental delivery; they may be preferred in cases of accidental dural puncture.

Intraspinal opioids do not cause motor blockade or maternal hypotension except pethidine, which has weak local anesthetic properties. Intrathecal morphine (0.5-1 mg) produces prolonged analgesia for 6-8 hours during first stage of labor. Onset of analgesia is slow (45-60 minutes) and associated with high incidence of side effects. Combining morphine (0.25 mg) with fentanyl (25 μg) or sufentanil (5-10 μg) results in rapid onset (5 minutes) and short duration (4-5 hours). Intermittent boluses of pethidine 10 mg, fentanyl 5-10 μg, sufentanil (3-10 μg) via an intrathecal catheter can also provide satisfactory analgesia.

Disadvantages

Single shot spinal with opioids provides analgesia for 1-3 hours, which may be inadequate to cover the full duration of labor. Other drawbacks include chances of cauda equina syndrome, incomplete analgesia, lack of perineal relaxation and side effects, such as pruritis, nausea, vomiting, sedation and respiratory depression.

Side effects improve with low dose naloxoane (0.2 mg/hour IV)

Epidural Opioids

Addition of opioids to local anesthetics, help reduce the dose of local anesthetic and improve the quality of analgesia. Currently, fentanyl and sufentanil are used (Table 4).

Morphine: A higher dose of more than 7.5 mg (high incidence of side effects) of morphine is needed during labor. Analgesia is more effective for early first stage of labor. It has a slow onset (30-60 minutes) but long duration (up to 24 hours) of effect.

Pethidine: Epidural pethidine 100 mg provides good but short duration analgesia (1-4 hours)

Epidural fentanyl (50-200 μg) or sufentanil (10-50 μg) produces rapid onset of analgesia (5-10 minutes) for short duration (1-2 hours) with few side effects. Combining low dose of morphine (2.5 mg) with fentanyl (25-50 μg) or sufentanil (10-20 μg) may result in rapid onset and prolongation of analgesia (4-5 hours) with fewer side effects. Single shot epidurals do not cause neonatal depression; however, caution should be exercised following repeated administration.

Local Anesthetics

Lumbar epidural anesthesia and spinal (intrathecal) anesthesia can be used during labor and delivery. Pain

Table 4: Narcotic dosages for relief of labor pain

Agent	Epidural	Intrathecal
Morphine	7.5–10 mg	0.5–1 mg
Pethidine	100 mg	10–20 mg
Fentanyl	50–200 μg	5–25 μg
Sufentanil	10–50 μg	3–10 μg

relief for first stage requires block of T10–L1 sensory level while second stage requires a T10–S4 block.

Continuous lumbar epidural is most versatile and most commonly used because it can be used for pain relief in the first stage of labor as well as anesthesia for subsequent vaginal delivery or cesarean section, if necessary.

Single shot epidural is used when pain relief is initiated just prior to vaginal delivery.

Epidural Drugs

Lignocaine and bupivacaine have been in use for a long time. Ropivacaine is a relatively new drug, which is being used for labor analgesia. Ropivacaine has less potential for central nervous system and cardiovascular toxicity than bupivacaine; in pregnant patients it produces less motor block than bupivacaine (Table 5).

Steps for Epidural Analgesia for Labor Pains

- Preanesthetic evaluation is done
- Explain the procedure to the parturient and record informed written consent
- Start IV fluids through 18 or 20 G IV catheter (preferably nondextrose containing crystalloids or colloids) and apply appropriate monitors [electrocardiogram (EKG), pulse oximeter and noninvasive blood pressure (NIBP)]
- Hydrogen (H_2) receptor antagonists (ranitidine 50 mg) + metoclopramide 10 mg + ondansteron 8 mg may be administered intravenously
- Ensure emergency drugs (ephedrine, atropine, etc.) and equipment for resuscitation is available
- Clean and prepare the back of the patient with antiseptic solution. Make a wheal with local anesthetic at site of puncture (preferably with 26/24 G hypodermic needle at L2/L3 or L3/L4 level) and inject into interspinous space
- Place epidural catheter taking aseptic precautions through Tuohy's needle. Secure catheter well and turn the patient supine
- Administer test dose of lidocaine 1.5% 2 mL or 1.0% 3 mL with epinephrine 1:200,000. Watch for signs of intravascular or intrathecal injection
- Once epidural placement of catheter is confirmed, administer initial dose of either lidoacine 1% or bupivacaine 0.125–0.25% or ropivacaine 0.125–0.175% + sufentanil 10–15 µg or fentanyl 20–25 µg
- Total volume of 10–15 mL may be required to provide good analgesia
- Subsequent analgesia options
  - Intermittent: every hourly 8–10 mL
  - Continuous infusion at the rate of 8–12 mL/hour of bupivacaine 0.125% alone or in combination with fentanyl 1–2 µg/mL
- Check blood pressure (BP) frequently every 2 minutes for initial 15 minutes and then every 5–10 minutes till block wears off
- Treat hypotension aggressively, if it occurs. Ephedrine 3–6 mg every 2–3 minutes till systolic BP is more than 90 mm Hg. Exaggerate uterus displacement towards left, rapid IV fluids; atropine 0.6 mg may be administered intravenously
- Maintain patient in lateral position. To avoid lateralization of epidural block turn the patient to the opposite side every 15–30 minutes
- Check sensory level prior to every top up and confirm correct placement of epidural catheter prior to top up.

Table 5: Combination of analgesic and opioid drug with their effects

Local anesthetics	Dose	Opioid	Comments
Bupivacaine 0.25%	10–15 mL	None	Good analgesia with slight motor blockade
Bupivacaine 0.125%	10–20 mL	Fentanyl 2–4 µg/mL	Excellent analgesia with no motor block
Bupivacaine 0.125%	10–20 mL	Sufentanil 0.5 µg/mL	Excellent analgesia with no motor block
Ropivacaine 0.2%	8–15 mL	Fentanyl 2–4 µg/mL may be added	Excellent analgesia with no motor block

Combined Spinal Epidural Analgesia (Ambulatory Labor Analgesia)

The aim is to provide analgesia while preserving motor function so as to permit ambulation and improve maternal satisfaction (Table 6).

- Locate the epidural place with a 16 Gauge Tuohy's needle
- Pass a 12 cm long, 26–27 Gauge spinal needle through it into the subarachnoid space
- Inject intrathecally, bupivacaine 2.5 mg (1 mL of 0.25%), fentanyl 25 µg or sufentanil 5 µg, saline 0.5 mL; withdraw the spinal needle
- Thread an epidural catheter via Tuohy's needle and leave it in epidural space; the needle is withdrawn. The catheter is well secured and used for later supplementation or institution of anesthesia via epidural route
- Observe the BP for 20 minutes, level of sensory and motor block.

Table 6: Drug doses for combined spinal-epidural analgesia in labor

Route	Local anesthetic	Opioid
Intrathecal injection	Bupivacaine 0.1–0.25%; 1–2.5 mg	Fentanyl 20–25 μg or sufentanil 3–10 μg
Epidural top-ups	Bupivacaine 0.1–0.125%; 10–15 mg first stage labor; usually adequate for second stage and assisted delivery. For operative delivery titrate the dose with bupivacaine 0.5% or xylocaine 2%	Fentanyl 20–25 μg or sufentanil 5–10 μg

If the block is adequate, the patient is allowed to walk.

If it is unilateral, turn the patient to unblocked side, give 5 mL of epidural mixture*; then further 10 mL in supine position (do not repeat dose of subarachnoid injection).

If inadequate, give epidural injection.

If there is rectal pressure, give fentanyl 100 μg in 10 mL saline via epidural catheter.

The subarachnoid block wears off in 90 minutes; give the first top-up of 15 mL of epidural mixture* via epidural catheter; subsequent top-ups of 10 mL as required.

Epidural mixture consists of:

Bupivacaine 50 mg (10 mL of 0.5%) + fentanyl 100 μg + saline to make up the volume to 50 mL.

Patient-controlled epidural analgesia (PCEA) is a relatively new method of maintaining labor analgesia (Table 7). PCEA has been compared with continuous epidural infusion (CEI). Patients who receive PCEA are less likely to require anesthetic interventions, require lower doses of local anesthetic, have less motor block and greater maternal satisfaction than those who receive CEI.

Most appropriate PCEA solutions are bupivacaine 0.0625–0.125% or ropivacaine 1 mg/mL, 10–15 mL with fentanyl 3 μg/mL. On demand boluses are 3–5 mL with 10–15 minute lockout interval.

Table 7: Drug doses for epidural analgesia maintenance techniques

Technique	Concentration and dosing schedule
Intermittent bolus	0.1–0.25% bupivacaine + fentanyl 3 μg/mL + adrenaline 1:200,000 (5 + 5 mL) boluses as needed.
Continuous infusion	0.044–0.125% bupivacaine + fentanyl 1.5–2 μg/mL at the rate of 8–14 mL/hour
PCEA with basal infusion	0.625–0.125% bupivacaine + fentanyl 2 μg/mL basal rate: 8–12 mL/hour; bolus 5 mL lockout 10 min; hourly limit 30 mL.
PCEA without basal infusion	0.125% bupivacaine + fentanyl 2 μg/mL 8 mL bolus dose; lockout 15 min; no hourly limit

Source: Gupta S, Kumar GS, Singhal H. Acute pain-labor analgesia. Indian J Anaesth. 2006;50(5):363-9.

Complications of Epidural Analgesia

1. *Maternal hypotension:* Maternal hypotension is one of the most common complications of epidural analgesia which can compromise uterine perfusion and oxygen transfer to fetus. It can be avoided by preloading with 750–1,000 mL of Ringer lactate; in presence of edema or partial exchange transfusion (PET) administration of colloid or less amount of crystalloid may be appropriate. The dose of local anesthetic is titrated to minimum dose necessary to achieve sensory block only.

   If hypotension occurs, it is treated aggressively with ephedrine 5–30 mg IV. Bradycardia, if observed, is treated with atropine 0.6–1.2 mg IV. If profound hypotension occurs following epidural, determine whether accidental intrathecal injection has occurred.
2. *Accidental dural puncture:* If it occurs, inject a small amount of fentanyl or sufentanil intrathecally, withdraw the needle and reinsert at another place.
3. *Intravascular injection:* "Every epidural injection is intravascular, until proved otherwise". "Every epidural dose should be a test dose."

   These two thoughts, if kept in mind, will prevent unintentional intravascular injection. Tachycardia immediately following epidural dose is indicative of intravascular injection.
4. *Accidental intrathecal blockade:* Usually intrathecal puncture is recognized by the appearance of cerebrospinal fluid (CSF). Occasionally, it is unrecognized and intrathecal injection of drug occurs resulting in dense motor and sensory block or the mother experiences unexpected rapid and complete pain relief; in worst case, scenario a total spinal may occur.
5. *Inadequate or failed block or atypical block:* These all can occur usually due to the drug being injected at a place other than the epidural or intrathecal space.
6. *Persistent neurological deficit:* This occurs in 1 in 20,000 cases; temporary deficit is more common. It is wise not to inject any solution epidurally, if pain results. Check the solution; reposition the needle or catheter.

7. *Epidural hematoma:* This is seen in conditions such as prior heparinization, preexisting coagulopathy, thrombocytopenia from any cause and use of low molecular weight heparin. Symptoms are segmental pain and paresis continuing after the epidural block is expected to wear off. A neurological consultation and surgery may be needed.

Other Regional Techniques

- Lumbar sympathetic block
- Pudendal nerve block
- Paracervical block.

These methods do not have the flexibility of epidural analgesia; they are technically difficult to perform and have more complications. They can be used in special circumstances, such as failed or inadequate neuraxial analgesia or in the presence of contraindications to neuraxial techniques such as deformity of spine or coagulopathy or in the absence of qualified anesthesiologist.

KEY POINTS

1. Among the current methods of obstetric analgesia, regional analgesia (mainly epidural analgesia) is the best because it is most effective and safe.
2. Walking epidural is the most acceptable method to mother and obstetrician and is associated with least side effects.
3. Systemic analgesia by parenteral opioids, nonopioid painkillers and inhaled anesthetic agents provide an alternative to regional analgesia but they are less effective and more hazardous.
4. Psychoprophylaxis and physical methods are not potent enough when used alone.
5. Communication and exchange of information between anesthesiologists, obstetricians and nurses in an ever-changing environment of labor and delivery are essential for a perfect outcome.
6. The safe labor analgesia or anesthesia requires appropriate staff, facilities and proper equipment for patient safety.

CHAPTER

8 Anesthesia for Obstetrics and Gynecology Surgery

Vinay Tiwari

The patient about to undergo surgery should be assessed by an anesthesiologist; in addition to taking a history, performing the relevant physical examination and writing up the drugs for premedication, the anesthesiologist should allow the patient to ask questions, state anxieties and be informed of the likely plan of anesthesia, surgery and the postoperative period.

PREOPERATIVE PREPARATION OF THE PATIENT

The immediate preoperative preparation of the patient includes a reassessment of the preoperative examination, laboratory reports and the plan of anesthesia. Anesthesiologists classify surgical procedures according to the risk of mortality. A dialogue between the surgeon and the anesthesiologist, taking into consideration the technical requirement of the operation, helps determine the best anesthesia for the individual case.

A povidone-iodine douche and a vaginal suppository of nitrofurazone inserted high into the vagina, the night before surgery, are useful for decreasing the incidence of cuff cellulites. Postmenopausal atrophic vagina can be prepared by using estrogen vaginal cream for 4–6 weeks preoperatively; this results in thickening of vaginal mucosa which eases dissection.

A light meal on the night before surgery is easily digestible, and prevents an overloaded alimentary tract and postoperative nausea and gas formation. Adequate night's rest before surgery is important for the patient; a mild sedative to overcome apprehension is usually given. Lower colon is cleansed by preoperative enema the night before and again in the morning of surgery.

A preoperative broad spectrum antibiotic is usually prescribed. New generation cephalosporins or semisynthetic penicillins or beta lactamase antibiotics are highly effective when given 2 hours before surgery.

THE DAY OF OPERATION

Food should be withheld for 6 hours and drink for 4 hours preceding operation; however, water is allowed till 2 hours before surgery. Excessive starvation and dehydration are to be avoided. Morphine premedication delays gastric emptying time, but diazepam 10 mg does not.

Lipstick, nail varnish and other cosmetics should be removed before the patient comes to theater so that the anesthetist can readily appreciate cyanosis, etc. Dentures, artificial limbs, artificial eyes, contact lenses, etc. should be removed before the journey to the theater. Hearing aids may often be retained by the patient so that communication can be restarted in the postoperative ward. The patient should not come to theater with a full bladder. The appropriate blood test results are inspected and crossmatching of blood may need to be confirmed.

An identification label is tied around the wrist or neck. This should state the name and case record number. The site of operation should be marked on the patient's skin with ink. The completed consent form and identity band are inspected, and the patient is asked to state her name and operation.

SUGGESTED ANESTHETIC PLAN

Two problems particular to vaginal surgery are related to the positioning of the patient and bleeding in the narrow confines of the vaginal surgical field. The patient is placed in the lithotomy position with a head down tilt, which results in a fall in vital capacity. A normal patient can withstand these changes comfortably but obese and cardiac patients can have their problems aggravated. Straightening of the table at the end of surgery should be gradual with a watch on the blood pressure (BP), especially under regional anesthesia. Lithotomy position is one of the causes of backache in the postoperative period.

For the surgeon to have a clear vision in the operative field, there should be as little bleeding as possible. Regional anesthesia offers good operating conditions because of the fall in BP, which accompanies the block. A hypotensive technique of anesthesia to reduce bleeding may be preferred by some.

PREMEDICATION

Drugs commonly used are:

- Anxiolytic to allay anxiety on the night before surgery
- Antiemetic to reduce postoperative nausea and vomiting (PONV)
- Hydrogen (H_2) blocker to reduce volume and pH of gastric secretions
- Pre-emptive analgesia with nonsteroidal anti-inflammatory drugs (NSAIDs)—no PONV as seen with opioids
- Deep venous thrombosis (DVT) prophylaxis, if necessary
- Atropine/glycopyrrolate to reduce secretions and vagal effects of anesthetic drugs
- Dexmedetomidine and clonidine are used in laparoscopic surgery to control tachycardia and rise in BP.

MONITORING

- Noninvasive blood pressure (NIBP)
- Pulse oximetry
- Electrocardiogram (ECG)
- Temperature
- Capnography.

The above are routinely monitored during surgery whereas arterial blood gases, S-T segment analysis, transesophageal echocardiography and invasive BP monitoring are usually reserved for severely ill patients. Entropy and bispectral index (BIS) can be used to monitor the depth of anesthesia.

Most gynecological procedures may be done under:

- General anesthesia (GA)
- Regional anesthesia which includes:
  - Spinal
  - Epidural
  - Combined spinal epidural.

Box 1 Advantages and disadvantages of general anesthesia (GA)

Advantages of GA
• Control of patient's airway is ensured
• Adequate oxygenation assured
• Better control of cardiovascular system
• Anesthetists are more familiar with GA
• Patient's preference
Disadvantages of GA
• Cardiovascular depression
• Protective reflexes depressed or lost
• Prolonged psychomotor impairment
• Nausea, vomiting, "groggy" patient
• Possibility of inadvertent awareness exists

***Abbreviation*:** GA, general anesthesia

GENERAL ANESTHESIA (BOX 1)

General anesthesia with endotracheal intubation and controlled ventilation provides good muscle relaxation, analgesia, protection from aspiration of gastric contents and optimal operative conditions.

Induction

Patients' condition permitting, a host of intravenous (IV) induction agents are available but sodium pentothal still remains the most commonly used drug. Of late, propofol has gained popularity as an induction agent because of clear headed recovery and an inherent antiemetic property resulting in less PONV. Ketamine is another agent that can be used in low general condition patient but avoided in young patients and patients with hypertension and cardiovascular disease.

Muscle Relaxants

For endotracheal intubation, succinylcholine ensures a quick onset of good intubating conditions but its property of muscular fasciculations leading to myalgia and rise in serum potassium levels are its drawbacks.

Rocuronium, vecuronium and atracurium, all nondepolarizer muscle relaxants, can be used for intubating the patients without the drawbacks of succinylcholine; moreover, they have the added advantage of being used for providing relaxation during the entire course of surgery. The disadvantage is that they take about 2–3 minutes before adequate intubating conditions are achieved, during which time, the airway is unprotected. Rocuronium provides good intubating conditions earlier than the other two.

Pancuronium causes tachycardia and may be avoided in hypertensive and patients with cardiovascular system involvement. Vecuronium and atracurium are newer relaxants, devoid of cardiovascular effects. Vecuronium is one-third more potent than pancuronium but it has shorter duration of action (25 minutes) and rapid recovery. With continuous infusion of more than 6 hours, recovery may be prolonged due to accumulation of active metabolites; onset time is decreased and duration prolonged with increasing doses. It does not have significant hemodynamic effects; a slight bradycardia may be seen when combined with potent opioids.

Atracurium has a duration of action one-third of pancuronium at equipotent doses; it undergoes rapid metabolism by Hoffman elimination and nonspecific enzyme hydrolysis; repeated doses and infusions have less cumulative effects on recovery rates than other muscle relaxants. Higher doses (> 0.5 mg/kg) may cause histamine release, decreased arterial pressure and tachycardia. Atracurium needs to be stored in a cold chain to retain its potency, hence may face storage difficulty in hot climate.

Maintenance

Anesthesia is maintained on nitrous oxide and oxygen (O_2) along with a muscle relaxant. An inhalation agent such as halothane or isoflurane can be added to deepen the level of anesthesia or a narcotic agent can be used in place of inhalation agent. Sevoflurane and desflurane are newer inhalation agents in use.

Concern on theater pollution has led to use of total IV anesthesia technique with propofol infusion along with O_2, fentanyl or a related opioid and use of muscle relaxant.

Trendelenburg position is unphysiological and should be maintained for as short a time as possible. It can lead to headache, regurgitation and steep rise in central venous pressure (CVP). Lesser the tilt, better it is for the patient's respiratory and cardiovascular function.

Pressure points need to be padded to prevent nerve compression in the lithotomy position. Maintenance of body temperature is important.

Intraoperative use of metoclopramide (5–10 mg) or ondansetron (4 mg) helps in reducing the incidence of PONV.

Reversal

Though relaxants such as atracurium need not be reversed, it is customary to reverse residual neuromuscular blockade with neostigmine (0.08 mg/kg) and atropine (0.04 mg/kg) at the end of surgery.

The patient is shifted to postoperative care unit when fully conscious and with return of protective reflexes. The patient should respond adequately to vocal commands, should be able to cough, move her limbs and raise her head off the pillow.

REGIONAL ANESTHESIA

Most gynecological procedures can be performed under spinal, epidural or combined spinal-epidural (CSE) block. One of the major advantages of regional anesthesia over GA is its safety and lack of serious complications.

Nerve supply of uterus can be summarized as follows:

- Sympathetic (motor to upper uterine segment) T6 down to L2
- Visceral afferents (sensory from uterus) T11-12 with possibly T10 and L1. Visceral afferent and efferent parasympathetic fibers (inhibitory to uterus and motor to cervix) come from S2, S3 and S4 dermatome.

It is evident from the nerve supply that complete blockade of uterus results from the spinal block extending to the T4 dermatome if the patient is not to feel the tug and pull that the surgeon exerts on the uterus during the surgery.

Drugs used for the following various regional blocks.

Spinal

- Lignocaine 5% (heavy) 1.6–2 mL
- Bupivacaine 0.5% (heavy) 3–4 mL
- Ropivacaine 0.75% 3–4 mL; maximum dose is 3 mg/kg.

Epidural

- Bupivacaine: 0.5% up to 20 mL (maximum dose 2 mg/kg).

Combined Spinal-Epidural

- Bupivacaine (spinal) 2.5–4 mL, 0.5% (epidural) 4–6 mL, 0.5%.

Advantages of Regional Anesthesia over General Anesthesia

- Decreased blood loss
- Decreased rate of DVT and pulmonary embolism
- Reduced stress response following surgery
- Better for patients with respiratory impairment
- Preserves airway
- CVS stability, if block is not too high
- Residual postoperative analgesia
- Allows verbal communication with patient
- No atmospheric pollution
- No GA complications, e.g. malignant hyperthermia, scoline-apnea
- Patient can eat/drink earlier than GA.

Advantages of Spinal over General Anesthesia

- Technical ease; high success rate
- Excellent operating conditions
- No need for deep anesthesia and muscle relaxation
- Preserves spontaneous respiration; lung functions better preserved
- No postoperative sore throat and coughing
- Analgesia continues into postoperative period
- Reduced blood loss during surgery
- Intestinal functions return early
- Minimal chance of aspiration of gastric contents
- Minimal upset of body chemistry
- Very cost effective.

Advantages of Spinal over Epidural

- Technically easy and safe even in inexperienced hands
- Quick onset of block
- Better muscle relaxation of abdominal wall
- Chances of drug toxicity negligible.

Disadvantages of Spinal Block

- Hypotension
- Postdural puncture headache (PDPH)
- Backache
- Transient neurological symptoms
- Motor paralysis continues into postoperative period
- Awake patient (apprehensive).

Advantages of Epidural Block

Because the dura is not punctured, there is no chance of PDPH.

With epidural catheter in place:

- The height of block can be controlled
- Easy to add "top-up" dose, if needed
- Excellent means of postoperative analgesia.

Disadvantages of Epidural Block

- Slow onset of block
- Large dose of drug used for block; can cause drug toxicity
- Accidental dural puncture with a large bore needle can be hazardous
- Epidural catheter has its own complications.

Combined Spinal-Epidural Block

Combined spinal-epidural block aims to provide the benefits of spinal block with the flexibility of an indwelling epidural catheter to extend the duration of analgesia into the postoperative period. The technique of sequential CSE involves injection of low dose of subarachnoid local anesthetic and then extension of the block by injecting the drug through the epidural catheter.

- Combined spinal-epidural is found to be better and superior alternative to epidural block. Advantages of CSE are faster onset of block, superior quality of analgesia, better muscle relaxation and less dose of local anesthetic required to reach the same level of block
- Combined spinal-epidural offers the best of both spinal and epidural techniques.

Contraindications of Regional Blocks

Absolute

- An unwilling patient
- Infection at site of injection and generalized sepsis
- Coagulation disorders
- Patients on anticoagulants
- Allergy to local anesthetic drugs.

Relative

- Hypovolemia
- Chronic backache and spinal deformities
- Diseases of central nervous system (CNS) and neuromuscular disorders
- Patients on platelets inhibiting drugs, e.g. aspirin, NSAIDs.

It would be fair to conclude that regional blocks offer a definitive advantage over GA as far as the lack of complications and patient safety is concerned, but acceptance of the technique by the patient is an absolute must before it is used.

8.1 ANESTHESIA FOR GYNECOLOGICAL ENDOSCOPIC SURGERY

Vinay Tiwari

LAPAROSCOPY AND HYSTEROSCOPY

Anesthesia for gynecological endoscopy concerns both hysteroscopic and laparoscopic procedures; these started as simple diagnostic procedures but have advanced to the present state of true surgical operations. This surgery requires the uterus or the peritoneum to be distended, which can result in significant changes due to the reabsorption of the gas or liquid used to distend the cavity; in the case of laparoscopic surgery, effect on the venous return and diaphragmatic movements due to increased intraabdominal pressure is substantial. The extent of these changes depends on the condition of the patient, the duration and specific conditions of the operation. There is considerable interdependence between the surgical procedure and the anesthetic management, which requires close collaboration between the anesthetist and surgeon.

PHYSIOLOGIC CHANGES RELATED TO PNEUMOPERITONEUM

Cardiovascular Changes

The hemodynamic changes seen during laparoscopy are due to the creation of pneumoperitoneum, the position of the patient and the effects of anesthetic agents used.

In Trendelenburg position mean arterial pressure (MAP) and systemic vascular resistance (SVR) are increased and the cardiac output falls. Cardiac index falls by 50% even in ASA (American Society of Anesthesiologists) class II patients. The fall in cardiac output is proportional to the intraperitoneal pressure. Very low intraabdominal pressures have no effect on cardiac output; in fact at intraabdominal pressure of 5 mm Hg, the venous return actually improves because the intraperitoneal pressure remains lower than the pressure in the vena cava which results in a flushing effect. When the intraperitoneal pressure rises above the intravascular pressure, it obstructs the venous return; a subdiaphragmatic narrowing of inferior vena cava occurs, which slows the flow of blood. The abdominal blood volume is reduced due to the pressure and a reflux into the venous system of the lower part of the body.

Systemic vascular resistance is increased considerably because of the splanchnic vascular compression due to pneumoperitonium; a hormonal factor has also been suggested. During the increase in intraperitoneal pressure there is a considerable rise in antidiuretic hormone (ADH); its vasopressive effects are well-known. The secretion of ADH is related to a drop in cardiac flow rate and a simultaneous rise in the level of plasma norepinephrine.

The use of the Trendelenburg position before starting peritoneal insufflations results in less hemodynamic disturbance because of the relative increase in venous return and the filling pressures in this position. This explains the importance of having an adequate circulating blood volume before beginning pneumoperitoneum.

Respiratory System Changes

Increased intraabdominal pressure because of pneumoperitoneum leads to upward displacement of diaphragm which results in increased airway pressure, increased physiological dead space, reduced lung compliance and reduced functional residual capacity (FRC). Reduction in lung volume and lung compliance results in ventilation-perfusion mismatch leading to hypoxia and carbon dioxide (CO_2) retention. Hypoxia is also due to reduced FRC. Increased airway pressure can lead to barotrauma during ventilation of lungs.

Peritoneal insufflation of CO_2 leads to increased end-tidal CO_2 (E_tCO_2) and increased partial pressure of CO_2 ($PaCO_2$) levels by 8–10 mm Hg because of CO_2 reabsorption from the peritoneal cavity which causes tachycardia, arrhythmias and increased myocardial O_2 consumption. In fact, this is a two phase phenomenon with absorption proportional to intraperitoneal pressure for low insufflation pressures, then a drop in the reabsorption rate due to the peritoneal circulation being crushed under the effect of the pressure. The variations in $PaCO_2$ observed during the second phase with high intraabdominal pressures are because of a change in the ventilation/perfusion ratio with an increase in the dead space.

The hypercapnia mechanism is different with extraperitoneal insufflation. In this case, the pressure effect limiting reabsorption from the peritoneum no longer applies. Reabsorption is directly proportional to the pressure and volume of CO_2 insufflated. Severe hypercapnia is thus possible. On the other hand, provided the hypercapnia is controlled, the circulatory repercussions of extraperitoneal insufflation are lower than those of intraperitoneal insufflation. The same is not true of acute hypercapnia, the sudden onset of which does not allow the physiological compensation mechanisms to come into play and which is thus accompanied by severe acidosis. This can be at the origin of noxious hemodynamic effects.

Apart from accidental leakage into the subcutaneous tissues connected with poor positioning of a trocar sleeve,

CO_2 is seen to spread outside the abdominal cavity during laparoscopic assisted hysterectomy and during bladder neck suspensions. In laparoscopic gynecological surgery, because this effusion originates in the pelvis, it mostly affects the sides and loins and generally remains hidden by the drapes until the end of the operation. Only a very large amount can be diagnosed by the anesthetist during the operation, when it shifts toward the upper part of the thorax. In this case, the capnographic signs of slow and regular increase in CO_2 expired, will provide an alert during the anesthesia.

During anesthesia, normocarbia is maintained by increasing minute volume by 25%. Intermittent positive pressure respiration (IPPR) will keep $PaCO_2$ within normal limits, avoid tachycardia and prevent gastric aspiration. Intraoperative respiratory problems commonly encountered are hypoventilation, increased airway pressure, endobronchial intubation and sometimes pneumothorax.

Postoperative lung function after laparoscopy is better preserved than after laparotomy; the changes in the lung-function return to normal values much earlier than laparotomy.

PATIENT SELECTION FOR LAPAROSCOPIC SURGERY

- Patients with cardiac pathology must be subjected to a preoperative assessment taking the particular hemodynamic conditions imposed by laparoscopic surgery into account
- The increase in SVR and the increased O_2 requirements of the myocardium make laparoscopy unsuitable for coronary patients. The postoperative benefits of laparoscopic surgery must be weighed against the peroperative risks. Preoperative investigations, especially for assessment of cardiac reserve, myocardial contractility and the ejection fraction must be done. The data provided by these investigations will also serve to indicate whether or not invasive monitoring is necessary
- Patients presenting with decompensated congestive cardiopathy cannot undergo laparoscopic surgery because the hemodynamic repercussions would be too difficult to manage, even with the help of invasive monitoring techniques
- The reduced venous return during peritoneal insufflation is one of the factors, which result in the drop in cardiac output during laparoscopic surgery. This reduced venous return is all the more important when the circulating blood volume is low. Creation of pneumoperitoneum should be delayed till the circulating volume has not been restored to normal. This is particularly important for ruptured ectopic pregnancy or during laparoscopic surgical exploration of abdominal injuries
- The variations in ventilation mechanics and intrathoracic pressure changes induced by the increase in intraabdominal pressure can be limiting factors for laparoscopic surgery in patients with lung diseases. Creation of the pneumoperitoneum results in a 30% decrease in pulmonary compliance and increased air way resistance. These changes can have adverse consequences for patients with emphysema; all those who suffer from dystrophy of the pulmonary parenchyma will find it difficult to cope with the considerable hyperventilation required to keep CO_2 levels within normal limits.

Monitoring

Monitoring of a laparoscopic surgical procedure has certain elements in common for all patients. Others are more specific to patients with cardiopathy. Ventilation monitoring is discussed in the section on reabsorption of CO_2.

Normal Monitoring

The stethoscope remains an important instrument enabling both lungs to be auscultated after any change in position and after insufflation of the pneumoperitoneum which, because it pushes back the tracheal carina, can deviate intubation to the right. The use of a stethoscope in the precordial position has also been recommended by certain authors in order to detect gas embolism, but requires continuous auscultation.

Electrocardiogram monitoring during laparoscopy enables arrhythmia, which may occur due to hypercapnia, to be rapidly detected. A sudden appearance of a microvoltage can be the sign of subcutaneous emphysema or pneumomediastinum. Automatic analysis of the ST segment is not of much use because the changes in axes brought about by changes in position and the pneumoperitoneum make any reference trace unusable; also the use of monopolar coagulation interferes with the trace.

Oximetry (SpO_2) is essential, especially because the dim lighting in the laparoscopic surgery theater make it difficult to recognize cyanosis. In any case, the latter is a late clinical sign of hypoxia. Variations in saturation are not specific during laparoscopic surgery. Desaturation is a late sign of complications such as gas embolism, pneumothorax, selective intubation or a shunt effect, due to excessively high intraperitoneal pressure.

During laparoscopic surgery, control of intraperitoneal pressure is an integral part of the anesthesia monitoring.

The insufflator must be equipped with automatic controls, even for high flow rates. Excessive intraperitoneal pressure must trigger an alert and an immediate halt in insufflation. As the majority of insufflators do not cater for a reduction in intraperitoneal pressure, this must be carried out by manual exsufflation via a trocar.

Monitoring of the neuromuscular block is especially important. Good muscle relaxation improves the laparoscopic surgeon's view and limits the peritoneal insufflation pressures. In addition, the wide range of operating times and the rapidity with which an operation is terminated, means it is essential to know exactly what the neuromuscular block situation is at any point of time.

Intraperitoneal insufflation of dry and unheated gas, possibly accompanied by irrigation with cold liquids results in heat loss during laparoscopic surgery. Temperature monitoring, associated with measures to combat heat loss, is essential during long procedures.

Cardiovascular Monitoring of High-risk Patients

Electrocardiogram and NIBP measurement do not permit variations in cardiac flow rate or the filling pressures induced by the pneumoperitoneum to be followed. These parameters can be important for adapting anesthesia and peroperative care of patients with limited circulatory reserve. But before the use of invasive monitoring, a risk versus benefit analysis of laparoscopic surgery in these situations must be done; the postoperative advantages for these patients often justifies this approach.

Intra-arterial BP monitoring enables arterial pressure to be monitored in real time. In addition, the appearance of cyclic variations in time with ventilation is an excellent indication of drop in preload, which prompt the intraperitoneal insufflation pressure to be limited to increase filling or even to accentuate the Trendelenburg position, when possible. Installation of an arterial entry point also helps with blood gas measurements.

Measurement of CVP is traditionally used to supervise the filling pressures in the right heart. This becomes difficult during laparoscopic surgery because of the changes in position and particularly because of the increase in intrathoracic pressure transmitted from the peritoneal area via the diaphragm. To get a true CVP, simultaneous measurement of intrathoracic pressure, which is obtained by esophageal pressure, is done and deducted from the measured CVP.

Catheterization of the right heart using a Swan-Ganz probe has been in widespread use for monitoring during laparoscopic surgery. An increase in pulmonary arterial pressure is an early sign of gas embolism. Aspiration of the gas bubbles by the proximal orifice placed in the right atrium is theoretically possible. Measurement of O_2 levels in mixed venous blood (SvO_2) is possible on certain Swan-Ganz catheters; a change in SvO_2 is often a sign of a change in cardiac flow rate.

The invasive and potentially dangerous nature of catheterization of the right heart has resulted in search of less invasive methods during laparoscopic surgery. Cardiac flow rate monitoring by transthoracic electrical bioimpedance which is low risk, noninvasive monitoring, easy, reliable and simple to use, is becoming popular. Transesophageal ultrasound cardiography and pulsed Doppler velocimetry are the other methods under evaluation.

Carbon Dioxide Monitoring

The CO_2 end tidal pressure ($PetCO_2$) provides a measure of CO_2 levels in the blood. A rapid increase in $PetCO_2$ is a complication:

- A rapid rise of a few millimeters of mercury returning to the base figures a few minutes later can be the sign of minimal CO_2 gas embolism
- A more gradual and persistent rise is often the sign of extraperitoneal diffusion of CO_2 (preperitoneal, subcutaneous, retroperitoneal, mediastinal, etc.) This increase in expired CO_2 continues after exsufflation of the pneumoperitoneum, often for several hours after the laparoscopic procedure, justifying monitoring of $PetCO_2$ in the recovery room
- The CO_2 is transported by the circulatory system from the peripheral areas toward the lungs. Any disturbance in the circulation will reduce the CO_2 expired. A rapid drop in $PetCO_2$ may be the sign of a drop in cardiac flow rate or a decreased venous return or pulmonary arterial obliteration. This is what happens in massive gas embolism, which shows up as a drop in $PetCO_2$ proportional in size and duration to the volume of the CO_2 embolus.

Classically, the $PetCO_2$ values are 2–6 mm Hg lower than that of $PaCO_2$. During anesthesia, the ventilation/perfusion ratio is often greater than 1, so a $PaCO_2$-$PetCO_2$ gradient of 10–15 mm Hg must be expected. However, during laparoscopic surgery, the change in the arterial CO_2-$EtCO_2$ gradient is very variable.

Changes in position such as the Trendelenburg or the lateral reclined position can modify the value of the $PetCO_2$.Furthermore, Wittgen et al. have shown that in cases of cardiovascular disease and obesity, the correlation between $PetCO_2$ and $PaCO_2$ was less good when compared to patients with no such pathology. A recent study confirms that in patients with respiratory impairment the increases in $PaCO_2$ are underestimated by $PetCO_2$. So, for these patients with respiratory or heart pathology, it is useful to duplicate the $PetCO_2$ measurement by arterial blood gases at the beginning of the operation and every time there is an important variation in $PetCO_2$.

In view of this uncertainty, transcutaneous CO_2 monitoring would give a better idea of $PaCO_2$, but this also raises a certain number of technical problems (heating of electrodes, difficulties with measurements in adults, etc.).

MANAGEMENT OF ANESTHESIA

The following must be kept in mind by everyone administering anesthesia for laparoscopic surgery:

- Maximum hemodynamic changes occur during insufflation of CO_2 for creating pneumoperitoneum. They settle down after 15–20 minutes of CO_2 insufflation but it is prudent to remain vigilant throughout the duration of surgery
- The hemodynamic changes are directly proportional to the intraabdominal pressure, which must be kept as low as possible
- The hemodynamic changes can be reduced by preloading with IV fluids but at the cost of volume overloading when the patient comes round. Having a moderate Trendelenburg position before starting creation of pneumoperitoneum is beneficial. In no case should a patient be tilted forward before the intraabdominal pressure has stabilized
- The hemodynamic modifications depend on time. Insufflation of the pneumoperitoneum must take place gradually to enable the circulatory adaptation mechanisms to counteract the effects of the pneumoperitoneum.

Day Case Surgery

Day case surgery can be carried out under local anesthetic, locoregional block or under GA.

Local Anesthesia

It is possible to use local anesthesia for procedures of short duration but it requires very quick and expert surgical technique and also a certain degree of cooperation from the patient. Sedation must be used very cautiously with the local anesthetic because it can encourage hypercapnia, because of the respiratory depression it induces.

Epidural Anesthesia

This anesthesia enables loss of consciousness and tracheal intubation to be avoided. Its use remains reserved for certain, very particular and exceptional situations such as:

- Where GA is not recommended
- When GA is refused
- When intubation is expected to be difficult
- Known and documented allergy to certain products used for GA (especially curare)
- When the vocal cords need to be protected (singers, etc.)
- In exceptional cases where the surgeon wishes to have peroperative verbal contact to keep the patient informed of surgical findings and maybe make a difficult decision immediately with the patient's consent.

In all these cases, a preoperative consultation concerning anesthesia is essential to explain the particular points about the regional technique, the need for good cooperation during the operation, and the possibility of GA, if the block is insufficient.

Apart from the risk of failure and the potential toxicity of local anesthetics, which are common to all epidural anesthesia, the use of this technique for laparoscopic surgery poses specific problems:

- A sensory block between T4 and S5 is usually necessary to obtain good quality anesthesia during laparoscopy. Upper level of the block must reach T4 to make pneumoperitoneum painless
- The association of a broad sympathetic T4-S5 block, the pneumoperitoneum (which can compress the lower vena cava whenever there is 10 mm Hg insufflation pressure or more), and a head-up position results in a drop in the venous return and also a drop in the cardiac output
- Locoregional anesthesia for laparoscopy is theoretically associated with several modifications in respiration. The T4-S5 sensory block is accompanied by a certain degree of paralysis of the intercostal muscles. In addition, the pneumoperitoneum using CO_2 associated with peroperative position of the patient results in the diaphragm being pushed up. All these changes, including the sedation which is often necessary, results in hypercapnia with a theoretical risk of hypoxia. Systematic administration of O_2 with spontaneous ventilation, is therefore, strongly recommended. However, it must be recognized that these are minor problems in reality than in theory, at least when used in young women with no past history of respiratory problems. Under these conditions, respiratory tolerance is good and the changes in respiratory parameters are only slight or moderate.
- Epidural techniques require a considerable time for installation, close monitoring and frequent contact with the patient; this is a major drawback for the use of epidural anesthesia under day surgery conditions.

General Anesthesia

Various anesthetic techniques have been proposed for outpatient laparoscopic surgery. There is, at present, no consensus concerning the anesthesia technique to use for outpatient laparoscopic surgery. At the very most, a few general remarks can be made, recommending products with suitable pharmacokinetics and being aware of the possibility of bradycardia associated with the use of propofol in patients who have not usually received any premedication.

Intubation is the reason for many cases of sore throat during the postoperative period. It may be a relatively minor discomfort but is more difficult to accept when the surgery itself results in little persistent pain. In the case of very short laparoscopies, ventilation with a face mask may be used. This opinion is far from being shared by everyone, if only for the risk of regurgitation due to the Trendelenburg position and raised intraabdominal pressure. The same arguments are applicable to the laryngeal mask airway recently proposed for outpatient laparoscopies with spontaneous ventilation.

The pneumoperitoneum must be evacuated as completely as possible and this is particularly important for the control of postoperative pain. In order to obtain correct exsufflation, the suprapubic trocar sheath must be kept under direct visual control to maintain it in just level with the peritoneum, with the patient in a slight Trendelenburg tilt, while gently pressing down on the abdomen. Installation of a drain for a few hours has also been suggested. Instillation of liquid into the abdominal cavity at the end of the laparoscopic operation has also proved to be an efficient technique.

When exsufflation is carried out correctly it is often possible to do without morphine-like substances, which are not easy to manage for outpatients, and the risk of nausea and vomiting involved with these drugs must also be borne in mind.

LENGTHY LAPAROSCOPIC PROCEDURES

Laparoscopic procedures, lasting more than 4 hours, are no longer exceptional in gynecological surgery. The management of these patients needs certain specific points to be taken into consideration.

They require special precautions when installing the patient and special care must be taken to avoid any risk of brachial plexus compression. Elongation of the plexus remains possible due to forced abduction of an upper limb. This might happen if a poorly tightened armrest gradually slips downward when the patient is in the Trendelenburg position. The increase in the number of onlookers during operations can also result in a limb slipping upward, if it is not correctly fixed alongside the body.

When the lower limbs are installed in leg sheaths or are fixed too tightly with straps, nerves can be compressed.

Considerable loss in body heat due to insufflation of cold gas and copious peritoneal irrigation justify the installation of a heated mattress. Venous stasis combined with the increase in intraabdominal pressure means there is a significant risk of thromboembolism. So, even if the patient is encouraged to get up and walk soon after the operation, prophylactic heparin should be given in the same way as for operations via laparotomy.

The anesthetic technique must be adapted to the constraints of long laparoscopic operations:

- The halogen anesthetics, and especially isoflurane, have vasodilator properties which enable the increase in vascular resistance which accompany peritoneal insufflation to be controlled. The use of halogen substances must however be reconsidered when the operation is to take place in the Trendelenburg position; changes in cerebral vasoregulation must be avoided in a patient who is going to lie with her head low down for several hours
- If peroperative ventilation is not used with a closed circuit, a heater-humidifier must be available on the respirator to avoid heat loss
- Correct muscle relaxation makes it possible to reduce the increase in intraabdominal pressure and its consequences on hemodynamics and ventilation. There is nothing specific to say about the use of central analgesics during the peroperative period compared with an equivalent procedure via laparotomy.

At the end of the procedure, SVR remains high even when intraperitoneal pressure has returned to normal. From the circulation point of view, this results in an increase in venous return, whereas the afterload remains high. An increase in arterial pressure is thus not unusual at this stage. In spite of all the precautions taken, patients often suffer from hypothermia at the end of a lengthy laparoscopic procedure. This is due at least in part to the reduction in pressure effect of the insufflated gases. The hypothermia means an increase in myocardial effort when the patient comes round because muscular shivering uses a lot of O_2. For all these reasons, the moment when exsufflation takes place and the period immediately after, are often a time of hemodynamic instability. Recovery should thus be calm and progressive, continuing to control all the parameters. Extubation should not take place too early. Mechanical ventilation should continue in the recovery room for about 30 minutes. Extubation will then take place in a patient who is awake, recovered from the neuromuscular block in a stable hemodynamic, ventilatory and thermal condition. Administration of high concentrations of O_2 using the high flow mask and monitoring of the various parameters is then initiated.

Extraperitoneal Laparoscopic Surgery

Certain procedures such as Burch vaginal suspensions or pelvic lymphadenectomies mean that the operating field is extended to include the preperitoneal or retroperitoneal space. Extraperitoneal insufflation of CO_2 is usually accompanied by hypercapnia due to the rise in pressure which increases the diffusion space and the surface through which CO_2 is reabsorbed. So reabsorption is directly proportional to the pressure and volume of CO_2 insufflated. Severe hypercapnia is therefore possible and may indeed be frequent in these situations. Because it occurs suddenly, the physiological compensation mechanisms do not have time to come into play and the hypercapnia is therefore accompanied by severe acidosis,which is what make this complication so important and requires certain steps to be taken:

- Auscultation of the patient to eliminate one sided intubation or a pneumothorax
- Hyperventilation to correct the hypercapnia
- Reduction of insufflation pressure. Good muscle relaxation usually enables this problem to be solved without reducing the surgeon's visibility. If surgical exposure is insufficient, the use of an abdominal wall suspension device must be considered
- If despite all these steps, the patient's carbon dioxide levels cannot be kept at acceptable levels (below 50 mm Hg), consider conversion to laparotomy.

COMPLICATIONS

Gas Embolism

Gas embolism is an unfamiliar subject to many due to its low incidence, estimated at between 0% and 0.6% of laparoscopic surgical procedures. In fact it is likely that the primitive forms, which give rise to nonspecific neurological problems or a simple delay in coming round, are far more frequent. They can also be mistaken for the various other hemodynamic complications of laparoscopic surgery such as acute obstacles to venous return or cardiac arrhythmia, not forgetting the delayed forms, which occur at the end of the operation when exsufflation of the pneumoperitoneum releases bubbles of CO_2 trapped in the mesenteric or portal circulation.

Mechanism

The entry point is most often in a large vein (iliac vein, inferior vena cava) punctured during insertion of the Veress' needle at the beginning of insufflation. Another entry point is the periumbilical venous plexus. Peroperative vascular injuries only lead to gas embolism if the pneumoperitoneum pressure is very close to venous pressure. If it is greater, as is most often the case in laparoscopic surgery, the vessels collapse, stopping any entry of gas. In the rare situations where the venous pressure is greater than the pneumoperitoneum pressure, the vascular opening results in hemorrhage and not in entry of gas.

Pollution of the intraabdominal CO_2 by nitrous oxide from the anesthetic circuit or by carbon monoxide from the diathermy probe worsens the repercussions of gas embolism because these gases are less soluble than CO_2. Similarly, the permeability of the foramen ovale in 30% of young subjects accounts for the high frequency of systemic embolus and neurological complications. In the same way, the lower solubility of nitrous oxide and air explain that these two gases are far more dangerous than CO_2 in case of gas embolism.

The volume of the gas embolus is the main factor governing the clinical symptoms. Only small flow rate emboli (less than 0.3 mL/kg/min in the dog) are accompanied by an increase in the $PetCO_2$, which shows the elimination of intravascular CO_2 via the pulmonary route. When the volume of the gas embolus increases, the $PetCO_2$ drops due to the decrease in exchanges at the pulmonary capillary bed and/or by circulatory arrest.

What to Do

Prophylactic measures are essential and must be applied systematically. These include not only the aspiration tests carried out when the Veress' needle is inserted, but also the use of open laparoscopy when a problem with insufflation can be expected (multiple abdominal operations). Generally speaking, it is important to limit the insufflation flow rate to 1 L/min for as long as the procedure remains blind. The use of esophageal or precordial Doppler, or failing this, a simple stethoscope is useful for early detection of gas embolism in high-risk situations.

What needs to be done in the presence of a gas embolism largely depends on the volume and thus the systemic effects. Whereas certain gestures must be systematic in the presence of massive gas embolism, installation of a central catheter in the right atrium to aspirate the CO_2 is of limited benefit, because only low volumes of gas are usually collected under these conditions.

The other treatments which follow the initial resuscitation are more debatable. Neuroprotection using barbiturates or hypothermia is not always beneficial, makes neurological monitoring more complicated and risks inducting noxious hemodynamic repercussions. The same is true for hyperbaric O_2 therapy, which is less useful than in cases of air embolism, because CO_2 is more soluble and there is a high pressure gradient between the blood and CO_2 bubbles (over 600 mm Hg), which encourages reabsorption. Use of this technique is only justified if the chamber is available within a short space of time and if it is possible to continue reviving the patient during the O_2 therapy session.

Cardiovascular Collapse

Etiology

A sudden drop in arterial pressure may occur during any of the various phases of laparoscopic surgery, indicating various etiologies:

- The first possibility of gas embolism is at the beginning of the procedure by direct insufflation of CO_2 into a vein during insufflation of the pneumoperitoneum. The second possible etiology is injury to a major vessel by the Veress' needle or a trocar. These injuries are often obvious but may also go undiagnosed immediately due to the retroperitoneal situation of the major vessels. A third cause of collapse at the time of insufflation is preoperative hypovolemia which magnifies the repercussions of the pneumoperitoneum on venous return
- During laparoscopic surgery, apart from gas embolism, cardiovascular collapse may result from faulty surgical hemostasis. This may be particularly difficult to achieve, especially in case of injury to the major vessels, because not all the vascular surgery instruments have yet been adapted for laparoscopic surgery. Sudden heart failure in a patient with coronary disease, for example, may also be a reason for this hypotension. This situation is becoming more common as laparoscopic surgery progresses to include older patients with past history of circulatory problems
- At the end of the operation, the two main causes of cardiovascular collapse are vascular injury, which has been overlooked, and delayed gas embolism.

Pneumothorax

This is an unexceptional complication, which has two very different etiologies. There may be passage of CO_2 through the pleura from the abdominal cavity. This effusion takes place gradually during the laparoscopy, is not usually suffocating and, in the moderately abundant forms, reabsorbs spontaneously. The usual explanation given to explain the mechanism of this complication is an anatomical malformation connecting the pleura and the peritoneal cavity. However, attempts to obtain hard evidence concerning this malformation, once a pneumothorax occurring during laparoscopy has abated, seem so far to be in vain. There is another objection to this hypothesis also in that the intrathoracic pressure in patients under controlled ventilation during laparoscopy is higher than the intraperitoneal pressure each time the respirator insufflates. It is thus difficult to see how CO_2 could accumulate in the pleural cavity even if there is an anatomical malformation.

Pneumothorax due to high pressure trauma is quite different. Abdominal insufflation is accompanied by an increase in intrathoracic pressures which can have detrimental effects in patients with bubbles of emphysema or a past history of recurring pneumothorax. In these cases the pneumothorax can be suffocating and must be drained immediately.

ANESTHESIA FOR HYSTEROSCOPY

Whereas diagnostic hysteroscopy can take place under simple sedation or with a paracervical block in the gynecologist's consulting rooms, anesthetic management is necessary when a surgical procedure is to be carried out by the endouterine route. This should be adapted to the patient's preoperative condition and how the procedure is to be carried out, this often being on a day surgery basis. GA or locoregional anesthesia may be used. The anesthetist must also bear potential complications in mind, such as vascular overloading or glycine intoxication, connected with re-absorption of the liquid used to distend and irrigate the uterine cavity.

Installation and Monitoring

Care must be taken, while installing the patients, that the external popliteal sciatic nerve is not compressed in the leg restraints.

Monitoring includes noninvasive measurement of arterial pressure, ECG, pulse oximetry and capnography. Given the considerable heat loss, which can occur with copious irrigation, temperature monitoring is also useful. When locoregional anesthesia is used, regular supervision of the patient's state of consciousness is also required.

Monitoring of the input and output of irrigation liquid is indispensable. If a deficit of 500 mL between input and output of irrigation liquid is noted, blood investigation for electrolyte levels is indicated. If this deficit reaches 1,000 mL, 20 mg frusemide should be administered intravenously and plasma electrolytes checked at the same time. If the deficit reaches 2,000 mL, the procedure must be interrupted immediately. Similarly, the anesthetist must pay careful attention to intrauterine pressure and check that this never exceeds 70 mm Hg.

Anesthetic Techniques

General Anesthesia

From the technical point of view, GA for hysteroscopy presents no specific problems. The choice of drugs will depend on the patient's preoperative condition, the expected duration of the procedure and whether it is on a day surgery basis or not. For a short procedure, ventilation can be provided by a face mask or by a laryngeal mask. For lengthy procedures or those which require an accentuated Trendelenburg position, tracheal intubation and controlled ventilation are indicated. The same applies to obese patients and those presenting hiatus hernia.

Locoregional Anesthesia

In order to ensure complete anesthesia during hysteroscopy, a block of the sensory levels from T8 to S5 is required. This can be achieved using epidural anesthesia or spinal anesthesia.

Spinal Anesthesia

The use of conical tipped needles (for example Whitacre type) limits the incidence of headache due to puncture of the dura mater during spinal anesthesia. Reducing the gauge of the needles has the same effect. The choice of local anesthetic drug (5% lidocaine or 0.5% bupivacaine) depends on how long the surgical procedure is expected to last.

Rapid installation of the sensory block enables surgery to commence quickly. The sympathetic nervous system block which takes place just as quickly, sometimes poses problems with respect to circulatory tolerance with sudden onset vasoparalysis. This is particularly true in older patients with doubtful circulatory conditions or in women presenting with preoperative hypovolemia. It is possible to ward off the effects of this vasoparalysis by prophylactic vascular filling (for example 1,000 mL crystalloids) and/or by using a vasoconstrictor agent such as ephedrine (30 mg in 250 mL, 5% glucose solution), with the flow rate adapted to the patient's BP.

Epidural Anesthesia

The main advantage of epidural anesthesia as compared with spinal anesthesia is the installation of a catheter which enables local anesthetics to be reinjected, if the surgical procedure is prolonged. The fact that the dura mater is not punctured also reduces the risk of postoperative headache. Finally, the epidural catheter can be left in place at the end of the operation in order to manage postoperative analgesia.

In fact, a hysteroscopic surgical procedure rarely lasts longer than the duration of the effects of a local anesthetic injected during spinal anesthesia, and the postoperative pain is usually easy to manage with non morphine-type analgesics administered systemically. So it is rarely justified to install an epidural catheter. Similarly, the argument of postspinal anesthesia headache has lost its importance since the arrival of the new conical tipped needles. All this considerably limits the indications for epidural anesthesia for hysteroscopy, and all the more so in that this anesthetic technique is longer and more complex than spinal anesthesia to use and is thus difficult to reconcile with the quick rotation of patients in a day surgery program.

COMPLICATIONS

Although still perhaps acceptable for diagnostic hysteroscopy, the use of CO_2 to distend the uterine cavity is no longer considered for endouterine surgery. The various solutions used for this surgery can induce nonspecific complications linked with reabsorption of the liquid. Some of them and more particularly glycine can be the origin of specific manifestations.

Nonspecific Complications

Endouterine surgery results in reabsorption of liquids by the broaching of endometrial or myometrial vessels, by a mechanism close to that described for prostate surgery. It would seem logical to carry out hysteroresection at the beginning of the cycle in order to limit reabsorption when the vessels are broached. This absorption can also take place via the peritoneal cavity when the solution injected into the uterus flows out through the tubes.

Supervision of the patient's weight before and after the hysteroscopy together with follow-up of input and output enable this reabsorption to be monitored (see above). Monitoring of intrauterine pressure and limiting it to 700 mm Hg is also essential. Massive reabsorption of dextran or glycine results in a drop in natremia, made evident by postoperative plasma electrolyte studies.

The clinical symptoms of massive reabsorption are associated with edema of the face, increase in diuresis and problems with consciousness after the patient has come round from the anesthetic, which can go as far as coma. Acute pulmonary edema can also complicate the situation. In this case, the CVP will be high. Symptomatic treatment of acute circulatory failure associating diuretics, inotropic support, O_2 and possibly controlled ventilation must be initiated.

Specific Complications

Acute intoxication with glycine is well-documented and is seen after large quantities of glycine have been reabsorbed. The toxicity is of dual nature:

- Intracellular hyperhydration and hyponatremia occurring when a hypo-osmolar and hypotonic liquid, i.e. 1.5% glycine penetrates the internal environment. This hyperhydration explains the majority of the circulatory signs seen

- The neurological symptoms would appear to be directly linked with neurological toxicity of glycine or one of its metabolites for the CNS. This amino acid which crosses the hematoencephalic barrier is also an inhibiting neurotransmitter at central level.

The clinical manifestations are neurological to begin with: problems with consciousness which range from simple confusion syndrome with agitation to coma. Signs are sometimes localized, such as a focal convulsive attack, or visual symptoms, such as a drop in visual acuity or even temporary blindness. The cardiovascular symptoms range from bradycardia to collapse with a broadening of the QRS complexes and modifications to the ST segment.

If these complications are to be prevented, the intrauterine pressure and volume of fluid injected must be checked. Treatment of the circulatory problems is the same as that for acute heart failure. The neurological signs can require intubation with controlled ventilation, combined with specific treatment for the epileptic manifestations.

CONCLUSION

Gynecological surgery, which saw the birth of laparoscopy, is still today, as in the past, a field of tremendous changes, where indications and new techniques continue to appear and develop. As anesthetists, we are called upon to accompany these changes whilst preserving the safety and well-being of the patients entrusted to us.

BIBLIOGRAPHY

1. Alahuhta S, Kangas-Saarela T, Hollmen AI, et al. Visceral pain during caesarean section under spinal and epidural anaesthesia with bupivacaine. Acta Anaesthesiol Scand. 1990;34:95-9.
2. Alexander GD, Wetchler BV, Thompson RE. Bupivacaine infiltration of the mesosalpinx in ambulatory surgical laparoscopic tubal sterilisation. Can J Anaesth. 1987;34:362-5.
3. Anathanarayan C, Paek W, Dhanidina K. Hysteroscopy and anaesthesia. Can J Anaesth. 1996;43:56-64.
4. Andel J, Grabner V, Zadrobilek E, et al. Cardiopulmonary effects of laparoscopic cholecystectomy. Anaesth Analg. 1992;74:S8.
5. Aoki T, Tanii M, Takahashi K, et al. Cardiovascular changes and catecholamine levels during laparoscopic surgery. Anesth Analg. 1994;78:S8.
6. Bard PA, Chen L. Subcutaneous emphysema associated with laparoscopy. Anesth Analg. 1990;71:101-2.
7. Barnes GE, Laine GA, Giam PY, et al. Cardiovascular responses to elevation of intra-abdominal hydrostatic pressure. Am J Physiol. 1985;248:R208.
8. Bayley PL, Streisand JB, Pace NL, et al. Transdermal scopolamine reduces nausea and vomiting after outpatient laparoscopy. Anesthesiology. 1990;72:977-80.
9. Bazin JE. Retentissement cardiovasculaire de la coelioscopie. In Anesthésie pour coelioscopie. Paris: JEPU; 1993.
10. Beattie WS, Linblad T, Buckley DN, et al. Menstruation increases the risk of nausea and vomiting after laparoscopy. A prospective randomized study. Anesthesiology. 1993;78:272-6.
11. Beilin B, Vatashsky E. Safe anaesthetic for laparoscopy with spontaneous respiration. Br J Anaesth. 1985;57:1041-2.
12. Benifa JL, Hauy JP, Guglielmina J, et al. Kystectomie percoelioscopique: découverte histologique fortuite d'un carcinome ovarien. J Gynecol Obstet Biol Reprod. 1992;21:45-9.
13. Berek J, Hacker N. Laparoscopy in the management of patients with ovarian carcinoma. Clin Obstet Gynaecol. 1983;10:213-22.
14. Blobner M, Felber AR, Gogler S, et al. Carbon dioxide uptake from pneumoperitoneum during laparoscopic cholecystectomy. Anesthesiology. 1992;77:A37.
15. Booker WM, French DM, Molano PA. Further studies on the acute effects of intra-abdominal pressure. Am J Physiol. 1947;149:92-8.
16. Brampton WJ, Watson. Arterial to end-tidal carbon dioxide tension difference during laparoscopy. Anaesthesia 1990;45:210-4.
17. Bridenbaugh LD, Soberstrom RM. Lumbar epidural block anesthesia for outpatient laparoscopy. J Reprod Med. 1979;23:85-6.
18. Bromberg N, Matuszak JP, Delecluze PH, et al. Fonction pulmonaire après cholécystectomie par voie laparoscopique chez l'obèse. Ann Fr Anesth Réanim. 1992;11:R20.
19. Bromberg N, Matuszak JP, Mahieu G, et al. Comparaison des mesures télé-expiratoires, transcutanées et artérielles du CO2 au cours de la cholécystectomie par laparoscopie. Ann Fr Anesth Réanim. 1992;11:R2.
20. Burchard KW, Ciombor DM, McLeod MK, et al. Positive end expiratory pressure with increased intra abdominal pressure. Surg Gynecol Obstet. 1985;161:313-8.
21. Calverly RK, Jenkins LC. The anesthetic management of pelvic laparoscopy. Can Anaesth Soc J. 1973;20:679-83.
22. Carroll GC. Capnographic trend curve monitoring can detect 1-ml pulmonary emboli in humans. J Clin Monit. 1992;8(2):101-6.
23. Chung F. Cancer, chemotherapy and anaesthesia. Can Anaesth Soc J. 1982;26:364-71.
24. Cigarini I, Joris J, Jacquet N, et al. Pain and pulmonary dysfunction after cholecystectomy under laparoscopy and laparotomy. Anesthesiology. 1991;75:A122.
25. Ciofolo MJ, Clergue F, Seebacher J, et al. Ventilatory effects of laparoscopy under epidural anesthesia. Anesth Analg. 1990;70:357-61.
26. Cohen SE, Woods WA, Wyner J. Antiemetic efficacy of droperidol and metoclopramide. Anesthesiology. 1984;60:67-9.
27. Cunningham AJ, Turner J, Grosso L, et al. Transesophageal assessment of hemodynamic function during laparoscopic cholecystectomy. Anesth Analg. 1993;76:S64.

28. Deeb RJ, Viechnicki MB. Laparoscopic tubal ligation under peritoneal lavage anesthesia. Regional Anesth 1985;10:24-7.
29. Degueldre M, Puissant F, Camus M, et al. Effets de l'insufflation de dioxyde de carbone pendant la coelioscopie sur la phase gazeuse des liquides de prélèvement d'ovocytes. In Anesthésie pour coelioscopie. Clermont-Ferrand: CARO; 1989. pp. 221-2.
30. deSousa H, Tyler IL. Can absorption of the insufflation gas during laparoscopy be hazardous? Anesthesiology. 1987;67:A476.
31. Diamant M, Benumof JL, Saidman LJ. Hemodynamics of increased intra-abdominal pressure: interaction with hypovolemia and halothane anesthesia. Anesthesiology. 1978;48:23-7.
32. Doyle DJ. Propofol bradycardia. Can J Anaesth. 1991;38:138.
33. Duale C, Bazin JE, Ferrier C, et al. Hemodynamic effects of laparoscopic cholecystectomy in patients with coronary disease. Br J Anaesth. 1994;76:A31.
34. Ekman LG, Abrahamsson J, Biber B, et al. Hemodynamic changes during laporoscopy with positive end-expiratory pressure ventilation. Acta Anesthesiol Scand. 1988;32:447-53.
35. Feig BW, Berger DH, Dougherty TB, et al. Pulmonary effects of CO_2 abdominal insufflation during laparoscopy in high-risk patients. Anesth Analg. 1994;78:S108.
36. Fitzgerald SD, Andrus CH, Baudendistel LJ, et al. Hypercarbia during carbon dioxide pneumoperitoneum. Am J Surg. 1992;163:186-90.
37. Fletcher R, Jonson B. Deadspace and the single breath test for carbon dioxide during anaesthesia and artifical ventilation. Br J Anaesth. 1984;56:109-19.
38. Fox LG, Hein HA, Gawey BJ, et al. Physiologic alterations during laparoscopic cholecystectomy in ASA III & IV patients. Anesthesiology. 1993;79:A55.
39. Freysz M, Timour Q, Bertrix L, et al. Propofol bradycardia. Can J Anaesth. 1991;38:137-8.
40. Ganansia MF, François TP, Ormezzano X, et al. Atrioventricular mobitz I block during propofol anesthesia for laparoscopic tubal ligation. Anesth Analg. 1989;69:524-5.
41. Goldiner P, Carlon GC, Cvitkovic E, et al. Factors influencing postoperative morbidity and mortality in patients treated with bleomycin. Br Med J. 1978;1:1664-7.
42. Goodwin APL, Rowe L, Ogg TW. Day case laparoscopy. A comparison of two anaesthetic techniques using the laryngeal mask during spontaneous breathing. Anaesthesia. 1992;47:892-5.
43. Hall D, Goldstein A, Tynan E, et al. Profound hypercarbia late in the course of laparoscopic cholecystectomy : detection by continuous capnometry. Anesthesiology. 1993;79:173-4.
44. Hamm P, Lang C, Fornecker ML, et al. Intubation bronchique sélective: répétition au cours d'une cholécystectomie coelioscopique. Ann Fr Anesth Réanim. 1993;12:67-9.
45. Hynes SR, Marshall RL. Venous gas embolism during gynaecological laparoscopy. Can J Anaesth. 1992;39:748-9.
46. Ivankovitch AD, Miletich DJ, Albrecht RF, et al. Cardiovascular effects of intraperitoneal insufflation with carbon dioxide and nitrous oxide in the dog. Anesthesiology. 1975;42:281-7.
47. Johannsen G, Andersen M, Juhl B. The effect of general anaesthesia on the haemodynamic events during laparoscopy with CO_2 insufflation. Acta Anaesthesiol Scand. 1989;33:132-6.
48. Johnson RV, Lawson NW, Nealon WH. Lower extremity neuropathy after laparoscopic cholecystectomy. Anesthesiology. 1992;77:835.
49. Joris J, Lamy M. Modifications hémodynamiques au cours de la coelioscopie. In: Schoeffler P (Ed.). Anesthésie pour coeliochirurgie. Paris: Masson Paris; 1993. pp.11-24.
50. Joris J, Ledoux D, Honore P, et al. Ventilatory effects of CO_2 insufflation during laparoscopic cholecystectomy. Anesthesiology. 1991;75:A121.
51. Joris JL, Noirot DL, Legrand MJ, et al. Hemodynamic changes during laparoscopic cholecystectomy. Anesth Analg. 1993;76: 1067-71.
52. Kashtan J, Green JF, Parsons EQ, et al. Hemodynamic effects of increased abdominal pressure. J Surg Res. 1981;30:249-55.
53. Kelman GR, Swapp GH, Smith I, et al. Cardiac output and arterial blood gas tension during laparoscopy. Br J Anaesth. 1972;44:1155-62.
54. Khan RM, Maroof M, Bhatti TH, et al. Correlation of end tidal CO_2 and hemodynamic variation following CO_2 insufflation during laparoscopic cholecystectomy. Anesthesiology. 1992;77:A464.
55. Kleinhaus S, Sammartano R, Boley SJ. Effects of laparoscopy on mesenteric blood flow. Arch Surg. 1978;113:867-9.
56. Kurer FL, Welch DB. Gynaecological laparoscopy: clinical experiences of two anesthetic techniques. Br J Anaesth. 1984; 56:1207-11.
57. Lamantia KR, Glick JH, Marshall BF. Supplemental oxygen does not cause respiratory failure in bleomycin-treated surgical patients. Anesthesiology. 1984;60:65-7.
58. Laville C, Magroian B, Lepage JY, et al. Hemodynamic changes and CO2 diffusion during retro and intraperitoneal CO2 insufflation for laparoscopic nephrectomy in the goat. Anesth Analg. 1994;78:S238.
59. Lenz RJ, Thomas TA, Wilking DG. Cardiovascular changes during laparoscopy. Anaesthesia. 1976;31:4-12.
60. Le Roith D, Bark H, Nyska M, et al. The effect of abdominal pressure on plasma antidiuretic hormone levels in the dog. J Surg Res. 1982;32:65-9.
61. Lister DR, Rudson-Brown B, Warriner CB, et al. Carbon dioxide absorption is not linearly related to intraperitoneal carbon dioxide insufflation pressure in pigs. Anesthesiology. 1994;80:129-36.
62. Lynch FP, Ochi T, Scully JM, et al. Cardiovascular effects of increased intra-abdominal pressure in newborn piglets. J Ped Surg. 1974;9:621-6.
63. Maiman M, Seltzer V, Boyce J. Laparoscopic excision of ovarian neoplasm subsequently found to be malignant. Obstet Gynecol. 1991;77:563-5.
64. Makinen MT. Dynamic lung compliance during laparoscopic cholecystectomy. Anesth Analg. 1994;78:S261.

65. Mann C, Colson P, Fabre JM, et al. Modifications hémodynamiques au cours de la coeliochirurgie digestive. Ann Fr Anesth Réanim. 1992;11:R67.
66. Marshall RL, Jebson PJ, Davie IT, et al. Circulatory effects of carbon dioxide insufflation on the peritoneal cavity for laparoscopy. Br J Anaesth. 1972;44:680-4.
67. Masey SA, Koehler RC, Buck JR, et al. Effect of abdominal distension on central and regional hemodynamics in neonatal lambs. Ped Res. 1985;19:1244-9.
68. McKenzie R, Kovac A, O'Connor T, et al. Comparison of ondansetron versus placebo to prevent postoperative nausea and vomiting in women undergoing ambulatory gynecologic surgery. Anesthesiology. 1993;78:21-8.
69. McKenzie R, Wadhwa RK, Bedger RC. Noninvasive measurement of cardiac output during laparoscopy. J Reprod Med. 1980;24:247-50.
70. McKinstry LJ, Perverseff RA, Yip RW. Arterial and end-tidal carbon dioxide in patients undergoing laparoscopic cholecystectomy. Anesthesiology. 1992;77:A108.
71. Melnick B, Sawyer R, Karambelkar D, et al. Delayed side effects of droperidol after ambulatory general anesthesia. Anesth Analg. 1989;69:748-51.
72. Monk TG, Despotis GJ, Hogue CW, et al. Hemodynamic and echocardiographic alterations during laparoscopic surgery. Anesthesiology. 1993;79:A54.
73. Morrisson LM, Davis J, Sumner D. Absorption of irrigating fluid during laser photocoagulation of the endometrium in the treatment of menorrhagia. Br J Obstet Gynecol. 1989;96:346-52.
74. Motew M, Ivankovich AD, Bienarz J, et al. Cardiovascular effects and acid base changes during laparoscopy. Am J Obstet Gynecol. 1973;115:1002-12.
75. Muchada R, Lavandier B, Cathignol D, et al. Surveillance hmodynamique non invasive dans la coelioscopie gyncologique. Ann Fr Anesth Ranim. 1986;5:14-7.
76. Mullet CE, Viale JP, Sagnard PE, et al. Pulmonary CO_2 elimination during surgical procedure using intra- or extraperitoneal CO_2 insufflation. Anesth Analg. 1993;76:622-6.
77. Myatt JK, Smith M, Plantevin OM, et al. Anaesthesia for day stay laparoscopy. Br J Anaesth. 1986;58:1200-1.
78. Nagai H, Kondo Y, Yasuda T, et al. An abdominal wall-lift method of laparoscopic cholecystectomy without peritoneal insufflation. Surg Laparosc Endosc. 1993;3:173-9.
79. Nyarwaya JB, Samii K, Mazoit JX, et al. Are pulse oximetric and capnographic monitoring reliable during laparoscopic surgery for cholecystectomy? Anesthesiology. 1991;75:A453.
80. Oester A, Madsen PO. Determination of absorption of irrigating fluid during transuretheral resection of the prostate by means of radio-isotopes. J Urol. 1969;102:714-9.
81. Osborne GA, Rudkin GE, Moran P. Fluid uptake in laser endometrial ablation. Anesth Intens Care. 1991;19:217-9.
82. Ovassapian A, Joshi CW, Brunner EA. Visual disturbances: an usual symptom of TURP reaction. Anesthesiology. 1982;57:332-4.
83. Pansard JL, Cholley B, Devilliers C, et al. Variation in arterial to end-tidal CO_2 tension differences during anesthesia in the "Kidney Rest" lateral decubitus position. Anesth Analg. 1992;75:506-10.
84. Pearce DJ. Respiratory acidosis and subcutaneous emphysema during laparoscopic cholecystectomy. Can J Anaesth. 1994;41: 314-6.
85. Perel A. The arterial pressure waveform during hypovolemia and congestive heart failure in mechanically ventilated patients. In: Balagny E, Cathelin M (Eds). La Pression artérielle en anesthésie, Anesthésie-Réanimation. Arnette: Pitié-Salpétrière; 1991. pp. 107-14.
86. Perry CP, Tombrello R. Effect of fluid instillation on postlaparoscopy pain. J Reprod Med. 1993;38:768-70.
87. Punnonen R, Viinamaki O. Vasopressin release during laparoscopy: role of increased intra-abdominal pressure. Lancet. 1982;16:75-176.
88. Puri GD, Singh H. Ventilatory effects of laparoscopy under general anaesthesia. Br J Anaesth. 1992;68:211-3.
89. Raemer DB, Francis D, Philip JH, et al. Variation in PCO_2 between arterial blood and peak expired gas during anesthesia. Anesth Analg. 1983;62:1065-9.
90. Rao PN. Absorption of irrigating fluid during transcervical resection of the endometrium. Br Med J. 1990;300:748-52.
91. Reid CW, Martineau RJ, Miller DR, et al. A comparison of transcutaneous end-tidal and arterial measurements of carbon dioxide during general anaesthesia. Can J Anaesth. 1992;39:31-6.
92. Richardson JD, Trinkle JK. Hemodynamic and respiratory alterations with increased intra abdominal pressure. J Surg Res. 1976;20:401-4.
93. Root B, Levy MN, Pollack S, et al. Gas embolism death after laparoscopy delayed by "trapping" in portal circulation. Anesth Analg. 1978;37:232-7.
94. Rothemberg DM, Parnass SM, Litwack K, et al. Efficacy of ephedrine in the prevention of postoperative nausea and vomiting. Anesth Analg. 1991;72:58-61.
95. Rubison RM, Vasko JS, Dopman JL, et al. Inferior vena cava obstruction from increased intra-abdominal pressure. Arch Surg. 1967;94:766-72.
96. Ruiz F. Cholecystectomie par coelioscopie chez 15 patients en mauvais état général (ASA III & IV): Etude hémodynamique. Clermont-Ferrand: Thèse Médecine; 1992.
97. Safran DB, Sgambadi S, Orlando R. Laparoscopy in high-risk cardiac patients. Surg Gynecol Obstet. 1993;176:548-54.
98. Safran DB. Physiologic effects of pneumoperitoneum. Am J Surg. 1994;167:281-6.
99. Salvo I, Calderini E, Casati A, et al. Surgical positions and dead spaces during general anesthesia. Anesthesiology. 1992;77:A1224.
100. Sarma VJ, Lunstr MJ. Epidural anaesthesia for day case surgery. Anaesthesia. 1989;44:683-5.
101. Sasaki J, Kikuchi H, Shinoda T, et al. The effects of position changes on $etCO_2$ and $PaCO_2$ in CO_2 intra-abdominal insufflation. In Abstracts, 10th World Congress of Anaesthesiologists. The Hague; 1992. p. 218.
102. Schoeffler P, Challier F, Gillart T. Anesthesie pour cøliochirurgie. In Conferences d'actualisation 1992, Paris: SFAR;1992. pp. 379-97.
103. Schoeffler P, Haberer JP, Manhes H, et al. Répercussions circulatoires et ventilatoires de la coelioscopie chez l'obèse. Ann Fr Anesth Réanim. 1984;3:10-5.

104. Scott BH, Vitkun SA, Poppers PJ. Effects of Trendelenburg position on serum catecholamines and hemodynamics in awake and anesthetized patients. Anesth Analg. 1972;74:S273.

105. Scott DB, Julian DG. Observations on cardiac arrhythmias during laparoscopy. Br Med J. 1972;1:411-4.

106. Scuderi P, Wetchler B, Sung YF, et al. Treatment of postoperative nausea and vomiting after outpatient surgery with the 5-HT3 antagonist ondansetron. Anesthesiology. 1993;78:15-20.

107. Selvin BI. Cancer chemotherapy: implications for the anesthesiologist. Anesth Analg. 1981;60:425-33.

108. Sha M, Katagiri J, Ohmura A, et al. Relationship between intra-abdominal pressure and airway resistance during laparoscopic cholecystectomy. Anesthesiology. 1994;81:A1450.

109. Shulman D, Aronson HB. Capnography in the early diagnosis of carbon dioxide embolism during laparoscopy. Can Anaesth Soc J. 1984;31:455-9.

110. Takata M, Wise RA, Robotham JL. Effects of abdominal pressure on venous return; abdominal vascular zone conditions. J App Physiol. 1990;69:249-56.

111. Torielli R, Cesarini M, Winnock S, et al. Modifications hémodynamiques durant la coelioscopie : étude menée par bioimpédance électrique thoracique. Can J Anaesth. 1990;37:46-51.

112. Wadhwa RK, McKenzie R, Wadhwa SR, et al. Gas embolism during laparoscopy. Anesthesiology. 1978;48:74-6.

113. Wallasvaara MT, Paloheimo M. Ventilation and body temperatures during laparoscopic vs. open cholecystectomy. Anesth Analg. 1992;74:S340.

114. Watcha MF, Simeon RM, White PF, et al. Effect of propofol on the incidence of postoperative vomiting after strabismus surgery in pediatric outpatients. Anesthesiology. 1991;75:204-9.

115. Wattiez A, Schoeffler P, Canis M, et al. Les insufflateurs pour endoscopie. Ann Chir. 1994;48:547-54.

116. Weingram J, Sosa RE, Stein B, et al. Subcutaneous emphysema (SCE) during laparoscopic pelvic lymph node dissection (LPLND). Anesth Analg. 1993;76:S460.

117. Westerband A, van de Water JM, Amzallag M, et al. Cardiovascular changes during laparoscopic cholecystectomy. Surg Gynecol Obstet. 1993;175:535-8.

118. Whiston RJ, Egger KA, Morris RW, et al. Tension pneumothorax during laparoscopic cholecystectomy. Br J Surg. 1991;78:1325.

119. White PF, Watcha MF. Are new drugs cost-effective for patients undergoing ambulatory surgery? Anesthesiology. 1993;78:2-5.

120. Whitesell R, Asiddao C, Gollman D, et al. Relationship between arterial and peak expired carbon dioxide pressure during anesthesia and factors influencing the difference. Anesth Analg. 1981;60:508-12.

121. Wieden TE, Wieden M, Foitzik, et al. Emphysem und akute hypercapnie während der laparoskopischen cholezystectomie. Eine methodenspezifische komplication? Minimal Invasive Chirurgie. 1992;1:20-5.

122. Wittgen CM, Andrus CH, Fitzgerald SD, et al. Analysis of the hemodynamic and ventilatory effects of laparoscopy cholecystectomy. Arch Surg. 1991;126:997-1001.

123. Yogasakaran N. Laparoscopy, surgical emphysema and ECG voltage. Anaesthesia. 1992;47:720.

8.2 ANESTHESIA FOR THE PREGNANT PATIENT UNDERGOING NONOBSTETRIC SURGERY

Vinay Tiwari

Approximately 2% of parturients will have surgery during their pregnancy. Surgery is needed to treat conditions such as traumatic injuries, ovarian cysts, appendicitis, cholelithiasis, breast biopsy, and cervical incompetence. However, major procedures such as craniotomy, cardiopulmonary bypass, may also be necessary in the pregnant patient, and usually result in good outcomes for mother and fetus. A pregnant patient requiring surgery is likely to present with extreme anxiety.

PHYSIOLOGY AND RISK ASSESSMENT

Anesthetic management now involves two patients and physiology specific to pregnancy. Alterations in maternal physiology involve many organ systems, but those most important to anesthetic management include the following:

- *Respiratory:* The pregnant woman will have increased O_2 consumption, decreased FRC, lower pCO_2 resulting from increased minute ventilation, greater likelihood of difficult intubation and increased mucosal vascularity with potential for bleeding. The pregnant patient is more prone to hypoxia and hypercarbia. Administer O_2 and monitor O_2 saturation by pulse oximetry. Normal CO_2 levels should be maintained during controlled ventilation because low CO_2 levels will compromise uteroplacental perfusion. Postoperative pain will cause rapid shallow respiration which will further decrease CO_2 levels, hence the need for good analgesia but without fetal depression
- *Cardiovascular:* Changes include increased blood volume and cardiac output, dilutional anemia, aortocaval compression when supine and decreased vascular responsiveness despite increased baroreceptor responsiveness. Any gravida with a coexisting heart disease has an increased risk of cardiac decompensation, especially those with mitral valve involvement. It needs aggressive medical treatment; if it fails, surgical correction is needed
- *Gastrointestinal:* Gastroesophageal sphincter tone is usually reduced and women often describe reflux symptoms
- *Central nervous system*: Local anesthetic requirements and minimum alveolar concentration (MAC) for inhalational agents are both decreased during pregnancy.

Maintenance of uterine perfusion with adequate maternal oxygenation is of utmost importance, to preserve fetal oxygenation during anesthesia in pregnant patient. Be aware of effects, anesthetic interventions may have on maternal cardiac output, O_2 delivery and uterine blood flow. Above all, avoid maternal hypoxia and hypotension.

Prevention and treatment of preterm labor is the most difficult problem to overcome and is the most common cause of fetal loss. It is probably not related to anesthetic management, but to the underlying disease and the surgery itself. Unfortunately, there are no reliable therapies to prevent or treat preterm labor in the perioperative period.

Teratogenic effects of anesthetics are probably minimal and have never been conclusively demonstrated in humans. The anesthetic drugs that usually generate the most concern are nitrous oxide and the benzodiazepines. No adverse effects of nitrous oxide have been demonstrated in human pregnancy despite extensive use. An association between benzodiazepine use and oral cleft anomalies was reported, but later case-control and prospective studies failed to demonstrate any relationship to benzodiazepine use during pregnancy. Opioids, IV induction agents and local anesthetics have a long history of safety when used during pregnancy. Studies on anesthetic exposure in the workplace concluded that a slight increased risk of miscarriage is the only potential obstetric problem for operating room (OR) personnel. The risk of smoking during pregnancy or ionizing radiation risks for pregnant personnel working in radiology are much higher than the potential risk for OR staff.

Of concern, however, is recent animal work on N-methyl-D-aspartate (NMDA) receptor blockers (for example, ketamine, nitrous oxide) and gamma amino butyric acid (GABA) receptor enhancers (for example, benzodiazepines, IV induction agents, volatile agents). All currently used anesthetics act by one of these mechanisms. In animal studies, fetal exposure to these agents results in widespread neurodegeneration and persistent memory/learning impairments. The relevance to human exposure is unclear; however, isoflurane has also been associated with postoperative cognitive deficits in human adults. At present, there is not enough information to change our clinical practice, and alleviation of pain and stress during surgery is obviously an essentially clinical goal.

ANESTHETIC MANAGEMENT

Preoperative assessment should include a pregnancy test if pregnancy status is doubtful or if the patient requests it. Every female patient should have the date of her last menstrual period documented on the anesthetic record. If possible, delay surgery to the second trimester or postpartum period, because risks of teratogenicity and spontaneous miscarriage are less. Preterm labor is not as common during second trimester as in the third trimester. The patient is counseled on anesthetic risks (or lack thereof) to the fetus and pregnancy, and told about symptoms of preterm labor and the need for left uterine displacement. Obtain obstetric consultation before performing nonobstetric surgery.

Administration of preoperative medications to allay anxiety or pain is appropriate because elevated maternal catecholamines may decrease uterine blood flow.

Consider aspiration prophylaxis with a combination of an antacid, metoclopramide, and/or H_2-receptor antagonist. Discuss perioperative tocolysis with the patient's obstetrician. Indomethacin (oral or suppository) and magnesium sulfate (by infusion) are the most commonly used perioperative tocolytics. Indomethacin has few anesthetic implications, but magnesium potentiates nondepolarizing muscle relaxants and attenuates vascular responsiveness, making hypotension difficult to treat during acute blood loss or volume shifts.

Intraoperatively, there is no evidence that any anesthetic technique is better than another as long as maternal oxygenation and perfusion are maintained. Monitoring should include BP measurement, pulse oximetry, end-tidal carbon dioxide ($EtCO_2$) and temperature measurement. $PaCO_2$ is decreased by approximately 10 torr during pregnancy resulting from increased minute ventilation. Maternal metabolic requirements are increased so desaturation occurs more quickly. If the procedure is prolonged, blood glucose should be checked to avoid hypoglycemia.

Use fetal monitoring, if necessary, to ensure optimal safety of the woman and her baby. If it will not interfere with the surgical field, intermittent or continuous fetal monitoring may be performed after approximately 24 weeks gestation to ensure that the intrauterine environment is optimized. This may be as simple as checking fetal heart tones before and after surgery or as complex as an attempt to do continuous fetal monitoring intraoperatively. If continuous monitoring is performed, loss of beat-to-beat variability is normal after GA medications or sedatives, but fetal bradycardia is not. Decelerations may indicate the need to increase maternal oxygenation, increase her BP, increase uterine displacement, change the site of surgical retraction or begin tocolysis. Fetal monitoring can help assess the adequacy of perfusion during induced hypotension, cardiopulmonary bypass or procedures involving large volume shifts. However, intraoperative fetal monitoring may be impractical in urgent situations or during abdominal surgery. Monitoring has not shown to improve fetal outcome. American College of Obstetricians and Gynecologists (ACOG) supports preoperative consultation with an obstetrician before any nonobstetric surgery during pregnancy, but states the need for fetal monitoring should be decided on a case-by-case basis.

General anesthesia should include full preoxygenation and denitrogenation, rapid sequence induction with cricoid pressure, a high concentration of O_2, and slow reversal of relaxants to prevent acute increases in acetylcholine that might induce uterine contractions. The pregnant airway is more edematous and vascular, and visualization may be more difficult during laryngoscopy. Propofol has recently been shown to reduce oxytocin-induced contractions of uterine smooth muscle in animals, although its value as a tocolytic is unknown. During first trimester, ketamine in doses greater than 2 mg/kg may cause uterine hypertonus, so lower doses are used. Inhalational agents should be kept less than 2.0 MAC to prevent decreased maternal cardiac output. Nitrous oxide may be used at the anesthesiologist's discretion.

Regional techniques have the advantage of minimizing drug exposure in early pregnancy and changes in fetal heart rate variability later in gestation. Prevent hypotension with adequate volume infusions and uterine displacement, and treat hypotension aggressively with vasopressors (phenylephrine or ephedrine), if needed. Decrease the neuraxial dose of local anesthetic by approximately one-third from that used in nonpregnant patients. Regional anesthetics provide excellent postoperative pain control, reducing the need for sedation; this is a major advantage because the patient can report symptoms of preterm labor, fetal heart rate variability is maintained and early mobilization can occur, reducing risk of thromboembolic complications.

Postoperatively, continue monitoring fetal heart rate and uterine activity. Preterm labor must be treated early and aggressively; parenteral pain medications will decrease fetal heart rate variability, so regional techniques should be used when possible. Pregnant patients are at high risk for thromboembolism and should be mobilized as quickly as possible—another reason for aggressive postoperative pain management. If mobilization is not possible, prophylactic anticoagulation should be considered. Maintain maternal oxygenation and left uterine displacement. Notify the pediatrics service if the fetus is of viable gestational age so they can provide counseling to the parents, if preterm labor occurs.

SPECIAL SITUATIONS

Cervical cerclage may be the most common surgical procedure during pregnancy. However, a recent study showed cervical cerclage does not substantially reduce the risk of early preterm delivery.

Trauma is a leading cause of maternal death. Fetal loss in these situations is the result of maternal death or placental abruption. An early ultrasound should be performed to determine fetal viability, and fetal monitoring should be continued. The mother should receive all needed diagnostic tests to optimize her management with shielding for the fetus, when possible. Exposure to less than 5 rad does not increase risk to the fetus. Ultrasound and magnetic resonance imaging are alternatives that do not use ionizing radiation.

There are few indications for an emergent cesarean delivery, but these would include:

1. A stable mother with a viable fetus in distress
2. Traumatic uterine rupture
3. A gravid uterus interfering with intra-abdominal repairs in the mother, and
4. A mother who cannot be saved with a fetus that is viable. If the fetus is previable or dead, optimize the mother's condition. She will tolerate vaginal delivery at a later time better than emergent laparotomy for cesarean delivery.

Neurosurgical procedures such as aneurysm clipping or arteriovenous malformation repair may be required in women of this age group. A variety of anesthetic agents have been administered successfully for neurosurgical procedures during pregnancy. Fetal monitoring may be helpful when controlled hypotension is planned, or if large volume shifts or blood loss are anticipated. Aggressive diuresis may reduce uterine perfusion if the mother's cardiac output is impaired. Hyperventilation reduces maternal cardiac output and decreases O_2 release to the fetus by shifting the maternal oxyhemoglobin dissociation curve to the left. Endovascular treatment of acutely ruptured intracranial aneurysms has been done successfully during pregnancy, thus avoiding craniotomy. Fetal shielding should be used whenever possible during radiology procedures.

Cardiac surgery requiring bypass has also been successfully performed during pregnancy. During pregnancy, the physiological increase in blood volume and cardiac output is maximal at 28–30 weeks, and this is a common time for cardiac decompensation in parturients with stenotic valvular lesions or pulmonary hypertension. Another high-risk period occurs immediately postpartum. After delivery, the release of aortocaval compression and autotransfusion of uteroplacental blood increases cardiac output to a maximum. Women who have severe cardiac symptoms during pregnancy, unresponsive to medical management, may benefit from surgery. If possible, surgery should be delayed until the second trimester when the major risk of teratogenicity (from cardiac drugs, X-rays, low-flow or hypoxic states) is past and preterm labor is less likely. If close to term, combined cesarean delivery and valve replacement has been done successfully. Do not withhold surgery if it is indicated for maternal reasons; maternal mortality during pregnancy is comparable to nonpregnant rates, although fetal morbidity may be high.

After 24 weeks gestation, monitor the fetus and maintain left uterine displacement to optimize uterine perfusion. Optimal pressures and flows on bypass are unknown and controversial, but higher flows and pressures may be beneficial to maintain uterine blood flow and fetal oxygenation. Fetal monitoring is a very sensitive measure of perfusion and can be used to optimize these values. Fetal bradycardia commonly occurs at the onset of cardiopulmonary bypass and slowly returns to a low normal rate with little or no beat-to-beat variability. Hypothermia has been used successfully, although some authors advocate warm bypass. Optimizing the mother's intraoperative and postoperative condition is the best way to ensure good fetal outcome.

Laparoscopic techniques avoid unnecessary laparotomy; fetal outcomes are similar with either laparotomy or laparoscopy, although maternal benefits of minimally invasive surgery are similar to nonpregnant patients. CO_2 pneumoperitoneum does induce fetal respiratory acidosis. Normalizing maternal $EtCO_2$ produces late and incomplete correction in the fetus. Whether this is biologically significant to the developing brain is unknown. Intra-abdominal pressure should be maintained as low as possible and operative time (i.e. insufflation time) kept to a minimum. Other technical considerations should include fetal shielding during cholangiograms, pneumatic stockings, left lateral table rotation and open trocar placement.

CONCLUSION

Surgery may be necessary during pregnancy. Anesthesiologists should reassure the mother that anesthetic drugs and techniques by themselves will not put her fetus or the pregnancy at risk. Prevention of preterm labor is the greatest concern and may require perioperative monitoring and tocolysis. Effective postoperative pain management without sedation will aid in early diagnosis and treatment of preterm labor and assist with early mobilization to prevent thrombotic complications.

BIBLIOGRAPHY

1. ACOG Committee on Obstetric Practice. Guidelines for diagnostic imaging during pregnancy. Obstet Gynecol. 2004; 104:647-51.
2. ACOG Committee on Obstetric Practice. Nonobstetric surgery in pregnancy. Obstet Gynecol. 2003;102:431.
3. Anand KJ, Soriano SG. Anesthetic agents and the immature brain: Are these toxic or therapeutic? Anesthesiology. 2004;101:527-30.
4. Boiven JF. Risk of spontaneous abortion in women occupationally exposed to anesthetic gases: A meta-analysis. Occup Environ Med. 1997;54:541-8.
5. Bouchard S, Johnson MP, Flake AW, et al. The EXIT procedure: Experience and outcome in 31 cases. J Pediatr Surg. 2002;37: 418-26.
6. Guidelines for laparoscopic surgery during pregnancy [Editorial]. Surg Endosc. 1998;12:189-90.
7. Ikonomidou C, Bittigau P, Ishimaru MJ, et al. Ethanol-induced apoptotic neurodegeneration and fetal alcohol syndrome. Science. 2000;287:1056-60.
8. Ikonomidou C, Bosch F, Miksa M, et al. Blockade of NMDA receptors and apoptotic neurodegeneration in the developing brain. Science. 1999;283:70-4.
9. Jevtovic-Todorovic V, Hartman RE, Izumi Y, et al. Early exposure to common anesthetic agents causes widespread neurodegeneration in the developing rat brain and persistent learning deficits. J Neurosci. 2003;23:876-82.
10. Khandelwal M, Rasanen J, Ludormirski A, et al. Evaluation of fetal and uterine hemodynamics during maternal cardiopulmonary bypass. Obstet Gynecol. 1996;88:667-71.
11. Koren G, Bologa M, Long D, et al. Perception of teratogenic risk by pregnant women exposed to drugs and chemicals during the first trimester. Am J Obstet Gynecol. 1989;160:1190-4.
12. Lo WY, Friedman JM. Teratogenicity of recently introduced medications in human pregnancy. Obstet Gynecol. 2002;100: 465-73.
13. Mazze RI, Fujinaga M, Baden JM. Halothane prevents nitrous oxide teratogenicity in Sprague-Dawley rats; folinic acid does not. Teratology. 1988;38:121-7.
14. Olney JW, Young C, Wozniak DF, et al. Anesthesia-induced developmental neuroapoptosis, does it happen in humans? Anesthesiology. 2004;101:273-5.
15. Piotin M, de Souza Filho CA, Kothimbakam R, et al. Endovascular treatment of acutely ruptured intracranial aneurysms in pregnancy. Am J Obstet Gynecol. 2001;185:1261-2.
16. Reedy MB, Kallen B, Kuehl TJ. Laparoscopy during pregnancy: A study of five fetal outcome parameters with use of the Swedish Health Registry. Am J Obstet Gynecol. 1997;177:673-9.
17. Reynolds JD, Booth JV, de la Fuente S, et al. A review of laparoscopy for non-obstetric-related surgery during pregnancy. Curr Surg. 2003;60:164-73.
18. Rosenberg L, Mitchell AA, Parsells JL, et al. Lack of relation of oral clefts to diazepam use during pregnancy. N Engl J Med. 1983;309:1282-5.
19. Shiono PH, Mills JL. Oral clefts and diazepam use during pregnancy [Letter]. N Engl J Med. 1984;311:919-20.
20. Strickland RA, Oliver WE, Chantigian RC, et al. Anesthesia, cardiopulmonary bypass and the pregnant patient. Mayo Clin Proc. 1991;66:411-29.
21. To MS, Alfrivecic Z, Heath VC, et al. Cervical cerclage for prevention of preterm delivery in women with short cervix: Randomized controlled trial. Lancet. 2004;363:1849-53.

8.3 ANESTHESIA FOR CESAREAN DELIVERY

Vinay Tiwari

GENERAL ANESTHESIA FOR CESAREAN SECTION

Cesarean deliveries now account for a large number of the deliveries. Anesthesia-related maternal mortality, although declining during the last few decades, still accounts for 3–12% of maternal deaths. General anesthesia (GA) for cesarean section (CS) is no longer the method of choice. Only about 15% of cases are performed under GA and the number is decreasing. The Practical Guidelines for Obstetrical Anesthesia from the ASA task force on obstetrical anesthesia observed that cesarean delivery can be successfully managed with all conduction techniques (spinal, epidural, CSE). The report also notes that GA may be associated with increased maternal mortality/morbidity as well as lower neonatal APGAR scores; hence, the use of any technique should be based on specific case-by-case assessments of clinical, laboratory, anesthetic and obstetric issues.

Complications related to anesthesia represent the sixth leading cause of peripartum maternal mortality with the risk of a maternal death being 16.7 times greater with general *versus* regional anesthesia. The problems associated with GA are related to failed intubations and aspirations. The physiological changes of pregnancy may increase the incidence of failed intubation and its associated maternal morbidity and mortality. The changes affecting the gastrointestinal tract (GIT) include delayed gastric emptying and reduced intestinal motility, reduced lower esophageal sphincter tone, increased intraabdominal pressure and increased gastric acid secretion. Most of the patients may not be fasting. All these contribute to the increased incidence of aspiration. As such, a risk/benefit analysis for the use of GA should be strongly considered before its use. In an acknowledgment of the risks associated with GA, ACOG has accepted that "cesarean deliveries for a nonreassuring fetal heart rate pattern do not necessarily preclude the use of regional anesthesia".

NEED FOR GENERAL ANESTHESIA

Anesthesiologists must be comfortable with their skills and treatment algorithms for the administration of GA to the parturient because the need for GA arises frequently. When time is the limiting factor, GA is sometimes necessary because it offers speed of induction, reliability, control and avoidance of sympathectomy-induced hypotension. Lack of time, contraindications to regional anesthesia, failed regional anesthesia, hemodynamic instability, maternal coagulopathy, sepsis and patient refusal are the most common causes responsible for administration of GA. Urgent GA may be requested for breech extraction or to provide uterine relaxation for intrauterine manipulation, particularly of a second twin, GA will usually be preferred for emergency CS following uterine rupture, antepartum hemorrhage (APH), placental abruption, acute fetal distress or cord prolapse. GA may also be requested in the presence of intrauterine fetal death. While lesser degrees of placenta previa can be satisfactorily managed under regional block, the method of anesthesia for a grade IV placenta previa remains controversial. Many anesthetists fear the combination of massive maternal hemorrhage and impairment of cardiovascular reflexes in an awake patient and prefer to give GA. GA may also be administered for removal of a cervical suture prior to labor, manual removal of the placenta, treatment of an acute inversion of the uterus and repair of a third-degree tear.

PREPARATION FOR GENERAL ANESTHESIA

Physical factors such as weight gain, enlarged breasts, edema of the upper airway may make endotracheal intubation difficult. It is prudent to evaluate the airway early so that the patient at risk can be identified. The most common critical incidents during GA are failure to ventilate: 70%, laryngoscope malfunction: 11%, premature extubation: 10% and problem with tracheal tube: 7%. Thirty three percent of these negative outcomes can be overcome by monitoring with pulse oximetry and capnography; of special importance is their use in the recovery area where 50% of cases of cardiac arrest and cerebral damage occur.

Prediction of Difficult Airway

- Teeth: Missing teeth, buck teeth, loose teeth and over riding of maxillary teeth over mandibular teeth contribute to difficulty in inserting the laryngoscope in the oral cavity. Loose teeth must be identified preoperatively and protected with a dental guard or occasionally removed
- If the patient can protrude the mandible beyond the maxilla, this signifies good temporomandibular joint function and good mouth opening, resulting in easy insertion of laryngoscope in the oral cavity
- Neck: A short and thick neck is difficult to maneuver and makes laryngoscopy difficult. Patients should be able to touch their chest with their chin and also be able to extend their neck, as far posteriorly as possible. Neck flexed on chest 35° and head extended on neck 80°

- Thyromental distance: If the distance between the notch of the thyroid cartilage and symphysis menti, with the neck fully extended, is more than three-finger breadths or greater than 5 cm, then intubation is easy
- Inter-incisor distance: If the distance between the upper and lower incisors on opening the mouth is more than two-finger breadths or greater than 3 cm, then laryngoscopy is easy
- A large tongue or a narrow, highly arched palate reduces the oropharyngeal volume and make visualization of the glottis difficult.

In cases of suspected difficult airway, the option of alternative methods such as awake intubation, fibroptic intubation, LMA and surgical airway should be available.

Aspiration Prophylaxis

Aspiration of the acidic gastric contents into the airway is one of the dreaded complications of GA. It occurs before or during endotracheal intubation when the airway is unprotected. Use of some drugs will greatly reduce the risks, although it cannot be guaranteed that the particular patient will not aspirate. Antacids are the mainstay of the treatment. 30 mL of 0.3 M sodium citrate is the drug of choice because it raises the gastric pH and being nonparticulate, does not cause airway obstruction, if aspiration at all occurs. Simultaneous use of H_2 blocking drugs will ensure prolonged intragastric alkalinization. Metoclopramide is also used to increase the lower esophageal sphincter tone and to reduce the residual gastric volume by promoting gastric emptying.

Preoxygenation

Filling the lungs with 100% O_2 will delay the onset of hypoxia which occurs as result of apnea during the induction of anesthesia. Administering 100% O_2 for 3 minutes or 4 maximal breaths is adequate; the partial pressure of oxygen (PaO_2) is about 375–400 mm Hg at this time.

Partial pressure of oxygen drops by about 80 mm Hg/min during induction. Maximal fetal oxygenation occurs at maternal PaO_2 of approximately 300 mm Hg.

Fetal Considerations

Blood gases and acid base status of babies born after GA or regional block are similar but babies born under GA have a higher percentage of neurobehavioral depression in the first 24 hours.

Optimal fetal outcome is ensured by:

- Maternal denitrogenation
- Left lateral tilt to prevent aortocaval compression
- Preinduction fluid loading to avoid maternal hypotension
- Prevention of maternal hypocarbia.

Uterine Incision to Delivery Time

It is important to deliver the fetus promptly after uterine incision within 3 minutes because babies born later have lower APGAR scores and acidotic blood gases.

CONDUCT OF GENERAL ANESTHESIA

Check the anesthesia machine, various monitors such as oximeter and capnograph, O_2 supply, laryngoscope with different sized blades, and different sized endotracheal tubes. Have a difficult intubation trolley ready; check suction machine and availability of suction catheters; see that the IV line is functional; have a skilled assistant ready. Check the tilting-movement of the operating table.

Lay the patient supine on the table with a wedge under the right hip.

Connect the ECG electrodes, oximeter and BP cuff.

Denitrogenation for 3 minutes with 100% O_2 by mask is done; this will raise maternal and fetal oxygenation. In an emergency, instruct the patient to take four deep maximal breaths with the O_2 mask in position on the face.

Induction

Thiopentone 3–5 mg/kg IV, ketamine 1–1.5 mg/kg IV, propofol 1–2.5 mg/kg are the most commonly used induction agents.

Thiopentone is the most commonly used agent while ketamine is used in cases of maternal hemorrhage and bronchial asthma. Ketamine in doses of more than 2 mg/kg is associated with fetal depression. Propofol has a rapid onset and rapid clear headed recovery but is associated with hypotension, crosses the placenta and can cause neurobehavioral changes. There is no significant advantage over thiopentone and is more expensive.

Intubation

Succinyl choline, 1–1.5 mg/kg, is still used to facilitate intubation because of its rapid and profound muscle relaxation. Rapacuronium, a new nondepolarizing muscle relaxant with a fast onset, may be an alternative to scoline.

Cricoid pressure is applied and trachea intubated; pressure is applied till the cuff of the tube is inflated and proper positioning is confirmed. If tracheal intubation fails, cricoid pressure is maintained till intubation is achieved or the patient awakens. There may be a small risk of esophageal rupture if pressure is applied in the presence of active vomiting. Some authorities have advocated the release of the applied pressure if vomiting occurs, but others disagree.

Maintenance

Nitrous oxide 50%, with 50% O_2 is used till delivery of the fetus; volatile agents are given only till delivery of the baby because longer use can cause uterine relaxation afterwards. They are needed to prevent maternal awareness when only 50% nitrous oxide is used. Isoflurane 0.5 MAC will prevent awareness in mother (incidence < 1%).

Sevoflurane and desflurane are safe to use but no advantage over isoflurane

After delivery, IV opioid and nitrous oxide 70% with O_2 are used to maintain anesthesia. Muscle relaxation can be provided by continuous scoline infusion or nondepolarizers.

Reversal

The stomach should be emptied via a nasogastric tube; scoline is allowed to be hydrolized or the nondepolarizing muscle blockade reversed with neostigimine and glycopyrolate. When patient is awake and ventilatory exchange adequate, extubation is done.

Intermittent intramuscular (IM) opioids are used to provide postoperative analgesia but this method is inferior to epidural opioids or IV patient controlled analgesia systems.

REGIONAL ANESTHESIA FOR CESAREAN SECTION

Of late, regional anesthesia has emerged as the method of choice for cesarean section (CS). It has resulted in a drop in maternal mortality rates and there are reports of neonates having better neurobehavioral scores under regional anesthesia. The indices of uteroplacental and fetal blood flow are either unchanged or slightly improved by regional anesthesia, provided maternal BP and cardiac output are maintained. The choice between epidural and spinal anesthesia is dictated by circumstances; there is very little difference between the two, regarding maternal and neonatal outcomes but spinal tends to give a better operative analgesia; it is a simpler technique with a definite end point and a lower drug dosage. Epidural anesthesia with the epidural catheter in place, has the advantage of being used for labor analgesia and if needed, for CS and postoperative analgesia. Spinal and epidural techniques both have advantages and disadvantages; CSE technique has been developed to combine the advantages of both without the disadvantages of either.

Choice between spinal and epidural anesthesia may be dictated by circumstances (urgency or pre-sited epidural catheter) or associated maternal disease such as valvular heart disease. The main differences between the two are rate of onset, drug dose and quality of block. Epidural requires a larger dose, has a delayed onset and is prone to patchy or incomplete block; epidural anesthesia requires a high concentration of local anesthetic and high volumes help in better spread of solution to nerve roots; spinal is more dependent on the dose of drug administered and volume does not affect the extent of blockade.

Absolute Contraindications to Regional Anesthesia

- Infection over injection site
- Bleeding diathesis; anticoagulant therapy
- Severe APH with hypovolemia and continued bleeding
- Sensitivity to local anesthetics
- Patient refusal
- Raised intracranial pressure.

Relative Contraindications

- Preexisting neurological disease
- Disorders of spine
- Cardiac diseases such as aortic stenosis, pulmonary hypertension, cyanotic lesions
- Severe infection.

Preoperative Preparation

Because there may be a sudden need of securing the airway and administering GA, preoperative preparation is the same as for GA, which includes preoperative fasting and antacid prophylaxis. Preoperative evaluation should include a history and examination, looking specifically for contraindications to regional anesthesia (coagulopathy, spinal deformity, infection, neurological disease and back pain) and potential hazards to GA and airway management.

Preoperative laboratory investigations are usually not needed in healthy females except for blood grouping and matching, and hemoglobin.

Before commencing regional analgesia, a wide bore IV cannula is put in, all equipment for GA checked and emergency drugs made available. In the absence of preoperative dehydration, large volume of fluids is unnecessary; large volume of dextrose solution is avoided as it may cause fetal acidosis and neonatal hypoglycemia. Ringer lactate is the solution most often used.

The regularly used local anesthetics are bupivacaine and lignocaine while the newer agents include ropivacaine and levobupivacaine. Bupivacaine is the most commonly used and most potent; 0.5% solution in a dose of 2 mg/kg provides adequate surgical anesthesia for 2–3 hours. The main problem is of slow onset and increased risk of cardiac toxicity. It is not possible to commence surgery before 20 minutes using unmodified 0.5% bupivacaine. Bupivacaine depresses the myocardium and also causes arrhythmias. It requires more prolonged resuscitative efforts before its effects can be reversed. The onset of action of local anesthetics can be quickened by adding sodium bicarbonate or by using a carbonated solution or by adding adrenaline just before use; but they all work well with lidocaine and less with bupivacaine. Lipid soluble opioids fentanyl and sufentanil have a rapid onset of action when given epidurally; they are given primarily to improve the quality of block but can quicken the onset of epidural anesthesia with bupivacaine.

Considerations during Surgery

All patients must have a left uterine displacement maintained at 20–30° by means of a wedge or a rolled blanket under the right hip. O_2 administration by face mask improves placental O_2 delivery. Onset and level of block is tested and it should extend till T4 level. Pain during surgery can occur because of incomplete or inadequate block; it usually occurs after delivery when the uterus is exteriorized. It is managed by IV fentanyl or fentanyl with a small dose of ketamine; administration of 50% nitrous oxide with O_2 or complete GA may be necessary. Nausea, vomiting and shivering occur frequently under regional anesthesia. Shivering can be controlled by warming the IV fluids, regulating the theatre temperature and use of drugs such as pethidine, tramadol or epidural fentanyl or sufentanil. Nausea and vomiting can occur because of hypotension or visceral pain sensation. After treating the cause, use of metoclopramide 10 mg, or droperidol 1 mg or ondansetron is effective.

Postoperative Care

The patient is shifted to the recovery area and handed over to the appropriately trained staff; they should be aware of any anesthetic or surgical problem occurring during the procedure. The patient should be kept warm, pain free and comfortable. In the absence of any complication, the patient is shifted to the ward when signs of recovery of sensory (two segment regression) and motor function are observed.

SPINAL ANESTHESIA

The choice of drugs is limited to two or three agents depending on duration of action and efficacy, and agent specific effects. Bupivacaine ideally fits the bill; it is a potent agent, the duration and extent of block are dose related. Dose requirement varies between 7.5 mg and 12 mg and usually a 0.5% solution is used.

Lidocaine has been popular choice for CS under spinal anesthesia. Usually a hyperbaric 5% solution in doses of 65–75 mg is used. Recently, it has fallen out of favor because of reports of transient neurological symptoms, cauda equina syndrome and radicular pain. If bupivacaine is available, it is clearly the agent of choice for CS under spinal anesthesia.

Extending the Duration of Spinal Anesthesia

Adrenaline and opiates are added to local anesthetic to increase the duration of block and also to improve the quality of intraoperative anesthesia. Fentanyl in doses of 6.25–15 μg added to intrathecal bupivacaine can significantly improve quality of anesthesia without maternal side effects; higher doses can prolong the duration of action but with increased sedation, decreased respiratory rate and pruritus. Sufentanil, 10 μg, can also be added to local anesthetic but causes more hypotension, O_2 desaturation and pruritus. Intrathecal morphine 0.2 mg, can improve intraoperative analgesia but it has a slower onset and a long duration of action.

Spinal Anesthesia Following Epidural Block

Occasionally, a patient with a unilateral or patchy epidural block presents for CS. If time is available, then other options exist like re-siting the epidural catheter or using the CSE technique with a very low spinal dose and using the epidural catheter for supplementation, if necessary. But in an emergency, single shot spinal or use of spinal catheter are the only options, other than GA. If a single shot spinal is given, a high sensory and motor block with apnea can occur. Several reasons have been given for this, such as expansion of epidural space compresses the spinal canal, causing higher spread of intrathecal drug; rapid transfer of epidural drug across the dural hole may occur and sufficient local anesthetic drug (given epidurally) may already be present in the nerve roots to decrease the requirement of the subsequent spinal dose of local anesthetic.

It has been suggested that the dose of intrathecal drug be reduced; also use a method to limit cephalad spread of drug by altering patient position to restrict the level of block below T4.

COMBINED SPINAL-EPIDURAL ANESTHESIA

Although used mostly for labor analgesia, it can be used for CS also. The advantage is that it provides rapid onset of anesthesia by one shot spinal anesthesia as well as flexibility of an epidural catheter, which allows extension of anesthesia in case of inadequate height of block or to prolong the duration in case surgery is prolonged and also can be used for postoperative analgesia. In this technique, a smaller dose can be used intrathecally, which may reduce the incidence of hypotension and inadvertent high motor block.

LOCAL INFILTRATION ANESTHESIA FOR CESAREAN SECTION

Rarely, local anesthesia may be the only viable option, e.g. severe kyphoscoliosis or when general and neuraxial anesthesia may be contraindicated or undesirable. Local anesthetic infiltration is performed using large volumes, 40–60 mL of diluted solution of local anesthetics. The injections are given in the various layers. 10 mL is injected immediately below the skin in the midline from the umbilicus to the pubis. Then 5 mL is injected into the rectus sheath at four points on either side, the needle should be felt passing through the anterior rectus sheath. 5–10 mL is infiltrated immediately below the linea alba after its exposure to anesthetize the parietal peritoneum. Once inside the peritoneal cavity, 5 mL is placed under the visceral peritoneum along the line of proposed lower segment cut into the uterus.

BIBLIOGRAPHY

1. ACOG Committee on Obstetrics: Maternal and Fetal Medicine. ACOG Committee Opinion No. 104. Washington, DC; 1992.
2. Confidential enquiry into maternal and child health: why mothers die 2000–2002. The sixth report of the confidential enquiries into maternal deaths in the United Kingdom. London: Royal College of Obstetricians and Gynaecologists; 2004.
3. Hawkins JL, Koonin LM, Palmer SK, et al. Anesthesia related deaths during obstetric delivery in the United States, 1979–1990. Anesthesiology. 1997;86:277-84.
4. Task Force on Obstetrical Anesthesia. Practice guidelines for obstetrical anesthesia: A report by the American Society of Anesthesiologists Task Force on Obstetrical Anesthesia. Anesthesiology. 1999;90:600-11.

8.4 POSTOPERATIVE CARE

Vinay Tiwari

Recovery from anesthesia should be ideally a smooth process but is often characterized by airway obstruction, shivering, agitation, delirium, pain, nausea, vomiting and hypothermia/hyperthermia.

Even patients receiving regional anesthesia can experience marked decrease in BP because the sympatholytic effects of regional blocks prevent compensatory reflex vasoconstriction when patients are moved.

ROUTINE RECOVERY

Vital signs and oxygenation should be checked immediately on arrival in the postoperative ward. BP, pulse and respiratory rate are routinely measured every 5 minutes for 15 minutes or until stable and then every 15 minutes. Pulse oximeter should be used to monitor O_2 saturation continuously in all patients recovering from anesthesia and at least one temperature recording is made.

All patients recovering from GA should receive 30–40% O_2; patients with pulmonary dysfunction will need O_2 supplementation for longer period. O_2 therapy can be guided by O_2 saturation percentage reading obtained from pulse oximeter. Patients with chronic obstructive pulmonary disease (COPD) and history of CO_2 retention have to be nursed in head up position and their O_2 intake needs to be carefully regulated (so as not to wipe out their respiratory drive). Deep breathing and coughing are encouraged periodically.

Patients recovering from regional anesthesia also need supplemental O_2 because they may be sedated or hemodynamically unstable. BP should be carefully monitored; bladder catheterization may be necessary after spinal/epidural anesthesia.

PAIN CONTROL

Pain can be managed with parenteral or intraspinal opioids, regional analgesia or specific nerve blocks. Adequate analgesia must be balanced against excessive sedation. When patient is fully awake, patient controlled analgesia can be instituted.

Opioids are most commonly used, titration of small IV doses is generally safe (morphine 2–4 mg or pethidine 10–20 mg). Analgesic effects usually peak within 4–5 minutes but maximal respiratory depression may not be seen till 20–30 minutes later. IM route suffers from delayed or variable onset (10–20 minutes) and delayed respiratory depression (up to 1 hour).

If an epidural catheter is in place, epidural fentanyl (50–100 µg) or morphine (3–5 mg) can provide excellent pain relief; however, delayed respiratory depression with morphine mandates monitoring precautions for 12–24 hours afterwards.

Mild to moderate pain can be managed with analgesics such as butorphanol 1–2 mg or ketorolac tromethamine 15–30 mg or diclofenac.

AGITATION

Before the patient is fully responsive, pain is often manifested as postoperative restlessness; other causes of restlessness are hypoxia, acidosis, or hypotension, marked anxiety, fear and adverse drug effects. Treat the cause; if agitation still persists, it can be treated with IV midazolam (0.5–1 mg).

NAUSEA AND VOMITING

Postoperative nausea and vomiting are common, following GA; they can also occur due to hypotension after spinal/epidural anesthesia. Highest incidence is seen in young women.

Droperidol IV 25 µg/kg, given intraoperatively reduces the incidence significantly; metoclopramide (0.15 mg/kg) or ondansetron (0.05–0.1 mg/kg) can also be used, if needed.

SHIVERING

It can occur because of intraoperative hypothermia or effects of anesthetic agents. Hypothermia can result from cold ambient temperature in operation theater (OT), cold IV fluids, cold gases and prolonged exposure. Shivering, in these cases, represents body's efforts to increase heat production and raise body temperature; it may be associated with intense vasoconstriction.

Shivering can follow epidural injection of local anesthetics; other causes can be sepsis, drug allergy or transfusion reaction. Shivering can result in metabolic acidosis, can increase O_2 consumption, CO_2 production and cardiac output significantly. These effects are poorly tolerated by patients with preexisting cardiac and pulmonary diseases.

Shivering is treated by keeping the patient warm and using warm IV infusions. Small doses of pethidine 10–20 mg IV, or tramadol can dramatically reduce or stop shivering.

HYPOTENSION

Hypotension results from surgical blood loss, third space sequestration of fluid, ongoing hemorrhage and inadequate volume replacement; failure of the myocardial pump (commonly due to arrhythmias or preexisting ischemic heart disease) may present as hypotension. It can also be an early sign of sepsis or anaphylaxis, both of which cause vasodilatation.

Hypotension is presumed to be due to hypovolemia until proved otherwise. Volume expansion is usually the first step in the resolution of hypotension in the immediate postoperative period because rapid fluid administration treats most causes and provides the necessary first step before vasopressor therapy. An indwelling bladder catheter is particularly useful in such circumstances to monitor urinary output. ECG will reveal irregularities of rhythm or ischemia.

Elevation of lower limbs augments venous return; colloids and crystalloids can be given at the rate of 10–20 mL/kg while hematocrit is assessed to guide further volume replacement. O_2 supplementation is always indicated.

HYPERTENSION AND TACHYCARDIA

Several causes of tachycardia and hypertension require intervention but not drug treatment. Bladder distention, hypothermia, shivering, carbon dioxide retention, emergence delirium are common and easily treated causes of postoperative hypertension. In many cases, BP elevation greater than 20% of baseline level in the absence of symptoms will resolve without further treatment. Postoperative pain is a potent stimulus for tachycardia and hypertension which will settle down with adequate analgesia. Tachyarrhythmias, pre-existing hypertensive disease, clonidine withdrawal, or compromised cardiac or renal function that may be adversely affected by elevated BP may demand primary treatment by drugs to reduce heart rate and BP.

Treatment options include beta-blockers, angiotensin converting enzyme (ACE) inhibitors, calcium channel blockers and direct vasodilators therapy.

HYPOXIA

The PaO_2 decreases after GA even when respiratory function appears to be normal; it is influenced by the site of operation, smoking, age, the presence of cardiorespiratory disease and obesity. The hypoxia is caused by mismatching of ventilation and perfusion and often corrected by O_2 administration.

Other causes of hypoxia in the early postoperative period are CNS depression because of sedatives or narcotics used as a part of anesthesia technique, residual neuromuscular paralysis because of incomplete reversal of the effect of muscle relaxant and respiratory obstruction due to tongue or presence of secretions, blood or vomitus. Clearing the airway, administration of O_2 and treating the cause is recommended.

POSTDURAL PUNCTURE HEADACHE

The incidence of postdural puncture headache (PDPH) is inversely related to the needle diameter; the use of fine 29 gauge needles is associated with low incidence of PDPH but requires more skill and experience and has a higher failure rate. PDPH may also be related to the design of the needle tip. With Quincke 25 or 26 gauge needles the incidence of PDPH is around 10% while with 22 gauge Whitacre and 22 and 24 gauge Sprotte spinal needles, the PDPH incidence is between 2% and 5%; a further reduction in PDPH incidence to between 1% and 3% may be expected with use of 25 gauge Whitacre needle. Most recently, 24 gauge Sprotte needle with pencil point with lateral hole reported 0.02% incidence of PDPH. Quincke point needle may cause dural tears to persist, while the blunt or non-cutting Whitacre and Sprotte needles may spread the dural fibers gently, allowing them to cinch closed after the needle is withdrawn.

Spinal needles must be inserted in such a manner as to orient their bevel parallel to longitudinal dural fibers. A paramedian approach and insertion of needle with the bevel parallel to longitudinal dural fibers may reduce the incidence of PDPH.

Clinical Presentation

Postdural puncture headache incidence is increased in younger age groups, is more common in females, especially during pregnancy. PDPH is related to posture—headache begins after assuming an erect posture and resolves quickly upon resumption of supine position.

The site of pain may be frontal, occipital or both; it may be associated with neckache, backache, nausea, blurred vision, photophobia, tinnitus and vomiting.

Severity of PDPH is increased by pressure on carotids and decreased by pressure on jugular veins. Headache may present immediately after dural puncture but will usually occur 24–72 hours later; it will rarely occur after 5 days. Seventy percent of PDPH will be relieved spontaneously within 7 days and 95% resolve within 6 weeks.

Treatment

Treatment includes analgesics, NSAIDs, steroids, tannic acid, abdominal binders, forced hydration, and lying prone. None of these have proven to be consistently beneficial. Most PDPH will resolve in less than 7 days. Bed rest, analgesics and hydration constitute accepted conservative treatment. Other methods include IV or oral caffeine, infusion of epidural saline and epidural blood patch (EBP).

One of the causes of PDPH is low cerebrospinal fluid (CSF) pressure, resulting in reflex vasodilatation of cerebral vessels, with the resultant pain. Caffeine relives headaches by reversing this vasodilatation because of its vasoconstrictor properties. Caffeine sodium benzoate 500 mg IV initially or 300 mg oral caffeine, repeated after 4 hours if symptoms are not relieved, was effective in 92% of cases. Side effects like flushing and dizziness are absent or very mild. Oral theophylline relieved symptoms of PDPH probably through its cerebral vasoconstrictor effects. Sumatriptan is a serotonin agonist and causes cerebral vasoconstriction; it is used for treating migraines and is found to be effective in PDPH.

Epidural blood patch or saline infusion either stops CSF leak or re-establishes normal CSF pressure; rarely patients will require surgical closure of dura. Epidural saline 10–20 mL is injected into epidural space; it is effective in about 60–80% of the cases but a high replace rate limits the technique. EBP is the gold standard for the treatment of PDPH, is safe, simple and efficient. Patients with PDPH are first hydrated with 500–1,000 mL of Ringer's lactate. Ten to fifteen milliliters of patient's blood is withdrawn aseptically and then injected into the epidural space till the patient complains of slightest discomfort in the legs or back. Patients are kept supine for 30 minutes. There is immediate and permanent relief of symptoms; failure to relieve PDPH with EBP is likely due to improper identification of epidural space or an error in diagnosis.

Epidural blood patch is remarkably safe; contraindications to EBP are septicemia, local infection of the back or active neurological disease. Blood injected into epidural space has not been reported to cause arachnoiditis or chemical meningitis. The most common complication is transient back pain during the first 72 hours. Some patients may have lower extremity pain or pain in the neck; a transient rise in temperature has been reported. Avoid giving EBP after injection of local anesthesia into epidural space because increased pressure in epidural space because of EBP will force the local anesthetic in the cephalad direction and may result in undesired high block.

DISCHARGE

All patients must be evaluated before being sent to the wards. They should have been observed for respiratory depression for at least 30 minutes after the last parenteral dose of narcotic (Box 1). Other discharge criteria for patients recovering from GA are easy arousability, full orientation, ability to maintain and protect the airway. All vital signs must be stable for at least 1 hour; the patients should have the ability to call for help, if necessary, and there should be no surgical complications. The patients should be pain free and normothermic. In addition to the above criteria, patients receiving regional anesthesia should show signs of resolution of both sensory and motor blockade.

Box 1 Postanesthetic recovery score

Color—O_2 saturation	
O_2 saturation >92% in room air	2
Needs O_2 to maintain O_2 saturation >90%	1
O_2 saturation <90% with O_2 supplement	0
Circulation	
BP within 20% of normal	2
BP within 20–50% of normal	1
BP deviating >50% from normal	0
Consciousness	
Awake, alert, oriented	2
Arousable but drifts back to sleep	1
No response	0
Respiration	
Can breathe deeply and cough	2
Shallow but adequate exchange	1
Apnea or obstruction	0
Activity	
Moves all extremities	2
Moves two extremities	1
No movement	0
Ideally the patient should be discharged when the score is 10	

Source: Aldrete JA, Kronlik D. A post-anesthetic recovery score. Anesth Analg. 1970;49:924.

BIBLIOGRAPHY

1. Cadanelli GP, Cavatorta E, Verrilli D. Chirurgia gynecologia e cardiopatie. Quad Clin Obstet Gynecol. 1967;22:911.
2. Cheng EY, Kay B. Manual of Anesthesia and the medically compromised patient. Philadelphia: Lippincott and Wilkins; 1990.
3. Foldes FF, et al. JAMA. 1963;183:672.
4. Gallagher EG, White M, Ward S, et al. Prophylaxis against acid aspiration syndrome : Single oral dose of H2-antagonist on the evening before elective surgery. Anesthesia. 1988;43:1011-4.
5. Goldberger AL, O'Konski J. Utility of routine ECG before surgery and on general hospital admission. Ann Intern Med. 1986;105:552.
6. Gold MJ, Helvich M. A study of the complications related to anesthesia in asthmatic patients. Anesth Analg (Cleve). 1963;42:283.
7. Heavey A. Learning to talk with patients. Br J Hosp Med. 1988;39:433-9.
8. Jackobsen CJ, Blom L, Brondbjerg M, et al. Effect of metoprolol and diazepam on pre-operative anxiety. Anesthesia. 1990;45: 40-3.
9. Mangano DT. Preoperative cardiac assessment. Philadelphia: Lippincott, 1990.
10. National study by R Coll. Radiol Lancet. 1979;2:83.
11. Nimmo WS. The promise of transdermal drug delivery. Br J Anaesth. 1990;64(1):7-10.
12. Olgivie C. Physician among surgeons: thoughts on preoperative assessment. Thorax. 1980;35:881
13. Owens WD, Felts JA, Spitznagel EL, et al. ASA physical status classifications: a study of consistency of ratings. Anesthesiology. 1978;49(4):239
14. Richards MJ, Skues MA, Jarvis AP, et al. Total i.v. anaesthesia with propofol and alfentanil: dose requirements for p,opofol and the effect of premedication with clonidine. Br J. Anaesth. 1990;65:157-63.
15. Roberts JG, Foex P, Clarke NS, et al. Haemodynamic interactions of high-dose propranolol pretreatment and anaesthesia in the dog. i: halothane dose-response studies. Br J Anaesth. 1976;48:315-26.
16. Sabrasez. Bordeaux Med J. 1902.

CHAPTER

9

Intraoperative Investigative Tools

Randhir Puri, V Chandra

INTRODUCTION

Newer technologies and advanced computer interface applications being introduced on a daily basis are providing newer vistas for evaluation of pelvic surgeries carried out conventionally. Endoscopy with ultrasonography has made it feasible to resect out, earlier thought inoperable tumors in pelvis. Additional masses not visible to naked eye can also be approached easily. In succeeding paragraphs, the available techniques and in combination one or more modalities are mentioned for intraoperative usage, in vogue more on experimental basis, today. They will be in common use in the near future.

Imprint Cytology

Cytology is the only method which gives intraoperative diagnosis of ovarian tumors within 20 minutes. It is helpful, especially in young patients who need conservative surgery in order to preserve fertility. It does not alter the quality of the biopsy specimen. Imprint cytology is a less expensive, simple and quick method of diagnosis, and is reliable in terms of accuracy, sensitivity, specificity and positive predictive value. It does not affect the utility of the specimen for histopathology.

Three-dimensional Sonography and Virtual Sonographic Cystoscopy

Cystoscopy is insertion of a rigid or flexible fiberoptic instrument into the bladder. It is used to help diagnose urologic disorders (e.g. bladder tumors or calculi), to manage urethral strictures and to access the bladder for ureteral X-rays or placement of JJ stents (stents with coiled ends placed in the renal pelvis and bladder). The main contraindication is active urinary tract infection (UTI). Cystoscopy is usually performed with local anesthesia or, when necessary, conscious sedation or general anesthesia. Prophylactic antibiotics are required. Complications include UTI, bleeding, and bladder and urethral trauma.

Three-dimensional (3D) sonography is a promising alternative noninvasive technique for use in detection of bladder tumors. With 3D sonography and virtual sonographic evaluation for bladder tumors, their localization, and perivesical spread is easy. The location, size and morphologic features of the tumors shown on 3D sonography agreed well with the findings of conventional cystoscopy. Moreover large pelvic mass, such as fibroids, ovarian tumors with extensive intrapelvic spread make it imperative on operating surgeon to evaluate course of ureters in suspected injuries. This can be done with preoperative or intraoperative ureteric catheterization. There are intraoperative infrared light illuminating systems also available during laparoscopic surgeries to delineate ureters, thus avoiding injuries to them.

Ureteric Injuries, Intraoperative

If the ureteral injury is noted intraoperatively and additional imaging is necessary to localize the lesion, the best imaging study is retrograde ureteropyelography. By placing a cystoscope in the bladder and cannulating the affected ureteral orifice with a ureteral catheter, dilute cystografin is injected into the ureter under fluoroscopy or taking a kidneys, ureters, bladder (KUB) image. If the dye is seen in the renal pelvis without any ureteral extravasation or significant narrowing along the ureter, the ureter is in continuity and may be managed conservatively, with either observation or stent placement.

If one is unsure whether a ureteral injury has occurred intraoperatively, intravenous (IV) administration of 10 mL of indigo carmine or methylene blue with 20 mg of furosemide may help localize a ureteral injury. Extravasations of blue dye indicate ureteral discontinuity. Intraoperative cystoscopy is a real-time imaging as well a diagnostic modality (Fig. 1).

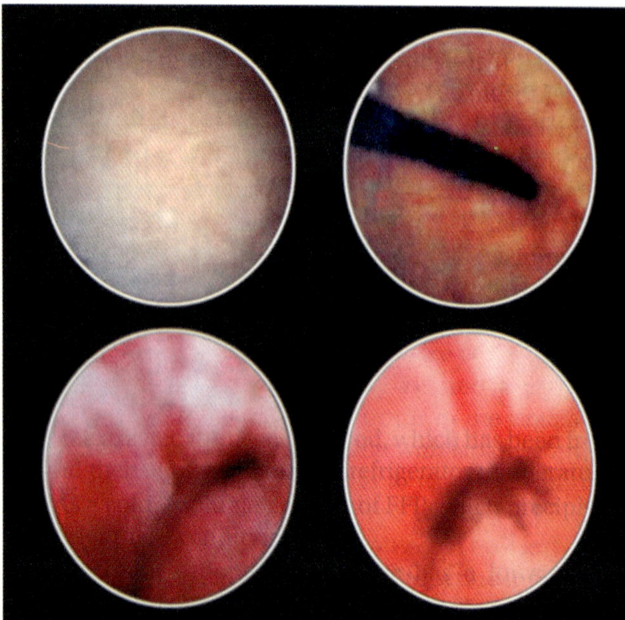

Fig. 1: Intraoperative cystoscoy: Images from a cystoscopy. The top two images show the interior of a bladder. The top left image shows the bladder wall, the top right shows the cystoscope passing into the bladder from the urethra. The bottom two images show an inflamed urethra

Real-time Textured 3D-models for Medical Applications

Realistic visualization becomes more and more important in medicine. Whenever a patient individual 3D-model was generated, the aim is to visualize the model as realistic as possible. 3D-models are used in diagnostic and therapeutic tools for intraoperative visualization, e.g. computed tomography (CT) scans. Most medical tools use surface-rendering or volume-rendering for virtual visualization. The coloration of a visualized model is normally done by using a convenient color for each surface. One of the approaches for 3D-models generated from motion in image series (e.g. video endoscopes) is to add textures to the 3D-model. The main problem is to handle the huge amount of video image-data (20 Mb/s) and render the model in real-time. This method is becoming a good intraoperative tool.

Computer-aided Tumor Resection in the Pelvis

Surgical treatment of large malignant tumors within the pelvis is a complex problem due to the anatomy and biomechanics. There are standardized preoperative diagnostic tools like CT or magnetic resonance imaging (MRI) that provide multidimensional information. However, this information cannot be transferred intraoperatively. Computer-aided surgery (CAS) may be a solution for precise intraoperative accuracy for these indications. A complete resection is possible with tumor-free resection margins. Navigation may be helpful in tumor surgery within the pelvis with computer aided tumor resection (CATS).

Intelligent Operating System

Many advances in technology has been achieved in diagnostic and operative tools, such as CT scan, MRI and positron emission tomography (PET) scan. In 20th century, however, intraoperative diagnostic tools are not sufficient for providing solid data. So, a new operating system has been developed for 21st century [intelligent operating theater (IOT)]. The IOT has an open MRI machine for intraoperative magnetic resonance (MR) imaging that provides objective anatomical data and the "real-time" navigation updated with iMRI that navigates surgeons to the target area. The IOT has contributed to the improvement of the resection rate in pelvic tumor cases. Real-time MRI can image soft tissue and may potentially guide therapeutic procedures without ionizing radiation. (Figs 2 and 3).

There is no question about the usefulness of intraoperative images for surgery. At the moment, ultrasonography, CT and MRI are used for intraoperative diagnostic imaging. Diagnostic ultrasound is cost effective and easy to use but provides images, which are not real-time during surgery. The image quality is also poor for depth. However, image quality is limited to conforming around the peripheral region of the cavity after tumor resection. To compensate for the poor image quality, integration of a navigation system using preoperative CT/W/MRI images with echograms has been attempted. However, this does not always overcome the problem of looking beyond the pelvic masses.

Natural Orifice Transluminal Endoscopic Surgery

Access to the abdominal cavity is required for diagnostic and therapeutic endeavors for a variety of medical and surgical diseases. Historically, abdominal access has required a formal laparotomy to provide adequate exposure. Natural orifice transluminal endoscopic surgery (NOTES) is an emerging experimental alternative to conventional surgery that eliminates abdominal incisions and incision-related complications by combining endoscopic and laparoscopic techniques to diagnose and treat abdominal pathology. During NOTES, commercially available flexible video endoscopes are used to create a controlled transvisceral incision via natural orifice access to enter the peritoneal cavity. Common incision-related complications such as wound infections, incisional hernias, postoperative pain, aesthetic disdain and adhesions could be minimized or eliminated by NOTES. NOTES has evolved from more

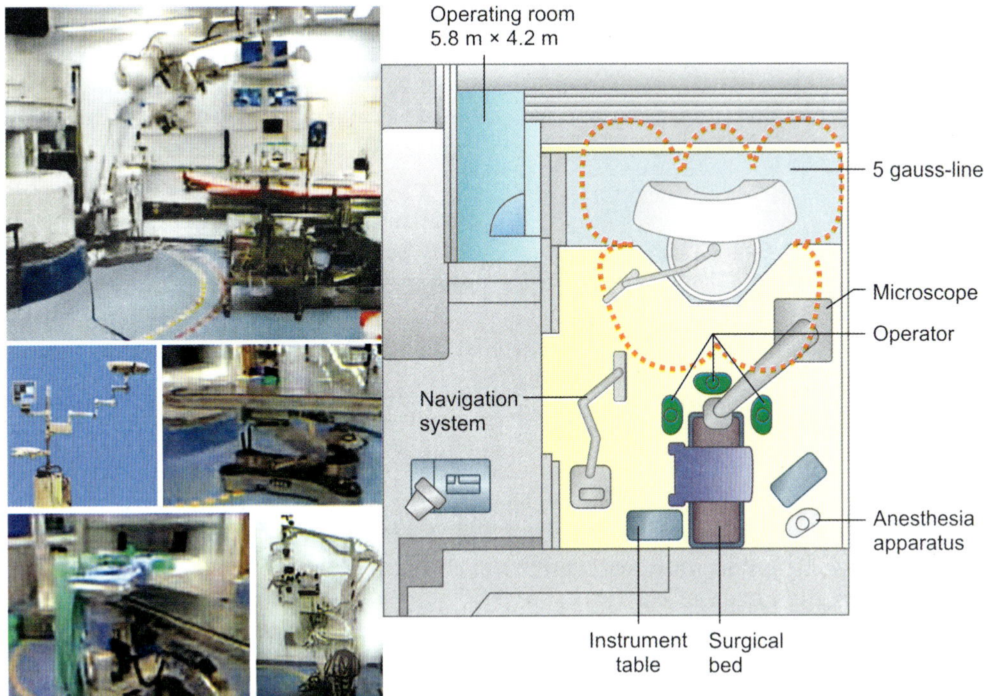

Fig. 2: Outline and surgical modalities and devices of intelligent operating theater

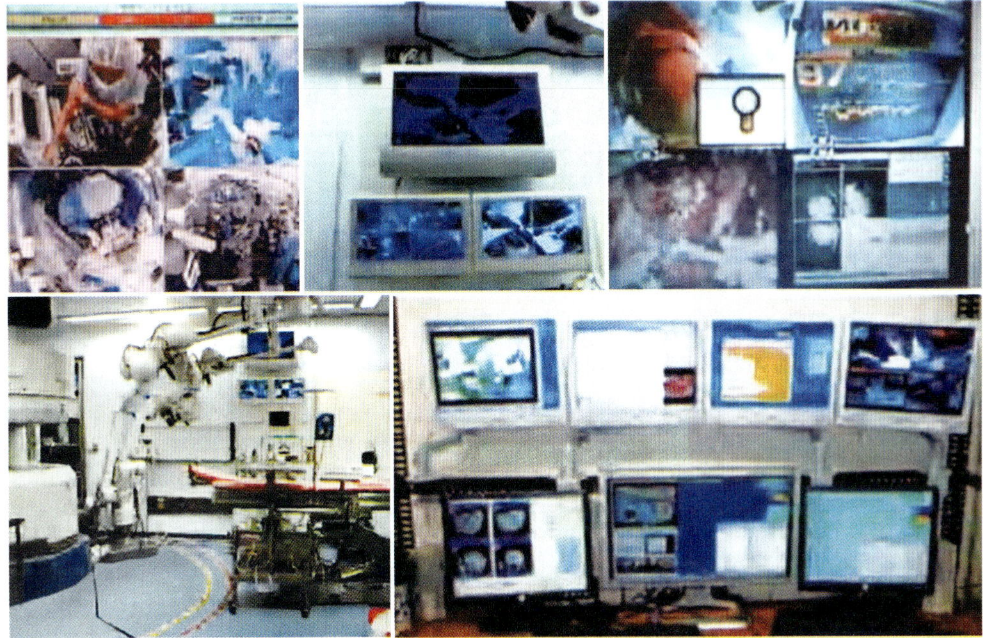

Fig. 3: Integrated surgical information on multiple displays during surgery

than two centuries of technological innovations and continued growth in the field of surgical endoscopy. Innovative surgical endoscopists have slowly developed means to surpass the constraints of the gastrointestinal lumen by using a flexible endoscope. The future of surgical endoscopy may be the shared entity of NOTES, which further integrates endoscopy, gastroenterology, and minimally invasive and general surgery. Although the promise of NOTES is electrifying to surgeons and endoscopists, several key issues need to be characterized prior to the incorporation of NOTES into routine practice (Fig. 4).

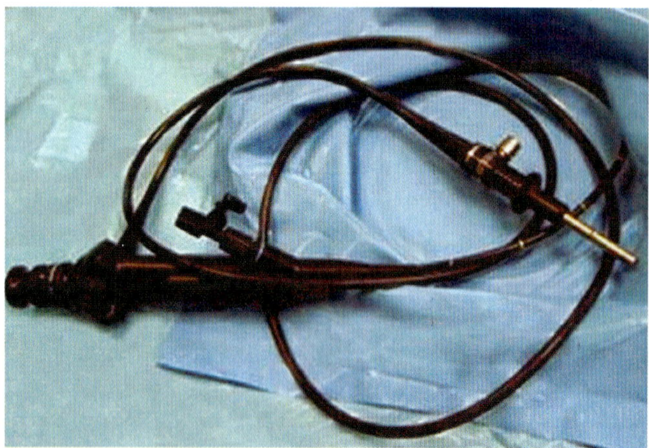

Fig. 4: Flexible endoscope for NOTES

Traditional flexible endoscopy has been limited to the confines of the gastrointestinal lumen; however, recent developments involving transluminal access to intra-abdominal structures hold the potential to revolutionize flexible endoscopy. Over the past few years, various studies have detailed techniques that intentionally breach the lumen and provide endoscopic access to the peritoneal cavity for diagnostic and therapeutic procedures. Unlike standard surgical approaches, which require incisions to be made in the abdominal wall, NOTES avoids the need for abdominal incisions and can offer specific advantages to select patient populations. Animal models have been used to demonstrate the possible applications of NOTES, including transgastric peritoneoscopy, tubal ligation, partial hysterectomy, oophorectomy, transcolonic exploration, liver biopsy and cholecystectomy.

Falloposcopy with Coaxial Catheter

A falloposcope is a fallopian tube microendoscope. Used in conjunction with a hysteroscope, laparoscope or catheter based system, falloposcopes visualize the fallopian tubes to diagnose and treat possible disorders.

This procedure is used to investigate and treat subfertility in women. Conventional investigation of subfertility in women often includes an examination of the fallopian tubes using hysterosalpingography (an X-ray test) or laparoscopy with dye injection to check the patency of the fallopian tubes. More rarely salpingoscopy is performed. This is the inspection of the inside of the fallopian tubes from the outer fimbrial end, at laparoscopy or laparotomy.

Falloposcopy is a technique that allows direct inspection of the inside of the fallopian tubes. The fallopian tubes are approached through the cervix and uterus.

There are two main types of falloposcope: coaxial and linear everting catheter. The coaxial technique involves inserting a narrow catheter over a guide wire through the cervix and uterine cavity into the fallopian tubes. The surgeon then passes a flexible endoscope through the catheter. Coaxial falloposcopy is usually carried out under local anesthetic and mild sedation.

The inability to access fallopian tubes easily and nonsurgically greatly impairs accurate diagnosis of the tubes health. The falloposcopy is a technology seeking a less invasive manner to create a more accurate diagnosis.

Intraoperative Sonography

Noninvasive imaging has developed rapidly resulting in increased accuracy for detecting primary and secondary tumors. Intraoperative ultrasonography (IOUS) was commonly considered to be the gold standard for ovarian pathology, but the current value of IOUS is unknown in view of more sophisticated radiologic tools (Figs 5A and B).

In one of the studies: Additional malignant lesions (AMLs) were first detected by inspection and palpation in 20 patients (13.4%). In another 18 patients (12.1%), IOUS revealed at least one AML. Overall, the findings obtained only by IOUS changed the surgical strategy in 34 cases (22.8%). It was concluded that IOUS, having undergone some refinement as well, still has immense diagnostic value in ovarian cancer of advanced stage in women. Frequently, avoiding palliative cytoreduction and occasionally disproving unresectability as assessed by preoperative imaging, IOUS is providing a significant impact on surgical decision making and should still be considered one of the gold standards.

Endoluminal Sonographic Evaluation

An endoluminal ultrasound system using a 12.5 or 20 MHz transducer housed in a 6.2 French catheter was used intraureterally in 38 patients being evaluated endoscopically for suspected tumors in the pelvis or ureter. The ultrasonographic, endoscopic and pathologic findings were evaluated. The location, size and sonographic characteristics of the tumors in the upper urinary tract were well demonstrated. The information obtained by this technique can be used to guide endoscopic biopsy and laser ablation of the tumor. Endoluminal ultrasonography also has proved helpful in defining the location of a tumor relative to an adjacent vessel and in identifying crossing vessels that cause extrinsic filling defects in the ureter. In a few pathologically correlated cases, endoluminal ultrasonography was accurate in assessing invasion in pelvic malignancy. A variety of nonneoplastic filling defects in relatively few cases have been evaluated successfully. Determination of the eventual usefulness of this technique awaits greater clinical experience and large clinical trials.

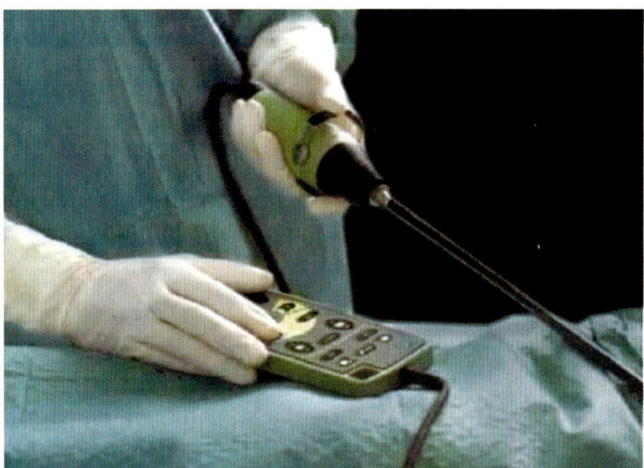

Fig. 5A: Intraoperative laparoscopic ultrasound system

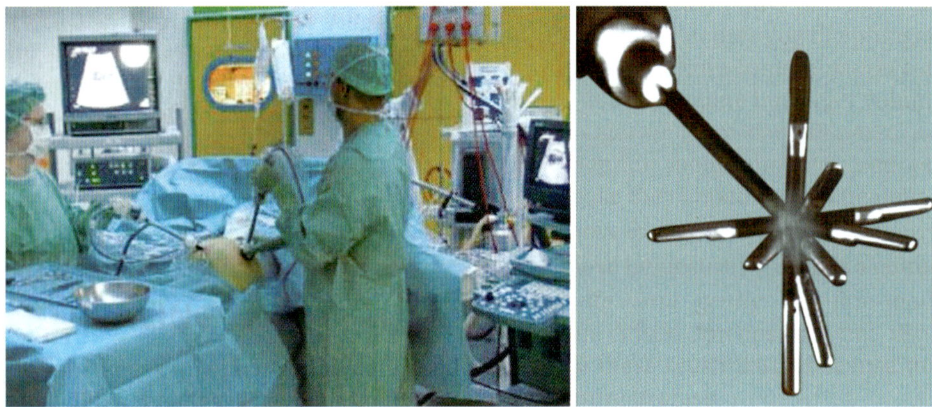

Fig. 5B: Intraoperative ultrasound and multidirectional ultrasonography probes

Flexible Transgastric Peritoneoscopy

Flexible transgastric peritonescopy is a novel approach to diagnostic and therapeutic interventions in the peritoneal cavity. A novel endoscopic peroral transgastric approach to the peritoneal cavity was tested in a porcine model in acute and long-term survival experiments. Transgastric peritoneoscopy was evaluated in 50 kg pigs. After upper endoscopy, the peritoneal cavity was accessed by needle-knife puncture of the gastric wall, followed by extension of the incision either with a pull-type sphincterotome or by balloon dilation. The peritoneal cavity was examined and a liver biopsy specimen was obtained. The gastric wall incision was closed with clips.

Twelve acute and five survival experiments were performed. Both techniques of gastric wall incision were without complication. The acute experiments demonstrated the technical feasibility of the approach. In the survival experiments, all pigs recovered and gained weight. The peroral transgastric approach to peritoneal cavity technically is feasible and has the potential to be an alternative to laparoscopy and laparotomy.

Culdoscopy

Culdoscopy is preferred in obese patients, when general anesthesia is contraindicated, and when fimbria and ovaries need visualization. Culdoscopy is not suitable if masses or pelvic or cervical inflammation are present. Laparoscopy is preferred for surgery and viewing of all peritoneal organs, particularly if the pathology is in doubt. Infertility cases can be examined by endoscopy to determine tubal patency; for example, culdoscopic sterilization and laparoscopy is comparable. Laparoscopy is indicated for patients in acute pelvic pain. The laparoscope offers better pelvic visualization. Laparoscopy can be performed in the presence of vaginal deformity, and laparoscopy is more easily learned than culdoscopy. Indications for culdoscopy include obese patients and patients with previous midline abdominal scars. Culdoscopy is cheaper to perform and takes less time than laparoscopy.

The number of endometriotic implants or adhesions is similarly counted for both operative techniques. The flexible 2.2 mm culdoscope provided a view of the pelvis similar to the laparoscope. Correlation between the procedures was 100%. The flexible scope achieved better visualization than the standard rigid posterior cul-de-sac culdoscope. Flexible culdoscopy is an excellent procedure for diagnostic endoscopy. It correlates well with office laparoscopy, requires less anesthesia and is better tolerated by patients. Several operative procedures are currently being tested through this mode of access.

Operative Culdolaparoscopy

It is a new approach combining operative culdoscopy and minilaparoscopy. It is a culdoscopy-assisted laparoscopic technique that utilizes a 12 mm trocar in the vagina as a multifunctional port in conjunction with laparoscopy and minilaparoscopy. The tendency is to use small cannulas for operative laparoscopy; however, working with these cannulas may have technical limitations. A new technique is emerging for performing appendectomy and other pelvic surgeries combining culdoscopy and minilaparoscopy. It uses 3 mm or 5 mm abdominal cannulas, and the large 10 mm or 12 mm cannula is inserted into the posterior vaginal fornix under laparoscopic surveillance. The vaginal port is used to introduce operative instruments and extract specimens, and for vision. Culdolaparoscopy avoids additional or large abdominal ports, thus overcoming limitations of small cannulas.

Culdolaparoscopy is not only exploratory but also concomitant surgeries, such as a cholecystectomy can also be undertaken. A cholecystectomy was performed utilizing the vaginal trocar as insufflations, visual and extracting port during a vaginal hysterectomy. Culdolaparoscopy, when performed during vaginal hysterectomy, can be used for exploration and operation in the abdominal cavity.

CONCLUSION

Time is not far when various modalities for evaluation and surgery will be available at same sitting to provide comprehensive treatment for complex masses while investigating the nature and pathology of such masses.

BIBLIOGRAPHY

1. Chak A, Soweid A, Hoffman B, et al. Clinical ultrasonography using through-the-scope catheter probes. Gastrointest Endosc. 1998;48(5):485-90.
2. Gulec SA, Hoenie E, Hostetter R, et al. PET probe-guided surgery: applications and clinical protocol. World J SurgOncol. 2007;5:65.
3. Henry-Suchet J, Loffredo V, Tesquier L, et al. Endoscopy of the tube (= tuboscopy): its prognostic value for tuboplasties. Acta Europ Fert. 1985;16:139-45.
4. Mohri T, Mohri K, Yamadori F. Tubaloscope. Flexible glass fiber endoscope for intratubal observation. Endoscopy. 1970;4:226-30.
5. Otto M, van Delden. Intraoperative Ultrasound, Presented at Practical Update in Radiology 2001.

CHAPTER

10

Operation Theater Setup

Nidhi Gupta, PL Gautam, Avtar Singh

Operation theater (OT) complex is the most important and critical area of the hospital. The patient's experience during hospital stay in this area, especially when he is under stress reflects on to quality of patient care and the reputation of the hospital. Moreover, the OT is crucial to emergency trauma and obstetric care (EmOC). For surgeons, anesthesiologists and other OT staff, there is no area more pious and holy other than OT suite (Fig. 1).

PLANNING AND DESIGNING OF AN OPERATION THEATER COMPLEX

Poorly planned, designed, constructed and organized OT complex can wipe out team's heroic efforts. Therefore, the ergonomically planned and designed OT complex will maximize patient comfort, technical and operational efficiency, and never the least will improve aseptic environment.

In addition, with fast evolving technology, it should hold flexibility to incorporate modifications of the changing trends.

To develop such an optimal design, it needs to involve all concerned in team.

- Administrators
- Surgeons
- Anesthesiologists
- Contractors
- Architects
- Civil engineers
- Clinical staff
- OT manager
- Equipment planners
- Biomedical personnels
- Infection control
- Hospital facilities maintenance.

Preferably, all theaters should be similar in design to have maximum utility and minimize time for orientation of OT personnel. Essential clinical input includes type of procedures to be undertaken, equipment used for that, and number of surgeons, staff and nurses needed. Early engagement of senior level staff of the team while line staff gets involved during the progress of the project is essential for the success. Patient needs, equipment, utilities, space and room size, telecom/data, air quality and infection control are the key guiding factors to help develop superior design, though each factor poses particular risks and challenges for the institution.

While preparing design, it is important to consider changing trends in patient sickness, procedures, equipment volume and increasing expectations of public

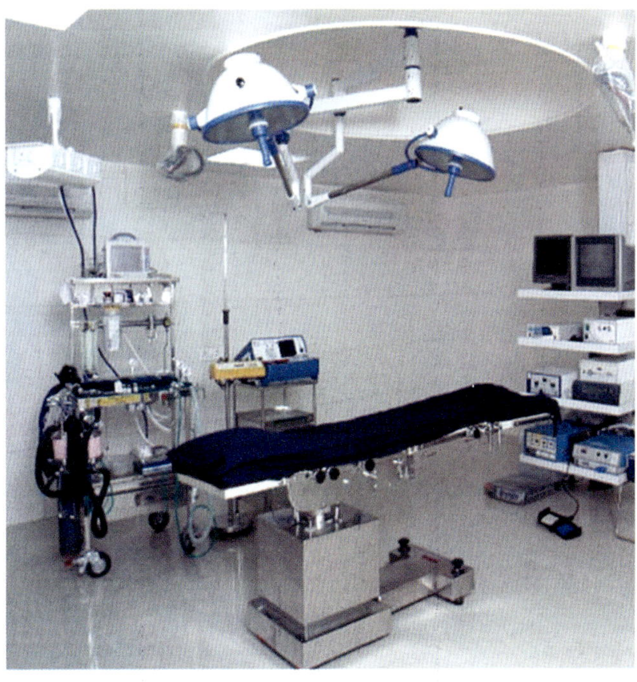

Fig. 1: Fully equipped theater

from healthcare providers. Organization structure must be congruent with the proposed function, cultural change and higher finish level.

NUMBER OF OPERATION THEATERS REQUIRED

For convenience, it is important to categorize the hospital on the basis of bed strength and type (Table 1).

Table 1: Hospital categorization on the basis of bed strength and type.

Category	Number of beds	OTs
A	25–50	1–2
B	51–100	2–3
C	101–300	4–6
D	300–500	7–10
E	> 500	1–1.5 OTs per 50 beds

Abbreviation: OTs, operation theaters

LOCATION

The OT complex is preferred to be located on the higher floors away from the hospital's general traffic area, i.e. corridors, to minimize the traffic and noise to maintain asepsis and provide quiet environment. It should have an easy access to surgical wards, emergency, intensive care unit, laboratory, blood bank and radiology department. It should have an efficient lift service. Obstetrical OT should be near to the labor room preferably within the same complex to facilitate wheeling in of the parturient without any inconvenience and delay. Total floor area of OT setup is given in detail in Table 2.

LAYOUT

The operating room complex has four main sections on the basis of cleanliness and asepsis.

1. *Protective zone (A)*: Theater supply, changing areas, preanesthetic room, waiting room.

Table 2: Total floor area required in an ideal operation theater building setup

OT complex	Area designation	Number	Area per room
1.	OTs	According to work load	35 m^2 per room
2.	OT incharge's room	1	17.5 m^2
3.	Doctors lounge	1–2	14 m^2
4.	Anesthesia rooms	1 for paired OTs	14 m^2
5.	Change rooms	2–4	17.5 m^2
6.	Store	1	28–34 m^2
7.	Staff support room	1	–
8.	Entrance lobby	1	–
9.	Preoperative room	1	28 m^2
10.	Postanesthesia care unit	1	87.5–109 m^2
11.	Sterile corridor	1	–
12.	Scrub station	1	10.5 m^2
13.	Preparation room	1	17.5 m^2
14.	Disposable corridor	1	–
15.	HS sterilizer	1	14 m^2
16.	Lift lobby	1	–
17.	AHUs	1	–
18.	Electrical room	1	10.5
19.	Portable X-ray room	1	14-–17.5 m^2
20.	Space for frozen section	1	17.5 m^2
21.	Anesthetist's room	1	14.5 m^2
22.	Trolley park	1	10.5 m^2
23.	Patients relatives waiting space with toilets	1	35 m^2
24.	Snack bar/coffee bay (optional)	1	10.5 m^2

Note: Rooms and areas need to be adjusted according to surgical workload, bed strength and occupancy

Abbreviation: OT, operation theater; AHUs, assistant hospitalo-universitaire

2. *Clean zone (B)*: Emergency OT, recovery room, theater packing room.
3. *Aseptic zone or sterile zone (C)*: It needs highest level of aseptic precautions. OTs, induction room, sterilizing room.
4. *Dirty zone (D)*: Used linen and instruments are transacted to washing and sterilization room through this corridor.

Entrance of OT suite through air lock curtains and separate rooms is helpful to create an efficient barrier. It is important to put barrier while crossing one area to another area. Various components and hospital in relation to OT are given in Figures 2 to 6.

Protective Zone (A)

Preoperative Area

From the patient's view-point of judgment, the intake waiting and registration space, the preoperative and to lesser extent the postoperative space are the most important. Under sized or poorly designed preoperative spaces will significantly affect the patient's experience through their journey to recovery, as it is he who is stressed, especially when the surgery is delayed. Therefore, it should be designed to provide patient comfort, minimize their anxiety and reduce the need for medication before surgery and enhance patient experience. Main features include:

- Adequate spaces for patients
- Privacy during examination and discussion with medical staff
- Finish, lighting and color to be soothing and refreshing
- Patient bays with hard walls on three sides
- Individually controlled lights in patient bays
- Sequestrated television areas
- Lockers big enough to even hold suitcases
- Convenient and comfortable waiting space for family/companions
- Children's play room.

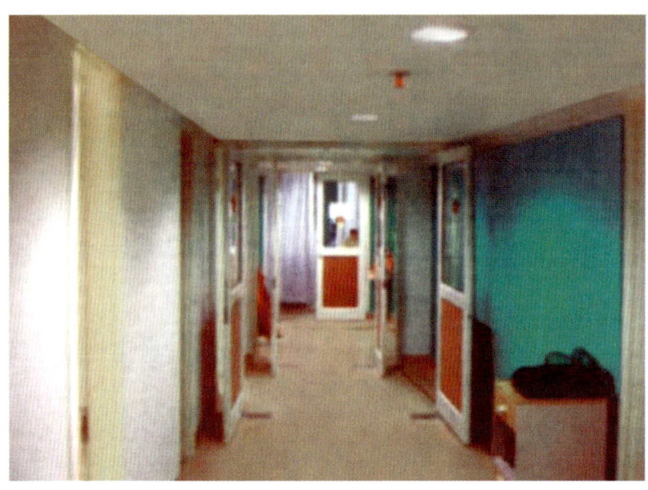

Fig. 2: Perfect illumination and ambience make a difference for the patient

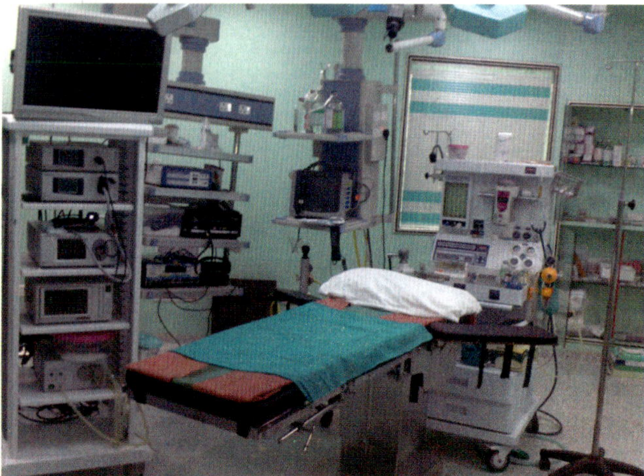

Fig. 3: View of the ward area

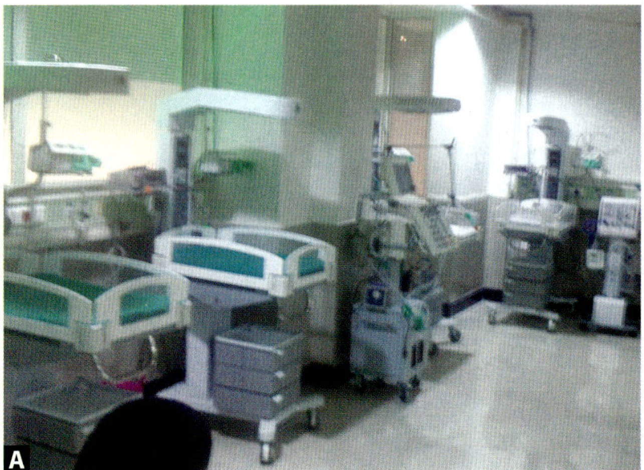

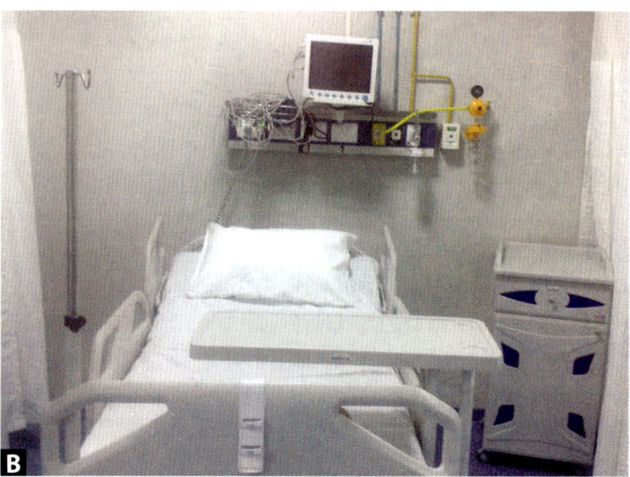

Figs 4A and B: (A) Neonatal intensive care unit; (B) Intensive care unit

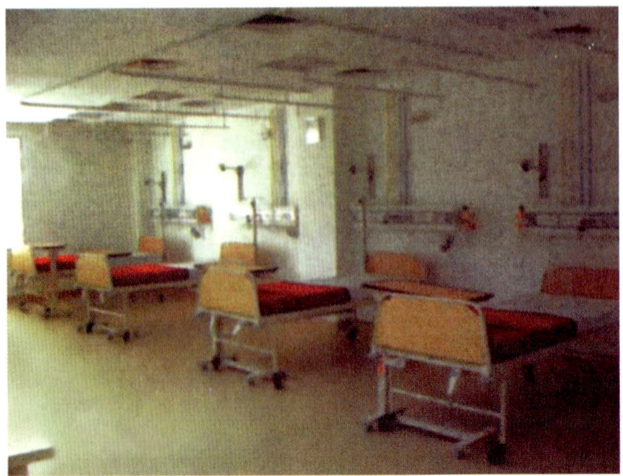

Fig. 5: Management of services is an important area for the planning

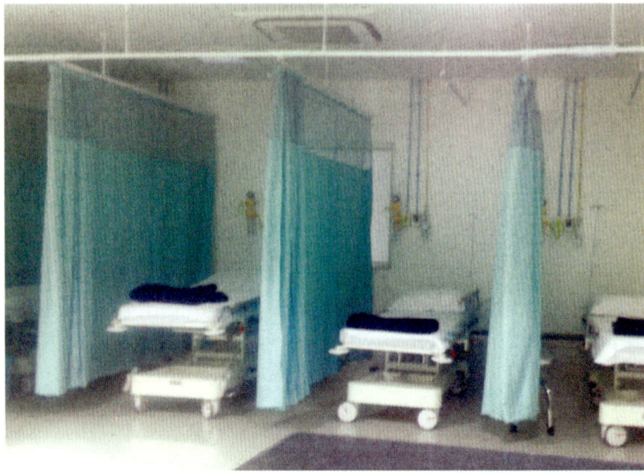

Fig. 6: Minor operation theater

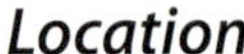

Location

Near main entrance of OT complex and away from OT personnel traffic (least disturbance area).

Size

- According to the number of operation rooms (at least one space per operation room)
- Provision to increase number of spaces as per need
- Bigger spaces for orthopedic beds if needed.

Configuration

- Nursing station to be located to minimize staff movements
- Curtains for privacy and flexibility
- Separate room to isolate patients with transmissible infections.

Lighting

- Indirect
- Additional lights to increase illumination for procedures.

Pipeline Outlets

- Oxygen supply port
- Suction port
- Ventilator port for ventilator dependent patients.

Electrical/Monitoring Outlets

- Adequate number of electrical outlets
- Electrocardiogram (ECG)
- Noninvasive blood pressure (NIBP).

Administration Area

- Computers
- Intercom
- Telephones
- Emergency call capability
- Data management
- Paperwork.

Changing Room

- For patients.

Rest Rooms

- For staff and visitors.

Store

- Space to store supplies.

Power Area

Many electrical and electronic appliances need uninterrupted power supply (UPS) service.

Pediatric Patients

- Space to accommodate child with family
- Spacious comfortable seating
- Provision of games.

The modern OT complexes have private preoperative suites where family members can stay with them until the patient is taken to the operating room. Changing trends of culture needs consideration of amenities such as business center with desk space to make calls, work on laptops, good sized lockers, refreshment bars and video consult booths.

Clean Zone (B)

Emergency Operation Theater

For minor surgery and comparatively less sterile patients a separate complex of emergency or casualty theater should be reserved. It should be near to emergency area with easy excess. It should also house septic OT for infected cases.

Recovery room: Adjoining to the OTs (main and emergency), there should be a recovery room or postanesthesia care unit with monitoring, oxygen and suction facility. The bed capacity depends upon the number of surgeries performed daily.

Theater packing room: It is workroom for preparing sutures, dressing material and other surgical items.

Aseptic Zone or Sterile Zone (C)

Operation Room Suites

General Considerations

- Control of entry and exit
- Quick transport between surgical floors
- Continuous progression through zones with increasing sterility
- Minimum 5–7 barriers with at least one air lock barrier prior to entering the sterile zone
- Wide corridors and doors
- Temperature 16–22°C
- Humidity 50%
- Ventilation 15–20 air changes per hour.

Hazards and Safety

- Fire-fighting systems
- Electroconductive flooring
- Concealed conduit wiring circuits.

Holding zone

It is an area where patients may be kept for a short while before taking them to the induction room. The ambience, quiet and serene environment of this place will help to lessen patient's anxiety and ensure comfort.

Operation Rooms

The number of OT will depend on the number of surgical beds in the hospital, the types of surgical procedures performed, and number of patients coming for ambulatory and emergency surgery. Rao Committee (1968) has recommended one OT for every 50 surgical beds.

Another way is computing through MaCaulay formula based on expected number of operations per day.

$$\text{Number of operations/day} = \frac{\text{Number of surgical beds} \times \text{\% of BOR} \times 365}{\text{ALS} \times 100 \times \text{Number of working days of hospital}}$$

where, ALS = average length of stay

BOR = bed occupancy rate

For example, 50 bedded surgical wing with 70% occupancy working 5 days a week

$$\text{Number of OTs} = \frac{50 \times 70\% \times 365}{7 \times 100 \times 5} = 3.6 \text{ or } 4 \text{ OTs}$$

Size

The reach and vision of the doctors and nurses is the most important factor. For the efficient use the surgical supplies, instruments and equipment needs to be immediately moved to the zone adjacent to the operating table, i.e. the reach zone. To achieve this flexibility, the practice of cart mounted equipment was introduced. This low density cart mounted equipment wastes the space within reach zone. Light source, cautery and IV stands, and suction apparatus wastes about one-third to half of the valuable space within reach. The need of more power supply, special circuits, data sheets and cables, communications, video and different medical gases for the OTs have increased considerably. Equipment congestion and a disarray of wires, tubes and lines (the *spaghetti syndrome*) is a common scenario in OTs. The radial arrangement of input and output signals and their interconnecting lines has been identified as the main source of clutter and congestion in this environment. Ceiling pendants with maneuverability and space for holding monitors, all gas and electrical outlets is essential to improve the work efficiency of OT personnel. The theater size has also increased to accommodate the latest surgical technologies and larger equipment. The average size operating rooms measure 400–500 ft^2. However, the modern OTs are bigger (600–650 ft^2) to meet the needs of technology oriented procedures. There is a sufficient space available to create three zones with high density arrangements immediately close to the operation table.

1. Central zone of operation table which ascertains that there is a purpose to approach this area.
2. Peripheral area of 30–36 inches along the walls for parking of carts and imaging equipment immediately not in use and also for students.
3. The annular zone between these two is a circulation area and should be clear of tripping hazards.

Scrub-up Area

- Single leaf door with self closing provision
- Viewing window to OT for communication
- A pair of sinks with elbow or knee operated taps.

Anesthesia Induction Room

- Very near to the OT
- Storage space sufficient for anesthesia workstation and other ancillary equipment
- Dust and moisture free.

Neonatal Resuscitation Room

- Adjoining to obstetrical OT with or without single leaf door
- Neonatal resuscitation trolley
- Gas and electrical outlets.

Flooring and Walls

The floors of the OT should be hard, seamless, easy to clean and able to withstand germicidal cleaning solutions. Wooden and cement floors are not suitable in the OT because contaminants can easily collect in the pitted and cracked surface. Walls with ceramic tiles are also not recommended in the OT because too many joints are difficult to keep clean. Laminated walls with three coats of polyethylene withstand wear and with an additional coat of epoxy paint, the problems of chipping, flaking or blistering are reduced. Mosaic is an excellent floor finish for the OT. It is recommended that the mosaic floor slopes toward a drain outlet. In this way, the floor can be easily kept clean. A very hard vinyl floor covering on a concrete base is acceptable for the OT providing that the seams are heat-sealed and the vinyl adheres to the concrete by a non-water-soluble adhesive. There should be no projections, pits, cupboards or other storing spaces to minimize the chances of holding dirt and dust.

Dirty Zone (D)

Used disposable and nondisposable items, linen and instruments are transacted to washing room and then sterilization room through separate corridor avoiding contamination of OT suite. The room should be provided with sinks, slop sink, bed pan sink, work bench and draining board, etc.

Ideal Obstetric Operating Theater Complex

In the ideal situation, the obstetric OT should be close to the labor room and delivery room. It should also have provision of neonatal resuscitation room, recovery room, dirty utility room, clean utility room with autoclave, clean storage room and toilets sinks. In the ideal situation, the

Flow chart 1: Showing operation theater traffic flow chart

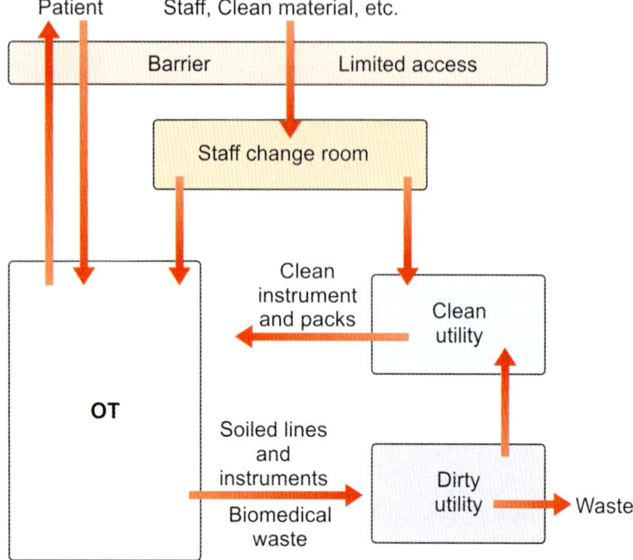

OT should be such that the "clean" and the "dirty" items do not cross paths (Flow chart 1). To best accomplish this, two distinct traffic patterns should be established. One traffic pattern should be dedicated to the two-way traffic flow (both "in" and "out") of patients, doctors and nurses. This route is also for clean items (instruments, equipment, supplies, etc.) being moved into the OT. And the other traffic pattern from the OT should be for the removal of all used dirty items, used disposables sponges, syringes, gloves, placental kit, etc. and biomedical wastes.

CONCLUSION

It has been said that the excellent is the enemy of the good. Predictions about the future OTs are neither accurate nor useful. However, ergonomic and human engineering principles remain the same and, their application along with consideration of the need while designing the OT are more useful. Flexibility to accommodate future technology is a fundamental of a robust design.

BIBLIOGRAPHY

1. Abreu E, Potter D. Recommendations for renovating an operating theater at an emergency obstetric care facility. Int J Gynecol Obstet. 2001;75:287-94.
2. Cathryn Bang. Optimal operating room design III. 2004. Available from: http://www.cbparch.com/optimal.pdf. [Accessed November, 2013].
3. Indian standard, recommendations for basic requirements of general hospital buildings. In: Medical services department buildings (Part 2). New Delhi: IS:10905; 1984. pp. 34-40.

CHAPTER

11

Operation Theater Protocols, Law and Administrative Requirement for Gynecological Surgeons

Nidhi Gupta , Sanjay Gupte, Nikhil Datar

INTRODUCTION

It is needless to say that the operation theater (OT) is one of the most important parts of the hospital/nursing home. The OT is a space intensive, capital intensive, equipment intensive entity and demands some very specific requirements which are different from other parts or rooms of the hospital.

Ideal Operation Theater

An ideal OT should have following requirements fulfilled:

1. Adequate space for rapid and swift movement of staff, equipment and patients
2. Adequate lighting
3. Continuous uninterrupted, stable electricity supply
4. Asepsis, a principal as suo moto
5. Optimal temperature and humidity regulation
6. Dedicated equipment and monitoring devices
7. Most importantly, systems to avoid mishaps and systems to record events.

These ideal requirements look simple. The ideal infrastructure for the OT can be created but maintaining ideal standards perpetually can be quiet difficult.

The level of asepsis depends on the kind of surgical work that is carried in the theater. Surgeries on reproductive tract have been classified as "clean contaminated". It need not be mentioned that level of asepsis shall differ from branch to branch. Thus there is a need to differentiate the needs depending on the nature of work.

Guidelines and Costing

Satisfying every requirement put above is a capital intensive proposition. The cost of health care delivered will be proportional to the capital invested.

Especially, in our country where cost of medical care is a major issue, a delicate balance between cost and necessity must be maintained.

It suffices to say that what strikes this balance is "minimum standards". Thus, two standards namely, "desirable" and "minimum", shall prevail in the subject matter.

Sources of Guidelines

The guidelines ultimately set the standard of care. These are the standards that shall be quoted in the court of law as well. The sources of the guidelines are:

- Laws of the land
- Government resolutions or rules
- Textbooks
- Recommendation from the professional bodies
- Accepted practices.

In the light of above, the authors have tried to look through various available guidelines in the literature, especially pertaining to India. The individual discretion has been used. The guidelines may not be applicable to all parts of the country as there is significant variation in the infrastructure and facilities available.

The chapter does not aim to set any standards universally acceptable all over the country.

Laws in the Country

Health is a subject of concurrent list of constitution. Hence, laws governing the health can be passed by union government as well as by the state. Most of states have their own enactments or ordinances governing the minimum requirements of the clinical establishments. The said enactments prescribe certain standards for the OT. The authors did not find any specific recommendations for gynecological OT per se. Some state legislations have categorically mentioned that the labor room and OT must be separate. The legislations prescribe the minimum area for the OT. Presence of shadowless lamp, adequate lighting, adequate equipment and drugs is what is prescribed by these legislations. It must be stated that the legal provisions appear to be grossly deficient.

Guidelines on Prevention of Infection in Operation Theater

There is no consensus on what is ideal formula for OT asepsis. There are no universally accepted guidelines.

The authors have drawn following inferences from "Consensus guidelines for the prevention of infections in the operating room" framed by "Hospital infection society" Mumbai forum.

Following things have been recommended:

- Preoperative bath
- Shaving immediately before operation or clipping or depilation before surgery
- Skin preparations by chlorhexidine gluconate 4%, povidone-iodine 10%, alcohol containing products
- For most gynecological surgeries, cephalosporins (cefazolin has been extensively tried) provide adequate antimicrobial cover. Anaerobic cover, if required, is achieved by metronidazole. Aminoglycosides are seldom required
- Clean surgical attire, caps, masks, shoes/shoe covers are recommended
- Various systems purifying the air such as high-efficiency particulate air (HEPA) filters, laminar airflows, ultraviolet (UV) germicidal irradiation has been found to be not very beneficial, especially considering the high cost for routine gynecological theaters.

Guidelines on Operation Theater Sterilization

Sources of microorganisms in OT are:

- Dust
- Lint
- Skin squames
- Aerosol
- Respiratory droplets

Thus, it is recommended that strategies to prevent dust accumulation, creation of barriers and maintaining that atmosphere where the growth of microorganisms will be less are the main stay of OT sterilization.

It is strongly recommended that repeated dusting and cleaning of environmental surfaces with antiseptic solutions such as sodium hypochloride, hydrogen peroxide (stabilized with silver) chlorhexidine gluconate is the main stay. Routine dusting of furniture, equipment, lights with special attention to flat surfaces with detergent is most important.

Fumigation/Fogging

This has been most popular method but has no longer been recommended.

Formalin is a proven carcinogen. It should be replaced by safer agent, such as hydrogen peroxide stabilized with a silver salt.

Atmospheric Conditions of Operation Theater

It is considered ideal to maintain temperature of 20–23°C and humidity of 30–60%.

Microbiological Sampling

This remains controversial due to several unresolved issues. Environmental swabs for organisms are of historic importance and should be abandoned. Settle plates are an insensitive means of air sampling.

Sterilization of Instruments

Surgical instruments should be soaked in germicidal detergent, thoroughly washed prior to steam sterilization. Use of biological indicators to check on microbial load is recommended. The authors would like to submit here that the biological indicators are difficult to procure in city like Mumbai as well.

Administrative Systems in Operation Theaters

Documentation

The staff of the OT must maintain a detailed and correct account of patients coming in the OT, nature of surgeries done, disposables and consumables required.

We recommend that register should be maintained giving:

- Account of patients
- Account of consumables
- Account of instrument and OT sterilization.

Avoiding Mishaps

- Identity of the patient and the operation
- Major centers where OT caters to multiple surgeries, a person should be designated to confirm the identity of the patient, surgery and whether valid consent has been taken or not.

Labeling the sample for histopathology

- This is another area where mere lack of communication may turn out to be disastrous
- Mop and instrument count
- The importance of mop and instrument count need not be stressed. In a study conducted by Association of medical consultants, Mumbai, through questionnaires that there is no set pattern or system in place to keep a check on mop and instrument count. We recommend that the every OT must have a black board on which pre- and postoperative counts are tallied
- The responsibility of checking the counts should be of the operating doctor when unqualified nursing staff is assisting. When qualified nursing staff is available the responsibility of checking must be of the nursing staff.

Routine Stock Checking and Instrument Check

This aims at:

- Checking the quantity
- Checking the expiry
- Checking the status of the instruments and assessing the need of service or repair.

It is difficult to set standard guidelines as far as the equipment and medicines in obstetrics and gynecology hospitals in our country are concerned. There are large ultramodern hospitals in metros, which are second to none of the advanced western medical centers. There are also large teaching hospitals with plenty of staff and good amenities. On the other hand, there are remote areas where essentials like oxygen, electricity, blood, anesthetists are not available. In between are the small hospitals up to 15 beds, owned by a single doctor who has to manage medical as well as nonmedical supplies.

In this scenario, we should aim at some basic minimum amenities keeping in view the patients' welfare and we should allow for some latitude according to the various localities.

We present to you the following guidelines keeping in view the small hospitals and doctors at moffusil areas who are the vulnerable people. We would hope that an apex body like the Federation of the Obstetric and Gynecological Societies of India would set up a committee to study, redefine, find and approve these guidelines.

MEDICINES

As far as the medicines are concerned, they would come under two main categories:

1. Emergency medicines
2. Medicines for routine use.

Emergency Medicines

1. Atropine
2. Adrenalin
3. Antihistamines
4. Corticosteroids
5. Aminophylline and deriphylline
6. Mephenitine and dopamine
7. Anticonvulsants
8. Antihypertensive
9. Digitals, furesemide (lasix) and mannitol
10. Oxytocins including prostaglandins.

Medicines for Routine Use

1. Narcotic analgesics
2. Nonnarcotic analgesics
3. Antispasmodics
4. Sodium bicarbonate
5. Calcium gluconates
6. Lignocaine
7. Antiemetics
8. Hydrogen (H_2) receptors, blockers (ranitidine)
9. Disinfectants like povidone-iodine, spirit, Savlon
10. Antibiotics
11. Etharcridine lactate.

Intravenous (IV) fluids like hemacel, 5% dextrose, Ringer's, normal saline, etc. of course form part of the emergency as well as standard armamentarium.

EQUIPMENT

As far as the standard equipment in obstetrics and gynecology nursing home are concerned, these can be grouped under:

1. Emergency equipment
2. Disposables
3. Standard equipment
4. Anesthesia equipment.

Emergency Equipment

1. Oxygen cylinders with all the accessories; minimum four cylinders would be advisable for a small hospital
2. Boyle's apparatus could now be considered as standard equipment (at least portable), but even at remote place ambulance bag or bellows apparatus should be a must
3. Suction machine-both electrical and foot operated
4. Blood pressure (BP) apparatus in working condition
5. Good emergency lamp or any alternative light source like generator should also be kept ready.

Disposables

1. Intravenous infusion sets
2. Blood administration sets
3. A few intracatheters and three-way cannulae
4. Disposable sterile syringes and needles

5. Sterile gloves
6. At least one set of emergency disposable linen.

Standard Equipment

Other standard equipment would of course include stethoscope, thermometer, BP apparatus, hammer, measuring tape, weighing machines (baby and adult), dressing drums, autoclave, sterilizer, standard linen, pads and bandages, operation table with instant head low facility, a good fumigation facility in working order, suture material of various type as required, Ryle's tube, urinary catheters (plain and Foley), standard operative instruments for common operations like dilatation (D) and curettage (C), medical termination of pregnancy (MTP), lower segment caesarean section (LSCS), hysterectomy, episiotomy, suturing as well as examination equipment, obstetric forceps or ventouse, baby receiving trays, kidney trays, facility to keep the baby warm, and pathology sample collecting bulbs.

All these have to be considered part and parcel of the standard equipment.

Anesthesia Equipment

Since anesthesia cannot be avoided in obstetrics and gynecology nursing home, anesthesia equipment, in addition to mentioned above, like laryngoscope, endotracheal tubes, connections and airways, various anesthesia drugs, muscle relaxants, spinal or epidural needles, 2% xylocaine jelly, and other adjuvant are required. All these anesthesia requirement will vary from place to place. A good fire extinguisher is also part of the standard equipment of any hospital.

FACILITIES

The physical facilities of an obstetric service should provide a safe and comfortable environment in which women can give birth and care for their infants. Ideally, the inpatient obstetric service should be consolidated in an area that is physically separate from rest of the hospital, such as on a separate floor or in a separate wing. The physical arrangement of the unit is determined by the patient load and the available space. Every effort should be put forth to make the facilities flexible and to meet local needs.

The following facilities should also be available:

1. Hospital beds and separate rooms
2. Consulting and examination room
3. Dressing and patient preparation room
4. Labor room
5. Dedicated OT
6. Sterilization equipment and area
7. Instrument clean up area
8. Secure area for storage of medications
9. Nurses station
10. Kitchen and pantry.

Even though, a lot of other facilities can be offered if the space permits, the above mentioned areas are bare minimum. A single room unit should provide comfort, privacy and protection against infection, as well as an atmosphere conducive to rest. Each patient unit should include the following items:

1. Beds with adjustable side rails
2. Adequate lighting
3. Bedside stand
4. Space for clothes and personal belongings
5. Signal or intercommunication device
6. Bathing, toilet and hand-washing facilities
7. Screening of beds in multiple bedrooms.

Among the intrapartum facilities, should be a separate area for patient examination and short-term observation (e.g., a labor lounge). A comfortable waiting area for families should be adjacent to the delivery suite; rest rooms should be nearby.

Labor-delivery-recovery rooms should be equipped with the following items:

1. Labor delivery bed
2. Operating room table
3. Emergency signal and intercommunication system (wherever feasible)
4. Fetal monitoring equipment
5. Anesthesia equipment for operative deliveries
6. Oxygen and suction facilities for mother and newborn
7. Adequate ventilation and temperature control for the newborn
8. Adjustable lighting system
9. Wall clock
10. Bedside stand
11. One or more comfortable chairs
12. Sink
13. Closet
14. Adjacent toilet facilities.

CONCLUSION

The OT is no doubt a place of worship for doctors and patients alike. This factory of surgeries needs to run like a clock-work with minimum room for mistakes or accidents. Towards this, all staffs have to follow the standard operating procedures laid down according to local laws and regulations in force, with ergonomic utilization of facilities available.

CHAPTER

12 Preoperative Management of the Gynecologic Surgery Patient

Sandhya Gupta, Suvarna Khadilkar, Madhu Nagpal, Rajni Sundar, C Kumar

12.1 PREOPERATIVE MANAGEMENT OF THE GYNECOLOGIC SURGERY PATIENT

Sandhya Gupta

INTRODUCTION

Patients about to undergo surgery present many challenges. The practice of medicine today is fraught with problems involving quality of care, availability of information, patient participation in her care and financial constraints. Technological advances have created challenges between the surgeon's desire to provide the best and most current modality of treatment and the high costs of newer technologies. As the population above 65 years increases, these problems are compounded by an increasingly larger group of geriatric patients, including many who have coexisting chronic diseases like diabetes mellitus, coronary artery diseases, hypertension, chronic obstructive pulmonary disease (COPD) and obesity.

Preoperative management is a dynamic process that is constantly aimed at enhancing outcome from a surgical procedure. Preoperative management must be thorough, streamlined, educational and cost-effective. Physician and patient satisfaction is the final goal.

Preoperative workup would therefore include patient evaluation, stratification of risk and risk factor modification. The gynecologic surgeon, thus is able to reduce delays in the preparation phase, enhance patient safety, recognize and treat complex medical problems, reduce evaluation costs, and minimize case delays and cancellations.

PREOPERATIVE EVALUATION

Preoperative evaluation of a patient is aimed at:

1. Evaluation of risks for anesthesia
2. Evaluation for confirmation of diagnosis requiring surgery
3. Evaluation to give a good surgical outcome.

Evaluation for confirmation of diagnosis is beyond the scope of this book. We shall, therefore discuss here in short the other two aims of preoperative evaluation.

ROUTINE INVESTIGATIONS FOR MAJOR GYNECOLOGIC SURGERIES

A good history and physical examination followed by review of patient's charts are undoubtedly the most important routine tests needed.

Preoperative Consultation

Medical consultation provides assistance with risk stratification, risk modification and planning perioperative patient management. Ideally, the medical consultants who are part of the perioperative evaluation should be the same individuals who provide continuing care for the woman.

Anesthesia Evaluation

The anesthesiologist's preoperative visit is a key in preparing the patient for the operating room. The method of anesthesia, the agents available, patient-controlled analgesia (PCA) or other modalities for postoperative pain relief are discussed.

The assignment of surgical risk is made using the American Society of Anesthesiologists (ASA) physical status classification. The letter E is added to any of the classes when an emergency surgical procedure is performed. Anesthesia and surgical morbidity increase as the physical status increases from status I through status V, as follows:

- Status I—A healthy patient
- Status II—Patient with mild-to-moderate systemic disease (e.g. anemia, morbid obesity)
- Status III—Patient with severe systemic disease that limits activity but not to the point of incapacitation [e.g. healed myocardial infarction (MI), diabetes with vascular complications]
- Status IV—Patient with incapacitating systemic disease that is life-threatening (e.g. advanced hepatic or renal insufficiency)
- Status V—Moribund patient who is not expected to survive (e.g. major cerebral trauma, massive pulmonary embolus).

Investigations

The use of laboratory tests before surgery became ingrained in clinical practice in the later half of the 20th century. However, the systematic evaluations of the clinical effectiveness and cost effectiveness of routine laboratory testing were often lacking. It also appears that the physicians are poor at evaluating the tests ordered.

Let us consider the various investigations a patient would require to do or not do before undergoing a major gynecologic surgery like a hysterectomy or myomectomy.

Complete Blood Count

There is no universally accepted minimum hemoglobin concentration for taking up a patient for surgery since the lowest hemoglobin tolerated depends on the patient's starting physiological status. However, a hemoglobin level of 10 g/dL is a widely accepted criterion that must be met before anesthesia is induced for elective surgical procedures. Obviously, this does not apply to patients with chronic conditions such as renal disease or sickle cell anemia. Thus, if a patient has hemoglobin less than 10 g/dL, performing an evaluation and treating her prior to surgery is prudent. Hemoglobin level is important not only in knowing the preoperative fitness of a patient, but it also gives us the basal preoperative value against which the postoperative hemoglobin, if required, can be compared, especially if there has been an appreciable intra- or postoperative blood loss. The prevalence of leukopenia or leukocytosis is extremely low and rarely leads to change in patient management. Also, thrombocytopenia is present in less than 1% of healthy elective surgery patients. Thus routine preoperative WBC or platelet count is not recommended unless indicated.

Therefore, complete blood count (CBC) would be indicated if:

- Evidence of recent blood loss
- Large predicted blood loss
- Symptoms of anemia
- Plethoric patient
- History of heart disease or chest disease.

Blood Sugar

The frequency of abnormal blood sugar result in an asymptomatic patient is up to 5.5% and may increase to 25% in patients above 60 years. Cardiovascular problems and poor wound healing are most common surgical risks. Therefore, assessment of blood sugar is necessary preoperatively.

Blood Grouping and Crossmatching

Knowing ones blood group is important for everyone and knowing it before a surgery is an absolute essentiality for both the surgeon and anesthetist. It helps one to keep adequate blood ready in cases of rare blood groups. Crossmatching and reserving of adequate blood is essential in surgeries where blood loss is anticipated, as in a myomectomy or a Wertheim's radical hysterectomy.

Creatinine

The prevalence of abnormal serum creatinine levels in asymptomatic patients is 0.2–2.4% and may increase to 9.8% in patients between 46 years and 60 years. Therefore, testing renal function with serum creatinine is only recommended for all patients above 40 years, those with diabetes mellitus or in whom use of nephrotoxic medication is anticipated. Serum creatinine as a measure of renal function assessment lacks sensitivity. Glomerular filtration rate (GFR) could be reduced by 50–70% without leading to an increase in serum creatinine concentration because the decrease in glomerular filteration of creatinine is balanced by the increased creatinine secretion by proximal tubular cells. Also, extra-renal variables like hemodilution, variable muscle mass and high metabolic rate affect serum creatinine levels. But creatinine greater than 2 mg/dL is an independent risk factor for cardiovascular morbidity and mortality.

Coagulation Studies

The prevalence of abnormal bleeding time (BT), prothrombin time (PT) and activated partial thromboplastin time (aPTT) in the absence of history of bleeding diasthesis is less than 1%. It has been shown that BT has no predictive value on the incidence of perioperative bleeding. Therefore BT, PT and aPTT are not routinely necessary unless indicated by history and examination.

Liver Function Tests

Since, most patients with elevated liver enzymes would be symptomatic and jaundice may be detected by physical examination, routine preoperative liver function test (LFT) is not recommended. However, in patients with history of jaundice in the recent past, those on drugs with possible hepatotoxic effects as with anti-tuberculous drugs or any other history suggestive of liver dysfunction, an LFT would be mandatory.

Electrolytes

Determination of serum electrolytes are only indicated in patients with:

- Diuretic therapy
- Pituitary or hypothalamic disease
- Renal disease
- Adrenal disease or corticosteroid use
- Fluid loss or shifts (e.g. bowel preparation)
- Digoxin therapy
- Central nervous system (CNS) disease
- Malignant arrhythmia.

Erythrocyte Sedimentation Rate

Though a test with poor specificity, erythrocyte sedimentation rate (ESR) assumes importance due to its markedly elevated levels in two common conditions encountered in practice—tuberculosis and malignancy.

Urine Analysis

The rationale for doing a urine analysis is to detect either asymptomatic renal disease or underlying urinary tract infection (UTI). It is unclear whether any relation exists between asymptomatic bacteriuria/UTI and surgical wound infection, but it would always be better if a urine analysis is done before all gynecologic surgeries since a gynecologist operates in close proximity to the urinary tract and also, since inadvertently, bladder injury may occur and an existing UTI in such cases would interfere with the healing process.

Electrocardiogram

Electrocardiogram (ECG) helps in preoperatively identifying high-risk patients with prior MI and arrhythmias since many studies have shown an association between preoperative MI and arrhythmias with surgical mortality. Therefore, ECG should be a mandatory test prior to any surgery, especially after the age of 40 years, though with the rising number of myocardial infarcts at an earlier age, it would be prudent to do ECG in all patients after the age of 30 years.

Chest X-ray

The incidence of abnormal chest X-rays in an otherwise healthy person is about 0.3% below 60 years of age and increases to nearly 20% in patients above 60 years. Therefore, routine chest X-ray is not advocated in healthy individuals preoperatively. However, X-ray chest should be done in all patients with respiratory (COPD, asthma) or cardiac dysfunction. Signs of associated complications like pneumonia, cardiac failure, etc. may be picked up. However, the author feels that in a country like India, where pulmonary tuberculosis is rampant, a chest X-ray would definitely be of help preoperatively not only to pickup signs of active tuberculosis, but also to see evidences of old, healed tuberculosis like scarring. Presence of active disease surely would require initiation of antituberculosis drugs much prior to surgery while presence of old lung scarring would require pulmonary function test (PFT) to be done if the area of scarring is large and the patient is symptomatic.

ROUTINE INVESTIGATIONS FOR MINOR GYNECOLOGIC SURGERIES

Going by the above discussion, minor surgeries like dilatation and curettage in a normal healthy patient with no positive history suggestive of vital organ dysfunctions rarely require any investigations. A baseline hemoglobin would be all that is required. But, if the patient does present with a history of specific organ dysfunction, necessary investigations may be performed. However, according to Rock JA, a CBC, hematocrit and urine analysis should be done in all gynecologic patients.

HIGH-RISK CASES

Cardiovascular

The cardiac evaluation of gynecologic patients should extend far beyond routine auscultation. A careful routine history and physical examination generally suffice in young, healthy, asymptomatic women with a benign cardiac history.

The gynecologic surgeons should be more concerned when their patients are older or have significant history or physical findings that require a more detailed cardiac evaluation.

Risk assessment is referenced differently depending on the specialty literature that is reviewed. The American Heart Association Task Force Report, perioperative cardiovascular evaluation for noncardiac surgery, is a commonly used modern reference for this type of assessment.

Myocardial hypoxia remains the major cardiac risk in any gynecologic surgery. The reported incidence rate of perioperative infarction is approximately 0.15–2%. However, patients with a history of previous MI have a 6.6% chance of having a second postoperative infarction. Furthermore, if surgery is performed within 6 months of infarction, these patients are at significant risk for reinfarction. Reinfarction rate of 27–37% was observed in patients undergoing surgery within 3 months of infarction, while it was 11–16% in those who underwent surgery within 3–6 months following an infarction. The reinfarction rate was just 5% when the surgery was performed 6 months after the infarction. Postponing elective open surgery for at least 6 months is thus advisable. Likewise, unstable angina of less than 3 months duration is an absolute contraindication to noncardiac surgery, except in a dire emergency. Such patients are an absolute contraindication for laparoscopic surgery.

Importantly, the gynecologic surgeon must pay attention to blood pressure (BP) control. As many as 28% of patients preparing for surgery are being treated for, or have, hypertension. Some authors report that as many as 4% of women have elevated BP from using oral contraceptives. Antihypertensive medication is taken up to the time of surgery and resumed early in the postoperative phase.

Key Aspects of Cardiac Assessment

According to the American College of Cardiology and American Heart Association (in 2002), there are three key aspects to assess:

1. Clinical predictors of perioperative risks
2. Functional capacity
3. Surgical risks.

Clinical Predictors of Perioperative Risks

- Major predictors—include unstable angina, recent MI, decompensated congestive cardiac failure (CCF), significant arrhythmias and severe valvular disease. The presence of these may justify a delay or cancellation of elective surgery or may require the patient to undergo preoperative coronary angiography, if the surgery is necessary
- Intermediate predictors—include mild angina, previous MI, compensated or previous CCF, diabetes and renal insufficiency. The presence of these requires a careful assessment of the patient's functional capacity when deciding whether preoperative cardiac testing is needed
- Minor predictors—include advanced age, abnormal results on ECG, any rhythm other than sinus rhythm on ECG, poor functional capacity, history of stroke and uncontrolled hypertension. The presence of these does not always require further cardiac testing unless the functional capacity is poor.

Functional capacity: The patient's functional capacity is expressed in terms of metabolic equivalents (MET), where one MET equals the oxygen consumption of a 70 kg. Fourty years old man in a resting state. The patients who cannot achieve 4 METs experience increased perioperative cardiac and long-term complications.

Surgical risks: The magnitude of the surgical procedure should be considered while assessing the preoperative cardiac risks. Cardiac death and nonfatal MI are highest in patients undergoing emergency surgeries and surgeries associated with significant fluid shifts and blood loss.

Noninvasive Testing

Women who would require cardiac evaluation and noninvasive testing have intermediate predictors and poor functional capacity or are undergoing high risk surgery.

Treadmill test (stress test)—is not recommended by American College of Physicians for preoperative prediction of cardiac risks, though according to a study, patients who can achieve 85% of their predicted maximum heart rate had 6% rate of cardiac complications whereas patients who could not achieve the same had 24% chance of cardiac complications.

Dipyridamole-thallium imaging (DTI) or dobutamine stress echocardiography have been used for further risk stratification, but their predictability is doubtful.

Beta-blockers Effect

Use of atenolol was found to reduce overall mortality (55% lower) and mortality due to cardiovascular complications (65% lower).

Hypertension

Patients with mild-to-moderate hypertension (systolic 140–180 mmHg and diastolic 90–110 mmHg) can proceed to surgery without changes in treatment as long as there are no changes in ECG.

There are limited studies on the risk of perioperative death or MI for patients with severe hypertension (systolic > 180 mmHg and diastolic > 110 mm Hg).

However, it is recommended that it would be advisable to delay surgery for better control of hypertension gradually, over a period of 6–8 months, to avoid exacerbating the effects of coronary stenosis.

Valvular Diseases

Systolic murmurs: Aortic stenosis is an independent risk for perioperative morbidity and mortality, and therefore the presence of a suggestive murmur always warrants further attention. Mitral regurgitation by itself is not a risk factor but may predispose to higher mortality due to its association with other independent risk factors.

Diastolic murmurs: Both aortic regurgitation and mitral stenosis are not in themselves independent risk factors for preoperative morbidity and mortality. Therefore, investigations are directed at detecting associated problems like CCF, arrhythmias or pulmonary hypertension.

Chronic Obstructive Pulmonary Disease

Many factors predispose patients to pulmonary complications postoperatively including advanced age, smoking, obesity and known pulmonary disease.

Chronic obstructive pulmonary disease, being a relative contraindication for laparoscopic surgery, require special attention. The incidence of postoperative pulmonary complications (PPC) varies in medical literature.

A proper preoperative counseling regarding possibility of disability or death along with a possible need of short-term postoperative mechanical ventilation should be given in all COPD patients.

A multispecialty team of consultants should be involved including a respiratory physician, anesthesiologist, physiotherapist and specially trained nurses. The preoperative visit should be planned well in advance of the surgery and those with stage II or III COPD should be admitted at least 24 hours in advance of the procedure and have their lung disease aggressively treated.

Patient should be taught breathing exercises and coughing techniques. Lung expansion methods like incentive spirometry and continuous positive air pressure may be used in extremely high-risk patients.

Blood gas analysis preoperatively is of help, especially in deciding postoperative ventilatory settings.

A preoperative chest X-ray is necessary for ruling out complications such as pneumonia or cardiac failure that may be associated with the pulmonary disease.

Pulmonary function tests characterize the type and severity of the underlying pulmonary disease, but are poor predictors of PPC. Studies show that there is little indication to perform pulmonary function tests (PFTs) to evaluate patients with mild-to-moderate COPD preoperatively.

Factors that lead to increased hypoxia in COPD patients include sedatives, narcotics and general anesthesia. Therefore, local or epidural anesthesia is preferred.

Using a preoperative management protocol is helpful prior to surgery. Using these protocols reduces postoperative complications. Features of the protocol may include an expectorant, a bronchodilator, adequate fluid volume, incentive spirometry, postural drainage and antibiotics for purulent sputum. If fewer pulmonary problems are present, cessation of smoking, use of incentive spirometry, chest physiotherapy and administration of a bronchodilator enhance pulmonary function before surgery.

For asthma, patients should be wheeze-free at the time of surgery. Patients with suboptimal control of asthma should have their surgery postponed.

Atelectasis and bronchitis remain the two most common complications postoperatively. These complications occur in approximately 10–20% of the healthy adult population. Knowledge of these complications requires the surgeon to remember to instruct the patient to use deep breathing exercises postoperatively.

The primary postsurgical risk is the development of bronchitis. In addition, at the time of endotracheal intubation, quiescent asthma can flare up, most likely secondary to irritation of airway receptors.

Postoperative pulmonary complications are more likely to occur in patients with predisposing factors like morbid obesity, cigarette smoking, chronic airway obstruction, heart disease and old age. Morbidity in these patients may reach 80% and mortality is about 3–5%.

Diabetes Mellitus

Diabetes mellitus is one of the most common endocrine diseases encountered in the preoperative evaluation. A proper management of diabetes is required to reduce operative risks including metabolic derangements, impaired wound healing and increased risk of postoperative infection.

Due to the contrasting pathophysiology of type I and type II diabetes, different perioperative strategies are required for each of them. Type I diabetics are prone to develop ketoacidosis in the absence of exogenous insulin on which they are completely dependent, whereas type II diabetics are resistant to development of ketoacidosis but are prone to more severe hyperglycemia and hyperosmolarity than type I diabetics.

Perioperative stress of any kind, whether psychological, due to anesthetic induction, intubation, surgical stimulation and postoperative pain responses can all cause an increase in the secretion of counter-regulatory hormones like glucagons, epinephrine, cortisol and growth hormone. Type I diabetics will respond to this with an exaggerated hyperglycemia and a five fold increase in serum ketone levels. Type II diabetics respond with an aggravating hyperglycemia.

Spinal and epidural anesthesias are associated with decreased levels of epinephrine and cortisol, respectively, and therefore have some advantage for diabetic patients.

Diabetic patients awaiting surgery are particularly prone to hypoglycemia, since they are fasting and because certain medications which may have been administered to them can potentiate the effects of oral hypoglycemics and insulin. In addition, sedatives and narcotics given during the course of anesthesia may mask the signs of hypoglycemia. Therefore, perioperative blood glucose management requires special attention with strict avoidance of hypoglycemia.

Blood Sugar Control

Even in the absence of end organ damage, diabetics are prone to impaired wound healing and postoperative infection. Animal studies have shown that blood glucose greater than 250 mg/dL is associated with impaired granulocyte phagocytosis, chemotaxis and bacterial killing as well as impaired procollagen and collagen synthesis. Hyperglycemia is also associated in humans with cerebral dysfunction. Blood glucose levels greater than 180 mg/dL in humans are associated with osmotic diuresis. Therefore, perioperative blood glucose monitoring should be aimed at a fine balance between prevention of hyperglycemia with its untoward CNS, renal and wound related complications, and prevention of hypoglycemia with its potential CNS malnutrition and permanent damaging effects.

A combination of various insulins with or without oral hypoglycemic agents are used in the perioperative blood glucose control.

Plain insulin due to its rapid onset of action and rapid clearance is the insulin of choice for intravenous (IV) route or for rapid control of hyperglycemia by subcutaneous route. Lente and neutral protamine hagedorn (NPH) insulins may be a part of patient's preoperative insulin doses. Oral hypoglycemic agents should be withheld on the day of the surgery due to their prolonged duration of action. Very long acting ones should be discontinued several days prior to surgery.

The aim of the treatment should be to maintain the blood glucose levels between 120 mg/dL and 200 mg/dL. Various protocols have been studied. The chosen approach should be easy to use, well monitored and cost effective.

Oral Hypoglycemics or Insulin?

It is found that up to 93% of type II diabetics can be managed perioperatively without insulin. Therefore, routine use of insulin is not required in these patients undergoing minor elective surgeries of less than 2–3 hours duration and whose diabetes is under reasonable control.

Oral hypoglycemics for management of type II diabetics with poor control is controversial. In such cases, it would be best to stop oral hypoglycemics on the day of surgery and switch over to IV insulin drip in 5% dextrose titrated against the blood sugar levels.

For type I diabetics, insulin is the main line of treatment. A back-up dose of intermediate acting insulin given subcutaneously is desirable to prevent ketosis, but should be in a dose just adequate to prevent hypoglycemia. About half of the daily dose of insulin is given as subcutaneous intermediate acting insulin and the blood glucose level is then titrated with plain insulin in 5% dextrose IV drip.

Obesity

In patients with morbid obesity it is essential to have a thorough clinical examination and a relevant history, looking for hypertension, with appropriate sized BP cuffs, signs of cardiac failure, diabetes with its associated complications and thorough respiratory assessment, especially for obstructive sleep apnea.

Apart from the routine investigations, ECG is mandatory. Echocardiography may provide information on eccentric left ventricular hypertrophy. Chest X-ray, PFT, baseline arterial blood gases may be essential.

Assessment of the airway and veins is essential to plan the approach and prevent last minute jitters. If peripheral lines are difficult to obtain, a central line should be established preoperatively.

Avoid narcotics and sedatives. Regional anesthesia should be used wherever possible.

Thyroid Dysfunction

Hyperthyroidism

Hyperthyroidism is usually caused by the multinodular diffuse enlargement associated with Graves's disease, but it also occurs in pregnancy, thyroiditis, thyroid adenoma, choriocarcinoma or with pituitary adenomas that secrete thyroid-stimulating hormone (TSH). Complaints usually observed include weight loss, diarrhea, warm moist skin, weakness of large muscle groups, menstrual abnormalities, nervousness, jitteriness, intolerance to heat, tachycardia, cardiac arrhythmias, mitral valve prolapse and heart failure.

When thyroid function is abnormal, the cardiovascular system usually is affected. The most concerning of these symptoms are tachycardia, irregular heart rhythm, atrial fibrillation, heart failure, and occasionally, papillary muscle dysfunction. Diarrhea does occur and can cause dehydration, which must be corrected preoperatively.

The prudent surgeon probably should operate on a woman with clinical hyperthyroidism only in a life-or-death situation. Otherwise, she should be made euthyroid prior to any surgical procedure. Antithyroid drugs are administered long-term and are continued till the morning of surgery.

If emergency surgery becomes necessary before the euthyroid state is achieved or if hyperthyroidism gets out of control during surgery, IV administration of esmolol and/or propranolol is titrated to restore normal heart rate. Intravascular fluid volume and electrolyte balance is maintained. However, administering propranolol or esmolol may not prevent thyroid storm.

Hypothyroidism

Hypothyroidism is a common disease in women. It occurs in as many as 5% of women. It usually is subclinical with serum thyroid hormones in the normal range and only serum TSH being elevated. Therefore, it may have little or no perioperative significance.

In women with overt hypothyroidism, however, relative lack of thyroid hormone results in slow mental functioning, slow movement, dry skin, periorbital edema, intolerance to cold, depression of the ventilatory responses to hypoxia and hypercarbia, impaired clearance of free water (with or without hyponatremia), slow gastric emptying and bradycardia. In extreme cases, cardiomegaly, heart failure, and pericardial pleural effusions manifest as fatigue, dyspnea and orthopnea.

A rising TSH level is the most sensitive laboratory indicator of a failing thyroid. Preoperative management of hypothyroidism consists of restoring normal thyroid status. A normal dose of triiodothyronine (T_3) or thyroxine (T_4) should be given on a long-term basis and orally on the morning of surgery.

Hematopoietic

The history generally uncovers abnormalities in the clotting cascade. Symptoms such as easy bruising and episodes of prolonged bleeding require determining PT, platelet count, BT and aPTT. Almost all bleeding abnormalities are discovered by some combination of these four tests. However, in the absence of an indicative history, suggestive of bleeding disorder, the above tests may not be done routinely.

If the patient needs blood transfusion, packed red blood cells are preferable. One unit should elevate the hematocrit by three points. Autologous transfusion is not practiced in India.

The chronic use of aspirin may create bleeding problems at the time of surgery. Aspirin inactivates platelet function for as long as 10 days after ingestion. Similarly, nonsteroidal anti-inflammatory drugs (NSAIDs), steroids and phenothiazines also interfere with platelet function.

Elective surgery should be postponed if the platelet count is less than 50,000/mm^3. Spontaneous bleeding usually is observed when the platelet count is close to 10,000/mm^3. Platelet transfusion may be given to these patients before and during surgery to raise the count above 50,000/mm^3.

OTHER CONSIDERATIONS

Antimicrobial Prophylaxis

A wound infection develops as a result of a complex interaction between the bacteria inoculated into the wound during surgery and the local and systemic resistance of the host to infection. The size of the bacterial innoculum is correlated directly with the risk of a postoperative wound infection. Factors such as prolonged preoperative hospital stay and the excessive use of antibiotics increase the risk of colonization with hospital-acquired pathogens. Alterations in the resistance of the host to infection may occur systemically or locally (i.e. within the wound).

Nutritional support and control of distant infection reduce the risk of wound infection. Achievement of optimal local resistance to infection is predominantly a surgical task. Various factors, such as the presence of blood, foreign bodies, ischemia or necrotic tissue, at the operative site may impair local host defenses and increase the risk of infection. Meticulous surgical technique helps avoid many of these contributing factors. The primary benefit of antibiotics is a reduction of the innoculum of viable bacteria in the wound.

Principles of Antibiotic Administration

Timing: Adequate concentrations of the drug must be present in the tissues at the onset and throughout the procedure. The latter problem is particularly significant when antibiotics with a short serum half-life are used, the operative procedure is prolonged, or both.

Route of administration: Intravenous administration of antibiotics is the optimal method to ensure adequate levels are present in tissues during most operative procedures. The exception to this principle is in bowel preparation. Preoperative oral administration of antibiotics is effective in preventing wound infections. Antibiotics administered orally prevent infection by reducing the high colonic bacterial innoculum rather than by achieving high concentrations in the wound.

Duration: A single dose of antibiotics immediately prior to surgery is sufficient for most procedures. If the procedure is going to last longer than 3 hours, consideration should be given to repeating the dose.

Choice of antibiotic regimen: The regimen chosen depends on the pathogens usually associated with wound infection in a given operation, the serum half-life of the antibiotic, the antimicrobial susceptibility patterns in the local hospital and the cost of the medication. The most important principle is that the antibiotic selected should be effective against the pathogens most frequently responsible for wound infection after the particular operation. The recommended regimen for women undergoing laparoscopically assisted vaginal hysterectomy/total laparoscopic hysterectomy (LAVH/TLH) or radical hysterectomy is a single IV dose of cefazolin (1 g) or cefotetan (1 g) at induction of anesthesia.

Antibiotics administered intravenously, immediately before surgery, ensure adequate levels in tissues throughout the surgical procedure. Therapy should last less than 24 hours and usually should consist of a single dose. The antibiotic regimen is chosen based on expected pathogens at the surgical site and local susceptibility patterns of these microorganisms. Appropriate use of antibiotics reduces wound infection rates and decreases morbidity and cost.

Patients on Medications for Acute and Chronic Medical Conditions

An increasing number of patients present to their surgeon's office taking medications used to treat multiple diseases. The average hospitalized patient receives more than 10 drugs. Many of these drugs have adverse effects that might make surgery more risky or patient management more difficult. One should always obtain a drug history including vitamins, herbs and alternative medicines.

In general, unnecessary drugs should be discontinued for at least three, preferably five, half-lives of the drugs. For essential or beneficial drugs, the optimal dose should be determined and maximized.

Anticoagulants

The use of anticoagulants poses additional problems in the management of routine and complicated gynecological cases. A frequent concern is the risk of perioperative or postoperative hemorrhage. Perioperative management of patients being treated with anticoagulants requires weighing the risks of increased surgical bleeding from residual anticoagulation versus potential thrombotic or embolic events from stopping the anticoagulant. An effective and safe plan for preoperative weaning from anticoagulant therapy and confirming the return of normal anticoagulation function must be determined prior to surgery. This decision is based, at least in part, on the type of operation and the indications for anticoagulation.

Heparin: Heparin is effective in reducing the risk of thrombosis; however, full anticoagulation can lead to increased bleeding and the risk for hematoma.

Warfarin: To minimize the risk of developing perioperative thromboembolism and surgical bleeding, the following recommendations are for the perioperative management of patients taking warfarin. If the INR is between 2 and 3, four scheduled doses of warfarin should be withheld to allow the INR to fall to 1.5 or less before surgery. Warfarin should be withheld for a longer period if the INR normally is maintained above 3 or if achieving a lower INR (<1.3) is necessary for the surgical procedure. The INR should be measured the day before surgery. If the INR is greater than 1.8, administering a small dose of vitamin K (1–2 mg) subcutaneously usually reduces the INR to less than 1.5 by the next morning. Mechanical methods of preoperative and postoperative prophylaxis against thromboembolism should be instituted for the period during which the INR is less than 2.

Patients undergoing emergency surgery who are receiving warfarin or those undergoing emergency surgery who are at high risk for venous thromboembolism may benefit by a rapid reversal of warfarin with the institution of heparin. Reversal of warfarin therapy may be accomplished rapidly with administration of a large dose (10 mg) of parenteral vitamin K (effective in 3–6 hours) or immediately with fresh frozen plasma.

Aspirin: Bleeding time has been suggested as the most reliable predictor of normal bleeding in patients receiving antiplatelet drugs; however, the BT for patients taking aspirin has not been proven to be a reliable indicator of platelet function nor predictor of surgical blood loss. BT quickly normalizes after aspirin ingestion, but it may take up to a week before platelet function completely normalizes.

Other NSAIDs, such as naproxen and ibuprofen, produce a shorter-term defect that normalizes within 3 days after discontinuation. Thus, platelet function is considered to be decreased for 1 week in patients taking aspirin and for 3 days in patients taking other NSAIDs.

Elective surgery generally should be avoided in the first month after an acute episode of venous thromboembolism. If this is not possible, IV heparin should be given both before and after the procedure while the patient is not anticoagulated with warfarin and the INR is below 2. The aPTT should be kept in the therapeutic range. One should stop IV heparin 6 hours before surgery. This provides sufficient time for heparin to be cleared, to minimize the risk of bleeding. Heparin therapy should not be restarted until 12 hours after most major surgeries and should be delayed even longer if any evidence of active bleeding is present or if the risk of any bleeding is life-threatening. The first aPTT is checked approximately 12 hours after restarting therapy, to allow time for a stable anticoagulant response.

Concerns with Regional Anesthesia and Anticoagulation

To lessen the possibility of complications for patients on long-term oral anticoagulation medications, the anticoagulant therapy must be stopped and the INR must be measured prior to initiation of neuroaxial block. Soon after discontinuation of warfarin therapy, factor VII levels rapidly normalize (within 24 hours), but normalization of coagulation and INR does not occur until factors II and X improve. An INR of 1.5 or less is considered safe enough to perform major regional blocks.

Summary of Anticoagulant Concerns

Testing of PT and aPTT should be performed prior to surgery of patients on long-term anticoagulation therapy in order to ensure that the anticoagulant effect of warfarin and heparin, respectively, is at a safe level for surgery. Measuring BT is not necessary before surgery in patients taking aspirin, unless they give a history of bleeding problems. Patients on long-term anticoagulation therapy with warfarin may stop warfarin several days before surgery and restart as soon as possible after surgery without excess risk of postoperative venous thromboembolism. Patients receiving anticoagulation for less than 1 month after an acute thromboembolic event should be brought in the day before surgery for heparinization and warfarin reversal, and should receive re-anticoagulation with heparin after surgery because they have a high risk of developing postoperative venous thromboembolism.

BIBLIOGRAPHY

1. Celli BR. Standards for the diagnosis and care of patients with chronic obstructive pulmonary disease. Am J Resp Crit Care Med. 1995;152(5):S77-121.
2. Cittanova ML. Is perioperative renal dysfunction of no consequence? British J Anaesth. 2001; 86(2):164-6.
3. Eagle KA, Berger PB, Calkin H, et al. Guidelines for perioperative cardiovascular evaluation for noncardiac surgery --executive summary a report of the American College of Cardiology/ American Heart Association Task Force on practice guidelines (committee to update the 1996 guidelines on perioperative cardiovascular evaluation for noncardiac surgery). J Am Coll Cardiol. 1996;15;27(4):910-48.
4. Jones J. Anaemia. In: Goldstone JC, Pollard BJ (Eds). Handbook of Clinical Anaesthesia, 7th edition. Philadelphia: Lippincott Williams & Wilkins; 1997. pp. 168-9.
5. Karnath BM. Preoperative cardiac risk assessment. Am Fam Physician. 2002;66(10):1889-97.
6. Owens WD, Felts JA, Spitznagel EL. ASA physical status classifications: A study of consistency of ratings. Anesthesiology. 1978;49(4):239-43.
7. Rao MS (2003). Morbid Obesity-Anaesthetic Management. [online] Available from: www.theiaforum.org/Article_Folder/ morbid-obesity-anaesthetic-management.pdf. [Accessed October, 2013].
8. Rock JA. Preoperative care. In: Thompson JD, Rock JA (Eds). Te Lind's Operative Gynaecology, 7th edition. Philadelphia: JB Lippincott; 1992. pp. 67-86.
9. Roizen MF. Anesthetic implications of concurrent diseases. In: Miller RD (Ed). Miller's Anesthesia, Philadelphia: Churchill Livingtone; 2000. pp. 903-99.
10. Roizen MF. Cost-effective preoperative laboratory testing. JAMA. 1994;271(4):319-20.
11. Supkis DE, Varon J. Anesthesia for the cancer patient: An overview. Anesthesiol Clin North America. 1998;16:524-5.
12. Van Norman GA. Preoperative assessment of common diseases in the outpatient settings. Ambul Anaesth Anaesthesiol Clin N Am. 1996;14(4):631-8.
13. Velanovich V. Preoperative screening electrocardiography: Predictive value for postoperative cardiac complications. South Med J. 1994;87(4):431-4.
14. Velanovich V. The value of routine preoperative laboratory testing in predicting postoperative complications: A multivariate analysis. Surgery. 1991;109(3 Pt 1):236-43.
15. Walton L. Preoperative Management. In: Sciarra JJ (Ed). Gynecology and Obstetrics. Philadelphia: Harper and Row; 1990. pp. 1-9.
16. Yamada D, Swietzer B, McHale MT. Preoperative assessment for gynaecologic surgery. Contemporary OB/GYN 2005.

12.2 POSTOPERATIVE MANAGEMENT

Suvarna Khadilkar

INTRODUCTION

Timely recognition of potential problems has a major impact on long-term outcome of patients. The postoperative management of women undergoing surgery, more often than not, gets less attention than preoperative and operative management. However, a well executed postoperative management brings about a significant reduction in morbidity, shorter and less expensive hospital stay, and more patient satisfaction.

The most critical period during a patient's postoperative course is within the first 72 hours of surgery. Precise monitoring of cardiovascular, renal and respiratory systems provide the most valuable information about the patient's postoperative condition. Of utmost importance is an appropriate preoperative evaluation of the surgical condition. Known risk factors ought to be identified at the time of preoperative assessment and postoperative care is planned so as to minimize the complications.

Gynecological surgical patients can differ in age, nutritional status and complexity of medical problems that they have. Stresses of surgery and an individual's complex response to that stress, needs to be understood.

OBJECTIVES

Postoperative management has three main objectives:
1. Postoperative care to assist rapid recovery.
2. Prevention of possible complications.
3. The early recognition and treatment of complications.

The first two points have a lot in common and are therefore dealt together.

Postoperative Care to Assist Rapid Recovery and Prevent Possible Complications

Correct Environment

For postoperative cases, a correct environment is one which has privacy, but at the same time has all facilities for close observation by adequate skilled nursing staff round the clock. It should be a place with facilities nearly equivalent to an intensive care unit.

Monitoring

Monitoring of a patient is the pillar of postoperative management. It helps not only in preventing complications by early detection of abnormal signs but also assists in early recovery. It is necessary that every patient be stabilized before transferring out of the recovery room. Every physician has his or her own set of routine postoperative orders and it is more effective to stick to a protocol which covers all aspects of monitoring. Monitoring should include evaluation of vital signs, catheter drainage including urinary catheter, nasogastric tubes and intraperitoneal drains, pulmonary status, abdominal examination, and looking for vaginal bleeding, if any.

Vital signs including pulse, blood pressure, temperature and respiratory rate should be monitored every 15 minutes till the patient is stable, then every 2 hours for the first 24 hours, and thereafter every 8 hours if the patient is stable.

Input/output chart: An input/output chart helps in monitoring fluid balance. In complicated cases, prolonged cases and in cases where there has been excessive loss of blood, an hourly output chart should be maintained. In uncomplicated cases, less frequent monitoring of output is sufficient.

Diet

Dieticians should be available in the ward. Proper nutritional status in pre- and postoperative periods has shown to improve the postoperative recovery. Preoperative nutritional status plays an important role in deciding the postoperative nutrition the patient must receive. Also, associated medical problems like diabetes, renal diseases, etc. have to be considered so as to give the patient an ideal diet and proper recovery. Most patients undergoing gynecologic majors like hysterectomy would go onto oral diet within 2 days postoperatively. However, in cases where oral intake is to be restricted for prolonged periods as in cases of surgeries for malignancies and those involving the bowel, total parenteral nutrition (TPN) may be required. When the period of TPN is going to be more than 7 days it should be given through a central venous line—subclavian vein being the most preferred access. If the TPN is to be given for less than 7 days than it may be given through peripheral lines. The osmolality of solutions used for peripheral lines is lower, about 800 mOsm, as compared with the one used for central line which is of higher osmolality, about 1800–2050 mOsm. The TPN solution should also have an ideal calorie:nitrogen ratio. Addition of lipids promotes positive nitrogen balance.

Prevention of Hypothermia

Maintenance of body temperature is of utmost importance, especially in old patients, since hypothermia leads to shivering which in turn causes increased oxygen demand. This requires increase in cardiac output and minute ventilation. Elderly patients and those with already compromised cardiac function may not be able to meet this demand resulting in hypoxemia and subsequent myocardial infarction.

Fluid Replacement

Proper management of fluids and electrolytes in gynecological surgical patients is of utmost importance. For patients undergoing major abdominal or vaginal surgery, intravenous (IV) fluid replacement is required to replace blood and fluid loss, and to allow for a period of decreased intake postoperatively, during recovery from anesthesia.

An average patient requires about 2.5-3 L of fluid per 24 hours, at least 75-100 mEq of sodium per day and 60 mEq of potassium per day in the immediate postoperative period of 24 hours. Potassium loss may be increased by persistent vomiting and replacement should be planned taking this into account.

There are patients who approach surgery in a depleted state, e.g. reduced intravascular volume in a case of hemorrhage from ruptured ectopic or a patient of radical surgery who has undergone bowel preparation prior to surgery. These increased losses should always be taken into account and additional fluid supplementation should be provided. Similarly, in cases with high fluid loss, as in those with pelvic drains, a long abdominal surgery, pyrexia (15% extra fluid should be given for each degree celsius rise in temperature) and in cases in which marked loss into 'third space' is suspected, e.g. following drainage of ascitis and debulking of ovarian tumor—although there may be no outward signs of fluid loss, adequate replacements have to be provided.

Postoperative Analgesia

Postoperative analgesia is an entity which till recent times was inadequately recognized and monitored. However, with recognition of disastrous effect of inadequate analgesia, namely, impaired oxygenation, reduction in deep breathing, risk of atelectasis and prolongation of hospitalization, more attention is being paid to individualize pain control in all gynecological surgery cases.

In cases of extended surgery, epidural analgesia is usually employed. This leads to a reduction in the depth of anesthesia required and is also beneficial by providing pain relief postoperatively.

Nonsteroidal analgesics are useful once acute pain has started to subside. Long acting preparations like diclofenac rectal suppositories provide very effective analgesia. Diclofenac skin patches are also now available which have an action over 24 hours.

Simple techniques such as infiltration of laparoscopy incision site with lignocaine may be of benefit. Adequate care is to be taken to remove as much gas as possible after the laparoscopic procedure is over, since retained gas can produce postoperative pain and discomfort.

Histamine receptors are involved in the development of inflammatory pain and hyperalgesia, and the use of antihistamines is advocated as an alternative for pain therapy and treatment of postoperative nausea and vomiting. Preoperative administration of promethazine 0.1 mg kg^2 reduces postoperative opioid analgesic consumption compared with postoperative placebo administration, and also reduces postoperative nausea and vomiting, and the number of patients asking for rescue antiemetic in the first 24 hours after surgery when compared with placebo. Centrally acting opioid analgesics like tramadol work well in combination with nonsteroidal antiinflammatory drugs (NSAIDs) to give pain relief.

Management of Drains

Drains may be inserted in cases with risk of hemorrhage and can be safely removed after 24 hours if loss is minimal. In cases of abscess or drainage of blood, after lymphadenectomy, they may be kept for longer periods. In such cases, dressing around the drain should be managed as per other wound management.

Management of Urinary Catheters

Most gynecologists use indwelling urinary catheters at the time of major pelvic surgery. It not only reduces the risk of bladder damage during surgery but is also important for the patient's comfort during recovery phase.

Following uncomplicated surgeries catheters should be removed. Once the patient can move out of bed, early removal of the catheter can also prevent the predisposition for urinary tract infection (UTI).

According to studies conducted, early removal of in-dwelling catheters after operation was not associated with an increased rate of febrile events, UTI or need for recatheterization. In addition, subjective pain assessment was significantly less in the early removal group. Early removal of an indwelling catheter immediately after operation was thus not associated with adverse events.

In cases where bladder has been opened during surgery, 7-10 days of in situ catheter is advised. Removal of catheter in such cases should always be preceded by clamping so that bladder tone and function is fully recovered.

Whatever the period of catheterization, care of the catheter is necessary to prevent infection and injury to the lower urinary tract. Simple measures such as strapping the catheter to the medial aspect of the thigh such that there is no strain on the inflated catheter bulb which is in the bladder, prevents injury to the bladder neck due to inadverent pulling of the catheter due to any cause. Cleansing of the vulva around the catheter and the exterior part of the catheter in immediate proximity to the vulva with antiseptic solutions helps in reducing chance of ascending infections.

Management of the Gastrointestinal Tract

Patients undergoing uncomplicated surgery, after tolerating clear liquids and passing flatus should be aggressively managed to go on to regular diet in a short time. Seriously ill or malnourished patients or those requiring extensive bowel dissection may require parenteral nutrition.

Extensive bowel manipulation requires introduction of nasogastric tube at the time of surgery, since return of the normal bowel function is delayed. A daily serum electrolyte level should be assessed in patients with nasogastric tube suction.

In case of delay in return of peristalsis, it is necessary to differentiate between postoperative illeus and postoperative obstruction so that proper treatment is given on time. Postoperative illeus will respond to conservative management of nasogastric tube, enema and cholinergic stimulation.

Postoperative nausea and vomiting has been dealt with separately in this book and therefore shall not be discussed here.

Mobilization and Physiotherapy

Early mobilization is useful in not only reducing risk of thromboembolic diseases and respiratory infection but also makes a substantial difference in return to normal activity.

A skilled physiotherapist, if available, is of great help. Physiotherapy plays a vital role in preventing complications and speeding up recovery.

Wound Care

After wound closure, a sterile dressing should be given which not only protects the suture line but also immobilizes the skin around the wound. In the initial phases, one has to be on the lookout for any seepage of blood or serum which may lead to infection and subsequent wound gape.

Suture or staple removal for transverse incisions may be done on day 7 while vertical wound may require 7–10 days to heal. Wound infection usually occurs on fifth postoperative day, and therefore this day should be scheduled for check dressing. One has to carefully look for induration and erythema which may be one of the first signs of infection.

If suspecting infection, the wound has to be probed and loculations of pus and necrotic material is to be removed. Wound swab should be sent for culture sensitivity before starting antibiotic therapy. Debridement and daily dressing is done if wound has gaped and healing by secondary intention is allowed. Appropriate antibiotic coverage should be given.

Subcutaneous drain helps in obese patients with several layers of subcutaneous fat. Some authors believe that routine subcutaneous drain helps in minilaparotomy incisions. However, some authors have not found it helpful as they found no statistically significant difference in wound complications as long as the patient received prophylactic antibiotic.

Place of Antibiotics in Gynecological Surgery

There is increasing evidence that intraoperative antibiotics, given intravenously, practically rule out the possibilities of postoperative infection. Also, further course of antibiotics can be avoided and hence can reduce the cost and discomfort of intramuscular injections. Microbes of all types should be tackled (Gram-positive, Gram-negative as well as anerobes).

Prevention of Bed Sores

Pressure sores over sacral promontory, greater trochanters and heels may occur in cases requiring prolonged immobilization. All efforts must be made to prevent these as they can lead to serious problems. Frequent change of posture, cleaning the pressure areas with alcohol and keeping them dry with talc and use of water beds will prevent the formation of bed sores.

Psychological Care

Postoperative care requires not only treatment of the body but also the mind. A postoperative patient is already under stress caused by the surgery, the pain associated with it, anesthesia and the fear of whether the recovery would be uneventful. Providing a cheerful homely environment, giving time to hear the patient's complaints and a few soothing words are of tremendous help in elevating the patient's mood which helps in early recovery.

Recognition and Treatment of Complications

Most of these complications have been discussed in detail in separate chapters in this book and have not been elaborated in detail here.

- Hemorrhage
- Pelvic hematoma

- Urinary complications
- Complications of GIT
- Cardiac complications
- Infection
- Thromboembolic diseases
- Wound dehiscence and incisional hernia.

Postoperative Bleeding/Hemorrhage

With proper surgical technique, postoperative hemorrhage is a rare occurrence. Every patient, however, has to be vigilantly monitored for signs of occult bleeding. Primary hemorrhage occurs in the immediate postoperative period while secondary hemorrhage is delayed. Distinction between the two is rarely clear. Rate of hemorrhage usually determines when the patient exhibits signs.

Fit patients can compensate for decreased intravascular volume and maintain blood pressure by causing tachycardia and peripheral vasoconstriction. The severity of the condition is not evident till the ability of the patient to continue compensation is exhausted and blood pressure falls suddenly. Such patients do not show any signs of bleeding in the recovery room. At times the vital signs may be stable for 12–18 hours after surgery and then suddenly hypotension, tachycardia, tachypnea, breathlessness, abdominal distension leads to diagnosis of intraperitoneal bleeding.

The peritoneal cavity has an enormous capacity for occult blood loss without appreciable abdominal distention. As much as 3,000 mL of blood (65% of blood volume) can be hidden in peritoneal cavity with only 1 cm increase in abdominal girth.

When massive blood loss occurs, a consumptive coagulopathy develops as all coagulation factors are exhausted. It is, therefore, mandatory to monitor the coagulation profile repeatedly during resuscitation. Even simple bedside observation of clot formation in a tube of blood eliminates this possibility.

Volume replacement: Large bore IV lines should be secured and fluid replacement started. Urine output should be monitored strictly. Broad spectrum antibiotics are started. Preoperative investigations should be obtained and reassessed. Operating room and anesthesia services should be notified. Interventional radiology team, if available, should also be informed.

Re-exploration: The earlier the bleeding presents, more likely it is that re-exploration will identify the bleeder. The original bleeding vessel, after more than 24 hours, may not be identified and only a generalize ooze may be encountered and hemostasis becomes difficult to achieve. In these cases angiographic embolization is the choice of management, if available.

Pelvic Hematoma

Vulval hematoma is a common complication after hysterectomy, especially by vaginal route.

One has to suspect the pelvic hematoma in the postoperative patient whose postoperative discomfort and anemia exceeds that which is normally expected and whose temperature is persistently increasing.

Definite diagnosis can be made by sonography or CT scan which is helpful in defining the exact site and location. Most people are of the school of thought that if the hematoma is drained, the patient's recovery is expedited. If the size of the hematoma as measured by sonography is found to be increasing in a patient whose vitals are also gradually deteriorating, then it is recommended that the hematoma be drained immediately. But in a few cases where the vitals are stable and the size of the hematoma is not increasing, drainage is difficult or contraindicated and if infection is not serious, it may be preferable to allow it to quietly resolve over a few months.

Abdominal wound hematoma is also common and tends to be self limiting. They may cause discomfort on mobilizing.

Laparoscopic port incisions which have been enlarged to remove samples contained in retrieval bags may lead to such hematomas.

Urinary Complications

Many of our patients undergoing gynecological surgery have pre-existing urinary dysfunction such as stress or urge incontinence, frequency, or incompetence of bladder. In any pelvic surgery, however, the most common complications of the urinary system are those related to catheterization.

The incidence of ureteric injury in gynecological surgery is 0.5–2.5%. Signs and symptoms such as flank pain, temperature elevation, retroperitoneal fluid collection and delay in return of bowel functions (ileus) ought to arouse suspicion. Sometimes, a pain similar to ureteric colic may be experienced by the patient immediately after the surgery which may mean a unilateral ligation of the ureter. Bilateral ligation of the ureter will lead to absent urinary output (anuria) which may arouse suspicion much earlier. The damage to the urinary tract at times is not apparent till several weeks after surgery. Postoperative ureteral obstructions may be discovered may years later as an incidental finding.

Vesicovaginal fistula (VVF) presenting in the 1st week may be because of trauma to the bladder during surgery. VVFs presenting late could be the end result of pelvic hematoma.

Whenever a urinary complication is suspected immediate postoperatively, the bladder should be catheterized to assess urine output and color of urine. This reduces the urine leak from bladder fistula. Fluid from abdomen drain should be analyzed for urea or creatinine contents. Three swab tests help to localize the fistula. Intravenous pyelography (IVP) helps in locating site of damage but small fistulas may not be seen.

Bladder repair: For cases that are voiding spontaneously with a small volume leak, catheterization for 7–10 days may be the only remedial measure required. If, however, leakage is significant, repair has to be performed in one or two layers with absorbable suture. Patient should remain catheterized for 7–10 days. Repair of ureter should be undertaken by an urologist.

Complications Related to the Gastrointestinal Tract

All complications affecting the bowel are due to surgery, but could be due to analgesic or anesthetic agents. Ileus following surgery will be due to handling and dissection of the bowel.

Abdominal distension after 24–48 hours is an early sign of either paralytic ileus or bowel injury. Every postoperative patient who is "not doing so well" should be vigilantly monitored and investigated before it is too late. Author strongly recommends an early ultrasound examination and a plain X-ray abdomen postoperatively in such patients. No hesitation should be there for re-exploration in cases with suspected bowel injury.

Late onset of distension could be due to intestinal obstruction and should be treated on individual merit of the case.

Cardiac Complications

Accurate fluid management will avoid fluid overload and cardiac failure. Stress of surgery can precipitate angina or myocardial ischemia in prone patients. Those at high risk, especially with previous history of angina or old infarction should be monitored intra- and postoperatively with a cardioscope so that the earliest changes are detected in the cardiac electrical activity and treatment started.

Infections

Fever and increased complete blood count (CBC) may be the indicators of infection. Subclinical tuberculosis may flare up after surgery.

Thromboembolism

Deep vein thrombosis in the lower extremities and pulmonary embolism are known complications that may prove fatal if not detected and treated in time.

Wound Dehiscence

Burst abdomen is a possibility in anemic patients and in presence of sepsis.

CONCLUSION

A comprehensive postoperative care carried out systematically helps in reducing postoperative morbidity and mortality by anticipation, prevention, early detection and prompt management of a multitude of postoperative complications which if unnoticed could lead to disastrous consequences.

BIBLIOGRAPHY

1. Al-Inany H, Youssef G, Abd ElMaguid A, et al. Value of subcutaneous drainage system in obese females undergoing cesarean section using pfannenstiel incision. Gynecol Obstet Invest. 2002;53(2):75-8.
2. Chia YY, Lo Y, Liu K, et al. The effect of promethazine on postoperative pain: A comparison of preoperative, postoperative, and placebo administration in patients following total abdominal hysterectomy. Acta Anaesthesiol Scand. 2004;48(5):625-30.
3. Dunn TS, Shlay J, Forshner D. Are indwelling catheters necessary for 24 hours after hysterectomy? Evid Based Nurs. 2004;7(2):45.
4. Horowitz IR, Rock JA. Postanaesthesia care and postoperative care. In: Thompson JD, Rock JA (Eds). Telindes Operative Gynecology, 7th edition. Philadelphia: Wolters Kluwer/ Lippincott Williams & Wilkins; 1992. pp. 87-122.
5. Panici PB, Zullo MA, Casalino B, et al. Subcutaneous drainage versus no drainage after minilaparotomy in gynecologic benign conditions: A randomized study. Am J Obstet Gynecol. 2003;188(1):71-5.

12.3 POSTOPERATIVE COMPLICATIONS

Madhu Nagpal

INTRODUCTION

Surgery is a unique experience in patient's life. The intraoperative surgical as well as anesthetic events leading to perioperative and postoperative complications can alter the outcome of surgery resulting in operative morbidity and mortality. Though surgeon is largely responsible yet the role of the anesthesiologist cannot be overlooked. They must counsel for choice of anesthesia, surgical options and facilities available. The informed consent is taken prior to any minor or major procedure. The procedural failures, residual sequelae and some unforeseen surgical mishaps are explained. A thorough preoperative clinical evaluation is jointly done.

Presently majority procedures are done as day care surgery or minimally access surgery where the hospital stay is considerably shortened. The endoscopic removal of uterus, myomas, ovarian cysts, tuboplasty operations, stress incontinence repair can be done with reasonable safety and ease. The medically compromised patient after conventional extensive gynecological surgery may need multispeciality intensive care management. The prime aim is to reduce operative morbidity and mortality.

An uneventful postoperative period is associated with minimal anesthetic complications and smooth convalescence. The pain is managed with simple analgesics or sedatives. The nausea and vomiting is treated with antiemetics. The vital signs remain unimpaired with complete hemodynamic stability. The fluid intake is sufficient to cover fluid and blood loss, maintain intravascular volume and provide calories requirement. The bladder function with adequate urine output of minimum 25-30 mL/hour and proper bowel function is ensured. Early ambulation is advocated to avoid complications like phlebothrombosis. Wound healing is checked. The sepsis is kept under control by the use of prophylactic/appropriate antibiotic cover. There is generalized sense of well being with optimum outcome of surgery.

Choice of Anesthesia

Various types of anesthesias used for gynecological surgery are local, regional (spinal, epidural or caudal) and general anesthesia. The complications of these methods and agents can be minor like local reaction due to extravasation of drug, anaphylaxis, headache, bronchospasm, hypotension or cardiorespiratory arrest. In a medically compromised patient pulmonary edema is fatal. The regurgitation of stomach contents carries the risk of aspiration as adult respiratory syndrome, Ryle's tube aspiration, metochlorpromide and ranitidine preoperatively prevent regurgitation. Epidural analgesia is beneficial as postoperative analgesic dose is repeated through indwelling catheter for pain relief in first 24 hours.

Recovery Period

While the patient is recovering from the effects of general anesthesia and regaining consciousness, the airway is maintained patent to avoid breathing difficulty. Until the patient is awake, semiprone position or left lateral position is helpful. Thereafter, position is changed frequently. The aspiration of the stomach contents or vomitus is avoided. An efficient nursing care is provided in the recovery suite under direct supervision of anesthesiologist and the surgeon.

EARLY COMPLICATIONS DURING PERIOPERATIVE PERIOD

Vital Signs Monitoring

Pulse/Blood Pressure

It is initially recorded every 15 minutes after a major operation and then every 30 minutes. Variations in pulse/blood pressure (BP) need to be registered. BP may be low due to anesthetic drugs. A rising pulse rate above 100/min, falling BP, air hunger, pallor or peripheral vasoconstriction indicate internal or external blood loss. The site and source of bleeding is secured by re-exploring the patient in the theater.

Respiration

It is second important information next to pulse/BP. It is deep and sighing due to air hunger following massive blood loss. The dyspnea with pulmonary edema due to overloading of circulation with fluids and blood transfusion should be recognized. In case of respiratory obstruction—ventilatory assistance is needed. The development of cyanosis in perioperative period is observed carefully.

A few days after surgery, dyspnea may occur due to chest complications like pneumonitis, atelactasis, pulmonary embolism or abdominal complications like peritonitis, paralytic ileus or abdominal distension.

Temperature

The rise of temperature up to 37–38°C in first 36 hours after surgery is usually seen after surgical trauma, especially in ectopic pregnancy with massive intraperitoneal hemorrhage.

In case of pyrexia, after 48 hours the site of infection should be localized. The fever due to urinary infection is associated with rigors, frequency of micturition and dysuria. There may be lung collapse in case of respiratory tract infection. If it is due to peritonitis, abdominal distension with paralytic ileus may be noteworthy. One should rule out wound hematoma, abscess or pelvic collection. There may be evidence of phlebothrombosis leading to pulmonary embolism.

To identify the site of infection and cause of fever, one should check abdominal wound area and vault in case of hysterectomy. The urine, pus from wound or vaginal swab is sent for culture and sensitivity. The ultrasound of abdomen is done to locate abdominal collection. The chest X-ray may indicate atelactasis or patchy consolidation or pleural effusion. The calf tenderness, if elicitable, signifies phlebothrombosis. The breasts may have engorgement, mastitis or breast abscess in lactating mothers.

The treatment is directed towards the cause by giving appropriate antibiotic and draining the collection, if present.

FLUID AND ELECTROLYTE IMBALANCE

Water Balance

Average daily intake of fluid is 750 mL in food and double the amount as drinks. Insensible loss through breath and sweating is about 1–1.5 L. The urinary excretion is nearly 1,500 mL per day and through stools the fluid loss is 150-200 mL per stool. The additional amount of loss through vomitus and drains also needs to be maintained.

Thus, proper fluid balance is maintained to avoid over infusion of fluids and the electrolyte imbalance. Multiple endocrinal and biochemical pathways work simultaneously after surgical trauma to counteract hypotension, preserve intravascular blood volume and tissue oxygenation. Antidiuretic hormone (ADH) results in water retention though aldosterone from adrenal cortex preserves sodium. Potassium follows the reverse pattern and is excreted in urine in increased amounts. The protein catabolism is accelerated due to operative trauma adding to increased urea excretion. If glucose 100 g orally or by intravenous (IV) route is given daily, then the protein loss can be spared. It is only in cases of paralytic ileus and peritonitis that sodium needs to be replaced. In case of poor muscle tone and lethargy potassium deficiency is replaced. Metabolic disturbances occur usually in septic abortion with renal failure, postoperative paralytic ileus or intractable diarrhea with pelvic peritonitis and pelvic abscess.

Sepsis

It is unusual to find high grade sepsis in an elective surgery patient but in an emergency situation with septic abortion or postpartum sepsis patient may suffer.

Wound Sepsis

It may be evident in previously scarred abdominal wall or in Pfannenstiel incision so local drainage may be preferred to allow serous effusion to flow out. An infected hematoma may present with fever, pain and tenderness. It needs drainage and appropriate antibiotic. Secondary suturing may be performed, if required.

Vaginal Vault Sepsis

Since vaginal suture line is naked, the ascending infection can occur. It is possible that patient may develop pelvic cellulitis or pelvic abscess. If residual collection exists in broad ligament, it may form infected hematoma of the vault. Patient presents with fluctuating high grade fever, raised pulse, pelvic pain, an ill defined mass and sometimes a foul smelling vaginal discharge. In cases of frank pelvic peritonitis and abscess, GI symptoms and diarrhea occurs. This usually happens from third to tenth postoperative day. The easy method of draining is by opening up the vault with finger.

Peritonitis

With the use of prophylactic or definitive appropriate chemotherapy, fortunately this complication is becoming rare. It appears after 48 hours by way of abdominal distension and paralytic ileus with evident signs and symptoms of febrile nature. Mostly it is seen when patient is already septic or when gastrointestinal tract (GIT) is simultaneously operated.

- *Pelvic peritonitis:* It is commonly seen after vaginal hysterectomy operation where residual broad ligament hematoma or infected fluid is collected in pouch of Douglas. This may present as tenderness in the lower abdomen but when frank pelvic abscess has formed it may extend beyond pelvic brim, point towards inguinal region, paracolic gutter, subphrenic area, perinephric region or burst into rectum.

  Ultrasound examination can detect the collection in the pouch of Douglas and early drainage is possible
- *General peritonitis*: This is evident usually on third postoperative day. The features are high grade pyrexia, tachycardia, persistent vomiting, abdominal distension, generalized pain and rigidity of abdomen. With the increasing discomfort and sense of ill

being, the patient looks toxic. The breathing is thoracic predominantly. The bowel sounds become absent when ileus is generalized. If the sepsis is far advanced, multiorgan involvement, especially renal function impairment occurs. The fluid and electrolyte imbalance occurs in association with GI dysfunction.

Patient requires multisystem support and close observation in critical care unit requiring daily input/output record maintenance, electrolyte assessment and renal function tests. Appropriate chemotherapy is instituted to reverse the phenomenon. IV fluids with electrolytes replacement is essential till patient accepts oral feeds. The surgical intervention is done, if indicated.

HEMORRHAGE

The ideal minimum hemoglobin (Hb) level at elective surgery should be 10 g/dL. In severely anemic subjects, blood should be transfused prior to surgery. In mildly anemic subjects, blood transfusion should be avoided, though arranged. Instead surgery should be carefully, quickly and gently performed to minimize blood loss and tissue damage. The ligatures on the pedicles should be properly secured. In case of wide spread ooze, the hemostasis is achieved with hot or cold sponges, tight packing or gelatin sponges or fibrin gels. In case of myomectomy operation tourniquet or myomectomy clamp is used.

The evaluation of blood loss can be made from the number of soaked sponges, weight of wet swabs, and variation of pulse and BP. The anesthesiologist can roughly estimate and requisite blood if there is massive blood loss. However, while doing Wertheim's operation or extensive ovarian cancer surgery blood should be infused in theater and is continued till the situation warrants.

Primary Hemorrhage

At the time of surgery, it may be arterial due to slipping of ligatures and retraction of vessels in it. One should tie double ligatures and avoid an unduly thick pedicle in single suture. Transfixation of suture is a promising step.

The venous blood loss is a widespread ooze from an ill defined area of dissection around a mass or adhesion. It is commonly seen in pelvic floor surgery. To prevent this, the dissection should be preferably blunt in the line of cleavage. If needed tight compression or vaginal packing may be done. In severe cases, packs may be left in for 24 hours with tail ends eggressing from abdominal or vaginal wounds. The risk of ureteric injury while re-exploration is high. Internal iliac ligation is recommended in case of intractable internal hemorrhage.

Reactionary Hemorrhage

It is a form of prolonged primary hemorrhage occurring on the operative day which is masked originally by the hypotensive effect of anesthetic drug or anesthesia. When BP reverts to normal, vasodilatation occurs and the ooze starts. It can be minimized by careful surgical technique without overlooking the factors of hypotension. At times simple packing fails. Reopening in theater to secure a small bleeding vessel is required after hematoma evacuation.

Secondary Hemorrhage

It occurs mostly from seventh to tenth postoperative day. The underlying cause is sepsis which erodes the vessel and bleeding starts from infected granulation tissue. The hemorrhage starts as dirty discharge and proceeds to form dark clots of recent past followed by fresh red profuse bleeding leading to hemodynamic instability and shock. The management is always vigorous. Broad spectrum IV antibiotic therapy is instituted with anerobic cover till culture sensitivity report is available. The sutures are ineffective due to infected tissue so tight compression achieves hemostasis to tide over the emergency till sepsis settles. Occasionally, descending cervical artery may require ligation through a deep bite.

Blood Transfusion

The properly crossmatched blood or its components are transfused in situations of hemodynamic instability, especially where intravascular volume is poor and patient is in collapsed state. In combating shock the blood transfusion is life saving. It increases the oxygen carrying capacity of the blood by the addition of red cells and restores blood volume, raises plasma proteins and thereby the osmotic pressure of circulating blood. It provides valuable clotting factors like platelets and prothrombin precursors.

Blood transfusion involves many risks. It should be used judiciously. While awaiting blood transfusion or where estimated requirement is one unit only, it is better to use Ringer lactate or plasma volume expander (Hemaccel or Hetastarch, a low molecular weight infusion). Overloading is avoided by noting any engorgement of jugular veins, increased pulse rate, cyanosis, dyspnea, dry cough and tightness in the chest.

The hemorrhage which is exteriorized, gets an early treatment but concealed intraperitoneal bleeding though insidious may be neglected till it becomes massive. Extra peritoneal hemorrhage is usually moderate leading to hematoma formation and presents as a boggy mass in the broad ligament, iliac fossa, renal fossa or abdominal wall.

Intra-abdominal hemorrhage can be massive presenting as abdominal pain which either localizes to lower abdomen or becomes generalized. Later on moderate ileus, vomiting and shock may result. When massive, it may ascend under diaphragm and irritate phrenic nerve to give shoulder pain. The ultrasonography can diagnose it early. The intraperitoneal hemorrhage affects pulse and BP much more than extraperitoneal hemorrhage which is self limiting. In that case, mass is localized with well defined boundaries or takes a definitive route of extension except for retroperitoneal hemorrhage which occurs quickly to produce shock.

Shock: It is a condition of collapse often due to various reasons.

Hemorrhagic shock: It is a hypovolumic shock that appears quickly after surgery. The temperature may remain subnormal. There are no GIT disturbances or toxic features. The response to IV fluid infusion and blood transfusion is good. The definite treatment is to control hemorrhage and restore intravascular volume. Adequate oxygen is given till breathing is normalized. There is risk of acute renal failure with irreversible shock becoming fatal.

Septic (endotoxic) shock: It is due to liberation of endotoxins from Gram negative bacteria into the blood stream from the septic foci. The generalized peritonitis in septic abortion cases is the common cause in gynecological field. There is typical livid gray hue with shallow respiration. The pallor is absent but looks are toxic resulting in hyperpyrexia. There is no recovery even if central venous pressure is maintained rather overinfusion aggravates cardiotoxic effect of septicemia. The blood culture reveals offending organisms. High doses of hydrocortisone and antibiotics are given. Where conservative methods to treat septic abortion or puerperal sepsis fail, emergency hysterectomy may be life saving. The risk of renal failure over infusion, electrolyte imbalance and disseminated intravascular coagulation is high. Clostridial infection is very fatal though not common.

Neurogenic shock: There is dyspnea with massive collapse associated with venous pooling and reduced cardiac output. The sweating is absent and limbs are warm. The modern anesthesia eliminates the risk of this shock.

Gastrointestinal Tract Complications

Slight postoperative nausea and vomiting (PONV) is due to anesthetic agent and is not alarming. The incessant vomiting due to paralytic ileus resulting from pelvic hematoma, peritonitis, bladder, rectal injury or hypokalemia is dangerous. It initially contains gastric contents, later on bile and lastly becomes offensive dark colored or fecal. It is effortless, associated with fall in BP. The patient becomes febrile. There occurs electrolyte imbalance due to depletion of water and electrolytes. The causative factor is treated vigorously. No bowel stimulant as soap water enema should be given till the condition has reversed and bowel sounds have reappeared. The lower bowel can be emptied of flatus by flatus tube and thereafter a small disposable enema can be given.

Intestinal Obstruction

It is due to kinking of gut or adhesions with the pelvic organs or due to involvement of gut in pelvic mass or hematoma or through herniation from a hole formed by adhesions or band. Mechanical obstruction needs immediate surgical intervention. This is clinically suspected when patient after surgery complains of severe colicky abdominal pain and has visible peristalsis with loud and exaggerated bowel sounds in gut proximal to the site of obstruction. Some degree of abdominal distension and vomiting of gastric or bilious contents is present. In case of partial obstruction the condition may settle down with time with expectant treatment. Postoperative acute dilatation of the stomach is, however rare, but very serious complication requiring immediate deflation of stomach with Ryle's tube and intensive management with restoration of fluid balance. The onset is heralded by upper abdominal distension and copious vomiting of dark colored fluid. The gynecologist should be well versed to do end to end anastomosis of gut after resection. The gastroenterological surgeon may be called for if needed.

In cases of intestinal injury, fecal fistula of the bowel and abdominal wall may be formed. If it is small bowel communication, local care and systemic support is required to limit peritonitis development till patient is fit to stand resection and end to end anastomosis in second phase by repeat surgery. Large bowel fistulas may spontaneously heal avoiding surgery unless patient is deteriorating. Fecal peritonitis is a real alarming situation requiring emergency laparotomy.

Pulmonary Complications

The upper respiratory tract infection such as acute/chronic bronchitis or pneumonitis should be treated vigorously prior to elective surgery, especially if planned under general anesthesia.

Postoperative bronchitis appears as severe and persistent cough with expectoration. The accompanying dyspnea is troublesome until treated with vigorous medical therapy.

Mendelson syndrome (adult respiratory syndrome) following inhalation of regurgitated gastric contents during anesthesia is diagnosed as acute respiratory distress with cyanosis due to bronchospasm and pulmonary edema. It may lead to hypotension, cardiovascular collapse and may be fatal.

Lung collapse due to blockage with tenacious mucous plug presents as dyspnea, constriction in chest and cyanosis of varying degree. The patient becomes febrile with resultant tachycardia. The chest on affected side has restricted movement with reduced air entry. The trachea and mediastinum may be displaced ipsilaterally. The diagnosis can be confirmed on chest radiography. Ventilatory support is required under good antibiotic cover.

Lung abscess, pleurisy and empyema are fortunately not common due to good case selection, improved anesthesia techniques and prophylactic antibiotic cover. Oxygen inhalation, suction, bronchodilators, bronchoscopy and lavage with normal saline or bicarbonate are advised. Heavy dose of hydrocortisone 200–800 mg is given immediately and repeated every 4 hours till acute phase is over.

Air embolism occurs usually when a bolus of air is pumped unintentionally into circulation that proves fatal within 10 minutes due to coronary or cerebral artery blockage or sudden cardiac arrest. This may happen while doing tubal patency test, creating pneumoperitoneum for laparoscopy, forcible pumping of blood or IV fluids, or criminal abortion cases.

Urinary Tract Complications

Urinary infection: It is commonly seen after vaginal surgery, prolonged or intermittent repeated catheterization, bladder surgery or extensive gynecological cancer surgery. The injury to the urethral mucosa while catheterization should be avoided as infection enters easily. In case of poor voiding after surgery or after extensive bladder dissection, residual urinary volume is increased resulting in cystitis. It presents as hypogastric pain, frequency of micturition and other lower urinary tract symptoms (LUTS). Urinary specimen reveals mostly *Escherichia coli* organisms. However, appropriate urinary antibiotic is instituted after culture/sensitivity report.

Occasionally, the infection may ascend to cause acute pyelonephritis. The patient is acutely ill with high fever with rigors, vomiting and anorexia. The pain is localized in loin and renal angle is tender to palpate. The management is conservative with hydration and appropriate antibiotics.

When residual volume of urine increases and detrusor action is weak, acute retention of urine may occur. This happens after pelvic floor dissection in prolapse, bladder dissection in cesarean section, hysterectomy for cervical fibroid or after tight vaginal packing after surgery. Catheterization with self retaining Foley catheter is recommended in these situations till ambulation of patient restores normal detrusor activity and micturition.

Retention of urine with overflow can be suspected when patient is voiding small amount of urine frequently over and above the full bladder. Urge incontinence due to abnormal detrusor activity is responsible for precipitancy and incontinence. It is caused by post-catheterization urethrotrigonitis.

Stress incontinence is a spill of small amount of urine during the acts of coughing and sneezing with raised intra-abdominal pressure. It may result after overzealous surgery on bladder neck while repairing anterior vaginal wall prolapse.

True incontinence of urine is a continuous dribbling due to bladder wall injury resulting in urinary fistula or urethral incompetence. Bladder drill is recommended for small capacity bladder while true vesicovaginal fistula should be repaired surgically.

Iatrogenic injuries to bladder and ureter are known to occur in gynecological practice.

Bladder injury, if recognized at the time of surgery, should be repaired immediately with continuous catheterization for 10–14 days under antibiotic cover. If unrecognized, urinary peritonitis occurs due to urinary leakage intra-abdominally. The catheterized specimen of urine from bladder is scanty and blood stained. Immediate laparotomy is indicated with repair of injury and peritoneal lavage followed by continuous catheterization per urethra for 14–21 days. It has fatal consequences, if neglected. Ischemic fistula formation is due to necrosis after denudation of blood supply while dissecting, especially during gynecological cancer surgery. The urinary leakage tracks down to trickle through vaginal vault from seventh to twelfth postoperative day and thus diagnosis is confirmed.

The same reasons apply to ureteric injury but eludes immediate recognition on many occasions. The surgeon must revise anatomical relationships in cases of high risk vulnerable situations and avoid ureteric involvement in incision, ligation (partial or complete) and excision of a segment. As a result of ischemic necrosis it may be ureterovaginal or ureterocervical fistula formation. If single ureter is involved patient passes the urine normally also in some amounts and leaks partially while in cases of bilateral involvement, bladder is empty.

If ureter is included in a ligature, ureteric obstruction causes back pressure changes as hydroureter and hydronephrosis which reverts once the obstruction is removed. The most likely surgery to involve ureters is for cervical fibroid or carcinoma cervix. The superadded urinary infection is prevented by antibiotic therapy.

The periureteric fibrosis as a result of spontaneous healing of ureteric fistula, urinoma or recurrent malignant infiltration is other cause of ureteric obstruction. It may silently progress towards hydronephrosis leading to renal atrophy.

Single ureter involvement is more common than bilateral involvement. In latter situation, there occurs complete anuria after surgery, so no urine is obtained on catheterization. The surgeon must review the operative steps to know the cause of anuria whether surgical or medical due to acute renal failure.

The preoperative evaluation of high-risk factors, IV pyelography and ultrasound of urinary tract provide reliable information for diagnosis of this complication.

Acute renal failure can occur due to shock of hemorrhagic or endotoxic variety. However, oliguria progressing toward anuria needs serial renal function tests for prognostic value. Nephrologist/urosurgeries help is co-opted for management of ACN or uretretic injuries.

PHLEBOTHROMBOSIS AND PULMONARY EMBOLISM

Pulmonary embolism is a dangerous complication leading to definite morbidity and mortality, if left unrecognized. Though small venous thrombi may pass unnoticed yet massive embolism may occur in 0.10% cases of abdominal hysterectomy (lesser with vaginal surgery). The factors contributing to this are venous stasis, recumbent position, lithotomy position with compression and angulation of veins at hip and knee joint, increased blood coagulability, elderly age and prolonged surgical trauma, as in cases of advanced cancer surgery.

The thrombus originates in deep veins of soleus muscle where there is a complex series of vascular arcades. Near the upper end of thigh there is a confluence of several large veins so local stasis is marked. The thrombus is friable, grows rapidly and has little or no local intimal anchorage. It travels rapidly into the blood stream to reach cardiopulmonary site.

There are no local signs unless suspected. The persistent small rise in temperature and pulse rate on 3rd day, aches or pain in lower limbs, calf tenderness, popliteal fossa pain or pain in thigh are elicitable. The flexion and extension of ankle joints may elicit pain (Homan's sign). The duplex ultrasound study of calf muscle blood flow can be done to reach at the diagnosis. Once the thrombus is dislodged, it passes via the vena cava and right heart to pulmonary arterial tree.

If clot is small, it produces small infarcts in the lungs. The diagnosis is eluded as pneumonitis with signs and symptoms of slight chest pain, moderate cyanosis, dyspnea or pleural effusion with blood stained sputum occurs.

If the clot is large, signs and symptoms are dramatic like intense pain in chest, acute dyspnea, cyanosis, rapid pulse and shock. If clot is massive, it is fatal in a very short time with profuse hemoptysis, gasping and collapse.

The prophylactic treatment recommended is low molecular weight dextran infusion or low molecular weight heparin. Early leg movements, ambulation, physiotherapy, avoidance of dehydration and tight binders for varicose veins are advocated.

Superficial Thrombophlebitis

It is an inflamed condition of superficial leg veins which are palpable as tender cord like structures. The clot formed in these veins has a firm internal anchorage and has no risk of detachment to form pulmonary embolism. There is risk of veins of wrist or elbow to be inflamed at the injection site for IV infusions.

WOUND COMPLICATIONS

Wound healing may be defective. The wound exudation may be serous, serosanguinous or purulent discharge continuing for days or months. The underlying unabsorbable suture is removed, if detected. The chronic sinus track needs exploration, granulation tissue scraping, excision and repeated antiseptic dressings. The sinuses may be multiple and nonhealing. Rare events of tubercular nonhealing sinuses responding to antitubercular therapy have been reported.

Wound sepsis may be the cause of burst abdomen in second postoperative week with gut and omentum peeping through the incision line for which emergency single layer closure and resuturing is performed.

A vigilant surgeon will observe precautionary measures against all the factors affecting wound healing like malnourishment, anemia, chronic disease, diabetes, malignancy, sepsis, especially in elderly patients who are obese and hypertensive. Massive corticoid therapy promotes sepsis and delays wound healing.

The surgical technique and suture material used for wound closure is improvised so that wound dehiscence, hematoma formation, stitch abscess and sinus formation is prevented.

Incisional hernia is due to herniation of abdominal contents, usually gut and omentum, through a gap of rectus sheath, as a result of partial or complete wound dehiscence. Postoperative complications like coughing, vomiting, etc. resulting in raised intra-abdominal pressure complicate the pre-existing poor wound healing. It is a major cause of discomfort rather than strangulation of gut. Repair of the hernia and strengthening with inlay or sublay of prosthetic mesh is indicated as an elective procedure at a later date.

Emphysema of abdominal wall occurring due to infiltration of gas in the layers of abdominal wall at the time of creation of pneumoperitoneum during laparoscopy needs observation as it gets absorbed spontaneously.

Vaginal vault disruption: A small rent in vaginal vault may be observed by local sepsis but usually healing occurs spontaneously. Herniation of gut into vagina in second postoperative week resulting in intestinal obstruction should be kept in mind as a rare complication. It warrants urgent laparotomy and reclosure of the vault. A fecal fistula through vaginal vault may close spontaneously. Rarely preceeding colostomy followed by definitive surgery may have to be undertaken.

NEUROLOGICAL COMPLICATIONS

Brachial, radial or ulnar palsy occurs due to faulty arm position. The lower limb nerves may be injured due to lithotomy position, exaggerated joint movements of knees and hips in old females who already suffer from osteoporosis. The backache occurs due to jerky positioning resulting in prolapsed intervertebral disc. The nerve entrapment can occur due to malignant infiltration or when surgical dissection is done to remove the obturator lymph nodes or dissect the bladder in the pelvic surgery. Thus femoral nerve, obturator nerve, lumbosacral plexus and bladder nerve supply from sacral two, three and four are at great risk of injury.

FOREIGN BODIES

A surgical mishap is recorded when a sponge, swab or an instrument is left unintentionally intra-abdominally. Patient presents with persistent fever and pain, localized pelvic abscess accompanied by foul smelling discharge per vaginum. Ultrasound examination may reveal a foreign body. An exploratory laparotomy is done to remove it.

Similarly, vaginal swab or pack may be forgotten in vagina. It presents as copious vaginal discharge. Digital exploration is done to remove it.

Late complications or residual sequelae include:

- Recurrent urinary tract infection
- Granulation tissue/prolapsed fallopian tube at vault
- Incisional hernia
- Vault prolapse
- Stress incontinence
- Stump carcinoma after subtotal hysterectomy
- Dyspareunia
- Postoperative psychosis/depression
- Menopausal syndrome
- Chronic pelvic pain
- Obstetrical problems like failed conception/recurrent miscarriage/preterm labor/ectopic pregnancy/sterilization failure
- General ill health and debility.

12.4 POSTOPERATIVE ANALGESIA

Rajni Sundar, C Kumar

INTRODUCTION

Pain is not just a sensory modality but an experience. The international association for the study of pain defines pain as "an unpleasant sensory and emotional experience associated with actual or potential tissue damage or described in terms of such damage".

The incidence of postoperative pain varies with individual patients but is largely governed by the site and nature of the operation. It is a consistent and predominant complaint of most individuals following surgery. The problems associated with pain are inadequate breathing, inadequate cough, and feeling of loss of control of oneself, fear and anxiety.

Postoperative pain is the most common form of acute pain, which is of two types; namely, somatic and visceral, which are differentiated based on origin and features.

Somatic pain arises from skin and deep somatic structures. It is constant, sharp and well-localized. Visceral pain arises from viscera and can be referred to somatic areas. It is colicky, dull to vague and poorly localized.

EFFECTS OF PAIN

Physiological effects of acute pain include various behavioral responses which range from withdrawal from interpersonal contact and reduced activity to seeking attention. It results in fear, anxiety, depression, anger, resentment and sleep deprivation.

Moderate to severe acute pain, regardless of site, can affect nearly every organ function and may adversely influence postoperative morbidity and mortality. Effective postoperative pain management is not only humane but a very important aspect of postoperative care.

Cardiovascular Effects

Pain can cause sympathetic nervous system stimulation with resultant tachycardia, hypertension, increased vascular resistance and increased cardiac output.

Respiratory Effects

Pain stimulates involuntary spinal reflexes causing increased skeletal muscle tone around injury site causing muscle splinting. There is a resultant decrease in respiratory muscle excursion, which indirectly causes reduced vital capacity, functional residual capacity and tidal volume and causes atelectasis. This along with a reduced ability to cough causes hypostatic pneumonia.

Gastrointestinal Effects

Pain-induced sympathetic activity causes increased secretions, increased smooth muscle sphincter tone and decreased gastrointestinal motility, leading to gastric stasis and paralytic ileus.

Genitourinary Effects

Urinary retention from increased bladder sphincter tone from sympathetic overactivity.

Immune Effects

Immune dysfunction leads to an increased occurrence of infective complications.

Metabolic Effects

Pain causes a transient initial hypometabolic phase, followed by a hypermetabolic phase which lasts for days to weeks. There is hyperglycemia, increased lipolysis and increased muscle protein catabolism.

Endocrine Effects

Pain induces an increased secretion of the catabolic hormones like adrenocorticotropic hormone (ACTH), cortisol, glycogen and decreases anabolic hormones like insulin and testosterone.

Hematological Effects

Pain induced stress causes increase in platelet adhesiveness, reduced fibrinolysis and hypercoagulability.

PAIN MEASUREMENT

Many a times pain is inadequately treated due to the lack of reliable objective signs and therefore, clinical assessment of severity of pain is difficult to measure. Assessment is usually the individual's "self report" of severity of pain they are experiencing. Recording of pain improves safety and effectiveness of acute pain management. Pain severity scores should be recorded along with heart rate, respiratory rate, blood pressure, and temperature and sedation score, to make them more effective.

- *Visual analogue scale:* It is a 10 cm line with the left anchor point depicting "no pain" and the right anchor point depicting the "worse possible pain". The patient is asked to mark on this line where the intensity of pain lies. Visual analogue scale (VAS) is simple, efficient and minimally intrusive method. Unfortunately, VAS assumes pain as one-dimensional. It describes intensity but not quality
- *Visual numerical rating scale:* In this scale, patients estimate their pain severity as a number "0" being no pain and "10" being the worst possible pain
- *Categorical rating scale:* It is a verbal method that can employ different predictions of pain—no pain, mild pain, moderate pain and severe pain.

MANAGEMENT

The goal in management of pain is to reduce pain to a tolerable level with minimal or no associated suffering or distress. Individual experience of pain can be reduced if intervention is applied before the application of noxious stimuli. This led to pre-emptive analgesia. The sensitization of nociceptors is reduced by this method. The advantages are that it reduces opioid requirement, allows earlier return to normal activities and results in fewer adverse outcomes.

ANALGESICS

Opioids are the most commonly used drugs for post-operative pain relief. The doses should be individualized and titrated to maximize analgesia and minimize side effects. The dose of the prototype opioid morphine is 0.1–0.2 mg/kg. The commonly used routes of administration are intramuscular or subcutaneous, both of which are safe and appropriate. The adverse effects of opioids are sedation, pruritus, nausea and vomiting, urinary retention, slowing of gastrointestinal function, respiratory depression, allergy tolerance, addiction and euphoria.

Opioid pumps: Infusion pumps are available with many manufacturers in India. Opioids/other drugs can be given at metered doses through the pump. This has the advantage of maintaining the serum drug level within the analgesic range and further attenuates fluctuations in level, resulting in improved analgesia and patient satisfaction without producing unwanted additional side effects.

Morphine: A loading dose of morphine (0.1%) 3–10 mg may be given at an infusion rate of 0.5–1.5 mg/hour.

Fentanyl (0.01%): Loading dose of 30–100 μg/h followed by a basal infusion of 10–20 μg/h.

Pethidine (1%): Loading dose 25–50 mg/h followed by an infusion rate 5–40 mg/h.

Precautions with opioid pumps: In renal insufficiency, decreased excretion of morphine glucuronide may result in increased sedation and respiratory depression. In pre-eclampsia, there is increased risk of sedation with morphine when patient is treated with magnesium sulphate. In hyperbilirubinemia, there is increased incidence of pruritis, possibly due to mast cell degranulation.

Acetaminophen is effective in mild to moderate pain and is usually used as an adjunct to opioids in severe pain. It acts by inhibiting the cyclo-oxygenase enzyme. It has analgesic and antipyretic effect. The dose is 10–15 mg/kg/dose. The usual dose is 325–1,000 mg every 4–6 hours as necessary, not to exceed 4 g daily. The usual routes of administration are oral or rectal. Anticonvulsants that induce hepatic microbial enzymes, including phenytoin, barbiturates and carbamazepine may aggravate acetaminophen-induced hepatotoxicity because of increased conversion of the drug to hepatotoxic metabolites. Usually, no dosage reduction is required in patients taking concomitant therapeutic doses of acetaminophen and anticonvulsants; however, patients should limit acetaminophen use while receiving anticonvulsants.

Nonsteroidal anti-inflammatory drugs (NSAIDs) are used in mild to moderate pain. It decreases opioid requirement and enhances opioid-based analgesia. It is rarely used as a sole agent after major surgery. The preferred routes of administration are oral or intramuscular. Adverse effects of NSAIDs are bronchospasm, gastric ulceration, renal dysfunction and inhibition of platelet function. Usually, administered adult doses are ketorolac 30 mg intramuscularly twice or thrice daily, dioclofenac 75 mg intramuscularly twice or thrice daily, oral diclofenac 50 mg thrice daily. Newer NSAIDs inhibits cyclo-oxygenase 2 enzyme system preferentially. As compared to nonselective NSAIDs, they have reduced gastrointestinal effects but comparable renal and hepatic effects.

Precautions: Conditions associated with dehydration increase the risk of renal toxicity and may impair cardiac function in some patients. All NSAIDs should be used with caution in patients who have impaired renal function, liver disease or congestive heart failure—especially those already receiving angiotensin-converting enzyme (ACE) inhibitors, angiotensin II receptors blockers (ARBs) or diuretics. NSAIDs should generally be avoided in patients who have a history of peptic ulcer disease (PUD) or gastrointestinal bleeding; if absolutely necessary, NSAID use should be limited to the lowest effective dose for the shortest treatment duration. Even without direct exposure, systemic cyclooxygenase type 1 (COX-1) inhibition compromises gastrointestinal protective mechanisms, including mucosal perfusion, bicarbonate production and mucus production, thus predisposing to PUD and upper gastrointestinal bleeding. Cytoprotective agents reduce the risk of NSAID-induced PUD. Proton pump inhibitors (PPIs) (e.g. omeprazole) have the best supporting evidence.

REGIONAL ANESTHESIA

Wound Infiltration

Wound infiltration is maximally effective in small adult wounds. Local anesthetics are used, usually 0.25% bupivacaine.

Ilioinguinal Block

Ilioinguinal and iliohypogastric nerve block is very useful for postoperative pain relief in cesarean section. Block is administered with 8 mL of 0.25% bupivacaine on both sides. A spinal needle is used and the ilioinguinal nerve is infiltrated 3 cm medial to and 3 cm inferior to the anterior superior iliac spine.

It produces excellent postoperative analgesia in postcesarean section patients with onset of analgesia being almost instantaneous. There is no need for supplemental analgesics for the duration of the block.

Neuraxial Blockages

Neuraxial blockages include epidural and intrathecal analgesic techniques which have the potential to improve postoperative analgesia and modify the physiological response to surgery. Neuraxial blocks have proven to reduce postoperative pulmonary morbidity and improve the overall patient outcome. If an epidural catheter is placed, it must be as close as possible to the dermatome affected by surgical incision. Pain relief via neuraxial technique needs safety measures. The patient should be reviewed by the anesthesiologist periodically, protocols should be followed, and nursing staff should receive specific training and education about potential adverse effects. The agents that are commonly used for neuraxial techniques are local anesthetics like 0.25% bupivacaine. Opioids like fentanyl, buprenorphine, butorphanol, etc. and non-opioids like clonidine can be used either alone or in addition with local anesthetics. Adverse effects of neuraxial techniques due to local anesthetics used are hypotension, cardiovascular and central nervous system toxicity. Adverse effects due to opioids are respiratory depression, pruritus, nausea and urinary retention. Problems related to technique are epidural hematoma, abscess formation, meningitis, neurological injury and total spinal.

Multimodal Analgesia

Multimodal analgesia is a balanced analgesia, where pain is managed with a combination of drugs with different modes of action, possibly administered by different routes. The main aim is to achieve improved pain relief with a reduction in side effects. The combination used is a regular acetaminophen with regular NSAIDs and a systemic opioid or a neuraxial technique.

BIBLIOGRAPHY

1. Ballan tyne JC. Use of NSAID for acute pain management probl. Anesth. 1998;10:23.
2. Budd K. Tramadol revisited. Br J Anaesth. 1999;82(4):493-5.
3. Dolin SJ, Cashman JN, Bland JM. Effectiveness of acute postoperative pain management. Br J Anaesth. 2002;89(3): 409-23.
4. Fleming BM, Coombs DW. A survey of complications documented in quality control analysis of PCA. J Pain Symptom Manage. 1992;7(8):463-9.
5. Lehmann LJ, DeSio JM, Radvany T, et al. Transdermal fentanyl in postoperative pain. Res Anesth. 1997;22(1):24-8.
6. Macintyre PE. Safety and efficacy of PCA. Br J Anaesth. 2001;87(1):36-46.
7. Moiniche S, et al. A qualitative and quantitative system review of pre-emptive analgesia for postoperative pain. Anesthesiology. 2002;96:725.
8. Schug SA, Torrie JJ. Safety assessment of postoperative pain management by acute pain service. Pain. 1993;55(3):387-91.
9. Souter AJ, Fredman B, White PF. Controversies in perioperative use of nonsteroidal anti-inflammatory drugs. Anesth Analg. 1994;79(6):1178-90.
10. Thomas V, Heath M, Rose D, et al. Psycological characteristic and effectiveness of patient-controlled analgesia . Br J Anaesth. 1995;74(3):271-6.
11. Tobias MD. Intravenous PCA. Probl Anesth. 1998;10:37.
12. Wu CL, Fleisher LA. Outcomes research in regional anesthesia and analgesia. Anesth Analg. 2000;91(5):1232-42.

CHAPTER

13

Postoperative Infections

Kavita N Singh

INTRODUCTION

Postoperative infections continue to be a significant risk in both the obstetrics and the gynecologic patient. Bacteria present in endogenous microflora of patient's lower genital tract are responsible for majority of pelvic and abdominal wound infections. Prevention requires increased education and awareness of its causes, use of meticulous technique and administration of prophylactic antibiotics. However, other factors which may contribute to the development of infection, such as chronic underlying medical illness, chronic subclinical infections and nutritional status of the patients. Therefore, postoperative infections cannot be entirely eliminated; there effective management in postoperative period demands various skills. Incidence of postoperative infections is 5–8% for all surgeries in obstetrics and gynecology.

RISK FACTORS

There are multiple reasons for postoperative infections which have been validated as risk factors.

PATHOGENS

In more than 90% of the cases, bacteria found among the endogenous microflora of the patient's lower genital tract cause the majority of pelvic and abdominal wound infections. On the basis of genus of bacteria, postoperative infections can be divided into two categories: unimicrobial and polymicrobial.

Unimicrobial infections are most frequently caused by *Streptococcus agalactiae, Escherichia coli, Gardnerella* and *Enterococcus faecalis*.

Polymicrobial infections involve 20% of aerobic Gram-positive cocci, 20% Gram-negative rods and 60% are anaerobes (Box 1).

Box 1 Pathogens responsible for postoperative infection

Aerobic Gram-positive cocci
- *Staphylococcus aureus*
- *Streptococcus viridans* group
- Group *B Streptococcus*
- *Enterococcus*

Aerobic Gram-negative bacilli
- Escherichia coli
- Proteus mirabilis
- Klebsiella species
- Gardnerella vaginalis

Anaerobes
- *Peptostreptococcus species*
- *Peptococcus species*
- *Bacteroides bivius*
- *Bacteroides disiens*
- *Bacteroides melaninogenicus*
- *Bacteroides capillosus*
- *Bacteroides fragilis* group
- *Bacteroides fragilis*
- *Bacteroides ovatus*
- *Bacteroides thetaiotaomicron*
- *Bacteroides distasonis*
- *Bacteroides vulgatus*
- *Clostridium perfringens*
- *Fusobacterium species*

(***Source:*** Bibliography 4)

The microflora of the vaginal ecosystem consists of an array of bacteria that includes Gram-positive and Gram-negative aerobic facultative and obligate anaerobic bacteria. The mean total bacterial counts in vaginal secretion actually approximate 10^8–10^{10} bacteria/mL.

THE VAGINAL ECOSYSTEM

A healthy vaginal ecosystem is characterized by the presence of *Lactobacillus acidophilus*, which is dominant and a major factor in maintaining healthy state. *Lactobacillus acidophilus* produces hydrogen peroxide, lactic acid and bacteriocin, which contribute to the survival of *Lactobacillus acidophilus* and supresses the growth of other pathogens.

The pH of healthy vaginal ecosystem is 3.8–4.2, whenever the vaginal pH is 5 or higher, the growth of *Lactobacillus* is inhibited and the growth of *Gardnerella* is enhanced. This results in further decrease in hydrogen ion and the oxygen concentration, eventually the pH reaches 5 and an anaerobic environment establishes which favors growth of obligate anaerobic bacteria. The pH value listed in Table 1 represents the acidity at which a specific condition is most likely to be present.

The bacteria that constitute the microflora, nonpathogens and pathogens of the healthy vaginal ecosystems most likely act antagonistically, and therefore, influence the growth of one another through the production of lactic acid, bacteriocins and hydrogen peroxide (*Lactobacillus* and *Gardnerella,* obligate anaerobes). Because of the large variety of bacteria, these organisms interact as commensals, synergistically or antagonistically towards one another. These relationships may have significant clinical implications (e.g. postpartum endometritis, pelvis abscesses). Laboratory experiments demonstrated that *E. faecalis* and *Provetella bivia*, placed in the intraperitoneal cavity of the rat, act synergistically to form abscesses. Other combinations of the bacteria, *E.coli* and *Bacteroides fragilis* have been shown to be abscessogenic in a similar model.

Thus, the variety and high numbers of bacteria found in the vaginal ecosystem pose a problem that could place the women's health in jeopardy. The significance lies in the potential for these bacteria to gain entrance to the upper genital tract without causing symptomatic infection. The potential for infection is gaining significance, and its importance lies in the fact that the upper genital tract is often asymptomatic. Recently, Korn and its associates demonstrated that 20% of women with bacterial vaginosis (BV) were found to have asymptomatic endometritis. According to Larson PG et al., whether BV is acquired from an edogenous or an exogenous source is subject to controversy, however, for women undergoing gynecology surgery such as therapeutic abortion, the relative risk of postoperative infections is clearly elevated. A weaker, association exits between *BV* and pelvic inflammatory disease (PID).

In consultation with clinical microbiologist for better results, simple issues like technique, transportation, temperature, and medium should be discussed prior to collection of the sample. Microbiological specimens for culture can be collected from urine, blood, pus, infected tissue or infected operative sites.

Other risk factors include age of the patient, socioeconomic status, type of surgery, site of incision, duration of surgery, use of implants, obesity, concurrent and comorbidities like diabetes mellitus, history of previous surgery, radiotherapy or chemotherapy, prolonged preoperative hospitalization, shaving of the skin, use of inappropriate antibiotic prophylaxis and dressing techniques.

Perioperative anemia appears not to play a large role. There is no support for transfusion to a certain hemoglobin level or hematocrit to promote wound healing. Likewise, there is no evidence that anemia increases the frequency of or severity of postoperative infection.

Table 1: Characteristics of the vaginal ecosystem

Characteristic	Healthy ecosystem	Bacterial vaginosis	Trichomoniasis	Candidiasis	GBS
Discharge color	White to slate gray	Dirty gray	Dirty gray to green	White	White to gray
Consistency	Homogeneous liquid to pasty	Liquid	Liquid	Pasty	Liquid
Odor	None	Fishlike	Foul	None	None
pH	3.8–4.2	≥5	≥5	<4.5	≥4.5
Whiff test	Negative	Positive	±	Negative	Negative
Clue cells	Absent	Positive	±	Negative	Negative

GBS, group B beta-hemolytic streptococci

PREVENTION

Prevention of postoperative infections relies on the following:

- *Preoperative screening of the vaginal ecosystem*: Prior to surgery along with respiratory, cardiovascular and urinary system, lower genital tract should be evaluated for presence of pathogenic bacteria. Screening for vaginitis and vaginosis is relatively simple and inexpensive process. The pH of vaginal system is accomplished by placing a pH indicator strip with color chart on the box or by Gram stained preparation. If diagnosis of bacterial vaginosis is established (by presence of clue cells, pH higher than 4.5) and WBCs are more than 5 per high power field, possibility of other infection should be considered. Once a specific condition is diagnosed, patient should be treated prior to surgery according to Rossaly V Starr et al. Preoperative vaginal scrub with povidone-iodine decreases the incidence of postcesarean endometritis, but does not decrease the overall risk of postoperative fever or wound infection
- *Prophylactic antibiotics usually 30 minutes prior to incision or at the time of induction of anesthesia*
- *Use of meticulous surgical technique*
- *Ensuring hemostasis and judicious use of cautery:* Drain should not be used as alternative to good homeostasis. The closed system of wound drainage is preferred where drainage is essential
- *Gentle handling of tissue, leaving small pedicle and use of fine nonreactive sutures*
- *Remove fat globules and bits of free tissues*
- *Operating theater sterilization* and high level disinfection of instruments, clean environment with adequate ventilation, disinfection of surgeon's hands and operating site are mandatory prior to surgery. In case of concurrent disease, delay operation till the disease is brought under control.

DIAGNOSIS AND TREATMENT

Common postoperative infections are classified in Box 2. Diagnosis of postoperative pelvic infection is difficult because the infected site cannot be sampled. Symptoms and signs of postoperative pelvic infections are listed in Box 3.

Box 2 Obstetric and gynecologic postoperative infections

Pelvic infections
- Pelvic cellulitis
- Vaginal cuff hematoma and/or abscess
- Septic pelvic vein thrombosis
- Postoperative adenexal abscess
- Ligneous cellulitis
- Osteomyelitis pubis
- Incisional wound infections
- Cystitis

Nonpelvic infections
- Pneumonia
- Bacteremia
- Pyelonephritis

(***Source:*** Bibliography 7)

Box 3 Symptoms and signs of a postoperative pelvic infection

Fever
- 100.4°F on two separate occasions measured at least 6 hours apart, or 101°F anytime
- Elevated WBC count >14,000
- Elevated immature polymorphonuclear leukocytes—10%

Postpartum endometritis
- Uterine tenderness
- Parametrial tenderness
- Cervix remains dilated
- Purulent uterine discharge may be present

Posthysterectomy pelvic cellulitis
- Vaginal cuff tenderness
- Mass may be present at vaginal cuff apex
- Purulent discharge from cuff apex

(***Source:*** Bibliography 7)

Pelvic Cellulitis

The patient presents with fever in second to fifth postoperative day after hysterectomy. Other findings are lower abdominal tenderness, peritoneal signs or ileus. Pelvic examinations reveal marked induration but no fluctuant mass. Treatment consists of systemic antimicrobial agents, bed rest, good hydration and other supportive measures.

Vaginal Cuff Hematoma and/or Abscess

The patient presents with fever in early postoperative period with rectal pressure or pelvic pain. Sometimes patients present with a purulent discharge or palpable collection at vaginal cuff.

Drainage by simple digital palpation or needle aspiration of vault responds rapidly. Antimicrobials are usually added along with drainage.

Septic Pelvic Thrombophlebitis

Septic pelvic thrombophlebitis is almost always diagnosis of exclusion in patient with postoperative febrile morbidity, not responding to antimicrobial therapy. Abdominal and pelvic findings are normal, there is no evidence of abscess on pelvic examination, ultrasonography or computed tomography (CT) scan, patients only presents with fever and tachycardia. A partial pressure of oxygen (PO_2), if less than 80 mm Hg in a nonsmoker, supports the diagnosis. Patient is treated by full heparin anticoagulation for a week, a dramatic response is observed within 24–48 hours of start of therapy.

If associated with pulmonary embolism, coumadin (warfarin sodium) is considered as additional long-term therapy, antimicrobial therapy mainly clindamycin, metronidazole, cefoxitin are used.

Postoperative Adnexal Abscess

Adnexal abscess presents with fever and abdominal pain late in the postoperative period along with a tender palpable adnexal mass.

Ultrasonography or CT scan confirms the diagnosis. Infection is mainly caused by *B. fragilis* in premenopausal women. Usually patients respond to clindamycin or metronidazole. In case of no response in 48–72 hours or mass increases in size, laparotomy is necessary for removal of the abscess.

A pelvic abscess can be drained by colpotomy if mass is fluctuant, adheres to parietal pelvic peritoneum and dissects into the midline of the upper one-third of the rectovaginal septum.

Ligneous Pelvic Cellulitis

A pelvic cellulitis with unremitting fever and widespread, tender induration of pelvis, which on examination is firm "woody on feel". Due to effective use of anaerobic antimicrobials, this condition is only of historical interest.

Osteomyelitis Pubis

Osteomyelitis of the pubis is a rare infection resulting from bacteremic seeding or extension of a contagious focus of infection. Usually, it occurs after surgeries like urethral suspension, radical vulvectomy or pelvic exentrations. Patient presents, with pubic bone pain, low grade fever, avoidance of ambulation and pain on abduction usually after 8 weeks of surgery, leukocytosis, elevated erythrocyte sedimentation rate and/or alkaline phosphatase level are present.

Antimicrobials covering *Staphylococcus aureus* and aerobic Gram-negative bacteria are used, oral quinolone group of antimicrobials are also used. Surgical debridement may be necessary.

Incisional Wound Infections

Incisional wound infections can be subclassified according to their clinical onset.

Early onset wound infection, is caused by group A β *hemolytic streptococci* or group B beta *hemolytic streptococci.* This rare infection responds to high dose of parenteral penicillin.

Late onset wound infection, most of these wound infections become apparent on fifth to seventh postoperative day. A fever with single high spike in afternoon or early morning is common presentation. Treatment consists of drainage, irrigation, dressing and systemic antimicrobials.

Necrotizing Fasciitis

Necrotizing fasciitis is also known as clostridial cellulitis, anaerobic cutaneous gangrene, synergistic necrotizing cellulitis, gangrenous erysipelas, hospital gangrene or acute dermal gangrene. Infection of subcutaneous tissues spreads in fascial clefts overlying deep fascia. Patient presents with pain and edema, skin is usually normal looking making early recognition difficult and causing fatal delaying appropriate treatment. A dishwater-like drainage from incision is typical of necrotizing fasciitis. In spite of minimal local findings, patients appear severely ill. Treatment includes broad spectrum antibiotic therapy and radical debridement to include removal of all necrotic and pale tissue. The reported mortality rate from necrotizing fasciitis is 21–76% more commonly seen in diabetics.

Cystitis

Cystitis usually takes place if appropriate care is not taken while catheterization or when urinary output is less than 2500 mL in 24 hours. Patient presents with fever with chills and rigor, pain and tenderness over hypogastrium. Antimicrobials should be started as per urine culture and sensitivity report. Methenamine hippurate prophylaxis effectively reduces postoperative urinary tract infection.

Early Onset Pyrexia

Noninfectious Causes

Most of the early postoperative fevers are noninfectious in origin. The cause of early, unexplained fever remains ill-defined. Possible causes are hypersensitivity reactions to anesthetic and other medications and pulmonary atelectasis. Physiologic response, intraoperative tissue trauma or hematoma formation causes release of pyrogenic substances into circulation. Extravasation of urine after unrecognized ureteral damage at surgery may result in high spiking fever in early postoperative period.

Infectious Causes

It includes pneumonia, contaminated intravenous infusions, *group B beta hemolytic streptococcal* wound infections, pelvic infections after manipulation, operative manipulation and early onset sepsis.

Late Onset Pyrexia

Febrile illness in late postoperative period is usually due to an adnexal abscess, wound infection or rarely osteomyelitis pubis. Transfusion associated infection in cases where patient has received blood transfusions (hepatitis B; non-A, non-B hepatitis, hepatitis C, malaria, brucellosis, human immunodeficiency virus (HIV), cytomegalovirus or Epstein-Barr virus).

Treatment Choice for Gynecologic Infections

Knowledge of appropriate, effective antimicrobial regimens is essential for treating these infections (Table 2).

Prophylactic antimicrobials have best results if given in well-defined short period beginning with the incision and lasting for about 3 hours. Earlier, administration is unnecessary and undesirable, but when surgery is delayed or prolonged, a second dose may be advisable. First generation cephalosporins have been widely used for prophlaxis in gynecologic surgery. Cefazolin, because of its longer half-life than other first generation cephalosporin, is the cephalosporin of choice.

Table 2: Treatment choices for gynecologic infections

Type of infections	Treatment choice		
	Recommended regimen		Penicillin allergy
Postoperative Mild to moderate	Extended-spectrum Cephalosporins or Extended-spectrum Penicillins	Clindamycin + Gentamicin	Clindamycin + Gentamicin
Severe	Clindamycin + Gentamicin	Clindamycin + Gentamicin	Clindamycin + Gentamicin
Pelvic abscess	Clindamycin + Gentamicin, or Metronidazole + Gentamicin	Reevaluate need for surgical drainage	Clindamycin + Gentamicin, or Metronidazole + Gentamicin
Staphylococcal infections (e.g. toxic shock syndrome or severe staphylococcal wound infection)	Nafcillin or oxacillin	Consultation indicated	Vancomycin

(*Source:* Bibliography 4)

BIBLIOGRAPHY

1. Korn AP, Bolan G, Padran N, et al. Plasma cell endometritis in women with symptomatic bacterial vaginosis. Obstet Gynecol. 1995;85:387.
2. Larson PG, Bargstorm M, Forsum U, et al. Bacterial vaginosis transmission role in genital tract infection and pregnancy outcome: an enigma: Apmis. 2005;113(4):233-45.
3. Martens MG, Fara S, Phillips Le, et al. Female genital tract abscess formation in the rate: use of pathogens including enterococci. J Reprod Med. 1993;38:719.
4. Mead PB. Postoperative Infections. In: Johnes HW, Rock JA (Eds). Telinde's operative gynecology, 9th edition. Lippincott Williams/ Wilkins Company; 2003. pp. 195-207.
5. Onderdonk AB, Kasper DL, Mansheim BJ, et al. Experimental animal models for anaerobic infections: Rev Infect Dis. 1979;1:291.
6. Schioz HA, Tanbo TG. Postoperative voiding, bacteriurea and urinary tract infection with Foley catheterization after gynecological surgery. Acta Obstetricia of Gynecolgic Scandinavia. 2006;85(4):476-81.
7. Sebastian F. Postoperative infections. In: Gershenson DM, Decherney AH, Curry, SL (Eds). Operative gynecology. WB Saunders; 2001. pp. 123-31.
8. Starr RV, Zurawski J, Ismail M. Preoperative vaginal preparation with povidone-iodine and the risk of postcesarean endometritis obstetrics and gynecology. Obstet Gynecol. 2005;105:1024-9.

CHAPTER

14

Sepsis

Randhir Puri, V Chandra, Umesh Gupta

14.1 SEPSIS IN OBSTETRICS

Randhir Puri, V Chandra

INTRODUCTION

Sepsis is an infection-induced syndrome defined as the presence of two or more of the following features of systemic inflammation: fever or hypothermia, leukocytosis or leukopenia, tachycardia, and tachypnea or supranormal minute ventilation. Sepsis is noted to be severe when the organ system begins to fail sequentially or collectively because of widespread inflammatory process. Worldwide, 30% of puerperal cases in some form will develop sepsis of which only 15% will go onto have severe sepsis with the shock syndrome, having mortality as high as 30–40%. The importance of this condition to be examined in detail comes from the fact that even in the United States more than 500,000 patients develop sepsis and only 55–65% survive.

HISTORICAL PERSPECTIVE

Sepsis is one of the earliest complications which began to glaringly show up during the initial phase of the concept of lying in hospitals. There were times in history when epidemics of sepsis set up in such hospitals in females after parturition. The first such epidemic recorded is the epidemic of puerperal fever occurred at the Hôtel-Dieu de Paris in 1646. At that point of time, the mortality due to sepsis in hospitals came to the tune of 25% with an almost 100% mortality on those this devil had set in.

Many physicians began to suspect lack of hygiene and contagion as a cause. In 1795, Alexander Gordon of Aberdeen, Scotland, suggested that the fevers were infectious processes, that physicians were the carrier and that "I myself was the means of carrying the infection to a great number of women". In 1843, Oliver Wendell Holmes published the controversial, "*The Contagiousness of Puerperal Fever*", stating the same. In 1844, Ignaz Semmelweis, an assistant lecturer in the first obstetric division of the Vienna hospital saw the connection between autopsies done in the hospital and the rise of sepsis. He ordered that all doctors and students working in the first division wash their hands in chlorinated lime solution before starting ward work and later, before each vaginal examination. The results were almost like magic: mortality rate from puerperal fever in the division fell from 18% in May, 1847 to less than 3% in June–November of the same year. Even with result saying on its face the effectiveness of his method, he was the subject of ridicule till his somewhat shocking death with the same devil he intend to eliminate: septicemia. His efforts were later used once people recognized his efforts. In 1879, Louis Pasteur showed that *Streptococcus* was present in the blood of women with puerperal fever. By the turn of the century, the need for antiseptic techniques was widely accepted and their practice along with the mid-century introduction of new antibiotics greatly diminished the rate of death during childbirth. In today's scenario, because of the precautionary measures taken, the arsenal of antibiotics sepsis is the exception than the rule in a well-governed hospital. Cases of sepsis mainly are caused by quacks and unhygienic home deliveries presently.

DEFINITION

Sepsis is considered to be present, if infection is highly suspected or proven and two or more of the following systemic inflammatory response syndrome (SIRS) criteria are met:

- Heart rate greater than 90 beats/min
- Body temperature less than 36°C (96.8°F) or greater than 38°C (100.4°F)
- Hyperventilation (high respiratory rate) greater than 20 breaths/min or, on blood gas, a partial pressure of carbon dioxide in the blood ($PaCO_2$) less than 32 mm Hg
- White blood cell count less than 4,000 cells/mm^3 or greater than 12,000 cells/mm^3 ($< 4 \times 10^9$ or $> 12 \times 10^9$ cells/L), or greater than 10% band forms (immature white blood cells).

RECENT UNDERSTANDING OF SEPSIS AND ITS PATHOPHYSIOLOGY (FLOW CHART 1)

The organisms causing sepsis can be endogenous or exogenous. Endogenous organisms are the normal inhabitants present in and around the reproductive region which attacks on alteration of environment or due to lowering of resistance in the case of trauma (uterus after birth can be considered as one huge gaping wound) or the presence of debris can lead to the attack by these otherwise silent organisms like the *Escherichia coli,* anaerobic streptococci, *Chlorella welchii,* etc. Exogenous, on the other hand, are those organisms who are being introduced into the site from external source by processes like repeated vaginal examinations. These organisms like the hemolytic Streptococci and the *Staphylococcus pyogenes* bask in the blood in the highly vascularized uterus and the adjoining areas causing sepsis.

Bacteriology of Sepsis

- Anaerobic Streptococci
- *S. pyogenes*
- Non-hemolytic Streptococci
- *Streptococcus viridans*
- *E. coli*
- Group A Streptococci
- *Cl. welchii*
- *Fecalis*
- Pneumococci
- Gonococci.

Predisposing Factors (Flow chart 2)

- Home birth in unhygienic conditions
- Low socioeconomic status
- Anemia
- Primiparity
- Prolonged rupture of membranes
- Prolonged labor
- Multiple vaginal examinations
- Obstetric maneuvers.

Flow chart 1: Pathophysiology of sepsis

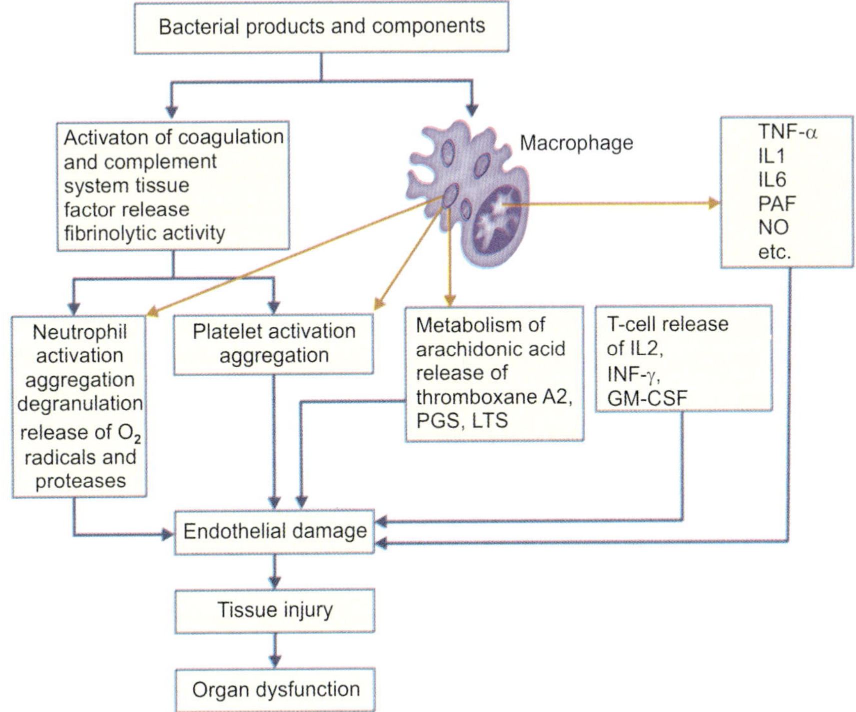

Changing bacteriology is a cause of concern in this Scenario, increased with the emergence of resistance due to exposure to inadequate dosage of antibiotics and multistep resistance over a period of time. An example to this is the increasing concern of *Staphylococcus* resistance. The stand of penicillins in today's management is somewhat expressed in the following lines "Fewer bugs are nowadays sensitive to penicillins and fewer patients that are not!"

The picture of sepsis is dependent on the following details:

- Patient general resistance
  - State of blood
  - State of anemia and malnutrition
  - State of general health.
- Initial state of tissues locally at beginning of puerperium (effects of trauma)
- Organism and their virulence, as well the nature of inflammatory response.

These days, sepsis is seen in the light of a proinflammatory and procoagulant response to invading pathogens. To understand this concept, we may probe further into the concept.

In our body, a potent enzyme cascade system exists, which enables us to protect ourselves from microbial invasions (Fig. 1). A deficient immunologic defense may

Flow chart 2: Predisposing factors in sepsis

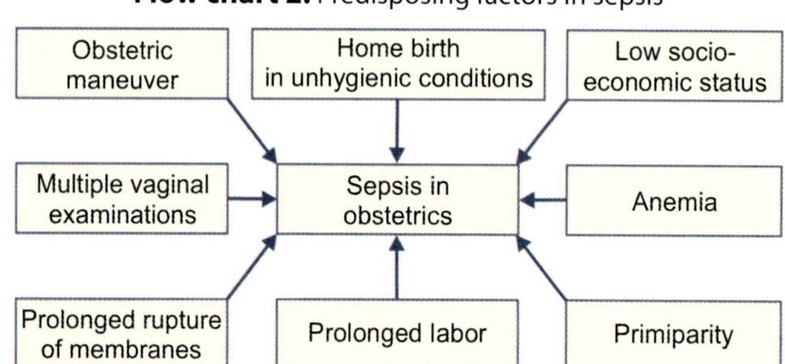

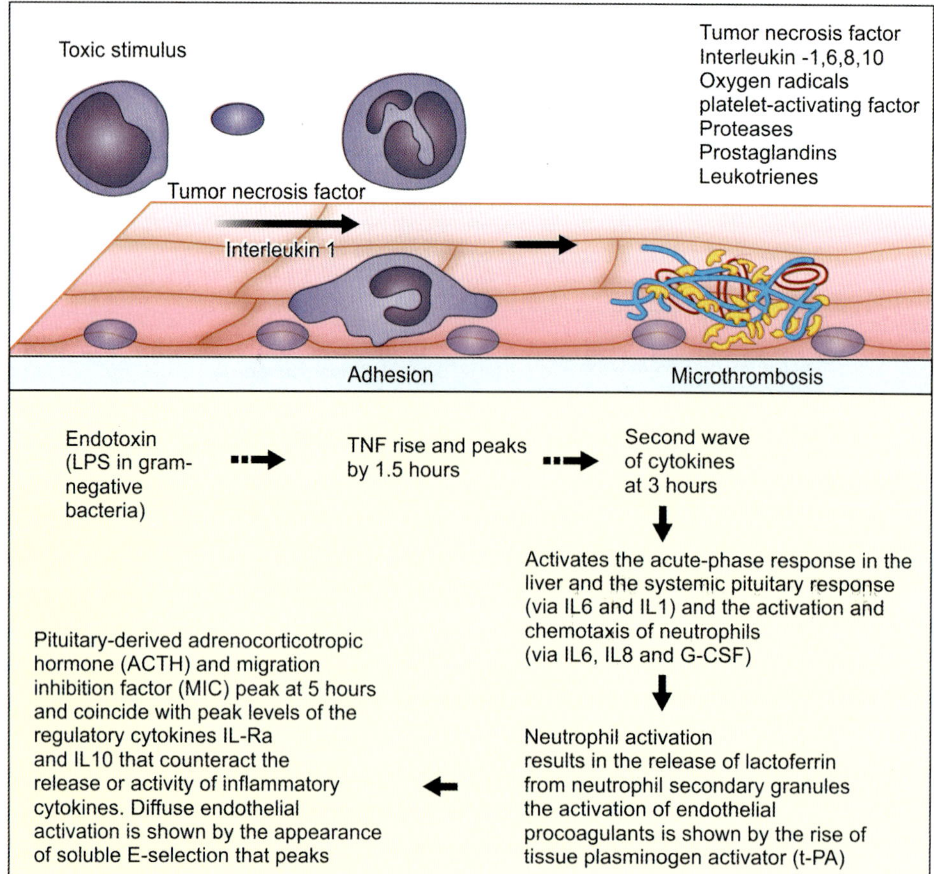

Fig. 1: Inflammatory cascade during sepsis

allow infection to get established; however, an excessive or poorly regulated response may harm the host through a maladaptive release of endogenously generated inflammatory compounds.

The key players in this game are cytokines which are:

- Host produced
- Pleomorphic
- Immunoregulatory peptides.

These cytokines can be divided into two kinds: *anti-inflammatory* and *proinflammatory*. In the anti-inflammatory category we have the *interleukin 6* and *interleukin 10,* while on the other side we have *tumor necrosis factor, interleukin 1* and *interleukin 8*. When a trigger, in this case a microbial toxin is introduced, tumor necrosis factor and interleukin 1 comes into play by initiating endothelial cell–leukocyte adhesion, release of proteases and arachidonate metabolites, and activation of clotting. Like adding oil to fire, the interleukin 8 comes into play as a neutrophil chemotaxin as well as perpetuating the inflammation. Interleukin 6 and interleukin 10, which are perhaps counter regulatory, inhibit the generation of tumor necrosis factor, augment the action of acute-phase reactants and immunoglobulins, and inhibit T-lymphocyte and macrophage function.

An excessive trip of balance in favor of the proinflammatory enzymes causes a severe reaction in the body in the form of sepsis, which on progression goes into organ failure simultaneously into a multiorgan manifestation finally into the exhaustion of the anti-inflammatory enzymes (especially, in protein C) leading to mortality.

With this understanding, we now will review sepsis in three stages:

- Stage 1: SIRS—the war cry of the body towards the sepsis
- Stage 2: Severe sepsis with organ failure predisposing to end organ failure
- Stage 3: Septic shock, where sepsis is present with refractory hypotension.

CLINICAL ASPECT OF SEPSIS

An interesting old dictum in the course of sepsis is that rather than the site from which it begins, it is the organism which gives the initial clinical picture. A few examples will explain this feature.

In case the initial organism which was causing the sepsis was Streptococci, the local response will not be overt. In this case, the increase in pulse rate will be much more when compared with the simultaneous increase in temperature. Moreover, in vessels of uterus infected thrombi are also seen. This is in sharp contrast to *E. coli* where a large abscess is seen locally.

S. pyogenes is notorious for multiple small abscesses, septicemia and metastatic infection while *S. viridans* gets more involved in vegetation formation in heart valves, especially in rheumatic or in heart with congenital heart disease.

Features that lead to anaerobic Streptococci as the culprit begins with history of trauma (e.g. laceration of cervix, opening up of tissues of parametrium, retained products of conception). An offensive lochia with induration of pelvic cellular tissue, consistency of which is being compared to that of plaster of Paris, is what we see. It also has the propensity of affecting the veins of pelvic organs leading to gross thrombophlebitis with a popular manifestation of pyemic abscess in lungs.

Clostridium welchii is an organism which is the natural inhabitant in a healthy vagina, starts acting only when there is traumatized and devitalized tissue present or when there is a dead fetus retained in utero. It leads to hemolysis and formation of gas with tissue emphysema and foamy liver.

Whatever be the organism and wherever be its site of action, in initiation, the real trouble begins when the body fails to regulate its inflammatory process. This process is seen in a majority of patients; to begin with lung dysfunction or shock. If it is the lung dysfunction which manifests, it occurs early and it persists in sharp contrast to shock, though can also occur early do resolve rapidly if the patient is to resolve from the sepsis. After several hours to days, there can be severe abnormalities of liver function, coagulation and central nervous system and these too may persist for intermittent periods.

Besides the number of organ failures, the severity of each failure affects the prognosis. For example, the lower the partial pressure of oxygen in the case of respiratory failure and the higher serum creatinine, in the case of renal failure, the prognosis certainly goes from bad to worse. This being the case, as a comfort for the treating physician, it is also seen that in survivors of sepsis, the majority of organ failures resolve within one month.

Now, we will take a close look into the actual compromises each system takes when it comes in the dark effects of sepsis; firstly, the lungs. Sepsis plays extreme demands on the lung requiring a high minute ventilation. The compliance of the respiratory system is diminished, airway resistance is increased and muscle efficiency is impaired. Even if arterial oxygen levels are shown to be normal, an increase of respiratory rate to 30 breaths/min or above is to be taken as impending ventilatory collapse. Radiographic evidence of pulmonary edema is at times mistaken for worsening pneumonia or heart failure.

Next in line is the cardiovascular system, which manifests as shock, leading to inadequate supply or inappropriate use of metabolic substrates resulting in lactic acidosis and tissue damage. The necessary circulation required for normal maintenance is decided by several indexes like mentation, urinary output, skin perfusion, and serum lactic dehydrogenase. Even though this is the case, we arbitrarily take blood pressure as the defining criteria for shock—a very imprecise method as the vasoactive drugs and fluids normalize blood pressure without correcting the defect.

Volume depletion results from reduced oral intake, increased losses (e.g. due to bleeding, vomiting, sweating, tachypnea and increased vascular permeability) and increased venous capacitance. Even if this volume is replete, hypotension can still persist due to the low systemic vascular resistance. Also, there can be reduction in myocardial contractility with the presence of myocardial depressant factors present in blood of patient.

Though not in line to any fixed organ, lactic acidosis do need a mention at this point. It can arise due to global ischemia or regional (i.e., organ specific) ischemia. Since, regional ischemia usually results from disordered local autoregulation or cellular dysfunction, it is unlikely to respond to an increase in oxygen delivery.

Oliguria, one of the signs of renal failure, occurs mostly due to the hypotension during shock. If urinary flow stops abruptly, then obstructive uropathy is to be ruled out. This oliguria can be at most times be reversed by the correction of volume deficits but doesn't necessarily revert the moderate levels of rise in creatinine level in serum. Renal failure requiring dialysis occurs in fewer than 5% of patients and eventual recovery is common.

Effect of Shock on Individual Organs (Fig. 2)

Pulmonary	Acute respiratory distress syndrome (ARDS), shunting with dysoxia and hypoxia
Cardiovascular blood pressure	Hypotension (vasodilatation)
Cardiac	Increased cardiac output with fluid replacement; myocardial depression with diminished output
Hematologic	Thrombocytopenia, Leukocytosis, coagulation activation
Renal	Oliguria, acute tubular necrosis
Gastrointestinal	Gastritis, hyperglycemia, toxic hepatitis
Central nervous system	
Cerebral	Confusion, somnolence, coma, irritability
Hypothalamic	Fever, hypothermia

Among other organ systems, liver, like the kidney, rarely goes into overt failure, ileus is seen in septic shock which can persists till 1 or 2 days after the hypoperfusion has been corrected. Another confusing and debated field is of the nutrition in these patients. Protein and caloric requirement are particularly high with underlying malnutrition further adding on to the already diminished resources of the body.

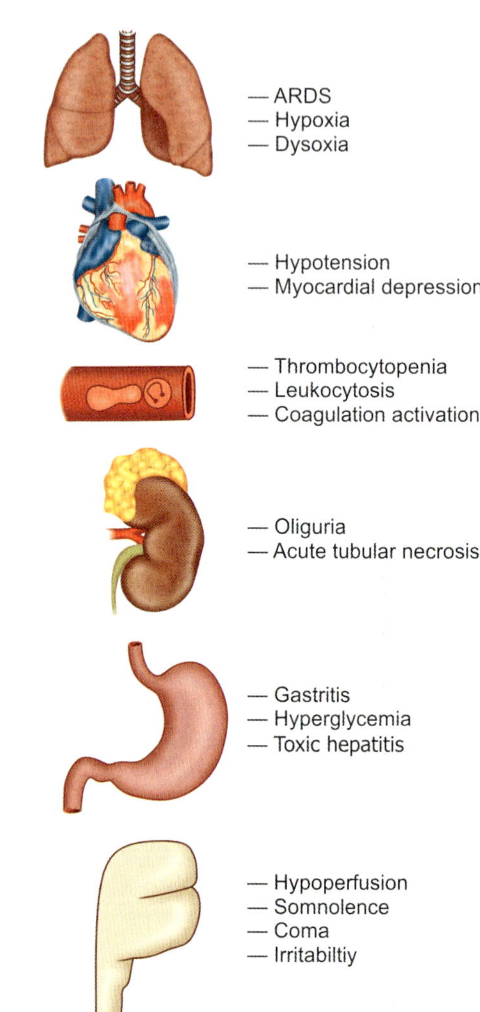

Fig. 2: Effects of sepsis on individual organs

ASSESSMENT AND MANAGEMENT OF SEPSIS

As a generalization, antibiotics and uterine evacuation are considered the definitive treatment, but when the sepsis has spread locally, surgical removal of dead tissue and abscess is also implicated. Hysterectomy may have to be done to salvage the patient. It goes without saying that the body has to be aggressively managed to tide over the crisis.

Signs

- Chills or sweats (rigors)
- Fever

- Foul-smelling vaginal discharge
- Distended abdomen
- Rebound tenderness
- Slightly low blood pressure (mild hypotension).

Symptoms

- History of interference with the pregnancy
- Abdominal pain
- Intrauterine device (IUD) in place
- Prolonged bleeding
- General discomfort; flu-like symptoms (malaise).

Besides this, also look for:

- Foreign material in the vagina
- Pus coming from cervix or mixed with blood in the vagina
- Signs of local pelvic infection: Uterine tenderness, tenderness when the cervix is moved, lower abdominal tenderness, or adnexal tenderness
- Foul odor to any blood or secretions
- Uterine subinvolution.

Risk Assessment for Sepsis

Low Risk

- First trimester abortion
- Mild to moderate fever (36.5–38.5°C or 99.5–101.5°F)
- No evidence of intra-abdominal injury
- Stable vital signs.

High Risk

- Second trimester abortion
- High fever (38.5 °C or 101.5 °F and greater) or subnormal temperature
- Any evidence of intra-abdominal injury
- Distended abdomen, decreased bowel sounds, rigid abdomen, rebound tenderness, nausea and vomiting
- Any evidence of shock: Low blood pressure (systolic less than 90 mmHg), anxiety, confusion, unconsciousness pallor (inner eyelids, around the mouth, palms), rapid, weak pulse (rate 110/min or more), rapid breathing (respirations 30/min or greater).

Immediate treatment with antibiotics is a life-saving measure for woman with pelvic infection and at risk for sepsis.

Signs of Critical Illness

Physiological

- *Signs of sympathetic activation:* Tachycardia, hypertension, pallor, clamminess and peripheral shutdown
- *Signs of systemic inflammation:* Fever or hypothermia, tachycardia and increased respiratory rate
- *Signs of organ hypoperfusion:* Cold peripheries, hypoxemia, confusion, hypotension and oliguria.

Biochemical

- Metabolic acidosis
- High or low white cell count
- Low platelet count
- Raised urea and creatinine concentrations
- Raised C-reactive protein concentration.

INVESTIGATIONS

Blood

- Hemoglobin or hematocrit
- Complete blood count for measure of infection
- Platelet count, if less, points to coagulopathy
- Peripheral smear for toxic granules and shift to left of neutrophils
- Blood culture for bacteremia and sensitivity tests.

Urine

Urine output and volume, if low:

- Low blood volume
  - Shock
  - Hemorrhage, and
  - Dehydration.
- Renal failure
- Proteinuria, as a measure of renal injury
- Pyuria, as a sign of infection.

Abdominal X-ray

- To assess the extent and severity of the infection
- Identify air or fluid levels in the bowel
- In the case of clostridial infection, gas may be seen in the tissues
- The presence of an IUD may also be confirmed
- Upright abdominal X-ray films will show air under the diaphragm from uterine or bowel perforation.

Ultrasound

- Bedside, a noninvasive investigation
- For fluid, abscesses, collections in the peritoneal cavity
- For retained products.

Computed Tomography Scan

- To differentiate gas in tissue planes
- To delineate the parametrial infections.

PRINCIPLES OF THERAPY

- Restore circulating volume to ensure adequate organ perfusion and correct acidosis
- Institute empiric antimicrobial therapy
- Surgically debride infected tissue; curette infected uterine contents and drain abscesses
- Monitor effects of therapy on vital functions and provide supportive care for organ system dysfunction.

Universal Measures

- Maintain airway; oxygen is not necessary if the woman is stable and is at low risk for shock. If she becomes unstable and oxygen is available then start oxygen at 6–8 L/min by mask or nasal cannulae
- Monitor vital signs and general condition with the insight that it can suddenly go worse with little time to act
- Do not give fluids by mouth to a woman
  - in shock
  - at high risk for shock
  - with an intra-abdominal injury,

  as she can vomit and inhale the vomit and/or she may require surgery.

MEDICINES

For women at high risk or in shock: Intravenous (IV) or intramuscular (IM) only (IV preferred). Consider starting a central venous pressure (CVP) line.

For women at low risk for septic shock, IV is preferred. If IV is not available, IM or oral is acceptable.

Antibiotics: IV preferred. Start antibiotics immediately. Give broad-spectrum antibiotics which are effective against Gram-negative, Gram-positive, anaerobic organisms and *Chlamydia*. Present trend is to give gentamicin, metronidazole 500 mg three times a day (tid) IV and ampicillin 500 mg four times a day (qid) IV or any first generation cephalosporins.

Tetanus Toxoid: IM. If there is a possibility that the woman was exposed to tetanus and there is any uncertainty of her vaccination history, then give her tetanus toxoid and tetanus antitoxin.

Pain control: Give as needed.

DEFINITIVE TREATMENT

Retained products of conception are often a source of infection. Uterine evacuation is an essential treatment for all women who are at risk for septic shock, who also have an incomplete abortion. If evacuation is not possible, then refer the woman once initial stabilizing steps have been taken. Intra-abdominal injury, pelvic abscess and peritonitis must be treated promptly, and surgery is often required for treatment of an intra-abdominal injury.

The most dangerous scenario complicating the entire picture is the onset of disseminated intravascular coagulation (DIC). Suspicion of DIC should come into mind when you see:

- Bleeding from oral mucosa (inside the mouth), bladder, injection site, or venipuncture site
- Blood in the urine
- Failure of patient's blood to clot (in the laboratory tube or on floor)
- Decreased platelet count
- Fragmented red blood cells under microscopic exam.

When DIC is suspected, the following has to be done:

- Treat source of infection
- Evacuate uterus without delay under cover of antibiotics
- Transfusion of fresh whole blood or plasma
- Antibiotics and fluid resuscitation
- Heparin 5,000–10,000 units subcutaneously every 6 hours
- If advanced facilities are not available transfer the patient to a tertiary care center.

After the initial management, she has to be further managed conservatively till signs of organ failure or other complications, which persist longer, subside.

Summary of sepsis in obstetrics is given in Flow chart 3.

THE FUTURE OF SEPSIS MANAGEMENT

Drotrecogin alfa is one drug which came as the new weapon in this fight against sepsis in 2001 after years of research into immunomodulatory therapies. It is a recombinant version of a natural anticoagulant protein, *activated protein C*. This is one drug which actually has shown to slow the onset of hematologic organ dysfunction, increase the speed of recovery from cardiovascular and respiratory dysfunction and improve organ function, besides this, it also has its effects beyond the 28 days end point. The main concern of using this modality is the risk of bleeding during the infusion of this drug. The instructions for the use of drotrecogin alfa (activated), therefore, clearly state that patients at high risk of bleeding should not be given the drug and it is contraindicated in patients with active internal bleeding, recent hemorrhagic stroke, intracranial or intraspinal surgery, severe head trauma, presence of an epidural catheter, intracranial

Flow chart 3: Summary of sepsis in obstetrics

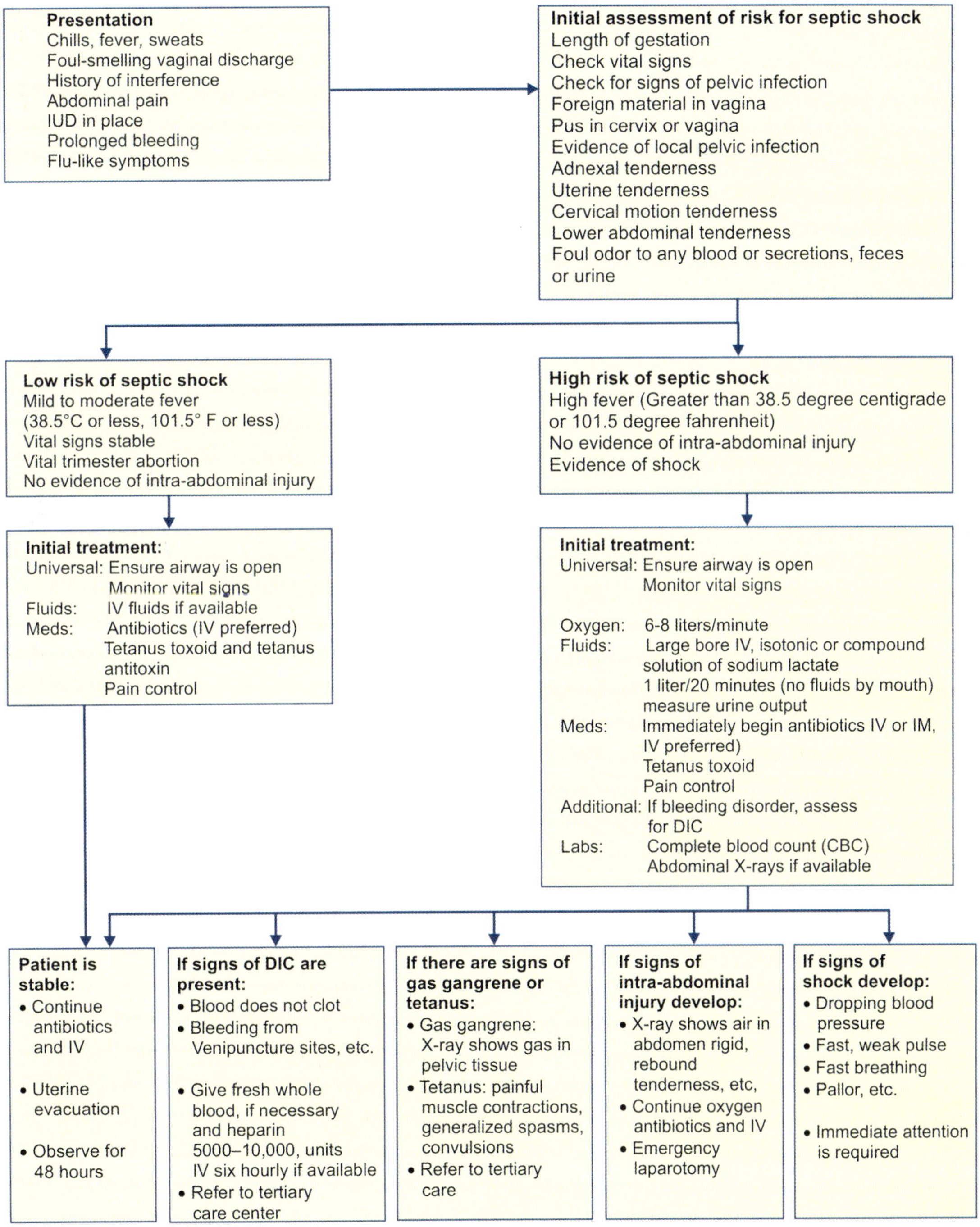

Presentation
Chills, fever, sweats
Foul-smelling vaginal discharge
History of interference
Abdominal pain
IUD in place
Prolonged bleeding
Flu-like symptoms

→

Initial assessment of risk for septic shock
Length of gestation
Check vital signs
Check for signs of pelvic infection
Foreign material in vagina
Pus in cervix or vagina
Evidence of local pelvic infection
Adnexal tenderness
Uterine tenderness
Cervical motion tenderness
Lower abdominal tenderness
Foul odor to any blood or secretions, feces or urine

Low risk of septic shock
Mild to moderate fever
(38.5°C or less, 101.5° F or less)
Vital signs stable
Vital trimester abortion
No evidence of intra-abdominal injury

Initial treatment:
Universal: Ensure airway is open
Monitor vital signs
Fluids: IV fluids if available
Meds: Antibiotics (IV preferred)
Tetanus toxoid and tetanus antitoxin
Pain control

High risk of septic shock
High fever (Greater than 38.5 degree centigrade or 101.5 degree fahrenheit)
No evidence of intra-abdominal injury
Evidence of shock

Initial treatment:
Universal: Ensure airway is open
Monitor vital signs
Oxygen: 6-8 liters/minute
Fluids: Large bore IV, isotonic or compound solution of sodium lactate
1 liter/20 minutes (no fluids by mouth)
measure urine output
Meds: Immediately begin antibiotics IV or IM, IV preferred)
Tetanus toxoid
Pain control
Additional: If bleeding disorder, assess for DIC
Labs: Complete blood count (CBC)
Abdominal X-rays if available

Patient is stable:
- Continue antibiotics and IV
- Uterine evacuation
- Observe for 48 hours

If signs of DIC are present:
- Blood does not clot
- Bleeding from Venipuncture sites, etc.
- Give fresh whole blood, if necessary and heparin 5000–10,000, units IV six hourly if available
- Refer to tertiary care center

If there are signs of gas gangrene or tetanus:
- Gas gangrene: X-ray shows gas in pelvic tissue
- Tetanus: painful muscle contractions, generalized spasms, convulsions
- Refer to tertiary care

If signs of intra-abdominal injury develop:
- X-ray shows air in abdomen rigid, rebound tenderness, etc,
- Continue oxygen antibiotics and IV
- Emergency laparotomy

If signs of shock develop:
- Dropping blood pressure
- Fast, weak pulse
- Fast breathing
- Pallor, etc.
- Immediate attention is required

neoplasm, or evidence of cerebral herniation. In addition, infusion should be interrupted for surgery or invasive interventions. Importantly, treatment with drotrecogin alfa (activated) seems to be most effective when started early, and it should not be reserved as a last-resort option. It is an expensive option so it is yet to gain widespread practice.

Common sense will explain the logic of having a research into blood purification systems which will remove the inflammatory substance thereby decreasing the effects and improving the outcome. But in practice it has been confronted by much difficulties.

Other modalities, similarly, under various phases of trials are new anti-endotoxins methods to regularize the apoptosis process disrupted by sepsis, thus keeping systems intact, medicines targeted against high mobility group B1 proteins—a late mediator of systemic inflammation released from endotoxin-stimulated macrophages.

CONCLUSION

Patient afflicted with sepsis additionally have some other major fatal illnesses or injuries. Exclusively only 50% of the sepsis modality is attributed to the septic processes. It is difficult to pin point a single cause for the fatality as septic shock syndrome or sepsis is a multiorgan system failure.

To treat the patient as a whole, besides specific treatment approaches, such as use of antibiotics, role of staff education for infection prevention, individualized aggressive support system modality, newer therapies keeping in view of the actual pathogenesis, will see decline in mortality due to sepsis, in time to come.

Acknowledgment

Dr Abhilash Unni Krishnan

BIBLIOGRAPHY

1. Bone RC, Balk RA, Cerra FB, et al. Definition for sepsis and organ failure and guidelines for the use of innovative therapies in sepsis. Chest. 1992;101:1644-55.
2. De Costa CM. The contagiousness of childbed fever: a short history of puerperal sepsis and its treatment. Med J Aust. 2002;177(11-12):668-71.
3. Schindler R, Mancilla J, Endres S, et al. Correlations and interactions in the production of interleukin-6 (IL-6), IL-1, and tumor necrosis factor (TNF) in human blood mononuclear cells: IL-6 suppresses IL-1 and TNF. Blood. 1990;75:40-7.
4. Vincent JL, Clausi CM, Bruhn A. Novel therapies in critically ill sepsis patients. In:Ortiz-Ruiz G, Perafán MA, Faist E (Eds). Sepsis, 2nd edition. Springer; 2006. pp. 25-33.
5. Wheeler AP, Bernard GR. Treating patients with severe sepsis. N Engl J Med. 1999;340(3):207-14.
6. www. who. int/reproductivehealthpublications/en/

14.2 PULMONARY EMBOLISM

Umesh Gupta

BACKGROUND

Pulmonary embolism (PE) is a common and potentially lethal disease; unfortunately, the diagnosis is often missed because patients with PE present with nonspecific signs and symptoms. If left untreated, approximately one-third of patients who survive an initial PE subsequently die from a future embolic episode. Most patients succumb to PE within the first few hours of the event. In patients who survive, recurrent embolism and death can be prevented with prompt diagnosis and therapy.

The mortality and morbidity rates from venous thromboembolism are best described by Ken Moser in two words: substantial and unacceptable. In the 1940s, Bauer performed fundamental studies that led to the current understanding of the pathogenesis of deep vein thrombosis (DVT). Subsequently, Savitt and Gallagher performed autopsy-based studies of the prevalence of venous thromboembolism in patients who had lower extremity fractures and other risk factors for PE. The most important conceptual advance that occurred over the last several decades is that PE is not a disease; rather, it is a complication of DVT.

Virtually every physician who is involved in patient care (e.g. internist, generalist, orthopedic surgeon, gynecologic surgeon, urologic surgeon, pulmonary subspecialist, cardiologist, etc.) encounters patients who are at risk of venous thromboembolism.

CASE HISTORY

Mrs RK, age 30 years, underwent abdominal hysterectomy and presented to the emergency with tender swelling of the entire left lower limb 2 weeks after surgery. With a high suspicion of DVT, she was immediately started on heparin infusion. The subsequent venous duplex confirmed thrombosis of the entire femoral vein with the thrombus extending into the common iliac vein. The patient developed shortness of breath despite being on adequate anticoagulation and a ventilation-perfusion scan confirmed PE. Being only 30 years of age and with no other risk factors for subsequent recurrence of DVT, we placed a temporary inferior vena cava (IVC) filter (fourth generation IVC filter) for 5 weeks. The filter was removed after 5 weeks and she was continued on oral anticoagulation (warfarin) for 1 year without further complications or recurrences.

PATHOPHYSIOLOGY

Natural History of Venous Thrombosis

In the 19th century, Virchow identified a triad of factors that lead to the pathogenesis of venous thrombosis: venous stasis, injury to the intima and changes in the coagulation properties of the blood. Thrombosis usually originates as a platelet nidus in the region of venous valves located in the veins of the lower extremities. Further growth occurs by accretion of platelets and fibrin and progression to red fibrin thrombus, which may either break off and embolize or result in total occlusion of the vein. The endogenous thrombolytic system leads to partial dissolution; then, the thrombus becomes organized and is incorporated into the venous wall.

Natural History of Pulmonary Embolism

Pulmonary emboli usually arise from the thrombi originating in the deep venous system of the lower extremities; however, rarely they may originate in the pelvic, renal, or upper extremity veins and the right heart chambers. After traveling to the lung, large thrombi lodge at the bifurcation of the main pulmonary artery or the lobar branches and cause hemodynamic compromise. Smaller thrombi continue traveling distally, occluding a smaller vessel in the lung periphery. These are more likely to produce pleuritic chest pain by initiating an inflammatory response adjacent to the parietal pleura. Most pulmonary emboli are multiple, and the lower lobes are involved more commonly than the upper lobes.

Respiratory Consequences

Acute respiratory consequences of PE include increased alveolar dead space, pneumoconstriction, hypoxemia and hyperventilation. Later, two additional consequences may occur: regional loss of surfactant and pulmonary infarction. Arterial hypoxemia is a frequent but not a universal finding in patients with acute embolism. The mechanisms of hypoxemia include ventilation-perfusion mismatch, intrapulmonary shunts, reduced cardiac output and intracardiac shunt via patent foramen ovale. Pulmonary infarction is an uncommon consequence because of the bronchial arterial collateral circulation.

Hemodynamic Consequences

Pulmonary embolism reduces the cross-sectional area of the pulmonary vascular bed, resulting in an increment in pulmonary vascular resistance, which in turn increases the right ventricular afterload. If the afterload is increased severely, right ventricular failure may ensue. In addition, the humoral and reflex mechanisms contribute to the pulmonary arterial constriction. Prior poor cardiopulmonary status of the patient is an important factor leading to hemodynamic collapse. Following the initiation of anticoagulant therapy, the resolution of emboli occurs rapidly during the first 2 weeks of therapy. Significant long-term nonresolution of emboli causing pulmonary hypertension or cardiopulmonary symptoms is uncommon.

Mortality/Morbidity

- Unexpected death from a massive PE is second only to the sudden cardiac death. Autopsy studies of hospitalized patients have shown approximately 80% of these patients died from massive PE
- Approximately 10% of patients who develop PE die within the first hour and 30% die subsequently from recurrent embolism. Anticoagulant treatment decreases the mortality rate to less than 5%
- The diagnosis of PE is missed in approximately 400,000 patients in the United States per year; approximately 100,000 deaths could be prevented with proper diagnosis and treatment.

Sex

- The risk of PE is increased in pregnancy and during the postpartum period; otherwise, sex is not a significant risk factor for PE.

Age

- In hospitalized elderly patients, PE is commonly missed and often is the cause of death.

HISTORY

The presentation of PE may vary from a sudden onset of catastrophic hemodynamic collapse to gradually progressive dyspnea. The diagnosis of PE should be sought actively in patients with respiratory symptoms unexplained by an alternate diagnosis. The symptoms of PE are nonspecific; therefore, a high index of suspicion is required, particularly when a patient has risk factors which include recent surgery, immobility or a hypercoagulable state.

The presentation of patients with PE can be categorized into four classes based on the acuity and severity of pulmonary arterial occlusion. These categories are: (1) massive PE, (2) acute pulmonary infarction, (3) acute embolism without infarction, and (4) multiple pulmonary emboli.

1. Massive pulmonary embolism
   - Large emboli compromise sufficient pulmonary circulation to produce circulatory collapse and shock
   - The patient has hypotension; appears weak, pale, sweaty and oliguric, and develops impaired mentation.
2. Acute pulmonary infarction
   - Approximately 10% of patients have peripheral occlusion of a pulmonary artery causing parenchymal infarction
   - These patients present with acute onset of pleuritic chest pain, breathlessness and hemoptysis
   - Although, the chest pain may be indistinguishable from ischemic myocardial pain, normal electrocardiogram findings and no response to nitroglycerine rules it out.
3. Acute embolism without infarction: Patients have nonspecific symptoms of unexplained dyspnea and/or substernal discomfort.
4. Multiple pulmonary emboli
   - This group consists of two subsets of patients
   - The first subset has repeated documented episodes of pulmonary emboli over years, eventually presenting with signs and symptoms of pulmonary hypertension and cor pulmonale
   - The second subset has no previously documented pulmonary emboli but have widespread obstruction of the pulmonary circulation with clot. They present with gradually progressive dyspnea, intermittent exertional chest pain, and eventually, features of pulmonary hypertension and cor pulmonale.

Most patients with PE have no obvious symptoms at presentation. In contrast, patients with symptomatic DVT commonly have PE confirmed on diagnostic studies in the absence of pulmonary symptoms. The most common symptoms of PE in the Prospective Investigation of Pulmonary Embolism Diagnosis (PIOPED) study were dyspnea (73%), pleuritic chest pain (66%), cough (37%) and hemoptysis (13%).

Patients with PE may present with atypical symptoms where strong suspicion in a high-risk patient often leads to consideration of PE in the differential diagnosis. These symptoms include the following:

- Seizures
- Syncope
- Abdominal pain
- Fever

- Productive cough
- Wheezing
- Decreasing level of consciousness
- New onset of atrial fibrillation.

Pleuritic chest pain without other symptoms or risk factors may be a presentation of PE.

Physical

The physical examination is quite variable in PE and, for convenience, may be grouped into four categories as follows:

1. Massive pulmonary embolism
   - These patients are in shock. They have systemic hypotension, poor perfusion to the extremities, tachycardia and tachypnea
   - Additionally, signs of pulmonary hypertension such as palpable impulse over second left interspace, loud P2, right ventricular S3 gallop, and a systolic murmur louder on inspiration at left sternal border (tricuspid regurgitation) may be present.
2. Acute pulmonary infarction
   - These patients have decreased excursion of involved hemithorax, palpable or audible pleural friction rub and even localized tenderness
   - Signs of pleural effusion, such as dullness upon percussion and diminished breath sounds, may be present.
3. Acute embolism without infarction
   - These patients have nonspecific physical signs that may easily be secondary to another disease process
   - Tachypnea and tachycardia frequently are detected, pleuritic pain sometimes may be present, crackles may be heard in the area of embolization and local wheeze may be heard rarely.
4. Multiple pulmonary emboli or thrombi
   - Patients belonging to both the subsets in this category have physical signs of pulmonary hypertension and cor pulmonale
   - Patients may have elevated jugular venous pressure, right ventricular heave, palpable impulse in the left second intercostal space, right ventricular S3 gallop, systolic murmur over the left sternal border that is louder during inspiration, hepatomegaly, ascites and dependent pitting edema
   - These findings are not specific for PE and require a high index of suspicion for pursuing appropriate diagnostic studies.

The most common physical signs in the PIOPED study were as follows:

- Tachypnea (70%)
- Rales (51%)
- Tachycardia (30%)
- Fourth heart sound (24%)
- Accentuated pulmonic component of the second heart sound (23%).

Fever of less than 39°C may be present in 14% of patients; however, temperature higher than 39.5°C is not from PE.

Chest wall tenderness upon palpation without a history of trauma may be the sole physical finding in rare cases.

CAUSES

The causes for PE are multifactorial and are not readily apparent in many cases. The following causes have been described in the literature:

1. Venous stasis
   - Venous stasis leads to accumulation of platelets and thrombin in veins
   - Increased viscosity may occur due to polycythemia and dehydration, immobility, raised venous pressure in cardiac failure or compression of a vein by a tumor.
2. Hypercoagulable states
   - The complex and delicate balance between coagulation and anticoagulation is altered by many diseases by obesity after surgery, or by trauma
   - Concomitant hypercoagulability may be present in disease states where prolonged venous stasis or injury to veins occur
   - Hypercoagulable states may be acquired or congenital. Factor V Leiden mutation causing resistance to activated protein C is the most common risk factor. Factor V Leiden mutation is present in up to 5% of the normal population and is the most common cause of familial thromboembolism
   - Primary or acquired deficiencies in protein C, protein S and antithrombin III are other risk factors. The deficiency of these natural anticoagulants is responsible for 10% of venous thrombosis in younger people.
3. Immobilization
4. Surgery and trauma
5. Pregnancy
6. Oral contraceptives and estrogen replacement
7. Malignancy.

Laboratory Studies

Clinical signs and symptoms are nonspecific; therefore, patients suspected to have PE must undergo diagnostic tests until the diagnosis is ascertained or eliminated or an alternative diagnosis is confirmed. Routine laboratory findings are nonspecific and are not helpful in PE, although they may direct towards another diagnosis.

Arterial Blood Gases

- Arterial blood gases (ABGs) characteristically reveal hypoxemia hypocapnia, and respiratory alkalosis; however, the predictive value of hypoxemia is quite low
- Both the PaO_2 and the calculation of alveolar-arterial oxygen gradient contribute to the diagnosis in a general population thought to have PE
- Nonetheless, in high-risk settings such as patients in postoperative states where other respiratory conditions can be ruled out, a low PaO_2 in conjunction with dyspnea may have a strong positive predictive value.

D-dimer

- D-dimer, a degradation product produced by plasmin-mediated proteases of cross-linked fibrin, is measured by performing a latex agglutination test or by performing an enzyme-linked immunosorbent assay (ELISA). The latex agglutination test is unreliable and has a sensitivity of 50–60%. The ELISA is more sensitive but does not carry a highly negative predictive value
- The D-dimer test misses 10% of patients with PE while only 30% of patients with positive D-dimer findings have a confirmatory diagnosis of PE. Therefore, the D-dimer test alone is not routinely recommended at present for aiding in a definitive diagnosis or in guiding the initiation of treatment in patients suspected to have PE.

Imaging Studies

Chest Radiograph

- Initially, the chest radiography findings commonly are normal. However, in later stages, the X-ray film may show radiographic signs that include a Westermark sign (dilatation of pulmonary vessels and a sharp cutoff), atelectasis, a small pleural effusion, and an elevated diaphragm
- Although chest radiograph findings may indicate an alternate diagnosis, this study alone is not sufficient to confirm the diagnosis of PE.

Ventilation-perfusion Scan

Ventilation-perfusion (V/Q) scanning of the lungs is an important diagnostic modality for establishing the diagnosis of PE. The PIOPED classification scheme allows the interpretation of the V/Q scan more meaningfully, in order to treat patients with anticoagulation. The scans should be interpreted primarily as a diagnostic or nondiagnostic pattern, indicating whether the patient has a high likelihood or does not have a high likelihood of having PE.

- Diagnostic pattern—Normal V/Q scan findings or findings indicating a high probability
  - Normal V/Q scan findings indicate an absence of any perfusion defects. Four percent of these patients still may have PE. Unless, the patient has features indicating very high clinical suspicion, these findings may be considered negative for PE
  - High-probability scan findings are two or more segmental or one larger perfusion defect in the presence of normal chest radiography findings and ventilation scan findings. Approximately, 87% of these patients were found to have PE. If accompanied by high pretest probability, the likelihood of pulmonary emboli increases to 95%.

Noninvasive Tests for Lower Extremity Deep Vein Thrombosis

- These may be helpful in the evaluation of patients who have nondiagnostic V/Q scan patterns of further intermediate and low probability
- Compression ultrasonography: Color-flow Doppler imaging and compression ultrasonography have a high sensitivity (89–100%) and specificity (89–100%) for detection of proximal DVT in symptomatic patients. However, compression ultrasonography has a low sensitivity (38%) and a low positive predictive value (26%) in patients without symptoms of DVT. Patients with positive findings for DVT can be anticoagulated, irrespective of their V/Q scan results; other patients must have more invasive investigations performed to definitely rule out PE.

Spiral Computed Tomography Scanning (Helical Computed Tomography Scan)

- The role of a spiral computed tomography (CT) scan for the diagnosis of PE has evolved over the last decade. Spiral CT can visualize main, lobar and segmental pulmonary emboli with a reported sensitivity of greater than 90%. The spiral CT scan can detect emboli as small as 2 mm that are affecting up to the seventh border division of the pulmonary artery. The only problem with spiral CT is that small subsegmental emboli may not be detected. The CT scan has another benefit; an alternate diagnosis may be suggested in up to 57% of the patients
- Sensitivity and specificity are discussed as follows:
  - The spiral CT scan has sensitivities for PE reported to be 53–100%
  - The specificity has been reported to be 78–96%
  - The negative predicted value is 81–100% and the positive predictive value is 60–100% for detecting emboli in segmental or larger arteries

- When one evaluates the clinical outcome following a negative result from a spiral CT scan, the outcome is favorable and the likelihood for subsequent thromboembolic events is extremely small
- Upon CT scan imaging, positive features include a central intravascular filling defect within the vessel lumen, eccentric tracking of contrast material around a filling defect and complete vascular occlusion. Smooth filling defects making an obtuse angle with a vessel wall may represent chronic thrombi or recent recanalization. The parenchymal findings of oligemia, pulmonary hemorrhage (ground-glass attenuation) and pulmonary infarction (peripheral wedge-shaped pleural-based opacification) may be seen.

Pulmonary Angiography

- Pulmonary angiography remains the criterion standard for the diagnosis of PE
- Following injection of iodinated contrast, anteroposterior, lateral and oblique studies are performed on each lung
- Positive results consist of a filling defect or sharp cutoff of the affected artery. Nonocclusive emboli are described to have a tram-track appearance
- Abnormal findings on V/Q scans performed prior to angiography guide the operator to focus on abnormal areas
- Angiography generally is a safe procedure. The mortality rate for patients undergoing this procedure is less than 0.5% and the morbidity rate is less than 5%
- Patients who have long-standing pulmonary arterial hypertension and right ventricular failure are considered high-risk patients
- Negative pulmonary angiogram findings, even if false-negative, exclude clinically relevant PE.

Magnetic Resonance Imaging

- Upon a magnetic resonance imaging (MRI), evidence of pulmonary emboli may be detected by using standard or gated spin-echo techniques
- Pulmonary emboli demonstrate increased signal intensity within the pulmonary artery. By obtaining a sequence of images, this signal that is originating from slow blood flow may be distinguished from PE. However, this remains a problem in pulmonary hypertension
- Presently, magnetic resonance angiography is performed following intravenous administration of gadolinium
- MRI has a sensitivity of 85% and specificity of 96% for central, lobar and segmental emboli; MRI is inadequate for the diagnosis of subsegmental emboli.

Echocardiography

- This modality generally has limited accuracy in the diagnosis of PE
- Transesophageal echocardiography may identify central PE, and the sensitivity for central PE is reported to be 82%
- Overall sensitivity and specificity for central and peripheral PE is 59% and 77%
- Echocardiography may demonstrate right ventricular dysfunction in acute PE, predicting a higher mortality and possible benefit from thrombolytic therapy.

Other Tests

Electrocardiogram

- The most common electrocardiogram (ECG) abnormalities of PE are tachycardia and nonspecific ST-T wave abnormalities. These findings are not sensitive or specific enough to aid in the diagnosis of PE
- The classic finding of right-heart strain demonstrated by an S1-Q3-T3 pattern is observed in only 20% of patients with proven PE.

MEDICAL CARE

Immediate full anticoagulation is mandatory for all patients suspected to have DVT or PE. Diagnostic investigations should not delay empirical anticoagulant therapy. Initial anticoagulation is performed with intravenous heparin which activates antithrombin III to slow or prevent the progression of DVT and reduces pulmonary emboli. Heparin does not dissolve the existing clot. The patient should be started simultaneously on oral anticoagulation with warfarin. After a therapeutic dose of warfarin is established, heparin is discontinued and warfarin therapy is maintained.

Thrombolytic Therapy

- Thrombolytic therapy should be considered for patients who are hemodynamically unstable, patients who have right-heart strain and high-risk patients with underlying poor cardiopulmonary reserve
- Although most studies demonstrate superiority of thrombolytic therapy with respect to resolution of radiographic and hemodynamic abnormalities within the first 24 hours, this advantage disappears 7 days after treatment. Controlled clinical trials have not demonstrated benefit in terms of reduced mortality rates or earlier resolution of symptoms when currently compared to heparin
- Until randomized clinical trials demonstrate a clear morbidity or mortality benefit, the role of thrombolytic

therapy in the management of acute PE remains controversial. The currently accepted indications for thrombolytic therapy include hemodynamic instability or right ventricular dysfunction demonstrated on echocardiography.

Goals of Anticoagulation Therapy

- The efficacy of heparin therapy depends on achieving a critical therapeutic level of heparin within the first 24 hours of treatment. The critical therapeutic level of heparin is 1.5 times the baseline control value or the upper limit of normal range of the activated partial thromboplastin time (aPTT)
- This level of anticoagulation is expected to correspond to a heparin blood level of 0.2–0.4 U/mL by the protamine sulfate titration assay and 0.3–0.6 U/mL by the antifactor Xa assay
- Each laboratory should establish the minimal therapeutic level for heparin, as measured by the aPTT, to coincide with a heparin blood level of at least 0.2 U/mL for each batch of thromboplastin reagent being used
- Heparin therapy generally is overlapped with warfarin for a minimum of 4–5 days
- A weight-based heparin dosing nomogram is an effective approach for achieving adequate anticoagulation. An initial bolus of 80 U/kg is followed by an infusion of 18 U/kg/hour. The heparin dose is further adjusted to maintain an aPTT in the therapeutic range.

Low Molecular Weight Heparin

- Low molecular weight heparins (LMWHs) have many advantages over unfractionated heparin. These agents have a greater bioavailability, can be administered by subcutaneous injections and have a longer duration of anticoagulant effect. However, for massive DVT or PE, standard heparin remains the standard choice.

Oral Anticoagulant Therapy

- The anticoagulant effect of warfarin is mediated by the inhibition of vitamin K-dependent factors, which are II, VII, IX, and X. The peak effect does not occur until 36–72 hours after drug administration and the dosage is difficult to titrate
- A prothrombin time ratio is expressed as an international normalized ratio (INR) and is monitored to assess the adequacy of warfarin therapy. The recommended therapeutic range for venous thromboembolism is an INR of 2–3. This level of anticoagulation markedly reduces the risk of bleeding without the loss of effectiveness. Initially, INR measurements are performed on a daily basis; once the patient is stabilized on a specific dose of warfarin, the INR determinations may be performed every 1–2 weeks or at longer intervals.

Duration of Anticoagulation

- A patient with a first thromboembolic event occurring in the setting of reversible risk factors such as immobilization, surgery, or trauma, should receive warfarin therapy for 3–6 months. In the absence of an identifiable risk factor, the first idiopathic thromboembolic event should be treated for a minimum of 6 months and 3 months of anticoagulation is insufficient in this setting
- Warfarin treatment for longer than 6 months is indicated in patients with recurrent venous thromboembolism or in those in whom a continuing risk factor for venous thromboembolism exists, including malignancy, immobilization, or morbid obesity
- Patients who have PE and pre-existing irreversible risk factors, such as deficiency of antithrombin III, protein S and C, factor V Leiden mutation, or the presence of antiphospholipid antibodies, should be placed on long-term anticoagulation.

SURGICAL CARE

Inferior vena cava interruption by the insertion of an IVC filter is indicated in the following settings:

- Patients with acute venous thromboembolism who have an absolute contraindication to anticoagulant therapy, e.g. recent surgery, hemorrhagic stroke, heparin-induced thrombocytopenia syndrome (HITS) or significant active or recent bleeding
- Patients with massive PE who survived but in whom recurrent embolism will be invariably fatal
- Patients who have objectively documented recurrent venous thromboembolism, adequate anticoagulant therapy notwithstanding.

IVC filters can be classified as permanent or temporary. Permanent IVC filters remain in the IVC through out the life and require lifelong anticoagulation. Till recently, all patients requiring an IVC filter received these types of filters. The availability of temporary IVC filters in India has broadened the indications for IVC filter placement. Temporary filters have the advantage that patients do not require to be on lifelong anticoagulation. Hence, all patients, in whom an IVC filter is indicated and do not have risk factors for recurrent DVT or PE, can benefit from temporary filters. On the other hand, patients of malignancy, protein C and S deficiency, paraplegics, etc. will benefit from a permanent filter.

Activity

Activity is recommended from day one as tolerated.

BIBLIOGRAPHY

1. Alpert JS, Smith R, Carlson J. Mortality in patients treated for pulmonary embolism. JAMA. 1976;236(13):1477-80.
2. Ballew KA, Philbrick JT, Becker DM. Vena cava filter devices. Clin Chest Med. 1995;16(2):295-305.
3. Brill-Edwards P, Ginsberg JS, Johnston M. Establishing a therapeutic range for heparin therapy. Ann Intern Med. 1993; 119(2):104-9.
4. Bulger CM, Jacobs C, Patel NH. Epidemiology of acute deep vein thrombosis. Tech Vasc Interv Radiol. 2004;7(2):50-4.
5. Carson JL, Kelley MA, Duff A. The clinical course of pulmonary embolism. N Engl J Med. 1992;326(19):1240-5.
6. Davey NC, Smith TP, Hanson MW. Ventilation-perfusion lung scintigraphy as a guide for pulmonary angiography in the localization of pulmonary emboli. Radiology. 1999;213(1):51-7.
7. Decousus H, Leizorovicz A, Parent F. A clinical trial of vena caval filters in the prevention of pulmonary embolism in patients with proximal deep vein thrombosis. Prevention du Risque d'Embolie Pulmonaire par Interruption Cave Study Group. N Engl J Med. 1998;338(7):409-15.
8. Deitelzweig S, Jaff MR. Medical management of venous thromboembolic disease. Tech Vasc Interv Radiol. 2004;7(2):63-7.
9. Drucker EA, Rivitz SM, Shepard JA. Acute pulmonary embolism: Assessment of helical CT for diagnosis. Radiology. 1998;209(1):235-41.
10. Egermayer P, Town GI, Turner JG. Usefulness of D-dimer, blood gas, and respiratory rate measurements for excluding pulmonary embolism. Thorax. 1998;53(10):830-4.
11. Ginsberg JS, Hirsh J. Use of antithrombotic agents during pregnancy. Chest. 1998;114(5 Suppl):524S-30S.
12. Ginsberg JS, Wells PS, Kearon C. Sensitivity and specificity of a rapid whole-blood assay for D-dimer in the diagnosis of pulmonary embolism. Ann Intern Med. 1998;129(12):1006-11.
13. Ginsberg JS. Management of venous thromboembolism. N Engl J Med. 1996;335(24):1816-28.
14. Goldhaber SZ. Pulmonary embolism. N Engl J Med. 1998; 339(2):93-104.
15. Hirsh J, Dalen JE, Anderson DR. Oral anticoagulants: mechanism of action, clinical effectiveness, and optimal therapeutic range. Chest. 1998;114(5 Suppl):445S-69S.
16. Hull R, Delmore T, Carter C. Adjusted subcutaneous heparin versus warfarin sodium in the long-term treatment of venous thrombosis. N Engl J Med. 1982;306(4):189-94.
17. Hull R, Delmore T, Genton E. Warfarin sodium versus low-dose heparin in the long-term treatment of venous thrombosis. N Engl J Med. 1979;301(16):855-8.
18. Hull RD, Raskob GE, Brant RF. The importance of initial heparin treatment on long-term clinical outcomes of antithrombotic therapy. The emerging theme of delayed recurrence. Arch Intern Med. 1997;157(20):2317-21.
19. Hull RD, Raskob GE, Ginsberg JS. A noninvasive strategy for the treatment of patients with suspected pulmonary embolism. Arch Intern Med. 1994;154(3):289-97.
20. Hull RD, Raskob GE, Rosenbloom D. Optimal therapeutic level of heparin therapy in patients with venous thrombosis. Arch Intern Med. 1992;152(8):1589-95.
21. Katz DS, Hon M. Current DVT imaging. Tech Vasc Interv Radiol. 2004;7(2):55-62.
22. Kovacs MJ, Anderson D, Morrow B. Outpatient treatment of pulmonary embolism with dalteparin. Thromb Haemost. 2000;83(2):209-11.
23. Levine M, Gent M, Hirsh J. A comparison of low-molecular-weight heparin administered primarily at home with unfractionated heparin administered in the hospital for proximal deep-vein thrombosis. N Engl J Med. 1996;334(11):677-81.
24. Levine M, Hirsh J, Weitz J. A randomized trial of a single bolus dosage regimen of recombinant tissue plasminogen activator in patients with acute pulmonary embolism. Chest. 1990;98(6):1473-9.
25. Mayo JR, Remy-Jardin M, Muller NL. Pulmonary embolism: Prospective comparison of spiral CT with ventilation-perfusion scintigraphy. Radiology. 1997;205(2):447-52.
26. Moser KM. Venous thromboembolism. Am Rev Respir Dis. 1990;141(1):235-49.
27. Mullins MD, Becker DM, Hagspiel KD. The role of spiral volumetric computed tomography in the diagnosis of pulmonary embolism. Arch Intern Med. 2000;160(3):293-8.
28. Ramzi DW, Leeper KV. DVT and pulmonary embolism: Part I. Diagnosis. Am Fam Physician. 2004;69(12):2829-36.
29. Ramzi DW, Leeper KV. DVT and pulmonary embolism: Part II. Treatment and prevention. Am Fam Physician. 2004;69(12): 2841-8.
30. Rathbun SW, Raskob GE, Whitsett TL. Sensitivity and specificity of helical computed tomography in the diagnosis of pulmonary embolism: A systematic review. Ann Intern Med. 2000;132(3):227-32.
31. Rosendaal FR. Venous thrombosis: Prevalence and interaction of risk factors. Haemostasis. 1999;29(Suppl S1):1-9.
32. Schulman S, Granqvist S, Holmstrom M The duration of oral anticoagulant therapy after a second episode of venous thromboembolism. The Duration of Anticoagulation Trial Study Group. N Engl J Med. 1997;336(6):393-8.
33. Simonneau G, Sors H, Charbonnier B. A comparison of low-molecular-weight heparin with unfractionated heparin for acute pulmonary embolism. The THESEE Study Group. Tinzaparine ou Heparine Standard: Evaluations dans l'Embolie Pulmonaire. N Engl J Med. 1997;337(10):663-9.
34. Stein PD, Hull RD, Saltzman HA. Strategy for diagnosis of patients with suspected acute pulmonary embolism. Chest. 1993;103(5):1553-9.
35. Stein PD, Saltzman HA, Weg JG. Clinical characteristics of patients with acute pulmonary embolism. Am J Cardiol. 1991;68(17):1723-4.
36. Tapson VF. Pulmonary embolism: the diagnostic repertoire. Chest. 1997;112(3):578-80.
37. Tibbutt DA, Davies JA, Anderson JA. Comparison by controlled clinical trial of streptokinase and heparin in treatment of life-threatening pulmonary embolism. Br Med J. 1974;1(904):343-7.
38. Wells PS, Ginsberg JS, Anderson DR. Use of a clinical model for safe management of patients with suspected pulmonary embolism. Ann Intern Med. 1998;129(12):997-1005.

CHAPTER

15

Postoperative Nutrition

Maninder Ahuja

INTRODUCTION

More recently, ensuring adequate nutritional intake has been a major focus of perioperative care and research has focused on the methods of delivering nutritional support, their comparative clinical benefits and minimizing the metabolic changes associated with surgical trauma.

Preoperative nutritional status of patients undergoing surgical procedures is very important and individuals with suboptimal nutritional parameters should be supplemented and replenished before elective surgery. In elective cases like obstetric surgery, antenatal care should be proper so that anemia and malnutrition is corrected beforehand, along with proper weight control and prevention of obesity. In case of malnourished cancer patients, presurgery nutrition should be preferably supplemented orally only, but if it is not feasible then enteral or parenteral route can be used.

The consequences of preoperative malnutrition were first recognized in the 1930s. Studley observed a direct relationship between preoperative weight loss and operative mortality rate, independent of factors such as age, impaired cardiorespiratory function and type of surgery. In midline laparotomies, malnutrition is one of the well known risk factors determining *wound dehiscence.*

Obesity has the same prognostic value as nutrition correlation also exists for postoperative mortality and it does not depend on whether the operation is performed in gastrointestinal tract or not, whether the primary disease is cancer or not.

EARLY POSTOPERATIVE NUTRITION

It is recommended to start early postoperative oral intake after both techniques *(laparoscopic surgery and open surgery).* Complication rate is not increased by starting early postoperative oral intake. Postoperative nutrition should be initiated as soon as possible. Preferred route for nutrient delivery is an oral diet; however, critically ill patients are unable to eat because of endotracheal intubation and ventilator dependence. Furthermore, oral feeding may be delayed because of impaired swallowing, anorexia induced by pain relieving medications or postoperative depression and traumatic shock. Patients who are able to eat may not be able to meet increased energy and nutrient requirement associated with metabolic stress and recovery and often oral nutritional supplementation or enteral tube nutrition or total parenteral nutrition (TPN) may be required.

Post Surgery Diet Progression

First Step: Clear liquids.

Second Step: Easy-to-digest foods and all foods in first step.

Third Step: Regular diet.

Solid oral feeding is often delayed for the first 24–48 hours following surgery to await the return of bowel sound or passage of flatus but there is no physiological reason why solid foods should not be introduced once the gastrointestinal tract is functioning and a few liquids are being tolerated.

Patients should avoid high-fat, greasy or deep-fat fried foods, which may not be well tolerated. Try to give smaller portions at frequent intervals.

In general, well nourished elective surgery patients are not considered to need nutritional support, unless postoperative complications prevent oral intake. The incidence of such complications (bowel obstruction, anastomotic disruption and pancreatitis) is low.

Protein and Caloric Requirements

Protein-energy malnutrition is a common problem in hospital patients. Studies have reported 40% of surgical and medical patients to be malnourished on admission to hospital. The majority of patients experienced nutritional depletion during the course of their hospital admission, which was more severe in those patients who were already depleted at the time of their admission.

- Daily protein turnover is 200–300 g After digestion, all amino acids are absorbed, save 1 g of nitrogen which is excreted in the stool. Proteolysis accounts for another 50–70 g of amino acids. In total, ingested amino acids contribute only 25 g to the free amino acid pool, whereas 250 g is provided by endogenous breakdown. *If adequate energy* is present, most of these amino acids are *resynthesized.* So, caloric supply is important. Carbohydrate increases muscle protein synthesis under the influence of insulin; *fat* increases hepatic and other visceral protein synthesis. The average normal requirement of a patient is 0.8 g of protein/kg/day. Any kind of trauma, including surgery, increases this requirement (Fig. 1).

Energy Requirement

After surgery, energy requirement depends upon type of surgery and is calculated as a factor of resting energy expenditure (REE) of that patient multiplied by stress factor. Stress factor is 1.35 for skeletal trauma, 1.6 for major sepsis, or another formula is 25–30 nonprotein calories/kg/day, but these methods may over estimate energy requirement in mechanically ventilated and sedated patients in whom neuromuscular paralysis has reduced calorie requirement by 30%.

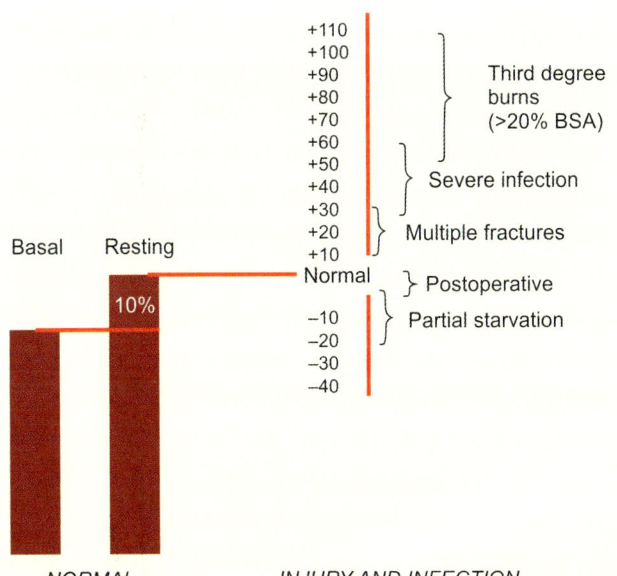

Fig. 1: The increases in resting energy expenditure that have been shown to occur during catabolic phase of trauma situations (injury and infection) when compared with the decreases that develop during partial starvation

Source: Sabiston Textbook of Surgery, 15th edition)

Protein Requirement

The average normal requirement of a patient is 0.8 g of protein/kg/day.

In cases of stress of surgery, it is 1.5 -2.0 g/kg/day.

Carbohydrates

Carbohydrates should constitute 60–70% of nonprotein calories.

Fat

Fat provides remaining 15–40% of nonprotein calories (Box 1).

Causes of Inadequate Nutrition or Increased Protein Loss

- Poor intake
- In-hospital malnutrition is poor food unappetizingly served, with timing for the benefit of hospital personnel rather than patients. Patients are given nothing by mouth for the most trivial reasons (chest or abdominal films;

Box 1 Total parenteral nutrition 24 hours

Basal Harris-Benedict Equation (Total daily caloric requirement):

Females: 65.5 + (9.6 × weight in kg) + (1.8 × height in cm) – (4.7 × age in years)

Males: 66.5 + (13.8 × weight in kg) + (5.0 × height in cm) – (6.8 × age in years)

Proteins: 1.0–1.5 g/kg body weight

Fat: 20–30% of total calories as continuous 24 hour infusion

Rest as carbohydrates: Fluid requirements are to be individualized

Daily trace elements: Zinc 4 mg, Copper 0.8 mg, Manganese 0.4 mg, Chromium 8 mcg Selenium 48 mcg

Vitamins: A: 3300 IU, D: 200 IU, E: 10 IU, C: 100 mg, Folic acid: 400 µg, Niacin: 40 mg, Riboflavin 3.6 mg, Thiamine 3.0 mg, B-6: 4 mg, B-12: 5 µg Pantothenic acid 15 mg, Biotin 60 µg

Maintain serum glucose 100–120 with glucocheck monitoring will be followed

other radiological exams). Diets are not advocated rapidly after minor operations, such as endometrial biopsy

- *Sepsis:* Proteolysis occurs in response to starvation, stress and sepsis; and it is mediated by glucagon, catecols and steroids, with a considerably smaller increase in insulin and (in trauma or sepsis) cytokines. There is rapid adaptation to resting starvation and proteolysis is minimal after as little as 4 days. The metabolic tragedy of sepsis is that this *adaptation to starvation does not occur,* and breakdown of protein continues to supply amino acids either for hepatic protein synthesis for host defenses or for gluconeogenesis for the energy needs of the individual.

Indications for Nutritional Support

The indications for nutritional support should consider the following:

- The premorbid state (healthy or otherwise)
- The current nutritional status
- Age of the patient
- Duration of starvation
- Degree of the anticipated insult
- The likelihood of resuming normal intake soon
- Weight loss of 15%
- A serum albumin value less than 3 g/100 mL.

METABOLIC CHANGES IN SURGICAL PATIENTS

Nutritional depletion is associated with changes in body composition.

Increased basal metabolic rate surgical trauma causes increase in sympathetic activity which causes increase in catecholamine secretion, followed by prolonged hyper metabolic state and then negative nitrogen balance and increase in basal metabolic rate (BMR) up to 10%.

Loss of Muscle Mass

If adequate nutritional support is not provided at this stage then excessive skeletal muscle proteolysis occurs with further depression of metabolism. Increased energy expenditure is associated with a range of hormonal responses that occur as a result of surgical trauma. Cytokines, including tumor necrosis factor (TNF) and interleukins (IL-1 and IL-6) have an important role in determining longer-term metabolic changes. These changes may not be clinically relevant unless postoperative sepsis or trauma follows surgery but in conjunction with preoperative starvation often results in a significant negative nitrogen balance.

Physiological Changes in Surgery

There is *increased intestinal permeability* two to four fold, in the immediate postoperative period and this is *aggravated by malnutrition.* This causes failure of the gut barrier function to exclude endogenous bacteria and toxins and *leads to sepsis and multiorgan failure.*

So malnutrition in perioperative period leads to:

- Delayed wound healing
- Reduced ventilatory capacity
- Reduced immunity and increased risk of infection.

Nutritional Assessment

How do we assess the nutritional level of a patient?

Clinical assessment is most superior parameter. We judge it by weight loss; if it is less than 10%, then it is mild malnutrition; and if it is greater than 30%, then it is severe malnutrition. Other important parameter is tumor necrosis factor (BMI).

Anthropometric assessment includes triceps skin fold thickness, mid-arm circumference and handgrip strength.

Blood indices are reduced serum albumin, prealbumin or transferin and lymphocyte count.

Benefits to Patients

Nutritional support leads to improved nutritional status and better clinical outcome.

It reduces morbidity and the stay in the hospital so it is cost-effective.

Routes of Nutritional Support

There is plethora of small clinical trials but no meta-analysis of data has been done so far about routes of administration of nutrient, i.e. enteral versus parenteral nutrition.

ENTERAL NUTRITION

Not routinely indicated in well-nourished patients:

Conventional treatment after bowel resection and all surgeries has typically entailed starvation with administration of intravenous fluids until passage of flatus, principally due to concerns over postoperative ileus. However, small intestinal motility recovers 6–8 hours after surgical trauma and moderate absorptive capacity exists even in the absence of normal peristalsis. It has since been shown that postoperative enteral feeding in patients undergoing gastrointestinal resection is safe and well tolerated even when started within 12 hours of surgery.

Clinical Benefits of Enteral Nutrition

- Reduces the incidence of postoperative infectious complications
- Improved wound healing response
- Alters antigen exposure and influences oxygenation of the gut mucosa, and villous depth is increased
- More research is required in this area to elucidate whether enteral nutrition truly modulates gut function or whether tolerance of enteral nutrition is predominantly indicative of a patient with healthy organ function.

Types of Oral Supplements or Enteral Feeds

These can be

- Home-blenderized tube feeding, or
- Commercially available formulas.

Home blenderized formula is about 1,800–2,500 kcal/day and it consists of:

- Strained meat 3.5 oz
- Strained vegetables 4.5 oz
- Strained fruits 4.5 oz
- Cup of dried skimmed milk powder
- Vegetable oil
- Corn syrup
- Water
- Whole milk
- Others.

(***Source:*** American dietetic association. Home enteral/parenteral nutrition therapy)

Commercially available formulas are primarily meant to augment the intake of solid foods. They generally provide 250 kcal/8 oz or 240 mL portion and about 8–14 gm of intact protein. Fat sources are mainly long chain triglycerides though some contain medium chain triglycerides (MCT) also.

Fluids

Fluid requirement per day are on an average 2–3 L/day and rarely exceeds 3–4 L/day.

Parenteral Nutrition

A large multicenter clinical trial has shown no significant reduction in morbidity or mortality when TPN was administered perioperatively to a heterogeneous group of surgical patients. Stratification of patients in this trial according to nutritional status showed that patients with mild malnutrition did not benefit from TPN but had more infectious complications. So, TPN should be limited to severely malnourished patients in the absence of other specific indications.

Alternative or Nonconventional Fuels

In addition to ongoing research ascertaining the specific benefits of the routes of delivery for nutritional support, more recent research has also focused on the composition of nutritional regimens. In particular, much attention has been paid to the potential for specific nutrients to influence the metabolic response to disease.

It has been demonstrated that the addition of *glutamine* to parenteral nutrition regimens given to patients after elective abdominal surgery results in a reduced length of hospital stay and reduced costs. This was accompanied by an improved nitrogen balance and quicker lymphocyte recovery. Glutamine has also been shown to maintain intestinal permeability in postoperative patients.

Nutritive solutions enriched with *arginine, ribonucleic acid (RNA) and omega-3 fatty acids* are also important fuels that influence positively the postoperative recovering of many plasma parameters which reflect patient's recovering from surgery. These "enriched solutions" are a better choice than standard diets in improving parameters such as prealbumin concentration, retinol binding protein concentration, delayed hypersensitivity responses, phagocytic ability of monocytes and concentration of IL-2 receptors. People who receive the enriched solution has the same risk of developing postoperative infections if compared with people who receive the standard diet, but the infections in the latter group tend to be much more severe and difficult to treat.

Vitamins and minerals are necessary and must be administrated within the nutritional support plan.

CONCLUSION

Wherever possible in malnourished patients oral route should be used for nutrient supplementation. Comparative studies show that in comparison to parenteral nutrition, enteral nutrition is well-tolerated and is associated with reduced septic morbidity, costs and length of stay. These studies form the basis of the current practice of the enteral feeding route being used, wherever possible. Further research is needed to elucidate whether alongside improvements in surgical technique and perioperative care, enteral nutrition will be associated with overall reductions in morbidity and mortality. A standardized and validated definition of nutritional depletion would enable nutrition support to be targeted to those surgical patients most likely to derive significant clinical benefit in terms of improved postoperative outcome. This would also facilitate direct comparison of trial data for large meta-analyses involving "malnourished" patients to provide robust, evidence-based guidelines for nutritional support of surgical patients.

CHAPTER

16 Physiotherapy in Postoperative Gynecological Surgery

Maninder Ahuja

Physiotherapy forms an integral part of postoperative care, as important as nutrition. Physiotherapy is needed:

- To prevent muscle loss or sarcopenia
- To prevent thromoembolic phenomenon
- To prevent pulmonary complications
- To help in better wound healing.

It should be started as soon as the patient comes out of anesthesia and consist of following components:

- Breathing exercises
- Exercises to increase circulation
- Exercises to prevent stiffness and increase flexibility
- Exercises to tone up muscles
- Exercises to strengthen abdominal muscles
- Exercises for back and shoulder muscles
- Exercises to tone up perineal muscles
- Progressive on strength and stamina building exercises.

DEEP BREATHING EXERCISES

Patient should sit with back supported and her knees bent. She should inhale slowly through her nose, feeling ribs expanding sideways. Then she should exhale. This should be repeated three times. This can be done lying down in bed also and several times a day.

When she comes out of her anesthesia, her sides should be changed to prevent pressure sores, and she should be asked to move her legs and arms by doing simple flexion and extension. Patients are advised to take 5–10 deep breathing exercises every waking hour after first postoperative day.

Coughing

- If she has any secretions (phlegm), she will need to cough effectively to clear her chest
- Ask her to sit forward with her knees bent and support her; wound with her hands or a pillow
- She should take 2–4 deep breaths then cough and spit any mucus into a tissue
- Repeat as often as she feels necessary.

Huffing

- This is useful if she find it difficult to cough effectively
- Take a medium size breath in and then breathe out
- Fast through an open mouth, using her stomach and chest muscles. This will squeeze sputum along the airways to a point where she can cough it up (imagine steaming up a mirror).

Day Two and Three

Patient should continue with deep breathing exercises and should start doing some stretching exercises.

She should lie comfortably on her back with her knees bent. She should put one hand under the small of her back and pull her tummy in and flatten her back onto her hand, and tilt her bottom off the bed slightly, then relax and repeat 5–6 times (Fig. 1).

Knee Rolling

She should lie in same position as above, with knees bent and feet together and pull her tummy in and gently roll

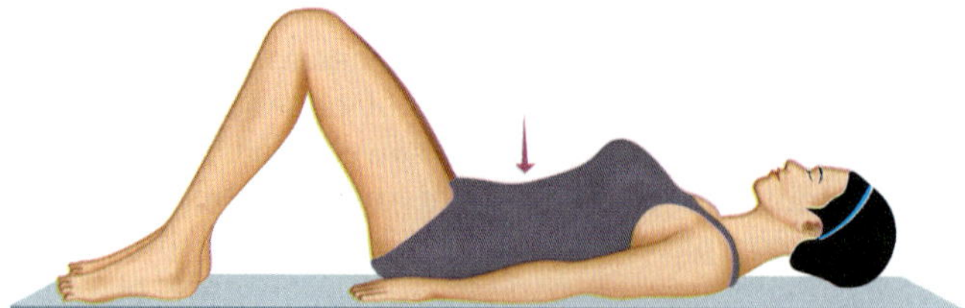

Fig. 1: Day two and three

her knees from side-to-side, a few inches to start with, gradually increasing. Repeat six times. This is a helpful movement to try if she is uncomfortable due to trapped wind (Fig. 2).

Circulation Exercises

Patient should bend and stretch her ankles briskly up and down 10 times and then move her feet at ankles inside and outside 10 times. This would increase circulation in her legs. Make 10 circles with her ankles clockwise and counter-clockwise (Fig. 3).

- Ankle circles can be done in different positions such as sitting, lying down, etc.

Abdominal Muscle Exercises

She may start to do these exercises from about after 2–6 weeks after surgery, however, people do recover at different rates, so it may vary from patient-to-patient.

Head Raising

She should lie flat on her back with her knees bent and her hands resting on her thighs. She should breathe in deeply, then pull her pelvic floor and deep tummy muscles in, and gently raise her head and shoulders, sliding her hands up her thighs towards her knees, whilst breathing out. Slowly lower head and shoulders back down and relax. Repeat five times (Fig. 4).

Leg Sliding

Lie on her back with her left knee bent (foot on the bed) and her right knee straight. Keeping the bent knee still, she should pull her tummy in and make the straight leg shorter by drawing up at the hip and waist. Then make it longer by stretching the leg down from the waist. Repeat with the other leg and do five times each side.

Transverse Abdominal Muscle

This is the layer of muscle that is closest to internal organs. Pulling this deep muscle in, places, all the other abdominal muscles in the correct position supporting the trunk and giving patient a less protruding abdomen. It is also vital in supporting the spine as it is the body's "natural corset". She can start this exercise after a few days. The best position to start doing this exercise is in Figure 5.

- She should let her tummy sag! breathe in gently
- She should breathe out through her mouth, at the same time as compressing and contracting her abdominal muscles, pulling her naval towards her spine. It may help to imagine that there is a gap in the front of her tummy, which she is trying to pull close
- She should hold this compression and breathe throughout. The breaths will be shallow and from the chest

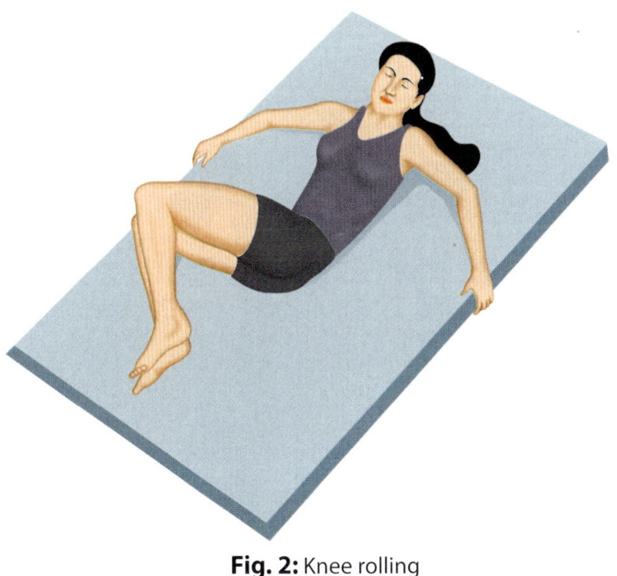

Fig. 2: Knee rolling

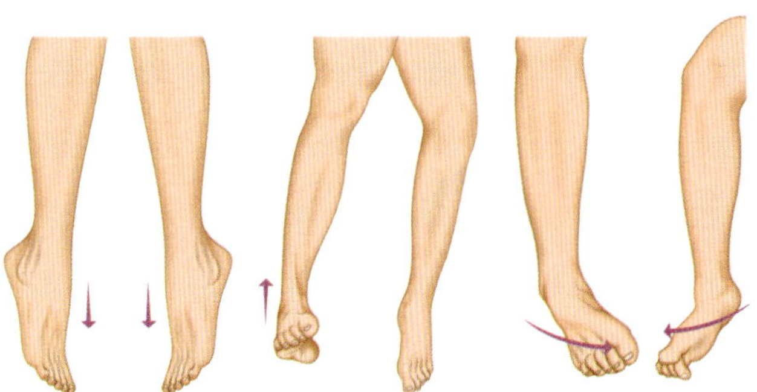

Fig. 3: Circulation exercises

Fig. 4: Head raising

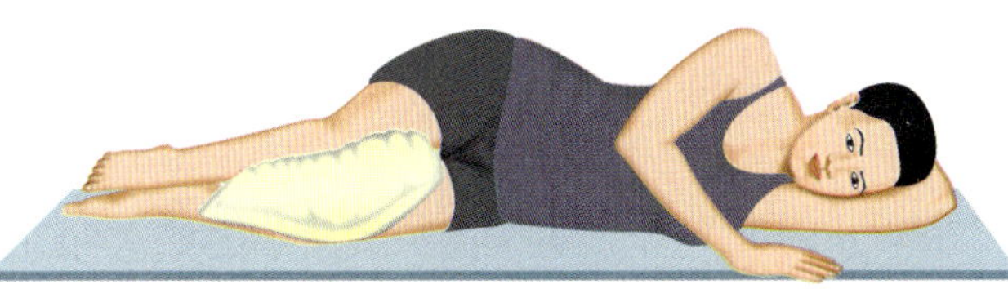

Fig. 5: Transverse abdominal muscle

- Once she can do this, she should try pulling up the pelvic floor muscles at the same time (gently to start with and only if she no longer have a catheter into her bladder), remembering to breathe throughout
- Try to gradually increase the amount of time she can hold this contraction, remembering to breathe. Start with 5 seconds, building up to about 20 or even 30 seconds after a few weeks of practice. However, long she decides to hold for, make sure she always feels comfortable and is not straining any of her muscles.

As these are postural muscles, they prefer to be exercised at least 6-7 times a day.

She should always rest, if:

- She feels that she is holding her breath
- The muscle contraction has gone or gets weaker
- She feels tired.

Back Care

- Whether patient is in bed or on chair, she should make sure that her back is well supported. Placing a small pillow or roll in the small of her back may increase her comfort and help to prevent backache
- When turning over in bed, her knees should be bent and she should try to roll over without twisting.

Getting in and Out of Bed

- When getting back into bed sit close to the bed's back support and reverse the above process (Fig. 6).

Walking

Patient can start walking for about 10 minutes daily and it should be a slow walk and she can just walk around house and this can be started after 1-2 weeks depending on patient's recovery, level of nutrition and will power.

While walking, standing posture should be maintained and there should not be any strain on her back (Fig. 7).

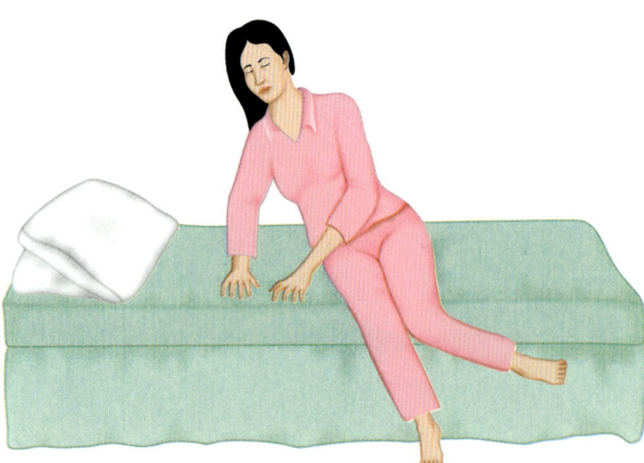

Fig. 6: Getting out of bed

Housework and Lifting (Fig. 8)

She should try to avoid any heavy lifting for several months after her operation. This includes heavy shopping bags, wet washing, full saucepans, the hoover, the ironing board, etc. While lifting she should:

- Bend her knees
- Keep her back straight
- Pull-in her tummy
- Pull-up her pelvic floor.

Advanced Abdominal Muscle Training Three Months After Surgery

Straight Curl-up

- Ask her to lie on her back with her knees bent and to breathe-in slowly through her nose
- Tuck in her chin and raise her head
- Point her hands toward her knees
- Exhale and lift her shoulders off the floor for a count of five
- Relax
- Repeat 3–5 times.

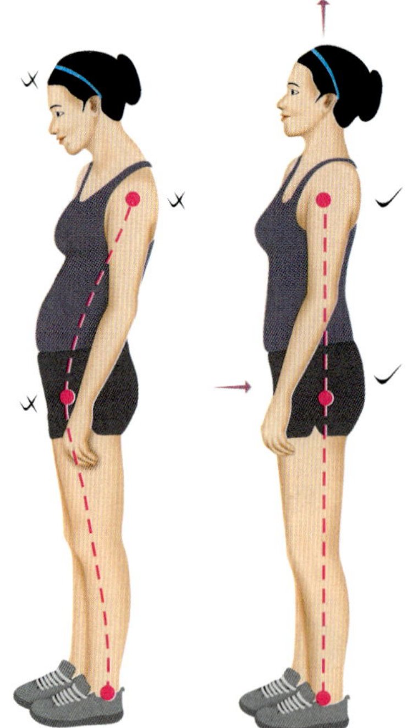

Fig. 7: Walking

As her strength and energy increases, she can begin more progressive abdominal sit-ups by:

- Folding her arms over her chest
- Placing her hands behind her head.

Sit-ups

- Elevate head with a pillow and bend knees
- Tuck chin, exhale and reach toward knees
- Hold for a count of five
- Inhale as your release
- Repeat 3–5 times.

Diagonal Sit-up (Waistline Exercise) (Fig. 9)

Ask her to:

- Lie on her back with her knees bent
- Exhale as she raises her head and right shoulder
- Point her right hand toward her left knee, keeping her heels on the floor and hold for a count of five
- Lower her head slowly for a count of five while breathing in through her nose
- Repeat using her other side pointing her left hand towards her right knee.

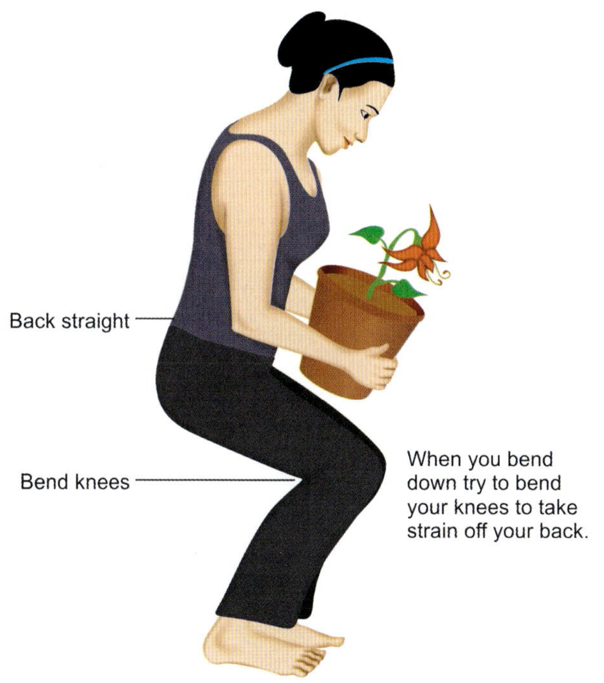

Fig. 8: Housework and lifting

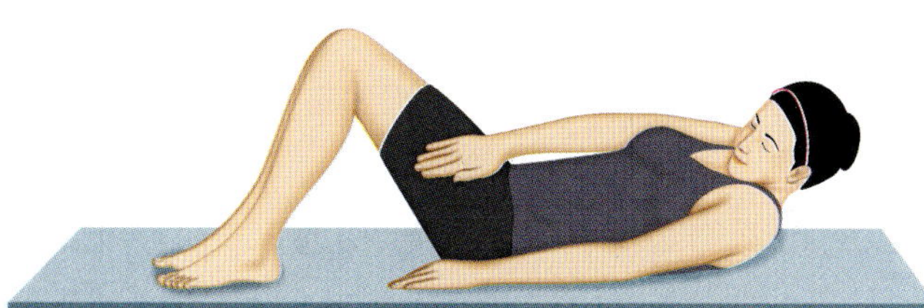

Fig. 9: Diagonal sit-up (waistline exercise)

PELVIC FLOOR MUSCLE EXERCISES

Kiegel Exercises

These exercises are very important for women of all stages and they strengthen pelvic floor muscles which make a sling from coccyx to pubis, and this sling is the support for bladder neck, urethra, vagina and rectum.

Women can start these exercises in the antenatal period and can continue throughout their life. These prevent urinary incontinence in the postpartum period and also in the perimenopause and menopause period. They help to improve fecal incontinence also.

Along with counseling and sex therapy these exercise also help women who have a problem reaching orgasm.

Technique of Doing Kiegel Exercises

It is very important to learn the correct technique of doing Kiegel exercises for them to be effective.

Find the Right Muscles

First patient has to identify the perineal muscles she has to contract. Ask her to go to toilet and pass urine and in between the process of urination she should try to hold the stream of urine and that is how she would learn how to contract these muscles. Secondly, ask her to put her finger in her vagina and to try to squeeze on it and she would be able to identify the muscles she has to contract. She would feel the contraction of vagina and feel the pelvic floor move upwards.

Then she should relax her muscles and feel her pelvic floor move down to the starting position. As the muscles become stronger—and patient becomes more experienced with the exercises—this movement will be more pronounced.

A cautionary note: Don't make a habit of starting and stopping her urine stream. Doing Kiegel exercises with a full bladder or while emptying her bladder can actually weaken the muscles. It can also lead to incomplete emptying of the bladder which increases her risk of a urinary tract infection.

Perfect the Technique

Once she has identified her pelvic floor muscles, then after emptying bladder and getting into a sitting or standing position she can do these exercises while doing her routine chores. Work up to keeping the muscles contracted for 10 seconds at a time, relaxing for 10 seconds between contractions.

Don'ts

Patient should not flex her *thigh, buttocks or abdominal muscles* while doing these exercises. She should breathe normally and should not hold her breath.

Biofeedback May Help

If she has trouble doing Kiegel exercises, biofeedback training may help. In a biofeedback session, a nurse, therapist or technician will either insert a monitoring probe into her vagina or place adhesive electrodes on the skin outside her vagina or rectal area. When she contracts her pelvic floor muscles, a measurement on a monitor will be seen and that lets her know whether she has successfully contracted the right muscles. She will also be able to see how long she can hold the contraction.

Another technique uses electrical stimulation to help one feel the muscles contract. The procedure is painless, although one will experience a buzzing feeling as a small electrical current is applied to patient's pelvic floor muscles, making them contract. Once women feel this sensation a few times, she will probably be able to duplicate the exercise on her own. Because simpler methods work for most women, this technique is rarely used.

When to Expect Results

If she does her Kiegel exercises faithfully, she can expect to see some results, such as less frequent urine leakage, within about 8–12 weeks. Her improvement may be dramatic—or at the very least, her problems can be prevented from getting worse. As with other forms of physical activity, you need to make Kiegel exercises a life-long practice to get life-long benefits.

Weight-bearing and Resistance Exercises

When recovered, patients must start proper strength and stamina building exercises by doing weight bearing and resistance exercises to build up their muscle mass and increase their bone mass density, especially when she has had her total hysterectomy along with bilateral oophorectomy. All the women above 40 should start doing these exercises along with other lifestyle modifications of proper diet, an adjuvant calcium and when needed, hormone therapy should be prescribed and she can do advanced abdominal muscles exercises. Women must do exercises for building back muscles like seated row because of increased risk of osteoporosis and silent spinal compression fractures leading onto "Dowager's hump" later on.

Driving

She should not drive until she feels confident to do an emergency stop! If she has had abdominal surgery, she is advised not to drive for 4 weeks.

Back to Work

It may be any time between 6 weeks and 12 weeks depending on the type of surgery she had, the rate of her recovery, the type of work she does and the amount of traveling involved.

CHAPTER

17

Grafts in Gynecological Surgery

Maninder Ahuja

INTRODUCTION

The role of graft materials in gynecologic surgery has undergone numerous modifications in the past 30 years. The growing interest in the use of graft materials stems from disappointing suboptimal cure rates obtained with traditional procedures. Pelvic prolapse is a common condition often leading to symptoms related to urinary, bowel and sexual dysfunction. According to an epidemiologic study performed by Olsen and colleagues, the estimated lifetime risk of undergoing a surgery up to 80 years for pelvic prolapse is 11% and approximately 30% of these patients will undergo a repeat prolapse surgery.

Traditional reconstructive repairs rely on placating tissue underlying a support defect. In theory, this tissue has become attenuated and damaged by childbirth/chronic trauma, or has defective collagen. Given current theories about the etiology of support defects, it is appealing to reinforce this tissue with graft materials during surgical intervention. Most of the long-term experience with mesh reinforcement stems from the general surgery literature and the experience with ventral and inguinal hernia repairs. In gynecologic surgery over the past two decades, mesh has been used for transabdominal prolapse repair, and more recently for suburethral slings and anterior and posterior repair of cystocele and rectocele.

BIOMECHANICS OF MATERIALS

Knowledge and understanding of the properties of the material are essential prior to its use. Despite advances in technology, the ideal biocompatible material has not yet been developed.

CLASSIFICATION OF GRAFTS

- Synthetic
- Autologous (tissue from the same person)
- Xenografts (tissue from an animal donor)
- Allografts (tissue from a human donor).

Autologous Grafts

These grafts are rectus fascia and fascia lata taken from the patient and harvested.

Advantage is of being native tissue with no risk for rejection and low risk for infection. However, the harvesting process can result in:

- Prolonged operative time
- Can lead to leg pain at the harvesting site
- In theory, this native tissue has the same propensity to tissue degradation in women who are predisposed to it
- The limited quantities available for harvesting limit its use to stress urinary incontinence (SUI) and is not routinely used for pelvic organ prolapse surgery.

Since the beginning of twentieth century, various autologous grafts have been used to perform the pubovaginal sling urethropexy, or "traditional" sling procedure. Overall success rate for the fascia lata pubovaginal sling urethropexy is 87%.

Abdominal retropubic urethropexy has the same results as traditional suburethral sling.

Traditional suburethral slings remain the gold standard for the treatment of SUI in the setting of intrinsic sphincter deficiency as well as for recurrent urinary incontinence with urethral hypermobility.

Complications

Postoperative voiding dysfunction in the form of urinary retention and urinary urge symptoms is the most commonly encountered complication after pubovaginal sling cystourethropexy. De novo detruss or instability occurs in 15–20% of patients.

Abdominal sacrocolpopexy (ASC) for the repair of apical prolapse has been well-established, with success rates ranging from 78% to 100%. This procedure entails the attachment of a graft material to the endopelvic fascia and vaginal wall, and suspending it to the anterior longitudinal ligament at about levels S2-S3 on the sacrum. The procedure secures apical support and provides a near-normal vaginal axis. There is no current agreement among pelvic surgeons as to the ideal material for this procedure. Autologous fascia provides an immunologically inert alternative without the risk for rejection and low risk for erosion.

Disadvantages of autograft:

- Morbidity resulting from the harvesting processing
- Limited amounts of available material
- Risk for hernia at the site of the harvesting, if rectus fascia is used.

Allografts

These are donor fascia lata and duramater, which have been used for many years, in an effort to avoid the morbidity that is associated with autologous tissue harvest. This tissue is cultured and sterilized with a freeze-dried technique as well as gamma radiation. Regardless of the sterilization techniques used in the preparation of these materials, small risk for transmission of infectious diseases is present.

Intact deoxyribonucleic acid (DNA) segments have been isolated from four commercial sources of processed human allografts. Although, the potential for transmission of infectious disease is a vital concern, so far there are no reported cases of disease transmission by this method. More importantly, however, is the emergence of increasing evidence that these materials are not as durable as autologous grafts or synthetic materials. Multiple reports have documented disappointing results with freeze-dried fascia lata as a result of tissue breakdown, which has been shown histologically.

In cases of a previously failed, either a fascia lata suburethral sling procedure or sacrocolpopexy, initial trials of *allogenic* slings were favorable, but more recently there have been reports indicating high failure rates (27% in one study, 52% in another) of freeze-dried and irradiated donor fascia lata in sling procedures for stress incontinence.

The explanation of failure rate of donor fascia lata includes:

- Host versus graft reaction
- Radiation-induced changes in tissue
- Variability in the quality of the donor tissue.

Xenografts

Xenografts provide yet another alternative to autologous tissue. Recent studies with porcine subintestinal mucosa and acellular porcine dermis show good short-term cure rates for SUI. However, there have been reports of postoperative tissue reactions to these materials, therefore prompting caution as to the tolerability and long-term outcomes with their use. There is also a possibility of transmission of infectious diseases with xenografts and allograft regardless of the processing techniques used.

There are insufficient data to comment on the use of xenografts as it applies to sacrocolpopexy. Until the ideal graft is developed, synthetic grafts continue to afford an excellent option for vaginal vault suspension.

Xenografts, such as acellular collagen matrix (*Pelvicol*) and porcine small intestinal mucosa (*Surgisis*, Cook Group, Inc., Bloomington, Indiana), have been reported as useful in the repair of rectovaginal fistulas. Although, the use of *Pelvicol* in the posterior compartment in small case series had a high risk for recurrence, the use of an acellular collagen matrix (*PelviSoft*, Biomesh, CR Bard, Inc., Cranston, Rhode Island) in mesh form has been reported to have promising anatomic results. In addition, a dermal graft (*Duraderm*, CR Bard, Inc., Covington, Georgia, or *Repliform*, Boston Scientific Corp., Natick, Massachusetts) has been reported to yield good anatomic results and a low rate of rectocele recurrence. It is difficult to compare these studies, because their study outcomes were not assessed in a standard fashion.

Synthetic slings gained popularity in the 1970s. The use of a synthetic permanent sling avoids the morbidity of harvesting fascia, as well as the risk for transmission of infectious disease present with allografts and xenografts. Other advantages of synthetic materials are that they are not absorbed or degraded and have good tensile strength.

Infection that occurs as a postoperative complication of the use of grafts is caused by infiltration and proliferation of bacteria behind the pores and interstices of the material. Chronic bacterial colonization is more likely to occur when either the interstices or pores are lesser than 10 μm. Therefore, there is an emphasis on using mesh with a pore size greater than 75 μm, which allows for the passage of leukocytes and macrophages and may be associated with fibrous healing. On the basis of this information, evidence favors the selection of a type I mesh, or macroporous

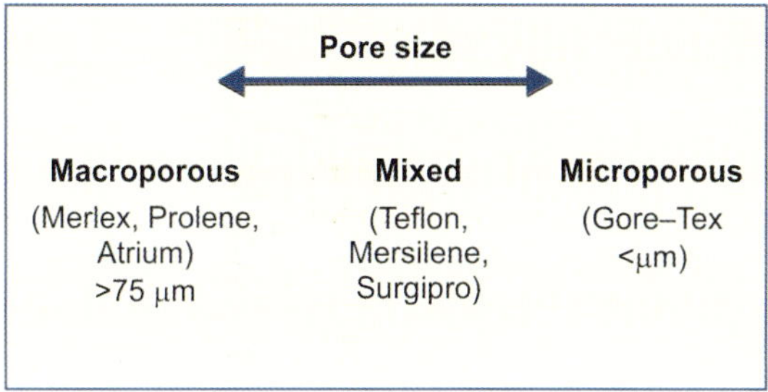

Fig. 1: Different types of mesh tapes with different pore sizes

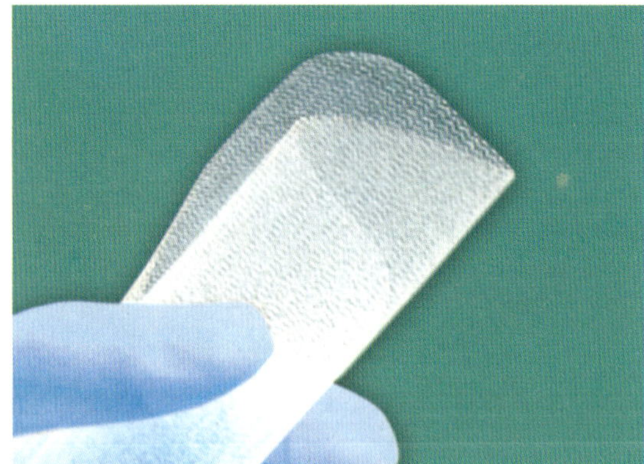

Fig. 2: Nonabsorbable polypropylene mesh

mesh, when selecting a synthetic material to use in pelvic surgery (Fig. 1).

Currently, most synthetic grafts are made of permanent fibers of:

- Polypropylene (Fig. 2)
- Polyester
- Polytetrafluoroethylene
- Polyethylene
- Nylon.

The elastic and mechanical properties depend on the synthetic material used and whether it is woven or knitted.

The stiffness and flexibility of the material will have an impact on all possible clinical complications.

Absorbable synthetic materials are also available. The two most commonly used absorbable synthetics are:

- Polyglycolic acid *(Dexon,* Davis and Geck, Inc., Norwalk, Connecticut)
- Polyglactin 910 (Vicryl; Ethicon, Inc., Somerville, New Jersey).

Both of these materials are generally well tolerated. They are mostly hydrolyzed at about 90 days and thus preclude the risk for erosion and infection, which makes their use appealing. However, studies performed on animals with these materials have shown that they provide insufficient strength before tissue healing is completed.

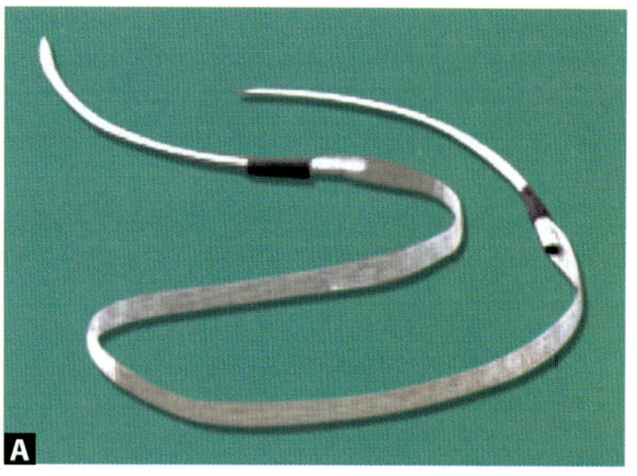

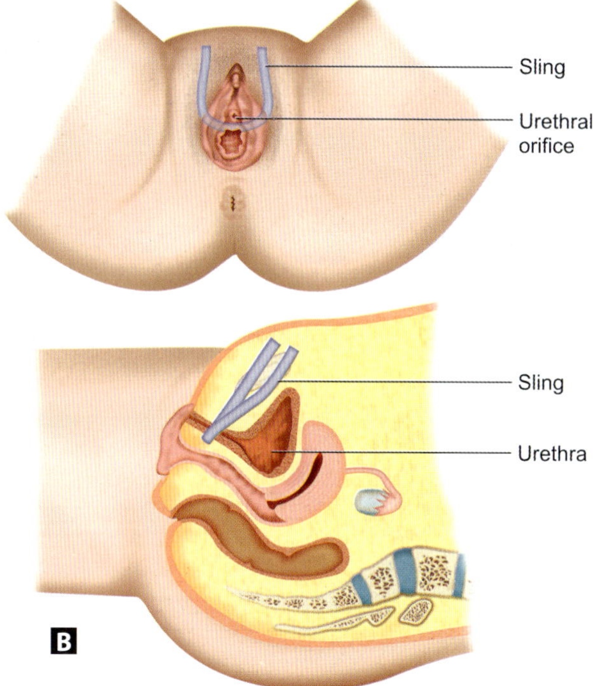

Figs 3A and B: Polypropylene tension-free vaginal tape with inserter and its diagrammatic representation of insertion and placement

The most popular material is a polypropylene sling (Fig. 3). This material is the one used in the tension-free vaginal tape (TVT) procedure, first introduced by Ulmsten and colleagues in 1996. The TVT procedure (Fig. 4) has prompted much enthusiasm because it is a minimally invasive procedure with low patient morbidity and mortality and high cure rates for SUI—up to 93% at a mean follow-up of 21 months.

TVT POLYPROPYLENE TAPE

Complications

- The rate of bladder perforations is about 5–34% and is inversely related to the expertise of the surgeon

- The overall rate of vaginal erosion of the TVT procedure is around 1%. Most cases of vaginal erosion with synthetic slings heal well with conservative management with estrogen cream or local excision of the mesh
- The two most common voiding-related complications of the polypropylene suburethral sling are de novo urge incontinence and postoperative voiding dysfunction requiring a temporary-indwelling catheter.

The transobturator approach (Fig. 5) to the placement of a suburethral sling was introduced in 2001 in an effort to avoid a blind passage of trochar through the retropubic space and thus decrease the risk for visceral injuries. This procedure has an 80% cure rate for SUI at 1 year.

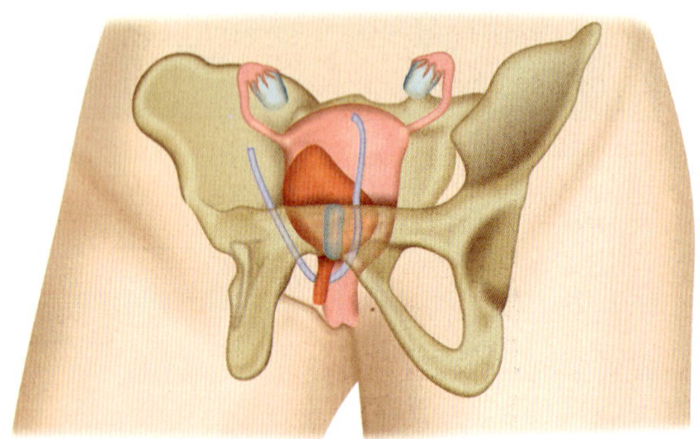

Fig. 4: TVT tape placement

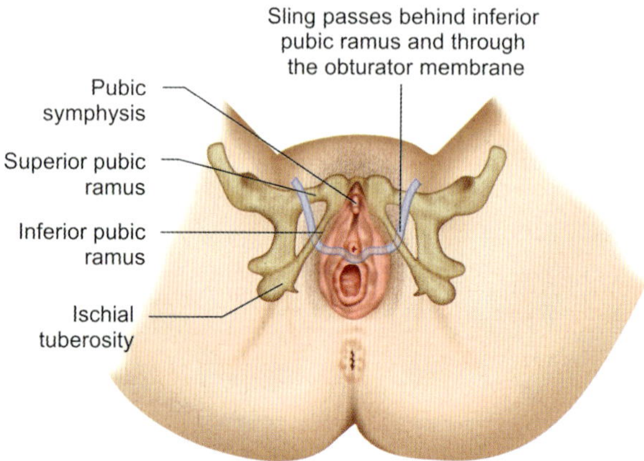

Fig. 5: Transobturator approach

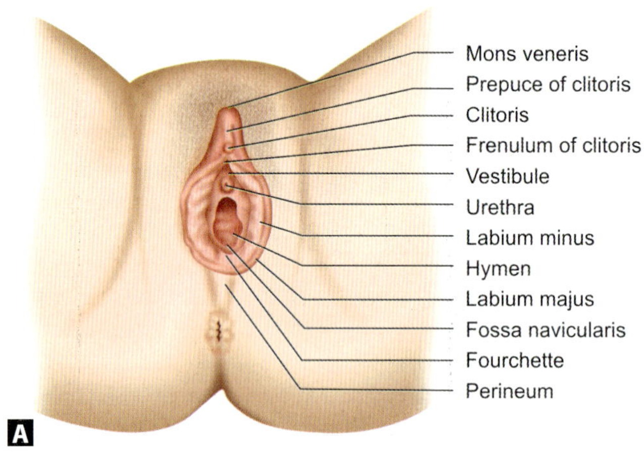

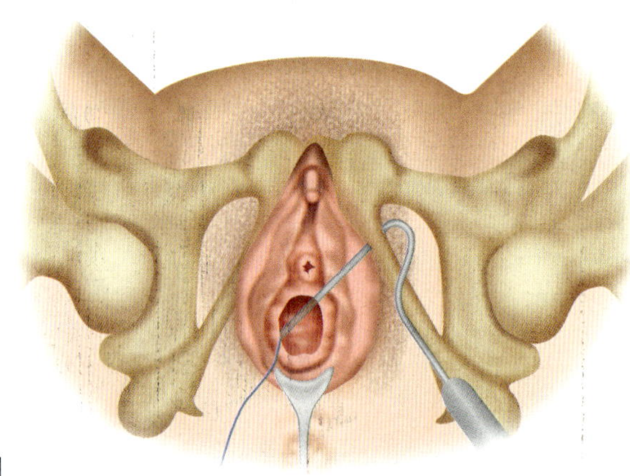

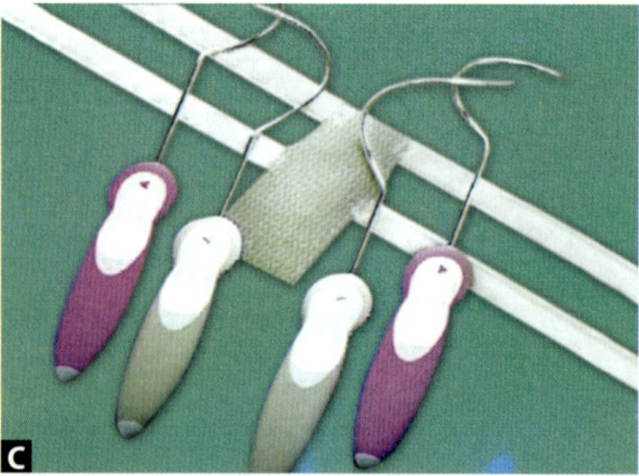

Figs 6A to C: Transobturator cystocele repair by mesh

Complications

- Bladder perforation rate of greater than 1%
- Urethral perforation rate of 2.5% (occurring during the learning phase of the procedure)
- Vaginal tape erosions
- Infected hematomas, and abscess formation
- Groin and leg pain
- Postoperative voiding dysfunction
- De novo urge incontinence as well as transient crural pain has also been reported.

Long-term follow-up is needed to assess the true incidence of complications with this technique.

SYNTHETIC GRAFTS IN ABDOMINAL SACROCOLPOPEXY

Synthetic grafts have been used in ASC procedures for decades with a high success rate. Albeit rare, serious complications, such as mesh erosion, infection and rejection, have been reported (Figs 7 and 8).

Complications

- A recent review of the literature reported the overall rate of synthetic mesh erosion to be 3.4% with a rate of reoperation of about 3%. The time to the detection of mesh erosion has been reported to range from 2 months to 33 months
- Other rare but serious complications, such as infection with sacral abscess formation
- Sinus tracts
- Sacral osteomyelitis

ANTERIOR AND POSTERIOR REPAIR

The most common site for recurrence of prolapse is in the anterior compartment, with recurrence rates of 20–37%. Several materials have been used to reinforce the anterior compartment, but the results are variable and the follow-up usually short-term. Permanent synthetic mesh, such as *Marlex* (Chevron Phillips Chemical Company LP, The Woodlands, Texas) and polypropylene mesh (*Atrium*, Atrium Medical Corporation, Hudson, New Hampshire; *Prolene,* Ethicon, Inc.), have been used to reinforce the anterior compartment with a reported success rate for cystocele repair up to 100% and it has been used in posterior compartment repair also with 92–100% success rate; complication of rectovaginal fistula requiring a Martius graft has been reported.

Complications

- Erosion rates ranging from 3% to 25%. Vicryl is being tried by some as an alternative but so far no consensus on its use
- Postoperative dyspareunia.

Xenograft such as acellular porcine dermis (*Pelvicol,* CR Bard, Inc., Covington, Georgia) shows a success between 81% and 93%.

In contrast, other xenografts, such as *AlloDerm* (fascia lata, LifeCell Corp., The Woodlands, Texas) have been reported to have no impact on the recurrence of cystocele.

Complication is unpredictable immune reaction to the graft during tissue healing, manifested as early postoperative superficial dehiscence.

Fig. 7: Sacrohysteropexy using mesh

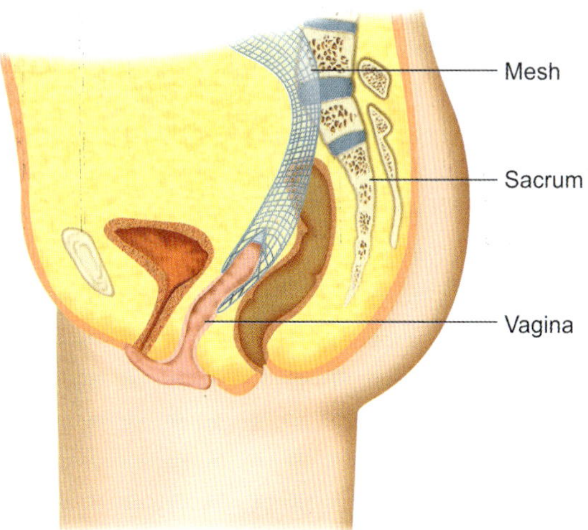

Fig. 8: Sacrocolpopexy using mesh to repair a vaginal vault repair

CONCLUSION

The ideal graft has not yet been developed. Two general categories of graft materials have promising results with respect to restoring anatomic and functional outcomes. On the one hand, the synthetic grafts prove to be durable and widely available. However, their application carries the risk for vaginal erosion, especially by the vaginal route. Biomaterials (xenografts) may provide a viable alternative to synthetics. However, their widespread tolerability and durability remain to be studied.

BIBLIOGRAPHY

1. Amid PK, Shulman AG, Lichtenstein IL, et al. Bio-materials for abdominal wall hernia surgery and principles of their applications. Langenbecks Arch Chir. 1994;379:168-71.
2. Amrute KV, Badlani GH. Female incontinence: a review of biomaterials and minimally invasive techniques. Curr Opin Urol. 2006;16:54-9.
3. Amundsen CL, Visco AG, Ruiz H, et al. Outcome in 104 pubovaginal slings using freeze-dried allograft fascia lata from a single tissue bank. Urology. 2000;56:2-8.
4. Babalola EO, Famuyide AO, McGuire LJ, et al. Vaginal erosion, sinus formation, and ischiorectal abscess following transobturator tape: ObTape implantation. Int Urogynecol J Pelvic Floor Dysfunct. 2005:1-4.
5. Cosson M, Debodinance P, Boukerrou M, et al. Mechanical properties of synthetic implants used in the repair of prolapse and urinary incontinence in women: which is the ideal material? Int Urogynecol J Pelvic Floor Dysfunct. 2003;14:169-78.
6. Culligan PJ, Blackwell L, Goldsmith LJ, et al. A randomized controlled trial comparing fascia lata and synthetic mesh for sacral colpopexy. Obstet Gynecol. 2005;106:29-37.
7. de Tayrac R, Picone O, Chauveaud-Lambling A, et al. 2-year anatomical and functional assessment of transvaginal rectocele repair using a polypropylene mesh. Int Urogynecol J Pelvic Floor Dysfunct. 2005;17:100-5.
8. Dwyer PL, O'Reilly BA. Transvaginal repair of anterior and posterior compartment prolapse with atrium polypropylene mesh. BJOG. 2004;111:831-6.
9. FitzGerald MP, Edwards SR, Fenner D. Medium-term follow-up on use of freeze-dried, irradiated donor fascia for sacrocolpopexy and sling procedures. Int Urogynecol J Pelvic Floor Dysfunct. 2004;15:238-42.
10. Flood CG, Drutz HP, Waja L. Anterior colporrhaphy reinforced with marlex mesh for the treatment of cystoceles. Int Urogynecol J Pelvic Floor Dysfunct. 1998;9:200-4.
11. Gandhi S, Goldberg RP, Kwon C, et al. A prospective randomized trial using solvent dehydrated fascia lata for the prevention of recurrent anterior vaginal wall prolapse. Am J Obstet Gynecol. 2005;192:1649-54.
12. Gomelsky A, Rudy DC, Dmochowski RR. Porcine dermis interposition graft for repair of high grade anterior compartment defects with or without concomitant pelvic organ prolapse procedures. J Urol. 2004;171:1581-4.
13. Hathaway JK, Choe JM. Intact genetic material is present in commercially processed cadaver allografts used for pubovaginal slings. J Urol. 2002;168:1040-3.
14. Huang YH, Lin AT, Chen KK, et al. High failure rate using allograft fascia lata in pubovaginal sling surgery for female stress urinary incontinence. Urology. 2001;58:943-6.
15. Julian TM. The efficacy of marlex mesh in the repair of severe, recurrent vaginal prolapse of the anterior midvaginal wall. Am J Obstet Gynecol. 1996;175:1472-5.
16. Kohli N, Miklos JR. Dermal graft-augmented rectocele repair. Int Urogynecol J Pelvic Floor Dysfunct. 2003;14:146-9.
17. Latini JM, Brown JA, Kreder KJ. Abdominal sacral colpopexy using autologous fascia lata. J Urol. 2004;171:1176-9.
18. Leboeuf L, Miles RA, Kim SS, et al. Grade 4 cystocele repair using four-defect repair and porcine xenograft acellular matrix (pelvicol): outcome measures using SEAPI. Urology. 2004;64:282-6.
19. Levin I, Groutz A, Gold R, et al. Surgical complications and medium-term outcome results of tension-free vaginal tape: a prospective study of 313 consecutive patients. Neurourol Urodyn. 2004;23:7-9.
20. McLennan MT, Melick CF. Bladder perforation during tension-free vaginal tape procedures: analysis of learning curve and risk factors. Obstet Gynecol. 2005;106:1000-4.
21. Moore RD, Miklos JR, Kohli N. Rectovaginal fistula repair using a porcine dermal graft. Obstet Gynecol 2004;104:1165-7.
22. Morgan JE, Farrow GA, Stewart FE. The marlex sling operation for the treatment of recurrent stress urinary incontinence: a 16-year review. Am J Obstet Gynecol. 1985;151:224-6.
23. Myers DL, LaSala CA. Conservative surgical management of mersilene mesh suburethral sling erosion. Am J Obstet Gynecol. 1998;179:1424-8.
24. Nygaard IE, McCreery R, Brubaker L, et al. Abdominal sacrocolpopexy: a comprehensive review. Obstet Gynecol. 2004;104:805-23.
25. Olsen AL, Smith VJ, Bergstrom JO, et al. Epidemiology of surgically managed pelvic organ prolapse and urinary incontinence. Obstet Gynecol. 1997;89:501-6.
26. Pye PK, Dada T, Duthie G, et al. Surgisistrade mark mesh: a novel approach to repair of a recurrent rectovaginal fistula. Dis Colon Rectum. 2004;47:1554-56.
27. Salomon LJ, Detchev R, Barranger E, et al. Treatment of anterior vaginal wall prolapse with porcine skin collagen implant by the transobturator route: preliminary results. Eur Urol. 2004;45:219-5.
28. Ulmsten U, Henriksson L, Johnson P, et al. An ambulatory surgical procedure under local anesthesia for treatment of female urinary incontinence. Int Urogynecol J Pelvic Floor Dysfunct. 1996;7:81-5.
29. Walter AJ, Hentz JG, Magrina JF, et al. Harvesting autologous fascia lata for pelvic reconstructive surgery: techniques and morbidity. Am J Obstet Gynecol. 2001;185:1354-8.

Section 2

Obstetrics

Section Outline

CHAPTER

18

Labor Room Operative Procedures

SN Daftary

INTRODUCTION

During the management of a parturient in active labor, the obstetrician may be called upon to perform several minor operative procedures to facilitate the process of labor and delivery. Some of these procedures are carried out in the labor room itself under strict aseptic precautions. For major obstetric interventions, the patient is best attended to in the regular operation theater.

ARTIFICIAL RUPTURE OF MEMBRANES

Definition

This is a procedure in which the attending obstetrician chooses to deliberately rupture the forewaters or the leading part of the bag of membranes.

Indications

- Induction of labor
- Augmentation of labor
- To observe the color of liquor amnii
- Prior to application of fetal scalp electrode for electronic fetal heart rate monitoring (EFHRM) during labor
- Prior to fetal scalp blood sampling in suspected fetal distress
- Prior to placement of intrauterine catheter for monitoring intrauterine pressure recordings
- Prior to placement of intrauterine catheters for amnioinfusion in cases of oligohydramnios or EFHRM revealing variable decelerations suggestive of fetal cord compression.

Advantages

- Amniotomy brings about wider contact between the presenting part and the cervix, encouraging release of endogenous prostaglandins and thereby augmenting labor and shortening its duration
- Amniotomy provides the opportunity of early detection of meconium staining of the liquor amnii and implementing closer observation of fetal well-being.

Disadvantages

- Reduction in amniotic fluid may result in cord compression
- The intensity of pains may increase to undesirable levels, adversely affecting the fetus
- Head compression may be excessive and harmful
- Danger of cord prolapse and limb prolapse
- Predisposes to a premature separation of the placenta
- The risk of ascending infection increases with time
- Amniotomy commits the obstetrician to accomplish delivery within reasonable time.

Procedure

The procedure is undertaken with the patient lying in the dorsal position with her feet widely parted. The vulva is cleaned with antiseptic lotion. The parts are isolated with sterile drapes. The obstetrician dons a pair of sterile gloves. After parting the labia, introduce the well lubricated examining fingers into the vagina to reach the membranes surrounded by the cervical rim. The membranes are tweaked with a Kocher's clamp (Drew-Smythe catheter, amniotomy forceps), preferably as posterior as possible, to prevent a sudden gush of amniotic fluid. Examine the patient carefully to exclude cord/limb prolapse. Examine the drained amniotic fluid for presence of meconium.

In case of difficulty to accomplish artificial rupture of membrane (ARM) successfully, consider placing the patient briefly in lithotomy position to accomplish the procedure.

EPISIOTOMY/PERINEOTOMY

Definition

It is an incision made into the perineum to enlarge the birth passage to facilitate the birth of the baby.

Types: The types of incisions made have been listed below (Fig. 1):

- Median or midline
- Mediolateral
- Mediolateral—J shaped
- Lateral.

Of these, the ones in common practice are the mediolateral, J-shaped, and midline episiotomies.

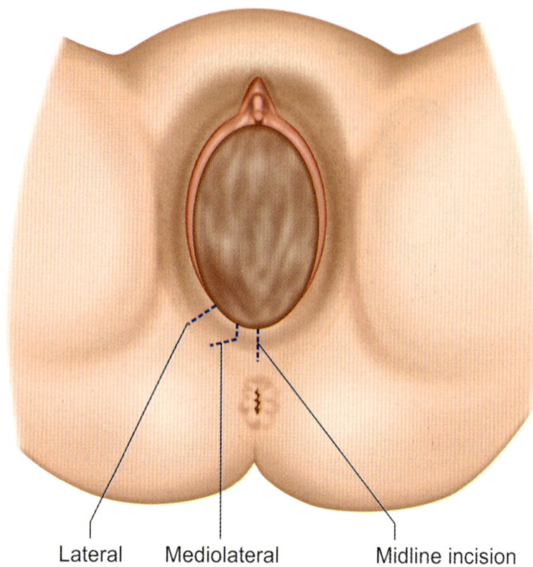

Fig. 1: Types of episiotomies

Maternal Benefits

The following have been claimed:

- A clean cut surgical incision is easier to repair than ragged perineal tear
- It prevents undue stretching of the vaginal walls which predispose to future cystocele, rectocele, uterine prolapse, deficient perineum, loose vaginal outlet, stress urinary incontinence, anal canal and rectal injuries, and periclitoral injuries.
- Shortens the duration of the second stage of labor
- Spares the mother bearing down efforts.

Fetal Benefits

- It spares the fetal head from the compressive forces prior to its exit
- It is of great benefit to preterm babies and high-risk babies.

Indications

These include:

- Prophylactic to spare strain on pelvic floor
- Arrest or progress of labor because of rigid perineum
- To facilitate instrumental assisted vaginal delivery
- Where large tears seem inevitable
- To prevent complete perineal tear when perineum is very short
- To spare prolonged compression of fetal head
- To shorten the second stage of labor in high-risk pregnancies
- Whenever the mother suffers from medical disorder—to reduce the strain of bearing down efforts.

Episiotomy Repair

- The surgical repair of an episiotomy should be undertaken with the same precautions as for any other surgical procedure (Figs 2A to C)
- Clean the parts with antiseptic
- Isolate the parts with sterile drapes
- Infiltrate the operation site with 1% xylocaine
- Examine the cervix, vaginal walls, vulvar outlet and paraurethral areas for any suspected injuries under a good light
- Place a sterile sponge in the vagina to pack away the cervix and prevent the trickle of blood into the operation field (Fig. 3)
- Identify the edges of the vaginal incision from its apex to the vulval outlet, commence suturing from the apex downward—approximating the cut edges of the vagina with a 2/0 continuous locking chromic catgut suture or with vicryl 2/0. The cut edges of the perineal muscle layer are approximated with interrupted suture of 1/0 chromic catgut, after ensuring proper hemostasis. Lastly, the skin edges are approximated with either interrupted 1/0 catgut or with 2/0 subcuticular suture. The wound is covered with antiseptic ointment (betadine) and covered with sterile gauze dressing
- The episiotomy is cleaned and a fresh dressing is applied every 8 hours and after every visit to the toilet.

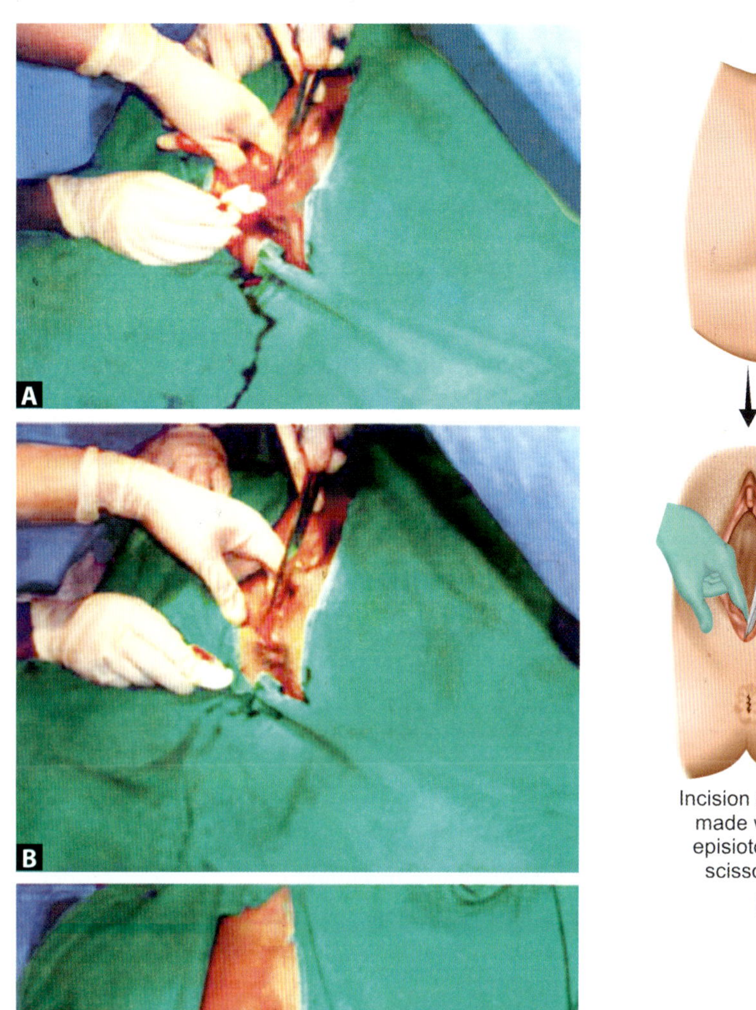

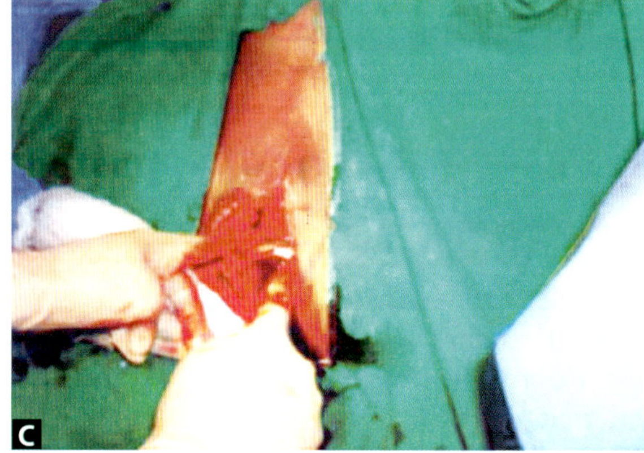

Figs 2A to C: Episiotomy being done and enlarging the fourchette

BLADDER CATHETERIZATION

Indications

These include the following:

- Retention of urine during pregnancy—retroverted gravid uterus, fibroid or pelvic mass in the pelvis impacting on the bladder neck
- In eclamptic patient—to monitor urinary output and to test urine for albumin

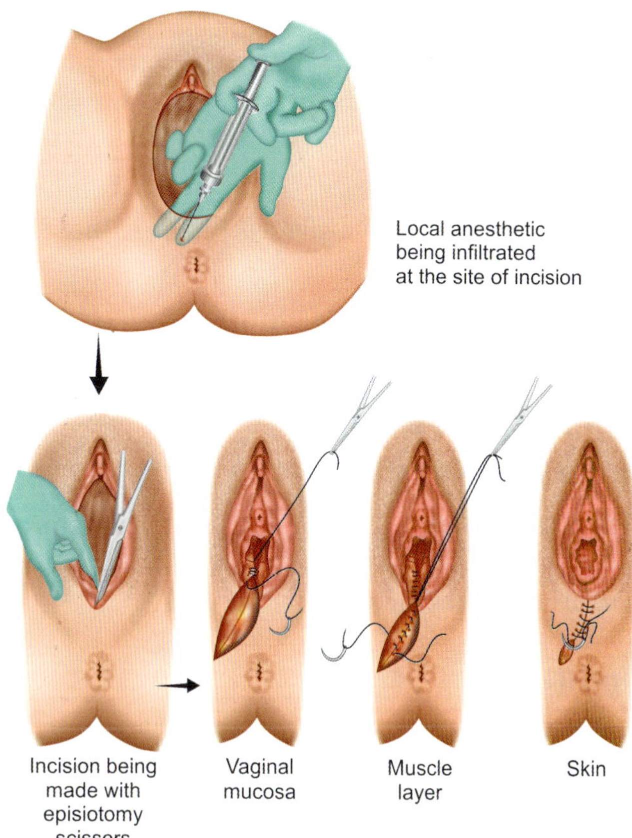

Fig. 3: Episiotomy being made and repaired

- Inability to void urine during advanced labor because of the deeply engaged fetal head
- Postpartum urinary retention because of the bladder insensitivity or due to reflex spasm as a result of pain from perineal site
- Prior to vaginal assisted instrumental delivery (forceps/ventouse)
- Prior to cesarean section.

Procedure

- Observe strict aseptic precautions
- Clean the vulva with antiseptic solution
- Part the labia digitally after wearing sterile gloves. Expose the external urinary meatus
- With the other gloved hand, pick up a sterile plastic disposable catheter, lubricate its tip with sterile jelly and direct it into the urethra, and advance it into the bladder cavity. If it is desired to retain the catheter—select a Foley catheter. After proper insertion, inflate its bulb with sterile saline and connect it to a sterile urobag

- During advanced labor, the advanced presenting part may render catheterization difficult. In such cases, the obstetrician pushes up the presenting part to facilitate introduction of the catheter.

Dangers

Catheterization carries the following risks:

- Trauma—bleeding
- False passage
- Ascending infection.

DILATATION AND EVACUATION (D & E)

Introduction

This is currently the most popular method of emptying the gravid uterus of its contents.

Indications

To terminate pregnancy for the following indications:

- First trimester medical termination of pregnancy (MTP)
- Incomplete abortion
- Inevitable abortion
- Missed abortion
- Vesicular mole.

Preoperative Preparation

- Counseling
- Informed consent
- Preoperative investigations: Hemoglobin, urine routine, ABO and Rh blood groups and blood sugar estimate
- Preoperative administration of prostaglandins help to soften the cervix and facilitate dilatation
- Shave and prepare private parts (not always observed)
- Inject 0.6 mg atropine half an hour before the procedure
- Preoperative sedation (pentazocine, diazepam/midazolam).

Procedure

- Patient in lithotomy position
- External genitalia cleaned with antiseptic solution (savlon/betadine)
- Parts isolated with sterile drapes
- Surgeon performs a bimanual examination observing strict aseptic precautions to determine the direction of the cervix and assess the size of the uterus
- The cervix is exposed after introduction of Sims speculum and an anterior vaginal wall retractor
- The anterior lip of the cervix is grasped with a tenaculum forceps
- A paracervical block is given
- The cervix gradually dilated with graduated cervical dilators (the silastic dilators are preferred) up to the number corresponding to the gestational size in weeks
- The suction cannula is introduced into the uterine cavity up to the fundus, it is connected through a suction tubing to a suction pump to achieve a suction force of 65 mm Hg. The cannula is gradually rotated inside the cavity as it is being withdrawn to aspirate the uterine contents. The procedure is judged to be complete when no further products are aspirated, the cervix begins to grip the cannula, and there is grating of the uterine walls all around. At this point, some surgeons request for the attending nurse to administer injections of 0.2 mg of methylergometrine maleate to ensure uterine contraction.

Complications

The major complications include:

Immediate Complications

- Continuation of pregnancy
- Incomplete evacuation
- Hemorrhage and shock
- Infection
- Perforation
- Visceral injuries
- Redo procedure.

Remote Complications

- Cervical trauma
- Incompetent cervix followed by repeated abortions
- Infertility (blocked tubal ostia)
- Oligomenorrhea due to synechiae
- Rh sensitization.

SYMPHYSIOTOMY

Definition

Division of the pubic symphysis to permanently enlarge the pelvic space in women with contracted pelvis.

History

- First performed by Signault in 1777
- Popularized by Zarate in Argentina in 1920

- Seedat and Crichton in Africa (1962) where women with previous cesarean section for cephalopelvic disproportion suffered uterine rupture as they failed to return to hospital in their future pregnancies.

Procedure

The simplified procedure of symphysiotomy can be accomplished by a trained obstetrician easily in the labor room itself without the need for transfer.

Advantages

- It can be accomplished in a short time
- It can be performed in the labor room itself
- Local anesthesia is sufficient
- The uterus is left unscarred
- The pelvic capacity is permanently enlarged for all subsequent deliveries.

Indications

- Poor surgical risks
- Moderate cephalopelvic disproportion in lower pelvic strait
- Difficult forceps delivery
- Difficulty with delivery of after coming head in breech delivery.

Prerequisites

- The uterus should be contracting
- The head should not be floating
- The cervix should be in an advanced state of dilatation (> 8 cm).

Contraindications

- Inefficient uterine contractions
- Cervix less than 8.0 cm dilated
- Previous cesarean scar
- Major disproportion
- Suspected uterine rupture
- Fetal macrosomia
- Maternal obesity (marked)
- Deformed pelvis, fetal malpresentation
- Experienced obstetrician not available.

Procedure

- Patient in lithotomy position
- Introduce Foley catheter to empty bladder
- The left hand is placed in the vagina to displace the urethra away from the midline
- The skin and subcutaneous tissues overlying the pubic symphysis are infiltrated with xylocaine. A sharp knife is introduced at the junction of middle and lower third of the symphysis in the midline, vertically in an anteroposterior direction with its blade pointing inferiorly. The lower third is divided
- The knife is withdrawn, reintroduced with its blade pointing superiorly to cut the upper part of the symphysis. During delivery, the patient's legs should be supported to permit controlled separation of the symphysis. A vacuum extractor should be used and the pull directed posteriorly. A liberal episiotomy spares undue strain on the anterior vaginal wall. After delivery, the skin over the symphysis is sutured with interrupted sutures.

Postoperative Care

- Bladder drainage continued for at least 5 days
- Antibiotics
- Pelvic elastic belt support
- Patient advised bed rest for 5 days followed by gradual ambulation over the next week
- Avoid physical strain for 6 weeks.

Complications

- Urinary tract problems—infection, fistula formation, stress urinary infection
- Hemorrhage
- Tears of anterior vaginal wall
- Postpartum hemorrhage
- Insecurity in the symphyseal joint rendering walking difficult (waddling gait).

CHAPTER

19

Induction and Augmentation Labor

Uday Thanawala, Kartik Bhagat

INTRODUCTION

Induction of labor is an intervention designed to artificially initiate uterine contractions followed by progressive dilatation and effacement of cervix culminating in the birth of a baby. The goal of induction of labor is to achieve a vaginal delivery by stimulating uterine contractions before the spontaneous onset of labor. It is to be considered only when vaginal delivery is deemed appropriate route of delivery.

Induction is indicated only when it is agreed that the mother or the fetus will benefit from the higher probability of better outcome than if birth is delayed. The benefits of labor induction must be weighed against the potential maternal and fetal risks associated with this procedure.

Man has always aspired to conquer nature. The wish to control birth has been the driving force of many great scientific researches. Some mechanical methods capable of forcibly dilating the cervix in order to initiate labor were used in the olden times. In 1948, Theobald and associates described the use of posterior pituitary extract for labor induction, which resulted in the synthesis of oxytocin, the first polypeptide hormone, by du Vigneaud and associates.

However, the synthesis of prostaglandins (PGs) and its introduction into clinical practice in 1968 by Karim and Embry, has revolutionized the concept of "Induction of Labor".

INCIDENCE

The incidence of induced labor has been increasing over the last few years and has almost doubled in the United States of America (USA) in the last 10 years. Almost 8–20% of labors are induced for a variety of reasons. The scope of induction is widening as the variety of reasons/indications for induction increase and the procedure becomes safer.

Prerequisites

Before induction is undertaken, the clinician should essentially discuss need for induction, end points of the process, need for lower segment cesarean section (LSCS) if induction fails, options of mode of delivery, neonatal outcomes and complications, with the patient. Women must be able to make informed choices regarding their care or treatment, and all relevant information should be made available to her. These choices should be recognized as an integral part of the decision-making process.

Before the induction is undertaken, it is imperative to do a complete examination including cervical assessment, pelvic assessment, assessment of the fetal size and presentation, and an attempt should be made to confirm the gestational age, fetal well-being and review investigations. Induction of labor is undertaken only if vaginal delivery is deemed possible by the clinician. Strict monitoring of the fetal heart and contractions is a must after induction. Maintaining a partogram is a healthy clinical practice in all labors, especially induced. Electronic fetal heart monitoring during labor is not mandatory but a helpful tool. Continuous care of the mother in labor has been shown to reduce cesarean section rates and the use of analgesia.

For women who are healthy and have had an otherwise uncomplicated pregnancy, induction of labor can be conducted in antenatal wards prior to the active phase of labor. The concept of ambulatory or domiciliary induction is still debatable. When undertaking induction of labor in women with recognized risk factors, the induction process should occur only in hospital setup.

Indications and Contraindications

There are no absolute indications for induction of labor. The most common indications for induction of labor are postdatism/post-term pregnancy, preeclampsia/eclampsia and premature rupture of membranes (PROM).

Other Indications

- Pregnancy complications like—intrauterine fetal death (IUFD), chorioamnionitis, abruptio placentae
- Maternal diseases like—diabetes mellitus, renal disease, chronic pulmonary disease, chronic hypertension
- Fetal conditions like—intrauterine growth retardation (IUGR), isoimmunization
- Labor may also be induced for social and practical reasons (like distance from the hospital, transport problems, availability of manpower) or psychological reasons.

Contraindications to induction of labor are the same as those for spontaneous labor and vaginal delivery—transverse lie, vasa previa, placenta previa, scarred uterus especially with the uterine cavity involvement. Certain special situations, which are not contraindications but demand discussion are previous LSCS, breech, multiple pregnancy, maternal heart disease, etc.

Cervical Ripening

The successful outcome of induction of labor depends to a great extent on the state of the cervix. A ripe cervix is associated with successful outcome in most cases, and induction fails in most cases if the cervix is unripe. If induction is indicated and the state of the cervix is unfavorable, agents for cervical ripening may be used. Cervical ripening involves a complex process where PGs achieve this by the breakdown of the cervical proteoglycan ground substance and dispersal of the collagen fibers. Cervical ripening is the first step to induce labor in a case with unripe cervix.

Even though other systems of evaluating the cervical status, like ultrasonography, are being resorted to, clinically, the status of the cervix can be determined by the Bishop scoring system (Table 1).

If the total score is more than 8, the probability of vaginal delivery after induction is similar to that after spontaneous labor. If the score is more than 6, the chances of successful delivery are good. A score of less than 5 usually requires cervical ripening before successful induction.

METHODS OF CERVICAL RIPENING AND INDUCTION OF LABOR

Induction does not generally involve just a single intervention, but is a complex set of interventions and, as such, presents a set of challenges for both clinicians and mothers. We shall discuss the methods of cervical ripening and induction of labor under one head because both form a continuum, one begins where the other ends. Acceptable methods of cervical ripening include nonpharmacological methods, mechanical cervical dilators and medications.

Pharmacological Methods

The most commonly used methods of cervical ripening include the administration of oxytocin, prostaglandin E1 (PGE1) or prostaglandin E2 (PGE2). Other pharmacologic methods include the use of extra-amniotic saline infusion, vaginal recombinant human relaxin, intracervical purified porcine relaxin and the use of isosorbide mononitrate (IMN).

Although parity does not appear to affect the choice of method of induction of labor it should influence the dosage of drugs used.

Prostaglandins

Prostaglandins have opened up a whole new world of labor management. Different PGs used for induction of labor are PGE2 (dinoprostone) and PGE1 (misoprostol) in different forms and formulations. PGs act on the cervix to enable ripening by a number of different mechanisms. They alter the extracellular ground substance of the cervix, and PGE2 increases the activity of collagenase in the cervix. They cause an increase in elastase, glycosaminoglycan, dermatan sulfate and hyaluronic acid levels in the cervix. A relaxation of cervical smooth muscle facilitates dilation. Finally, PGs allow for an increase in intracellular calcium levels causing contraction of myometrial muscle.

Risks associated with the use of PGs include uterine hyperstimulation, and maternal side effects, such as nausea, vomiting, diarrhea and fever.

Table 1: Bishop's score

Score	Dilation (cm)	Effacement	Station	Cervix consistency	Cervix position
0	Closed	0–30	–3	Firm	Posterior
1	1–2	40–50	–2	Medium	Midposed
2	3–4	60–70	–1, 0	Soft	Anterior
3	5–6	80	+1, +2	—	—

Dinoprostone, a synthetic PGE2 analog, is commercially available as two preparations—a gel available in a 2.5 mL syringe containing 0.5 mg of drug and a vaginal insert containing 10 mg of the drug (in India only gel is available as yet). Both the preparations are approved by the United States Food and Drug Administration (US FDA) for cervical ripening at or near term. The vaginal insert releases PGE2 at a very slow rate of 0.3 mg/h compared to the gel. Both the preparations are reported to not only shorten the induction—delivery interval, but also decrease the total and maximum dose of oxytocin needed to augment labor. If there is inadequate cervical change with minimal uterine activity after a single dose of intracervical PGE2 gel, a second dose may be administered 6–12 hours later, till maximum dose of 1.5 mg or 7.5 mL of gel within 24 hour period.

Technique of Application

The intracervical PGE2 gel administration (0.5 mg) has a 1% rate of hyperstimulation, while the intravaginal PGE2 gel (2–5 mg) or vaginal insert is associated with a 5% rate. (Rayburn WF. Obstet Gynecol. 1992; Witter FR. Am J Obstet Gynecol 1992, J Matern Fetal Med 1996). Hyperstimulation typically begins within 1 hour of the PGE2 instillation but may occur up to 9½ hours after the vaginal insert placement. Removing the vaginal insert will usually help reverse the effect of hyperstimulation. Vaginal or cervical irrigation is not beneficial. Maternal side effects (fever, vomiting, diarrhea) are quite uncommon with the low-dose PGE2. Caution should be exercised while using PGE2 in patients with glaucoma, severe hepatic or renal dysfunction, and asthma. PGE2 is a bronchodilator and there are no reports of bronchospasm or significant blood pressure (BP) changes after administration of low-dose gel.

Method

- *Patient selection, counseling, initial maternal and fetal assessment*
- Bring gel to room temperature before application
- Monitor fetal heart rate (FHR) and uterine activity continuously starting before gel introduction and continuing for 30–120 min after gel insertion
- Introduce the gel into the cervix, care being taken to avoid its placement above the internal os
- After application of the gel, the patient should remain recumbent for 30 minutes before being allowed to ambulate
- A second dose may be repeated after 6–12 hours, up to a maximum of three doses in 24 hours
- End points for ripening include strong uterine contractions, a Bishop score of greater than or equal to 8, or a change in maternal or fetal status
- Maximum recommended dosage is 1.5 mg of dinoprostone (three doses) in 24 hours
- Do not start oxytocin for 6–12 hours after placement of the last dose, to allow for spontaneous onset of labor and protect the uterus from overstimulation
- Intravaginal application also works, but the effect is slower to start with and of low intensity when induction of labor is undertaken with vaginal PGE2 preparations; vaginal tablets should be considered in preference to intracervical gel formulations as they are equally effective and administration1 of vaginal PGE2 is less invasive.

Recommended Regimens for Vaginal PGE2 Preparations

PGE2 tablets: 3 mg PGE2 6–8 hourly. The maximum total dose is 6 mg for all women.

PGE2 gels: 2 mg PGE2 in nulliparous women with an unfavorable cervix (Bishop's score less than 4), 1 mg for all other women.

- In either, a second dose of 1–2 mg can be administered 6 hours later
- The maximum dose is 4 mg PGE2 for nulliparous women with an unfavorable cervix and 3 mg for all other women
- Vaginal PGE2 tablets seem to be as effective as gel formulations.
- In the absence of clinical benefit, prostaglandins PGE2 tablets offer financial savings when compared with PGE2 gel
- Vaginal PGE2 gel and tablets appear to be more effective than pessary formulations
- Sustained-release formulations of PGE2 do not appear to be more effective than other PGE2 preparations
- There are limited data regarding the use of different dose regimens and the timing of administration of PGs.

When cervical ripening has been induced by PG gel, the process of ripening imperceptibly merges into induction of labor in 30–50% of cases.

Oral PG tablets are more effective when the cervix is unfavorable (Usha Krishna, 1990).

Since, the effect of the drug cannot be reversed easily, the antidote, injection terbutaline SC, should always be kept ready.

Oxytocin

Oxytocin is the most commonly used drug for induction of labor. As pregnancy progresses, the number of oxytocin receptors in the uterus increases (by 100-fold at 32 weeks and by 300-fold at the onset of labor). Oxytocin activates

Table 2: Injection pitocin induction rate of flow and dosage

Regimen	Starting dose	Incremental increase (mU/min)	Dosage interval (min)
Low-dose	0.5–1	1	30–40
	1–2	2	15
High-dose	6	6	15
	6	6, 3, 1*	20–40

*Incremental increase is reduced to 3 mU/min in presence of hyperstimulation and reduced to 1 mU/min with recurrent hyperstimulation

the phospholipase C-inositol pathway and increases intracellular calcium levels, stimulating contractions in myometrial smooth muscle. Oxytocin is the preferred pharmacologic agent for inducing labor when the cervix is favorable or ripe. Numerous randomized, placebo-controlled studies have focused on the use of oxytocin in labor induction. It has been found that low-dose (physiologic) and high-dose (pharmacologic) oxytocin regimens are equally effective in establishing adequate labor patterns (Table 2).

The side effects of oxytocin are dose related and it is to be used with great caution as fetal distress can occur from hyperstimulation, and rarely, uterine rupture or abruptio placentae can occur. Multiparous women are at higher risk for uterine rupture. If hyperstimulation occurs with abnormal FHR tracings, the oxytocin infusion has to be decreased or discontinued to correct the pattern along with left lateral position, nasal oxygen (O_2) and intravenous (IV) fluids. Water intoxication can occur with high concentration of oxytocin infused with large quantities of hypotonic solutions. The antidiuretic effect is usually observed only after prolonged administration with at least 40 mU/min of oxytocin. Hypotension may occur following a rapid IV infusion of oxytocin.

The effective dose of oxytocin varies greatly between women. A numeric value for the maximum dose of oxytocin has not been established.

Oxytocin is cautiously administered in IV fluids (Ringer lactate or normal saline), gradually increasing the rate of infusion until good labor is established (three contractions in 10 min, each lasting more than 40 seconds). This rate is maintained until delivery. To reduce error, a standard dilution should always be used. Suggested standardized dilutions and dose regimens include: 30 IU in 500 mL of normal saline; hence 1 mL/h = 1 mU/min or 10 IU in 500 mL of normal saline; hence, 3 mL/h = 1 mU/min. As a routine practice, a partogram is maintained. The uterus is felt to relax between contractions and the fetal heart sounds should remain normal throughout labor.

Method

- Infuse oxytocin 2.5 units in 500 mL of Ringer's lactate (or normal saline), starting at 8–10 drops/min. This is approximately 2.5 mU/min
- Increase the infusion rate by 8–10 drops/min every 30 minutes until a good contraction pattern is established (contractions lasting more than 40 seconds and occurring three times in 10 minutes)
- Maintain this rate until delivery is completed
- If *hyperstimulation occurs* (any contraction lasts longer than 60 seconds), or if there are more than four contractions in 10 minutes, stop the infusion and relax the uterus using tocolytics:
  - Terbutaline 250 µg IV slowly over 5 minutes
  - Salbutamol 10 mg in 1 L IV fluids (normal saline or Ringer's lactate) at 10 drops/min.
- If there are *not three contractions in 10 min*, each lasting more than 40 seconds with the infusion rate at *60 drops/min*:
  - Increase the oxytocin concentration to 5 units in 500 mL of Ringer's lactate (or normal saline) and adjust the infusion rate to 24–30 drops/min (15 mU/min)
  - Increase the infusion rate by 8–10 drops/min every 30 minutes until a satisfactory contraction pattern is established or the maximum rate of 60 drops/min is reached.
- If labor still has not been established using the higher concentration of oxytocin:
  - In *multigravida* and in *women with previous cesarean scars,* induction has failed; deliver by LSCS
  - In *primigravida,* infuse oxytocin at a higher concentration (rapid escalation)
  - Infuse oxytocin 10 units in 500 mL dextrose (or normal saline) at 30 drops/min
  - Increase infusion rate by 8–10 drops/min every 30 minutes until good contractions are established
  - If good contractions are not established at 60 drops/min (60 mIU/min), deliver by LSCS.
- Most women should have adequate contractions at 12 mIU/min
- If regular contraction not established after total of 5 IU (5 hours on suggested regimen) then induction should be stopped
- Do not use oxytocin 10 units in 500 mL (i.e. 20 mU/mL) in multigravida and women with previous cesarean section
- In women with intact membranes, amniotomy should be performed where feasible, prior to commencement of an infusion of oxytocin
- Oxytocin augmentation, after the use of 1.5 mg intracervical or 2.5 mg intravaginal PGE2, should not

be started within 6–12 hours because the effect of PGE2 may be heightened
- After the use of sustained release PGE2, delaying oxytocin induction by 30–60 min after removal is sufficient.

Misoprostol (Cytotec), a synthetic PGE1 analog, is currently approved by the US FDA for the prevention of peptic ulcers and not for cervical ripening or induction of labor. However, there is quite a literature available on the intravaginal or oral use of 25–50 μg of PGE1 for cervical ripening/induction of labor. It is currently available as a 100–200 μg tablet which is not scored. The broken tablet may not contain the desired amount of the drug creating problems. Clinical trials indicate that the optimal dose and dosing interval is 25 μg intravaginally every 4–6 hours. Higher doses or shorter dosing intervals are associated with a higher incidence of side effects, especially hyperstimulation syndrome, defined as contractions lasting longer than 90 seconds or more than five contractions in 10 min. Risks also include tachysystole, defined as six or more uterine contractions in 10 min for two consecutive 10 min periods, and hypersystole, a single contraction of at least 2 min duration. Finally, increase in uterine rupture in women with previous cesarean section is a possible complication, limiting its use to women who do not have a uterine scar.

Also, an increase in the meconium stained fluid has been reported with PGE1 use. In hyperstimulation not responding to routine measures and subcutaneous terbutaline, emergency cesarean should be considered.

Oral misoprostol administration is associated with lower incidence of side effects compared to vaginal administration. Complications appear to be dose related.

The review of literature shows that use of misoprostol resulted in an overall lower incidence of cesarean section, a higher incidence of vaginal delivery within 24 hours of application and a reduced need for oxytocin (pitocin) augmentation.

Method

- Place misoprostol 25 μg in the posterior fornix of the vagina. Repeat after 6 hours, if required;
- If there is *no response after two doses of 25 μg*, increase to 50 μg every 6 hours
- Do not use more than 50 μg at a time and do not exceed four doses (200 μg)
- Do not use oxytocin within 8 hours of administration of PGE1.

Although PGE1 appears to be safe and effective in inducing labor in an unripe cervix, further studies are needed to establish a detailed safety profile.

A DISCUSSION ON THE RELATIVE MERITS OF PROSTAGLANDINS AND OXYTOCIN FOR INDUCTION OF LABOR

Prostaglandins are More Successful than Oxytocin in Inducing Labor:

Prostaglandins should be used in preference to oxytocin when induction of labor is undertaken in either nulliparous or multiparous women with intact membranes, regardless of their cervical favorability.

Either PGs or oxytocin may be used when induction of labor is undertaken in nulliparous or multiparous women who have ruptured membranes, regardless of cervical status, as they are equally effective.

Prostaglandin induced labors have a shorter rupture of membrane (ROM)-delivery interval compared to oxytocin-amniotomy when the cervix is ripe.

PGE1 is a more effective method of cervical ripening than either intravaginal or intracervical PGE2 or oxytocin.

Misoprostol is significantly cheaper than currently recommended PGE2 preparations.

The safety issues concerning the use of vaginal misoprostol are unclear.

PGE1 and PGE2 are equally effective for cervical ripening and induction of labor but PGE1 was associated with increased incidence of hyperstimulation.

Intracervical or intravaginal PGE2 use is superior to placebo or no therapy in promoting cervical ripening. Intravaginal use of PGE2, though appears safe and effective in patients with ruptured membranes, has not been approved by the FDA.

Mechanical Methods

All mechanical modalities share a similar mechanism of action—namely, some form of local pressure that stimulates the release of PGs. The risks associated with these methods include infection (endometritis and neonatal sepsis), bleeding, ROM, placental disruption. Hygroscopic dilators absorb endocervical and local tissue fluids, causing the device to expand within the endocervix and providing controlled mechanical pressure. The products available include natural osmotic dilators (e.g. *Laminaria japonicum*) and synthetic osmotic dilators. The main advantages of using hygroscopic dilators include outpatient placement and no FHR-monitoring requirements. Balloon devices like the 24/26-French Foley's balloon and the double balloon device (Atad Ripener device) provide mechanical pressure directly on the cervix as the balloon is filled.

Currently, several randomized controlled trials (RCTs) are comparing use of a balloon device with administration of an extra-amniotic saline infusion, laminaria or PGE2. Results from these trials indicate that each of these methods is effective for cervical ripening and each has comparable cesarean section delivery rates in women with an unfavorable cervix.

Surgical Methods

Stripping of the Membranes/ Sweeping of Membrane

Stripping the amniotic membrane is one of the most common methods of induction used in clinical practice. Stripping of the membranes causes an increase in the activity of phospholipase A_2 and prostaglandin F_{2a} as well as causing mechanical dilation of the cervix, which releases PGs. The membranes are stripped by inserting the examining finger through the internal cervical os and moving it in a circular direction to detach the inferior pole of the membranes from the lower uterine segment (Evidence level C, consensus opinion). Risks of this technique include infection, bleeding, accidental rupture of the membranes and patient discomfort. Stripping of the membranes alone does not seem to produce clinically important benefits, but when used with another method, it does seem to be associated with a lower mean dose of oxytocin needed and an increased rate of normal vaginal deliveries (Evidence level A, RCT).

Membrane sweeping is associated with a reduction in the length of time between treatment and spontaneous labor; it increased the likelihood of both: Spontaneous labor within 48 hours and birth within 1 week. Sweeping of the membranes reduces the incidence of not only prolonged pregnancy but also the need for the use of other formal methods of induction of labor. However, the risk of operative delivery is not changed by this intervention and the risk of maternal infection or neonatal infection does not rise.

Amniotomy

Artificial rupture of membranes (ARM) is used as a method of induction only if the cervix is favorable. The result may be unpredictable and the induction-onset interval long if not followed by oxytocin augmentation. It is hypothesized that amniotomy increases the production of, or causes a release of PGs locally. Membrane rupture, whether spontaneous or artificial, often sets off the following chain of events: amniotic fluid is expelled; uterine volume is decreased; PGs are produced stimulating labor; uterine contractions begin (if the woman is not in labor) or become stronger (if she is already in labor). Risks associated with this procedure include umbilical cord prolapse or compression, maternal or neonatal infection, FHR deceleration, bleeding from placenta previa or low-lying placenta, and possible fetal injury. Only two well-controlled trials studied the use of amniotomy alone, and the evidence did not support its use for induction of labor (Evidence level A, systematic review of RCTs).

If the *membranes are intact,* it is recommended practice in both induction and augmentation of labor to first perform ARM. In some cases, this is all that is needed to induce labor.

Method

- Check the FHR
- Perform the ARM using proper aseptic technique
- Note the color of the liquor. If *thick meconium is present,* suspect fetal distress
- After ARM, listen to the FHR during and after a contraction. If the *FHR* is abnormal (less than 100 beats/min or more than 180 beats/min), suspect fetal distress
  - If delivery is not anticipated within 18 hours, give prophylactic antimicrobial to reduce the Group B *Streptococcus* infection in the neonate: penicillin G 2 million units IV or ampicillin 2 g IV, every 6 hours until delivery.
- If there are no signs of infection after delivery, discontinue antibiotics
- If good labor is not established 1 hour after ARM, begin oxytocin infusion
- If labor is induced because of severe maternal disease (e.g. sepsis or eclampsia), begin oxytocin infusion at the same time as ARM
- PGE2 may also be used.

OTHER PHARMACOLOGICAL METHODS OF INDUCTION OF LABOR

Mifepristone

Mifepristone (Mifeprex) is an antiprogesterone agent. Progesterone inhibits contractions of the uterus while mifepristone counteracts this action. Currently, seven trials are underway involving 594 women using mifepristone for cervical ripening. Results have shown that women treated with mifepristone are more likely to have a favorable cervix within 48–96 hours when compared with placebo. In addition, these women were more likely to deliver within 48–96 hours and less likely to undergo cesarean section. However, little information is available about fetal outcomes and maternal side effects; thus, there is insufficient information to support the use of mifepristone for cervical ripening.

Relaxin

The hormone relaxin is thought to promote cervical ripening. Cochrane reviewers evaluated results of four studies involving 267 women and concluded that there is insufficient support for the use of relaxin at this time. As with many of the other methods described in this review, further trials are needed.

Isosorbide Mononitrate

An agent that ripened the cervix without stimulating uterine activity would be the ideal cervical ripening agent for outpatient use. The need to carry out preinduction cervical ripening on an outpatient basis and concerns about the use of PGs has resulted in identification of this drug. PGs are known to induce uterine contractions that may lead to fetal hypoxia. IMN in the dose of 40 mg at 48 hours, 32 hours and 16 hours vaginally before scheduled hospital admission is both effective in inducing cervical ripening at term and is associated with no associated FHR abnormalities. In contrast to PGs, nitric oxide donors inhibit rather than stimulate uterine contractions and promote rather than restrict uterine blood flow. Thus, nitric oxide donors such as IMN appear to be the ideal cervical ripening agent for outpatient use.

Outpatient IMN will reduce the time from hospital admission to delivery, reduce the costs of induction of labor and improve women's experience of induction of labor (with no increase in operative delivery rates).

Breast Stimulation

Breast massage and nipple stimulation have been shown to facilitate the release of oxytocin from the posterior pituitary gland. The most commonly prescribed technique involves gently massaging the breasts or applying warm compresses to the breasts for 1 hour, three times a day. Occasionally an abnormal FHR tracing similar to that occurring in oxytocin challenge test is seen. Two poorly designed studies conducted in the 1970s and 1980s demonstrated a difference in the intervention groups, but the poor study design suggests that evidence is lacking to support breast stimulation as a viable method of inducing labor.

Acupuncture/Transcutaneous Nerve Stimulation

Acupuncture involves the insertion of very fine needles into designated locations with the purpose of preventing or curing disease. In the Chinese system of medicine, it is thought that acupuncture stimulates channels of qi, or life energy. This energy flows along 12 meridians with designated points along these meridians. Each point is given a name and a number and is associated with a specific organ system or function. In Western medicine, it is thought that acupuncture and transcutaneous nerve stimulation (TENS) may stimulate the release of PGs and oxytocin. Most of the studies involving acupuncture were poorly designed. A well-designed RCT is needed to evaluate the role of acupuncture and TENS in labor induction.

Partogram, Fetal Surveillance and Induction of Labor

- All labors should be monitored with a partogram
- Wherever induction of labor occurs, facilities should be available for continuous uterine and FHR monitoring
- Fetal well-being should be established immediately prior to induction of labor
- Following induction of labor, fetal well-being should be established once contractions are detected or reported. Once normality is confirmed, intermittent monitoring can be used
- Continuous electronic fetal monitoring is not a norm, intermittent auscultation is equally effective
- In cases of uterine hypercontractility with a suspicious or pathological cardiotocograph (CTG), secondary to oxytocin infusions, the oxytocin infusion should be decreased or discontinued
- In the presence of abnormal FHR patterns and uterine hypercontractility (not secondary to oxytocin infusion), tocolysis should be considered. A suggested regimen is subcutaneous terbutaline 0.25 mg
- In cases of suspected or confirmed acute fetal compromise, delivery should be accomplished as soon as possible, taking account of the severity of the FHR abnormality and relevant maternal factors. The accepted standard has been that, ideally, this should be accomplished within 30 minutes
- Prolonged use of maternal facial O_2 therapy may be harmful to the fetus and should be avoided.

Though induction and augmentation of labor appear to be mere extensions of the same process, merging imperceptibly one into another forming a continuum, there are categorical differences between the two entities. At times, it is difficult to know where one ends and another begins. On one hand, induction is an attempt to interrupt the course of ongoing pregnancy and augmentation is to accelerate the course of labor as a physiological process which has already begun on the other hand. Induced labors are generally slow or prolonged, there is a sharp increase in the rate of operative interference and the demand for pain relief is more pronounced. On the other hand, accelerated labors are shorter; the operative interference is reduced and need for pain relief is less. Delivery by propulsive forces is almost always preferable to delivery by traction.

Duration is the kernel of the problem of management of labor. More than any other measurable factor, duration determines the impact not only on the mothers, but also on the babies and the healthcare providers. Duration of labor is generally equated with the number of hours spent in the delivery unit. The overall duration of labor is determined by the length of first stage because the number of hours taken for the cervix to dilate represents approximately 90% of the entire birth process. The second stage is short by comparison and contributes little to the duration of prolonged labor. The impact of labor on the mother should be evaluated not only in physical but also emotional terms, both of which are related ultimately to the number of hours spent in the delivery unit. Prolonged labor is invariably associated with dehydration, ketoacidosis or salt depletion and extreme exhaustion. The profound emotional disturbance caused by prolonged labor may haunt the mother for lifetime. The morale of the average mother begins to deteriorate perceptibly after 6 hours. After 12 hours the deterioration accelerates rapidly—almost in geometric rather than arithmetic proportions—"until eventually a stage is reached when an adult is reduced to pleading for deliverance from passers by unless she is rendered semiconscious with drugs or lulled into a false sense of security with epidural anesthesia". Prolonged labor invariably is associated not only with increase in the incidence of instrumental deliveries and cesarean sections but also increase in the perinatal and maternal morbidity. Prolonged labor was defined at the National Maternity Hospital in Dublin as more than 36 hours in 1963, reduced to 24 hours in 1968 and finally to 12 hours in 1972. By contrast there is total abolition of dehydration, ketosis, salt depletion and a dramatic reduction in demand for analgesia which is evident in shorter labor. There is a parallel decline in the need for instrumental delivery, especially rotational forceps, because women are better able to cope and eventually deliver themselves with shorter labor.

The armamentarium we have to accelerate labor is not different than the one we use for induction of labor. All we need to do is qualify their use with certain safety precautions. The easily available methods of acceleration of labor are ARM/oxytocin/PGs: PGE2, PGF2α, PGE1.

Amniotomy

Amniotomy is performed once the diagnosis of labor is confirmed. The nature of liquor is checked and FHR noted. Nature/color of liquor provides vital evidence about the fetal well-being which should be known before proceeding further. Rupture of membranes alone may be sufficient to accelerate labor in quite a few cases.

Six relatively unbiased trials, including two multicentric studies from Canada and the United Kingdom, with over 2,000 participants, showed a modest decrease in the duration of labor in the group randomized to membrane rupture, but meta-analysis failed to show a substantive effect on maternal or fetal outcomes. The trials, as performed, provide a good test of a policy of routine early amniotomy compared with relatively late amniotomy and show that such a policy is associated with a small decrease in the duration of labor, is probably not harmful to the fetus, but does not lower the rate of cesarean sections or operative vaginal deliveries.

Oxytocin

Oxytocin is the most commonly used drug to accelerate labor all over the world. Oxytocin is not nearly as predictable in initiating labor as it is in accelerating the progress when labor has already begun. Uterus in labor is almost uniformly responsive to oxytocin, provided the forewaters are ruptured. Oxytocin is to be used on a woman in labor with singleton pregnancy in cephalic presentation (vertex) after confirming the diagnosis. Rupture of membrane is recommended before starting an oxytocin infusion as it may be ineffective with intact membranes and it may not be used or used with extreme caution in presence of meconium stained liquor. Theoretically, oxytocin with intact membranes may increase the risk of an amniotic fluid embolism. Oxytocin is to be used with extreme caution in multigravidae as they are prone to rupture, malpresentations and twins.

In order to prevent inadvertent complications of the drug, certain very effective series of safeguards are recommended by the Dublin experience. It is to be used in a standard concentration in all circumstances. The standard concentration recommended is 5 units in 500 mL or 10 units in 1,000 mL of Ringer's lactate, the total dose of oxytocin not to exceed 10 units, the rate of infusion not to exceed 60 drops, i.e. 40 mU/min and the total volume infused not more than 1,000 mL.

The oxytocin infusion is started at 8–10 drops/min with the standard IV set (16–20 drops = 1 mL) and the rate increased by 8–10 drops every 15 minutes to a maximum of 60 drops/min the rate of increase is titrated against uterine activity till optimum uterine activity is achieved. The optimum contractions are 3–4 in 10 minutes, each lasting for 35–40 seconds. Care is taken to see that number of contractions do not exceed 4–5 in 10 min or 7 in 15 min to safeguard against hyperstimulation. A strict check is kept on the FHR throughout the process. Acceleration should stop at the first evidence of fetal distress.

The only direct toxic effect of oxytocin is water intoxication. The possibility of water intoxication arises when more than 3L of salt-free fluid is administered intravenously. Limiting the volume of IV infusion to 1,000 mL provides reasonable guarantee against water intoxication.

An overall increase in the incidence of neonatal jaundice in cases treated with oxytocin is seen, but seems to be confined to the cases in which oxytocin was used to induce labor. This may be a "product of the relative state of immaturity that results from interruption of the pregnancy before the natural conclusion and not a direct toxic effect of the drug".

Four randomized studies have examined the effects of oxytocin as a single intervention in spontaneous labor. Oxytocin had a modest effect on reducing the duration of labor in only one of the four trials. The only statistically significant differences shown in the meta-analysis were in side effects: an increased incidence of hyperstimulation and of pain in the group given oxytocin. There was no significant reduction in the incidence of cesarean section or instrumental vaginal delivery with use of oxytocin and fetal condition was the same in both groups.

Prostaglandins

Prostaglandins have been used mainly for induction of labor since 1975. PG induced labors have a shorter interval between ROM and delivery compared to oxytocin and amniotomy when the cervix is ripe; however, with unripe cervix, PGs are more successful than oxytocin in inducing labor. In the most commonly used regime, PGE2 tablets (0.5 mg each) have been used in the dose of 2 tablets orally every hour until labor is established, followed by 1 tablet orally every hour if necessary to augment labor. Oral PG tablets help to augment labor pains and accelerate the progress of labor whenever desired. PGE2 gel has also been used to accelerate labor even at a later stage.

Prostaglandins induced labors permit ambulation, the labor contractions are less painful, the risk of postpartum hemorrhage (PPH) is reduced and there is no danger of fluid overload and neonatal jaundice.

Oxytocin infusion used to augment labor is easier to control with continuous monitoring of the uterine activity and FHR compared to PG. The rate of infusion is controlled by the healthcare provider and can be stopped or reduced any moment whenever the need arises. However, once a PG tablet has been consumed orally or PG gel instilled, the effect of the drug cannot be as easily reversed unlike oxytocin.

Misoprostol

Misoprostol has been used to induce labor and has been successful in achieving more vaginal deliveries in 24 hours compared to other drugs. The most commonly used dosage regimen advocates vaginal administration of 25 μg misoprostol every 4–6 hours. Vaginal route is more effective than the intracervical or oral route. Compared with PGE2, it is cheaper, can be stored at room temperature and easy to administer. Tachysystole, hyperstimulation and meconium stained liquor are associated with misoprostol use. Birth asphyxia, meconium aspiration, cervical tear and even rupture uterus may occur when the drug is not used in proper doses. In obstetrics, misoprostol is only approved for use in termination of pregnancy up to 7 weeks. Its use for induction/augmentation of labor is not advocated till it gets approval, which may come quite soon.

No discussion on acceleration or augmentation of labor can be complete without reference to partograms, FHR monitoring and pain relief during labor.

No labor should be left unattended. High risk labors are anyway well supervised but it is in normal women that most of the problems of labor arise. It is our firm belief that rather than being called to perform an emergency operation at the last moment in an attempt to redeem a situation which could have been foreseen much earlier, it is better to get involved with the labor from the beginning to be able to take remedial measures at an appropriate stage.

Partogram

The progress of labor is monitored with the help of a partogram. The partogram (or partograph) is a simple, inexpensive tool to provide a continuous pictorial overview of labor. Many hospitals now use a partogram to assist them in the detection of prolonged labor.

The first obstetrician to provide a tool for the assessment of individual labors was Friedman. He plotted the graph of cervical dilation against time producing a slope resembling a sigmoid curve (starting with a gentle incline and rising more steeply as time passes). This was known as the cervicograph. He demonstrated that the cervix dilates at the rate of 1 cm/h. In 1972, Philpott and Castle modified the original cervicograph for use in a hospital in Zimbabwe, where doctors were in short supply and tertiary care was at least 2–4 hours away from primary health centers. Their objective was to provide a practical tool with which midwives and assistants could record all intrapartum details, not just cervical dilation. Unlike Friedman study, women were only included if the cervix was already 3 cm dilated on admission, recognizing that progress would be slower if women were not in established labor. They added the "alert line" and the "action line" on the partogram. The alert line was straight, not curved, and was a modification of the mean rate of cervical dilatation of the slowest 10% of primigravid women who were in the active phase of labor. This line represented a progress rate of 1 cm/h. The "action line", 2 hours to the right of the alert line was developed on the premise that correction of primary inefficient uterine action would lead to a vaginal birth. It also showed a lowered incidence of prolonged labor and a reduction in cesarean sections. John Studd became an advocate of the partograph following his visit to Zimbabwe and promoted its use in the United Kingdom. Studd developed the "nomogram" by finding the mean for cervical dilation during normal labor for a British population. Studd concluded that the partogram could aid in the early recognition of prolonged labor and routine use of the partogram in Britain is attributed to him and his work. Daftary et al. developed the Indian nomogram in 1977.

Routine use of partorgam is strongly recommended for all labors. The patient's partogram is charted alongside the standard nomogram. Should the patient's partogram stray to the right of the nomogram, the clinician is alerted to a tardy labor and prompted to augment contractions with oxytocin or PGs in absence of other problems. If the partogram still remains to the right of the nomogram and crosses the action line, remedial action is warranted to affect a timely delivery.

The endpoint of each labor is a healthy newborn which cries lustily. Monitoring the fetal condition throughout the labor is equally essential for optimal obstetric outcomes. Intermittent auscultation is as effective as the continuous electronic FHR monitoring. Any change in the FHR will warrant a re-evaluation and quick delivery. Acceleration of labor should stop immediately if the FHR abnormality is detected.

The most disturbing aspect of labor to the mother is the fear of isolation and pain. Pain relief during labor spells a humane approach to delivery. Labor analgesia allays fear and anxiety, relieves pain, prevents maternal hyperventilation and undue muscular efforts which cause maternal exhaustion, provides periods of restful sleep between contractions and controls alterations of placental function. All these favor a shorter and less traumatic labor requiring less obstetric interventions and hence an improved obstetric outcome. Pain relief is given with the use of analgesics/antispasmodic drugs or the epidural anesthesia. Pain relief provided by epidural anesthesia is more pronounced compared to the use of drugs but it involves an invasive procedure with inherent risks, increases the incidence of instrumental deliveries and may increase the duration of labor.

Indian Prospective

Daftary et al. in 2001 advocated an indigenously developed protocol for management of labor with the dual objective of providing pain relief during labor and reaching the goals of safe motherhood by optimizing obstetric outcome. The protocol developed rests on three pillars:

1. Ensuring adequate uterine activity—active management of labor.
2. Providing optimum pain relief—use of analgesics and antispasmodics.
3. Close clinical monitoring of labor events—maintaining a partogram.

The parturient is put on the protocol once the inclusion criteria have been satisfied only when she is in active labor, i.e. with a single viable pregnancy in cephalic presentation at 3 cm dilation with 3 contractions in 10 minutes, each lasting for at least 35–40 seconds. If the uterine activity is not adequate, oxytocin infusion or PGE2 tablets are used following amniotomy to optimize uterine activity. Progress of labor is monitored on the partogram. Combination of drugs—analgesics and antispasmodics which help cervical softening, yielding and dilatation—is used to provide effective pain relief. The use of multiple drugs provides synergism at the same time restricts the dose of each drug to minimal amount and hence safeguards the mother and fetus against major side effects. Pain relief is provided with a bolus of injection pentazocine 6 mg and diazepam 2 mg (one-fifth ampoule of Fortwin and one-fifth ampoule of Calmpose diluted in 10 mL of distilled water) IV slowly. Injection tramadol in the dose of 1 ng/kg body weight is given intramuscular (IM) along with any of the antispasmodics: injection drotin/anafortan/epidocin in the dose of 1 ampoule IM. The labor is monitored on the partogram. The patient experiences considerable pain relief till the head pushes the perineum. At around 7–8 cm dilatation, if she complaints of unbearable pain, injection ketamine in the initial dose of 0.5 mg/kg body weight is used IV in diluted form. The pain relief is quite prompt and considerable. Thereafter, if the pain persists, a top up of half the initial dose is used every half hour till delivery. After delivery active management of the third stage is used by using injection PGF2α IM and the baby is given to the mother for the breast crawl and skin-to-skin contact.

To conclude, we must remember that induction is an attempt to interrupt the course of ongoing pregnancy and augmentation is to accelerate the course of labor as a physiological process, which has already begun. Inefficient uterine action is by far the most common problem of childbirth and is why long and difficult labor occurs more often in primigravidae. A shorter labor, by contrast, is associated with total abolition of dehydration, ketosis, salt depletion and a dramatic reduction in demand for analgesia. There is also parallel decline in the need for instrumental delivery, especially rotational forceps and cesarean section rates because women are better able to cope and eventually deliver themselves with shorter labor.

BIBLIOGRAPHY

1. ACOG Practice Bulletin: Clinical Management Guidelines for Ob-Gyn Number 10, November 1999.
2. Adair CD. Nonpharmacologic approaches to cervical priming and labor induction. Clin Obstet Gynecol. 2000;43:447-54.
3. American College of Obstetricians and Gynecologists. (1999). Induction of labor with misoprostol [online]. Available from www.cytoteccase.com/Excerpts%20for%20Cytotec%20 Bulletin%20w%20Mark%20Bower%20commentary.pdf. Accessed November, 2013.
4. Arias F. Pharmacology of oxytocin and prostaglandins. Clin Obstet Gynecol. 2000;43:455-68.
5. Barrett JR, Savage J, Phillips K, et al. Randomised trial of amniotomy in labor versus the intention to leave membranes intact until the second stage. Br J Obstet Gynaecol. 1992;99:5-9.
6. Beal MW. Acupuncture and acupressure. Applications to women's reproductive health care. J Nurse Midwifery. 1999;44:217-30.
7. Bhasin A. Comparison of maternal complications in patients induced with oral PGE2 and oxytocin. J Obst Gynaecol India. 1993;43:553.
8. Bollapragada S, Mackenzie F, Norrie J, et al. IMOP: randomised placebo controlled trial of outpatient cervical ripening with isosorbide mononitrate (IMN) prior to induction of labour – clinical trial with analyses of efficacy, cost effectiveness and acceptability. BMC Pregnancy Childbirth. 2006;6:25.
9. Bricker L, Luckas M. Amniotomy alone for induction of labor. Cochrane Database Syst Rev. 2002;2:CD002862.
10. Buccellato CA, Stika CS, Frederiksen MC. A randomized trial of misoprostol versus extra-amniotic sodium chloride infusion with oxytocin for induction of labor. Am J Obstet Gynecol. 2000;182:1039-44.
11. Buser D, Mora G, Arias f. A randomized comparison between misoprostol and dinoprostone for cervical ripening and labor induction in patients with unfavorable cervices.. Obstet Gynaecol. 1997;89(4):581-5.
12. Caldeyro-Barcia R, Hech E. Effect of rupture of the membranes on fetal heart rate patterns. Int J Gynaecol Obstet. 1972;10: 169-72.
13. Daftary SN. Cervicographs in the management of labors in primigravida. J Obst Gynaecol India. 1977;27:687.
14. Daftary SN. Modern management of labor. In: Desai P, Malhotra N, Shah D (Eds). Principles and Practice of Obstetrics and Gynecology for Postgraduates, 3rd edition. New Delhi: Jaypee Brothers Medical Publishers; 2003. pp. 209-307.
15. du Vigneaud V Ressler C, Swan JM. The synthesis of an oct apeptide am ide with the hormonal activity of oxytocin. J Am Chem Soc. 1953;75:4879-80.
16. Fraser WD, Marcoux S, Moutquin JM, et al. Effect of early amniotomy on the risk of dystocia in nulliparous women. N Engl J Med. 1993;328:1145-9.
17. Fraser WD. Amniotomy to shorten spontaneous labor. In: Enkin MW, Keirse MC, Renfrew MJ (Eds). Pregnancy and childbirth module, Cochrane Database of Syst Rev. 1992.
18. Fraser WD. Early oxytocin to shorten spontaneous labor. In: Enkin MW, Keirse MC, Renfrew MJ, Neilson JP (Eds). Pregnancy and Childbirth Module. Cochrnane Database of Syst Rev. 1992.
19. Friedman EA. Labor, clinical evaluation and management, 2nd edition. New York: Appleton-Century-Crofts; 1978.
20. Goldberg AB, Greenberg MB, Darney PD. Misoprostol and pregnancy. N Engl J Med. 2001;344:38-47.
21. Goldman JB, Wigton TR. A randomized comparison of extra-amniotic saline infusion and intracervical dinoprostone gel for cervical ripening. Obstet Gynecol. 1999;93:271-4.
22. Guinn DA, Goepfert AR, Christine M, et al. Extra-amniotic saline, laminaria, or prostaglandin E(2) gel for labor induction with unfavorable cervix: A randomized controlled trial. Obstet Gynecol. 2000;96:106-12.
23. Hadi H. Cervical ripening and labor induction: Clinical guidelines. Clin Obstet Gynecol. 2000;43:524-36.
24. Hofmeyr GJ, Gulmezoglu AM. Vaginal misoprostol for cervical ripening and induction of labor. Cochrane Database Syst Rev. 2002;2:CD000941.
25. Keirse MC. Augmentation of labor. In: Chalmers I, Enkin M, Keirse MC (Eds). Effective care in pregnancy and childbirth. Oxford: Oxford University Press; 1989. pp. 951-66.
26. Kelly AJ, Kavanagh J, Thomas J. Relaxin for cervical ripening and induction of labor. Cochrane Database Syst Rev. 2002;2:CD003103.
27. Lin A, Kupferminc M, Dooley SL. A randomized trial of extra-amniotic saline infusion versus laminaria for cervical ripening. Obstet Gynecol. 1995;86(4 part 1):545-9.
28. Lydon-Rochelle M, Holt VL, Easterling TR, et al. Risk of uterine rupture during labor among women with a prior cesarean delivery. N Engl J Med. 2001;345:3-8.
29. Neilson JP. Mifepristone for induction of labor. Cochrane Database Syst Rev. 2002;2:CD002865.
30. O'Driscoll K, Meagher D, Robson M. Active Management of Labour: The Dublin Experience; Mosby; 2003.
31. Philpott RH, Castle WM. Cervicographs in the management of labor in primigravidae. BJOG. 1972;79(7):599-602.
32. Rayburn WF. Prostaglandins E2 gel for cervical ripening and induction. Am J Obstet Gynaecol. 1989;160(3):529-34.
33. RCOG evidence-based Clinical Guideline Number 9, June 2001.
34. Rouben D, Arias F. A randomized trial of extra-amniotic saline infusion plus intracervical Foley catheter balloon versus prostaglandin E2 vaginal gel for ripening the cervix and inducing labor in patients with unfavorable cervices. Obstet Gynecol. 1993;82:290-4.
35. Sanchez-Ramos L, Gaudier FL, Kaunitz AM. Cervical ripening and labor induction after previous cesarean delivery. Clin Obstet Gynecol. 2000;43:513-23.
36. Sawai SK. Sequential outpatient application of intravaginal PGE2 gel in the management of post-term pregnancies. Obstet Gynaecol. 1991.
37. Schreyer P, Sherman DJ, Ariely S, et al. Ripening the highly unfavorable cervix with extra-amniotic saline instillation

or vaginal prostaglandin E2 application. Obstet Gynecol. 1989;73:938-42.

38. Sherman DJ, Frenkel E, Pansky M, et al. Balloon cervical ripening with extra-amniotic infusion of saline or prostaglandin E2: A double-blind, randomized controlled study. Obstet Gynecol. 2001;97:375-80.

39. Stubbs TM. Oxytocin for labor induction. Clin Obstet Gynecol. 2000;43:489-94.

40. Theobold GW. The use of posterior pituitary extract in obstetrics. BMJ. 1948.

41. UK Amniotomy Group. Comparing routine versus delayed amniotomy in spontaneous first labor at term-a multicentre randomized trial. Online J Curr Clin Trials. 1994;3:122.

42. Ventura SJ. Births: Final Data for 1997. In: National Statistics Reports. National Center for Health Statistics; 1999.

43. Witter FR. Prostaglandin E2 preparations for preinduction cervical ripening. Clin Obstet Gynecol. 2000;43:469-74.

44. Zeeman GG, Khan-Dawood FS, Dawood MY. Oxytocin and its receptor in pregnancy and parturition: Current concepts and clinical implications. Obstet Gynecol. 1997;89(5 pt 2):873-83.

CHAPTER

20

Operative Principles of Fetal Malpositions and Malpresentations

Shyam Desai

INTRODUCTION

Fetal malpositions and malpresentations comprise of a set of variable position adopted by fetus near term, which if not recognized well in time, will result in severe maternal and neonatal morbidity and mortality, and hence needs to be recognized.

Principles involved in management of malpresentation at labor are as follows:

- Identification and confirmation of malpresentation
- Immediate steps at rectification
- Facilitating safe vaginal delivery
- Preparation for laparotomy—Cesarean section/other interventions.

Consider the possibility of fetal malpresentations and malpresentations in the following subjects. Antenatal suspicion of malpresentations should mandate sonographic confirmation of the same and prompt the clinician to undertake efforts to exclude contracted pelvis as a possible contributory factor.

- Women of short stature or with skeletal deformities
- Elderly primigravida
- Grand multipara
- Women with pendulous abdomen
- Antepartum hemorrhage suspected of placenta previa
- Multiple pregnancy
- Hydramnios and oligohydramnios
- Women with bad obstetric history
- History of previous malpresentation.

ANTENATAL PRECAUTIONS

- Confirmation of clinically suspected fetal malpresentations with timely sonography is the first step in management of fetal malpresentations
- Some malpresentations tend to get corrected spontaneously as pregnancy advances, e.g. breech presentation, oblique lie. In case of some malpresentations like mentoposterior presentations, persistent brow presentation and breech presentations at term in a primigravida, or with additional complications like stargazing appearance of the fetus, the decision for elective cesarean section is an accepted norm. Persistent transverse lie and abnormal presentation in the first of twins constitute valid indications for elective cesarean section
- Malpresentations in the presence of any other additional high risk obstetric factor like contracted pelvis, placenta previa or intrauterine growth retardation (IUGR) goes in favor of cesarean section.

However, an obstetrician as faced with an unexpected malpresentation during the course of labor, there are situations which put to test and tax obstetric judgment and skills to maximum.

MANAGEMENT OPTIONS

Occipitoposterior Positions

In practice, about 5–10% of women admitted in labor with cephalic presentations present with occipitoposterior presentations. Given time and patience, many of these will rotate and get corrected to occipitoanterior position and deliver normally. However, about 10% of these will fail to rotate. The partogram in labor provides guidance in noting satisfactory progress. Some of these will rotate posteriorly to persistent occipitoposterior position (POP) with good contractions. These babies deliver face to pubes spontaneously or with assisted vaginal instrumental delivery (forceps/ventouse), a wide episiotomy is recommended to prevent bad perineal injuries. Others will

rotate partially and get arrested at the midpelvic station, as deep transverse arrest of the head. After evaluating the lower pelvic strait, if clinically adequate, optimizing uterine contractions with oxytocin infusion and applying the ventouse often accomplishes complete rotation of the fetal head followed by a vaginal delivery. When in doubt, transfer the patient to the operation theater—with full readiness to proceed for a cesarean section—a trial vacuum extraction may be attempted. If the descent of the fetal head continues, proceed to deliver the patient vaginally. In case of unsatisfactory progress, desist from attempts to deliver the baby vaginally, proceed to a cesarean section in time to prevent obstetric complications.

Face and Brow Presentations

Mentoanterior presentations are known to progress satisfactorily and vaginal delivery may be confidently awaited in the absence of other obstetric abnormalities. Mentotransverse positions may get corrected to mentoanterior presentations, however, in the presence of good uterine contractions—if the mentotransverse position persists and in all cases of mentoposterior presentations—it is wise to perform a cesarean section before the fetal head get jammed in the mentoposterior position deep in the pelvis. In all cases of extended cephalic presentations, be on the look out for cord presentation/prolapse. Should these be detected—then proceed cesarean section forthwith. Brow presentations are often transient in nature, with good uterine contractions, these often get converted to vertex or face presentations and progress to vaginal delivery, but in those cases wherein the presentation persists as brow, when the patient enters in the active phase of labor, it may be judicious to proceed to cesarean section. High index of suspicion is mandatory for cord complications.

Transverse Lie

This is encountered in 1:400 to 1:600 pregnancies. If it is often detected antenatally, complications like contracted pelvis or placenta previa should be looked for, cord complications are not uncommon. In modern day practice, elective cesarean section is the chosen mode of delivery. In India, transferred cases of transverse lie continue to challenge obstetrician. In case, fetus is alive and mature, a cesarean section continues to be a better option. In women presenting with obstructed labor with threatened rupture of the uterus, cesarean section is indicated in maternal interest, irrespective of the condition of the baby. Occasionally, a multiparous patient may present in advanced labor with hand prolapse and recently ruptured membranes. If the uterus is found to be relaxing well in between the pains, trained obstetricians still perform internal podalic version successfully under general anesthesia. When in doubt, proceed to cesarean section. Transverse lie in the second of twins can be successfully delivered by internal podalic version, provided fetus is not big in size.

Multiple Pregnancies

There is an increasing trend to deliver triplets and higher order births by cesarean section. However, when dealing with twin pregnancy—the consensus of opinion is that if both twins are in cephalic presentation—consider vaginal delivery. If the first twin is in an abnormal presentation, consider cesarean section, but the controversy arises when the second baby is in an abnormal presentation. Some obstetricians prefer attempting vaginal delivery. After the birth of the first twin, the lie of the second twin is corrected by external version and the second twin delivered as vertex or breech. However, the perinatal risk for the second of twins is somewhat enhanced. The patient should be counseled about perinatal risks and the proposed mode of delivery accordingly and her wishes given due weightage in the decision-making process.

Cord Presentation and Cord Prolapse

The incidence is about 1:500 pregnancies. The predisposing factors include malpresentations, contracted pelvis, hydramnios, low insertion of cord, long cord, placenta previa, prematurity and multiple pregnancy. Suspect its possibility in presence of any of the above causes or if there is sudden severe fetal distress or the electronic fetal heart rate machine (EFHRM) tracing shows sudden decelerations. It can be detected on bimanual examination as a cord like pulsating structure. If the membranes are intact, the condition is diagnosed as cord presentation, and after rupture of membranes it is called cord prolapse.

Unless prompt delivery is accomplished, the perinatal risks are very high. If the patient is in advanced labor and the presenting part is low down in the pelvis, consider facilitating delivery with forceps/vacuum. If the cervix is not adequately dilated in the meantime, to avoid cord compression, consider the following options:

- Placing the patient in the knee chest or Trendelenburg position
- Manually lifting off the presenting part away from the brim
- Fill the urinary bladder with 200 mL of sterile saline to displace the presenting part and avoiding pressure on the cord. An infusion with tocolytic agent helps to relax the uterus. In the meanwhile, prepare for an emergency cesarean section.

Compound Presentation

Compound presentation is defined as one in which there is prolapse of one or more limbs along with the fetal head or the breech, Footling breech and shoulder presentations are excluded. Associated cord prolapse has been reported in 15–25% cases. The incidence of compound presentations has been estimated to be about 1:1,000 to 1:1,500 deliveries. Often a compound presentation detected in early labor tends to get spontaneously corrected with passage of time. It is observed in preterm deliveries, in multipara and following spontaneous rupture of the membranes and in twin pregnancies. The condition is suspected when the partogram shows that there is delay in progress of the active phase of labor, when the presenting part fails to engage. Observation often reveals that as the presenting part descends, the associated fetal limb recedes leading to spontaneous correction. If dystocia occurs, the baby remains high and operative treatment is needed. Cesarean section is preferred to any vaginal intervention procedures.

CHAPTER

21

Operative Delivery

Subhas Nargolkar, Mitra Sexena

INTRODUCTION

The ability to perform operative vaginal delivery using forceps or vacuum is important to those who provide maternity care because as many as 25% of nulliparous women have operative vaginal delivery. Increasing use of operative vaginal delivery is one means suggested to help reduce cesarean delivery rates.

An operative delivery is performed if a spontaneous birth is judged to pose a greater risk to mother or child than an assisted one. Operations are divided into abdominal methods (cesarean section) and vaginal assisted deliveries (forceps delivery and vacuum extraction).

Preparations for Operative Delivery

- Discuss operative delivery with the woman and her partner (if time is short, at least outline what will happen)
- Follow the woman's wishes; no operative delivery can proceed without her consent even if the doctors think that the baby will die, if it is not done
- Get written consent for elective procedures
- A pediatrician should attend any delivery, where problems are anticipated; local guidelines should be drawn up and followed for all operative deliveries.

FORCEPS

When spontaneous vaginal delivery is not possible, instrumental delivery may be attempted.

A pair of curved blades can secure a purchase on the rounded head and so apply traction to alter the speed of progress. Usually this is to hasten delivery, but occasionally it is to slow it down, as when delivering the after-coming head in a breech delivery.

Use

Forceps deliveries are performed in 5–10% of deliveries depending on the indication, the availability of trained obstetricians and the population served. In Britain, use of vacuum extraction is now greater than use of forceps because of reduced maternal trauma; both forms of vaginal delivery, however, are giving way to cesarean section.

Indications for Using Obstetric Forceps

- Fetal distress in second stage of labor
- Maternal distress in second stage of labor
- Lack of advance in second stage of labor
- Prophylactic shortening of second stage, for example in heart disease
- Control of after-coming head in a breech delivery.

Indications

All indications are relative and depend on the facilities for diagnosis and the attitudes of the professional staff.

Types of Instruments

There are two types of forceps those with a pelvic curve, and those without (Figs 1 to 4). Kielland's forceps are for rotation and extraction; Simpson's forceps are for mid-cavity assisted delivery without the need for rotation when the maximum diameter of the fetal head is about 5–8 cm above the vulva. Short forceps (Wrigley's) are for low extraction when the maximum diameter is about 2.5 cm above the vulva. These were designed for use by general practitioner obstetricians with the safety feature that they could not reach high into the pelvis.

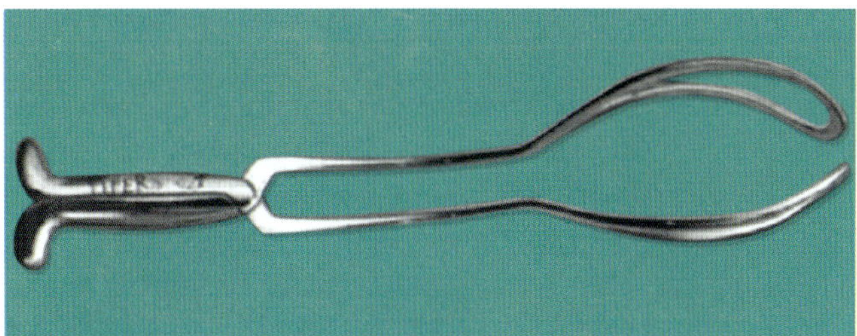

Fig. 1: Curved Simpson's forceps

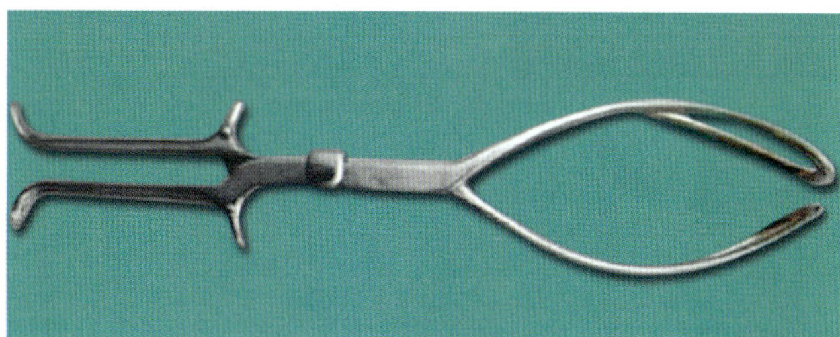

Fig. 2: Kielland's forceps

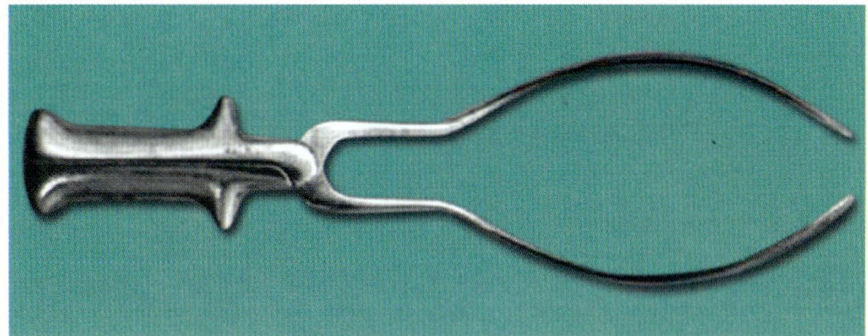

Fig. 3: Delee Simpson type forceps

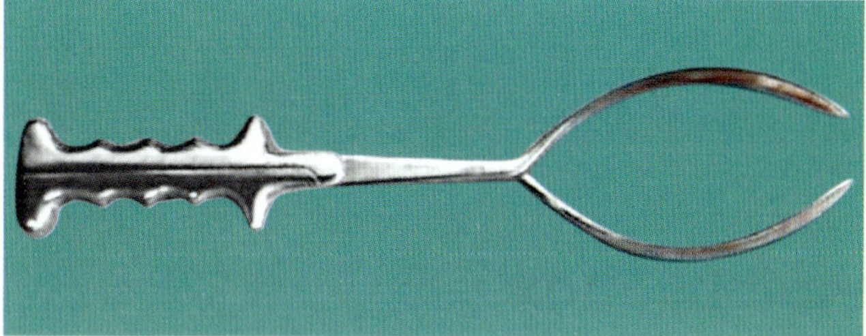

Fig. 4: Elliott type forceps

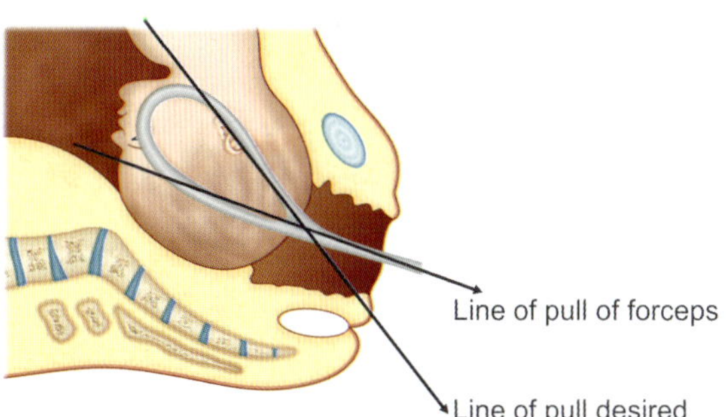

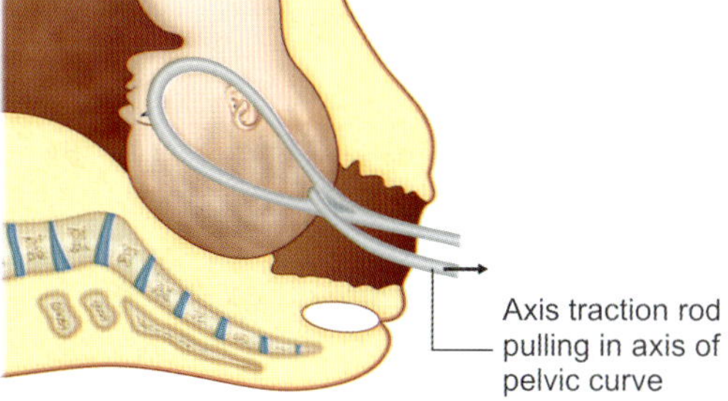

Fig. 5: Forceps, direction of pull, along the curve of Carus

Correct line for pull of forceps is along the curve of Carus (Fig. 5). The line of pull is the resultant of two lines of forceps in mid-cavity. As the head descends, the line of pull needs to become more anterior to negotiate the pelvic curve.

ANATOMY OF FORCEPS

A. Two separable arms: right and left
   1. Shank, can be
      a. Parallel
      b. Overlapping

   Types of forceps used in Britain: straight Kielland's forceps for rotation (left); curved Wrigley's forceps for lower cavity traction (center).
   2. Arm locks, types are:
      a. Sliding
      b. English (scissors)
      c. French lock (set screw).
   3. Handle.

B. Blade (tow and heel)
   1. Blade curves
      a. Pelvic curve: Blades follow birth canal curve
      b. Cephalic curve: Blades apply well to fetal head.
   2. Blade shape
      a. Fenestrated
      b. Semi-fenestrated
      c. Solid.

Directions (Figs 6 to 10)

A. Station (*See* fetal descent)
   1. Level of fetal head to maternal ischial spines

B. High forceps (Kielland's forceps)
   1. Vertex not engaged
   2. No longer used (historical reference only)

C. Mid-forceps (Anderson's or Simpson's forceps) (Figs 9A to F)
   1. Head engaged (above +2 station)
   2. Rarely used

D. Low forceps or outlet forceps (Wrigley's forceps) (Figs 10A to F)
   1. Below +2 station
   2. Rotation required, lesser than 45°.

Low forceps

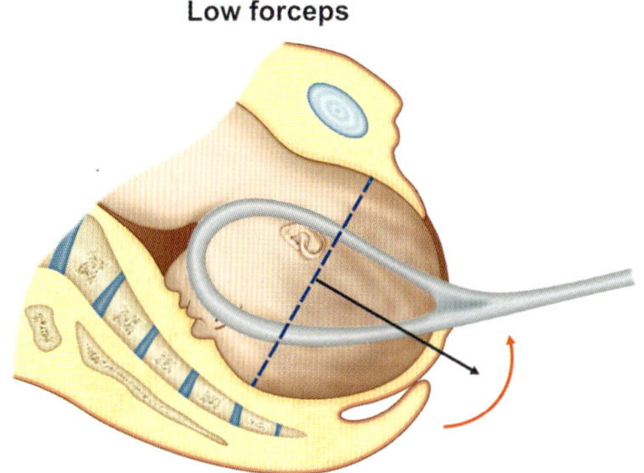

Mid forceps

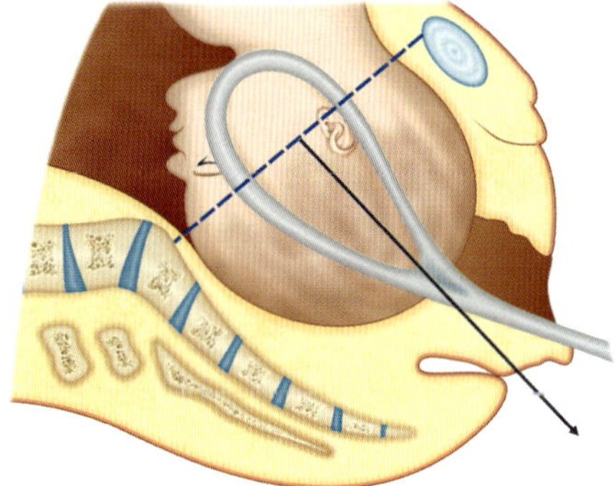

Fig. 6: Forceps, direction of pull

Indications

A. Maternal distress
   1. Cardiac disease
   2. Pregnancy-induced hypertension
   3. Chorioamnionitis
   4. Acute pulmonary edema
   5. Maternal exhaustion, in second stage
B. Fetal distress
   1. Cord prolapse
   2. Abruptio placentae
C. Prolonged second stage of labor
   1. Inadequate contractions
   2. Ineffective maternal effort
   3. Malrotation of the fetal head (occiput posterior)
   4. Perineal rigidity
   5. Epidural anesthesia.

Preparation for Assisted Delivery

A. Preconditions
   1. Head engaged
   2. Vertex presentation
   3. Head position known
   4. Complete cervical dilation to 10 cm
   5. Rupture of membranes
   6. No cephalopelvic disproportion
   7. Bladder empty
   8. Adequate anesthesia, analgesia.

TECHNIQUE

How to use forceps is again best learned by watching and doing the procedure under skilled tutelage. The woman should receive an explanation of what will happen. The bladder is catheterized and regional anesthesia is given. Each blade is slipped beside the fetal head, the vagina being guarded by the operator's hand. When correctly sited, the handles should lock, and gentle traction in the correct line of pull will help delivery. An episiotomy is usually required to achieve a line of pull sufficiently posterior. Once the head is crowned, the blades can be removed and the rest of the baby delivered normally.

Steps of Forceps Delivery (Box 1)

Simpson's forceps, commonly used forceps:
1. Forceps applied across ears to mandible region
2. Apply forceps flat against head, then rotate
3. Posterior fontanel is 1 cm anterior to plane of shank
4. Sagittal suture bisects longitudinal axis
5. Handle closes easily
6. Traction to head until under symphysis pubis
7. Rotate handle up
8. Do not rotate greater than 45° forceps; at delivery, scalp visible at introitus.

Complications

A. Maternal complications
   1. Vaginal lacerations or cervical lacerations
   2. Postpartum hemorrhage
   3. Maternal infection
B. Fetal complications: Birth trauma
   1. Cephalohematoma
   2. Facial nerve palsy
   3. Depressed skull fracture.

Box 1 Documentation: Operative forceps delivery note, an example

A. Indication: Maternal exhaustion
B. Instrument: Simpson's forceps
C. Operation: Outlet forceps
D. Anesthesia: Local 2% xylocaine (Fig. 7)
E. Bladder: Via straight catheter
F. Blood loss: <500 cc
G. Infant: Apgars of 8 and 9
H. Maternal: Small episiotomy repaired with 2–0 vicryl

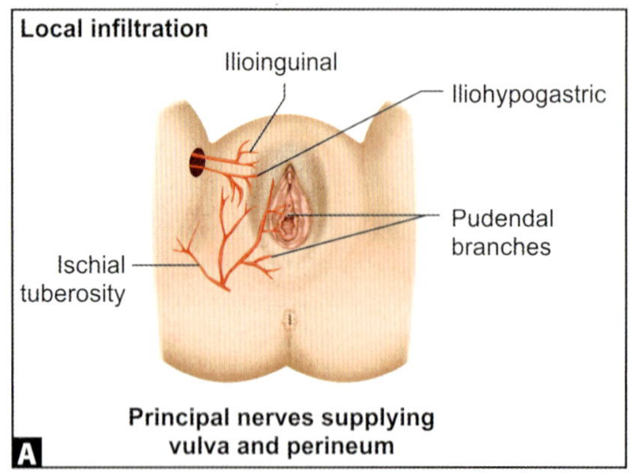

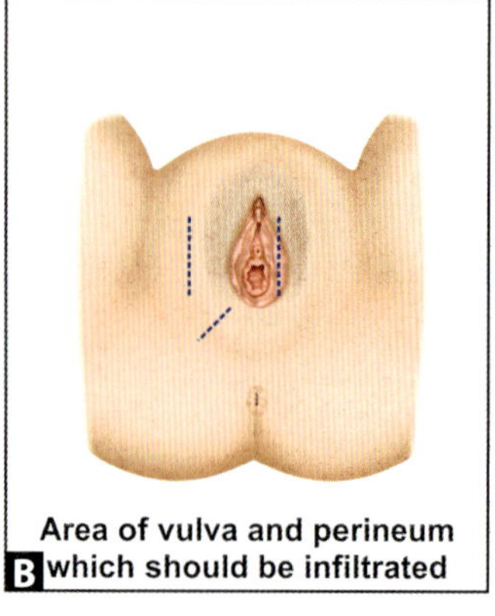

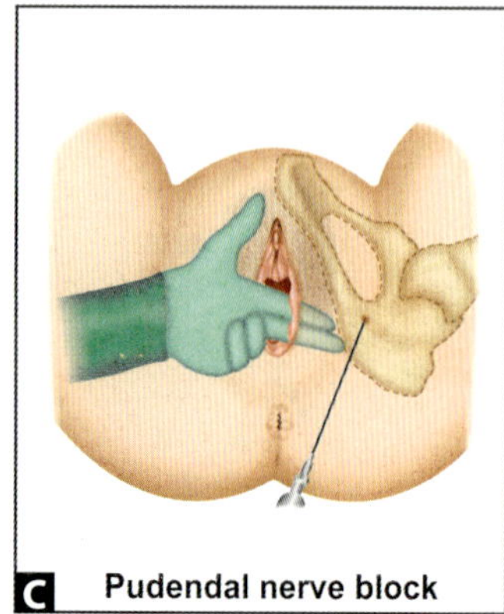

Figs 7A to C: Local anesthesia for forceps application

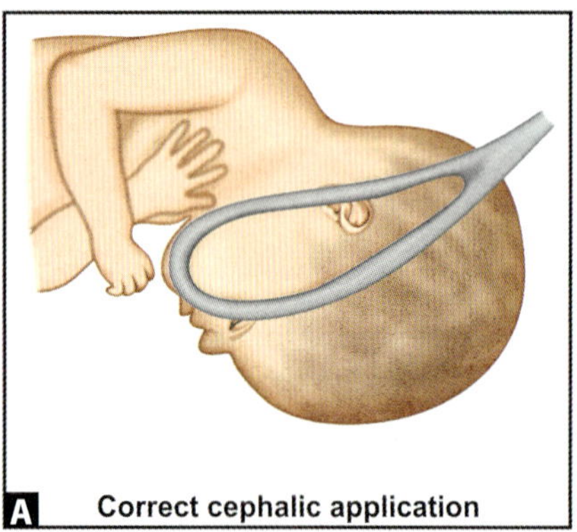

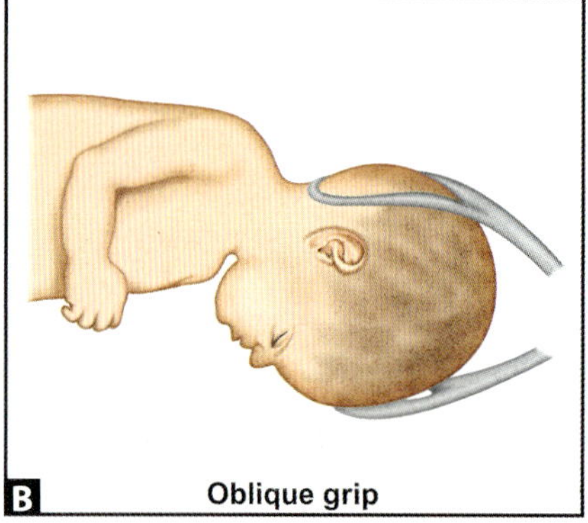

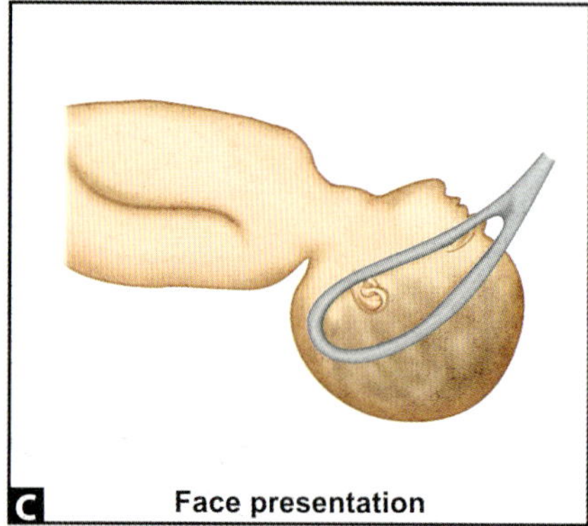

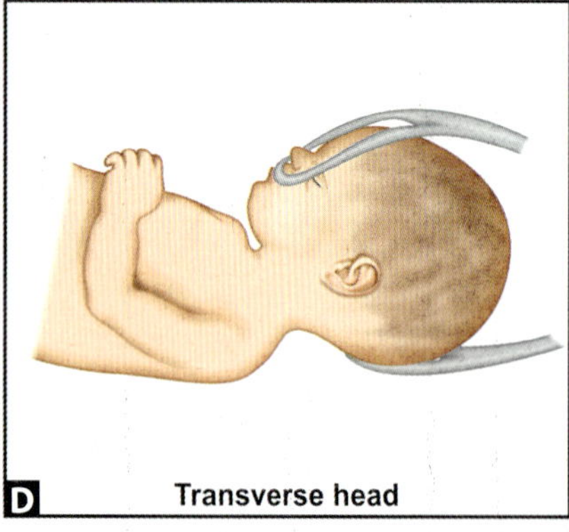

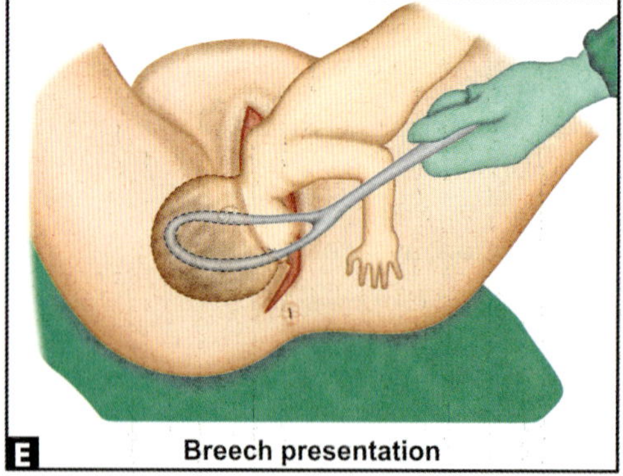

Figs 8A to E: Different forceps grips

ASSISTED VAGINAL DELIVERY USING THE VACUUM EXTRACTOR

When spontaneous vaginal delivery is not possible, instrumental delivery may be attempted. In 1705, Yonge described an attempted vaginal delivery using a cupping glass. In 1848, the developer of the Simpson forceps devised a bell-shaped device called an "air tractor vacuum extractor". Multiple innovations followed, and a metal-cup extractor was developed by Malmström in 1953. More recently, bell-shaped and hemispheric silicone rubber cups (Fig. 11) have come into use. Following procedure discusses the two basic types of vacuum extractors and their use in vaginal deliveries.

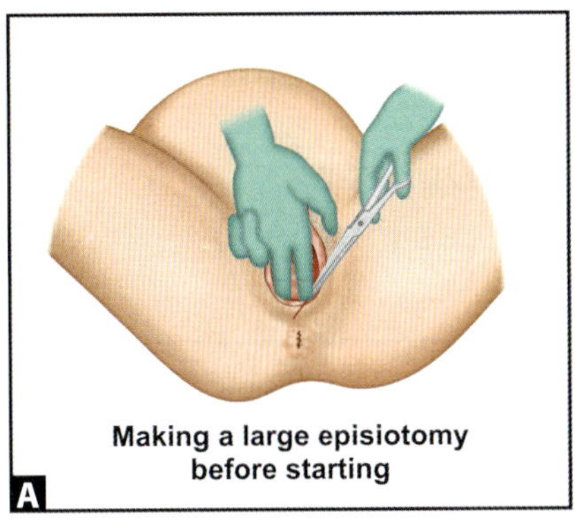

A — Making a large episiotomy before starting

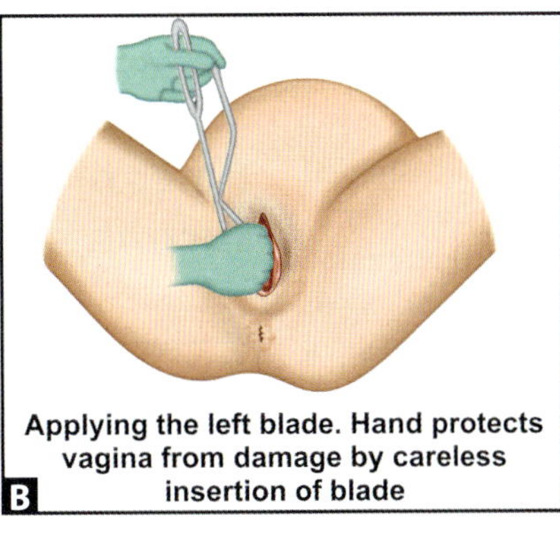

B — Applying the left blade. Hand protects vagina from damage by careless insertion of blade

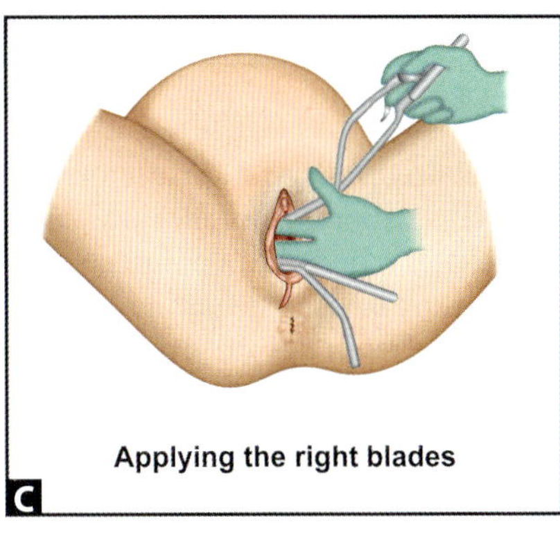

C — Applying the right blades

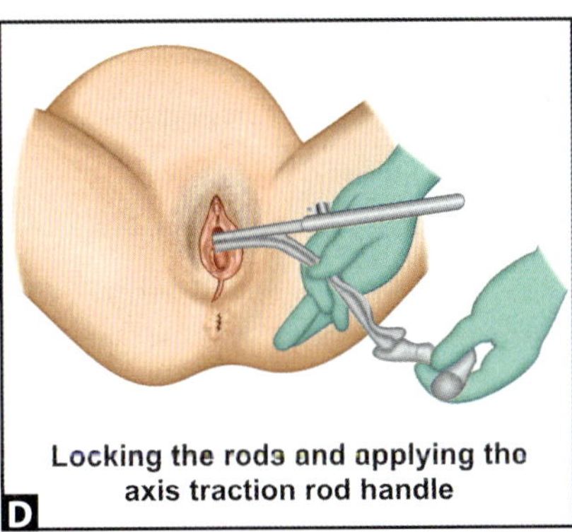

D — Locking the rods and applying the axis traction rod handle

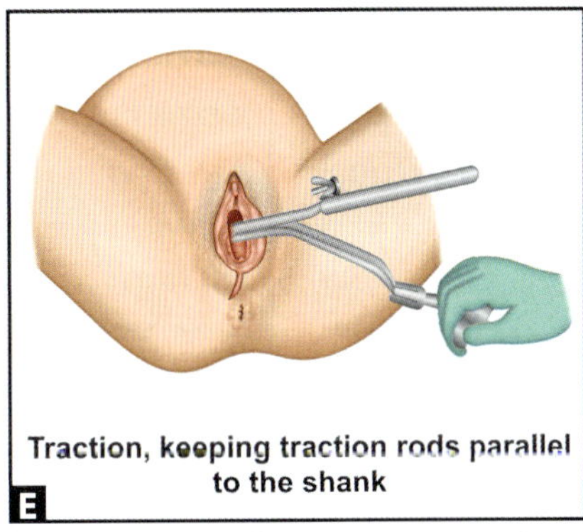

E — Traction, keeping traction rods parallel to the shank

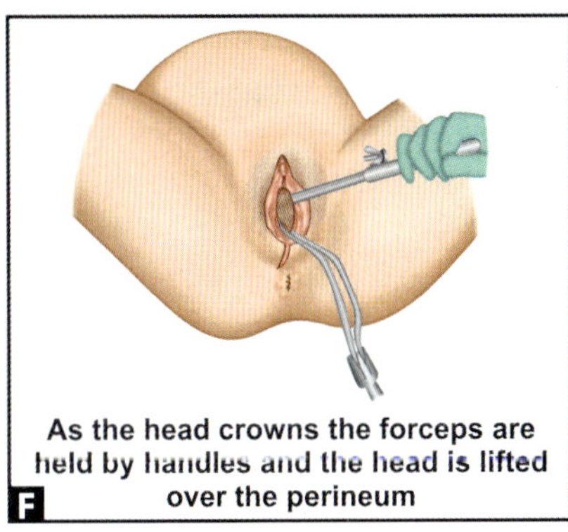

F — As the head crowns the forceps are held by handles and the head is lifted over the perineum

Figs 9A to F: Mid-forceps application

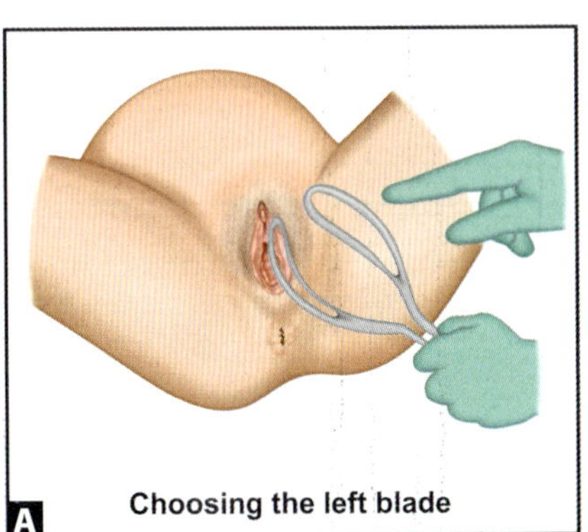

A — Choosing the left blade

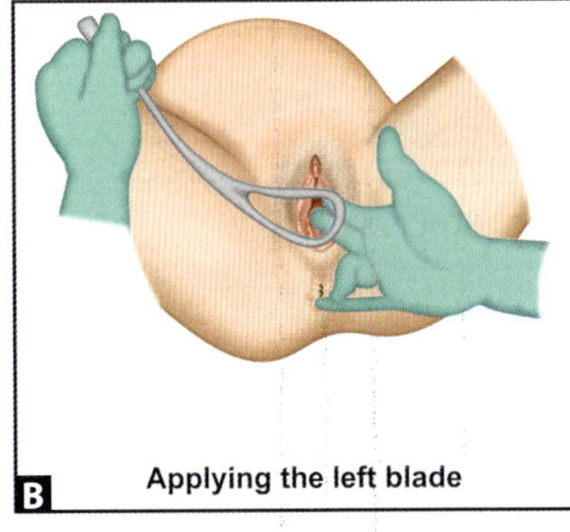

B — Applying the left blade

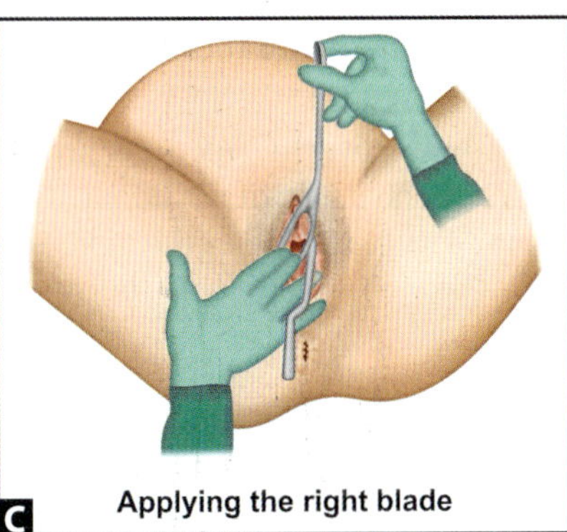

C — Applying the right blade

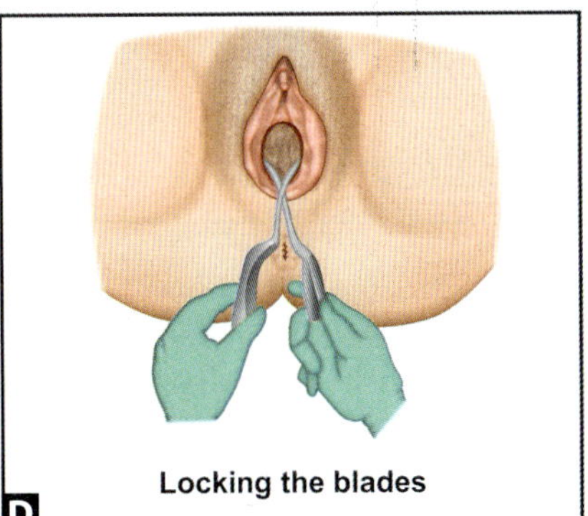

D — Locking the blades

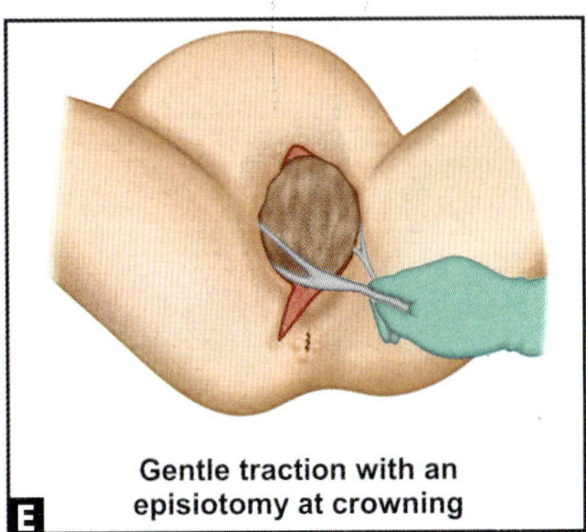

E — Gentle traction with an episiotomy at crowning

F — The correct cephalic application (in the mentovertical line)

Figs 10A to F: Low-forceps application

TYPES OF VACUUM EXTRACTORS

Metal Cup

The metal-cup vacuum extractor is a mushroom-shaped metal cup varying from 40 mm to 60 mm in diameter. A centrally attached chain connects the cup to a detachable handle that is used to apply traction. A mechanical or electrical suction device is attached to the metal cup via a peripherally located vacuum port.

The advantages of metal-cup vacuum extraction over soft-cup extraction include a higher success rate and easier cup placement in the occipitoposterior (OP) position, especially when an OP cup is used. Unfortunately, the rigidity of metal cups can make application difficult and uncomfortable, and their use is associated with an increased risk of fetal scalp injuries. Metal-cup vacuum extractors are rarely used in the United States.

Soft Cups

Compared with metal-cup devices, soft-cup vacuum extractors cause fewer neonatal scalp injuries. However, these instruments have a higher failure rate.

Soft-cup instruments can be used with a manual vacuum pump or an electrical suction device. Some have a built-in vacuum-release valve that allows pressure to be rapidly attained and accurately controlled. This results in easy maneuverability and simplicity of operation. Soft-cup vacuum extractors may be disposable or reusable.

Traditionally, the soft cups are bell or funnel-shaped (Fig. 12). A newer variety, the mushroom-shaped vacuum cup, or M-cup, combines the advantages of soft and metal cups. The soft sidewall of the M-cup minimizes infant scalp trauma compared with the Malmström metal cup (Figs 13 and 14).

Types of Vacuum Delivery Suction-cup Devices (Table 1)

Table 1: Types of vacuum delivery suction-cup devices

Name	Size	Material
Soft cups (silicone or plastic)		
Gentle Vac	60 mm	Soft rubber
Kiwi ProCup	65 mm	Soft plastic
Mityvac Bell	60 mm	Soft silicone
Secure Cup	63 mm	Rubber
Silc Cup	50–60 mm	Silicone rubber
Soft Touch	60 mm	Soft polyethylene
Tender Touch	60 mm	Soft silicone
Vac-U-Nate	65 mm	Soft silicone
Rigid "anterior" cups (plastic or metal)		
Flex Cup	60 mm	Polyurethane
Kiwi Omnicup	50 mm	Rigid plastic
Malmström (Fig. 15)	40–60 mm	Metal
Mityvac "M" Style	50 mm	Rigid polyethylene
Rigid "posterior" cups (plastic or metal)		
Bird posterior cup (Fig. 16)	40–60 mm	Metal
Kiwi Omnicup	50 mm	Rigid plastic
Mityvac "M" Select	50 mm	Rigid polyethylene

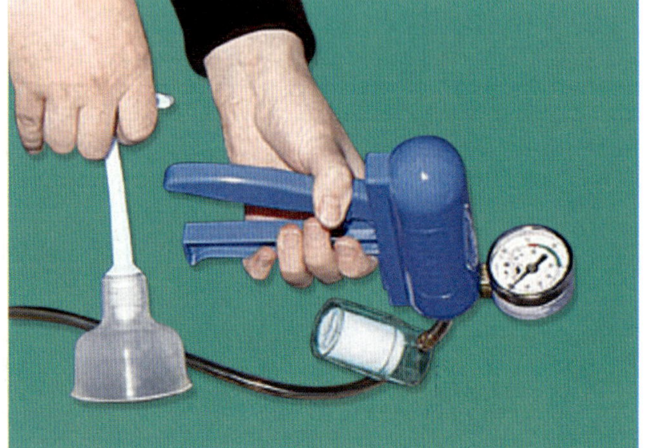

Fig. 11: Equipments for soft-cup vacuum extraction: cup with traction handle, fluid trap, vacuum gauge and manual vacuum pump

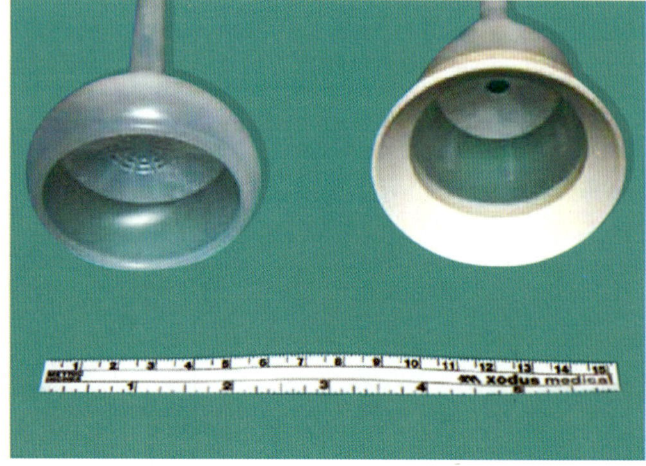

Fig. 12: Soft cup vacuum extractors

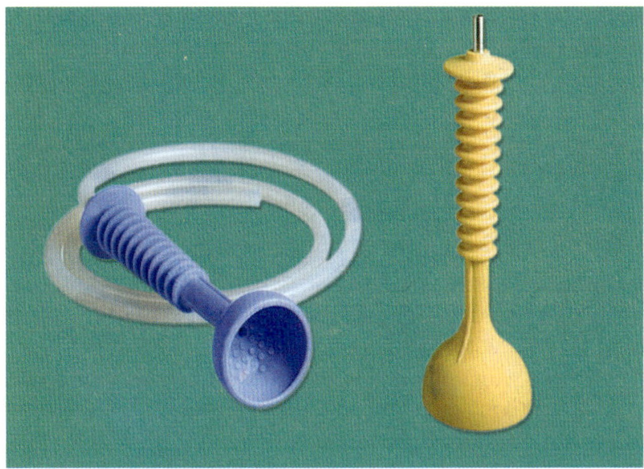

Fig. 13: Autoclavable silicone cup

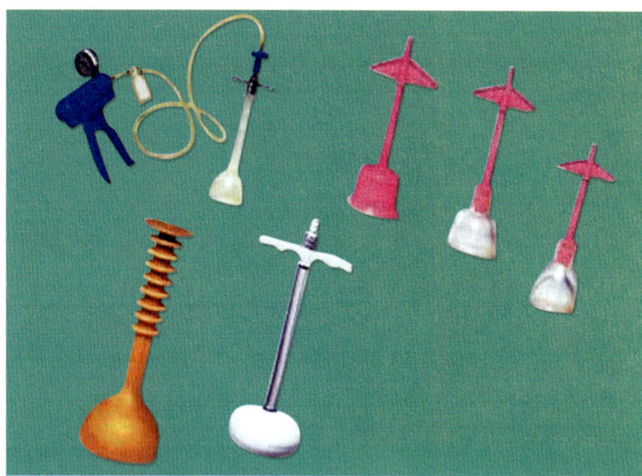

Fig. 14: Disposable polyethylene bell-shaped cups (disposable mushroom-shaped cups, reusable silicone bell-shaped cups, manual vacuum pumps, adapters)

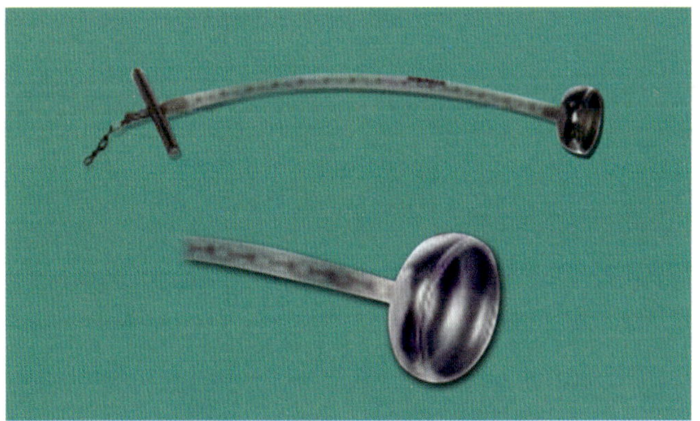

Fig. 15: Malmström suction cup

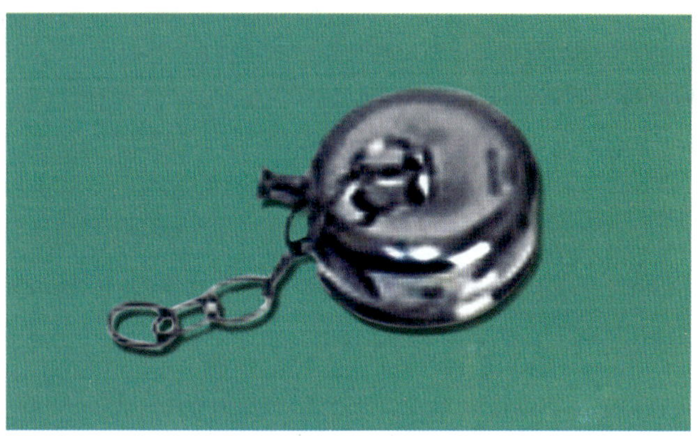

Fig. 16: Bird suction cup

VACUUM EXTRACTORS AND FORCEPS

In Europe, the vacuum extractor has long been the instrument of choice for assisted vaginal delivery. In the United States, the forceps had been preferred, although the vacuum extractor is becoming increasingly popular. The advantages and disadvantages of vacuum extractors and forceps are listed in Table 2. A recent Cochrane review found that the risks and benefits of the two forms of assisted delivery are comparable. Often, the delivery instrument is selected based on the training and experience of the individual physician.

Table 2: Comparative advantages of vacuum extractors and forceps

Vacuum extractors	Forceps
Easier to learn Quicker delivery Less maternal genital trauma Less maternal discomfort	Fewer neonatal injuries, including cephalohematoma, retinal hemorrhage, and transient lateral rectus palsy
Fewer neonatal craniofacial injuries Less anesthesia required	Higher rate of successful vaginal delivery

INDICATIONS AND CONTRAINDICATIONS FOR VACUUM EXTRACTION

Maternal and fetal indications for vacuum-assisted delivery are listed in Table 3. Relative contraindications for vacuum extraction are given in Table 4.

The exact gestational age at which a fetus is considered too premature for vacuum-assisted delivery has been debated. Many authors use a gestational age of 34 weeks as the cutoff point. One review found no significant difference in neonatal morbidity rates following vacuum extraction of preterm infants (birth weights of 1,500–2,499 g) and full-term infants.

Table 3: Indications for vacuum-assisted delivery

Maternal indications	Fetal indications
Need to avoid voluntary maternal expulsive efforts (e.g. the mother has cardiac or cerebrovascular disease)	Nonreassuring fetal heart tracing
Inadequate maternal expulsive efforts	Prolonged second stage of labor
Maternal exhaustion or lack of cooperation	Failure to progress in second stage of labor

Table 4: Relative contraindications for vacuum extraction

Fetal prematurity (<34 weeks of gestation)	Nonvertex presentation or other malpresentation
Fetal scalp trauma	Cephalopelvic disproportion
Unengaged head	Delivery requiring rotation or excessive traction
Incomplete cervical dilatation	Inadequate anesthesia
Active bleeding or suspected fetal coagulation defects	
Suspected macrosomia	

Soft-cup vacuum extractors cause fewer neonatal scalp injuries than metal-cup devices, but they have a higher failure rate.

Some authors now consider vacuum-assisted deliveries to be possible before full cervical dilatation and at higher locations (stations) of the occiput in the birth canal.

The decision to proceed with a vacuum-assisted delivery when a relative contraindication exists must be based on a comparison of the risks of the vacuum-assisted delivery and the risks of other delivery options. In these situations, consultation is generally advisable.

PROCEDURE USING SOFT-CUP VACUUM EXTRACTION

After the patient has emptied her bladder, she is placed in the dorsal lithotomy position without strapping or taping of her legs. Adequate anesthesia can be obtained with an epidural, spinal or pudendal block. The fetal presentation, position and station are then confirmed.

Avoiding undue stretch on the perineum, the physician applies the soft cup by spreading the patient's labia, compressing the cup and inserting it gently by pressing inward and downward with the inferior edge over the posterior fourchette.

When contact is made with the fetal scalp, the center of the cup should be over the sagittal suture and about 3 cm (1.2′′) in front of the posterior fontanel. As a practical guide, the cup is generally placed as far posteriorly as possible (Figs 17A and B). This cup placement maintains flexion of the fetal head and avoids traction over the anterior fontanel. In positioning the cup, the physician should be careful to avoid trapping maternal soft tissue between the cup and the fetal head.

Where should the cup be applied on the fetal head?

Whether the infant presents with the occiput anterior, posterior or some degree of transverse, major causes of difficulty with the second stage of labor and failure of assisted vaginal birth are deflexion of the fetal head and acyclitism. Goals of cup positioning are, therefore, maintenance or improvement of flexion and cyclitism. To optimize these factors, the cup should be placed on the "flexion point", the center of which is located directly over the sagittal suture and about 6 cm behind the anterior fontanel (Fig. 18). In occiput transverse positions, autorotation of the fetal head occurs during assisted delivery without any intentional twisting motion by the operator.

After the cup is properly positioned, the physician places the fingers of one hand against the suction cup and grasps the handle of the instrument with the other hand. Once vacuum is applied, the cup should not be twisted. Twisting the cup may lead to "cookie-cutter" or semi-circumferential laceration of the fetal scalp, although this is less likely to occur with the soft cup than with the metal cup.

The degree of vacuum determines the traction forces (Fig. 19). Effective traction usually requires a pressure of at least 0.6 kg/cm^2 (440 mm Hg). Although more negative pressures reduce the risk of cup detachment, lowering the pressure beyond 0.8 kg/cm^2 (588 mm Hg) increases the risk of fetal scalp and cerebrocranial trauma.

Traction should be in line with the pelvic axis and coordinated with maternal expulsive efforts. The traction can be relieved or maintained between contractions with no difference in maternal or fetal outcome. Some authors suggest that continued moderate traction may aid in maintaining gained progress in descent of the fetal vertex.

If the cup is dislodged, it is reapplied only after careful inspection of the fetal scalp for injury.

Traction is repeated with each contraction until the head is crowned. As the head clears the pubic symphysis, the vertex is pulled upward at an angle of 45° to the floor. Once the head is delivered, suction is released and the cup is removed (Figs 20A to D). Delivery then proceeds as usual.

Vacuum extraction should not be attempted for more than 20 minutes. The procedure should be abandoned if delivery is not achieved or the labor does not progress. Under ordinary circumstances, the procedure should be abandoned after three cup detachments. The procedure

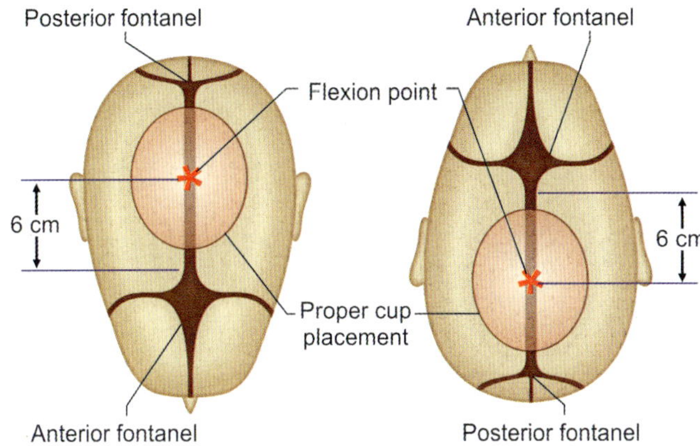

Fig. 17A: Proper placement of the cup used in vacuum extraction. The center of the cup should be over the sagittal suture and about 3 cm (1.2´´) in front of the posterior fontanel. The cup is generally placed as far posteriorly as possible

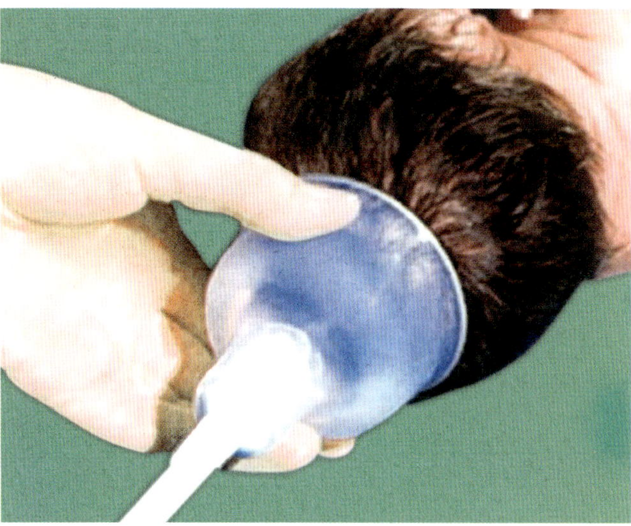

Fig. 17B: Proper placement of cup

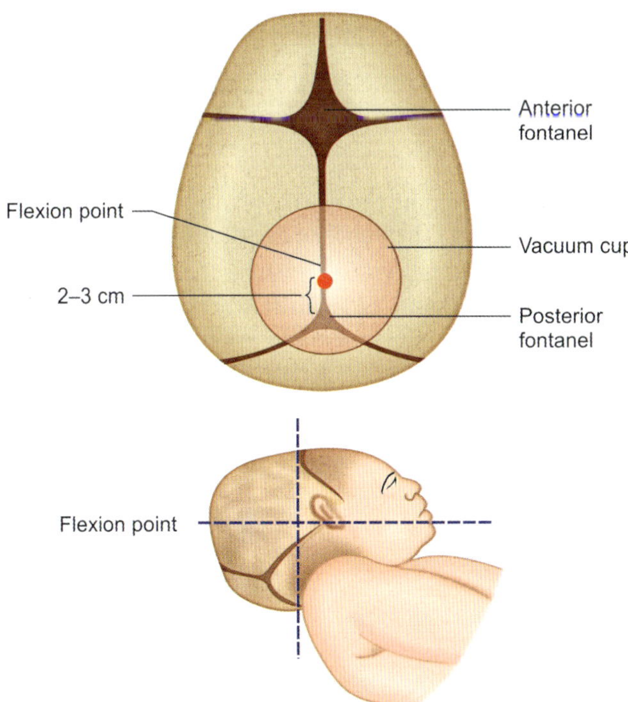

Fig. 18: Flexion point in relation to fetal skull landmarks

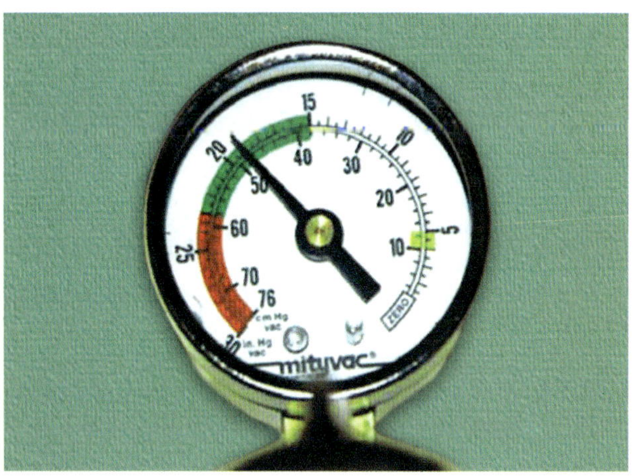

Fig. 19: Suction gauge. Suction should be generated until the long arm points to the green zone

should also be stopped if there is any evidence of fetal trauma.

MATERNAL AND FETAL COMPLICATIONS

Maternal complications associated with vacuum extraction are comparable to those associated with spontaneous deliveries. Complications do not vary with the type of vacuum extractor used.

Subgaleal hemorrhage should be suspected in infants delivered by vacuum extraction who have a boggy scalp, swelling crossing the suture lines and an expanding head circumference. These infants may also have signs of hypovolemia, pallor, tachycardia and a falling hematocrit.

Subgaleal hemorrhage is a serious neonatal complication of vacuum extraction. This complication occurred in 1.0–3.8% of vacuum extractions in one series but has been much less common in more recent studies.

Cephalohematoma is another fetal complication of vacuum extraction. This complication has a mean incidence of 6% (range: 1–26%) in vacuum-assisted deliveries.

Intracranial hemorrhage has been found to occur in one of every 860 vacuum-assisted deliveries compared

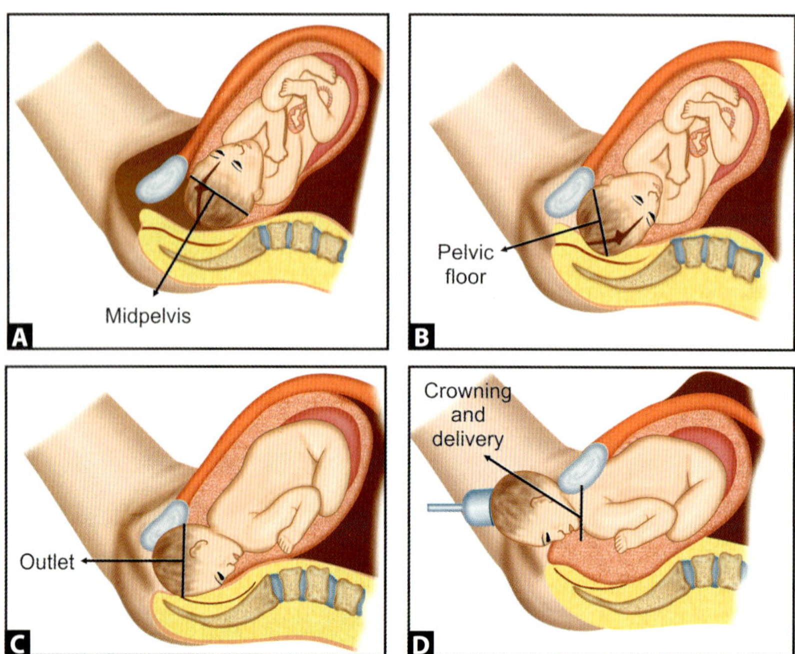

Figs 20A to D: The axis of traction is more toward the rectum for higher head stations. As the head descends and crowns, traction is directed increasingly upward along the pelvic curve and autorotation of the head occurs

with one of every 1,900 spontaneous deliveries (a statistically significant difference). Yet, the comparative rate of intracranial hemorrhage is not statistically different when vacuum extraction, forceps delivery and cesarean section during labor are compared. It is possible that the abnormal labor that necessitated the assisted delivery may be an underlying cause for a portion of the morbidity attributed to operative deliveries.

Retinal hemorrhages may be more common in vacuum-assisted deliveries but are most often associated with duration of labor. Because these hemorrhages resolve within several weeks, they are unlikely to be associated with long-term morbidity.

Transient neonatal lateral rectus paralysis has been found to occur more frequently in vacuum-assisted deliveries (3.2%) than in forceps deliveries (2.4%), normal spontaneous vaginal deliveries (0.1%) and cesarean sections (0%). Because the paralysis resolves spontaneously, it is unlikely to be of clinical importance.

Vacuum extraction has not been found to result in significant intellectual or neurologic disability.

Medicolegal Concerns

Before vacuum extraction is initiated, the parents should be given a clear explanation of the risks and benefits of vacuum extraction for the mother and fetus. Advising the patient that an attempt at instrumental delivery may not result in vaginal delivery may avoid unrealistic expectations. Avoiding the use of vacuum extraction when the fetus is high in the pelvis or the mother is not pushing can reduce the risk of complications.

Following vacuum-assisted delivery or an attempted assisted delivery, documentation should include the indication for the procedure, a record of the discussion with the patient and a detailed description of the procedure itself.

CONCLUSION

Assisted vaginal delivery is an integral part of obstetric care worldwide.

It may be performed as infrequently as in 1.5% of deliveries (Czechoslovakian Republic) or as often as in 15% (Australia and Canada) (Stephenson 1992). Discrepant rates may be related to differences in labor management. In general, maternal outcome may be improved by a reduction in instrumental delivery rates. Various techniques may help to achieve lower rates of assisted delivery, e.g. companionship in labor, active management of the second stage of labor with syntocinon, upright posture with use of the birth cushion or undertaking fetal scalp blood sampling rather than expedited delivery when fetal heart rate decelerations occur. When epidural analgesia is used, allowing time for the analgesic effect to wear off, or having a more liberal approach to the length of the second stage also reduces the need for assisted delivery.

BIBLIOGRAPHY

1. ACOG committee opinion. Delivery by vacuum extraction. Number 208, September 1998. Committee on Obstetric Practice. American College of Obstetricians and Gynecologists. Int J Gynecol Obstet. 1999;64(1):96.
2. Bofill JA, Martin JN, Morrison JC. The Mississippi Operative Vaginal Delivery Trial: lessons learned. Contemp Ob Gyn. 1998;43:60-79.
3. Bofill JA, Rust OA, Schorr SJ, et al. A randomized prospective trial of the obstetric forceps versus the M-cup vacuum extractor. Am J Obstet Gynecol. 1996;175:1325-30.
4. Bofill JA, Rust OA, Schorr SJ, et al. A randomized trial of two vacuum extraction techniques. Obstet Gynecol. 1997;89:758-62.
5. Chadwick LJ, Pemberton PJ, Kurinczuk JJ. Neonatal subgaleal haematoma: associated risk factors, complications and outcome. J Paediatr Child Health. 1996;32:228-32.
6. Johanson R, Menon V. Soft versus rigid vacuum extractor cups for assisted vaginal delivery. Cochrane Database Syst Rev. 2000;2:CD000446.
7. Johanson R. Choice of instrument for vaginal delivery. Curr Opin Obstet Gynecol. 1997;9:361-5.
8. Johanson RB, Menon BK. Vacuum extraction versus forceps for assisted vaginal delivery. Cochrane Database Syst Rev. 2000;2:CD000224.
9. Kuit JA, Eppinga HC, Wallenburg HC, et al. A randomized comparison of vacuum extraction delivery with a rigid and a pliable cup. Obstet Gynecol. 1993;82:280-4.
10. Lucas MJ. The role of vacuum extraction in modern obstetrics. Clin Obstet Gynecol. 1994;37:794-805.
11. Meniru GI. An analysis of recent trends in vacuum extraction and forceps delivery in the United Kingdom. Br J Obstet Gynaecol. 1996;103:168-70.
12. Morales R, Adair CD, Sanchez-Ramos L, et al. Vacuum extraction of preterm infants with birth weights of 1,500-2,499 grams. J Reprod Med. 1995;40:127-30.
13. OBG Management. (1999). Cutting your legal risks with vacuum-assisted delivery. [online] Available from: www.obgmanagement.com/cutrisk/vacuum.html. [Accessed January, 2014].
14. Operative vaginal delivery. ACOG technical bulletin number 196—August 1994 (replaces number 152, February 1991). Int J Gynaecol Obstet. 1994;47:179-85.
15. O'Grady JP. Modern instrumental delivery. Baltimore: Williams and Wilkins; 1988. pp. 155-85.
16. Ross MG. Vacuum delivery by soft cup extraction. Contemp Obs Gyn. 1994;39:48-53.
17. Towner D, Castro MA, Eby-Wilkens E, et al. Effect of mode of delivery in nulliparous women on neonatal intracranial injury. N Engl J Med. 1999;341:1709-14.
18. Vacca A. Birth by vacuum extraction: neonatal outcome. J Paediatr Child Health. 1996;32:204-6.
19. Williams MC. Vacuum-assisted delivery. Clin Perinatol. 1995;22:933-52.

CHAPTER

22

Repair of Tears: Vaginal, Perineal and Cervical

Alka Kriplani, Sumana G

INTRODUCTION

Perineal and vaginal tears are not uncommon associates of vaginal delivery. Morbidity due to vaginal delivery is due to postpartum hemorrhage and damage to pelvic floor. Appropriate repair of perineal tears is therefore important, not only to avoid immediate morbidity due to blood loss but also due to long-term morbidity in the form of anal incontinence and prolapse.

Obstetric trauma at vaginal delivery is the major cause of anal incontinence in women. The incidence of anal sphincter injuries (third and fourth degree tears) is 0.5–5% of vaginal deliveries in centers practicing mediolateral episiotomies and 17% in centers where midline episiotomies are in use. Anal incontinence occurs in 40% of women following vaginal deliveries. With obstetric litigation on the rise, the last decade has addressed several issues about perineal tears and evidence-based guidelines are now emerging. The focus should hence be on understanding perineal anatomy and physiology, using standardized classification systems, recognizing perineal trauma at delivery, anatomic re-approximation of tissues and most importantly preventing their occurrence. Proceedings are to put forth evidence-based issues to aid better understanding and management of perineal tears.

SURGICAL ANATOMY

The perineum is a diamond-shaped aperture corresponding to the pelvic outlet. It is bounded by the lower margin of the pubic symphysis anteriorly, the coccyx posteriorly and the ischial tuberosities laterally. It is divided into an anterior urogenital triangle and a posterior anal triangle.

The central perineal tendon forms the posterior support of the lower aspect of the anterior vaginal wall. It lies at the base of the urogenital diaphragm between the vaginal and anal orifices. It is formed by the convergence of the tendinous attachments of the bulbocavernosus, external anal sphincter (EAS) and the superficial transverse perinei muscles. Its superior border represents the point of insertion of the rectovaginal fascia (Fig. 1).

The bulbocavernosus muscle surrounds the orifice of the vagina and covers the vestibular bulbs. They insert anteriorly into the corpora cavernosa clitoridis and are called "sphincter vaginae".

The superficial transverse perinei is a small strip that arises from the medial side of each ischial tuberosity and joins its fellow in the central perineal tendon. The deep transverse perineal muscles are the most posterior fibers of the sphincter urethrae. They get attached to the vaginal walls.

Anal continence is maintained by the EAS and the internal anal sphincter (IAS). EAS has three parts that are indistinctly separated from each other. It is supplied by the pudendal nerve.

1. Subcutaneous part with no bony attachment.
2. Superficial oval part: Fibers arise from the coccyx and anococcygeal ligament and pass anteriorly around the anus to insert into the perineal body.
3. Deep part arises from the perineal body, encircles the lower half of the anal canal and is fused with the puborectalis.

Internal anal sphincter is involuntary, formed by the circular smooth muscle of the rectum. It is innervated by sympathetic fibers from the presacral ganglia (L5) and parasympathetic fibers from sacral segments (S2–S4). The central tendon plays an important anchoring role in the musculofascial support of the pelvic floor. Its tearing or stretching during vaginal delivery removes support from the posterior wall of the vagina. This results in anal incontinence or prolapse of the uterus.

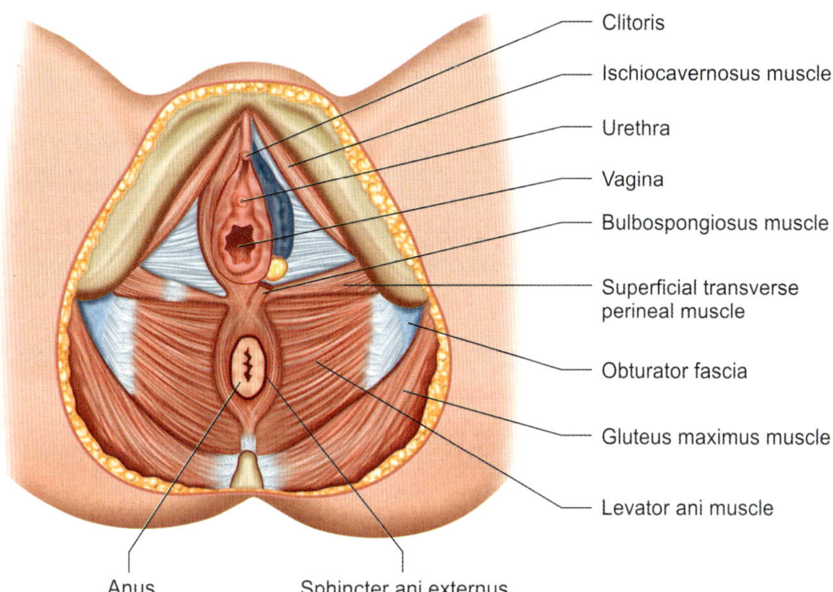

Fig. 1: Anatomy of the perineum

Physiology

When the introitus stretches beyond its elastic capacity or expands too rapidly, tissues tend to tear resulting in perineal trauma. Restoration of anal continence in third or fourth degree tears require a sound understanding of its physiology. Anal continence is the result of the coordinated action of anatomic and physiological elements. It requires normal rectal sensation and compliance, a competent and innervated anal sphincter and an intact recto-anal inhibitory reflex. The IAS maintains sphincter tone at rest and its disruption causes passive insensible incontinence of feces. The voluntary EAS maintains the resting tone of the anal canal. It reflexly contracts when there is rise in intra-abdominal pressure and its disruption causes urge incontinence. The pudendal nerve that innervates the external sphincter runs along the pelvic side wall and is susceptible to traction injury or direct trauma during childbirth.

Anal continence may be disturbed by disruption of sphincter muscle, traction pudendal neuropathy or a combination of both. Pudendal neuropathy is a much ignored entity that occurs secondary to demyelination caused by traction during delivery. Rarely complete axonal disruption also occurs. It usually recovers in the 1st year after delivery.

Classification

There is a wide variation in classification of perineal injury used by obstetricians worldwide. It is recommended that a uniform classification system is required to be followed to avoid under-reporting, allow proper documentation, audit and to assess treatment outcomes.

First degree: Injury to vaginal mucosa not involving the muscle.

Second degree: Injury to the perineum involving perineal muscles but not involving the anal sphincter.

Third degree: Injury to perineum involving the anal sphincter complex (EAS and IAS):

- 3a: Less than 50% of EAS thickness torn
- 3b: More than 50% of EAS thickness torn
- 3c: IAS torn.

Fourth degree: Injury to perineum involving the anal sphincter complex (EAS and IAS) and rectal mucosa.

Injury to the anal sphincter results in incontinence to flatus, liquid/solid stool, passive soiling, fecal urgency, rectovaginal fistula, pelvic pain and dyspareunia. These symptoms are a social taboo, often preventing women from availing medical assistance and thus resulting in under-reporting.

Risk Factors

A number of obstetric risk factors for occurrence of major degree tears have been identified. Recognition of risk factors may probably minimize the development of sphincter injuries.

Vaginal Delivery

Perineal tears and anal incontinence are the consequences of vaginal delivery. Anal incontinence (of some form) is known to occur in 40% of women undergoing vaginal delivery. Transient symptoms may occur in intrapartum cesareans, especially those done late in labor, but prelabor cesareans avoid the risk altogether.

Instrumental Deliveries

Instrumental vaginal delivery, particularly with the use of episiotomy, increases the risk of laceration significantly. A failed vacuum followed by a forceps application carries with it the highest risk of perineal trauma.

Epidural Anesthesia

This may contribute by prolonging second stage of labor that often calls for instrumentation and episiotomy, which are each by themselves risk factors for perineal trauma.

Parity

Primigravid uterus more often than not suffers inefficient contractility leading onto prolonged labor, receives epidural analgesia and have a rigid perineum that predisposes to perineal trauma.

Episiotomy

Episiotomy originated to prevent lacerations and thus prevent pelvic floor damage. But evidence till date reveals that a midline episiotomy places the sphincter at greatest risk and today there is no scientific justification for its performance. Technically inept and ill-directed episiotomies do more harm than good. Episiotomy is the greatest risk factor for a sphincter tear. An appropriately performed mediolateral episiotomy may cause fewer tears. A study showed a 50% relative reduction in risk of sustaining a third degree tear for every 6° away from the perineal midline that an episiotomy was cut. In other words, a larger angle of episiotomy is associated with a lower risk of third degree tear and mediolateral episiotomy incisions should be made at as large an angle as possible to minimize the risk of sphincter disruption. Restrictive use of episiotomy appears to reduce the likelihood of perineal lacerations. Episiotomy has not been found to be associated with reduced risk of incontinence to stool or flatus, urinary incontinence or prolapse. Women with episiotomy had less recovery of postpartum perineal muscle function than those without episiotomy.

Other Intrapartum Risk Factors

Macrosomia (weight >4 kg), shoulder dystocia, occipito-posterior positions, midline episiotomy (10% chance of third degree tear), history of third degree tear in previous delivery, prolonged second stage, upright or lateral position (compared with supine or lithotomy positions), fundal pressure and Indian/Asian descent are all independent risk factors. A short perineum and anterior displacement of the anus is associated with traumatic vaginal delivery in primigravidae.

Preoperative Preparation and Tests

Recognition of Perineal Trauma

Maternal anal sphincter tears after vaginal delivery are frequently not diagnosed clinically and are associated with subsequent fecal incontinence. Endoanal ultrasonography with a high frequency 10 MHz probe has been found to be the best imaging modality for diagnosis of perineal trauma. The actual reported prevalence of sphincteric defects on ultrasound is 35–41%. Clinically undiagnosed tears are the major cause of subsequent anal incontinence. This calls for enhanced training of obstetricians at a resident level. Though endoanal ultrasound sounds promising, intraoperative ultrasound has been found to have no role. Disrupted tissues can be opposed under vision.

Timing of Repair

Primary repair immediately or within hours is the best time. This decreases patient inconvenience but expertise at emergency hours is often lacking. Delayed repair after 12 hours till more surgical expertise arrives has also been proposed by some, but not very acceptable.

Operative Technique

The principles of repair as in aseptic technique, attention to hemostasis and anatomic re-approximation of muscular and fascial supports of rectum and perineum should be followed. Individual reconstruction of each muscle group is necessary for cosmetic and functional results.

Steps

1. The perineum should be cleaned and draped with sterile drapes. If soiled with stool or in third or fourth degree tears, the area should be well irrigated with antiseptic solution.
2. The extent of trauma should be assessed with adequate light and retraction. In deep tears, involvement of the anal sphincter should be looked for. A gloved finger is placed in the anus and gently lifted. One should feel for the tightness or tone of the sphincter (Fig. 2).
3. If no sphincter tear is found, suturing is proceeded with. Small first degree tears that are not actively bleeding may not be sutured.
4. One percent lignocaine is infiltrated locally.
5. Any tear in the vaginal mucosa is sutured with continuous suture up to the level of the introitus (2–0 vicryl rapide or chromic catgut). Care should be taken to suture the apex under vision; the first suture taken

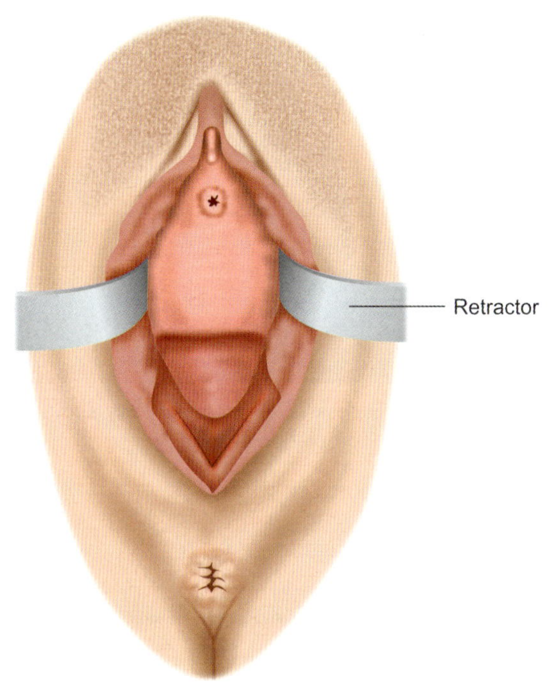

Fig. 2: Exposure of a perineal tear

1 cm above the proximal end of the tear. Most bleeding that continues to occur or occurrence of vulval hematoma is often because of an ignored apex.

6. The perineal muscles are difficult to identify individually and tend to be closed *en masse*. They are approximated by interrupted 2-0 sutures with adequate attention paid to hemostasis.
7. The skin is then closed using interrupted mattress sutures or subcuticular sutures.
8. At the end, a perrectal examination is done to ensure no ligatures through the mucosa.

Repair of Third and Fourth Degree Tears (Figs 3 to 6)

1. Identification of injury to the sphincter and rectal mucosa are primary concerns.
2. The area is well irrigated with saline and antiseptic solution. The most experienced obstetrician available should be called for.
3. Prophylactic antibiotics are administered.

Fig. 3A: Complete perineal tear, is not evident unless vulva is separated, as is clear in succeeding photograph

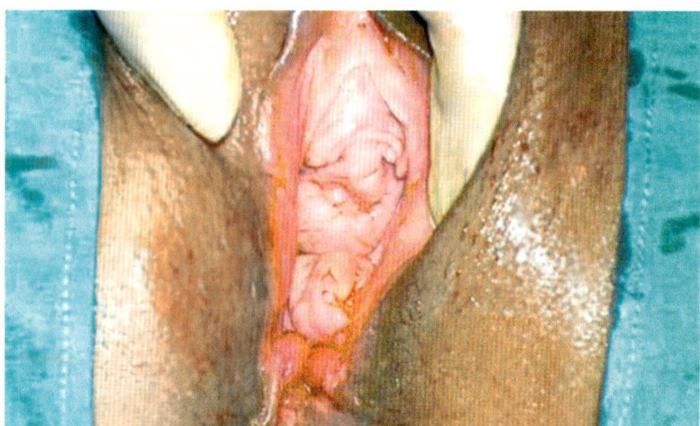

Fig. 3B: Complete perineal tear showing rectal mucosa defect and from sphincter

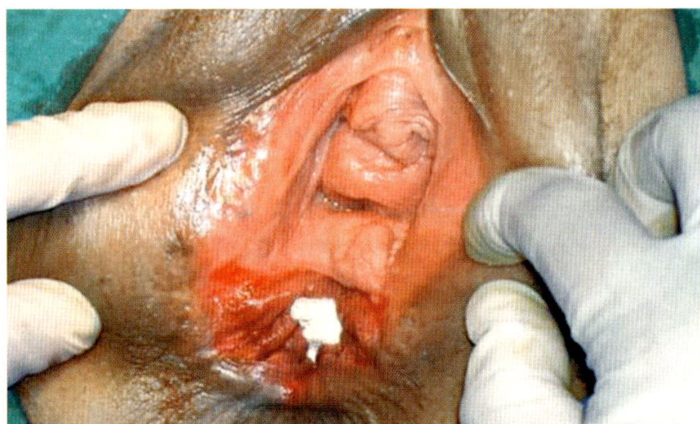

Fig. 3C: Padding of cotton gauze swab in rectum to avoid soiling and delineation of mucocutaneous junction

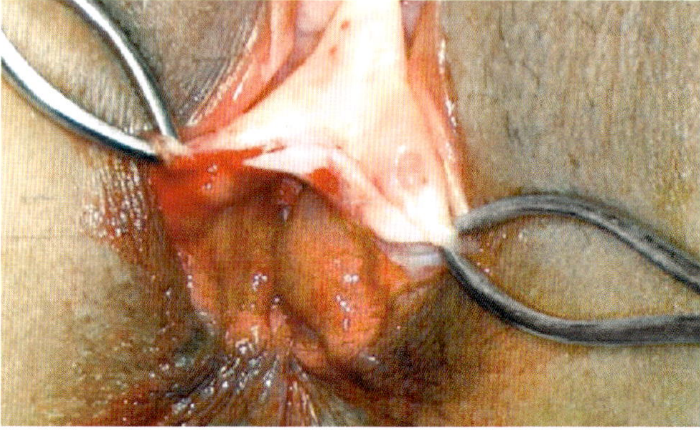

Fig. 3D: Separation of rectal mucosa from vaginal mucosal layer

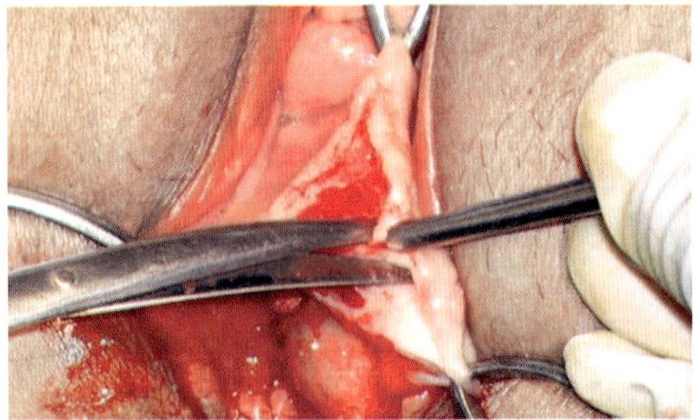

Fig. 3E: Using scissors, sharp dissection to create planes for sphincteric area

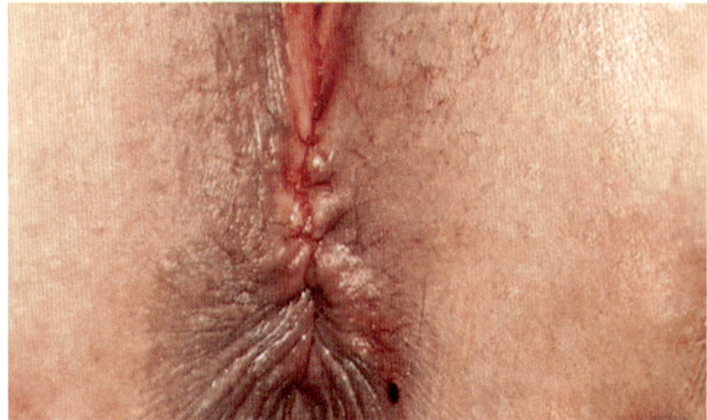

Fig. 3F: Repair of mucosal layers, perineal body, sphincter after completion of surgery

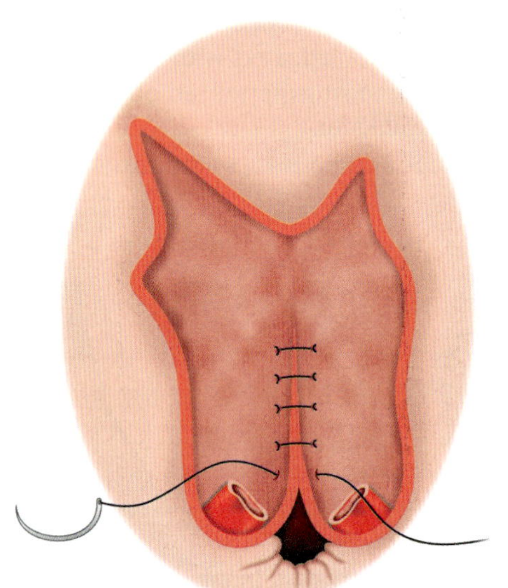

Fig. 4: Repair of fourth degree tear of rectal mucosa

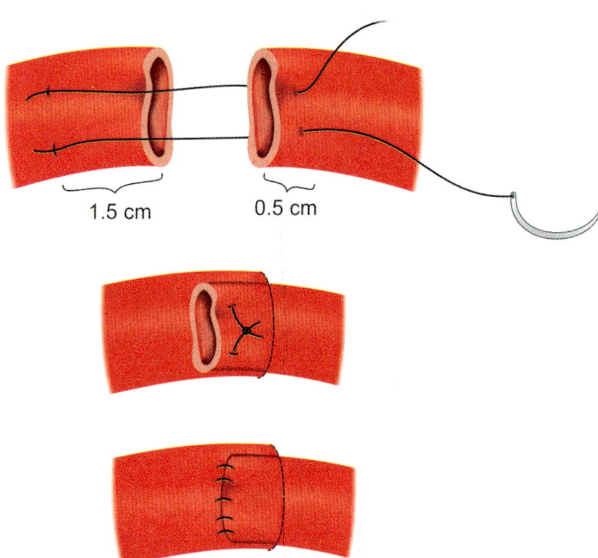

Fig. 5: Overlap method of suturing anal sphincter

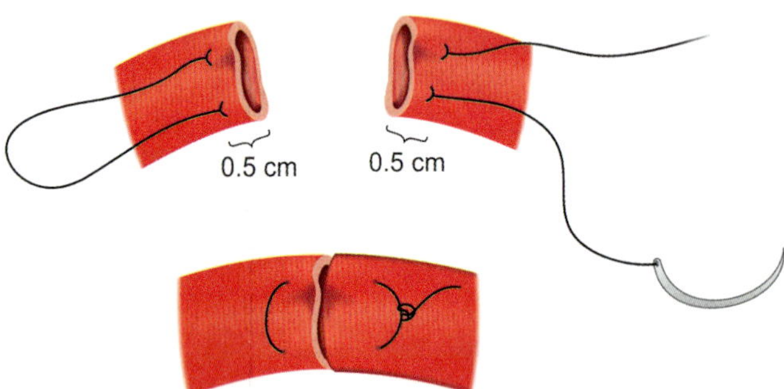

Fig. 6: End-to-end repair of anal sphincter

4. The rectum is closed with 3-0 or 4-0 interrupted vicryl sutures to bring the mucosa together. The sutures are placed in the muscularis avoiding the mucosa.
5. The IAS is approximated using interrupted 3-0 vicryl sutures.
6. The torn ends of the sphincter are held with Allis forceps. It is to be remembered that the torn ends often retract.
7. There are two methods of repairing the sphincter: end-to-end repair and overlap method
   - End-to-end repair: The sphincter ends are approximated with two or three interrupted 2-0 vicryl sutures
   - Overlap method: Two sets of suture are taken. The first row of sutures is taken 1.5 cm from the edge on one side and 0.5 cm on the other side. On tying, the two ends overlap one another. The free end is then sutured to the rest of the sphincter.

Compared to immediate primary end-to-end repair, early primary overlap repair appears to be associated with lower risks for fecal urgency and anal incontinence symptoms.

Complications

- Wound breakdown
- Hematoma: If observed, the repair has to be opened and hematoma drained. If no evidence of infection exists and hemostasis is secured, the wound can be closed
- Infection: Prevention by adherence to aseptic technique and prophylactic antibiotics. The earliest evidence of infection warrants beginning antibiotics and opening the wound and debridement, if required. Severe deep infection may even result in necrotizing fasciitis
- Persistent incontinence for 6 months calls for repeat surgery. Augmented biofeedback physiotherapy can be done to restore sphincteric function and muscle bulk
- Superficial dyspareunia, perineal pain
- Perineal granulation tissue, skin bridges, atrophy, local scarring injection of hyaluronidase or local application of steroid may be beneficial
- Psychosocial dysfunction
- Rectovaginal fistula: Repair done 3 months postpartum.

Postoperative Care

Evidence supports administration of prophylactic antibiotics in fourth degree tears. The World Health Organization (WHO) recommends ampicillin 500 mg oral and metronidazole 400 mg oral at the start of procedure. But these recommendations can be individualized considering the degree of facilities available.

- Daily follow-up should be done to look for evidence of wound infection
- Stool softeners should be given for 2 weeks
- The patients should be advised fluid diet for a day and gradual resumption of low residue diet for a week
- Visual rectal or vaginal examinations should not be done for 2 weeks till complete healing.

VAGINAL TEARS

These tears usually occur along with perineal tears; isolated vaginal tears are uncommon. They may occur following a spontaneous vaginal delivery but more commonly following instrumental or difficult deliveries.

They tend to bleed profusely and are diagnosed only after thorough exploration with an index of suspicion. They are usually longitudinal and lateral, deep extension into underlying tissue being common.

They should be sutured with adequate attention to the apex. Anterior and posterior tears should be repaired keeping in mind the close relation to the urethra and rectum, respectively.

CERVICAL TEARS

Minor tears in the cervix lesser than 0.5 cm occur in more than half of the vaginal deliveries.

- Most tears are small, less than 0.5 cm
- Deep tears may extend to the upper vagina, lower uterine segment, uterine arteries
- Predisposing factors:
  - Instrumental deliveries (forceps/ventouse)
  - Instrumental deliveries with an undilated cervix
  - Delivery of large babies
  - Scarred cervix: Old tears, amputation, conization
- Annular or circumferential or bucket handle tears are tears that occur along the circumference of the cervix often detaching the cervix from the vagina. These occur mainly due to instrumental deliveries, and forceps blades that may be applied before full dilatation over the cervix and traction applied. These also occur after scarred tissue from McDonald's suture.

Diagnosis

Small cervical tears that do not bleed, do not usually require repair (Figs 7 to 9). They heal rapidly, but on healing may considerably widen the cervical opening or cause ectropion.

Cervical or vaginal tears should be suspected when there is excessive bleeding per vaginum and a well retracted uterus. It should be a routine practice in the labor room to explore the cervix after every instrumental or difficult delivery.

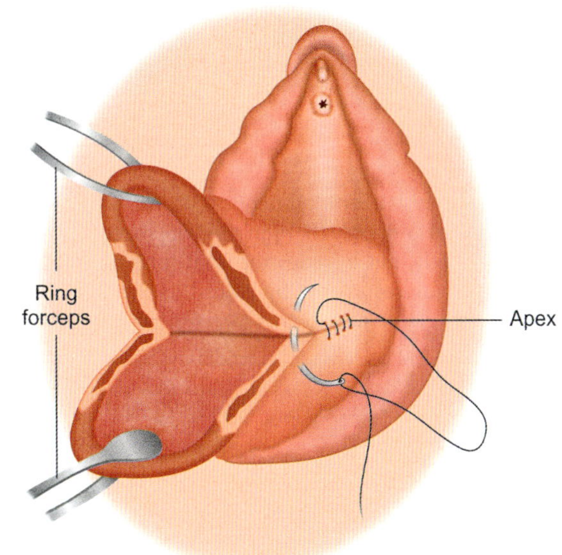

Fig. 7: Repair of cervical tear

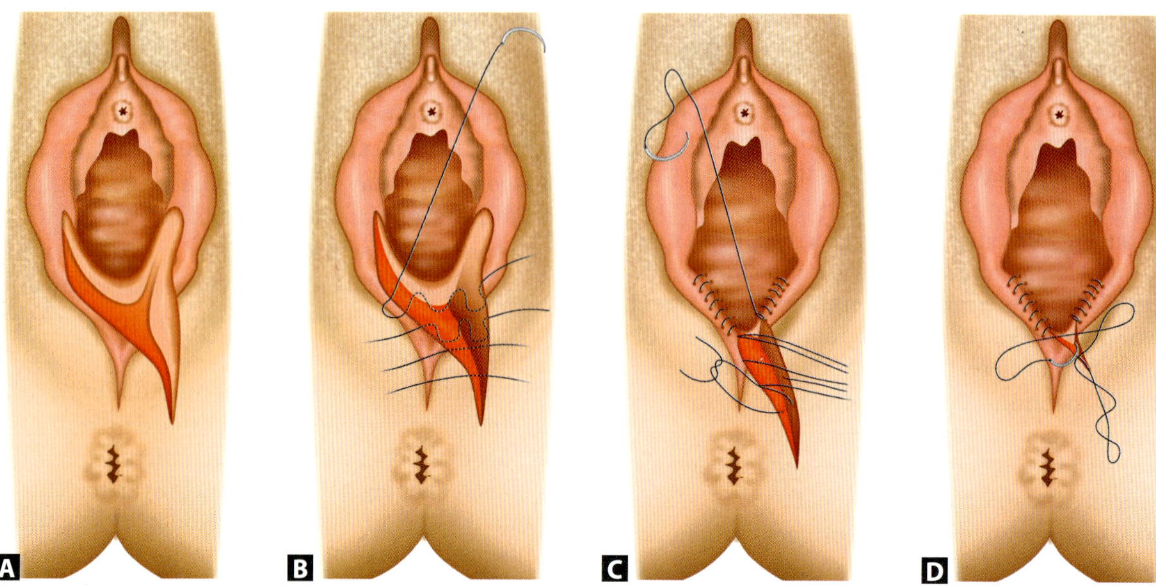

Figs 8A to D: A second-degree laceration involves the fourchette, the perineal skin and the vaginal mucous membrane. A second-degree laceration also includes the muscles of the perineal body. The rectal sphincter remains intact

Source: Reproduced with permission from: Gabbe SG, Niebyl JR, Simpson JL. Closure of 2nd degree laceration. Obstetrics: Normal and Problem Pregnancies, 3rd edition, New York: Churchill Livingstone Inc; 1996.

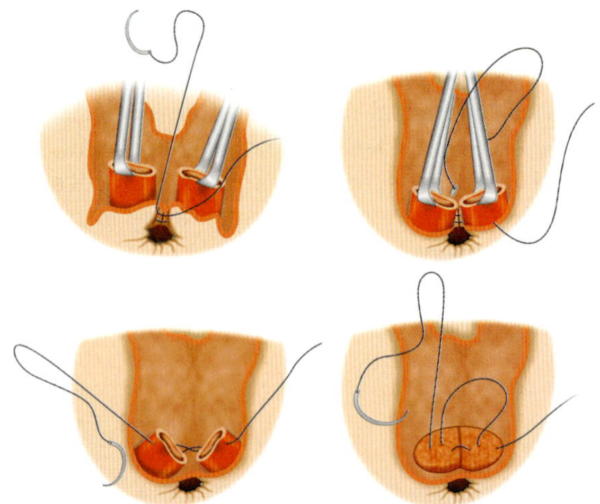

Fig. 9: Repair of superficial perineal layers. A third-degree laceration extends not only through the skin, mucous membrane and perineal body, but includes the anal sphincter. Interrupted figure-of-eight sutures should be placed in the capsule of the sphincter muscle.

Source: Reproduced with permission from: Gabbe SG, Niebyl JR, Simpson JL. Closure of 2nd degree laceration. In: Obstetrics: Normal and Problem Pregnancies, 3rd edition, New York: Churchill Livingstone Inc; 1996.

Cervical Exploration

The cervix cannot be assessed on palpation. It has to be well visualized with adequate lighting and retraction of vaginal walls to rule out any trauma.

This procedure requires a Sim's speculum, three sponge holding forceps and an assistant. The speculum and a right angled retractor are inserted into the vagina and the cervix is exposed. The assistant applies slight fundal pressure to aid visualization of the cervix. The cervix is held at 12 o'clock position with one sponge forceps and this remains constantly held. The second and third forceps are applied serially at 3 o'clock, 6 o'clock, and 9 o'clock, visualizing each quadrant of the cervix individually.

Treatment

1. Before beginning to suture a cervical tear, its extent should be clearly known. Any suspected extension into the lower uterine segment, involvement of uterine arteries, broad ligament hematoma, retroperitoneal or intraperitoneal bleeding may warrant a life-saving laparotomy.
2. The anterior and posterior margins of the torn edges of the cervix are held with a sponge forceps and traction applied gently.
3. The first suture is applied about 1 cm above the apex. The rest of the tear is repaired by interrupted mattress or continuous sutures taken from inside out.
4. Cervical tears are notorious in being deep and highly inaccessible. If the apex of the tear cannot be visualized easily, a suture is taken in the most accessible upper limit of the tear. Gradual downward traction on this suture will gradually bring the more proximal tissues into view and allow suturing of a deep apex.

Complications

Undiagnosed upward extension involving uterine vessels can be catastrophic.

Tears which are not repaired can lead to ectropion, cervical incompetence in future pregnancies. Overzealous repair causes stenosis.

BIBLIOGRAPHY

1. ACOG. ACOG practice bulletin number. 71: Episiotomy. Obstetrics and Gynecology. 2006;107(4):956-62.
2. Andrews V, Sultan AH, Thakar R, et al. Risk factors for obstetric anal sphincter injury: A prospective study. Birth. 2006;33(2):117-22.
3. Buppasiri P, Lumbiganon P, Thinkhamrop J, et al. Antibiotic prophylaxis for fourth-degree perineal tear during vaginal birth. Cochrane Database Syst Rev. 2005;4:CD005125.
4. Carroli G, Belizan J. Episiotomy for vaginal birth. Cochrane Database Syst Rev. 2000;(2):CD000081.
5. Cornelia L, Stephan B, Michel B, et al. Trans-perineal versus endo-anal ultrasound in the detection of anal sphincter tears. Eur J Obstet Gynecol Reprod Biol. 2002;103(1):79-82.
6. Eogan M, Daly L, O'Connell PR, et al. Does the angle of episiotomy affect the incidence of anal sphincter injury? BJOG 2006;113(2):190-4.
7. Faltin DL, Sangalli MR, Roche B, et al. Does a second delivery increase the risk of anal incontinence? BJOG. 2001;108(7):684-8.
8. Fernando R, Sultan AH, Kettle C, et al. Methods of repair for obstetric anal sphincter injury. Cochrane Database Syst Rev. 2006;3:CD002866.
9. Fernando RJ, Sultan AH, Kettle C, et al. Repair techniques for obstetric anal sphincter injuries: A randomized controlled trial. Obstet Gynecol. 2006;107(6):1261-8.
10. Gupta JK, Hofmeyr GJ. Position for women during second stage of labor. Cochrane Database Syst Rev. 2004;1: CD002006.
11. Jones KD. Incidence and risk factors for third degree perineal tears. Int J Gynaecol Obstet. 2000;71(3):227-9.
12. O'Herlihy C. Obstetric perineal injury: Risk factors and strategies for prevention. Semin Perinatol. 2003;27(1):13-9.
13. Rizk DE, Thomas L. Relationship between the length of the perineum and position of the anus and vaginal delivery in primigravidae. Int Urogynecol J Pelvic Floor Dysfunct. 2000;11(2):79-83.
14. Royal College of Obstetricians and Gynecologists. Third- and Fourth-degree Perineal Tears, Management. [online]. Available from: www.rcog.org.uk/womens-health/clinical-guidance/management-third-and-fourth-degree-perineal-tears-green-top-29. [Accessed November, 2013]

CHAPTER

23 Manual Removal of Placenta

Nidhi Gupta

INTRODUCTION

The operation to remove the placenta manually was once considered a very formidable procedure, was undertaken with great reluctance and undertaken after prolonged attempts made to express the organ failed. In a great majority of patients the placenta is completely separated within a few minutes after delivery of the baby. It may not be delivered for a considerable period of time because of uterine atony, contraction of the cervix or because of injudicious conduct of the third stage of labor. In other instances and for reasons that are poorly understood, the organ may remain attached to the uterus over part of its surface.

It has been observed that many of the serious complications attributed to attempted manual removal were due to associated hemorrhage rather than due to the actual operation. For this reason, it is illogical to wait, in the absence of bleeding for more than 30 minutes before removing the placenta. It has also been seen that the cervix contracts soon after delivery, especially if oxytocin has been administered. For this reason, it is beneficial to perform manual removal of the placenta at an earlier time following delivery under local anesthesia, sedation than after general anesthesia, but if bleeding (from the uterus) exceeds 400 mL, the obstetrician must proceed with the operation immediately.

PHYSIOLOGY OF PLACENTAL SEPARATION

Separation of the placenta and the greater part of the membranes does not normally occur until the third stage.

At the beginning of this stage the uterus measures about 20 cm vertically and 10 cm anteroposteriorly. The reduction in the area of the placental site, on an average, from 20 cm to 7 cm in diameter is far greater than that which can occur in the placenta and in consequence a *shearing force* is instituted between the placenta and the placental site, which brings about their almost immediate separation.

The plane of cleavage runs through the cavernous layer of the decidua basalis.

The placenta is separated in one of the two following ways.

Schultze's Method

A portion of the placenta near its center becomes separated due to buckling of the placenta after the birth of the baby due to the decrease in size of the uterus leading to hemorrhage from the torn uterine sinuses at that spot.

As more blood is effused, an increase in the area of separation occurs by the formation of a retroplacental hematoma. The center of the placenta is then forced down towards the cervix, where its fetal surface, with the umbilical cord attached presents.

It then passes through the aperture in the membranes formed by the passage of the fetus and enters the vagina, pulling the membranes off behind it and turning them inside out.

Mathew-Duncan Method

When retraction occurs after the expulsion of the child, the area of the uterine surface is much diminished; the placenta, being a relatively inelastic organ, cannot follow this diminution to any great extent and therefore becomes detached, the uterine wall tearing itself away from the placenta. This process begins at the lower pole, because there the edge is entirely unsupported. Separation thus begun is advanced by each recurring contraction.

When the Placenta has Separated Fully, Expulsion Occurs

It is gradually forced down, first into the passive lower segment and thence through the open cervix by recurring uterine contractions and retractions.

Once in the vagina, it is expelled either by the patients own expulsive efforts (bearing down) alone or aided by the doctor.

Signs of Placental Separation

- Uterus becomes globular and firmer (this sign is the earliest to appear)
- A sudden gush of blood
- The uterus rises and becomes more mobile in the abdomen
- The umbilical cord protrudes further out of the vagina causing "true lengthening of the cord".

These signs usually appear within 5 minutes after delivery of the fetus.

INDICATIONS OF THE PROCEDURE

- Placenta is separated but not expelled (simple retention)
  - Uterine inertia
  - Mismanaged third stage of labor
  - Constriction ring
  - Bicornuate uterus
- Placenta is not separated/adherent placenta
  - Simple adhesion
  - Morbid adhesion
- Placenta accreta
- Placenta increta
- Placenta percreta.

RETENTION OF THE PLACENTA

When the third stage of labor is allowed to take its natural course, the placenta separates and descends to a lower level in the genital tract in about 10–15 minutes. This time is noticeably shortened if an oxytocic is given at the end of the second or early in the third stage.

If after half an hour in the third stage of labor the signs of separation and descent of the placenta have not eventuated, the placenta should be regarded as retained and measures should be instituted without further delay to promote its delivery.

Measures Instituted to Promote Delivery of Placenta

The Brandt-Andrews maneuver of cord fixation combined with uterine elevation after rubbing up a contraction should be tried and repeated, if necessary (Figs 1 and 2).

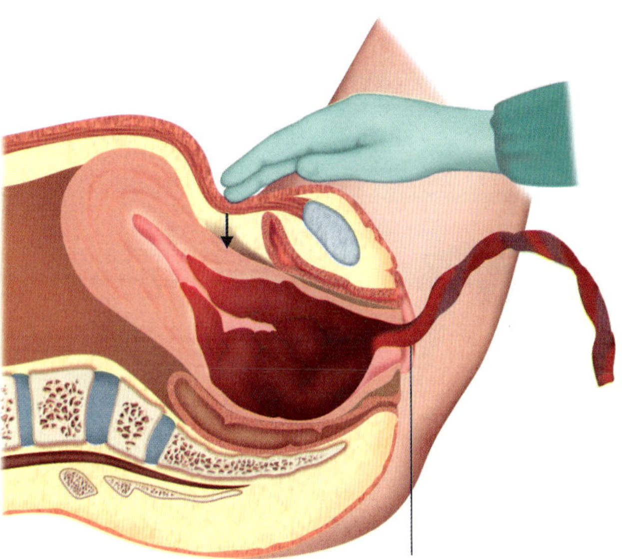

Fig. 1: Brandt's method of expression of placenta

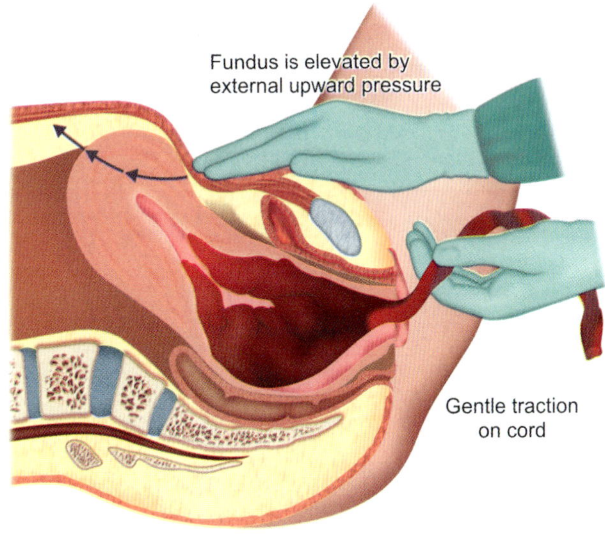

Fig. 2: Fundus is elevated by external upward pressure combined with Gentle cord traction—Modified Brandt-Andrews method

If unsuccessful, a vaginal examination under aseptic conditions is done, and if the placenta is found partly separated through the cervix, a Crede's type of abdominal expression should be tried by rubbing up a contraction and then compressing the uterus from before backward and from above downward to express the uterine contents into the vagina (Fig. 3).

It must not be repeated if it fails because it is apt to cause shock.

If neither of these measures proves effective, especially if the cervix is found to have closed down, proceed at once to a manual removal of the placenta under anesthesia.

Two further points deserve consideration.

In the first place, postpartum hemorrhage may occur before the placenta is expelled and in this event active measures to control it must be adopted at once. As a temporary measure, further oxytocic intravenously or intramuscularly will control the rate of blood loss.

Secondly, if the patient is already under an anesthetic—as for instance when a forceps or assisted breech delivery has been carried out, it is pointless and indeed harmful to wait as long as half an hour, especially if ergometrine has been given intravenously with the birth of the child.

If retention of the placenta is due to a contraction ring and descent does not appear in the next few minutes, internal manual removal of the placenta should be proceeded with.

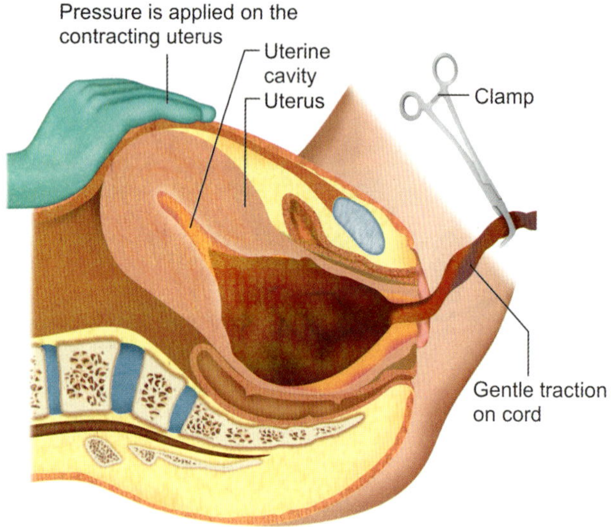

Fig. 3: Expression of placenta—Crede's method

Types of Placental Retention

1. The placenta, though completely detached, is not expelled. This is known as simple retention and may be either due to uterine inertia, the uterus being too feeble to complete the third stage, or to the formation of a contraction ring (hour-glass contraction) (Figs 4A and B).
2. Adherent placenta, of which two varieties must be distinguished:
   a. In *"simple adhesion"* or *"simple nondetachment",* the placenta remains in union with the uterine wall although its attachments are not abnormal
   b. In *morbid adhesion* or *placenta accreta*—on the other hand, a very rare condition—the attachments are definitely abnormal, the chorionic villi being attached directly to the muscle.

This condition results from deficiency of the decidua basalis, in consequence of which the uterine muscle is exposed to invasion by the trophoblast and to penetration by the chorionic villi. The union between the placenta

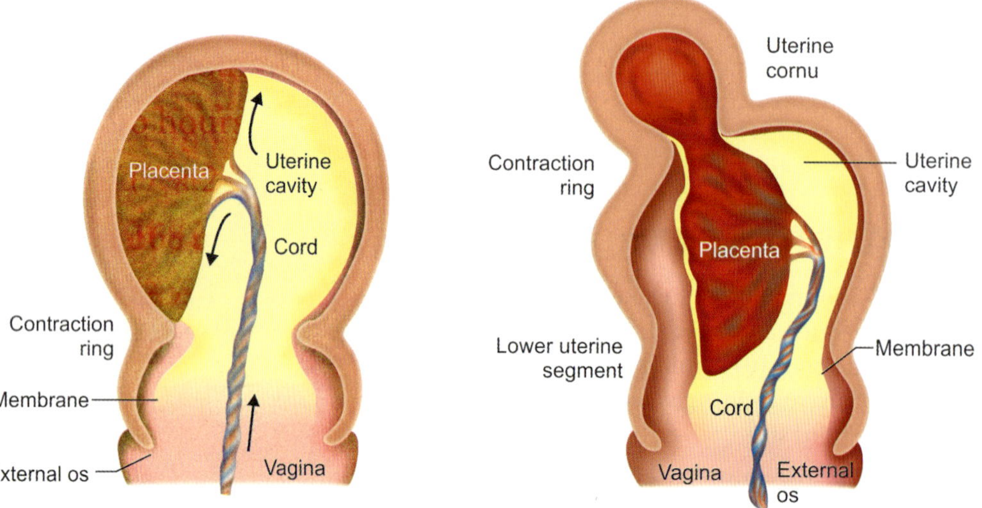

Figs 4A and B: Retained placenta. (A) Contraction ring below the placenta; (B) Contraction ring in upper segment

and uterine wall is very intimate. Its etiology is unknown. Fortunately, it is rare when the placenta is in its normal position but is seen more often in placenta previa. Depending on the propinquity of the villi and the uterine muscle, three degrees of morbid adherence are described:

1. *Placenta accreta* when the villi are merely in contact with the myometrium.
2. *Placenta increta* when the villi penetrate the muscle.
3. *Placenta percreta* when invasion by the villi has reached the serosal layer of the uterus.

Clinically, it must be distinguished from simple adhesion of the placenta and this cannot be done except when attempting manual removal.

In simple adhesion, a line of cleavage is easily found and separation presents no difficulty, whereas in placenta accreta the line of cleavage is not nearly so definite and the placenta can only be separated by the fingers working slowly and methodically. More often the morbidity affects only a part of the placenta and then full attention must be given to avoiding incomplete removal.

When the placenta is found actually to have invaded the uterine muscle as revealed by a complete failure in defining any line of cleavage, unless it affects a very small area, one of two policies may be adopted—the placenta may be allowed to remain in situ in the hope that it will gradually disappear by lysis or hysterectomy may be done. The latter would be chosen if the patient is fit and is a successful multipara reproductively or if persistent bleeding has been provoked.

The dangers of morbid adherence arise from persisting in manual attempts at removal.

These are:

- Hemorrhage
- Uterine rupture
- Damage to intestines
- Sepsis.

Dangers of leaving the placenta in situ are:

- Infection
- Secondary hemorrhage.

ANESTHETIC TECHNIQUES

Regional versus General Anesthesia

Usually, the operation of manual removal is carried out under general or regional anesthesia, but with care and gentleness it can at times be carried out under a pudendal block; in an emergency, without anesthesia at all.

Because epidural and subarachnoid anesthesia cause peripheral vasodilation, they can exacerbate hypotension and shock in women with postpartum hemorrhage. For some years, an informal debate took place between leading obstetric anesthesiologists as to whether regional anesthesia should be initiated or extended in mothers with postpartum bleeding.

When bleeding is controlled and vital signs are stable, judicious institution of epidural or subarachnoid anesthesia is acceptable. However, persistent bleeding, uncontrolled by pharmacologic agents and uterine massage, associated with signs of shock contraindicates the establishment of regional anesthesia. In mothers with an epidural block in situ, augmentation of the block to provide uterine analgesia (T8–T10 level) is reasonable if vital signs are stable and resuscitation is in progress.

General anesthesia inevitably carries risks, notably the unexpected difficult intubation and pulmonary aspiration. The delayed gastric emptying, which results from narcotic analgesia in labor, further compounds this risk. Therefore, the choice of technique becomes a matter of weighing the immediate and remote risks against the benefits. One advantage of general anesthesia is the tocolytic effect of volatile anesthetic agents, should it prove impossible to explore the uterus (e.g. in retained placenta).

Preoperative Management

- Careful assessment of the maternal vital signs is mandatory
- With two intravenous (IV) lines in situ, immediate resuscitation should begin with crystalloid and colloid till blood is available for replacement
- Blood sample should be sent for grouping and crossmatching
- Preoxygenation by the rapid 3–4 breath technique is normally effective, except in cases of significant hypovolemia and reduced cardiac output, preoxygenation should be prolonged to allow for equilibration
- Bladder should be evacuated just before starting the procedure
- A broad spectrum antibiotic cover should be given to the patient
- An informed consent regarding the risks of anesthesia and the operation per se must be taken
- Routine blood studies, blood volume determination and coagulation screening should be done wherever necessary
- All these formalities must be expedited, especially if the patient is in a low general condition.

Positioning of the Patient/Draping

If the mother has delivered in the lithotomy position, her legs should be placed flat before induction of anesthesia. This has a dual effect:

- It enables re-evaluation of the mother's vital signs, since any "autotransfusion" from the legs may obscure significant hypovolemia

- It avoids the increased intragastric pressure that accompanies the lithotomy position.

Anesthesia should be induced using a rapid sequence technique and an appropriate choice of induction agent.

When the airway is secure, the patient may be placed in the lithotomy position with legs supported to permit uterine exploration.

The most scrupulous antiseptic precautions must be taken.

The vulval region and the vagina are recleansed and the patient is redraped with sterile towels, and the operator prepares himself as for any other surgical operation. Fresh sterile long cuffed gloves should be worn taking all aseptic precautions.

Operative Steps (Figs 5 to 7)

1. The patient should be in the lithotomy position.
2. The left hand placed on the abdomen should steady the fundus and push the uterus downwards, shoving it, as it were on to the right hand, which is steadily pressed through the constricting muscle into the upper portion of the uterus.

   The fingers and thumb of the right hand are bent into the shape of a cone and the whole hand gently introduced through the introitus, the labia being separated with the fingers of the other hand.

   When the fingers first encounter the relaxed cervix and lower uterine segment, the inexperienced operator may mistake this for the uterine cavity proper. To enter the latter, however, the barrier of the retraction ring has to be overcome. In some instances, the obstruction may be pronounced, and in attempting to force the hand through the ring, injury may very readily be done to the thinned-out lower segment. If however, the internal hand guided by the cord is carefully insinuated through the retraction ring and the external hand presses down the uterus on to it, the risk of doing injury to the wall of the lower segment is negligible.

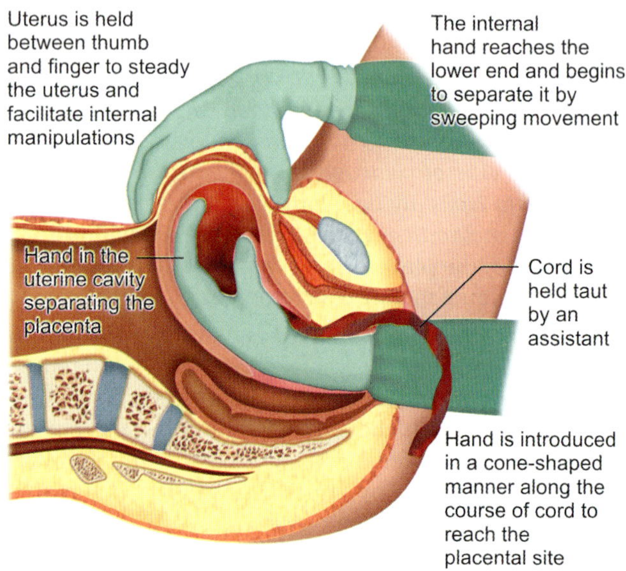

Fig. 5: Manual removal of placenta

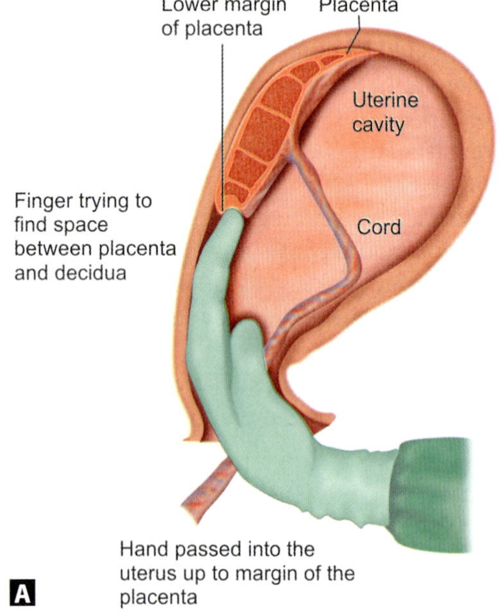

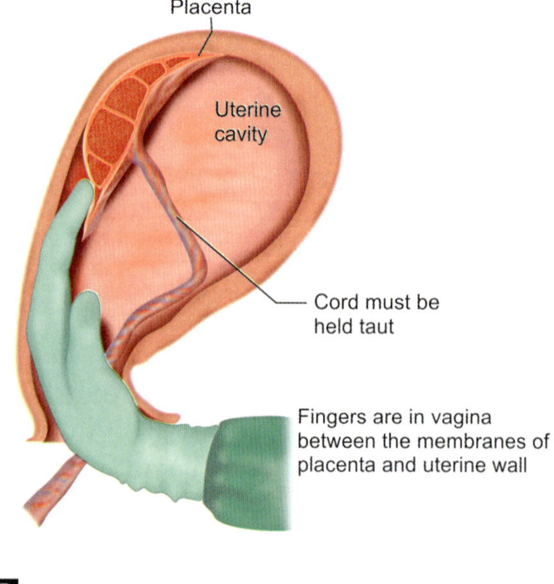

Figs 6A and B: Manual removal of placenta. Internal hand passes into uterus up to the margin of placenta and fingers invaginate the membranes between the placenta and uterine wall

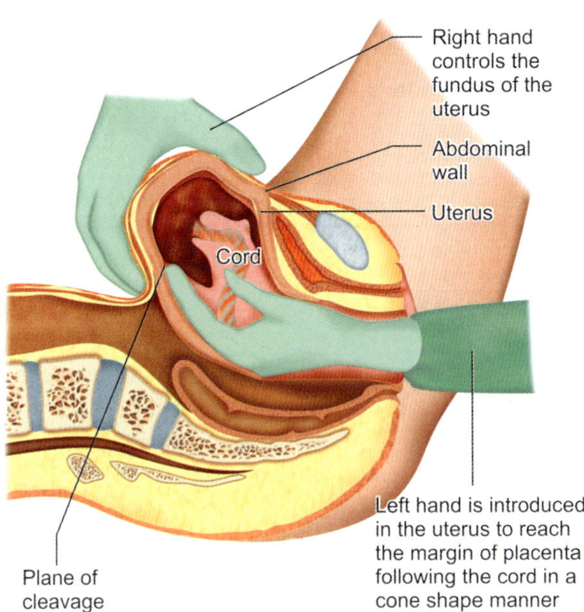

Fig. 7: Manual removal of placenta

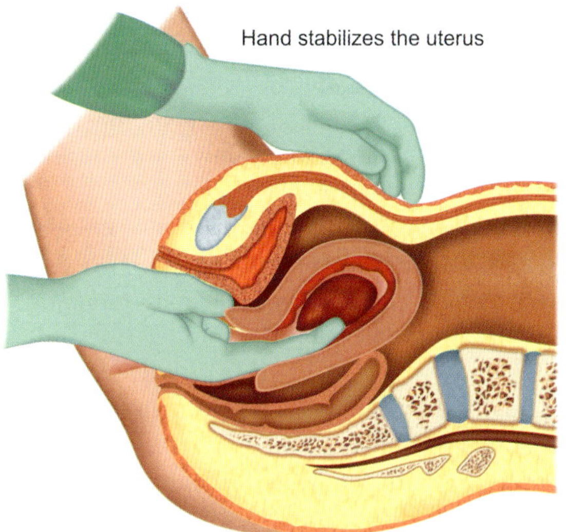

Fig. 8: Digital separation of placental tissue

3. The cord should be held taut by the nurse while the hand is introduced into the uterus along the course of the cord in a cone shaped manner; this guides the operator to the placental site and ensures that he passes his hand into the upper segment.
4. Having reached the lower margin of the placenta, the operator should begin to detach the latter by a sweeping movement of the hand using the external hand to move the fundus and facilitate these internal manipulations (Fig. 8).
5. The placenta having been separated as described, it should be withdrawn by gentle traction. It is most undesirable and adds to the risk of infection, if the hand has to be reintroduced. With this in mind, the placenta should be maneuvered into the palm of hand, and then by pulling on the cord to slide it out alongside the wrist, leaving the hand in position to feel for any possible remnants of placenta and any significant damage to the uterine wall.

Immediately after the placenta has been removed it should be examined, and if it is incomplete, the retained portions must be removed [look for placenta succenturiata (Fig. 9)].

Introduction of the hand to remove the placenta often has the effect of temporarily paralyzing the uterus, and the completion of the operation should always be followed without withdrawing the hand from the vagina, by bimanual compression, until firm contraction is felt. It must be remembered, however, that it is quite normal for the uterus to contract and relax in the third stage, as in the first and second, and that as long as there is effective retraction proved by the absence of bleeding, it is harmful and dangerous to squeeze and knead a uterus in such a state. By doing so, the all-important clots forming in the placental bed sinuses are apt to be disturbed and the safeguard against bleeding when retraction passes off, removed. Nevertheless vigilance must be maintained. During or after the removal of the placenta, syntometrine should be administered. A copious low-pressure hot antiseptic (chlorhexidine) intrauterine douche reduces the bacterial contamination incident to manual removal of the placenta as suggested by some obstetricians (optional).

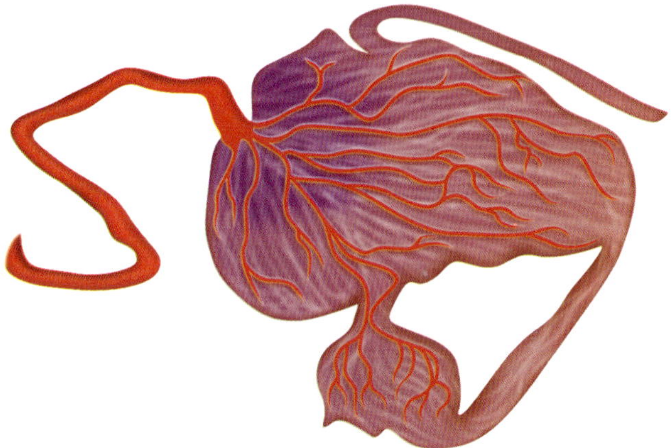

Fig. 9: Placenta succenturiata

After the operation is completed, the patient should be given ergometrine 0.5 mg by intramuscular injection. A blood transfusion is also advisable and should always be given if there has been much hemorrhage with hypovolemia.

Postoperative Care

After evacuation of the atonic uterus, the patient who underwent general anesthesia may need increased oxytocic drug administration to achieve uterine contraction.

She should be extubated awake in the left lateral position in the operating room only when she is clearly able to maintain her airway.

Uterine massage and additional oxytocic agents may be required in the recovery room.

Fresh blood after proper blood grouping and crossmatching must be infused according to the individual requirement.

Broad spectrum antibiotics should be given parenterally.

Strict postoperative progress charting is mandatory, especially the vitals, input/output and evidence of fresh bleeding.

Complications (Box 1)

Carelessness in performing this operation may result in perforation of the uterus, incomplete removal of the placenta or troublesome hemorrhage; in spite of precautions, some uterine infection is almost unavoidable and a wide spectrum antibiotic cover should be given for at least 5 days.

The chorion may also be morbidly adherent inside the uterus and may get expelled later.

Box 1 List of complications

- Perforation/uterine rupture
- Incomplete removal
- Hemorrhage
- Infection
- Secondary postpartum hemorrhage

CONCLUSION

In earlier days manual removal of placenta was taken as a very formidable procedure, but later it was observed that many of the serious complications attributed to attempted manual removal were due to associated hemorrhage rather than to the actual operation. With better anesthetic techniques and antibiotics this procedure is undertaken today without much hesitation. Routine manual removal of the placenta immediately after delivery, as advocated by some writers, must not be undertaken. An exception to this rule may be made if prompt separation and expression do not occur and where intrauterine exploration is indicated, e.g. vaginal delivery after a previous cesarean section, version and extraction. A further objection to manual removal is suggested in the situation, where potential isoimmunization can occur.

BIBLIOGRAPHY

1. Barker GH. Munro Kerr's Operative Obstetrics, 10th Edition. London: Bailliere Tindall; 1983.
2. Cunningham FG, MacDonald PC, Gant NF . Williams Obstetrics, 18th edition. Dallas, Texas: Prentice-Hall International Inc; 1989.
3. Datta S (Ed). Anesthetic and Obstetric Management of High-Risk Pregnancy, 2nd Edition. Florida: Mosby, Inc; 1996.
4. Donald I. Practical Obstetric Problems, 5th edition. PG Pub; 1983.
5. Holland EL, Brews A, Percival R. Holland Brew's Textbook of Obstetrics, 14th Edition. Churchill Livingstone; 1980.

CHAPTER

24

Uterine Rupture, Scar Dehiscence and Uterine Inversion

Saroj Singh, Mohita

INTRODUCTION

Uterine rupture is a catastrophic tearing/opening of the uterus into the abdominal cavity. The onset is often marked only by sudden fetal bradycardia and treatment requires immediate surgical attention for good neonatal and maternal outcomes. Its incidence depends upon the standards of obstetric care and varies between 1:500 and 1:4,000.

INCIDENCE

The rate of true uterine rupture with one prior low transverse scar has been reported by American Congress of Obstetricians and Gynecologists (ACOG) in 2003 to be between 0.2% and 1.5% (1:67 to 1:500 women); other studies report an average of 0.6%.

In woman with two or more prior cesareans, the rate of rupture rises as high as 3.9%. A history of successful prior vaginal delivery was found to reduce the risk of rupture from 1.1 to 0.2%.

Between less common incisions, classic and T-shaped uterine incisions are reported in 4.9% cases while low vertical incisions carry a rupture risk of 1–7%. In comparison, rupture of an unscarred uterus occurs in 1:8,000 to 1:17,000 deliveries.

Scar dehiscence is subperitoneal separation of scar, with chorioamniotic membranes visible through the peritoneum of lower uterine segment. Scar rupture is defined as a complete separation of uterine scar resulting in complete communication of uterine and peritoneal cavities (Fig. 1).

In the majority of cases rupture begins in the lower uterine segment, the reason being that this part of the wall is thinnest and is also most liable to overdistension. The rupture may be confined to the lower segment or may extend upwards into the uterine body, or even to the fundus, or downwards into the vaginal fornices. Tears of the anterior wall occasionally extend into the bladder.

Uterine rupture may be:

- Incomplete
- Complete.

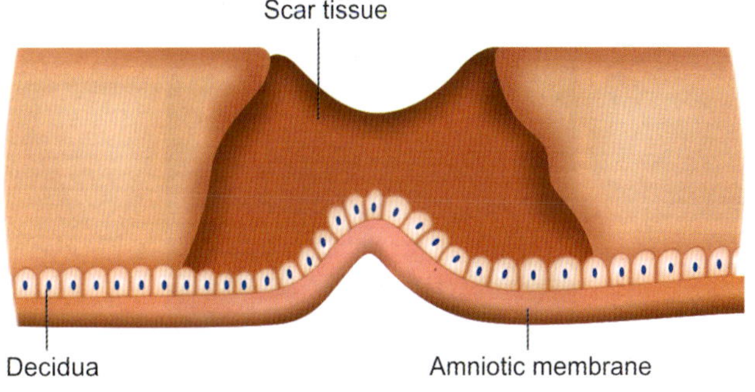

Normal scar

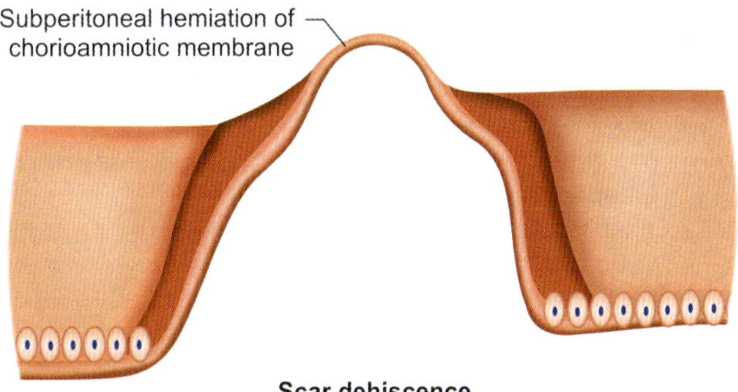

Scar dehiscence

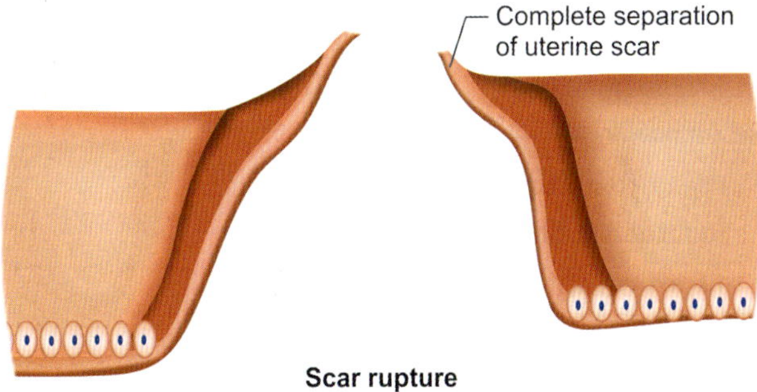

Scar rupture

Fig. 1: Involvement of various uterine wall musculatures during scar dehiscence and scar rupture

Rupture of the uterus is said to be complete when all the walls including the peritoneum are torn and, incomplete when this is not the case. Rupture of the lateral wall of the uterus, which in pregnancy is uncovered by peritoneum may include the whole thickness of muscular wall and still be incomplete, as it only open up the broad ligament but does not tear the peritoneum (Fig. 2).

Many clinical conditions have been associated with uterine rupture. One-third of ruptures in patients with a previous classical uterine incision occur before the onset of labor (Box 1).

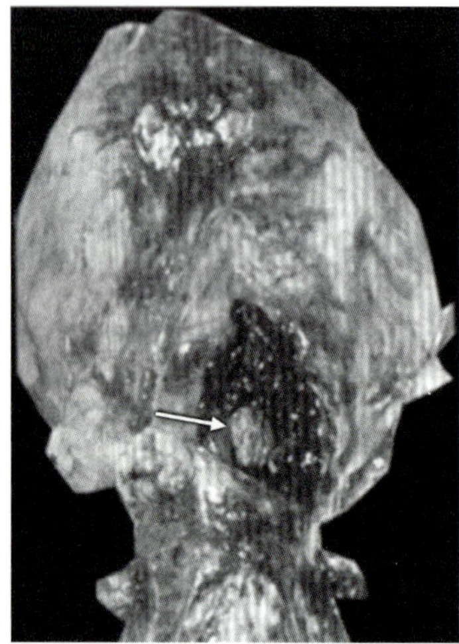

Fig. 2: Complete scar rupture (arrow)

Box 1 Predisposing factors for rupture of uterus (*ACOG practice bulletin*)

- Uterine scars:
  - Prior cesarean section
  - Prior rupture
  - Trauma
  - Injury from instrumentation during abortion
  - Myomectomy
  - Any cause of uterine perforation
- Uterine anomalies (i.e. undeveloped uterine horn)
- Prior invasive molar pregnancy
- History of placenta percreta or increta
- Difficult forceps delivery
- Malpresentation
- Fetal anomaly
- Obstructed labor
- Induction of labor
- Excessive uterine stimulation
  - Prostaglandin E1
  - Prostaglandin E2
  - Oxytocin
  - Alkaloids (cocaine abuse)

Abbreviation: ACOG; American Congress of Obstetricians and Gynecologists

DIAGNOSIS

Timely management of uterine rupture depends on prompt detection. In the past, caregivers were taught to look for classic signs such as sudden tearing uterine pain, vaginal hemorrhage, cessation of uterine contractions and regression of fetus. Recent experience has shown that these signs are unreliable and often absent. Instead fetal distress has been found to be the most reliable presenting clinical sign. Prolonged late and variable decelerations, and bradycardia seen on fetal heart rate monitoring are the most common and often the only manifestation of uterine rupture. Ridgeway and co-workers found that bradycardia was the only finding that differentiated uterine rupture from a successful trial of labor (Table 1 and Box 2).

Preoperative Preparation

1. It includes careful assessment of women and fetus. Complicating conditions or illnesses, hemodynamic stability and coagulation status are particularly important. The blood bank is asked to prepare appropriate blood replacement products. Blood transfusion usually begins before surgery in unstable

Table 1: Presenting manifestation of uterine rupture

Manifestation	Incidence
Bradycardia (sole manifestation)	5 of 5 rupture (100%)
Bradycardia, fetal distress	9 of 11 ruptures (82%)
Abnormal fetal heart rate tracing	23 of 70 ruptures (33%)
Failure to progress	15 of 70 ruptures (21%)
Pain	13 of 99 ruptures (13%)
Vaginal bleeding	11 of 99 ruptures (11%)

Box 2 ACOG selection criteria for vaginal birth after cesarean section candidate

Candidate for trial of labor

- One or two prior low transverse cesarean deliveries, clinically adequate pelvis
- No other uterine scars or previous rupture
- Obstetrician immediately available throughout active labor, capable of monitoring labor and performing emergency cesarean delivery
- Availability of anesthesia and personnel for emergency cesarean delivery

Circumstances under which a trial of labor should not be attempted

- Prior classical or T-shaped incision or other transfundal uterine surgery
- Contracted pelvis
- Medical or obstetrics complication that precludes vaginal delivery

patients, however, surgical hemostasis must not be delayed if bleeding continues.

2. An experienced surgical team is assembled consisting of a nurse circulator, surgical technician, anesthesiologist, assistant surgeon and principal surgeon.
3. The situation is discussed with the woman and her family, and informed consent is taken.
4. Prophylactic antibiotics are ordered before or during surgery.
5. Indwelling Foley catheter with a large balloon is placed to empty the bladder and monitor urine output.
6. Instruments and sutures can be chosen before the operation begins.
7. Prior to and during surgery, whole blood should be transfused. Volume of blood depends on the amount lost. Overcorrection is just as hazardous as underplacement.

Anesthesia

Conservation of time is essential, therefore, inhalation anesthesia after induction with intravenous agents and coupled with muscle relaxants is preferable to any other type.

Position, Incisions and Evaluation

Patient is laid in supine position on the table. Abdomen is painted and draped under all sterile precautions. Surgery can be performed through either vertical or transverse abdominal wall incisions. Adequate visualization of operative site is essential. The fastest method is vertical incision below the umbilicus. It offers good exposure to explore the entire abdomen and is easily extended. The dissection is carried down to the peritoneal cavity promptly. Bleeding vessels are clamped but may not be tied immediately.

Anatomical Alterations Causing Problems During Surgery

There are a number of changes, both anatomic and physiologic, in a pregnant woman that increase the likelihood of intraoperative problems.

- The uterus is markedly enlarged and pelvic blood vessels are large and tortuous. The bulky uterus is difficult to manipulate during obstetric surgery. It cannot be safely manipulated by means of clamps on friable adnexal structures
- Collateral circulation enlarges vessels that are normally of little concern during gynecologic surgery
- Pelvic tissues are edematous and more friable than in nonpregnant woman. Rapid control of all vascular supply to the uterus is essential. Dilated vessels and multiple collaterals require careful dissection. Extra clamps are necessary to avoid retrograde blood loss from severed blood vessels. All pedicles should be inspected several times for hemostasis
- The bladder wall becomes edematous and friable during labor and is easily injured by blunt dissection
- There are often dense adhesions between the bladder and lower uterine segment in woman with previous cesarean scars. Metzenbaum scissors with the curve turned downwards away from the bladder can be used to accomplish meticulous sharp dissection
- The ureter is dilated and sluggish. The surgeon should be aware of the proximity of the ureter at all phases of operation
- The vaginal wall is friable and edematous. Firm traction on clamps attached to the vagina will tear the tissues.

Operation

- Repair of the uterus
- Subtotal hysterectomy
- Total hysterectomy.

REPAIR OF UTERUS

Indications

- Repair is mostly applicable to a scar rupture where the margins are clean
- Repair is mostly considered in young woman desirous of further childbearing
- Repair is a poor option in an elderly multigravida with a completed family and a poor risk patient
- In the event of incomplete rupture (peritoneal window) of a previous cesarean section scar, we prefer to repair the wound.

Procedure

- The torn edges of the wound are meticulously debrided and all scar tissue removed
- Interrupted sutures of 1-0 delayed absorbable suture are then placed through the myometrium down to the endometrium. The sutures do not completely penetrate the lateral structure of the wound and are held for traction purpose. Subsequently, they are independently tied without undue tension in order to avoid necrosis at the suture site
- A second continuous inverting suture is then placed. The serosa of the uterus (or uterovesical fold of peritoneum as the case may be) is then approximated

with continuous suture. With slight modification, technique is same as closure of cesarean wounds
- In event of uncontrollable bleeding, it may be advisable to ligate the hypogastric arteries or other large vessels supplying the uterus. Before closure of parietal peritoneum, a careful search should be made for bleeding. This is of importance when there has been a trauma in the broad ligament and to the paracervical and paravaginal tissues
- Bladder should be carefully inspected for rupture and tear in bladder is repaired in two layers by 2-0 delayed absorbable sutures
- Postoperative care of patient includes a careful check of the hematocrit at intervals and blood replacement if needed
- Urinary output is held in constant surveillance and electrolyte balance is maintained.

Subtotal Hysterectomy

It is indicated if the patient is in poor condition and if supracervical amputation of the cervix is sufficient to control bleeding.

Total Hysterectomy

- Satisfactory exposure is best obtained by cephalic traction on the uterus. The bladder flap is deflected down to the level of the cervix, if possible
- After cesarean delivery and placental removal, if the hysterotomy wound is bleeding appreciably it can either be sutured or a sponge forceps can be applied for hemostasis
- The round ligaments are divided between two Kochers clamps placed close to the uterus and doubly ligated
- The incision in the vesicouterine serosa, that was made to mobilize the bladder, is extended laterally and upwards through the anterior leaf of the broad ligament to reach the incised round ligament (Fig. 3A). The posterior leaf of the broad ligament adjacent to the uterus is perforated just beneath the uterovarian ligament, fallopian tube and ovarian vessels (Fig. 3B). These vessels are then doubly clamped and divided, and the lateral pedicle is doubly ligated. The posterior leaf of the broad ligament is divided inferiorly towards the uterosacral ligament (Fig. 3C)
- Next, the bladder and the attached peritoneal flap are again deflected and dissected from the lower uterine segment and retracted out of the operative field (Fig. 3D)
- The ascending uterine vessels on either side are identified near their origin. These pedicles are then doubly clamped immediately adjacent to the uterus, divided and doubly suture ligated (Fig. 3E)
- In case of profuse hemorrhage, it may be advantageous to rapidly doubly clamp and divide all the vascular pedicles between the clamps to gain hemostasis and then return to suture ligate all the pedicles
- It may be technically easier to amputate the uterine fundus and placing Kochers clamp on the stump for traction and hemostasis. To remove the cervix, it is necessary to mobilize the bladder much more extensively in the midline and laterally
- The cardinal ligaments, uterosacral ligaments contain many large vessels and these ligaments are doubly clamped as close to the cervix as possible, taking care not to include excessive tissue in each clamp (Fig. 3F). Tissue in between the clamps is incised and distal pedicle ligated. These steps are repeated till the level of the lateral vaginal fornix is reached
- Immediately below the level of the cervix a curved clamp is placed across the lateral vaginal fornix and the tissue is incised medial to the clamp. The entire cervix is then excised from the vagina and is inspected to ensure complete removal (Fig. 3G)
- Each of the angles of the lateral vaginal fornix is secured to the cardinal and uterosacral ligament. Following this the vagina may be closed either by figure-of-eight or running lock of stitches (Fig. 3H). The open vagina may promote drainage of fluid that would otherwise accumulate and contribute to hematoma formation and infection
- After ensuring adequate hemostasis, reperitonization of the pelvis is done followed by closure of the abdomen. A drain may be left in the abdominal cavity if required.

COMPLICATIONS

Emergency obstetric hysterectomies historically have the maximum complications and highest mortality rate.

Operative Complications

- Hemorrhage—it may be caused by:
  - Loss of control of uterine/adnexal pedicle
  - Refraction bleeding from severed pedicles
  - Adnexal bleeding may also occur due to torn ovarian vessels being pierced by sutures.
- Urinary tract injury:
  - Bladder injury may occur during dissection or inclusion of the bladder in the suture or clamp
  - Ureter may be injured during dissection.

Postoperative Complications

- Febrile morbidity
- Vaginal cuff abscess or hematoma
- Urinary tract infections
- Wound abscess or dehiscence
- Pulmonary complications
- Postoperative bleeding requiring surgery—vaginal pack or suture at laparotomy
- Urinary fistulas; vesicovaginal, ureterovaginal and others
- Thromboembolism
- Intestinal obstruction.

PREVENTION OF SCAR DEHISCENCE

Unfortunately, uterine rupture cannot be adequately predicted among women desiring a trial of labor for vaginal birth after cesarean section (VBAC), so constant preparedness is needed. Screening patients is helpful in some cases. Prophylaxis begins much earlier; it starts

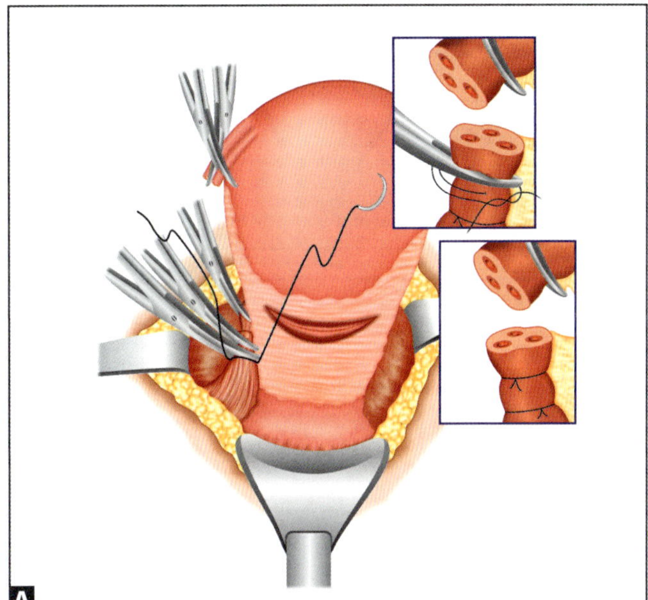

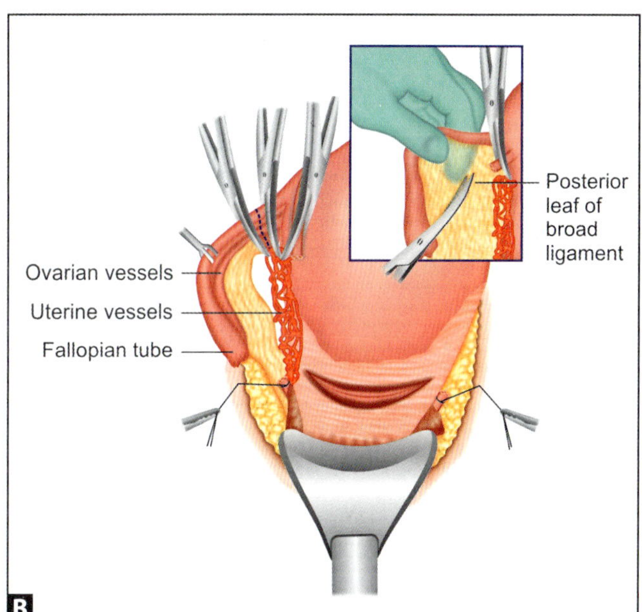

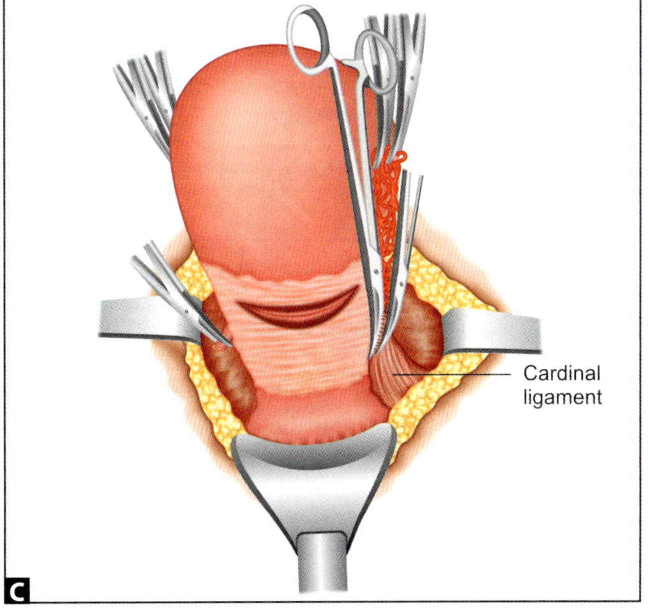

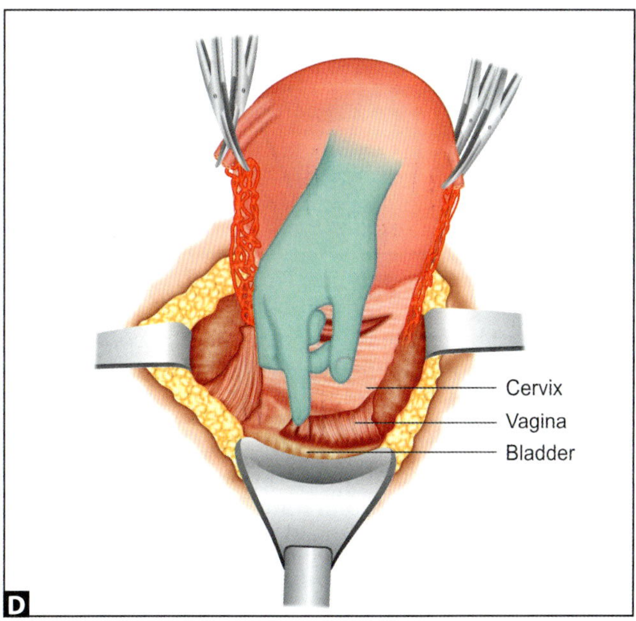

Contd...

Contd...

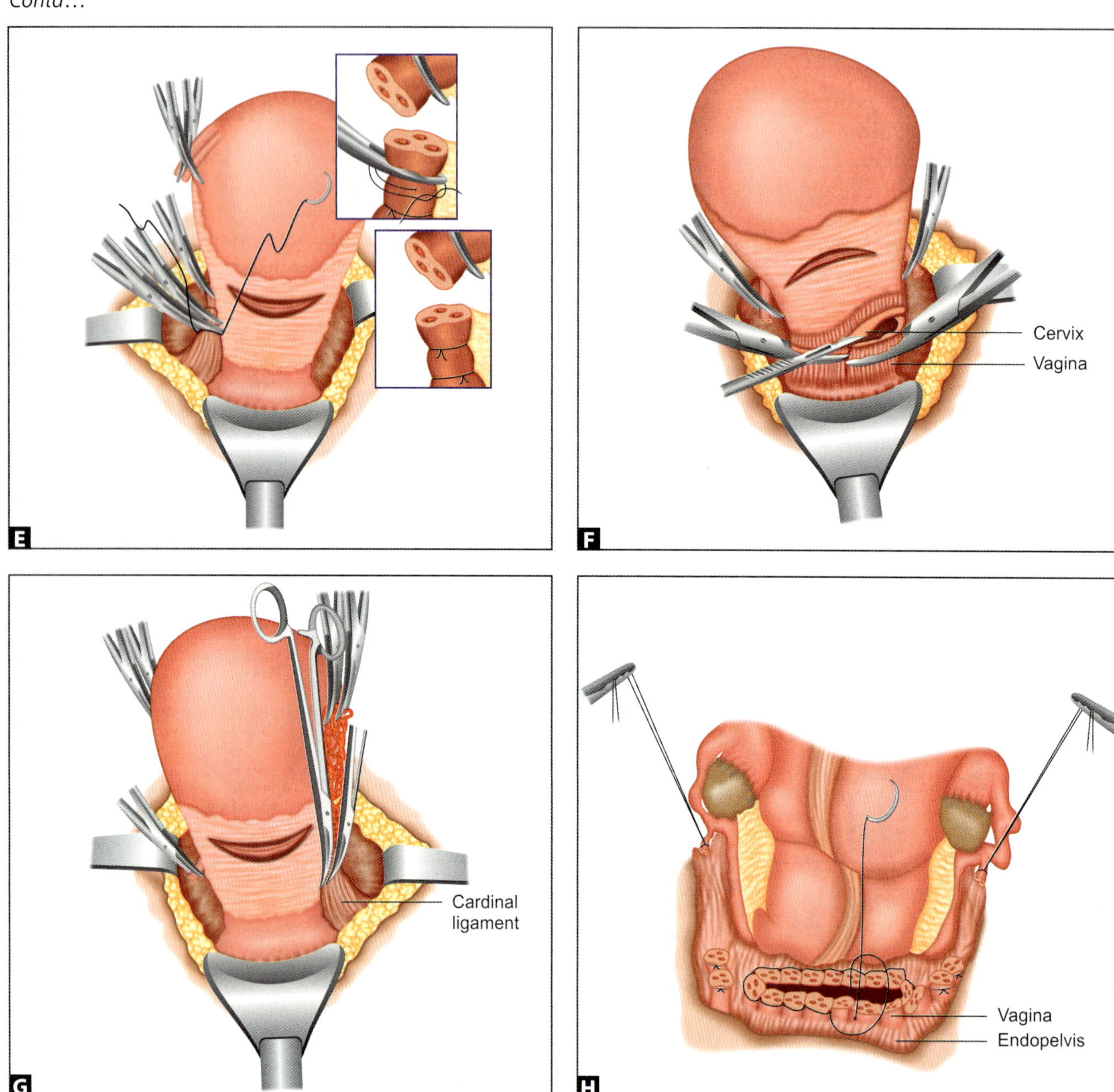

Figs 3A to H: Steps of peripartum total hysterectomy for ruptured uterus; steps are explained in text and referred therein

with thorough antenatal assessment and condition of pelvis. Presentation of fetus and size of fetus should be determined.

In case of scarred uterus, various imaging modalities have been used to determine the integrity of scar and assess the risk of intrapartum rupture or dehiscence.

Hysterography in interconception period 6 months after operation may reveal defcct on scar (<5 mm or >5 mm).

Ultrasonography has been used in antenatal period in patients with previous cesarean. In ultrasonography (USG), lower uterine segment reveals a homogenous acoustic reflection of three layered structure that consist of amniotic membrane, a decidualized endometrial layer, middle myometrial layer and outer visceroparietal peritoneal layer of lower uterine segment. Any thinning, wedge defect, ballooning or abnormal thick wall should be noted.

Patient with previous lower segment cesarean section (LSCS) should be admitted at 38 weeks to assess the case and decide the line of treatment. Patients with previous hysterotomy or classical cesarean should be admitted at 36th week because chance of scar rupture is more during last week of pregnancy.

Judicious selection of cases and careful watch should be done during oxytocin infusion for either induction or acceleration of labor. Before full dilatation of cervix, forceps applications or breech extraction should be avoided. Skilled personnel should perform destructive vaginal operation and manual removal of morbid adherent placenta. Exploration of uterus should be done as a routine following delivery.

Signed documentation of this discussion and the patients wishes should be placed in medical record.

During trial of labor, continuous fetal heart rate monitoring is imperative because this can be the only indication of an impending rupture. Patients with previous scar should be instructed to go promptly to the hospital at the onset of contractions and should not be allowed to labor unmonitored at home.

Physician are also advised to carefully review their hospital resources for handling emergent complications such as uterine rupture. An important aspect of prevention is arranging for and confirming prompt surgical back up before emergencies such as uterine rupture, access or referring the patient to a center where more intensive care can be provided.

BIBLIOGRAPHY

1. American College of Obstetricians and Gynecologists. Vaginal Birth after previous caesarean delivery: Practice Bulletin. 1998;2.
2. Toppenberg KS, Block WA. Uterine rupture: What family physicians need to know. Am Fam Physician. 2002;66(5):823-9.
3. American College of Obstetricians and Gynecologists. Vaginal birth after previous cesarean delivery. Int J Gynecol Obstet. 1999;66:197-204.
4. Oh W, Gilstrap L (Eds). Guidelines for Perinatal Care, 5th edition. Elk Grove Village, IL: American Academy of Pediatrics, American College of Obstetricians and Gynecologists; 2002.
5. Ridgeway JJ, Weyrich DL, Benedetti TJ. Fetal heart rate changes associated with uterine rupture: Study of 19 patients. Obstet Gynecol. 2004;103:506-12.
6. Rageth JC, Juzi C, Cerossenbacher H. Delivery after previous cesarean: a risk evaluation. Swiss working care of obstetric and gynaecologic institution. Obstet Gynaecol. 1999;93:332-7.
7. American College of Obstetricians and Gynecologists. Vaginal Birth after previous caesarean delivery: Practice Bulletin No. 54.2004.
8. Munro MG. Supracervical hysterectomy: A time for reappraisal. Obstet Gynecol. 1995;85:412.
9. Plauche WC. Peripartum hysterectomy. In: Plauche WC, Morrison J, O'sullivan MJ (Eds), Surgical Obstetrics. Philadelphia: WB Saunders; 1992b. p. 447.

CHAPTER

25 Postpartum Hemorrhage—Surgical Interventions

Pankaj Desai, Hemant Deshpande

INTRODUCTION

Postpartum hemorrhage (PPH) is the leading cause of maternal mortality. All women who carry a pregnancy beyond 20 week's gestation are at risk for PPH and its sequelae. Although maternal mortality rates have declined greatly in the developing as well as developed countries, PPH remains a leading cause of maternal mortality. In developed countries, PPH usually ranks in the top three causes of maternal mortality, along with embolism and hypertension. In the developing world, several countries have maternal mortality rates in excess of 450 women per 100,000 live births, and WHO statistics suggest that 25% of maternal deaths are due to PPH, accounting for more than 100,000 maternal deaths per year.

Incidence of PPH is estimated to occur in 5–10% of deliveries. Moreover, PPH remains the leading cause of maternal mortality worldwide, contributing to a greater proportion of maternal deaths than in other comparable causes. According to the National Committee on Maternal Mortality, more than 80% of deaths due to PPH are avoidable deaths, involving unrecognized diagnosis, delay in providing care and underestimation of the severity of blood loss and availability of trained anesthetists, blood transfusion. These factors suggest weaknesses in the capacity for providing adequate care in cases of PPH. On the other hand, although some specific clinical and surgical interventions have proved their value in decreasing postpartum blood loss, integration of these guidelines into clinical practice is still to be achieved.

DEFINITION

The definition of PPH is somewhat arbitrary and problematic. PPH is defined as blood loss of more than 500 mL following vaginal delivery or more than 1,000 mL following cesarean delivery.

Blood loss of these amounts within 24 hours of delivery is termed early or primary PPH; it is termed late or secondary PPH, if they occur 24 hours after delivery till the end of puerperium.

Clinically, any amount of blood loss after delivery that causes tachycardia, hypotension and signs of hypovolemic hemorrhagic shock is PPH. A severe PPH is defined as a PPH that is associated with one or more of the following:

- Peripartum hemoglobin drop greater than 4 g/dL
- Sign of hypovolemic hemorrhagic shock
- Shock
- Need for more than five blood transfusions and components therapy, arterial embolization, surgical procedures, such as hysterectomy or arterial ligation and transfer of the mother to intensive care unit.

MANAGEMENT OF POSTPARTUM HEMORRHAGE

Patients with PPH require aggressive measures to restore and maintain the circulating blood volume. Management of massive obstetric hemorrhage outlines a protocol for PPH and implement with the same attention to details and documentation. It is advised to conduct periodic reviews and practice emergency drills. The diagnosis of PPH is established. The amount of bleeding and the patient's clinical status, level of consciousness and vital signs are continually assessed. Once the diagnosis is made call for help immediately. Specialized personnel are called; two obstetricians and one anesthetist are necessary. Designate an experienced person to document critical information and time slot. Ensure the availability of an operation theater. The speed with which PPH occurs, becomes life-threatening, though can be successfully managed with relatively simple interventions.

Fluid Therapy

Fluid replacement is sometimes conservative. Possible reasons for this include:

- Blood loss being generally underestimated both in volume and rapidity
- Women initially compensate well for losses because of their good health and the hemodynamic changes of pregnancy
- Over resuscitation may lead to pulmonary edema.

Raising the legs improves venous return and is consistent with the positioning used to diagnose and treat the underlying causes of bleeding. Administer oxygen and obtain intravenous access. Intravenous lines is started with wide bore cannula. Twice as much fluid can be infused through a 14-gauge intravenous line compared with an 18-gauge intravenous line over the same time period. During labor, place at least one intravenous line in women at risk for PPH.

The initial replacement is with crystalloids, either normal saline (NS) or Ringer's lactate solution. Central venous access is not routinely required. Take blood sample for baseline lab measurements. Five percent dextrose or dextrose with normal saline (DNS) has no role in the management of PPH. The loss of 1 L of blood requires replacement with 4–5 L of crystalloid and the blood volume changes last for 40 minutes. PPH of up to 1,500 mL in a healthy woman can usually be managed with crystalloid infusion alone, if the cause of bleeding is arrested completely. Blood loss in excess of this usually requires the addition of colloids and blood transfusion.

Because a large portion of crystalloid fluid volume is lost to the interstitial space, the use of colloids in resuscitation is used. These solutions are largely retained within the intravascular space and include albumin, dextran, hydroxyethyl starch and modified fluid gelatin. Colloid solutions of 1,000 mL can be given after initial crystalloids; starch preparations are preferred over gelatinous one as they do not interfere with crossmatching and do not cause anaphylactic reactions. The blood volume hemodynamic changes by colloids last for 4 hours.

Blood Transfusion

Blood transfusions are indicated if blood loss is continuous and more than 2,000 mL or if the patient is developing shock despite aggressive resuscitation. Active management of third stage reduces requirement of blood transfusion. Whole blood is available in most settings in India, and, packed red blood cells (PRBCs) and blood components are given, if indicated.

Rapidly transfuse 2–4 units (U) of PRBCs to replace lost oxygen-carrying capacity and to restore circulating volume and this is preferred over whole blood. Administer the blood transfusion through a set with an integrated filter, rapid infusion set with an integrated warmer or a pressure cuff may be used to increase the infusion rate.

Dilutional coagulopathy is not usually observed until approximately 80% of the original blood volume has been replaced. If there is continuous bleeding or oozing from puncture sites, mucous surfaces, or wounds, hematuria, coffee brown aspirates from stomach, additional blood component products are required. Infuse fresh frozen plasma (FFP), beginning with 4 U and following with additional units to normalize the coagulation test findings. It is recommended that addition of 1 U of FFP for every 5 U of PRBCs or 4 U of whole blood be practiced.

Thrombocytopenia is likely complication; keep the platelet count more than $50 \times 10^9/L$ by using platelet transfusion. Each unit of platelets increases the platelet count by approximately $10 \times 10^9/L$ (platelets are usually given in packs of 5–6 U). Platelet preparations contain some RBCs, and the administration of anti-D immunoglobulin is recommended for Rh-negative women after the crisis has passed.

Disseminated intravascular coagulation (DIC) may also develop if shock has led to marked hypoperfusion of tissues, causing tissue damage and release of tissue thromboplastin, laboratory investigations reveal that the D-dimmer levels are elevated and serum fibrinogen levels are less with a prolonged thrombin time. Restoration and maintenance of circulating volume along with blood product replacement is necessary. Cryoprecipitate may be given with FFP in hypofibrinogenemia. Cryoprecipitate provides a more concentrated form of fibrinogen and other clotting factors VIII, XIII and von Willebrand factor.

Monitoring Response to Resuscitation

Monitor level of consciousness, pulse, blood pressure (BP) and urine output during the course of the management of massive hemorrhage. Minimum 30 mL/h urine indicates adequate renal perfusion. Keep a watch on complete blood count (CBC), coagulation, and blood gas values and acid-base status. Adequate tissue perfusion and oxygen saturation is detected by pulse oximetry. Pulmonary edema is the risk in fluid replacement, hence periodic auscultation of the lung fields is needed for the diagnosis and also to find out development of adult respiratory distress syndrome.

Management of Massive Obstetric Hemorrhage

The word "ORDER" is a useful mnemonic for remembering the basic outline:

O—Organization

- Call for help, obstetrician and anesthetist
- Call for adequate blood
- Record vital signs, urine output, and fluids and drugs administered
- Keep operation theater ready.

R—Resuscitation

- Start oxygen by mask
- Start two large bore intravenous lines
- Take blood for crossmatch and for CBC, coagulation profile, urea level, creatinine value, and electrolyte status
- Fluid replacement with NS or Ringer's lactate solution
- Transfuse blood.

D—Defective Blood Coagulation

- Coagulation profile
- Give FFP if coagulation test results are abnormal
- Give cryoprecipitate
- Give platelet concentrates if the platelet count is less than 50×10^9/L
- Give cryoprecipitate and platelet concentrates before surgical intervention.

E—Evaluations

- Monitor pulse, BP, blood gas status, and if possible central venous pressure
- Measure urine output hourly.

R—Remedy Treats the Cause

- Give oxytocin, methylergometrine prostaglandin
- Explore and empty the uterine cavity
- Examine the cervix and vagina, ligate any bleeding vessels, and repair trauma
- Devascularization of uterus (i.e. uterine, ovarian, and/or internal iliac arteries)
- Arterial embolization
- Obstetric hysterectomy.

SURGICAL MANAGEMENT

Surgical management is necessary, if the uterus is still flabby and bleeding persists despite all treatment.

Packing of the Uterus

Packing of the uterus may be an option until preparation for surgery. Uterine packing may hide the ongoing blood loss, and increasing the risk of infection. The uterus and vagina tightly packed with continuous, layered, 2 to/or 4-inch gauze under direct visualization using a speculum and retractors, packing may be useful in some cases. The packing is usually removed in 24–48 hours, preferably in operation theater.

Intrauterine Tamponade

Intrauterine tamponade for bleeding have also been used. In the past, large bulb Foley catheters or Sengstaken tubes have been used. More recently, experience has been gained using special catheters specifically designed for PPH. Antishock garments used in military emergencies may be used in available settings for both the definitive treatment of uterine atony as well as a method to allow time to bring other treatments to bear.

Foley Catheter Procedure

The technique is simple. A Foley catheter with a 30 mL balloon capacity is easy to acquire and may routinely be stocked in labor room. Using a no. 22–24 Foley catheter, the tip is guided into the uterine cavity and inflated with 60–80 mL of saline. Additional Foley catheters can be inserted, if necessary. If bleeding stops, the patient can be observed with the catheters in place and then removed after 12–24 hours.

Intrauterine Condom Packing

With aseptic precautions, a sterile rubber catheter fitted with a condom was introduced into the uterus. The condom was inflated with 250–500 mL NS, according to need. The condom catheter was kept for 24–48 hours, depending upon the initial intensity of blood loss, and gradually deflated when bleeding ceased.

- Ability of condom catheter to stop bleeding
- Time required to stop bleeding after the tamponade was applied
- Subsequent morbidity in terms of infection, despite use of prophylactic antibiotics.

The hydrostatic condom catheter can control PPH quickly and effectively. It is simple to use, inexpensive, and safe. In developing countries where PPH remains a primary cause of maternal mortality, any health care provider involved in delivery may use this procedure for controlling massive PPH to save the lives of patients. Oxytocin was administered along with introduction of the condom catheter.

The steps are as follows:

1. Under aseptic precautions, a sterile rubber catheter was inserted within the condom and tied near the mouth of the condom by a silk thread.

2. Urinary bladder was kept empty by indwelling Foley catheter.
3. After putting the patient in the lithotomy position, the condom was inserted within the uterine cavity.
4. Inner end of the catheter remained within the condom.
5. Outer end of the catheter was connected with a saline set and the condom was inflated with 250–500 mL of running NS.
6. Bleeding was observed, and when it was reduced considerably, further inflation was stopped and the outer end of the catheter was folded and tied with thread.
7. Uterine contraction was maintained by oxytocin drip for at least 6 hours after the procedure.
8. The uterine condom was kept tight in position by ribbon gauze pack .
9. The condom catheter was kept for 24–48 hours and then was deflated gradually over 10–15 minutes and removed.

Patient was kept under triple antibiotic coverage [Ampicillin (500 mg every 6 hours) + Metronidazole (500 mg every 8 hours) + Gentamycin (80 mg every 8 hours)] administered intravenously for 7 days.

Selective Arterial Embolization

Angiographic embolization may be useful in situations in which desire to restore fertility is needed, when surgical options have been unsuccessful in managing bleeding or hematoma. An additional advantage of embolization is uterine preservation with the possibility of future pregnancy.

Angiography is to be performed in the angiography suite using a right transfemoral approach (Figs 1A and B). This was followed by either selective embolization of a single bleeding vessel, arteries or by embolization of the anterior divisions of the internal iliac arteries, if the source is bilateral. Embolization material used includes Gelfoam pledgets and/or metallic platinum tufted coils. Embolization was defined as completed when cessation of flow, in the affected vessel(s) and distal branches, was identified. In the presence of an abnormal coagulation profile, an access sheath to be left in the common femoral artery until coagulation is normalized (<24 hours). Patients are to be managed in the intensive care unit.

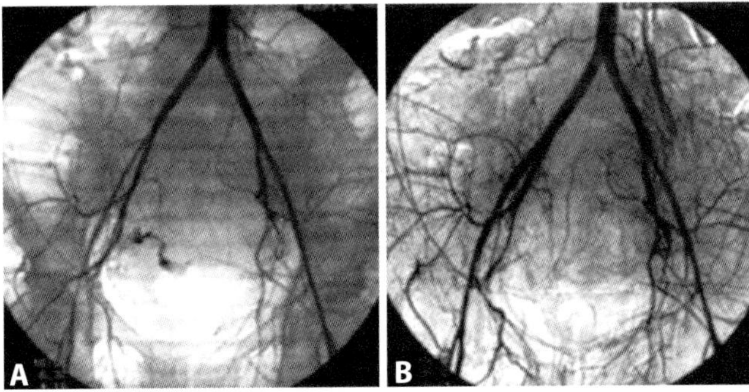

Figs 1A and B: Angiography pictures following uterine artery embolization

Both hypogastric arteries are rapidly occluded with small pledgets of Gelfoam. Gelfoam is a temporary occluding agent, which dissolves in 1–3 weeks. The pledgets are carried distally by the blood flow, occluding small arteries and preventing continued bleeding from collaterals. Frequently, the diagnostic arteriography identifies a specific arterial bleeding point, which can be selectively embolized avoiding the need for more widespread occlusion. The extent and number of vessels that need to be occluded determine the embolic agent(s) selected.

Complications include local hematoma formation at the insertion site; infection; ischemic phenomena, including uterine necrosis sometimes and dye-related adverse effects. Complications associated with uterine artery embolization in obstetric patients are rare; these include transient fever, transient buttock ischemia, transient foot ischemia, rarely iliac artery perforation and abscess.

Genital Tract Trauma

Genital tract trauma is the most likely cause if bleeding persists or is present despite a well-contracted uterus. Use appropriate analgesia along with good lighting and positioning, which facilitates excellent exposure. If not already initiated, moving the patient to an operating room is necessary at this time. Experienced assistants are essential. Directly visualize and inspect the cervix with the aid of two sponge-holding forceps. The anterior lip is grasped, and the cervix is inspected by using a second forceps placed at the 2 o'clock position, followed by progressively "leap-frogging" the forceps ahead of one another until the entire circumference has been inspected. Small, non-bleeding lacerations of the cervix do not need to be sutured. Suture any bleeding lesions longer than 2 cm and with a bleeding vessel. Each side of the laceration can be grasped with a sponge-holding forceps from the torn edge and gentle traction can be used to have good exposure.

Use an absorbable needle chromic catgut, give continuous interlocking stitches, and use round body needles for all repairs except for the perineal skin. Ensure that the stitch begins 1 cm above the apex of the tear, as with vaginal lacerations and episiotomies. If the apex cannot be visualized, place the stitch as high as possible and then use it to apply gentle traction to bring the apex area into view. Catgut especially on needle may be somewhat less likely to tear the friable tissues of the cervix and vaginal vault and may thus be useful in repairing lacerations in these areas. The laceration must be observed for bleeding after the torn edges of the cervix are approximated.

Lacerations of the vaginal vault must be well visualized to their full extent for repair. Lacerations high in the vaginal vault and those extending up from the cervix may involve the uterus or lead to broad ligament or retroperitoneal hematoma. The proximity of the ureter to the lateral vaginal fornices, and the base of the bladder to the anterior fornix, must be kept in mind when repair is undertaken in these areas. Deeply placed stitches can lead to genitourinary fistulas. An absorbable, continuous interlocking stitch is used. The stitch must start and finish beyond the apices of the laceration. Great care must be taken because the tissue is usually devitalized and friable.

Take a good amount of tissue thickness and adequate depth (Fig. 2). Ongoing bleeding and hematoma formation are possible if small bites are taken and they cut through.

Lacerations must be observed for bleeding after the repair is complete. Pressure or packing over the repair may achieve homeostasis or allow for better placement of further hemostatic stitches. Cervical and vaginal vault lacerations that continue to ooze or those that are associated with hematoma may be amenable to selective arterial embolization.

Traumatic hematomas are rare and may be related to lacerations or may occur in isolation. They include vulvar and paravaginal hematoma in the lower genital tract and broad ligament and retroperitoneal hematomas adjacent to the uterus. Patients with lower genital tract hematoma usually present with intense pain and localized, tender swelling and tachycardia. Broad ligament hematoma may be palpated as

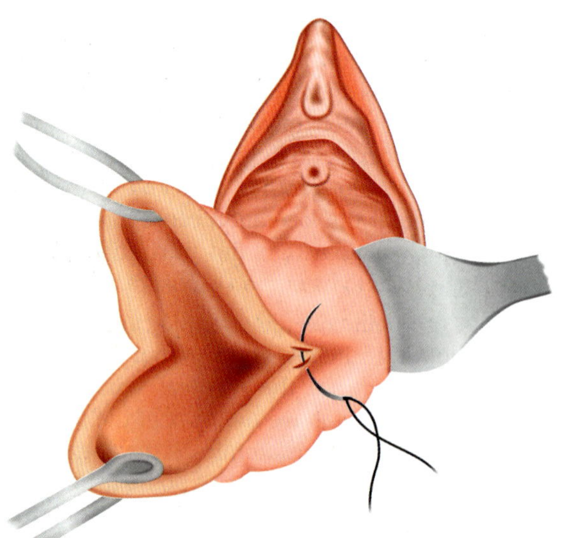

Fig. 2: Suturing of cervical tear devitalized and friable

masses by the side of the uterus. All may result in significant concealed blood loss that requires treatment.

Lower genital tract hematomas are usually managed by incision and evacuation and under general anesthesia; although expectant management is acceptable if the lesion is not enlarging. Any bleeding vessels are tied off, and oozing areas may be over sewn. Place a Foley catheter because reflex urinary retention can occur because of pain and tissue distortion. Vaginal packing may be useful following drainage and repair of paravaginal hematoma. Remove the pack in 24–48 hours.

Broad ligament and retroperitoneal hematomas are initially managed expectantly if the patient is stable and the lesions are not expanding. Ultrasound, computed tomography (CT) scanning and magnetic resonance imaging (MRI) all may be used to assess the size, site, extent and enlargement of these hematomas. Consider involving a surgeon with extensive experience operating in the retroperitoneal space. Selective arterial embolization may be the treatment of choice if intervention is required in these patients.

If manual exploration has excluded uterine rupture or retained placental fragments, bleeding from a well-contracted uterus is most commonly due to a defect in homeostasis. A review of the history and risk factors along with coagulation test results clarifies this diagnosis. Proceed with blood product replacement in order to correct abnormalities of homeostasis. If the coagulation status is normal and bleeding is ongoing despite a well-contracted uterus, then the possibilities of uterine rupture or an inadequately repaired uterine incision if the patient had a lower segment cesarean section must be considered.

Ongoing bleeding secondary to an unresponsive and atonic uterus, a ruptured uterus, or a large cervical laceration extending into the uterus, cervical, perineal tears, vaginal tears, paraurethral and paraclitoral tears warrants surgical treatment.

Adequately resuscitate the patient before surgery. This includes optimizing hemoglobin and coagulation status. Fully inform anesthetist the nature of the case. Sustained bimanual compression and massage and uterine packing may be used to gain time to mount a surgical response. Military antishock trousers provide the equivalent of an approximately 500–1,000 mL autotransfusion and potentially gain time during resuscitation. Only the leg portion of the trousers is inflated in the setting of PPH. Direct compression of the aorta may be performed for a short period while the operating room is prepared in critical cases.

LAPAROTOMY

The choice between a subumbilical vertical incision and a Pfannenstiel's incision for entry into the abdomen is left to the individual surgeon. The vertical incision is recommended for more exposure and extension. Broad-spectrum antibiotic coverage is advised.

Upon entry, remove any free blood and inspect the uterus and surrounding tissues for evidence of rupture or hematoma. If uterine rupture is found, a rapid decision must be made concerning the feasibility and viability of repair versus hysterectomy. Bleeding may be reduced in either instance by grasping bleeding points on the torn edges with clamps. The number of layers used for any repair is dictated by the thickness of the tissue and the hemostatic response to suturing. Delayed absorbable suture material is used to stitch the uterine trauma. Principles are similar to those of cesarean delivery incision repair. Ensure that bleeding is stopped and not merely internalized because this would result in ongoing vaginal bleeding or hematoma formation. Any repair must be carefully observed for homeostasis before abdominal closure is performed. Uterine exteriorization may improve exposure and decrease operating time, but great care must be taken to not worsen uterine trauma and to keep the uterus warm and well perfused to avoid worsening atony.

Homeostasis must be reassessed after the uterus is returned to the abdominal cavity. Consider placement of a suction drain.

If the uterus is intact upon entry and the bleeding has been caused by atony, then direct bimanual massage and compression may be performed while systemic uterotonic is continued. Direct injection of oxytocin, carboprost and/or ergometrine may be successful in overcoming atony.

BLEEDING AT CESAREAN DELIVERY

Most cases of intractable PPH followed vaginal delivery and were due to uterine atony; however, more cases are now associated with cesarean delivery. Cesarean delivery for placenta previa, obstructed labor, deep transverse arrest, carries a relative risk for peripartum hysterectomy, with many patients having a diagnosis of placenta accreta. High-resolution ultrasound with color Doppler may detect antenatal placenta accreta.

Uterine rupture has also become a more common cause of severe PPH necessitating hysterectomy. The vast majority of these cases occur in patients with a previous cesarean. Counsel all women with placenta previa, and especially those with a previous lower segment uterine scar, in the antenatal period regarding the risk of severe PPH and the possible need for transfusion and even hysterectomy.

The management of bleeding at cesarean delivery or following uterine rupture is not greatly different from that following vaginal delivery. Aggressive resuscitation is performed with attention to restoration of circulating volume and oxygen-carrying capacity and correction of hemostatic defects. Direct bimanual compression may be used in the case of atony. Retained tissue may be removed under direct visualization. Abnormally adherent tissue is a concern; leave it in situ if it cannot be easily removed.

Direct intramyometrial injection of uterotonic may be undertaken for atonic uterus, care to be taken to avoid intravascular injection. Individual vessels in the placental bed may be ligated. Simple or box stitches may be placed where continuous oozing is present. In cases of placenta previa, the lower uterine segment may be temporarily packed; leaving a pack in the uterus is also an option. The end of the pack is fed through the cervix and into the vagina for easy removal and is removed 24–36 hours later. Uterine rupture or extension of a uterine incision requires excellent visualization and careful repair with attention to adjacent structures.

The stepwise surgical approach described above may be used if these measures are unsuccessful and preservation of fertility is desired. Strongly consider immediate hysterectomy if further reproduction is not an issue or if bleeding or damage to the uterus appears severe. Embolization may be considered in this setting. Its successful use has been described both intraoperatively to preserve the uterus and after hysterectomy for continued bleeding. Embolization may also be used for continued postoperative vaginal bleeding.

Persistent bleeding following hysterectomy may also be managed by packing with gauze brought out through the vagina or by a pelvic pressure pack composed of gauze in a sterile plastic bag brought out through the vagina and placed under tension. This pack is also known as a parachute, mushroom, or umbrella pack. Place a Foley catheter to monitor urine output and prevent urinary retention. The placement of a suction drain may be useful to monitor losses in cases of ongoing oozing. Consider coagulopathy in patients with continued slow blood loss.

Postoperatively continue resuscitation, and repeat laboratory tests. Monitor vital signs, urine output and any bleeding. Shift patient to an obstetric intensive care unit. The patient must be monitored for complications.

Follow-up Care

Full documentation of the case is imperative, and a careful explanation of events and interventions must be given to the patients and relatives.

Most patients with PPH are quickly identified and successfully treated before major complications develop. The most common problem is anemia and loss of iron stores, which results in fatigue in the postpartum period. Clinicians and patients are more tolerant of low hemoglobin levels, mild postural light headedness, and fatigue because of current concerns over blood transfusion. Not surprisingly, many of the complications of severe PPH are related to massive blood loss and hypovolemic shock. Damage to all major organs is possible; respiratory (adult respiratory distress syndrome) and renal (acute tubular necrosis) damage are common but rare.

Renal failure is usually self-limited, and renal function recovers fully within 7–10 days. Temporary dialysis is seldom required. Pulmonary edema is uncommon in this previously healthy group; however, it may develop acutely or during the recovery phase because of fluid overload or myocardial dysfunction. Response to standard therapy is usually prompt.

Pregnant women are at increased risk of venous thrombosis and embolic events. Many of the risk factors for PPH are also risk factors for venous thrombosis and embolic events, including operative vaginal delivery, cesarean delivery and pelvic surgery. Venous stasis due to shock and immobility also contribute to morbidity.

Hypopituitarism following severe PPH (Sheehan's syndrome) is due to critical ischemia of the hypertrophied pituitary. This condition should be considered if a failure to lactate occurs, other features are loss of axillary and pubic hair, amenorrhea.

Evidence suggests that prophylaxis against gastrointestinal ulceration is useful in critically ill patients, especially those requiring ventilation. The recommended agents are sucralfate and histamine 2 blockers. Both are effective at reducing the risk of ulcers. Sucralfate may be associated with a lower incidence of pneumonia.

Christopher B-Lynch Suturing in PPH

The Christopher B-Lynch suturing technique, uterine brace suture, is particularly useful because of its simplicity of application, lifesaving potential, relative safety, and its capacity for preserving the uterus and thus fertility. Satisfactory hemostasis is assessed during application only. Advantage of this innovative technique is a right alternative to major surgical procedures to control pelvic arterial pulse pressure or hysterectomy. This suturing technique has been successfully applied with no apparent complications.

B-Lynch Sutures and Variants

The use of transmural uterine compression sutures helps in rapid control of bleeding. The initial procedure described, the B-Lynch technique, which involves opening the lower segment and passing a suture through the posterior uterine wall and then over the fundus to be tied anteriorly. A similar technique has been described without opening the uterus. A long, straight needle is passed anterior to posterior through the lower uterine segment; the suture is passed over the fundus and then tied anteriorly. Both techniques use bilateral stitches. The most recent variant uses multiple stitches passed transmural and tied anteriorly at various points over the uterine body. This technique is focused in the area of the placental bed in cases of abnormal placentation. All of these procedures effectively produce tamponade by compressing together the anterior and posterior walls and placental sinuses (Figs 3A to C).

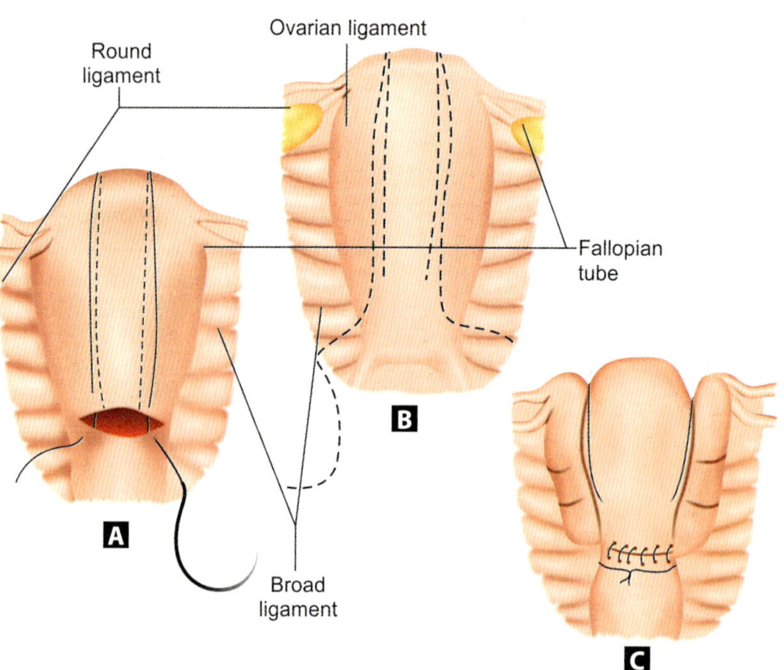

Figs 3A to C: Placement of sutures in B-Lynch procedure.
A: Anterior view; B: Posterior view; C: Anterior view

The effectiveness of the suture can be tested by prior bimanual compression of the uterus.

If the compression controls bleeding, it is likely that suture will work. Effect can be seen immediately on application of the suture.

Steps

1. General anesthesia, urinary catheter in place and the patient in the Lloyd-Davies position.
2. Pfannenstiel's incision given to open the abdomen.
3. Lower segment uterine incision as for cesarean section made after dissecting off the bladder but of small size. The advantages of this window are:
   a. Uterine evacuation
   b. To see any bleeding after compression of uterus, this assesses the efficacy of stitch.
4. Bimanual compression of the uterus to assess the potential chance of success of the suture.
5. A suture on needle number 2 (round body needle), chromic catgut is used to puncture the uterus about 3 cm below the right hand corner of the lower segment incision and brought about 3 cm.
6. Above the same corner (as one would place the first suture when closing this corner of the incision). From this point, the suture is passed over the right cornu of the uterus, approximately 3–4 cm medial to the right cornual border, where it may be fixed to prevent it from slipping of the fundus and then fed posteriorly and vertically down to the same level, where the suture has previously left the uterine cavity from the anterior. The suture is then placed through the posterior uterine wall into the cavity under the direct vision of the surgeon and back through the posterior wall about 4–5 cm left of the previous entry site. With the suture outside and posterior of the uterine cavity at this stage, it is now passed over the left cornu, approximately 3–4 cm medial to the left cornual border, where again it may be fixed to the fundus, then fed anteriorly and vertically down to the level of the left corner of the lower segment incision. The needle is then passed through the left corner in the same fashion as on the right hand side, to emerge below the incision margin on the left side.
7. With the suture now in place, the assistant bimanually compresses the uterus while the surgeon pulls the chromic suture taught. If a third person confirms that the bleeding is controlled (as observed vaginally), the surgeon ties the suture to keep it in position and closes the lower segment uterine incision.
8. The author's modification of B-Lynch stitch is anchoring the stitch to uterus at six places so as to achieve symmetrical, nonslippable stitch with good efficacy. The stitch is anchored over anterior wall of uterus exactly in the middle of lower segment incision and fundus, then at fundus 3 cm medial to uterotubal junction, on posterior wall in the center of fundus and posterior transverse bite. This makes stitch not to slip or loose and maintains symmetrical compression. As number 2 on needle catgut is used and it dissolves within a few weeks, there is no risk of intrauterine adhesions.

INTERNAL ILIAC, UTERINE ARTERY LIGATION/DEVASCULARIZATION OF UTERUS

Uterine Artery Ligation

Uterine artery ligation is a relatively simple procedure and can be highly effective in controlling bleeding from uterine sources (Fig. 4). These arteries provide approximately 90% of uterine blood flow. The uterus is grasped and tilted to expose the vessels coursing through the broad ligament immediately adjacent to the uterus. Ideally, place the stitch 2 cm below the level of a transverse lower uterine incision site. A large atraumatic (round body) needle is used with a delayed absorbable suture. Include almost the full thickness of the myometrium to anchor the stitch and to ensure that the uterine artery and veins are completely included. The needle is then passed through an avascular portion of the broad ligament and tied anteriorly. Opening the broad ligament is unnecessary. Perform bilateral uterine artery ligation. While the uterus may remain atonic, blanching is usually noted and blood flow is greatly diminished or arrested.

Local oozing may be controlled with compression. Stepwise approach is after initial uterine artery ligation, subsequent stitches to be placed 2–3 cm below the initial stitches following bladder mobilization for cervical branch

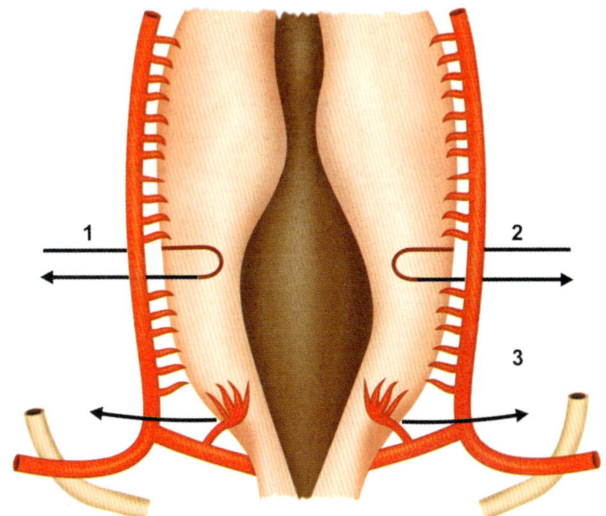

Fig. 4: Stepwise devascularization of uterus

ligation, and, finally, ovarian artery ligation should be performed, if required. Menstrual flow and fertility does not get adversely affected.

VAGINAL TECHNIQUE OF UTERINE ARTERY LIGATION

This procedure, which is quickly learned, can be performed with minimal preparation, with or without bladder retraction. A 2-cm horizontal incision is made in the anterior cervix 1 cm below the estimated vaginocervical fold and the bladder reflected in the natural plane. Firm but gentle downward traction on the uterus to the contralateral side of the intended ligature maximizes cephalic and lateral access, permitting bilateral uterine artery ligation from laterally under direct vision or by transcervical palpation (Fig. 5).

The vaginal route offers a novel, simple, effective and minimally invasive technique for treating intractable puerperal hemorrhage by uterine artery ligation. Timely intervention avoids hysterectomy and consumption coagulopathy and preserves reproductive potential.

The procedure itself can be performed with bladder retraction. The anterior and posterior cervical lips are clamped with sponge-holding forceps. A 2-cm horizontal incision is made in the anterior cervix about 1 cm beneath the estimated vaginocervical fold, and the bladder is reflected as much as possible in the natural plane using a swab on a holder. Gentle but firm traction is then used to pull the uterus downward and sideways, towards the contralateral side of the intended ligature, to maximize cephalic and lateral access.

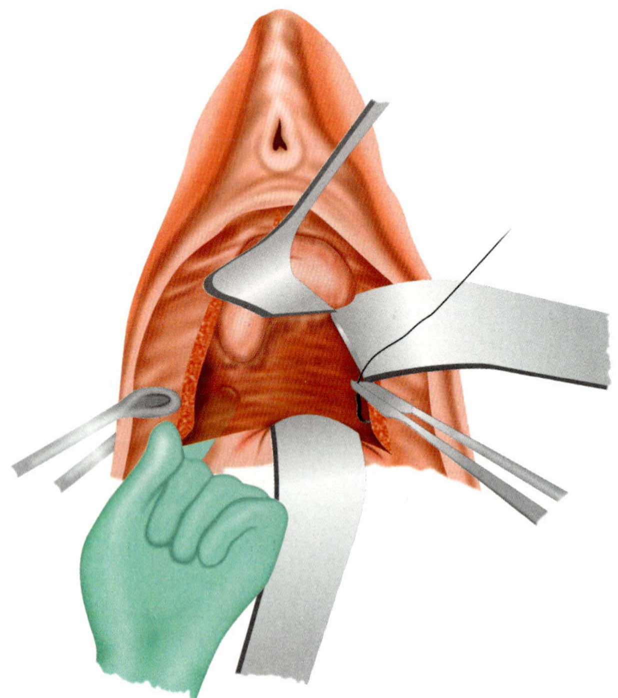

Fig. 5: Vaginal technique of uterine artery ligation

From cephalic end a curved needle is led towards the myometrium under the guidance of the index finger placed in the cervical canal and lower uterine segment. The uterine artery whose pulsation is readily palpable and sometimes visible laterally, then encircled with the artery and vein and a layer of uterine tissue and ligated. Fingertip injury is avoided by retracting the finger after palpation and immediately before applying the stitch. It is very important to pull the uterus gently towards the contralateral side to allow for ample working space and visualization of the vessel bundle. The synthetic absorbable thread is clamped using artery forceps and the vessel bundle pulled caudally. Additional one or two ligatures, depending on the anatomical variations of the uterine artery applied to secure the ligation, using the same technique. The whole procedure is then repeated with the contralateral vessel bundle. The anterior vaginal wall and anterior cervical lip are reunited with a few interrupted stitches. Delayed absorbable on needle suture material is used for this procedure. Vaginal ligation of the uterine arteries should not be performed in women with known or suspected human immunodeficiency virus and/or hepatitis B or C virus. This procedure is highly effective if performed in time. It is quickly learned as it resembles the part of preparation for vaginal hysterectomy.

Ovarian Artery Ligation

The ovarian artery arises directly from the aorta and ultimately anastomoses with the uterine artery in the region of the uterine aspect of the utero-ovarian ligament near cornu. Ligation is performed just inferior to this point in a manner similar to that of uterine artery ligation. The amount of uterine blood flow supplied by these vessels may increase following uterine artery ligation. The procedure is easy to perform.

Internal Iliac (Hypogastric) Artery Ligation

Bilateral internal iliac artery ligation/hypogastric artery ligation to control pelvic hemorrhage was first supposedly performed by Kelly in 1894. Since then, many reports have emerged describing its diverse indications, surgical technique and effectiveness in controlling pelvic hemorrhage.

Internal iliac artery ligation can be effective to reduce bleeding from all sources within the genital tract by reducing the pulse pressure in the pelvic arterial circulation. It is indicated that pulse pressure was reduced by 77% with unilateral ligation and by 85% with bilateral ligation (Clark, 1985). Hypogastric artery ligation is not much more difficult to perform, but may be associated with damage to nearby structures.

Prerequisites for the procedure include operator experienced in the procedure and a desire of patient to maintain reproductive potential.

The retroperitoneal space is entered by incising the peritoneum between the fallopian tube and the round ligament. The ureter must be identified and reflected medially with the attached peritoneum. The external iliac artery is identified on the pelvic sidewall and followed proximally to the bifurcation of the common iliac artery. The ureter passes over the bifurcation. The internal iliac artery is identified and followed distally approximately 3–4 cm from its point of origin. This site is ideal for ligation as posterior division arises within 3 cm of bifurcation. The loose areolar tissue is carefully dissected from the artery. A right-angle clamp (mixture) is passed beneath the artery at this point, with great care to avoid damage to the underlying internal iliac vein.

With a sound knowledge of anatomy (Fig. 6), the dissection is safe and easy if we pass the clamp from lateral to medial in order to minimize the chance of damage to the adjacent external iliac vessels and internal iliac vein. Gentle elevation of the artery with clamp and separating 1 cm area is needed to pass the suture material.

Ligate the artery with no. 2 chromic catgut (absorbable suture) at two sites 1 cm apart, but do not divide it. Palpate the femoral and distal pulses dorsalis pedis before and after the ligation to ensure that the external or common iliac artery was not inadvertently ligated. Place the ligation distal to the posterior division of the artery because this decreases the risk of subsequent ischemic buttock pain. Identification of the posterior division may be difficult, and ligation 3 cm from the internal iliac artery origin usually ensures that it is not included.

After ligature, circulation in the parts supplied by the internal iliac artery would be carried on by the anastomoses of:

1. The uterine and ovarian arteries
2. The middle and the superior vesical arteries
3. The iliolumbar with the last lumbar
4. The lateral sacral with the middle sacral arteries (Fig. 6). The mechanism responsible for controlling pelvic hemorrhage following ligation of internal iliac artery without compromising blood supply is that the ligation of internal iliac artery greatly dampened the pulse pressure and transformed the pelvic arterial system into a venous like system with slow and sluggish blood flow. The "trip hammer effect" of the arterial pulsation was lost. The blood clots, which were formed distal to the ligation, therefore, remain in place.

After the bilateral ligation, the drop in pulse pressure was 85% whereas with unilateral ligation it was 77% on the same side and 14% on the opposite side. The mean arterial pressure decreased to 24% with bilateral ligation and with unilateral ligation the decrease was 22% on the

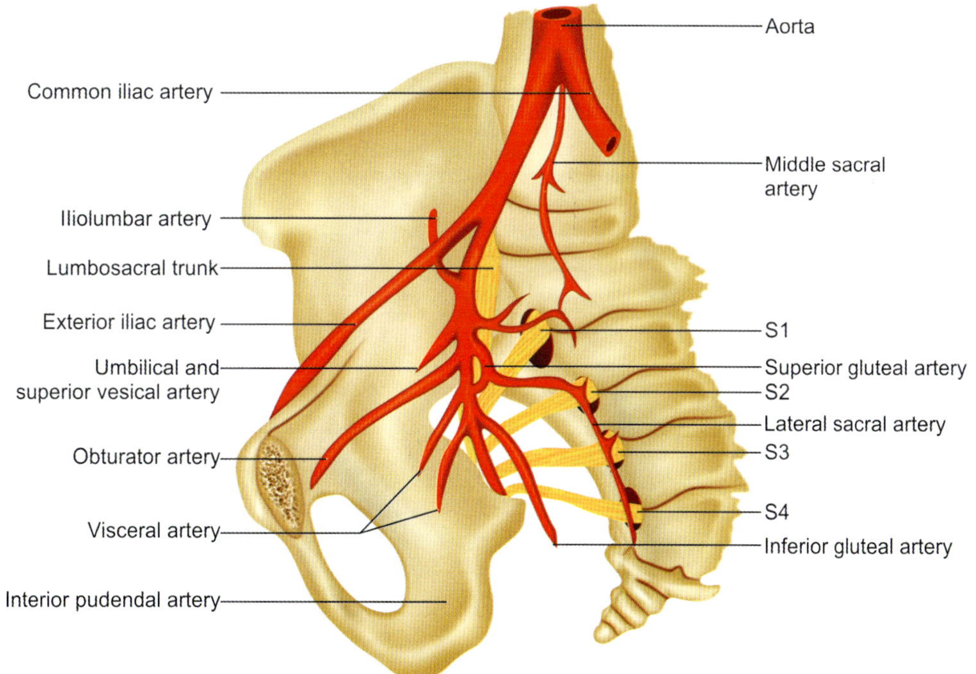

Fig. 6: Anatomy of internal iliac artery

same side and 10% on the opposite side. The rate of blood flow dropped to about 48% on the same side after ligation.

Delayed complications like ischemic necrosis, paresthesia of gluteal region or bladder atony, injury to the iliac vein and bladder necrosis may be seen in a few patients. Internal iliac ligation is a valuable surgical procedure and should be the first line of treatment where conservation of the uterus is desired. The complications encountered are few if the procedure is performed carefully and with knowledge of pelvic anatomy.

Internal iliac artery ligation is a highly effective method of stemming uterine hemorrhage which is grossly under used in obstetrics. Bilateral iliac artery ligation is mainly indicated in PPH due to uterine atony, ruptured uterus and placenta accreta. The main advantage of procedure is effectiveness and preserving future fertility in women who had internal iliac ligation for control of life-threatening obstetric hemorrhage.

OBSTETRIC OR CESAREAN HYSTERECTOMY

The procedure was originally developed in an attempt to reduce the mortality from hemorrhage and sepsis that accompanied abdominal delivery. In modern obstetric practice, emergency cesarean and postpartum hysterectomy are still critical lifesaving procedures in cases of intractable obstetric hemorrhage. The cesarean hysterectomy in which both mother and infant survived was reported by Dr Eduardo Porro in 1876. Porro's success prompted other obstetricians to perform peripartum hysterectomy as a lifesaving measure. By the early 1900s, the technique had been refined and obstetricians were more comfortable performing the surgery. Modern times have seen a return to using peripartum hysterectomy almost solely for management of obstetric emergencies.

Details of the procedure are available in other Chapters.

SUMMARY

Postpartum hemorrhage is a common complication of childbirth and a leading cause of maternal morbidity and mortality. Clinicians should identify risk factors before and during labor so that care may be optimized for high-risk women. However, significant life-threatening bleeding can occur in the absence of risk factors and without warning. All caregivers and facilities involved in maternity care must have a clear plan for the prevention and management of PPH. This includes sound resuscitation skills and familiarity with all medical and surgical therapies available.

BIBLIOGRAPHY

1. Abouzahr C. Antepartum and postpartum haemorrhage. In: Murray CJ, Lopez AD (Eds). Health Dimensions of Sex and Reproduction. Boston, Mass: Harvard University Press; 1998. pp.172-4.
2. Atoyebi W, Mundy N, Croxton T, et al. Is it necessary to administer anti-D to prevent RhD immunization after the transfusion of RhD-positive platelet concentrates? Br J Haematol. 2000;111(3):980-3.
3. B-Lynch C, Coker A, Lawal AH, et al. The B-Lynch surgical technique for the control of massive postpartum haemorrhage: an alternative to hysterectomy? Five cases reported. Br J Obstet Gynecol. 1997;104(3):372-5.
4. Baskett TF. Complications of the third stage of labour. Essential Management of Obstetrical Emergencies, 3rd edition. Bristol, England: Clinical Press; 1999. pp. 196-201.
5. Kelly H. Ligation of both internal iliac arteries for haemorrhage in hysterectomy for carcinoma uterus. John Hopkins Med J. 1894;5:53-4.
6. Prendiville WJ, Elbourne D, McDonald S. Active versus expectant management in the third stage of labour. Cochrane Database Syst Rev. 2000;(2):CD000007.

CHAPTER

26

Peripartum Hysterectomy

Alka Saraswat

INTRODUCTION

Peripartum hysterectomy may be an emergency procedure or may be planned, often in conjunction with cesarean delivery. Obstetric hysterectomy refers to surgical removal of the pregnant or recently pregnant uterus with the pregnancy in situ or due to complications of delivery. It is an indispensable lifesaving procedure for management of intractable obstetric hemorrhage unresponsive to other treatments.

INCIDENCE

The incidence of peripartum hysterectomy is from 0.05 to 0.1% of deliveries, but there is a considerable difference in its incidence in different parts of the world depending upon modern obstetrical services, standard and awareness of antenatal care, and effectiveness of family planning activities of a given community.

RISK FACTORS FOR PERIPARTUM HYSTERECTOMY

In many instances, the obstetrician can anticipate the possible need for peripartum hysterectomy and the woman can be apprised of this risk in the antenatal period. The indications for peripartum hysterectomy, her chances of needing the procedure, and the possible outcome should be discussed and documented when obtaining informed consent prior to labor and delivery.

INDICATIONS

Severe Uterine Hemorrhage

Certain hemorrhages cannot be controlled by conservative measures. Such hemorrhage may be due to abnormally implanted placenta (e.g. accreta, increta, percreta):

- Uterine atony
- Uterine rupture
- Coagulopathy
- Laceration of a pelvic vessel
- Uterine inversion.

The relative frequency of these conditions varies among series and is dependent upon patient population and practice patterns. Hysterectomy is usually a last resort to save the life of a woman with persistent bleeding.

Uterine Infection

Infection that is unresponsive to antibiotics.

Stage I Cervical Carcinoma

This can be treated by a cesarean delivery followed by radical hysterectomy.

SURGICAL ANATOMY

Anterior view of female pelvis and vascular supply is shown in Figure 1.

Superior view of female pelvis with detailed right uterus vascular supply is shown in Figure 2.

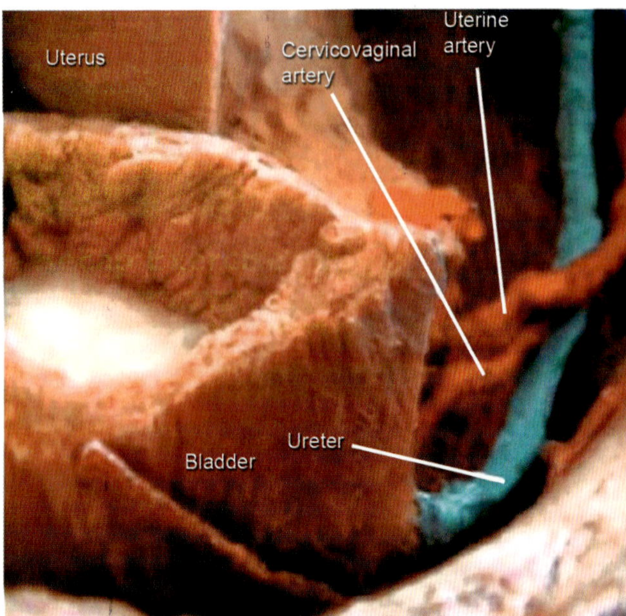

Fig. 1: Uterine artery and ureter crossing, anterior view

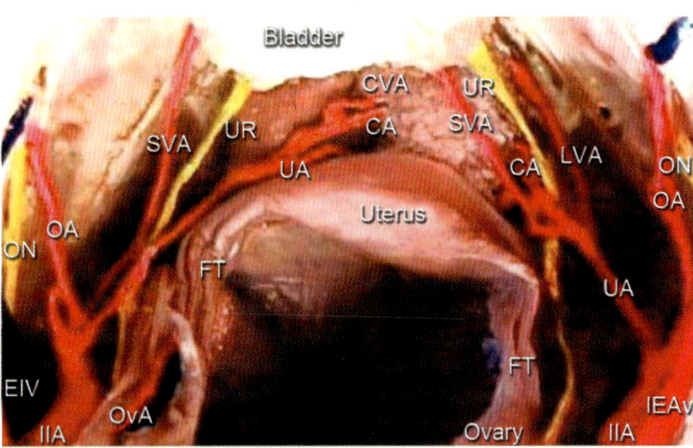

Fig. 2: Uterus blood supply, right vascular pedicle

Abbreviations: IIA: iliac internal artery; IEV: iliac external vein; IEA: iliac external artery; OvA: ovarian artery; OA: obturator artery; ON: obturator nerve; SVA: superior vesical artery; UR: ureter; FT: fallopian tube; UA: uterine artery; CA: cervical artery; CVA: cervicovaginal artery; LVA: Large vesical artery.

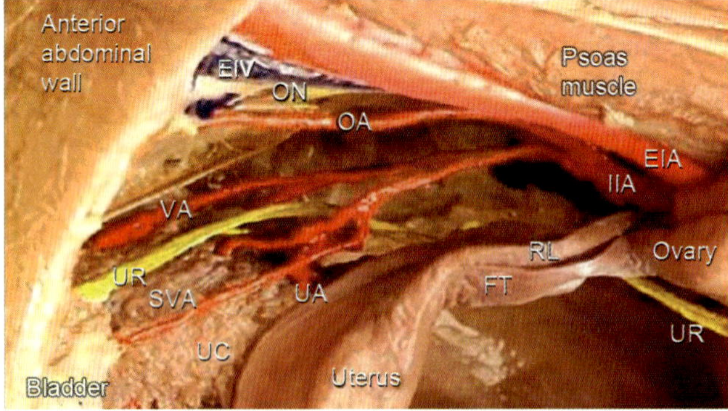

Fig. 3: Female pelvis, vascular supply, left uterine pedicle and left ureter

Abbreviations: IIA: iliac internal artery; EIV: external iliac vein; IEA: iliac external artery; OvA: ovarian artery; OA: obturator artery; ON: obturator nerve; SVA: superior vesical artery; UR: ureter; FT: fallopian tube; UA: uterine artery; CA: cervical artery; CVA: cervicovaginal artery; VA: vesical artery; UC: uterine cervix.

Left uterine pedicle and left ureter are shown in detail in Figure 3.

Classification of Peripartum Hysterectomy

- Circumstances
- Emergency
- Indicated
- Elective.

Extent

- Supracervical
- Total
- Radical.

Clinical Context

- Planned cesarean birth
- Emergency cesarean birth
- Postpartum.

Salpingo-oophorectomy

- None
- Unilateral
- Bilateral.

Elective hysterectomy at the time of delivery is a controversial procedure because of the increased morbidity related to surgery on highly vascular pelvic organs. It has been advocated for parturients with gynecologic disorders such as leiomyomas or high-grade cervical intraepithelial neoplasia, but surgery usually can be safely delayed until the pelvis returns to its pre-pregnant state.

Timing is the key to an optimal outcome; the procedure should not be performed too early or too late. A sequence of conservative measures to control hemorrhage should be initiated before resorting to hysterectomy. If an intervention does not succeed, the next treatment in the sequence must be swiftly instituted. Indecisiveness delays therapy and results in excessive hemorrhage, which eventually causes dilutional coagulopathy. This will make control of hemorrhage more difficult and will increase the risks of hysterectomy, major morbidity from hemorrhagic shock and death.

In some cases, and most often because of emergent complications such as intractable hemorrhage, abdominal hysterectomy is indicated following delivery. When performed at the time of cesarean delivery, the operation is termed cesarean hysterectomy. If done within a short time after vaginal delivery, it is termed postpartum hysterectomy.

Postpartum hysterectomy can be subtotal unless the cervix and lower uterine segment are involved. Total hysterectomy may be necessary in the case of a tear of the lower segment that extends into the cervix or bleeding after placenta previa.

Concurrent follow-up for:

- Review for indications
- Review operative care principles and start an intravenous (IV) infusion
- Give a single dose of prophylactic antibiotics:
  - Ampicillin 2 g IV
  - Cefazolin 1 g IV
- If there is uncontrollable hemorrhage following vaginal delivery, keep in mind that speed is essential to open the abdomen.

ANESTHETIC CONSIDERATIONS

Peripartum hysterectomy is often associated with substantial blood loss and fluid requirement. Airways in pregnant patients are susceptible for developing tissue edema as a result of IV infusion of fluids that produce a decrease in the colloid osmotic pressure which is already decreased in pregnant subjects. The airway changes from class 2 to class 4 are shown in Figures 4A to D. Postoperative diuresis gradually results in normalization of the airway in the next 48 hours.

A change in airway status has two important clinical implications in the management of parturient for peripartum hysterectomy. First, intraoperative induction of general anesthesia may be required in patients undergoing peripartum hysterectomy under regional anesthesia any time during the course of the procedure, and secondly, general anesthesia may be required to facilitate reoperation to explore and control excessive postoperative hemorrhage. Although it is not a contraindication to perform cesarean hysterectomy under regional anesthesia, one should carefully take into consideration that the airway may worsen during the course of surgery. The relative risk of experiencing a difficult intubation in comparison to an uncomplicated class I airway increases by four times when the airway class changes from class 2 to class 4 airway. The risk may increase further if the patient has other risk factors such as obesity, protruding upper teeth, short thyromental distance and increased weight gain in the pregnancy. In addition, the laryngeal edema that may accompany upper airway edema can also contribute to a difficult intubation. It may be prudent to induce general anesthesia and secure the airway as soon as substantial hemorrhage, requiring large volume infusion/transfusion, is anticipated. On the other hand, if the airway is not secured, periodic assessment of the airway during the course of surgery is recommended to determine worsening of the airway. If this approach is chosen, contingency plans to deal with a challenging airway should be readily available in case a difficult intubation is encountered during intraoperative induction of general anesthesia.

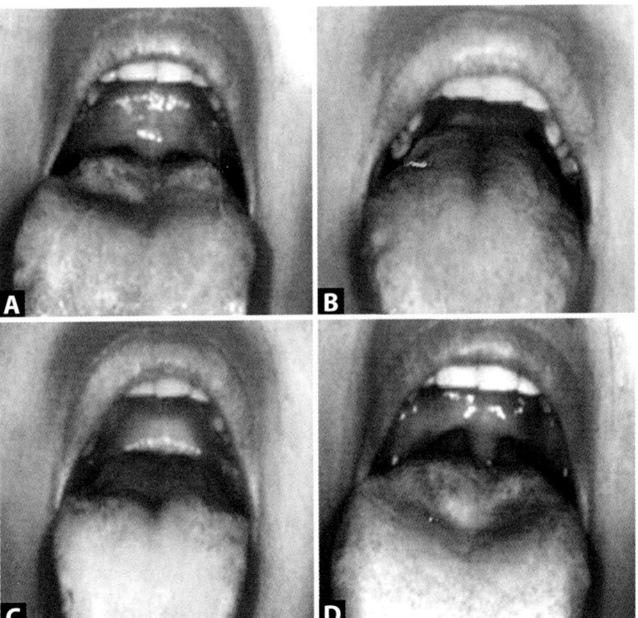

Figs 4A to D: Airway changes during cesarean hysterectomy. (A) Preoperative (airway class 2); (B) Immediate postoperative (airway class 4, lips and tongue are swollen); (C) 24 h postoperative (airway class 3); (D) 48 h postoperative (airway class 2)

OPERATIVE STEPS

- Make a midline vertical incision below the umbilicus to the pubic hair, through the skin and to the level of the fascia
- Make a 2–3 cm vertical incision in the fascia
- Hold the fascial edge with forceps and lengthen the incision up and down using scissors
- Use fingers or scissors to separate the rectus muscles (abdominal wall muscles)
- Use fingers to make an opening in the peritoneum near the umbilicus. Use scissors to lengthen the incision up and down in order to see the entire uterus. Carefully, to prevent bladder injury, use scissors to separate layers and open the lower part of the peritoneum
- Place a bladder retractor over the pubic bone and place self-retaining abdominal retractors
  - If the delivery was by cesarean section, clamp the sites of bleeding along the uterine incision
- In case of massive bleeding, have an assistant press fingers over the aorta in the lower abdomen. This will reduce intraperitoneal bleeding.
  - Extend the skin incision, if needed.

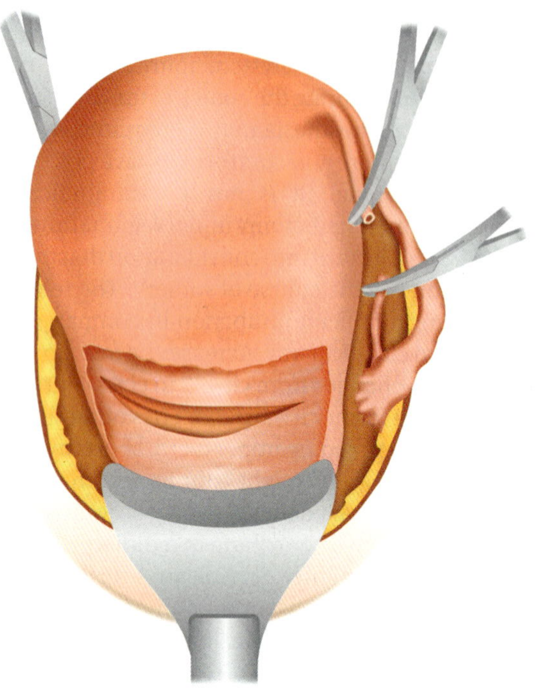

Fig. 5: Dividing round ligaments

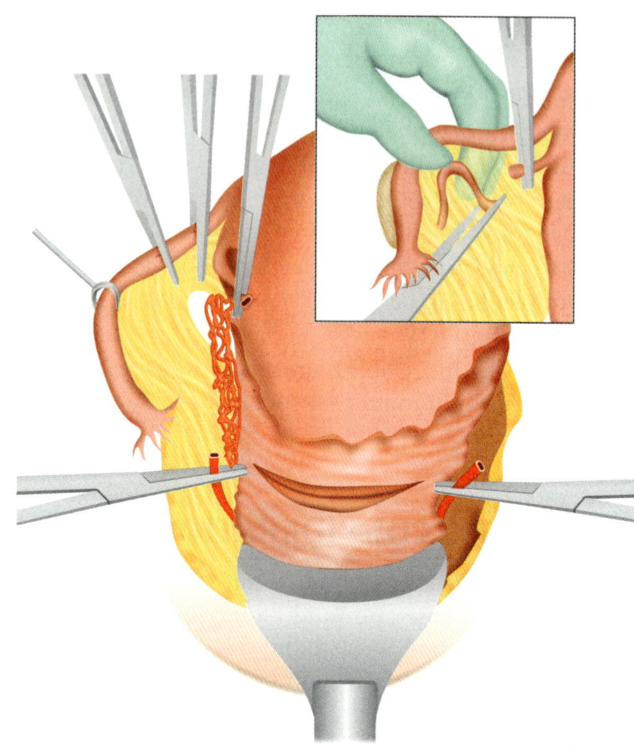

Fig. 6: Cutting the tubes, the ovarian ligaments and broad ligament

SUBTOTAL (SUPRACERVICAL) HYSTERECTOMY

- Lift the uterus out of the abdomen and gently pull to maintain traction
- Doubly clamp and cut the round ligaments with scissors (Fig. 5). Clamp and cut the pedicles but ligate after the uterine arteries are secured to save time.

Dividing the Round Ligaments

- From the edge of the cut round ligament, open the anterior leaf of the broad ligament. Incise to:
  - the point where the bladder peritoneum is reflected onto the lower uterine surface in the midline; or
  - the incised peritoneum at a cesarean section
- Use two fingers to push the posterior leaf of the broad ligament forward, just under the tube and ovary, near the uterine edge. Make a hole of the size of a finger in the broad ligament using scissors. Doubly clamp and cut the tube, the ovarian ligament and the broad ligament through the hole in the broad ligament (Fig. 6).

The ureters are close to the uterine vessels. The ureter must be identified and exposed to avoid injury during surgery or including it in a stitch.

Dividing the Tube and Ovarian Ligaments

- Divide the posterior leaf of the broad ligament downward towards the uterosacral ligaments using scissors
- Grasp the edge of the bladder flap with forceps or a small clamp. Using fingers or scissors, dissect the bladder downwards off the lower uterine segment. Direct the pressure downward but inward, towards the cervix and the lower uterine segment
- Locate the uterine artery and vein on each side of the uterus. Feel for the junction of the uterus and cervix
- Doubly clamp across the uterine vessels at a 90° angle on each side of the cervix. Cut and doubly ligate with 0 chromic catgut (or polyglycolic) suture (Fig. 7).

Dividing the Uterine Vessels

- Observe carefully for any further bleeding. If the uterine arteries are ligated correctly, bleeding should stop and the uterus should look pale
- Return to the clamped pedicles of the round ligaments and tubo-ovarian ligaments and ligate them with 0 chromic catgut (or polyglycolic) suture
- Amputate the uterus above the level where the uterine arteries are ligated, using scissors (Fig. 8).

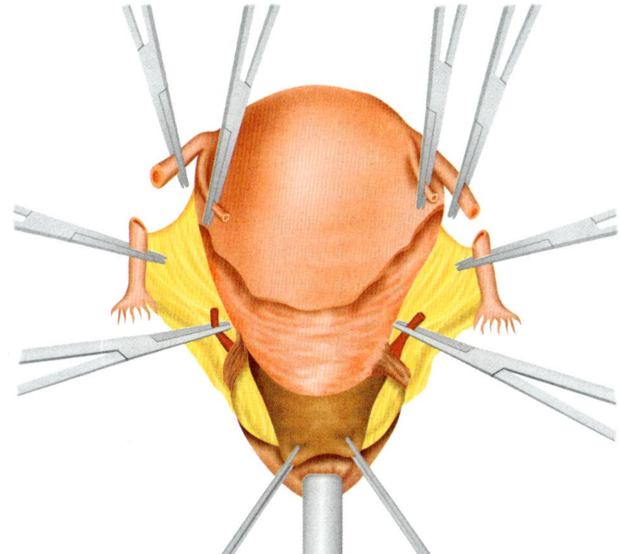

Fig. 7: Clamping and cutting uterine arteries

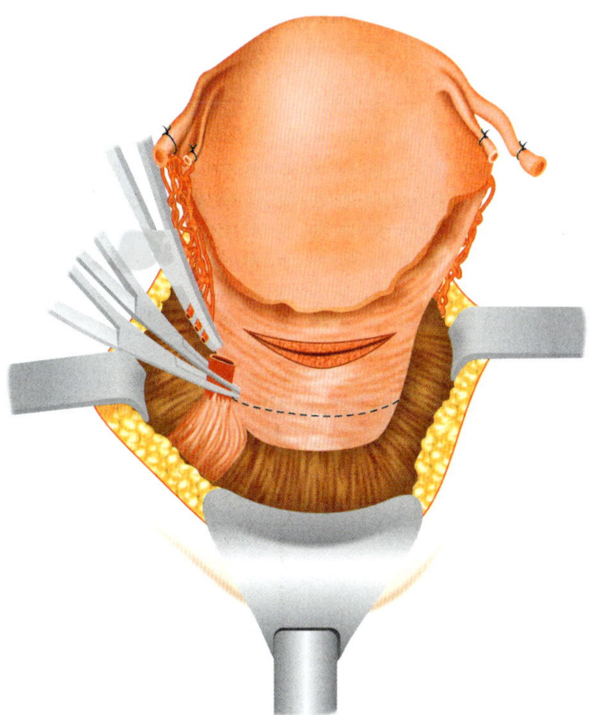

Fig. 8: Supracervical amputation of uterus above uterine arteries

Line of Amputation

- Close the cervical stump with interrupted 2-0 or 3-0 chromic catgut (or polyglycolic) sutures
- Carefully inspect the cervical stump, leaves of the broad ligament and other pelvic floor structures for any bleeding
- If slight bleeding persists or a clotting disorder is suspected, place a drain through the abdominal wall. Do not place a drain through the cervical stump as this can cause postoperative infection
- Ensure that there is no bleeding. Remove clots using a sponge suction
- In all cases, check for injury to the bladder. If a bladder injury is identified, repair the injury
- Close the fascia with continuous 0 chromic catgut (or polyglycolic) suture.

  Note: There is no need to close the bladder peritoneum or the abdominal peritoneum.
- If there are signs of infection, place suction drain and place not too tight 0 catgut (or polyglycolic) sutures. Close the skin with a delayed closure after the infection has cleared
- If there are no signs of infection, close the skin with vertical mattress sutures of 3-0 nylon (or silk) and apply a sterile dressing.

TOTAL HYSTERECTOMY

The following additional steps are required for total hysterectomy:

- Push the bladder down to free the top 2 cm of the vagina
- Open the posterior leaf of the broad ligament
- Clamp, ligate and cut the uterosacral ligaments
- Clamp, ligate and cut the cardinal ligaments, which contain the descending branches of the uterine vessels. This is the critical step in the operation:
  - Grasp the ligament vertically with a large-toothed clamp (e.g. Kochers clamp).
  - Place the clamp 5 mm lateral to the cervix and cut the ligament close to the cervix, leaving a stump medial to the clamp for safety.
  - If the cervix is long, repeat the step two or three times as needed.

The upper 2 cm of the vagina should now be free of attachments.

- Circumcise the vagina as near to the cervix as possible, clamping bleeding points as they appear
- Place hemostatic angle sutures, which include round, cardinal and uterosacral ligaments
- Place continuous interlocking sutures on the vaginal cuff to stop hemorrhage
- Close the abdomen (as above) after placing a drain in the extraperitoneal space near the stump of the vault.

POSTOPERATIVE CARE

- Review postoperative care principles
- If there are *signs of infection* or the woman *currently has fever*, give a combination of antibiotics until she is fever-free for 48 hours:

  - ampicillin 2 g IV every 6 hours;
  - plus gentamicin 5 mg/kg body weight IV every 24 hours;
  - plus metronidazole 500 mg IV every 8 hours
- Give appropriate analgesic drugs
- If there are no signs of infection, remove the abdominal drain after 48 hours.

COMPLICATIONS

Intraoperative Complications

- Urinary bladder injury
- Adnexal bleeding
- Retroperitoneal hematoma.

Postoperative Complications

- Coagulopathy
- Pneumonia
- Re-exploration laparotomy
- Vaginal cuff cellulitis
- Acute renal failure
- Urinary tract infection
- Wound infection.

Peripartum hysterectomy is a major operation, and in current times almost always an emergency with high risk for significant blood loss. The obstetrician should be ready to do it, and an early decision should be to save blood and prevent complications. Postoperative complications, mostly bleeding and infections may be severe. Early intervention and proper technique facilitate good outcomes.

BIBLIOGRAPHY

1. Aleem M, Bashir A. Caesarean and postpartum hysterectomy. Specialist (Pak J Med Sci). 1994;10(3): 233-7.
2. Baker E. Caesarean section birth and hysterectomy. Clin Obstet Gynecol. 1994; 37:806-15.
3. Barclay DL. Caesarean hysterectomy at charity hospital in New Orlean, 1000 consecutive operations. Clin Obstet Gynecol. 1969;19:635.
4. Bowman EA, Barelay DS, White LC. Caesarean hysterectomy: an analysis of 1000 consecutive operations. Bull Tulane Med Faculty. 1964;23:75.
5. Castaneda S, Karrison T, Cibil LA. Peripartum hysterectomy. J Perinat Med. 2000;28(6):722-81.
6. Clark SL, Koonings PP, Phelan JP. Placenta previa accrete and prior caesarean section. Obstet Gynecol. 1985; 66:89-92.
7. Deppe G, Baumann P, Malviya VK. Emergency postpartum hysterectomy. Wien-Klin-Wochenschr. 1994;106(18):581-3.
8. Engelsen IB, Albrechtsen S, Iversen OE, et al. Peripartum hysterectomy incidence and maternal morbidity. Acta Obstet Gynecol Scand. 2001;80(5):409-12.
9. Farmer RM, Kirschbaum T, Potter D, et al. Uterine rupture during trail of labour after previous caesarean section. Am J Obstet Gynecol. 1991;165:996-1001.
10. Gardeil F, Daly S, Turner MJ. Peripartum hysterectomy. Rev Fr Gynecol Scan. 1995;90(10):431-4.
11. Miller DA, Diaz F, Paul RH. Vaginal birth after caesarean: A 10 year experience. Obstet Gynecol. 1994;84:255-8.
12. Nasrat HA, Youssef MH, Marz Koongi A, et al. "Near Miss" Obstetric morbidity in an inner city hospital in Saudia Arabia. East Mediterr Health J. 1999;5(4):717-26.
13. Ogyunniyi SO, Esen UI. Obstetric hysterectomy in Tieife, Nigeria. Intern J Gynecol Obstet. 1990;32:23-7.
14. Osefo NJ. Caesarean and postpartum hysterectomy. Int J Gynecol Obstet. 1989;30:93-7.
15. Park EH, Sachs BP. Postpartum haemorrhage and other problems of third stage. In: James DK, Steer PJ, Weiner CP, Gonik B (Eds). High Risk Pregnancy: Management Options, 2nd edition. Philadelphia: WB Saunders; 1999. pp. 1231-46.
16. Patterson SP. Caesarean hysterectomy. Am J Obstet Gynecol. 1970;107:729.
17. Platt LD, Druzin ML. Acute peurperal inversion of uterus. Am J Obstet Gynecol. 1981;141:187-90.
18. Saxhdev PS, Munir A. Obstetric hysterectomy at Liaqat Medical College Hospital. Pak J Obstet Gynecol. 1996;9(1):31-4.
19. Shah Hosseini R, Errard JR. Peurperal uterine inversion. Obstet Gynecol. 1989;73:567-70.
20. Stanco LM, Schrimmer DB, Paul RH, et al. Peripartum hysterectomy. Am J Obstet Gynecol. 1993;168:879-83.
21. Suner S, Tagminash, Piepert JF, et al. Fatal spontaneous rupture of a gravid uterus. Case report and literature review of uterine rupture. J Emerg Med. 1996;14:181-5.
22. Zelop CM, Harlow BL, Frigoletto FD, et al. Emergency peripartum hysterectomy. Am J Obstet Gynecol. 1993;168:43.
23. Zorlu CG, Turan C. Emergency hysterectomy in modern practice changing clinical perspective in time in Turkey. Acta Obstet Gynecol Scan. 1998;77(2):186-90.

CHAPTER

27 Bladder Injuries and Other Complications

MS Agrawal, Sumit Bansal

INTRODUCTION

The close embryologic development and anatomic proximity of the urinary and genital organs predisposes the urinary tract to injury during surgical procedures in the female pelvis (Figs 1A and B). Though it is difficult to estimate the true incidence of such injuries, the quoted incidence of ureteral injury in gynecological operations is 0.43% (0.2–0.5%) and of bladder injury is 0.5–1%. The reported incidence of ureter and bladder injury in obstetric operations is 0.25% and 0.3% respectively.

URETERAL INJURIES

Surgical Anatomy of the Ureter

The ureters descend retroperitoneally, lateral to the transverse processes of the vertebrae, over the anterior surface of the psoas muscles to pass dorsal to the ovarian vessels and then cross the pelvic brim and enter the true pelvis. Within the pelvis they descend anterior to the bifurcations of the common iliac vessels, forming the posterior boundary of the ovarian fossae. They then pass under the uterine arteries and turn anteriorly, medial to

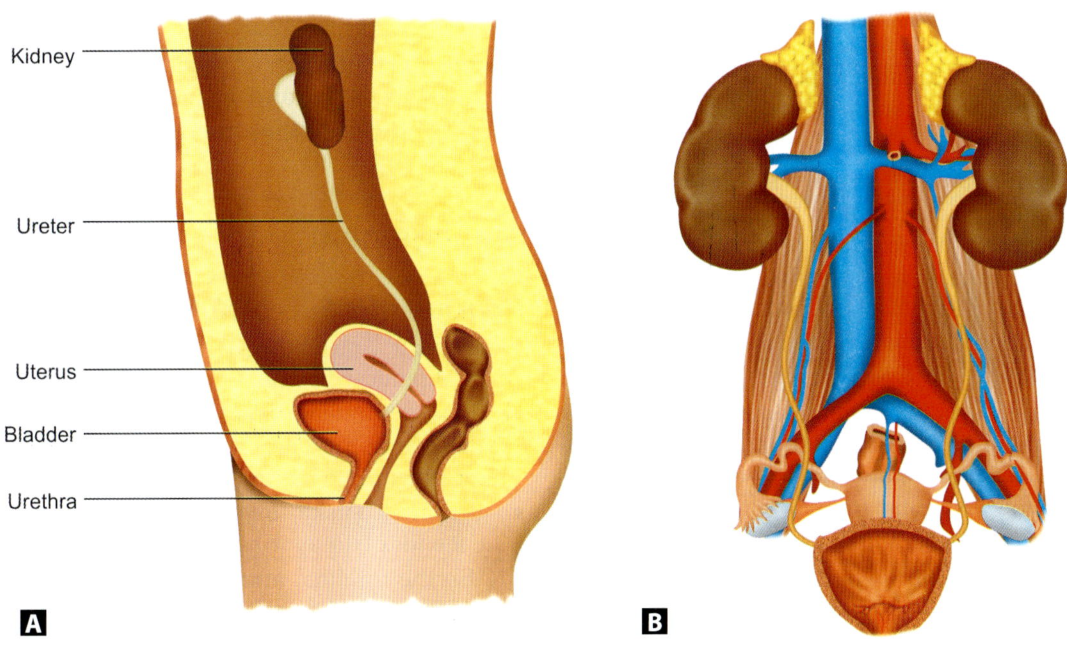

Figs 1A and B: Anatomical proximity of female genitalia to urinary tract

the obturator vessels and nerve, to pass about the cervix and upper vagina to enter 1.5–2.0 cm intramural tunnel within the base of the bladder. The ureters open into the bladder on either end of the interureteral ridge (Mercier's bar) that forms the base of the trigone of the bladder.

Incidence of Ureteral Injury

The surgical literature has historically attributed gynecologic procedures as a most common cause of ureteral injuries. Recent reviews have reported that urological procedures are more common cause of ureteral injuries (42%) followed by gynecologic procedures (34%) and general surgical procedures (24%).

Ureteral injury is much more likely to occur during an abdominal hysterectomy than during a vaginal hysterectomy. Other procedures associated with ureteral injuries are periaortic node dissections, obstetric procedures (e.g. cesarean section and cesarean or postpartum hysterectomy), and operative laparoscopy.

Pelvic surgery will never be free of ureteral injuries. However, it is possible to minimize the risk of ureteral injury by identifying the course of the pelvic ureters and vigilant surgery. Unfortunately, most surgical injuries to the ureter are not recognized at the time they occur. It is important for the surgeon to demonstrate the integrity of the ureter by surgical dissection whenever there is suspicion of ureteral injury during surgical procedure.

Diagnosis

Intraoperative

During surgery, if there is reason to suspect that ureteral injury has occurred, a number of procedures can be used to determine the location and extent of the injury. These include the following:

Ureteral dye injection: 5 mL of indigo carmine or methylene blue is injected through a 22-gauge needle into the ureter above the suspected site of injury. Resistance to the injection suggests ureteral obstruction, leakage of dye into the operative field below the injection site indicates ureteral injury, and excretion of dye in the urine suggests ureteral patency.

Intravenous (IV) dye injection: Injection of IV indigo carmine (5 mL) should be followed in 5–10 minutes by the excretion of blue urine. Complete bilateral ureteral obstruction prevents urine from reaching the bladder. Unilateral ureteral obstruction cannot be detected by the IV administration of indigo carmine unless ureteral excretion is observed via cystotomy or cystoscopy. Leakage of blue urine through an injured ureter into the operative site identifies an area of ureteral injury.

Intraoperative ureteral catheterization: The ureter(s) can be catheterized during surgery by ureterostomy, cystotomy or cystoscopy. A linear ureterotomy above the site of suspected injury permits catheter passage down the ureter and into the bladder. A cystotomy may be performed in the anterior wall of the bladder to visualize the ureteral orifices and to pass ureteral catheters. During an abdominal procedure, transurethral cystoscopy is a somewhat cumbersome method of ureteral catheter placement, unless the patient is in lithotomy position.

Dissection of the ureter: When there is concern about the integrity of a ureter, there is no substitute for dissecting the retroperitoneal space and visualizing the ureter throughout its course. Ureter can be easily identified on table by observing its peristalsis.

Postoperative

Approximately two-thirds of the cases are diagnosed postoperatively. Ureteric trauma can easily be missed, particularly in the case of unilateral injury. If the contralateral kidney is healthy, it will compensate for the loss with only a transient rise in serum creatinine. Eventually, the affected kidney will lose its function. The patients may complain of loin pain due to hydronephrosis. Pyrexia is common. A urinary fistula may arise at any time during the first 4 weeks after the operation communicating with vagina or uterine cavity (ureterovaginal/ureterouterine fistula) or with the skin (ureterocutaneous fistula).

If the urine is unable to escape, it will accumulate as a localized urinoma, which can present as abdominal distension, swinging pyrexia, or urinary ascites with ileus or peritonitis. Anuria develops in cases of bilateral ureteric obstruction (5–10% cases are bilateral). Early postoperative diagnosis of ureteric injury typically takes place 7–10 days after surgery. It is, however, important to remember that unilateral ureteric injury can be asymptomatic and may remain undetected.

Management

Principles for Successful Ureteral Repair

- Perform meticulous ureteral dissection using atraumatic instruments
- Preserve ureteral blood supply and microvasculature by leaving the peritoneal attachment and dissecting outside the adventitial sheath
- Perform a tension-free anastomosis with spatulation of cut ends of ureter to prevent stenosis
- Use the minimal amount of the smallest absorbable suture needed to obtain a watertight anastomosis
- Surround the anastomosis with retroperitoneal fat or omentum to assist healing
- Drain the retroperitoneal anastomotic site to prevent accumulation of urine, lymph or blood

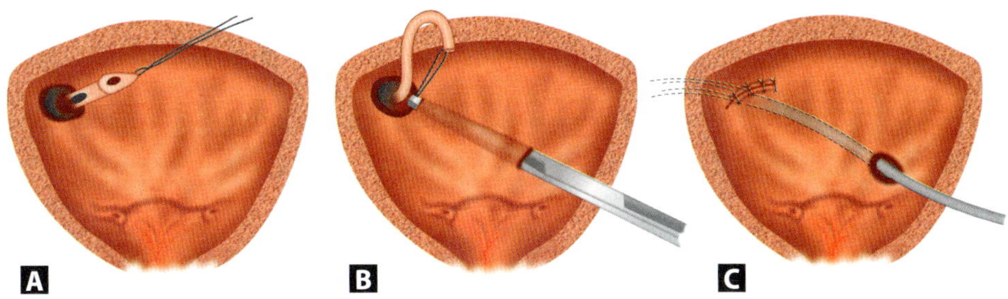

Figs 2A to C: Ureteroneocystostomy

- Ureteral stenting, using a "double J" (self-retaining) ureteric stent preferably, with or without proximal urinary diversion.

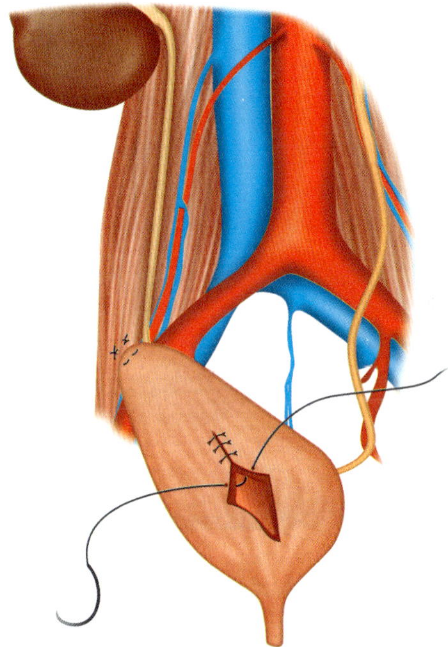

Fig. 3: Psoas hitch procedure

MANAGEMENT OF SPECIFIC INJURY TYPES

Ureteral Ligation

Complete ureteral ligation is an uncommon event. It is much more common that the ureter will be angulated or kinked by the placement of a suture that is either within the paraureteral tissue or partially placed through the ureter. In the first instance, which is probably much more common than has been recognized, simple ureterolysis, making sure that one stays out of the adventitial sheath, is all that is necessary. In those instances where the ureter has been either partially or totally ligated, management begins by removing the suture. Viability of ureter can be assessed by noticing blanching and blood flow through the vessels in the adventitial sheath, ureteral peristalsis and lack of discoloration. If there is any question about viability, the segment of the ureter must be resected and handled as outlined in the following section. A ureteral stent is placed once binding has been affected.

Partial Ureteral Transection

Repair of a partial transection is probably the easiest and fastest of all the ureteral injuries to manage. Because the ureterotomy already has occurred (although inadvertently), the ureteral stent is placed up and down through the ureterotomy. The ureter is repaired using 4-0 or 5-0 interrupted absorbable sutures over the ureteral stent. Excessive suture placement should be avoided.

Total Transection

Lower Third of Ureter

Following a ureteral transection of the lower third of the ureter, the standard for repair in these situations is ureteroneocystostomy with antireflux procedure over a ureteral stent (Figs 2A to C).

In case a tension-free anastomosis is not possible, psoas hitch procedure (Fig. 3) is undertaken in which bladder wall is brought close to the transected ureter by fixing to ipsilateral psoas muscle with nonabsorbable sutures.

If the length of ureter still falls too short for tension-free repair then there is a choice of doing Boari flap operation (Figs 4A to C). A broad based bladder wall flap is raised by which a tube is formed and this tube is anastomosed to the cut end of proximal ureter. Boari flap can be carried up to bridge long defects, even up to middle one-thirds of ureter.

Upper and Middle Thirds

Transection of the ureter in the upper and middle thirds in gynecological operations is uncommon. When this type of injury occurs, an ureteroureterostomy over a ureteral stent (Figs 5A to C) or transureteroureterostomy (Fig. 6) is the recommended method of repair. Both proximal and distal cut ends of the ureter are spatulated (to cut along the length of ureter to make flap closure) to prevent stricture formation

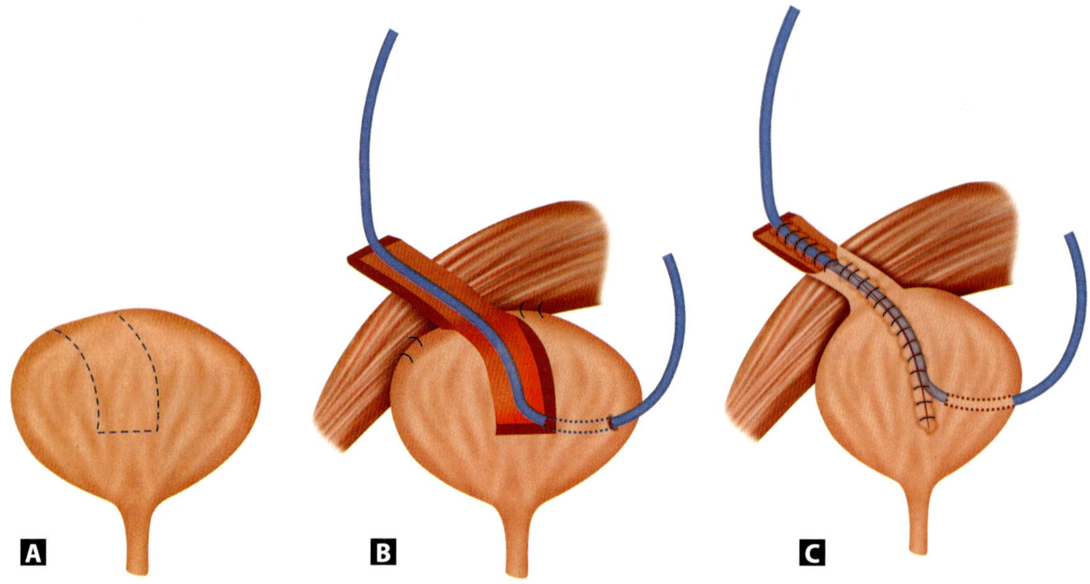

Figs 4A to C: Boari flap operation

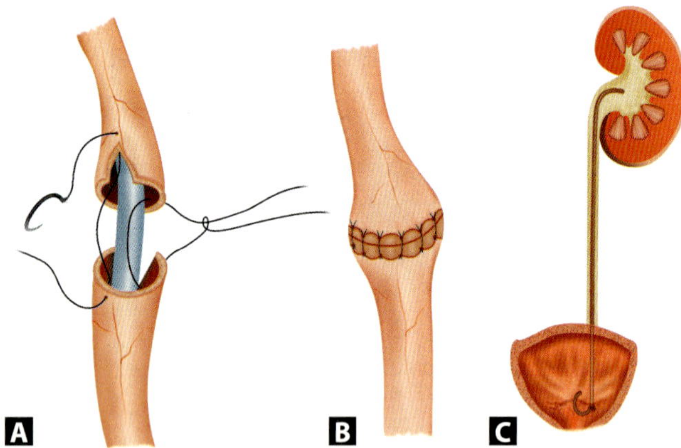

Figs 5A to C: Ureteroureterostomy over a double-J stent

at the anastomotic site. Extra length of the proximal segment of ureter can be obtained by mobilizing the kidney to make the anastomosis completely tension-free.

In cases where the divided ends of ureter cannot be brought together in a tension-free fashion using either proximal or distal mobilization, ureteroileal interposition (Fig. 7) or ileal replacement of ureter is the final approach for salvaging in these injuries.

PREVENTION OF URETERAL INJURY

Preoperatively, IV urograms may assist in detecting congenital anomalies of the urinary tract and in documenting involvement by disease processes. However, routine preoperative urograms have not been shown to lower the overall incidence of operative ureteral injuries.

Preoperative placement of ureteral catheters to assist in the identification and the dissection of the ureters during surgery is not always practical or desirable. Ureteral catheterization cannot be expected to reduce the overall incidence of ureteral injuries, most of which occur in patients for whom there is no indication that their use is needed. It has been suggested that during dissection of a ureter, an unyielding ureteral catheter may, in fact, cause mucosal injury or predispose the ureter to devascularization or laceration.

The most effective way to prevent ureteral injury during pelvic laparotomy is to identify the ureters as they enter the pelvis over the bifurcations of the common iliac arteries and to trace the pelvic course of each ureter during dissection of the retroperitoneal spaces. Every effort should be made to protect the blood supply to each ureter and the network of the microvasculature within the adventitial sheath of ureter.

BLADDER INJURIES

Intraoperative Recognition

Intraoperative injury to bladder is recognized by spillage of urine in the operative field. These injuries can be managed in the form of immediate bladder repair in single or double layer using 2-0 or 3-0 continuous absorbable sutures with catheter drainage of urinary bladder (Fig. 8). Prognosis is excellent.

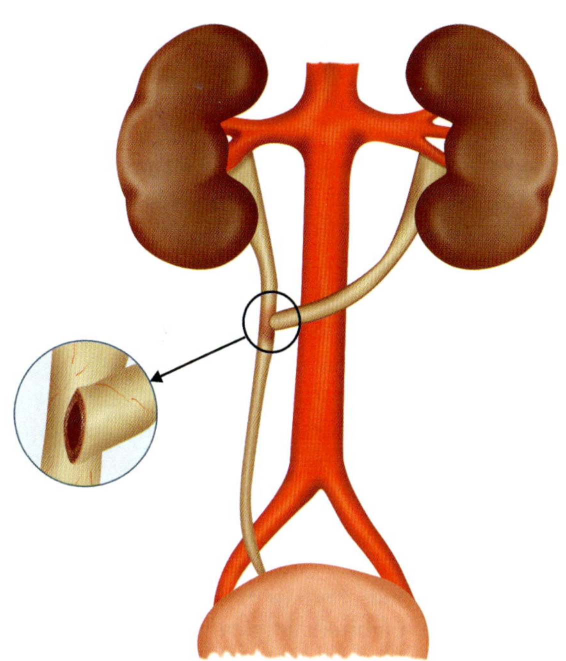

Fig. 6: Transureteroureterostomy

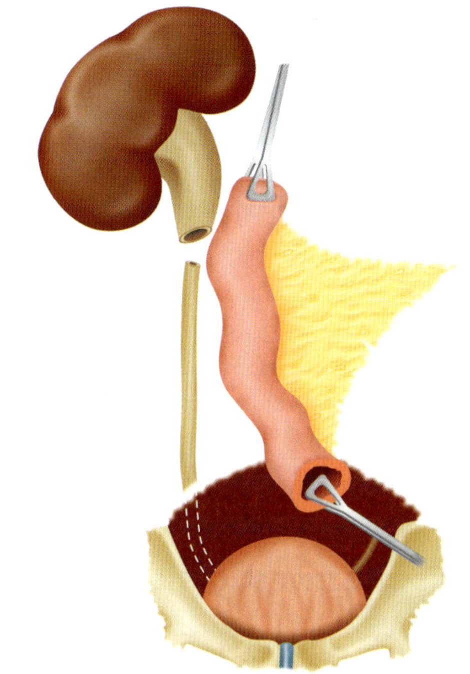

Fig. 7: Ureteroileal interposition

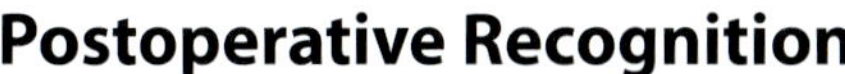

Postoperative Recognition

Postoperatively bladder injuries usually present as urinary fistula. In the western world, it usually results from pelvic surgery or pelvic malignancy and its treatment. In third world countries, obstructed labor leading to pressure necrosis continues to be a common cause. The duration of obstruction and the level at which descent of the presenting part is arrested determine the extent of tissue damage. Not only the bladder but sometimes the urethra and ureters together with the rectum and cervix may be involved in the sloughing process.

A fistula first recognized after hysterectomy is usually the result of unrecognized penetration or laceration at the time of the primary operation, the result of trauma recognized but inadequately repaired, or sometimes the result of postoperative necrosis of an area of bladder wall devascularization by a suture placed into or immediately adjacent to the bladder wall.

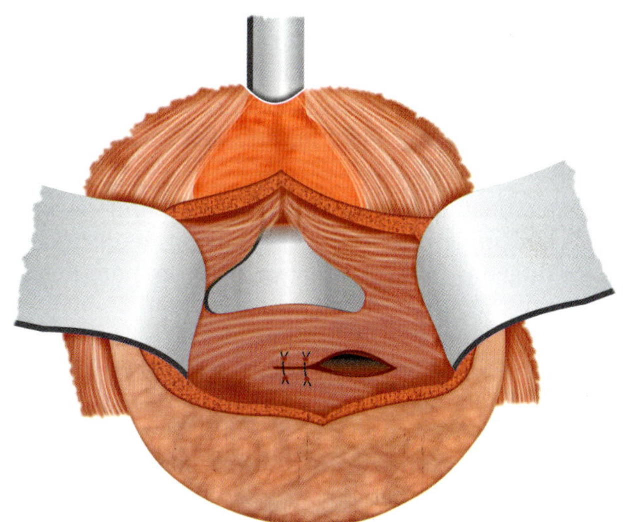

Fig. 8: Immediate bladder repair

Clinical Presentation

The presenting feature of vesicovaginal fistula (VVF) is continuous leakage of urine from the vagina. In both obstetric and gynecological fistulae, urinary leakage is most commonly recognized in the first 10 days after operation and less commonly, between the 10th and 20th postoperative day.

In obstetric fistula, leakage usually starts after sloughing of tissues affected by pressure necrosis, whereas in the case of posthysterectomy VVF, onset of symptoms and early diagnosis may be delayed by postoperative vaginal cuff edema. In rare cases, it may be difficult to distinguish urine loss secondary to a VVF and other forms of urinary incontinence, like severe stress incontinence.

The size and location of the fistula determines the degree of leakage. Patients with small fistulae may void normal amounts of urine and may experience leakage only at maximal bladder capacity. Women with larger fistulae may not be able to collect enough urine intravesically in order to void normally. Irritation of the vagina, vulvar mucosa, and perineum follows and women complain of a foul ammoniacal odor. As urea is split by vaginal flora, the vaginal pH becomes alkaline, which precipitates greenish-gray phosphate crystals in the vagina and on the vulva. Large vaginal encrustations are seen with fistulae secondary to neglected vaginal foreign bodies.

Fistula Site

The clinical grouping of fistulae involving the urinary bladder system is as follows (Fig. 9):

- Vesicovaginal fistula without urethral involvement
- Vesicovaginal fistula with partial or complete urethral destruction
- Vesicocervical or vesicouterine fistula.

Diagnosis and Investigations

Even though a diagnosis is obvious in many patients, a thorough urologic investigation is mandatory, especially to rule out coexistent fistulae. Evaluation begins with a history and physical examination facilitated by use of a speculum, good lighting and positioning. A history of large-volume vaginal leakage with no voided urine suggests a sizable VVF, whereas lesser vaginal fluid drainage associated with regular voiding raises the possibility of an ureterovaginal fistula or, perhaps, a very small or intermittent VVF. Leakage from the vagina during and after voiding suggests a urethrovaginal fistula.

Differentiation between a VVF and an ureterovaginal fistula is of primary importance. In making this distinction, many surgeons find that the two swab tests are helpful. Two swabs are inserted into the vagina, and 25–50 mL of methylene blue or indigo carmine solution is then injected into the bladder. The patient is instructed to walk around for 10 or 15 minutes, after which the swabs are examined. If only the lower swab is wet and blue, the patient presumably has urinary stress incontinence or detrusor instability; if the upper swab is wet and blue, the patient probably has a VVF; if the upper swab is wet but not blue, the diagnosis is a ureterovaginal fistula. Vaginal fluid may be collected for measurement of urea concentration, and a urinalysis and urine culture may identify the presence of a concomitant infection. IV urography and ultrasonography are used to exclude concomitant ureterovaginal fistula. A ureterovaginal fistula is associated commonly with hydronephrosis and hydroureter because stenosis of the ureter occurs at the site of the injury. Scarring at the edges of a VVF in the region of the ureteral orifice also may lead to ureteral stenosis and proximal dilatation.

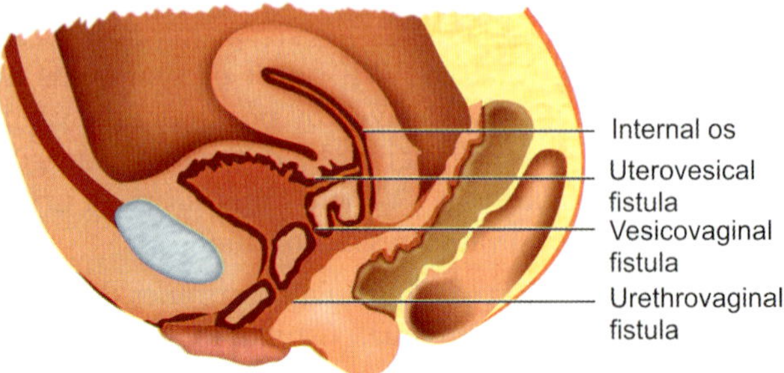

Fig. 9: Sagittal section showing different fistulae

Urethrovaginal fistulae usually are easily distinguished on examination. Small fistulae can be identified more easily if a probe can be passed through the fistula from the vagina into the bladder.

Cystoscopy is a crucial adjunct to demonstrate the location and size of the fistula as well as proximity to one or both ureteral orifices. This also assesses the bladder mucosa for edema and persistent necrosis, which may complicate planned surgical repair. A retrograde ureteropyelogram may also be done to fully evaluate the ureter.

The surgeon must always consider the possibility of multiple fistulae when investigating a recognized fistula. Obviously, the surgical correction of the recognized fistula will not eliminate incontinence resulting from an unrecognized and thus unrepaired coexistent fistula.

Treatment

Optimal results for fistula closure are obtained when surgery is performed on a mature fistula tract. It is generally agreed that the first effort at surgical fistula closure is the most likely to succeed. Results approximating 90% are obtainable on the first operative intervention in women who have not undergone radiation and do not have active carcinoma as the cause of the fistula. Multiple factors affect the success of fistula repair, including the etiology, duration of fistula, the presence of necrotic tissues, and surgical technique and experience of the operating surgeon.

Surgical Principles in Bladder Fistula Surgery

- Obstetrical fistula should be repaired after a minimum of 3 months from the time of fistula formation to buy time for local necrosis and edema to settle down
- The bladder and vaginal walls should be closed in different planes so that as little as possible of one suture line is superimposed on the other
- Postsurgical fistula can be treated in the early postoperative period as soon as fistula is diagnosed as

the tissue margins are usually healthy and there is not much of tissue necrosis

- To avoid intraoperative injury to ureter, ureteric catheter should be placed before starting surgery
- Tissue interposition should be undertaken whenever possible to achieve better results and reduction in risk of recurrence
- Cystourethroscopic examination during the course of an operation should be done to determine the proper eversion of healthy tissue and mucosa-to-mucosa approximation within the bladder.

Surgical approaches used for VVFs include vaginal, abdominal or combined abdominovaginal. The approach chosen is contingent on several factors, including location of fistula (position related to trigone and ureteric orifices), quality of tissue and surgical experience.

Vaginal surgery is more rapid and results in less morbidity and more rapid recovery; however, the vaginal route is difficult in patients with a significant degree of fibrosis, with pelvic immobility, or with large fistulae in close proximity to the ureteral orifices.

The abdominal approach should be used for patients with a poorly visualized or highly placed tract or a narrow or immobile vagina or in whom there is close proximity to a ureteral orifice. All approaches should lend themselves to the possibility of interposition grafts, which should be used liberally by the operative surgeon.

Vaginal Approach

The vaginal approach uses the creation of an anterior vaginal wall mucosal flap. Subsequently, a tension-free closure is performed using a long-acting (polyglycolic acid or polydioxanone) suture and nonoverlapping closure lines. Interposition tissue may be mobilized from labia, peritoneum, or vaginal advancement flaps.

A suprapubic catheter should be placed. Urinary drainage should also be supplemented with a urethral catheter. If the fistula communication occurs in proximity to the ureteral orifices, ureteral catheterization should be performed with cystoscopic assistance before fistula closure. Optimal visualization is dependent on tissue mobility. The use of lateral relaxing incisions may help operative visualization and approach to the fistulous tract.

To assist dissection, vaginal retraction is obtained with a self-retaining retractor, and a small balloon catheter (Fogarty or Foley) should be placed in the fistula tract. A vaginal incision is accomplished utilizing either a U- or a J-type incision incorporating the base of the fistula tract in the flap. The flap is usually oriented anteriorly for fistulae located at the cuff; however, posterior flaps may also be used, depending on the location of the fistula. The fistula tract is circumscribed but should not be widely excised. In contradistinction to the abdominal approach, the excision of the fistula tract may result in a large defect that may compromise the integrity of the closure.

Complete mobilization of the vaginal wall away from the edges of the fistulous tract is performed, and the vaginal wall opposite the flap is excised to allow advancement of the vaginal flap beyond the fistula's repair site once the fistula itself is closed. Some debridement of the fistula edges may be required to avoid a "bunching" effect on the tissue with closure. The tract itself is closed using a 2-0 to 3-0 polyglycolic suture. This layer incorporates the fistula tract and full thickness of the bladder wall. A second closure layer is completed vertically to the first suture line using similar suture in the perivesical tissue. The integrity of the closure may then be tested using fluid placed into the bladder followed by re-examination of the fistula tract vaginally. A third closure layer is then completed by advancing the vaginal wall over the fistulous closure site using absorbable suture (either polyglycolic acid or chromic gut).

Vaginal pack is placed, and continuous catheter drainage with both suprapubic and urethral catheters is maintained. If the fistula repair is tenuous or there is concern regarding apposition of suture lines, a Martius interpositional graft may be used. If this is not obtainable, alternative graft sources include a peritoneal flap or an interposition graft using gracilis muscle tissue. The peritoneum can be freed from the posterior aspect of the bladder and easily advanced to cover the layers of the closure as well.

Martius interposition uses the fibrofatty tissues of the labia majora, which are well vascularized (Fig. 10). The fat pad may be mobilized using either anterior or posterior based pedicle because of the constancy of blood supply. After mobilization of the fat pad, the graft is tunneled under the vaginal wall from labia to vaginal incision and is sutured in place over the fistula repair site with absorbable sutures. The vaginal mucosal flap is then closed over the site. A small Penrose drain is usually placed in the harvest site (the labia) to prevent hematoma accumulation.

In patients who are poor operative candidates, the Latzko technique of proximal vaginal fistula repair may also be attempted. This technique involves excision of the vaginal epithelium around the fistula site and colpocleisis, with several layers of absorbable sutures from anterior to posterior wall obliterating the upper vagina. No actual excision of the fistula tract occurs during this procedure.

Abdominal Approach

All bladder fistulae (except those extending into the urethra) may be approached using the abdominal approach, and this is the preferred approach in those

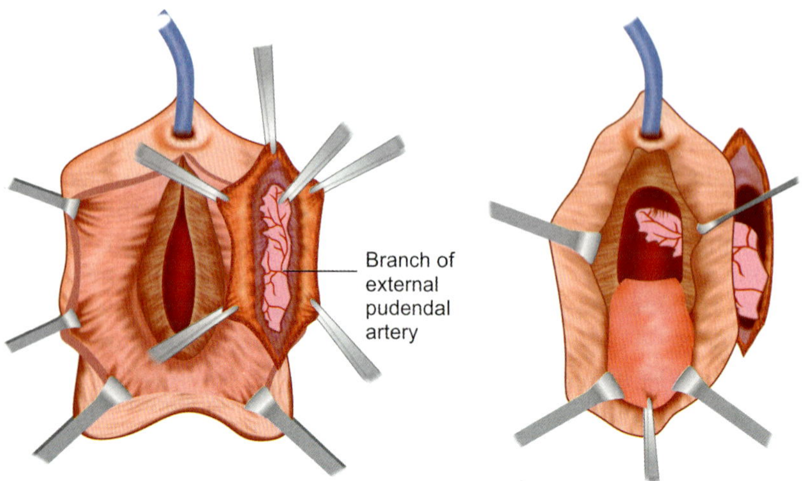

Fig. 10: Martius interpositional graft (vaginal approach)

patients requiring bladder augmentation or ureteral reimplantation. This technique requires placement of ureteral catheters to localize the ureteral orifices. An abdominal incision is then performed (midline or Pfannenstiel) and anterior wall of bladder is opened. The bladder and vaginal walls are mobilized and separated from each other by dissecting along the vesicovaginal septum. A complete excision of the fistula tract is completed. If the tract is extensively indurated, a posterior bladder flap may be mobilized to repair the defect. Separate closure of the vagina and bladder is performed using absorbable sutures (polydioxanone or polyglycolic).

In difficult cases and with large fistula, bisection of the bladder to the level of the fistula is done, fistula is excised in toto and vagina and bladder closed in separate layers with omental interposition.

This technique is most expeditiously performed intraperitoneally, although an extraperitoneal approach may be used. The intraperitoneal technique allows for harvesting of the omentum, whereas the extraperitoneal approach relies on perivesical or extraperitoneal fibrofatty tissue interposition. The omentum is secured between the bladder and the vagina with 3-0 polyglycolic acid sutures (Fig. 11).

In general, the vaginal approach avoids the potential morbidity associated with abdominal surgery and is believed to provide a quicker recovery and a more cosmetic result. It does not require a laparotomy so it is considered to be easier, safer and more comfortable for the patient.

In large complex fistulae, a combined vaginal and abdominal approach may be helpful.

Postoperative Care

Patient management after vaginal, abdominal or combined fistula repair approach is similar. Uninterrupted urinary drainage with large urethral and suprapubic catheters is crucial, as is bladder paralysis obtained with either oral or intrarectal anticholinergics. IV or oral antibiotics may be used as long as the urinary catheters are in place. Catheter drainage should be used for 10–14 days postoperatively before a voiding cystourethrography (VCUG) to confirm fistula tract closure. Anticholinergics should be discontinued for approximately 24–48 hours before performing the VCUG. If the closure is confirmed and the patient is able to void once the urethral catheter is removed, then the suprapubic catheter may be subsequently removed.

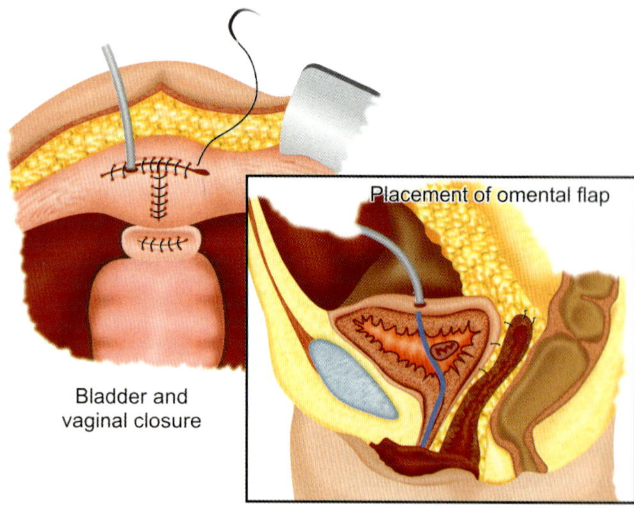

Fig. 11: Vesicovaginal fistula repair (abdominal approach)

Estrogens both orally and topically should be used preoperatively as well as perioperatively to promote healing. Vaginal manipulation should be avoided for the first 2 months postoperatively to avoid creating undue tension on the suture lines.

Complications

Complications pertinent to the surgery include fistula recurrence, injury to surrounding structures including ureters and dyspareunia resulting from cicatricial vaginal stenosis. Recurrent fistulae identified immediately postoperatively should be managed conservatively; however, if a fistula persists, a secondary repair should be undertaken after postoperative mucosal inflammation has resolved. If ureteral obstruction supervenes, the possibility of endoscopic and percutaneous management should be considered. In those patients who develop significant vaginal stenosis, use of relaxing interpositional vaginal grafts should be considered to improve vaginal dimensions.

RARE FISTULAE

Vesicouterine and Vesicocervical Fistulae

Vesicouterine and vesicocervical fistulae are suspected if urine escapes through the external cervical os. A standing lateral cystogram or hysterogram will confirm the diagnosis. Urinary incontinence does not always occur with vesicocervical fistula, the sole symptom is sometimes menstrual hematuria, erroneously suggesting endometriosis of the bladder. Vesical endometriosis should be excluded by careful cystoscopic examination.

Menouria, which may consist of cyclic hematuria, a vesicouterine fistula above the level of the internal cervical internal os, and apparent amenorrhea in the presence of a patent cervix but without coincident urinary incontinence has come to be known as Youssef's syndrome.

Vesicocervical fistula has been reported as a result of a cesarean section during which a suture used in the repair of the uterine incision compromising the integrity of the bladder. Occasionally, such a fistula develops after uterine rupture as a result of precipitate labor.

Surgery involves the anatomic dissection and separation of the bladder from the uterus at the site of the fistula, freshening of the edges and separate repair of each organ with absorbable suture. Catheter decompression of the bladder for at least 10 days after surgery is desirable.

Such a fistula may be repaired preferably abdominally and the option of coincidental hysterectomy considered according to the patient's wishes for future reproduction. Normal subsequent pregnancy and delivery have been reported in patients in whom the uterus was retained.

Urethrovaginal Fistulae

Urethrovaginal fistulae may present with a variety of complaints, depending on the location of the fistula. Patients with distal fistulae may be asymptomatic or complain of spraying of urine or an otherwise abnormal urinary stream. Midurethra fistulae may present with stress incontinence, recurrent cystitis or no symptoms. Fistulae involving the proximal urethra and bladder neck present similar to VVF.

The repair of urethrovaginal fistulae is more difficult than for VVF. Extensive urethral loss and lack of viable tissue may make conventional layered closures difficult. Tissue interposition in the form of Martius flap is extremely useful in these cases. It is generally reported that the success rate of urethrovaginal fistula repair is 73–100%. The surgical principles of VVF repair also apply to the correction of urethrovaginal fistulae.

BIBLIOGRAPHY

1. Al-Juburi A, Aloosi I, Khundra S. Unusual vesicovaginal fistulas. Obstet gynaecol. 1984;4:264.
2. Assimos DG, Patterson LC, Taylor CL. Changing incidence and etiology of iatrogenic ureteral injuries. J Urol. 1994;152:2240-6.
3. Ball TL. Gynecologic Surgery and Urology, 2nd edition. St Louis: Mosby; 1963.
4. Chan JK, Morrow J, Manetta A. Prevention of ureteral injuries in gynecologic surgery. Am J Obstet Gynecol. 2003;188:1273-7.
5. Cruikshank SH. Surgical method of identifying the ureters during total vaginal hysterectomy. Obstet Gynecol. 1986;67:277-80.
6. Hurd JK. Vaginal repair of vesicovaginal fistula. In: Libertino JA, Zinman L (Eds). Reconstructive Urologic Surgery. Baltimore: Williams and Wilkins; 1977.
7. Mattingly RF, Thompson JD. Te Linde's Operative Gynecology, 6th edition. Philadelphia: JB Lippincott Co; 1985.
8. Park RC, Duff WP. Role of cesarean hysterectomy in modern obstetric practice. Clin Obstet Gynecol. 1980;23:601-20.
9. Piscitelli JT, Simel DL, Addison WA. Who should have intravenous pyelograms before hysterectomy for benign disease? Obstet Gynecol. 1987;69:541-5.
10. Symmonds RE. Ureteral injuries associated with gynecologic surgery: prevention and management. Clin Obstet Gynecol. 1976;19:623-44.
11. Thompson RH. Ureteral injuries in pelvic surgery. Bull Dept Gynecol Obstet Emory U. 1980;11:93.
12. Youssef AF. Menouria following lower segment cesarean section; a syndrome. Am J Obstet Gynecol. 1957;73:759-67.

CHAPTER

28

Cesarean Section

Sukumar Barik, Narayan Jana, Ashis Kumar Mukhopadhyay

INTRODUCTION

Rising trend of cesarean section (CS) rate is a major public health concern worldwide. There appears no indication of reversal of this trend in the foreseeable future, and the procedure continues to be associated with increased rate of maternal morbidity and mortality, compared to vaginal delivery. It is of paramount importance that evidence based, sound, safe and most effective techniques are adopted in each step of this operation. Better anesthetic techniques, availability of wide-spectrum antibiotics, improvement in transfusion medicine and significant development of neonatal care have also made obstetric practice safer. Furthermore, optimum preoperative preparation and postoperative care has also produced a palpable impact on the safety record of CS leading to more demand of the procedure "on request". A recent guideline has provided two-pronged approach to this complex issue of CS—adopting steps, which can reduce the likelihood of CS and identification of those interventions, which can reduce morbidity from CS (Box 1). Surgical techniques of CS have undergone many modifications in recent years. In spite of being practiced for more than several centuries, very few procedures have generated so much of controversies right from the indications through operative steps to the postoperative care.

Box 1 Interventions should be used to decrease morbidity from cesarean section

- Regional anesthesia
- Antibiotic prophylaxis
- Thromboprophylaxis
- Antacids
- Antiemetics

Source: Adopted from clinical guidelines on cesarean section. National Institute of Clinical Excellence. 2004.

INDICATIONS

Cesarean delivery is appropriate when the risk to the fetus and/or the mother is considered to be greater than that of vaginal delivery. Common indications are fetal distress, failure to progress, malpresentation and previous CS (Box 2). Cultural changes, expectations of the general population and the obstetricians' fear of litigation have an important impact on the changing rate and indication for CS. Economic incentive and lack of time in singularly managed obstetric care have also contributed to some extent.

Maternal wish/request/demand as a sole indication (in absence of any traditional obstetric indication) has received much attention in recent years. Primary elective cesarean performed on a patient's request now comprises 4–18% of all cesareans and 14–22% of elective cesareans in reported series. Patients most commonly choose cesarean because of tocophobia or fear of childbirth. This is a debatable issue and has its own advantages and disadvantages. Obstetricians are also widely divided in this issue.

Box 2 Major indications for cesarean section

- Dystocia—37.5%
- Fetal distress—33.4%
- Repeat section—29%
- Malpresentation—14.5%
- Pregnancy-induced hypertension—12.5%

PREOPERATIVE PREPARATION

Prevention of gastric content/acid aspiration is extremely important during CS. Use of hydrogen (H_2)-receptor blocker (ranitidine 150 mg); antiemetic (metoclopramide 10 mg) and nonparticulate antacid (sodium citrate 0.3 molar solution 30 mL) should be administered at least 2 hours before CS.

Position and Draping

A lateral tilt of 15° of the operating table is currently practiced to reduce maternal hypotension. Modifications of disposable draping have been found to be no more effective than conventional draping in reducing infective morbidity from the procedure.

Anesthesia

Cesarean section can be performed under either general or regional anesthesia. In the recent years, regional anesthesia is favored. Spinal anesthesia is currently being preferred in most cases of CS both in elective and emergency procedures. Although, benefits of regional anesthesia are several, recent Cochrane review has concluded effective anesthesia for CS can be provided by both spinal and epidural techniques. Both techniques are associated with moderate degrees of maternal satisfaction. Spinal anesthesia has a shorter onset time, but hypotension is more likely. There is no evidence from this review to show that regional anesthesia is superior to general anesthesia in terms of major maternal or neonatal outcomes. Further research is needed to evaluate neonatal morbidity and maternal outcomes including satisfaction with anesthetic technique.

OPERATIVE STEPS

- Checking lie, presentation, position and fetal heart sound
- Insertion of Foley catheter: In and out plain rubber catheter before CS is an alternative to insertion of Foley catheter. Proponents suggest that CS without urethral catheterization does not compromise with the safety or ease of surgery and it may reduce the risk of urinary infection. Current guidelines suggest that women undergoing CS under regional anesthesia require an indwelling catheter to prevent over distension of bladder because the anesthetic block interferes with normal bladder function
- Antiseptic dressing and draping
- Skin incision and opening abdomen: The choice of skin incision depends upon the indication of the operation, maternal body habitus, history of previous surgery, choice of the mother, and also on skill and preference of the surgeon. Like any other procedure, individualization is important, so that the choice gives the maximum benefit.

Transverse suprapubic incision is the most commonly practiced skin incision. Although there are several methods of entry into abdominal cavity, two main methods are discussed in details and other areas are discussed as alternative procedures.

In cases of Pfannenstiel's incision, skin incision is placed about 2–3 cm above the symphysis pubis (Fig. 1). Then the subcutaneous tissue is incised. Hemostasis is obtained using diathermy. Rectus sheath is incised in the middle and the incision is extended on both sides by the scissors (Fig. 2). Rectus sheath is held in both sides by Allies tissue forceps (Fig. 3) and dissected upward; hemostasis is again achieved with diathermy. The parietal peritoneum is identified and is held by two artery forceps. The incision is placed in between the two artery forceps after checking that no other structure is held by the artery forceps. The incision is extended upward and downward using scissors and taking care of the bladder.

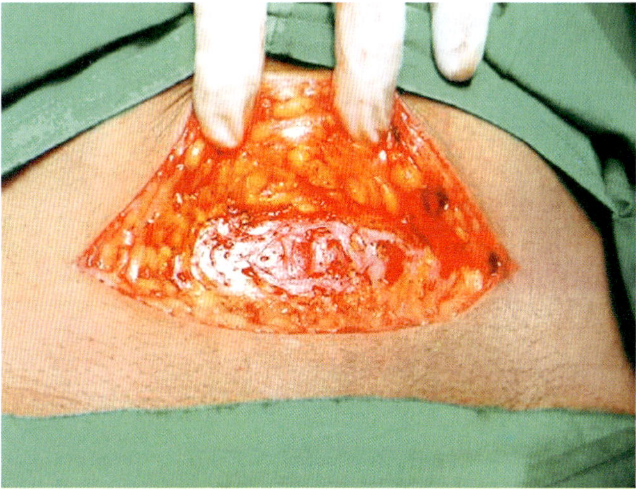

Fig. 1: Skin incision

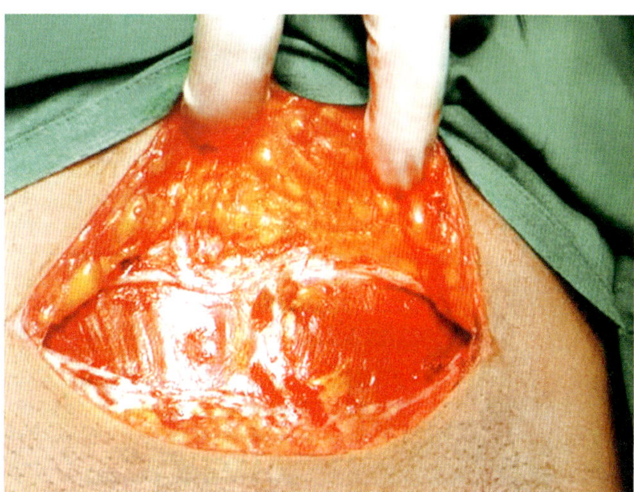

Fig. 2: Opening rectus sheath

In cases of modified Joel-Cohen incision, the skin incision is placed slightly higher. This is also a transverse suprapubic skin incision placed about 3 cm below the line joining the anterior superior iliac spines. About 3 cm area in the midline is incised into the rectus sheath and then the sheath is stretched laterally using both index fingers. The upper flap of the rectus sheath is held by index and middle finger and pulled upward. Parietal peritoneum is identified and finger dissection is done, and hole is made in the parietal peritoneum. The opening of the parietal peritoneum is extended by the pull by the surgeon and the assistant (Fig. 4). Hemostasis is obtained by use of diathermy. Recently, further modification of the technique has been known as finger-assisted stretching technique (FAST) and shown to be equally safe and faster than the traditional method. A recent Cochrane review concluded that the Joel-Cohen incision has advantages compared to the Pfannenstiel's incision. There is less fever, pain and analgesic requirements; less blood loss; shorter duration of surgery and hospital stay. These advantages for the mother could be extrapolated to savings for the health system. However, these trials do not provide information on severe or long-term morbidity and mortality.

- Insertion of Doyen's retractor (Fig. 5)
- Checking rotation of uterus by the round ligaments, identification of lower segment, presenting part and loose fold of peritoneum
- Incision and division of uterovesical fold of peritoneum (Fig. 6)
- Pushing the bladder down: The lower flap of the peritoneum is held by a tissue forceps and the loose areolar tissue can be pushed down by finger dissection. Care must be taken to keep the finger toward the uterine side rather than the bladder side.

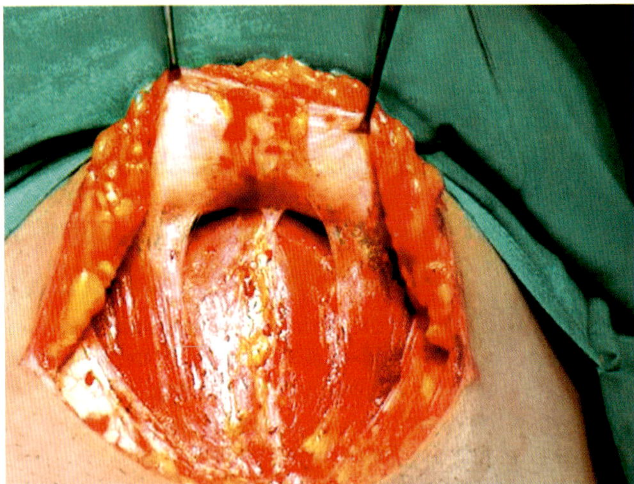

Fig. 3: Separating rectus sheath upward

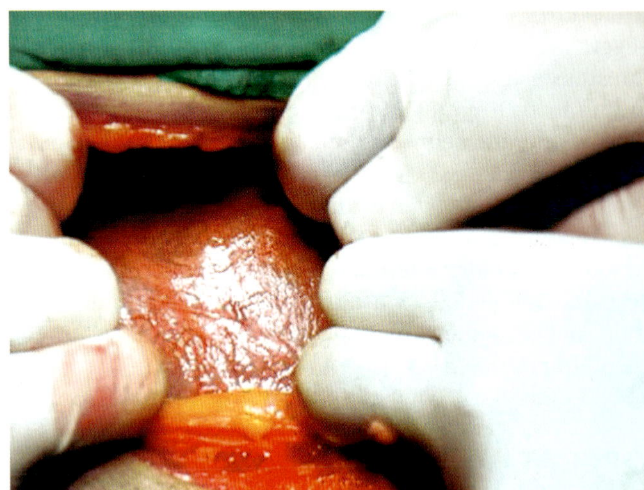

Fig. 4: Stretching abdominal wall laterally

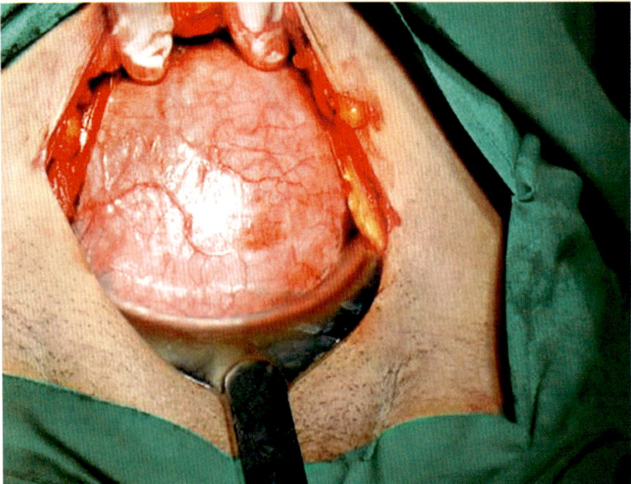

Fig. 5: Insertion of Doyen's retractor and identification of lower segment

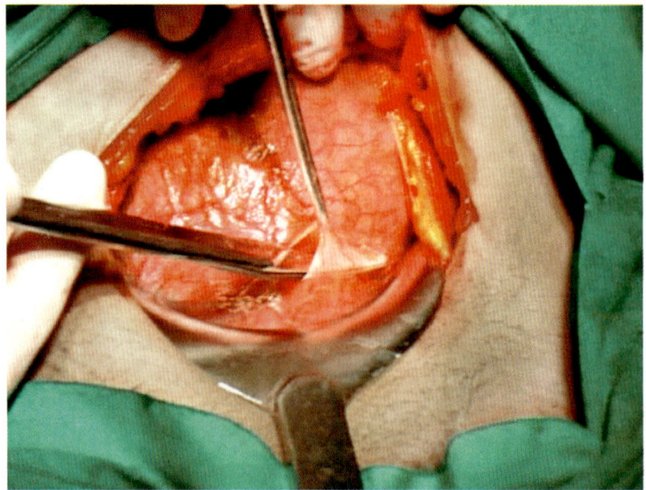

Fig. 6: Incising uterovesical fold of peritoneum

- Identification and placement of incision at uterine wall: Commonly practiced lower segment transverse incision is usually placed about 2–3 cm above the bladder base (Fig. 7). It is very important to remember that during CS in advanced labor or in second stage, the lower segment usually is very much stretched and incision is placed relatively higher to avoid the extension laterally and towards the vagina. Thick lower segment may pose a problem. There are several alternatives like making J-shaped, U-shaped or T-shaped incision. Occasionally, low midline incision may have to be considered. Placing a single silk suture just below lower segment for easier identification is a good practice
- Rupturing the membranes (Fig. 8)
- Extending uterine incision in two ways: the uterine incision is extended—either by finger stretching or placing the index and middle finger inside the incision line and dividing by the scissor (Fig. 9)
- Delivering fetal presenting part: Placing the right hand below the presenting part and once the fetal presenting part is held properly the Doyen's retractor is taken out and fundal pressure is applied by the assistant. The hand of the surgeon usually works as a fulcrum (Fig. 10). In cases of high floating head, application of low forceps may be necessary
- Clamping the cord and handing over baby to the assistant of the pediatrician (Figs 11A and B)
- Delivering the placenta: Waiting for spontaneous separation (technique similar to controlled cord traction) is usually preferred (Figs 12 and 13) over manual removal of placenta. The evidence suggests that manual removal of the placenta at CS may do more harm than good by increasing maternal blood loss and increasing the risk of infection
- Cleaning the uterine cavity: This procedure is not practiced routinely. Those who practice it explain that remaining bits of decidua or membranes can be

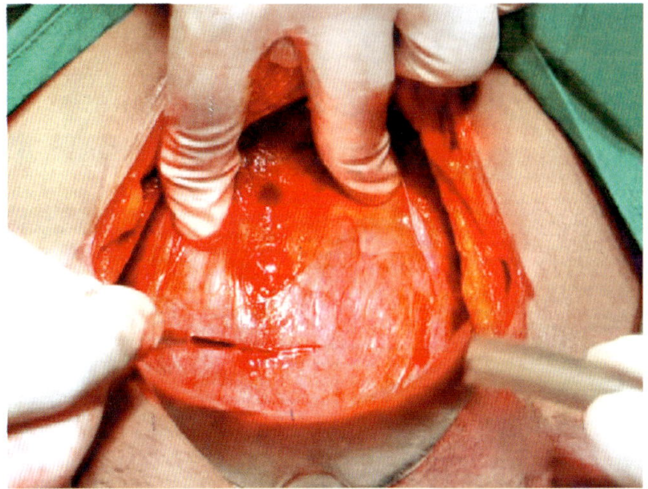

Fig. 7: Transverse incision on lower uterine segment

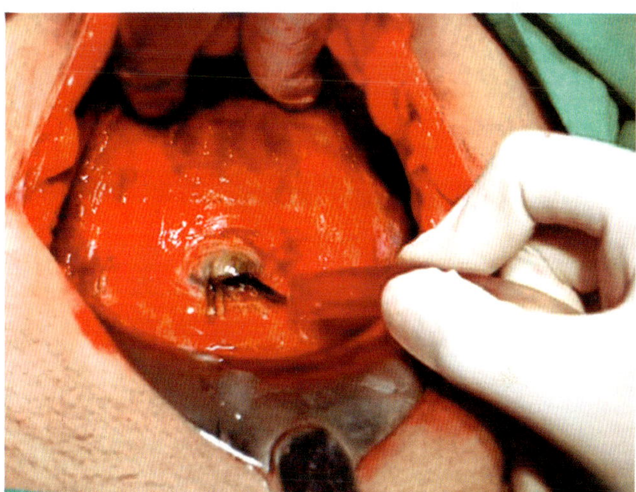

Fig. 8: Rupture of amniotic sac

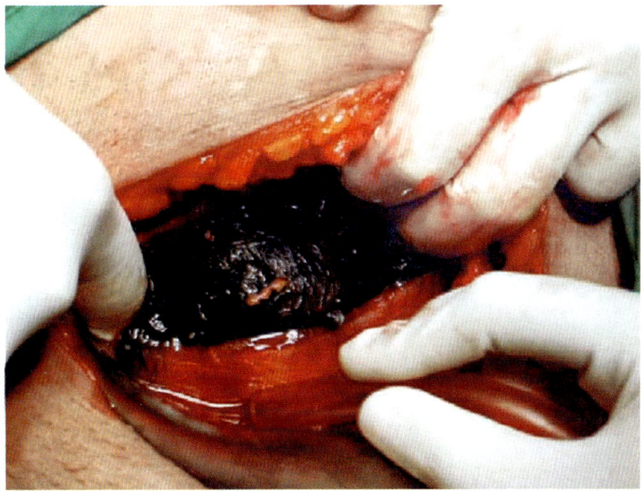

Fig. 9: Finger stretching of uterine incision

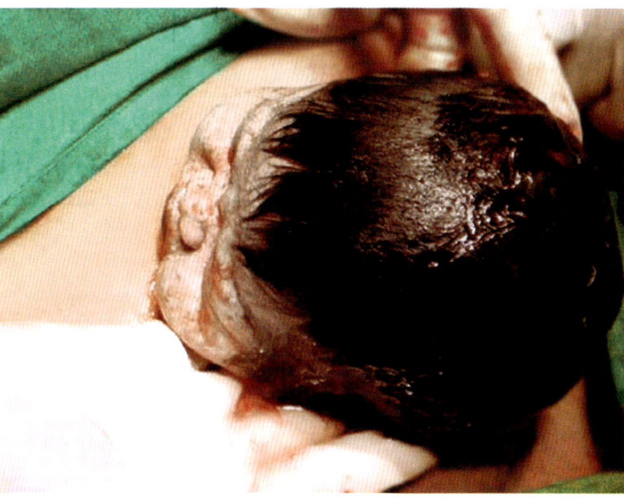

Fig. 10: Delivery of the fetus

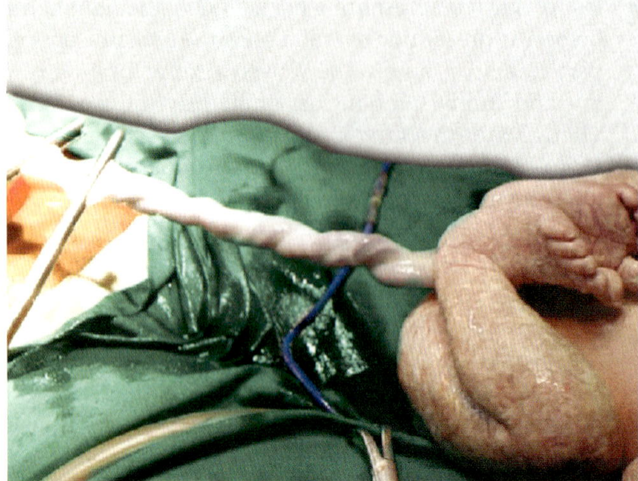

Fig. 11A: Clamping the cord

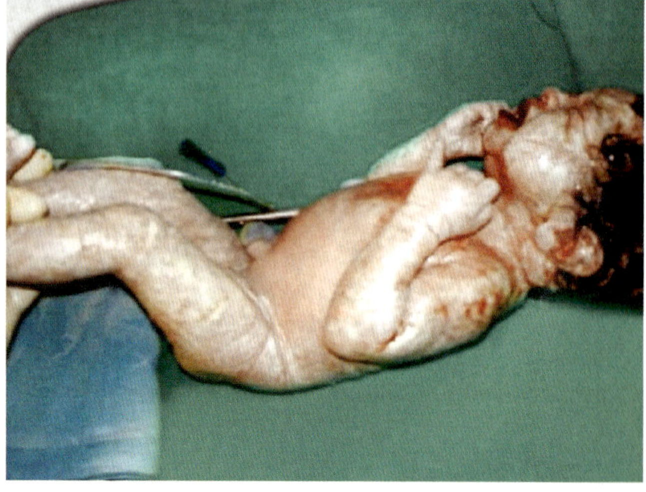

Fig. 11B: Handing over the baby to the assistant

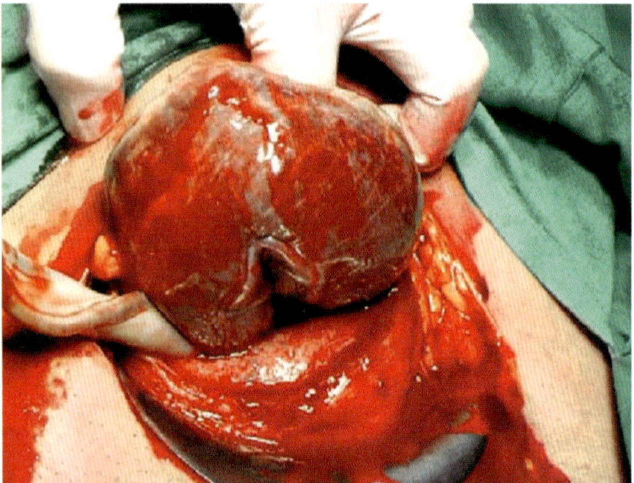

Fig. 12: Delivery of placenta

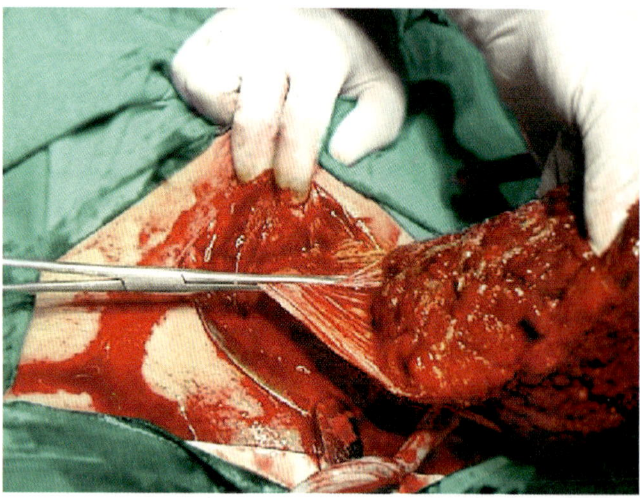

Fig. 13: Delivery of membranes

wiped out (Fig. 14). Those who do not, explain that this procedure is not performed during normal delivery, so why practice it? In addition, infective morbidity may increase rather than decreasing

- Identification of margins and application of hemostatic clamps: Application of hemostatic clamp is usually helpful not only for hemostasis but also for identification of the margins. Opinion varies about the type of hemostatic clamps used for this purpose. Green Armytage clamp (Fig. 15) is one of the commonly used one but some prefer the Allis's tissue forceps
- Dilating the internal os: Sometimes practiced, particularly during planned CS with the view of better drainage of lochia. Those who do not practice it is in the opinion that if menstrual blood can drain without much dilatation of the os then why to dilate it during

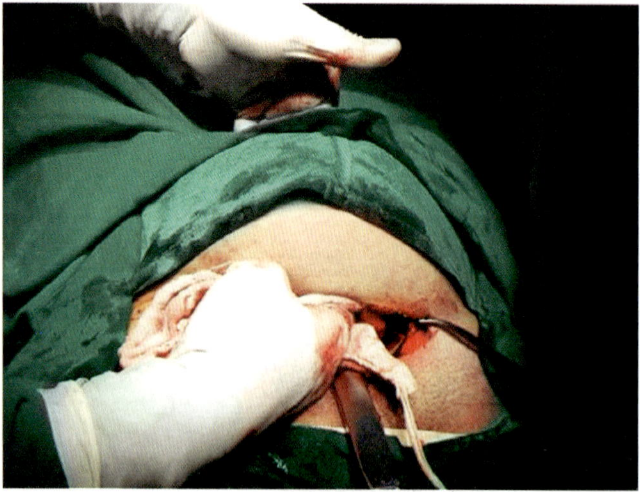

Fig. 14: Wiping the uterine cavity

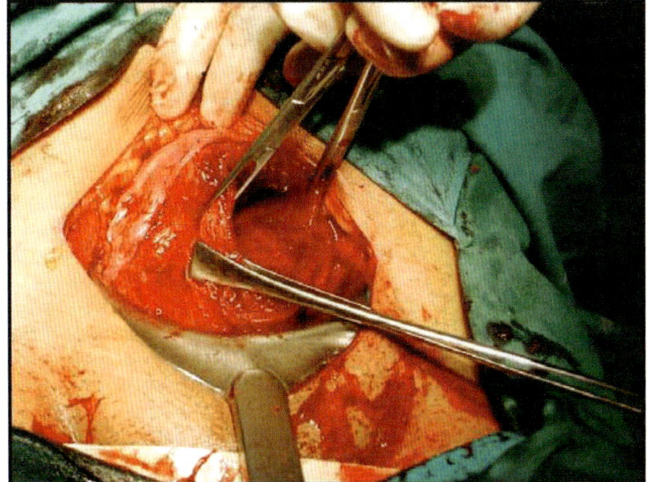

Fig. 15: Application of hemostatic clamps

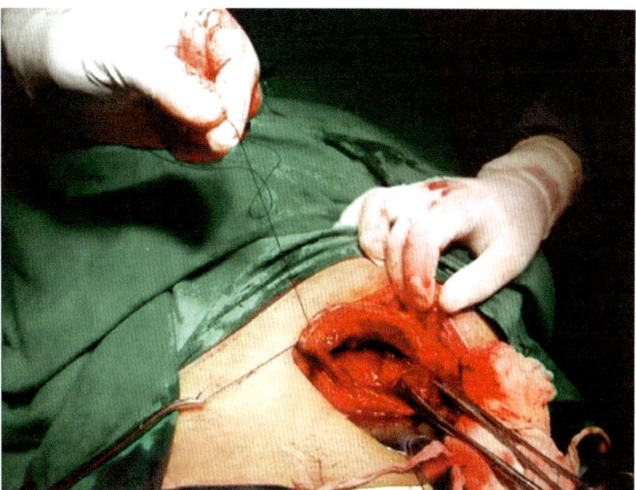

Fig. 16: Application of stay knot

section? A small study concluded that intraoperative cervical dilatation during elective CS did not reduce the risk of postoperative maternal fever, wound infection or change in hemoglobin concentration

- Repair of uterine incision: Approximation and hemostasis are the basics of any repair of the wound. There is considerable debate about the single layer closure versus double layer closure (Figs 16 to 19). The Cochrane review concluded that the only benefit of single layer closure is reduction in operative time. In a recent study of women on trial for vaginal delivery after CS, of the 948 subjects identified, 913 had double layer closure and 35 had single layer closure. The uterine rupture rate was significantly higher in the single-layer closure group (8.6% vs 1.3%, p = 0.015). The authors concluded that single-layer uterine closure may be more likely to result in uterine rupture
- Exteriorization of the uterus is also a topic of controversy. Exteriorization may cause more nausea and vomiting but the proponents describe the technical advantage of the repair and less bleeding. The Cochrane review concluded that there is no evidence from this review to make definitive conclusions about which method of uterine closure offers greater advantages, if any. However, these results are based on too few and too small studies to detect differences in rare, but severe complications
- Visceral peritoneum: Currently, repair of visceral peritoneum is not practiced
- Cleaning the paracolic gutter: Ideally should be done with suction whenever more than average amount of blood loss is found; but caution should be exercised in not being too vigorous and rubbing of the area with mops should be avoided. Only removal of large clots is recommended, not a thorough cleaning
- Inspection of adnexa: It is a good practice and sometimes may identify unsuspected adnexal mass, and can be dealt with at the same time of the operation (Fig. 20)
- Checking bladder margin
- Parietal peritoneum: Closure of parietal peritoneum is currently disfavored as we understood from animal experimentation that adhesion formation may be more if it is repaired with sutures. Several recent publications again are putting some doubts on this practice. Parietal peritoneal closure at primary cesarean delivery was fivefold protective against all adhesions (odds ratio 0.20, 95% confidence interval: 0.08–0.49) and threefold protective against dense adhesions (odds ratio: 0.32, 95% confidence interval: 0.13–0.79). Omental-fascial adhesions were decreased most consistently. This study concluded that parietal peritoneal closure at primary cesarean delivery was associated with significantly fewer dense and filmy adhesions. The practice of nonclosure of the parietal peritoneum at cesarean delivery should be questioned
- Inspecting/checking hemostasis below the rectus sheath is a must
- Sheath closure should be done taking care of identifying the angles properly. Stay knot in contralateral side is a good technique. No 1-0 polydioxanone suture (PDS) is preferred by some; vicryl 1-0 is a compromising alternative. No good study is available which has addressed this issue
- Checking hemostasis in subcutaneous layer (Fig. 21)
- Closure of subcutaneous layer: After securing satisfactory hemostasis, routine approximation of subcutaneous tissue is not practiced at present. A meta-analysis demonstrated that suture closure of subcutaneous fat during cesarean delivery results in

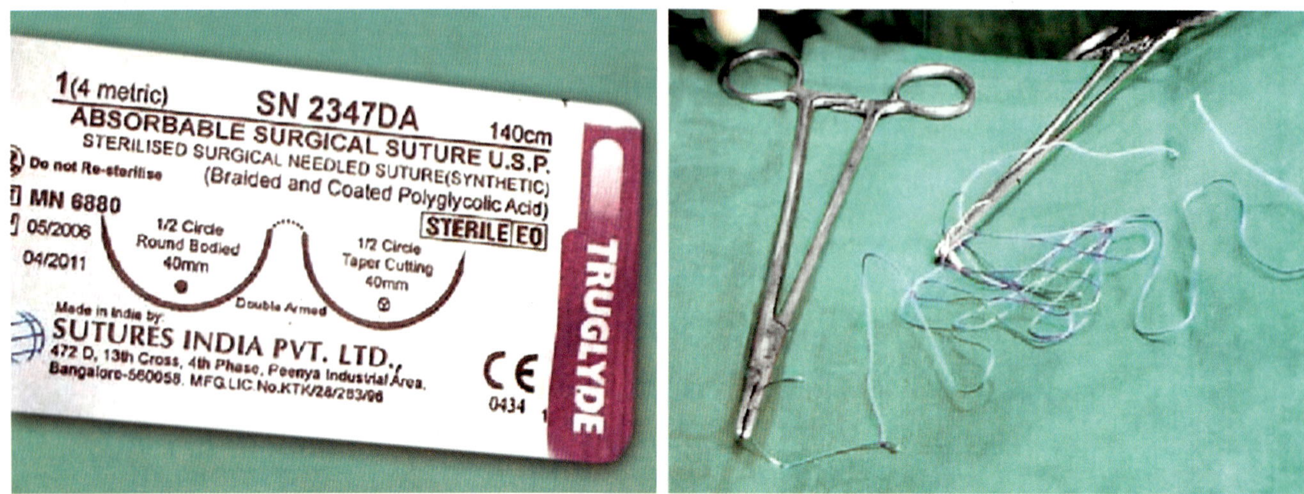

Fig. 17A: Single double needle polyglycolic acid suture for uterine wound closure

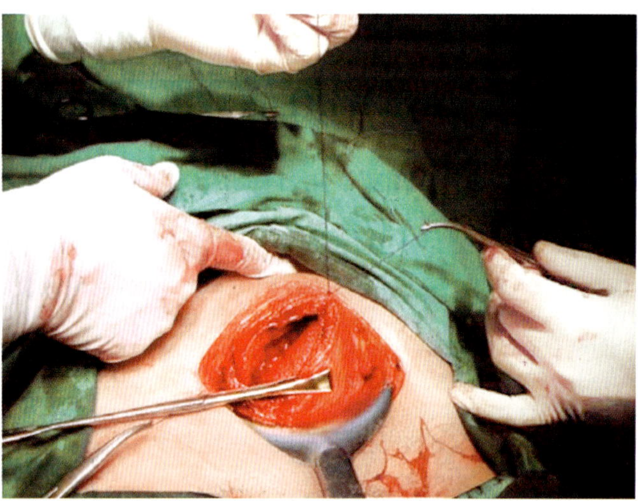

Fig. 17B: Suturing of first layer of uterine incision

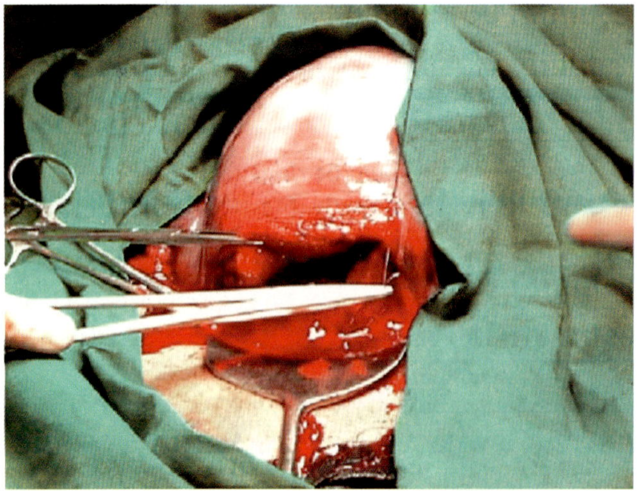

Fig. 18A: Continuous interlocking suture of uterine wound

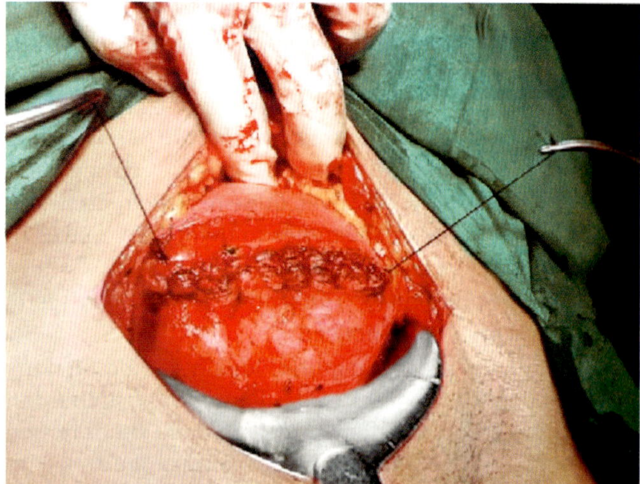

Fig. 18B: Completion of first layer suture

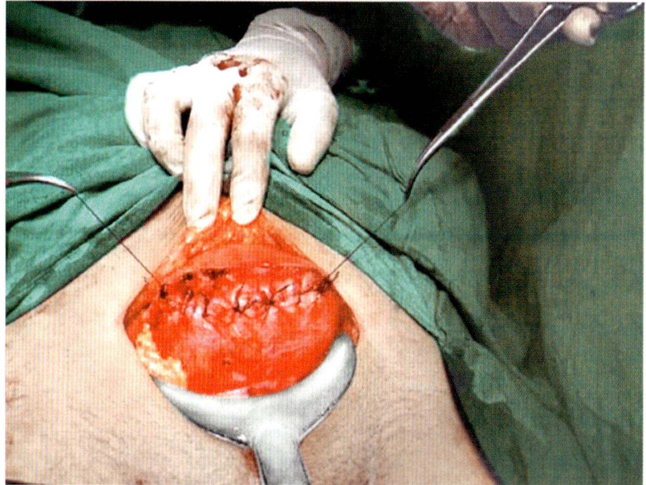

Fig. 19: Completion of second layer suture

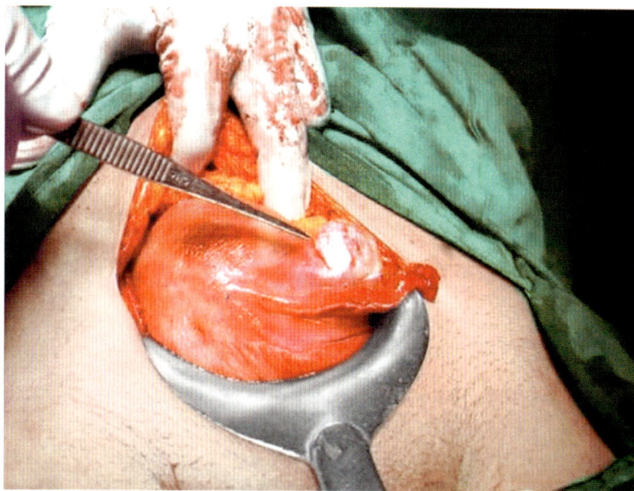

Fig. 20: Inspection of adnexa

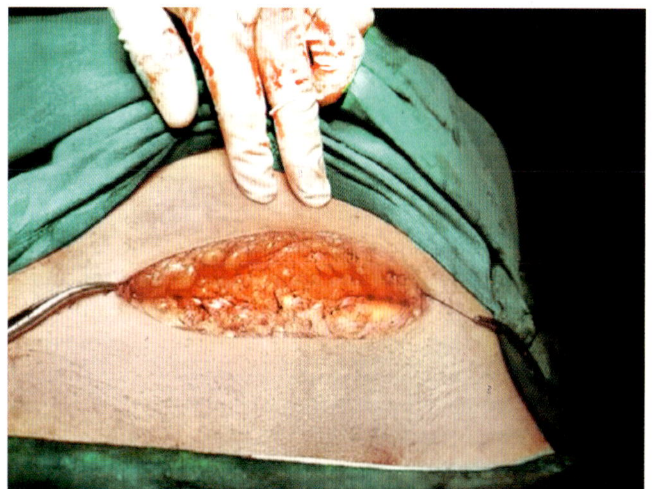

Fig. 21: Checking hemostasis in subcutaneous layer

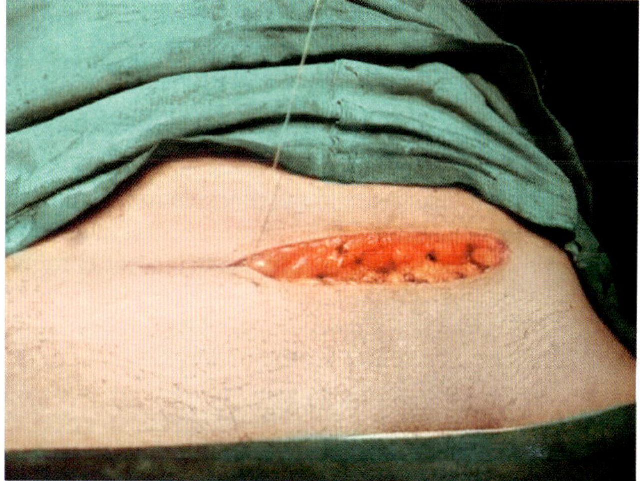

Fig. 22: Subcuticular skin suture

a 34% decrease in risk of wound disruption in women with fat thickness greater than 2 cm

- Skin closure: Currently, three methods of skin closure are in practice—subcutaneous repair using absorbable or nonabsorbable sutures, interrupted stitches using nonabsorbable sutures or staples (Figs 22 and 23). There is no conclusive evidence about how the skin should be closed after CS. Questions regarding the best closure technique and material and the outcomes associated with each remain unanswered. The appearance and strength of the scar following CS is important to women and the choice of technique and materials should be made by the woman in consultation with her obstetrician (based on the limited information currently available)
- Vaginal swabbing, practiced by few
- Application of dressing to the wound.

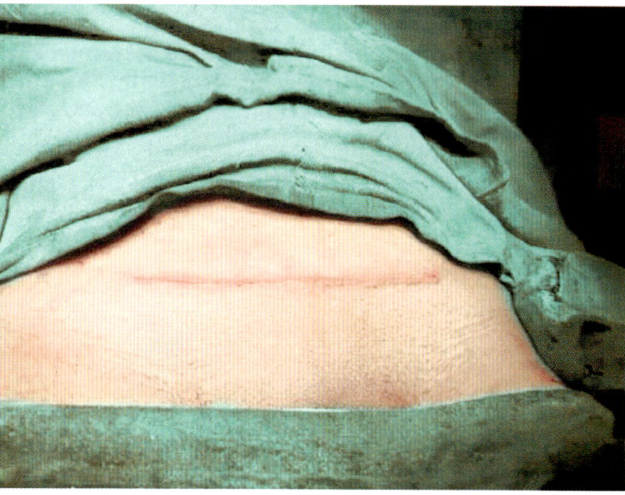

Fig. 23: Completed skin suture

Midline Abdominal Incision

In rare circumstances that a midline abdominal incision is used at CS, mass closure with slowly absorbable continuous sutures should be used because this results in fewer incision hernias and less dehiscence than layered closure.

Alternative Techniques

Pelosi Technique

A Pfannenstiel abdominal incision is used. Electrocautery is used to divide the subcutaneous tissues and the fascia transversely. The rectus muscles are separated by blunt dissection to provide space for both index fingers, which free the fascial layer vertically and transversely. The peritoneum is opened by blunt finger dissection and all the layers of the abdominal wall are stretched manually to the extent of the skin incision. The bladder is not reflected inferiorly. A small transverse lower segment incision is made through the myometrium and extended laterally, curving upward with blunt finger dissection or scissors. The baby is delivered with external fundal pressure, oxytocin is administered and the placenta removed after spontaneous separation. The uterus is massaged. The myometrial incision is closed with a single layer chromic catgut continuous locking suture. Neither peritoneal layer is sutured. The fascia is closed with a continuous synthetic absorbable suture. If the subcutaneous layer is thick, interrupted 3-0 absorbable sutures are used to obliterate the dead space. The skin is closed with staples.

Misgav-Ladach Technique

This technique is a modified Joel-Cohen technique. The Joel-Cohen abdominal incision is used. The uterus is opened as for the Joel-Cohen method. The placenta is removed manually. The uterus is exteriorized. The myometrial incision is closed with a single layer locking continuous suture. The peritoneal layers are not sutured. Continuous suture is used to close the fascia. The skin is closed with two or three mattress sutures. The skin edges are approximated with Allis forceps between these sutures, and are left in place for about 5 minutes while the drapes are being removed.

Classical Cesarean Section

The classical CS is a vertical incision into upper uterine segment and infrequently practiced in modern obstetrics. Large fibroid in the lower segment, pregnancy with invasive carcinoma cervix, dorsoinferior transverse lie, inaccessible lower segment are few indications where upper segment incision may be necessary. There are many disadvantages of classical uterine incision. The incision is more complicated and time consuming to repair, incidence of infection is higher, and adhesion formation is common. The risk of uterine rupture is higher, may occur before term and resultant bleeding is much more than rupture of relatively less vascular lower segment.

Complications and its Management

Complications of CS can be anesthetic, operative and postoperative. Operative procedure complications are as follows.

Hemorrhage

Excessive bleeding at CS can be because of bleeding from the uterine vessels, venous sinus from the margins, and venous sinus from the placental bed or atonic uterus. Bleeding from the uterine vessels can be managed by appropriate identification and placement of sutures. Sometimes exteriorization of uterus may be helpful; placing the finger behind the broad ligament before putting the sutures may be helpful. Bleeding from the venous sinus of the margin can be tackled by application of hemostatic clamp and then appropriate suture. The placental bed bleeding is controlled by compression of warm pack or occasionally figure-of-eight sutures. Atonic uterus needs uterine massage and oxytocic agents including prostaglandins.

Injury to the Bladder

Occasionally, in spite of appropriate preventive measures, inadvertent damage to the bladder happens. Proper identification and then repair in two layers and keeping the Foley catheter for 7–10 days is necessary.

CONCLUSION

Obstetric practice has undergone significant changes over the years. Controversies still exist in technical aspects of different steps of CS, although practiced for several centuries. Systematic reviews have addressed few controversial areas but in other areas evidence is still evolving. Individualization is important in managing a patient but we should keep our mind open to accept the changing trend in practice evolving from robust evidence.

BIBLIOGRAPHY

1. Afolabi BB, Lesi FE, Merah NA. Regional versus general anaesthesia for cesarean section. Cochrane database Syst Rev. 2006;(4):CD004350.
2. Ahmed B, Abu Nahia F, Abushama M. Routine cervical dilatation during elective cesarean section and its influence on maternal morbidity: a randomized controlled study. J Perinat Med. 2005;33:510-3.
3. Alderdice F, McKenna D, Dornan J. Techniques and materials for skin closure in caesarean section. Cochrane Database Syst Rev. 2003;2:CD003577.
4. Barik S, Jones MH, Meniru GI. Obstetric intervention and economic imperative (correspondence). Br J Obstet Gynaecol. 1994;101:88.
5. Chelmow D, Rodriguez EJ, Sabatini MM. Suture closure of subcutaneous fat and wound disruption after cesarean delivery; a meta-analysis. Obstet Gynecol. 2004;103:974-80.
6. Dickinson JE. Cesarean section. In: James DK, Steer PJ, Weiner CP, Gonik B (Eds). High Risk Pregnancy—Management Options, 3rd edition. Philadelphia: Elsevier; 2006. pp. 1543-56.
7. Enkin MW, Wilkinson C. Single versus two layer suturing for closing the uterine incision at caesarean section. Cochrane Database Syst Rev. 2000;2:CD000192.
8. Gyamfi C, Juhasz G, Gyamfi P, et al. Single versus double - layer uterine incision closure and uterine rupture. J Matern Fetal Neonatal Med. 2006;19:639-43.
9. Jacobs-Jokhan D, Hofmeyr G. Extra-abdominal versus intra-abdominal repair of the uterine incision at caesarean section. Cochrane Database Sust Rev. 2004;(4):CD 000085.
10. Kambo I, Bedi N, Dhillon BS, et al. A critical appraisal of cesarean section rates at teaching hospitals in India. Int J Gynaecol Obstet. 2002;79:151-8.
11. Lyell DJ, Caughey AB, Hu E, et al. Peritoneal closure at primary caesarean delivery and adhesions. Obstet Gynecol. 2005;106: 275-80.
12. Malo S, Barik S, Kundu P, et al. Trends of anesthetic practice for cesarean sections in a semi-rural tertiary care hospital. In: Book of Abstract, 50th All India Congress of Obstetrics and Gynaecology. Kolkata; 2007. pp. 51.
13. Mathai M, Hofmeyr G. Abdominal surgical incisions for caesarean section. Cochrane Database Syst Rev. 2007;24:CD004453.
14. National Institute of Clinical Excellence. (2004) Cesarean section: Clinical guideline 13 [online]. Available from www.nice.org.uk/nicemedia/pdf/cg013niceguideline.pdf. [Accessed November, 2013].
15. Penn Z, Ghaem-Maghami S. Indications for cesarean section. Best Pract Res Clin Obstet Gynecol. 2001;15:1-15.
16. Senanayake H. Elective Caesarean section without urethral catheterization. J Obstet Gynaecol Res. 2005;31:32-7.
17. Song SH, Oh MJ, Kim T, et al. Finger-assisted stretching technique for cesarean section. Int J Gynecol Obstet. 2006;92:212-6.
18. Wax JR, Cartin A, Pinette MG, et al. Patient choice cesarean section: an evidence-based review. Obstet Gynecol Surv. 2004; 59:601-16.
19. Wilkinson C, Enkin MW. Manual removal of placenta at caesarean section. Cochrane Database Syst Rev. 2000;2:CD000130.

CHAPTER

29

Ectopic Pregnancy—Surgical Management

Sadhana Desai, Partha Guha Roy

INTRODUCTION

Ectopic pregnancy occurs when the conceptus implants outside the uterine cavity. The most common implantation site is within the Fallopian tube, usually in the ampullary portion. Other less common sites include the ovary, the cornual segment of the uterus, the cervix and rarely, other peritoneal or serosal surfaces within the abdominal cavity. Women of childbearing age has 2% incidence of ectopic pregnancy. It is a life-threatening situation if not timely diagnosed and treated and her future ability to reproduce may be adversely affected.

RISK FACTORS

The reasons for development of an ectopic pregnancy are probably multifactorial, and proportion of women who develop ectopic pregnancies do not seem to have any identifiable risk factors (Box 1). The main risk factors are previous ectopic pregnancy, tubal damage from either infection or previous abdominal or pelvic surgery, history of infertility, treatment for in vitro fertilization (IVF), increased age and smoking.

Box 1 Risk factors for development of ectopic pregnancy

- History of pelvic inflammatory disease or acute salpingitis
- Tubal factor infertility
- Previous ectopic pregnancy
- Previous tubal surgery
- Assisted reproduction
- Previous acute appendicitis
- History of peritonitis
- History of previous pelvic or abdominal surgery
- Smoking
- Female sterilization
- Current use of an intrauterine contraceptive device (IUCD)

PRESENTATION

Most women with an ectopic pregnancy present early. The average gestation of presentation of an unruptured pregnancy is 6.9 weeks, and 7.2 weeks if the tube is ruptured. Fifty percent of patients present with the classic clinical triad of pain, amenorrhea, and vaginal bleeding (Box 2). One should have a high index of suspicion for ectopic pregnancy in any woman who presents with these symptoms and who presents with physical findings of pelvic tenderness, enlarged uterus, adnexal mass, or tenderness. History and presenting symptoms of ectopic pregnancy and nonspecific and may be confused with those of miscarriage, ovarian torsion or pelvic inflammatory disease. Fortunately, using modern diagnostic techniques, viz laparoscopy, quantitative beta human chorionic gonadotropin (βhCG) assay, and high resolution ultrasonography (USG) with color Doppler, most ectopic pregnancies can be diagnosed prior to rupture.

Box 2 Percentage occurrence of history and presenting signs with ectopic pregnancy

- Abdominal pain (97%)
- Vaginal bleeding (79%)
- Abdominal tenderness (91%)
- Adnexal tenderness (54%)
- History of infertility (15%)
- Use of an intrauterine contraceptive device (IUCD) (14%)
- Previous ectopic pregnancy (11%)

Numerous conditions may have a presentation similar to an extrauterine pregnancy. The most common of these are appendicitis, salpingitis, ruptured corpus luteum cyst or ovarian follicle, spontaneous abortion or threatened abortion, ovarian torsion, and urinary tract disease. Intrauterine pregnancies with other abdominal or pelvic problems such as degenerating fibroids must also be included in the differential diagnosis.

MEDICAL THERAPY

Medical therapy of ectopic pregnancy is appealing over surgical options for a number of reasons, including eliminating morbidity from surgery and general anesthesia (GA), potentially less tubal damage, and less cost and need for hospitalization. Methotrexate is the common drug being used today. It can be used in multiple doses or a single dose.

Factors to be Considered for Medical Therapy

She must be hemodynamically stable, with no signs or symptoms of active bleeding or hemoperitoneum, she must be reliable, compliant, and able to return for follow-up and another factor is size of the gestation, which should not exceed 3.5 cm at its greatest dimension on USG measurement. She should not have any contraindications to the use of methotrexate.

A βhCG level of greater than 15,000 IU/L, fetal cardiac activity, and free fluid in the cul-de-sac on US (presumably representing tubal rupture) are contraindications. Contraindications to the use of methotrexate include:

- Documented hypersensitivity to methotrexate
- Breastfeeding
- Immunodeficiency
- Alcoholism
- Alcoholic liver disease or any liver disease
- Blood dyscrasias
- Leukopenia
- Thrombocytopenia
- Anemia
- Active pulmonary disease
- Peptic ulcer disease
- Renal, hepatic, or hematologic dysfunction.

However, in each case, the risk of surgery must be weighed against any relative contraindication.

The single dose injection is the more popular regimen today. It involves injection of methotrexate as 50 mg/m^2 intramuscular (IM) or intravenous (IV) in a single injection or as a divided dose. With smaller dosing and fewer injections, fewer adverse effects are anticipated and the use of leucovorin can be abandoned.

Two to three days after the injection two-thirds of the patients experience at least one episode of increased abdominal pain. It can be differentiated from tubal rupture in that it is milder, of limited duration (lasting 24–48 hours), and is not associated with signs of acute abdomen or hemodynamic instability.

Patients should be advised to avoid alcoholic beverages, vitamins containing folic acid, nonsteroidal anti-inflammatory drugs (NSAIDs), and sexual intercourse until advised otherwise. A signed written consent demonstrating the patient's comprehension of the course of treatment must be obtained. Information pamphlet to be given to all patients receiving methotrexate and it should include a list of adverse effects, a schedule of follow-up visits, and a method of contacting the physician or the hospital in case of emergency.

Before initiating therapy, draw blood to determine baseline laboratory values for renal, hepatic, and bone marrow function, as well as a baseline β-hCG level. Determine blood type, Rhesus (Rh) factor, and the presence of antibodies. Patients who are Rh negative should receive Rh immune globulin. Obtain repeat β-hCG levels between 4 days and 7 days after the methotrexate injection. An initial increase in β-hCG levels often occurs by the 3rd day and is not a cause for alarm. A decline in β-hCG levels of at least 15% from days 4 to 7 postinjection indicates a successful medical response. Monitor the patient's β-hCG levels weekly until they become undetectable.

Failure of medical treatment is defined when β-hCG levels increase, plateau or fail to decrease adequately by 15% from days 4 to 7 postinjection. At this time, surgical intervention may be warranted. A repeat single dose of methotrexate can also be a viable option after re-evaluation of the patients' indications and contraindications (including repeat USG) for medical therapy.

Treatment with methotrexate is an especially attractive option when the pregnancy is located on the cervix, ovary, or in the interstitial or the cornual portion of the tube. Surgical treatment in these cases is often associated with increased risk of hemorrhage, often resulting in hysterectomy or oophorectomy.

Preliminary reports of use of oral methotrexate show promising result. However, efficacy remains to be established. Direct local injection (salpingocentesis) of methotrexate into the ectopic pregnancy under laparoscopic or USG guidance has also been reported in the literature; however, reports from these studies have yielded inconsistent results, and its advantage over IM injection remains to be established.

Mifepristone

Mifepristone has been used in combination with methotrexate for the medical treatment of ectopic pregnancy. In a randomized controlled trial (RCT) comparing methotrexate combined with mifepristone and methotrexate alone in 50 women with unruptured tubal ectopic pregnancy, the ectopic pregnancy resolved faster in women given the combined treatment. The effect of the combined treatment was also more pronounced in women with higher serum concentrations of hCG.

Expectant Management

Candidates for successful expectant management are asymptomatic and have no evidence of rupture or hemodynamic instability. Furthermore, they should portray objective evidence of resolution, such as declining βhCG levels. They must be fully compliant and must be willing to accept the potential risks of tubal rupture.

Rupture despite low and declining serum levels of βhCG has been reported, making close follow-up and patient compliance of paramount importance.

SURGICAL THERAPY

Within the last 2 decades, a more conservative surgical approach to unruptured ectopic pregnancy using minimally invasive surgery has been advocated to preserve tubal function. The conservative approaches include linear salpingostomy and milking the pregnancy out of the distal ampulla. The more radical approach includes resecting the segment of the Fallopian tube that contains the gestation with or without reanastomosis.

Laparoscopy has become the recommended approach in most cases (Figs 1 and 2). Laparotomy is usually reserved for patients who are hemodynamically unstable or patients with cornual ectopic pregnancies. It also is a preferred method for surgeons inexperienced in laparoscopy and in patients where laparoscopic approach is difficult (e.g. secondary to the presence of multiple dense adhesions, obesity or massive hemoperitoneum). Multiple studies have demonstrated that laparoscopic treatment of ectopic pregnancy results in fewer postoperative adhesions than laparotomy. Furthermore, laparoscopy is associated with significantly less blood loss and a reduced need for analgesia. Finally, laparoscopy reduces cost, hospitalization, and convalescence period.

In a patient who has completed childbearing and no longer desires fertility, in a patient with a history of an ectopic pregnancy in the same tube, or in a patient with severely damaged tubes, total salpingectomy is the procedure of choice. The presence of uncontrolled bleeding and hemodynamic instability warrants radical surgery over conservative methods.

Follow-up Care

After surgical excision of the ectopic gestation, weekly monitoring of quantitative β-hCG levels is necessary until the level is zero to ensure that treatment is complete. This is especially true following treatment with conservative surgery, i.e. salpingostomy, which carries a 5–15% rate of persistent trophoblastic tissue. The average time for βhCG to clear the system is 2–3 weeks, but up to 6 weeks can be required.

TREATMENT SUCCESS RATES AND FUTURE REPRODUCTIVE OUTCOME

Data in the literature have failed to demonstrate substantial and consistent benefit of either salpingostomy or salpingectomy in improving future reproductive outcome. Despite the risk of persistent ectopic pregnancy, some studies have shown salpingostomy to improve reproductive outcome in patients with contralateral tubal damage.

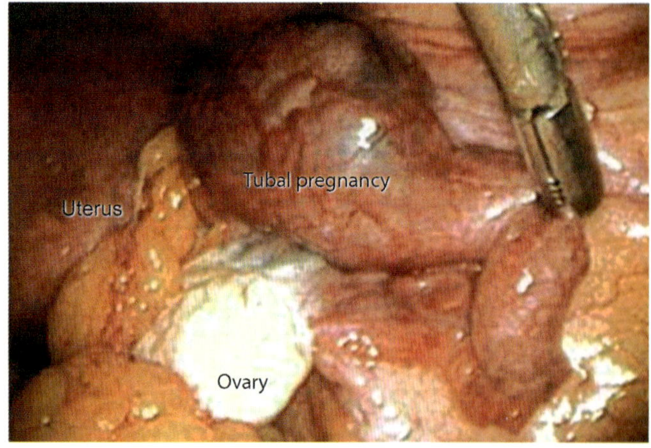

Fig. 1: Laparoscopic view of ectopic pregnancy

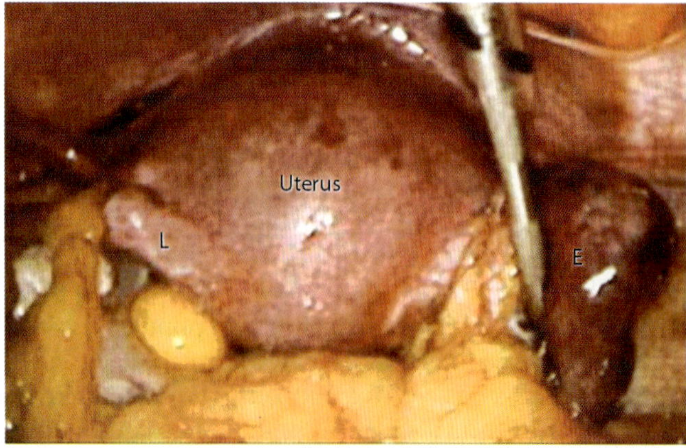

Fig. 2: Laparoscopic view of periampullary ectopic pregnancy

In 1997, Yao and Tulandi concluded from a literature review that laparoscopic salpingostomy had equal or slightly better reproductive performance than salpingectomy; however, slightly higher recurrent ectopic pregnancy rates were noted in the salpingostomy group.

Parker and Bistis (1997) concluded that when the contralateral Fallopian tube is normal, the subsequent fertility rate is independent of the type of surgery.

Future fertility rates are similar in patients who were treated surgically by laparoscopy or laparotomy.

The success rates after methotrexate are comparable with laparoscopic salpingostomy, assuming the selection criteria mentioned above are observed. The average success rates using the multiple-dose regimen are in the range of 91–95%, demonstrated by multiple investigators. One study of 77 patients desiring subsequent pregnancy showed intrauterine pregnancies in 64%, and recurrent ectopic pregnancy occurred in 11%. Other studies have demonstrated similar results, with intrauterine pregnancy rates ranging from 20% to 80%.

The average success rates for the single-dose regimen are reported to be from 88% to 94%. In a study by Stovall and Ling (1992), 113 patients (94%) were treated successfully, 4 (3.3%) of whom needed a second dose. No adverse effects were encountered. Furthermore, 87.2% of these patients achieved a subsequent intrauterine pregnancy, whereas 12.8% experienced a subsequent ectopic pregnancy. Other studies have reported similar results with some mild adverse effects and lower reproductive outcomes.

CONCLUSION

As the ability to diagnose ectopic pregnancy improves, physicians will be able to intervene sooner, preventing life-threatening sequelae and extensive tubal damage, which could preserve future fertility. Already, with improving technology, physicians are treating ectopic pregnancies with minimally invasive surgery or no surgery at all. Physicians have been able to reduce the mortality rate secondary to ectopic pregnancy despite its growing incidence. Also, effective vaccination against *Chlamydia trachomatis* is under investigation. Once clinically available, it should have a dramatic impact on the frequency of ectopic pregnancy, as well as on the overall health of the female reproductive system.

BIBLIOGRAPHY

1. Ankum WM, Mol BW, Van der Veen F, et al. Risk factors for ectopic pregnancy: a meta-analysis. Fertil Steril. 1996;65(6):1093-9.
2. Barnhart K, Mennuti MT, Benjamin I. Prompt diagnosis of ectopic pregnancy in an emergency department setting. Obstet Gynecol. 1994;84(6):1010-5.
3. Bengtsson G, Bryman I, Thorburn J, et al. Low-dose oral methotrexate as second-line therapy for persistent trophoblast after conservative treatment of ectopic pregnancy. Obstet Gynecol. 1992;79(4):589-91.
4. Breen JL. A 21 year survey of 654 ectopic pregnancies. Am J Obstet Gynecol. 1970;106(7):1004-19.
5. Bruhat MA, Manhes H, Mage G, et al. Treatment of ectopic pregnancy by means of laparoscopy. Fertil Steril. 1980;33(4):411-4.
6. Centers for Disease Control and Prevention. Ectopic pregnancy–United States, 1990–1992. JAMA. 1995;273(7):533.
7. Chi IC, Potts M, Wilkens L. Rare events associated with tubal sterilizations: an international experience. Obstet Gynecol Surv. 1986;41(1):7-19.
8. Chow WH, Daling JR, Cates W, et al. Epidemiology of ectopic pregnancy. Epidemiol Rev. 1987;9:70-94.
9. Clausen I. Conservative versus radical surgery for tubal pregnancy. A review. Acta Obstet Gynecol Scand. 1996;75(1): 8-12.
10. DeStefano F, Peterson HB, Layde PM, et al. Risk of ectopic pregnancy following tubal sterilization. Obstet Gynecol. 1982;60(3):326-30.
11. Diquelou JY, Pia P, Tesquier L, et al. The role of *Chlamydia trachomatis* in the infectious etiology of extra-uterine pregnancy. J Gynecol Obstet Biol Reprod (Paris). 1988;17(3):325-32.
12. Dor J, Seidman DS, Levran D, et al. The incidence of combined intrauterine and extrauterine pregnancy after in vitro fertilization and embryo transfer. Fertil Steril. 1991;55(4):833-4.
13. Doubilet PM, Benson CB, Frates MC. Sonographically guided minimally invasive treatment of unusual ectopic pregnancies. J Ultrasound Med. 2004;23(3):359-70.
14. Dubuisson JB, Morice P, Chapron C, et al. Salpingectomy-the laparoscopic surgical choice for ectopic pregnancy. Hum Reprod. 1996;11(6):1199-203.
15. Emerson DS, Cartier MS, Altieri LA, et al. Diagnostic efficacy of endovaginal color Doppler flow imaging in an ectopic pregnancy screening program. Radiology. 1992;183(2):413-20.
16. Fernandez H, Coste J, Job-Spira N. Controlled ovarian hyperstimulation as a risk factor for ectopic pregnancy. Obstet Gynecol. 1991;78(4):656-9.
17. Fylstra DL. Tubal pregnancy: a review of current diagnosis and treatment. Obstet Gynecol Surv. 1998;53(5):320-8.
18. Gazvani MR, Baruah DN, Alfirevic Z, et al. Mifepristone in combination with Methotrexate for the medical treatment of tubal pregnancy; a randomised, controlled trial. Human Reprod. 1998;13:1987-90.
19. Goldner TE, Lawson HW, Xia Z, et al. Surveillance for ectopic pregnancy-United States, 1970-1989. Mor Mortal Wkly Rep CDC Surveill Summ. 1993;42:73-85.

20. Gracia CR, Brown HA, Barnhart KT. Prophylactic methotrexate after linear salpingostomy: a decision analysis. Fertil Steril. 2001;76(6):1191-5.
21. Graczykowski JW, Mishell DR. Methotrexate prophylaxis for persistent ectopic pregnancy after conservative treatment by salpingostomy. Obstet Gynecol. 1997;89(1):118-22.
22. Kadar N, Bohrer M, Kemmann E, et al. The discriminatory human chorionic gonadotropin zone for endovaginal sonography: a prospective, randomized study. Fertil Steril. 1994;61(6):1016-20.
23. Langer R, Raziel A, Ron-El R, et al. Reproductive outcome after conservative surgery for unruptured tubal pregnancy-a 15-year experience. Fertil Steril. 1990;53(2):227-31.
24. Levin AA, Schoenbaum SC, Stubblefield PG, et al. Ectopic pregnancy and prior induced abortion. Am J Public Health. 1982;72(3):253-6.
25. Lipscomb GH, Bran D, McCord ML, et al. Analysis of three hundred fifteen ectopic pregnancies treated with single-dose methotrexate. Am J Obstet Gynecol. 1998;178(6):1354-8.
26. Lundorff P, Hahlin M, Sjoblom P, et al. Persistent trophoblast after conservative treatment of tubal pregnancy: prediction and detection. Obstet Gynecol. 1991;77(1):129-33.
27. Lundorff P, Thorburn J, Lindblom B. Fertility outcome after conservative surgical treatment of ectopic pregnancy evaluated in a randomized trial. Fertil Steril. 1992;57(5):998-1002.
28. Majmudar B, Henderson PH, Semple E. Salpingitis isthmica nodosa: a high-risk factor for tubal pregnancy. Obstet Gynecol. 1983;62(1):73-8.
29. Marchbanks PA, Annegers JF, Coulam CB, et al. Risk factors for ectopic pregnancy. A population-based study. JAMA. 1988;259(12):1823-7.
30. Maymon R, Shulman A, Halperin R, et al. Ectopic pregnancy and laparoscopy: review of 1197 patients treated by salpingectomy or salpingotomy. Eur J Obstet Gynecol Reprod Biol. 1995;62(1):61-7.
31. McCausland A. High rate of ectopic pregnancy following laparoscopic tubal coagulation failures. Incidence and etiology. Am J Obstet Gynecol. 1980;136(1):97-101.
32. Nieuwkerk PT, Hajenius PJ, Van der Veen F, et al. Systemic methotrexate therapy versus laparoscopic salpingostomy in tubal pregnancy. Part II. Patient preferences for systemic methotrexate. Fertil Steril. 1998;70(3):518-22.
33. Ory SJ, Nnadi E, Herrmann R. Fertility after ectopic pregnancy. Fertil Steril. 1993;60(2):231-5.
34. Parker J, Bisits A. Laparoscopic surgical treatment of ectopic pregnancy: salpingectomy or salpingostomy? Aust N Z J Obstet Gynaecol. 1997;37(1):115-7.
35. Perkins JD, Mitchell MR. Heterotopic pregnancy in a large inner-city hospital: a report of two cases. J Natl Med Assoc. 2004;96(3):363-6.
36. Pouly JL, Chapron C, Manhes H, et al. Multifactorial analysis of fertility after conservative laparoscopic treatment of ectopic pregnancy in a series of 223 patients. Fertil Steril. 1991;56(3):453-60.
37. Pulkkinen MO, Talo A. Tubal physiologic consideration in ectopic pregnancy. Clin Obstet Gynecol. 1987;30(1):164-72.
38. Ransom MX, Garcia AJ, Bohrer M, et al. Serum progesterone as a predictor of methotrexate success in the treatment of ectopic pregnancy. Obstet Gynecol. 1994;83(6):1033-7.
39. Robertson JN, Hogston P, Ward ME. Gonococcal and chlamydial antibodies in ectopic and intrauterine pregnancy. Br J Obstet Gynaecol. 1988;95(7):711-6.
40. Rulin MC. Is salpingostomy the surgical treatment of choice for unruptured tubal pregnancy? Obstet Gynecol. 1995;86(6):1010-3.
41. Saraiya M, Berg CJ, Kendrick JS. Cigarette smoking as a risk factor for ectopic pregnancy. Am J Obstet Gynecol. 1998;178(3):493-8.
42. Savare J, Norup P, Grove Thomsen S, et al. Heterotopic pregnancies after in-vitro fertilization and embryo transfer-a Danish survey. Human Reprod. 1993;8:116-8.
43. Shalev E, Peleg D, Tsabari A, et al. Spontaneous resolution of ectopic tubal pregnancy: natural history. Fertil Steril. 1995;63(1):15-9.
44. Shepherd RW, Patton PE, Novy MJ. Serial beta-hCG measurements in the early detection of ectopic pregnancy. Obstet Gynecol. 1990;75(3):417-20.
45. Sivin I. Dose- and age-dependent ectopic pregnancy risks with intrauterine contraception. Obstet Gynecol. 1991;78(2):291-8.
46. Stock RJ. Persistent tubal pregnancy. Obstet Gynecol. 1991;77(2):267-70.
47. Stovall TG, Ling FW, Buster JE. Outpatient chemotherapy of unruptured ectopic pregnancy. Fertil Steril. 1989;51(3):435-8.
48. Stovall TG, Ling FW, Carson SA, et al. Serum progesterone and uterine curettage in differential diagnosis of ectopic pregnancy. Fertil Steril. 1992;57(2):456-7.
49. Stovall TG, Ling FW, Gray LA. Single-dose methotrexate for treatment of ectopic pregnancy. Obstet Gynecol. 1991;77 (5):754-7.
50. Stovall TG, Ling FW. Single-dose methotrexate: an expanded clinical trial. Am J Obstet Gynecol. 1993;168(6): 1759-62.
51. Trio D, Strobelt N, Picciolo C, et al. Prognostic factors for successful expectant management of ectopic pregnancy. Fertil Steril. 1995;63(3):469-72.
52. Tuomivaara L, Kauppila A. Radical or conservative surgery for ectopic pregnancy? A follow-up study of fertility of 323 patients. Fertil Steril. 1988;50(4):580-3.
53. US Department of Health and Human Services, Public Health Services. National Center for Health Statistics: advanced report of final mortality statistics, 1992. Washington, DC; 1994.
54. Vermesh M, Silva PD, Rosen GF, et al. Management of unruptured ectopic gestation by linear salpingostomy: a prospective, randomized clinical trial of laparoscopy versus laparotomy. Obstet Gynecol. 1989;73(3):400-4.
55. Vermesh M, Silva PD, Sauer MV. Persistent tubal ectopic gestation: patterns of circulating beta-human chorionic gonadotropin and progesterone, and management options. Fertil Steril. 1988;50(4):584-8.
56. Westrom L, Bengtsson LP, Mardh PA. Incidence, trends, and risks of ectopic pregnancy in a population of women. Br Med J (Clin Res Ed). 1981;282(6257):15-8.
57. Yao M, Tulandi T. Current status of surgical and nonsurgical management of ectopic pregnancy. Fertil Steril. 1997;67(3):421-33.
58. Ylostalo P, Cacciatore B, Sjoberg J, et al. Expectant management of ectopic pregnancy. Obstet Gynecol. 1992;80(3):345-8.

CHAPTER

30

Laparoscopy and Obstetrical Practice

Col Krishan Kapur

We are living in an era when minimal access surgery is seen to dominate every surgical discipline. The advantages of minimal access surgery are unequivocal and laparoscopic surgery is being used for various indications. As the years go by, surgeons and gynecologists are gaining great experience in this procedure, and technological advances by the manufacturers of laparoscopic equipment as far as imaging, electrocautery and other instrumentation is concerned, is making this procedure easier with better visualization.

The advantages of the laparoscopic technique are so great that there is no reason why a pregnant woman should not be allowed to enjoy the benefits of this procedure, should it be required to be done for a condition in her pregnancy. Apart from the usual advantages of laparoscopic surgery, the advantages of laparoscopic surgery over laparotomy during pregnancy include less postoperative narcotic requirements, lower risk of wound complications, shorter hospital stays and decreased thromboembolic events due to early mobilization. Laparoscopy also reduces the risk of uterine irritability by decreasing the need for uterine manipulation because of improved visualization, and decreased uterine irritability results in lower rates of spontaneous abortion and preterm delivery.

Earlier concerns about the performance of laparoscopic surgery on pregnant women centered around the potential risk to the fetus due to trocar insertion, carbon dioxide (CO_2) insufflation and the technical ability to obtain good operative exposure with the gravid uterus, making laparoscopy to be traditionally avoided in pregnancy. However, as the wheel of time has turned, this procedure is being routinely used in pregnancy for various intra-abdominal disorders.

Pregnancy is characterized by changes in physiological and abdominal anatomy. Intra-abdominal diseases requiring surgical intervention during pregnancy present unique challenges in diagnosis and management. In addition these changes make laparoscopic surgery technically more difficult. During pregnancy it is important that the gestational age and viability of the pregnancy must be determined and risks related to pregnancy and surgery be explained to the patient.

INDICATIONS FOR LAPAROSCOPIC SURGERY IN PREGNANCY

Approximately 1 in 500 to 1 in 635 women will require nonobstetrical surgery during their pregnancy.

Intra-abdominal disorders encountered in pregnancy which require laparoscopic intervention can be divided into gynecological and nongynecological. The gynecological problems frequently encountered are persistent ovarian cysts, twisted adnexal masses, ectopic pregnancies and heterotopic pregnancies. The nongynecological indications for laparoscopy in pregnancy are commonly acute appendicitis, gallbladder disease and some cases of acute abdomen where laparoscopy may be used for diagnosis. Other rarer indications for laparoscopic surgery in pregnancy are adrenal tumors, splenic disorders, symptomatic hernias and complications of inflammatory bowel disease.

It has been reported that maternal abdominal disorders and its laparoscopic management is associated with a fetal loss rate of 2–24% according to recent literature.

Laparoscopy can be safely performed during any trimester of pregnancy. There was earlier a concept of delaying surgery till the second trimester as surgery in the first trimester was associated with a spontaneous abortion rate as high as 12% and surgery in the third trimester was associated with preterm labor of up to 40%. This experience has not been reproduced in recent literature reporting on laparoscopic cases. Several studies have shown that pregnant patients may undergo laparoscopic surgery safely during any trimester without any appreciable risk to the mother or fetus, and if surgery is delayed in patients with symptomatic gallstone disease during pregnancy, there may be complications of gallstone disease such as acute cholecystitis and gallstone pancreatitis and these complications can lead to a higher spontaneous abortion rate and preterm labor.

Generally 26–28 weeks is taken as gestation age for successful completion of laparoscopic surgery, but laparoscopic cholecystectomy and appendectomy have successfully been performed late in the third trimester. Some important indications for laparoscopic surgery in pregnancy are:

- Diagnostic laparoscopy for pain abdomen is safe and effective when used selectively in the workup and treatment of acute abdominal processes in pregnancy. Although, enough data is not available to recommend laparoscopy as a primary diagnostic approach in a pregnant patient, it is certainly a reasonable alternative
- *Ectopic pregnancy:* The details have been covered in another chapter in the book. Today with the rampant use of assisted reproductive technologies, not only is the incidence of ectopic pregnancy rising but we frequently see heterotopic pregnancies, which were seen very rarely in the past. Here, it is important that the ectopic pregnancy is removed without harming the intrauterine pregnancy commonly by doing a laparoscopic salpingectomy. Although a salpingostomy can be done, a salpingectomy is preferable for a heterotopic pregnancy as it is better to have the shortest possible operative time, and after salpingostomy it becomes difficult to follow-up the case with serum beta human chorionic gonadotrophin (HCG) levels in view of the intrauterine pregnancy
- *Gallbladder disease*: Some authorities recommend nonoperative management for symptomatic cholelithiasis in pregnancy. Other workers prefer surgical management as the recurrence rate of symptoms due to gallstones is 92%, 64% and 44% for those managed nonoperatively in first, second and third trimester respectively. Apart from recurrence, delay in surgical management results in significant morbidity including increased hospitalization, spontaneous abortion and preterm labor in those patients not undergoing cholecystectomy. Improved outcomes with decreased risk of spontaneous abortion and preterm labor have been reported in laparoscopic cholecystectomy when compared to laparotomy
- *Laparoscopic appendectomy:* Laparoscopic appendectomy is considered by many to be the standard of care in a gravid patient with appendicitis. Although, the anatomic changes and leukocytosis of pregnancy is thought to make the diagnosis of appendicitis difficult in pregnancy, a recent article has shown that the majority (> 83%) of pregnant patients with appendicitis present with classic right lower quadrant pain. When the diagnosis of appendicitis with ultrasound is equivocal, promptly proceeding to diagnostic laparoscopy will allow early identification and intervention in appendicitis decreasing the rate of perforation. It has been reported that 66% of cases will have a perforation when surgery is delayed by more than 24 hours compared to 0% incidence when surgical management is initiated within 24 hours.

Adnexal masses: Laparoscopy is safe and effective in gravid patients with symptomatic cystic masses. Observation is acceptable for all cystic lesions lesser than 6 cm provided tumor markers are normal and ultrasound is not suspicious of malignancy. The incidence of adnexal masses is 2%. Masses less than 6 cm have a spontaneous resolution rate of 82–94% and can be observed. Persistent masses are commonly functional cysts or mature cystic teratomas, with incidence of malignancy reported at 2–6%. Previously, masses that were persistent at 16 weeks of pregnancy and greater than 6 cm in diameter were taken up for surgery for fear of malignancy, but recent literature supports the safety of close observation of these patients, if they are asymptomatic, tumor markers are normal and ultrasound findings are not suspicious of malignancy.

If surgery is indicated, the laparoscopic approach is generally preferred in every trimester.

Laparoscopic approach is recommended for both diagnosis and treatment of adnexal torsion unless clinical severity warrants laparotomy. About 10–15% of adnexal masses can undergo torsion and multiple case reports have confirmed the safety and efficacy of laparoscopy for adnexal torsion in pregnant patients. In fact, laparoscopy is the preferred method of diagnosis and treatment of adnexal torsion in a gravid patient.

If diagnosed early the patient may be treated by laparoscopic adnexal detorsion, but with late diagnosis there may be adnexal infarction which can lead to peritonitis, spontaneous abortion, preterm delivery and death, and in this condition the gangrenous adnexa should be completely resected. Laparotomy may be indicated by the patients' clinical severity and intraoperative findings.

Solid organ resection: Laparoscopic adrenalectomy, nephrectomy and splenectomy are safe procedures in pregnant patients when indicated and standard precautions are taken.

Laparoscopic adrenalectomy during pregnancy has been proven to be effective in the management of primary hyperaldosteronism, Cushing's syndrome and pheochromocytoma.

Laparoscopic splenectomy is also becoming an increasingly accepted modality in pregnancy for conditions like hereditary spherocytosis and autoimmune thrombocytopenic purpura.

Two cases of laparoscopic nephrectomy have recently been reported in first and second trimester of pregnancy without any associated complications in mother and fetus.

TECHNICAL CONSIDERATIONS WHILE PERFORMING LAPAROSCOPY IN PREGNANCY

Patient Positioning

When a pregnant patient beyond the 16–18 weeks of pregnancy is placed in the supine position the gravid uterus presses on the inferior vena cava (IVC) resulting in decreased venous return to the heart, maternal hypotension, reduction in cardiac output by 10–30% and decreased placental perfusion during surgery. Pregnant patients should be placed in the left lateral recumbent position to minimize compression of the vena cava and aorta, thus improving venous return and cardiac output.

Initial Port Placement

In pregnancy, as the uterus enlarges there has been concern about the risk of injury to the uterus with the Veress needle and at the time of insertion of the primary trocar. Injury to the uterus could result in bleeding, infection, gas embolism or ruptured membranes. Such complications can easily be avoided by using an appropriate site for entry of the Veress needle and trocar. One of the methods used to overcome this risk is that, as the uterus enlarges, the access site is shifted from the umbilicus to the subcostal region and the abdominal wall is lifted at the time of insertion. Many workers place the first trocar just below the xiphisternum and all other trocars are placed under direct vision. Other workers have used optical trocars that allow the surgeon to see tissue planes and intra-abdominal organs as the trocar is advanced. Another technique used to avoid injury to bowel, uterus or vessels is to use Hassan's open laparoscopic technique for port placement and this is probably the safest way to place the primary trocar in advanced pregnancy. Ultrasound guided trocar placement has also been described in literature as an additional method to visualize trocar placement. With the above precautions both the open (Hassan) technique and the Veress needle technique can be safely performed.

Stomach and bowel injury from needle and trocar have been reported but a large number of their injuries go unrecognized because of the ability of the stomach and intestines to heal small injuries. Undetected bowel injury is a major factor of postoperative mortality and morbidity. These patients usually present late in sepsis, peritonitis, and this could lead to fatal maternal mortality and morbidity. The most life threatening complication of laparoscopy is injury to the large retroperitoneal vessels like aorta, IVC and iliac vessels. Early recognition and prompt treatment is of essence if these vessels are injured.

Insufflation Pressure

During pregnancy, as the diaphragm is pushed upwards by the growing fetus, there is decreased residual lung volume and functional residual capacity making her more susceptible to arterial desaturation. With pneumoperitoneum, the diaphragm is pushed further up, further compromising the respiratory physiology. Most workers recommend that intra-abdominal pressures be maintained at less than 12 mm Hg to avoid worsening pulmonary physiology. Others have argued that less pressure does not give adequate visualization and a pressure of 15 mm Hg is acceptable.

As CO_2 exchange occurs with intraperitoneal insufflation, there have been concerns over the effect on the fetus, especially the effects of acidosis. As has been brought out later in the chapter, there is no evidence to support long-term detrimental effects resulting from CO_2.

Venous Thromboembolic Prophylaxis

Pregnancy is a hypercoagulable state with 0.1–0.2% incidence of deep venous thrombosis. CO_2 pneumoperitoneum increases venous stasis and this may further increase the risk of deep venous thrombosis in pregnancy even if the insufflation pressure is left at 12 mm Hg. As there is an increased risk of thrombosis, prophylaxis with pneumatic compression devices both intraoperatively and postoperatively, along with early ambulation are strongly recommended in pregnancy. Unfortunately, there is a paucity of research on prophylaxis for deep venous thrombosis in a pregnant patient and there is no data on the use of low molecular weight heparin in pregnant patients undergoing laparoscopy but its use has been suggested in patients undergoing major surgery.

Intraoperative CO_2 Monitoring

Fetal acidosis with CO_2 pneumoperitoneum has not been documented in the human fetus but concerns over the potential detrimental effects of acidosis have led to the recommendation of maternal CO_2 monitoring. There was debate over maternal blood gas monitoring of arterial CO_2 versus end-tidal CO_2 ($ETCO_2$) monitoring, but the less invasive capnography has been demonstrated to adequately reflect maternal acid base status in humans and several large studies have demonstrated the safety and efficacy of $ETCO_2$ measurement in pregnant women making routine blood gas monitoring unnecessary.

FETAL RISKS OF LAPAROSCOPY IN PREGNANCY

There are several mechanisms which can possibly contribute to increased fetal morbidity and mortality as a result of laparoscopic surgery in pregnancy. Some of the important points to be remembered are listed below.

Decreased Uterine Blood Flow

It has been hypothesized that decreased uterine blood flow and oxygen delivery to the fetus during laparoscopic surgery may occur due to increased intra-abdominal pressure and due to position of the patient where the uterus presses on the great vessels. However, the question of decreased uterine blood flow due to pneumoperitoneum is unlikely to be a major concern as there are frequent intra-abdominal pressure alterations induced during valsalva, coughing, straining, which do not adversely affect uterine blood flow, and further retraction by pneumoperitoneum may be safer than manual uterine retraction. As has already been brought out, the pressure of the gravid uterus can be taken off the great vessels by proper positioning of the patient.

Effect of Increased Intra-abdominal Pressure

During laparoscopic surgery, the abdomen has to be distended with CO_2 for adequate visualization. High intra-abdominal pressures (greater than 15 mm Hg) adversely affect cardiac and respiratory physiology, and during laparoscopic surgery intra-abdominal pressures should be kept as low as possible and a pressure of 12 mm Hg is generally sufficient for adequate visualization.

If the intra-abdominal pressure is raised above 15 mm Hg, not only is the cardiac and respiratory system compromised, but the risk of gas embolism is also increased which can be a lethal complication for both mother and fetus.

Some workers use gasless laparoscopy where a laprolift raises up the abdominal wall and no gas is used but the procedure is cumbersome and conversion rate to laparotomy is higher than conventional laparoscopy.

As pregnancy is a hypercoaguable state and as pneumoperitoneum enhances lower extremity venous stasis, the risk of thromboembolic complications is increased in pregnancy. To prevent these complications, pneumatic compressor devices may be used along with early ambulation after surgery.

Effect of CO_2 Pneumoperitoneum

Although laparoscopic surgery in pregnancy is gaining wider acceptance for a number of intra-abdominal surgical disorders, there is great concern over the effect of CO_2 pneumoperitoneum on the fetus. Hunter et al. reported fetal respiratory acidosis during CO_2 pneumoperitoneum in a pregnant Ewe model. Fetal hemodynamic abnormalities like tachycardia and hypertension were noted and attributed to fetal hypercarbia. This was later reversed by maintaining mild respiratory alkalosis. Limited animal studies have suggested that fetal acidosis and tachycardia induced by CO_2 pneumoperitoneum is due to short-term acidosis, which even if severe, may not lead to deleterious effects. However, at present the short-term and long-term effects of this are not known. Should there be maternal acidosis, the pneumoperitoneum should be released and patient hyperventilated to expel CO_2 gas before continuing the procedure. It should always be remembered that the fetus will be more academic than the mother.

A number of studies have shown that if the intra-abdominal CO_2 pressure is kept below 15 mm Hg, the effect of fetal perfusion and blood gases is negligible.

Effect of Anesthesia and Anesthetic Drugs

In a recent study published in 2004, the authors concluded that CO_2 pneumoperitoneum produces respiratory acidosis but does not decrease fetal oxygenation. In contrast, the findings of other studies suggest that in the preterm fetus insufflation induced hypercapnia and acidosis are accompanied by prolonged fetal hypoxia and cardiovascular depression. The results suggest that additional work should be conducted to confirm the presumed safety of doing laparoscopic procedures during the second trimester.

Apart from CO_2, anesthetic drugs administered during the first trimester of pregnancy may cause abnormalities during the period of organogenesis. Such objections are contraindicated by a Swedish registry study for the years 1973–1983, covering 720,000 pregnant women of which 5,405 underwent surgery, mainly diagnostic laparoscopy. It appears that in general pregnancy, causes no increase in stillbirth or birth defects and does not result in any difference in time or type of delivery compared with controls, but it leads to increased infant mortality and lower birthweight. The authors concluded that the causes are related more to mother's illness that required surgical treatment than surgery or anesthesia.

Fetal Effects During Laparoscopy

As far as the long term fetal consequences of laparoscopic surgery in pregnancy are concerned, one study shows that successful laparoscopic surgery was performed in 10 cases with one conversion to an open procedure. Intraoperative and postoperative fetal monitoring was performed for at least 24 hours. No fetal distress or demise occurred nor were any tocolytics used. The resultant children were followed-up for 1–8 years with no evidence of developmental and physical abnormalities during the study period. The authors concluded that laparoscopic surgery is now proving to be as safe as open surgery in pregnancy.

Although surgical intervention either open or laparoscopy is safe in pregnancy especially with advances in anesthetic, perinatal and perioperative care, the fact remains that surgical intervention during pregnancy may still result in spontaneous abortion (especially in first trimester) or preterm labor (especially in third trimester). There is also an increase in low birthweight infants and growth restricted babies with surgical intervention in pregnancy and whenever possible surgery should be deferred until after delivery. Unfortunately, urgent surgical intervention in a gravid patient is occasionally necessary.

CONCLUSION

Laparoscopic surgery has been widely used in the last three decades by both gynecologists and general surgeons because of its major advantages. With the advancement in anesthesia, laparoscopic surgery has been used in the three trimesters of pregnancy for different intra-abdominal obstetrical and nonobstetrical pathologies. Laparoscopic surgery can be performed safely during pregnancy but possible complications such as uterine injury, difficulty during procedure, increased intra-abdominal pressure and CO_2 absorption by the fetus and the mother should be considered seriously.

The primary underlying disease and not the surgery appear to be the most important factor in determining the fetal and maternal outcome.

Most of the data available today are case reports and small series and these are not enough to make conclusions about the safety of the procedure and its complication rate. Larger controlled and randomized studies will be required to assess the superiority of laparoscopy in pregnancy.

BIBLIOGRAPHY

1. Affleck DG, Handrahan DL, Egger MJ, et al. The laparoscopic management of appendicitis and cholelithiasis during pregnancy. Am J Surg. 1999;178(6):523-9.
2. Allen JR. Helling TS, Langefeld M. Intraabdominal surgery during pregnancy. Am J Surg. 1989;158(6):567-9.
3. Allran CF, CA Weiss, Park AE. Urgent laparoscopic splenectomy in a morbidly obese pregnant woman: case report and literature review. J Laparoendosc Adv Surg Tech A. 2002;12(6):445-7.
4. Amos JD, Schorr SJ, Norman PF, et al. Laparoscopic surgery during pregnancy. Am J Surg. 1996:171(4):435-7.
5. Arvidsson D, Gerdin E. Laparoscopic cholecystectomy during pregnancy. Surg Laparosc Endosc. 1991;1(3):193-4.
6. Barone JE, Bears S, Chen S, et al. Outcome study of cholecystectomy during pregnancy. Am J Surg. 1999;177(3): 232-6.
7. Bhavani-Shankar K, Steinbrook RA, Brooks DC, et al. Arterial to end-tidal carbon dioxide pressure differences during laparoscopic surgery in pregnancy. Anesthesiology. 2000;93 (2);370-73.
8. Boschert S. Low insufflation key to laparoscopy in pregnancy, try to avoid surgery in first trimester. Obgyn news December 1: 2003.
9. Bozzo M, Buscaglia M, Ferrazzi E. The management of persistent adnexal masses in pregnancy. Am J Obstet Gynecol. 1997;177(4):981-2.
10. Clark SL, Cotton DB, Pivarnik JM, et al. Position change and central hemodynamic profile during normal third-trimester pregnancy and post partum. Am J Obstet Gynecol. 1991;164(3):883-7.
11. Comitalo JB, Lynch D. Laparoscopic cholecystectomy in the pregnant patient. Surg Laparosc Endosc. 1994;4(4):268-71.
12. Costantino GN. Laparoscopic cholecystectomy in pregnancy. J Laparoendosc Surg. 1994;4(2):161-4.
13. Curet MJ. Special problems in laparoscopic surgery. Previous abdominal surgery, obesity, and pregnancy. Surg Clin North Am. 2000;80(4):1093-110.
14. Elkayam U, Norbert G. Cardiovascular physiology of pregnancy. In: Elkayam U, Norbert G (Eds.). Cardiac problems in pregnancy: diagnosis and management of maternal and fetal disease. New York: Liss;1982. p.5.
15. Fatum M. Rojansky N. Laparoscopic surgery during pregnancy. Obstet Gynecol Surv. 2001;56(1):50-9.

16. Geisler JP. Non-gynecologic laparoscopy in second and third trimester pregnancy: obstetric implications. JSLS. 1998;2(3): 235-8.
17. Graham G, Baxi L, Tharakan T. Laparoscopic cholecystectomy during pregnancy: a case series and review of the literature. Obstet Gynecol Surv. 1998;53(9):566-74.
18. Guidelines for laparoscopic surgery during pregnancy. Society of American Gastrointestinal Endoscopic Surgeons (SAGES). Surg Endosc. 1998;12(2):189-90.
19. Hunter JG, Swanstrom L, Thornburg K. Carbon dioxide pneumoperitoneum induces fetal acidosis in a pregnant ewe model. Surg Endosc. 1995;9:272-79.
20. Iwase K, Higaki J, Yoon HE, et al. Hand-assisted laparoscopic splenectomy for idiopathic thrombocytopenic purpura during pregnancy. Surg Laparosc Endosc Percutan Tech. 2001;11(1): 53-6.
21. Kammerer WS. Nonobstetric surgery during pregnancy. Med Clin North Am. 1979;63(6):1157-64.
22. Kenichiro U, McClaine RJ, de la Fuente SG, et al. Maternal insufflation during second trimester equivalent produces hypercapnia, acidosis and prolonged hypoxia in fetal sheep. Anesthesiology. 2004;101(6):133-8.
23. Kort B, Katz VL, Watson WJ. The effect of nonobstetric operation during pregnancy. Surg Obstet Gynecol. 1993;177(4):371-6.
24. Kort B, VL Katz, WJ Watson. The effect of nonobstetric operation during pregnancy. Surg Gynecol Obstet. 1993;177(4):371-6.
25. Mage G, Canis M, Manhes J, et al. Laparoscopic management of adnexal torsion. A review of 35 cases. J Reprod Med. 1989;34(8):520-4.
26. McKellar DP, Anderson CT, Boynton CJ, et al. Cholecystectomy during pregnancy without fetal loss. Surg Gynecol Obstet. 1992;174(6):465-8.
27. Melnick DM, Wahl WL, Dalton VK. Management of general surgical problems in the pregnant patient. Am J Surg. 2004;187 (2):170-80.
28. Morice P, Louis-Sylvestre C, Chapron C, et al. Laparoscopy for adnexal torsion in pregnant women. J Reprod Med. 1997;42(7):435-9.
29. Mourad J, Elliott JP, Erickson L, et al. Appendicitis in pregnancy: new information that contradicts long-held clinical beliefs. Am J Obstet Gynecol. 2000;182(5):1027-9.
30. Muench J, Albrink M, Serafini F, et al. Delay in treatment of biliary disease during pregnancy increases morbidity and can be avoided with safe laparoscopic cholecystectomy. Am Surg. 2001;67(6):539-42; discussion 542-3.
31. O'Connor JP, Biyani CS, Taylor J, et al. Laparoscopic nephrectomy for renal-cell carcinoma during pregnancy. J Endourol. 2004;18(9):871-4.
32. Pucci RO, Seed RW. Case report of laparoscopic cholecystectomy in the third trimester of pregnancy. Am J Obstet Gyneco. 1991;165(2):401-2.
33. Reedy MB, Galan HL, Richards WE, et al. Laparoscopy during pregnancy. A survey of laparoendoscopic surgeons. J Reprod Med. 1997;42(1):33-8.
34. Rizzo AG, Laparoscopic surgery in pregnancy, long-term follow up. J Laparoendosc Adv Surg Tech. 2003;13(1):11-5.
35. Rollins MD, Chan KJ, Price RR. Laparoscopy for appendicitis and cholelithiasis during pregnancy: a new standard of care. Surg Endosc. 2004;18(2):237-41.
36. Sainsbury DC, Dorkin TJ, McPhail S, et al. Laparoscopic radical nephrectomy in first-trimester pregnancy. Urology. 2004;64(6):1231.e7-8.
37. Sherard GB, Hodson CA, Williams HJ, et al. Adnexal masses and pregnancy: a 12-year experience. Am J Obstet Gynecol. 2003;189(2):358-62; discussion 362-3.
38. Soriano D, Yeifet Y, Seidman DS, et al. Laparoscopy versus laparotomy in the management of adnexal masses during pregnancy. Fertil Steril. 1999;71(5):955-60.
39. Tamir IL, FS Bongard, SR Klein. Acute appendicitis in the pregnant patient. Am J Surg. 1990;160(6):571-5; discussion 575-6.
40. Tazuke SI, Nezhat FR, Nezhat CH, et al. Laparoscopic management of pelvic pathology during pregnancy. J Am Assoc Gynecol Laparosc. 1997;4(5):605-8.
41. Visser BC, Glasgow RE, Mulvihill KK, et al. Safety and timing of nonobstetric abdominal surgery in pregnancy. Dig Surg. 2001;18(5):409-17.
42. Visser BC, Glasgow RE, Mulvihill KK, et al. Safety and timing of nonobstetric abdominal surgery in pregnancy. Dig Surg. 2001;18(5):409-17.
43. Wang CJ, Yen CF, Lee CL, et al. Minilaparoscopic cystectomy and appendectomy in late second trimester. JSLS. 2002;6(4):373-5.
44. Yuen PM, Chang AM. Laparoscopic management of adnexal mass during pregnancy. Acta Obstet Gynecol Scand. 1997;76(2):173-6.

CHAPTER

31 Prenatal Diagnostic Procedures

Nutan Agarwal, Deepika Deka

INTRODUCTION

Prenatal diagnosis is one of the major evolutions in the field of obstetrics. It helps in detection of structural, chromosomal and genetic fetal diseases while fetus is in utero. Major structural malformation can be detected by ultrasound (USG), whereas USG-guided prenatal diagnostic procedures are required to get the fetal tissues to diagnose various chromosomal, genetic, metabolic disorders in the fetus. Commonly used prenatal diagnostic procedures are chorionic villus sampling (CVS), amniocentesis and fetal blood sampling.

Any of the sample obtained by different procedures can be used for cytogenetic, molecular or biochemical tests. Overall CVS sample is a desired sample for deoxyribonucleic acid (DNA) based test, whereas amniotic fluid for cytogenetic analysis. Fetal blood by cordocentesis can be used for all testing including hematological, infections, etc. Decision of the doing the particular test depends on type of disease to be diagnosed and period of gestation when procedure is being performed. CVS is done earlier at 10–12 weeks, amniocentesis at 16–18 weeks and cordocentesis after 18–24 weeks of gestation.

PREGNANCIES WHICH MAY REQUIRE PRENATAL DIAGNOSES

Prepregnancy Factors

- Advanced maternal age more than 35 years at delivery
- Consanguinity
- Family history of chromosomal anomalies
- Multiple abortions, stillbirths
- Genetic diseases like thalassemia and hemophilia
- Previous baby with malformation.

Factors Identified During Pregnancy

- Congenital anomalies on USG
- Abnormal maternal biochemical screening
- Severe early onset intrauterine growth restriction (IUGR) or oligohydramnios
- Polyhydramnios
- Maternal congenital infection
- Exposure to teratogens.

Pregnancies at risk are identified. Patient is counseled regarding method available, severity of disorder, treatment availability of disorder, acceptability of termination if fetus is affected. Pretest counseling is very essential prior to performing procedures. Here we are going to discuss various diagnostic procedures, their indications, techniques and their complications.

Procedures

- Chorionic villus sampling
- Amniocentesis
- Cordocentesis.

CHORIONIC VILLUS SAMPLING

Prenatal diagnosis by CVS allows early diagnosis, hence earlier and safer abortion can be performed if fetus is found affected. Cells of villi and fetus originate from fertilized egg and are identical. So, cytogenetic information of villi is same as fetus except in rare cases of mosaicism.

Indications of CVS

- DNA analysis for diagnosis of genetic disorder without prior culture
  - Single gene disorder

- Thalassemia major
- Hemophilia
- Duchene muscular dystrophy (DMD)

  – Inherited disorder of metabolism
  – Determination of paternity

- Early karyotype is required
  – Increased maternal age
  – Previous aneuploidy
  – Parental balanced translocation
  – Fragile X syndrome.

In our center, thalassemia and DMD are most common indications of CVS.

Timing of CVS

Chorionic villus sampling has been described as early as 8–9 weeks of gestation. However, it is safer to perform CVS 10 weeks onward to minimize the teratogenic effect of CVS. Transcervical CVS is not beyond 12 weeks as the chorion laeve and frondosum fuse; whereas transabdominal CVS can be performed later also. However, 11–12 weeks is considered optimum time to perform the procedure.

Technique of CVS

Ultrasound-guided transcervical and transabdominal aspiration techniques are the most commonly used methods.

Ultrasound evaluation should be done to rule out multiple gestation and to assess gestational age, viability, uterine position, placental position. Point of insertion and accessibility of trophoblastic tissue should be assessed. Whatever route is selected, sampling should be taken in strictly sterile conditions.

Transabdominal Aspiration Technique

The transducer is placed in a sterile bag. The sampling site is localized on the USG screen. Needle guide may be attached to transducer head to predetermine the needle pathway. A long 18 gauge (G) needle is used. We use disposable spinal needle for this purpose. Needle is introduced in desired direction through skin, then uterus to the edge of the trophoblast under USG guidance and continuous observation (Fig. 1). Thicker part of placenta which is away from the cord insertion is chosen. The needle is accurately introduced into the placental tissue, taking care not to pierce the amniotic sac. A 20 mL syringe containing 1–2 mL of culture media is attached to it. Vacuum is created in the syringe by pulling the plunger up and keeping it steady. Syringe should be very tightly fitted over the needle so that vacuum is created adequately. Needle can be rotated to loosen the villi and then up and down movements are made in placenta three to four times, along the length of the placenta depending on the placental thickness, and villi are slowly aspirated. It is essential to visualize the needle by USG continuously. Villi with culture media in syringe are flushed into a Petri dish and examined. Figure 1 depicts transabdominal (TA)-CVS procedure.

Transcervical CVS

Transcervical (TC)-CVS is performed if placenta is located posteriorly in lower uterine part, as the abdominal approach may be difficult in such cases. After cleaning, cervix is held with tenaculum. USG is placed on suprapubic area in order to give a longitudinal view of cervix and uterus. Sampling site is identified in the thickest area of trophoblast. Flexible catheter is introduced slowly into the cervical canal and directed to the placental area (anterior, posterior, or lateral). USG allows continual guidance of catheter. The stellate is withdrawn, and a 20 mL syringe (containing 3 mL of heparinized culture media) is attached to free end of catheter with gentle back and forth movements of the catheter, villi are aspirated, then catheter is removed. Contents of catheter and syringe are flushed into a sterile Petri dish, and examined. Figure 2 depicts TC-CVS procedure.

Trophoblastic tissues are cleaned and specimen immediately transported to laboratory. Aspirated tissue needs to be separated carefully under dissection microscope in order to exclude maternal cells contamination. After sampling, USG examination is done to ensure viability and absence of hematoma at the site of sampling. Rhesus (Rh) negative patient should receive 100 μg of anti-D immunoglobin.

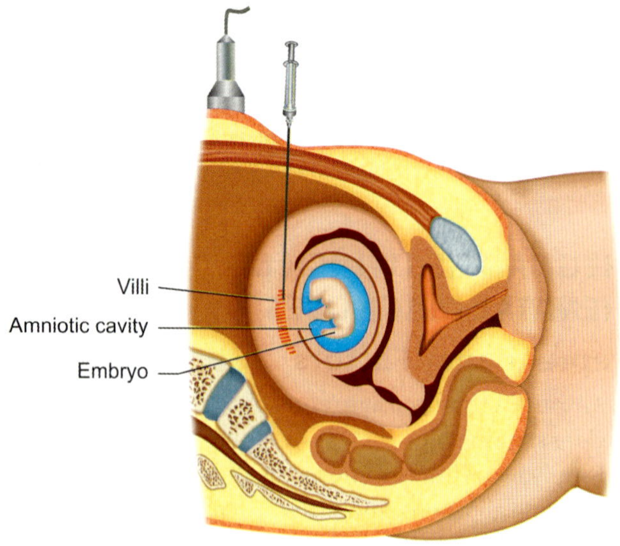

Fig. 1: Transabdominal chorionic villus sampling (TA-CVS)

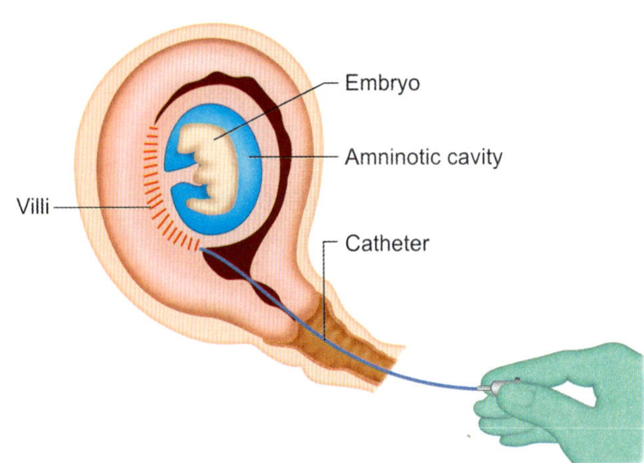

Fig. 2: Transcervical chorionic villus sampling (TC-CVS)

Transabdominal versus Transvaginal

Both routes are comparable and performed between 10 weeks and 12 weeks. TC-CVS is associated with potential risk of ascending infection. Threatened abortion and vaginal bleeding are also frequent. TC-CVS is opted for in cases where the placenta is posterior and approach through anterior route does not seem to be feasible. If period of gestation is more than 12 weeks then also only TA-CVS is performed.

Complications

Procedure-related complications:

- Mild transient uterine cramps
- Failure to obtain adequate sample
- Risk of abortion is 2.3% at 10 weeks of gestation and 1–1.5% once 12 weeks are crossed
- Limb reduction defects, 0.1% cases where sampling is done between 56 days and 63 days
- Infection, bleeding, leaking per vagina.

Other complications like IUGR, prematurity, intrauterine fetal death and neonatal death are equal to those observed in general population.

Diagnosis-related complications:

- Maternal cell contamination
- Mosaicism and other placental variant 1%.

Failure Rate of CVS

Success rate depends on experience of the team, at first attempt success is 80% and at second attempt about 95%. More than two attempts at same sitting are not recommended. Nonetheless transcervical sampling technique is associated with a slightly lower sampling failure rate. It may be due to flexibility of plastic catheter and movement may occur more easily.

In a study of 203 cases where TA-CVS was done in 129 (63%) and transcervical in 24 (36.5%) cases, no statistical significant difference was found in complications.

Advantage

CVS can provide early information to patients who want to make reproductive decision. Early amniocentesis can be performed but pregnancy loss rate is significantly higher after early amniocentesis than after CVS.

Disadvantage

Limb defects after CVS, if occurs, are reported only before 10 weeks. There is no evidence to suggest an increased risk of congenital malformation when CVS is performed after 10 weeks.

AMNIOCENTESIS

Amniocentesis has been used regularly since 1960s for Rh isoimmunized pregnancies but in 1966, Steele and Breg demonstrated the feasibility of performing chromosomal analysis of amniotic fluid cells. Now, it is the most commonly performed procedure. It poses the least risk to fetus among all prenatal diagnostic procedures.

Amniocytes obtained from amniotic fluid, are cells used for cytogenetic and molecular genetic studies. Biochemical analysis of fluid permits test for fetal lung maturity, open neural tube defects, etc. It is also used to assess for various viral and bacterial perinatal infections.

Indications

As prenatal diagnostic procedure for karyotype analysis:

- Maternal age more than 35 years at delivery
- Parental balanced translocation
- Previous aneuploid offspring
- Previous birth defect and unknown karyotype
- Dysmorphology on fetal USG evaluation
- Increased risk of aneuploidy on maternal serum screening result
- Rh isoimmunization for Rh typing, spectrophotometry
- Congenital infections.

Timing of Amniocentesis

Traditionally amniocentesis is performed between 16 weeks and 18 weeks when ratio of viable to nonviable amniotic fluid cells is greatest and amount of amniotic fluid is also sufficient (200–250 mL), so that up to 15–20 mL can be aspirated easily. Early amniocentesis prior to 15 weeks (11–14 weeks) evolved as a result of desire to provide an earlier prenatal diagnosis so that if a woman elects to undergo pregnancy termination after abnormal results, it can be done easily.

Early versus Late Amniocentesis

Early amniocentesis may be technically different. Amniotic fluid volume is less so removal of fluid is of greater concern. There are lesser number of amniocytes in early pregnancy fluid and it may lengthen the time necessary to grow an adequate number of cells to obtain result. So, it potentially decreases the advantage of an earlier procedure. Moreover, there is an increased rate of membrane tenting and less or chance of resealing of membrane if fluid leak occurred. There is a 6% risk of neonatal pulmonary complication after early amniocentesis. There is also an increased risk of spontaneous abortion in early amniocentesis versus traditional (4% vs 1%, which is more than CVS, 2%).

Increased risk of hip dislocation, respiratory distress, and neonatal pneumonia is reported with amniocentesis less than 15 weeks. Relative safety of early amniocentesis is not established, hence, preferred time of amniocentesis is 16–18 weeks.

Procedure

Abdomen is prepared for asepsis. Optimum pocket of amniotic fluid is located by USG. A thin 22–23 G spinal needle is used for aspiration of amniotic fluid. There is no need for local anesthesia. Under continuous USG guidance after localization of amniotic fluid pocket, needle is inserted through the abdomen. Selection criteria for choosing needle insertion site ideally includes the presence of relative large fluid pocket away from the fetus. Insertion through placenta is avoided. Needle tip should be kept away from fetal face and cord. On entering the amniotic fluid pocket, stylet is withdrawn and a 2 mL syringe is connected to the hub of the needle. Initial 1–2 mL fluid aspirated is discarded. Then 15–20 mL of amniotic fluid is obtained in a different syringe and transferred to transportation tubes or vacutainers. Figure 3 shows needle tip in amniotic fluid. Figure 4 shows withdrawal of amniotic fluid.

Complications of Amniocentesis

- Procedure related infection as a cause of pregnancy loss is reported in 0.1–0.3%
- Amniotic fluid leak is reported to be 1.2%
- Procedure related loss is approximately 0.5%
- Preterm premature rupture of membranes (PPROM) is reported in 3% and preterm delivery risk is about 8%
- Amniocentesis is not associated with increased risk of abruption
- Amniotic fluid culture failure is reported in 0.5% of specimen. Repeat amniocentesis or cordocentesis may be required in such cases.

CORDOCENTESIS

Fetal blood sampling was performed in 1974 by fetoscopy for the first time for diagnosis of hemoglobinopathies. Transabdominal USG-guided cordocentesis was first performed by Daffos in Paris in 1983.

Indications of Cordocentesis

Diagnostic

- Chromosomal analysis (rapid karyotype)
  - Advanced gestation for prenatal diagnosis
  - Fetal structural malformation on USG
  - Severe early onset fetal growth restriction or oligohydramnios
  - Failed diagnosis by amniocentesis or CVS
  - Chromosomal mosaicism on amniocentesis or CVS

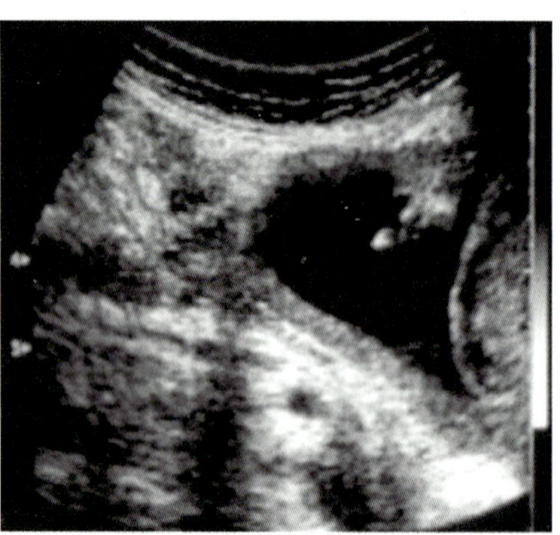

Fig. 3: Needle tip in amniotic fluid

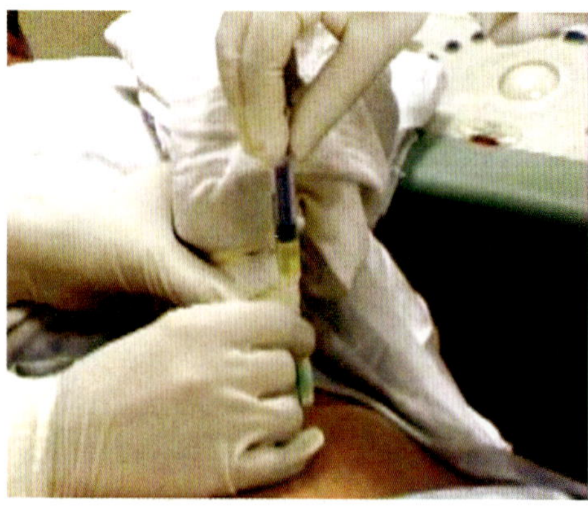

Fig. 4: Withdrawal of the amniotic fluid

- Single gene defect like
  - Thalassemia, hemophilia, DMD (molecular defect has not been identified)
- Other hematological disorders like thrombocytopenia
- Congenital infection, rubella, cytomegalovirus (CMV), toxoplasmosis, parvovirus, varicella by estimation of IgM—one specific genomic genetic material for polymerase chain reaction (PCR)
- Hemoglobin and hematocrit estimation in fetal anemia like Rh isoimmunization, nonimmune hydrops
- Fetal blood gas analysis.

Therapeutic Cordocentesis

- Intrauterine transfusion
- Drug therapy—fetal arrhythmias
- Stem cell transplant.

About 5-6% of cordocentesis are reported to be performed due to failure of amniocentesis.

Timing of Cordocentesis

It is generally performed after 18 weeks period of gestation. Before that, cord being of small size, procedure is difficult. As the period of gestation increases, cord vessel diameter increases and so the procedure becomes easier. But most of the time, diagnosis is required earlier than 20 weeks so that termination can be offered, if results are abnormal.

Procedure

After abdominal part preparation, USG evaluation is done for placental localization and placental origin of cord as this is the best site for cordocentesis. Cord is comparatively fixed at its origin and so needle entry is less likely to slip, and be successful at this site. Color Doppler may also sometimes facilitates the localization of cord insertion. If the site is not accessible or feasible then free loop of cord can be selected for puncture. Fetal side of cord should be avoided as there is increased risk of needle displacement and fetal bradycardia. Needle length is decided on the basis of distance from skin to site of puncture. Spinal or Chiba needle depending on need of length of needle, with size of 21-22 G can be used. Under continuous USG guidance needle is inserted through abdomen. Confirmation of the site of entry on the abdomen is done by assessing the planned needle tract. Needle tip is advanced towards puncture site avoiding injury to fetal structures. Pancuronium 0.1 mg intramuscular (IM) can be given to fetus if there are excessive fetal movements or placenta is posterior. It is more likely to be required when needle has to be kept in position for a longer time like as in intrauterine transfusions.

When needle tip reaches the cord, a sharp and quick puncture is made over the wall to achieve penetration into vessel. Tip of needle can be visualized inside the lumen of vessel. Stylet is withdrawn, syringe attached, 2-4 mL of fetal blood is aspirated. After obtaining blood, needle and stylet are withdrawn. Fetal heart activity is then checked for any abnormality. Figure 5 shows cordocentesis—needle tip in the lumen of vessel.

Problems During Procedure

- Localized uterine contraction may occur immediately. Such contractions alter the course or decrease the visualization of needle. Operator can wait for contraction to pass away or remove the needle and readjust its direction
- Blood in amniotic fluid. About 0.1 mL heparin can be added quickly to prevent clotting and trapping of amniocytes in the clot. The procedure may have to be repeated after 1-2 weeks
- Discolored amniotic fluid: It may be due to old intra-amniotic hemorrhage. It indicates high chances of pregnancy loss.

Postprocedure Observation

- Observe for any bleeding from puncture site which is usually self-limiting, lasting 1-2 minutes
- Fetal bradycardia may be transient, fetal heart rate (FHR) should be monitored; atropine 0.6 mg to be given IM may improve FHR. In rare instances, emergency cesarean section may be needed
- Patient may not perceive fetal movement for 2 hours if pancuronium is given to fetus
- Anti-D is to be given, if patient Rh negative, nonimmunized pregnancy
- Prophylactic antibiotic may be given.

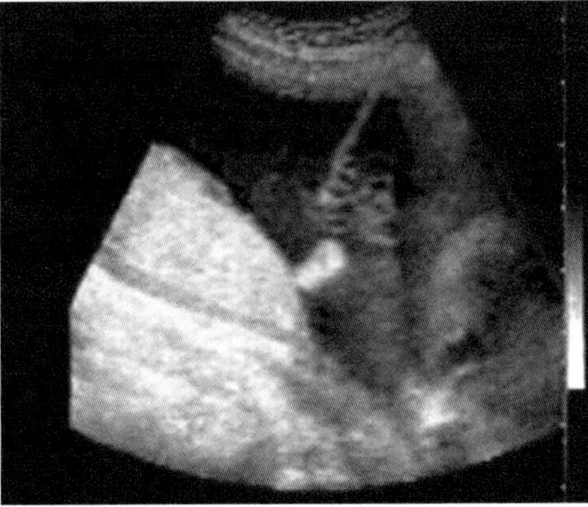

Fig. 5: Cordocentesis—needle tip in the lumen of vessel

Limitations of Cordocentesis

- Occasionally there may be inability to visualize the cord insertion site. Fetal position or movement may interfere with optimal cord visualization and needle placement
  Placental position influences the likelihood of success or occurrence of complications associated with procedure
  - *Anterior placenta:* Cordocentesis is easier but as the needle is transversing the placental villi, there are higher probabilities of maternal contamination in the specimen or it may worsen Rh immunization in Rh negative women
  - *Posterior placenta:* Attempting cordocentesis in posterior placenta is more likely to be difficult because interposed fetus may obstruct the optimal pathway for needle.

Complications of Cordocentesis

Complications of procedure depend on indication for the procedure itself. Higher fetal loss may be expected if it is performed for severe IUGR, nonimmune hydrops, or structural anomalies compared to cordocentesis for confirmation of genetic diseases. Overall procedure related risk is less than 2%.

Fetal Complications

- Transient bleeding from puncture site (10–20%), cord hematoma
- Fetal bradycardia
- PPROM.

Maternal Complications

- Chorioamnionitis
- Bleeding
- Risk of emergency—lower segment cesarean section (LSCS)
- Needle injury to maternal intra-abdominal organs.

CONCLUSION

Recently four-dimensional ultrasonographic guidance for needle placement in prenatal diagnostic procedures has been reported to decrease or eliminate errors in the techniques.

Detection of fetal cells or fetal DNA in maternal blood may evolve to prenatal diagnosis by noninvasive methods in future.

BIBLIOGRAPHY

1. Alfirevic Z, Gosden CM, Neilson JP. Chorion villus sampling versus amniocentesis for prenatal diagnosis. Cochrane Database Syst Rev. 2000;(2):CD000055.
2. Cederholm H, Haglund B, Azalsson D. Maternal complications following amniocentesis and chorionic villus prenatal karyotyping. BJOG. 2003;110(4):392-9.
3. Cederholm M, Haglund B, Axelsson O. Infant morbidity following amniocentesis and chorionic villus sampling karyotyping. BJOG. 2005;112(4):394-402.
4. Deka D, Arora S, Kabra M, et al. Amniocentesis for Rh grouping by PCR: a major breakthrough in anti-D prophylaxis and management of Rh negative pregnancies. J Obst Gynaecol India. 2004;54(2):151-4.
5. Dunn LK, Godmillard L. A comparison of less rates for first trimester CVS, early amniocentesis and need trimester amniocentesis in a population of women of advanced age. Am J Hum Genet. 1990;47:A273.
6. Kino SK, Cho DJ, Kim JW, et al. Adverse pregnancy outcome following post-chorionic villus sampling compared to chorionic villus sampling. J Obstet Gynecol Res. 2000;26(3):209-13.
7. Kriplani A, Agarwal N, Sharmila K, et al. Evaluation of efficacy, fetal loss and pregnancy outcome in patients undergoing transabdominal vs. transcervical chorionic villus sampling. Asian J Obstet Gynecol Prac. 2004;(8)1:9-13.
8. Kuliev AM, Modell B, Jackson L, et al. Risk evaluation of CVS. Prenat Diagn. 1993;13:197.
9. Laperrelle J, Senal MV, Picone O, et al. Amniocentesis practice assessment of south-west Francilians. J Gynecol Obstet Bio Reprod. 2008;37(2):135-42.
10. Mathur R, Dubey S, Hamilton S, et al. Rapid prenatal karyotyping using fetal blood obtained by cordocentesis. Natl Med J India. 2002;15(2):75-7.
11. Nicolaides K, Brizot M, Patel F, et al. Comparison of chorionic villus sampling and amniocentesis for fetal karyotyping at 10-13 weeks gestation. Lancet. 1994;344:435.
12. Penso CA, Sandstrom MM, Garber F, et al. Early amniocentesis report of 407 cases with new born follow-up. Obstet Gynecol. 1990;76:1032.
13. Ranjan R, Biswas A, Kannan M, et al. Prenatal diagnosis of haemophilia A by chorionic villus sampling and cordocentesis: All India Institute of Medical Science experience. Vox Sang. 2007;92(1):79-84.
14. Smidt-Jensen S, Permin N, Philip J. Sampling success and risk by transabdominal chorionic villus sampling versus chorionic villus sampling and amniocentesis: a randomized study. Ultrasound Obstet Gynecol. 1991;1(2):86-90.

CHAPTER

32

Fetal Surgery

Deepika Deka

INTRODUCTION

It is now routine to perform ultrasound (USG) for fetal congenital structural malformations. Complications such as polyhydramnios, oligohydramnios or growth restriction leads to performance of more USG scans than for anomalies. Most of the times, the 2D scan shows a structurally normal fetus, but in 2–5% cases, a fetal anomaly or multiple anomalies may be identified. A lethal anomaly such as bilateral renal agenesis, anencephaly need to be managed by termination of pregnancy (TOP). An anomaly detected late, with mild organ damage such as mild ventriculomegaly, hydronephrosis may be left alone and the newborn managed after birth by a team of neonatologists or pediatric surgeon/nephrologist/cardiologist/neurologist, etc. depending on the case. However, if continuation of the pregnancy is desired in a case with fetal structural defect which could cause grave organ damage, morbidity or mortality if left alone in the expectation of treatment after birth, the option of therapeutic intervention during fetal life in utero—"fetal surgery" seems to be the only viable alternative. Research and rapid growth of the new subspecialty of Fetal Diagnosis and Therapy has increased access to treatment for women with fetal anatomic defects as they became available. The ultimate goal of research in congenital malformation diagnosis has always been Fetal Management, not just the ability to make the diagnosis. The topic is now of intense focus and increasing demand as we may have something better to offer beyond a defeated course, i.e. TOP.

EVOLUTION OF FETAL SURGERY

In the initial years, fetal surgery was performed by hysterotomy, followed by the fetal procedure with partial extrusion of fetus from uterus. The fetus was returned into the uterine cavity, amniotic fluid replaced and water-tight closure of the uterine rent performed. Premature uterine contractions usually followed soon after and the problems of a scarred uterus thwarted fulfilling results. Less invasive techniques were sought, and simultaneous marvelous advances in interventional USG and endoscopy were taken advantage of. Endoscopic modification from experiences of open fetal surgery paved the way for fetal endoscopic surgery (FETENDO).

In the 1990s, the merger of fetoscopy and advanced video-endoscopic surgery formed the basis for endoscopic fetal surgery. The first clinical fetoscopic surgeries were interventions on the umbilical cord and the placenta, often referred to as Obstetrical Endoscopy. At present, most experience has been gathered with fetal tracheal occlusion as therapy for severe congenital diaphragmatic hernia. As in other fields, minimally invasive surgery has pushed back boundaries and now allows safe operations to be performed on the fetus, the patient. Whereas minimal access seems to solve the problem of preterm labor, all procedures remain invasive, and carry a risk to the mother and a substantial risk of preterm prelabor rupture of the membranes (PPROM). The latter problem may prove to be a bottleneck for further developments, although treatment modalities are currently being evaluated. Thus, fetal surgery may offer an alternative to abortion, intrauterine death, or a life with disability. Expertise is limited, however, to a few treatment centers worldwide, and there are many technical hurdles to overcome, including requirements for miniaturized instrumentation, real-time high-resolution imaging, and harmless fetal access. While the number of potential patients is low, research for implementation of robotics in the field of fetal surgery is justified by the morbidity rates of current procedures, proven favorable outcomes with intervention, and the educational value with potential for extension to other medical disciplines. In India, very few centers such as the All India Institute of Medical Sciences, New Delhi, India, are involved in research and patient care in this exciting, rapidly advancing field.

PRINCIPLES OF FETAL SURGERY

Since fetal structural abnormalities have a wide spectrum of clinical severity and prognosis, a thorough and accurate assessment of fetal status and management plan should be defined in consultation with team of ultrasonologist, geneticist, neonatologist, pediatric surgeon, and if necessary cardiologist, microbiologist, etc. depending on the case, at a specialized tertiary care center.

The biochemical screen report should be checked to correctly define the type and severity of abnormality. Detailed targeted USG should be done for other associated abnormalities or syndromes. If the structural defect is suggestive of a chromosomal abnormality, a fetal karyotype is performed by amniotic fluid or cord blood sampling.

Parents should be counseled regarding the maternal and fetal risks, the interventions possible, cost involved and length of expected hospital stay and ultimate fetal or neonatal prognosis.

INDICATIONS

The primary indication is that, otherwise, the progressive fetal structural malformation disease process would lead to severe damage to fetal vital organs by the time of birth or eventual neonatal therapy.

As yet, only few malformations in well selected cases appear to have a good benefit from in utero surgery. A lot more procedures are still being developed in animal experiments. A system wise comprehensive list is given in Table 1, with details of each therapy featured subsequently. Conditions and malformations which may benefit from fetal surgery are described below.

Pertinent aspects of some defects and corrective fetal surgical procedures are also described.

Table 1: Various in utero fetal malformation amenable to fetal surgery

Fetal structural defect	Natural fetal outcome	Recommended treatment
• Urinary tract obstructive defects - Pelviureteric junction obstruction - Ureterovescical junction obstruction - Urethral obstruction - Ureterocele	Renal failure Renal failure hypoplasia Oligohydramnios	Vesicocentesis Vesicoamniotic shunt Fetoscopic vesicostomy and Laser ablation
• Lung defects - Cystic adenomatoid malformation - Pleural effusion - Pulmonary sequestration	Pulmonary hypoplasia Respiratory failure	Pleuroamniotic shunt Thoracoamniotic shunt Open pulmonary lobectomy
• Diaphragmatic hernia	Pulmonary hypoplasia	Open complete repair Temporary tracheal occlusion
• Multiple pregnancy - Twin-twin transfusion syndrome - Acardiac twins	Hydrops fetalis Intrauterine death	Laser ablation Cord occlusion
• Sacrococcygeal teratoma	Hydrops fetalis	Resection of tumor Radiofrequency ablation Fetoscopic vascular occlusion
• Ovarian cysts	Torsion	Cyst aspiration
• Placenta or amnion - Chorioangioma of placenta - Amniotic band syndrome	Polyhydramnios Amputation of limb	Vascular occlusion
• CNS defects - Aqueductal stenosis - Dandy Walker - Myelomeningocele	Brain damage Paralysis	Ventriculoamniotic shunt Open ventriculo-peritoneal shunt Fetoscopic coverage Open repair
• Facial defects - Cleft lip and palate	Facial deformity	Fetoscopic coverage Open repair

Abbreviation: CNS; central nervous system

URINARY TRACT OBSTRUCTIVE DEFECTS

Obstructive renal disease is defined as the need for surgical treatment, while nonobstructive disease includes those cases that require no therapy. Renal pelvis dilatation was the primary postnatal sonographic finding in 66.4% of cases of congenital renal anomalies.

Ureteropelvic Junction Obstruction

There is dilatation of the renal pelvis and calyces leading to hydronephrosis due to accumulation of urine. It is unilateral in 70% cases, more common in males. Back pressure resulting from obstruction to flow of urine from renal pelvis to proximal ureter by ureteral valves, a dysfunctional or adynamic ureteric muscle segment or stricture, external pressure by crossing vessels or fibrous band may cause renal cortical thinning. In severe cases, there are renal parenchymal dysplastic changes in the cortex, with associated oligohydramnios.

On USG, hydronephrosis is defined as dilatation of renal pelvis, anteroposterior (AP) diameter more than 10 mm, while lesser dilatations of more than 3 mm in second trimester or more than 6 mm after 32 weeks are termed "pyelectasis".

Fetal surgery is usually not indicated for unilateral disease or mild bilateral disease without oligohydramnios. Even if unilateral ureteropelvic junction (UPJ) obstructed kidney is severely damaged, provided the other kidney is normal, the risk of in utero management does not warrant intervention. USG should be done every 3–4 weeks for renal pelvis dilatation.

Catheter placement is indicated if liquor is decreasing and severity of calyceal dilatation is increasing. Presence of lung hypoplasia and deficient renal function are poor prognostic factors.

Ureterovesical Junction Obstruction

This may result from presence of ureteral valves, ectopic ureter or due to dynamic distal ureteral segment. The ureterovesical junction (UVJ) obstruction causes accumulation of urine in the proximal ureter resulting in a megaureter and subsequently to hydronephrosis. Fetal ureters visible on USG, is termed "hydroureter".

Urethral Obstruction

Posterior urethral valve (PUV) is the most common cause in male fetuses. Other causes are megalourethra, atresia, ureterocele, cloacal dysgenesis. Fetal bladder enlargement or "megacystis" is one which reaches above the abdominal wall insertion of the umbilical cord.

For fetuses less than 32 weeks with oligohydramnios, evaluation of underlying renal function is done by sequential USG-guided "vesicocentesis" in which the fetal bladder is completely drained at 48–72 hour intervals on a minimum of two to three occasions. The urine is analyzed for electrolyte and protein values as a reflection of the level and severity of damage to the fetal kidneys. Fetuses that demonstrate progressive hypotonicity on sequential urine samples and have final values which fall below recommended thresholds have been shown to benefit from in utero intervention.

Fetal urine evaluation parameters showing good prognosis are:

Sodium	≤ 100 mg/dL
Osmolality	≤ 200 mOsm/L
Chloride	≤ 90 mg/dL
Calcium	≤ 8 mg/dL
Total protein	≤ 20 mg/dL
β-2 microglobulin	≤ 6 mg/L

Fetal Vesicocentesis

Under continuous USG guidance with color Doppler visualization to prevent inadvertent umbilical vessel injury, a 22 gauge or 23 gauge needle is inserted into the fetal bladder. The bladder is completely emptied of urine by aspiration with 20 mL syringe or continuous rapid suction, while constantly maintaining the needle tip placement within the cavity of the shrinking bladder. The urine is sent for required analysis.

Aspirated "old" urine may be concentrated, as water is absorbed through bladder wall. However, if urinary values are normal, renal dysplasia is not present. In unilateral disease also, the values may not reflect specific kidney function because of normal contralateral kidney. If values are high, repeat vesicocentesis should be done after 48 hours, and if still above normal, a third sampling can be performed. Cord blood sampling for renal parameters can also be useful (creatinine, beta 2-microglobulin).

Percutaneous Vesicoamniotic Shunt

This is performed if kidney functions are normal, the karyotype is normal and there are no major malformations. It can be performed under local, regional or general anesthesia, usually local.

The location and position of the placenta and fetus are identified on USG to avoid passing through the placenta. Since most of these fetuses have oligohydramnios, amnioinfusion may be carried out using warmed Ringer lactate solution, and is helpful in placement of proximal part of shunt in the uterine cavity and not in the myometrium. The ideal fetal site of entry is chosen very carefully—it should be below the umbilicus, avoiding vessels as seen by color Doppler. Fetus is first given analgesia (0.2 μg/kg pancuronium, 10 μg/kg/fentanyl).

Once the appropriate approach is chosen, the maternal skin is anesthetized with 1% lignocaine and a small 3–5 mm stab wound is made to allow easy passage of the shunt trocar. The shunt trocar is then carefully introduced into the amniotic space near the lower fetal abdomen into a fetal amniotic pocket and is quickly inserted into the fetal bladder using sharp, shift movement and positioned centrally. Urine sample is aspirated, sent for culture and renal function. The double pigtail "Rodeck" or "Harrison" shunt catheter is now gently straightened and threaded into the trocar sheath prior to removal of internal stylet wire. Using push rods, the proximal segment of the catheter is pushed into the fetal bladder and the distal end of the catheter is positioned in the amniotic space.

Percutaneous Fetal Cystoscopy

This new technique has set a unique, diagnostic and therapeutic standard.

Standard fetal endoscopy: A 3 mm or 3.9 mm trocar with 2.7 mm or 3.3 mm operating endoscope is used. The fetal bladder is entered as in shunt procedure, and ablation of ureteral valve or ureterocele wall lysis is done using contact yttrium aluminum garnet (YAG) laser.

Endoscopic Fetal Cystotomy—Fetal Hydrolaparoscopy

Similar to adult laparoscopy, access into the fetal peritoneal cavity by the endoscope is achieved and the bladder is identified. Dome is incised using 20 W laser, 3.3 mm endoscope is inserted inside the bladder and posterior urethral valve (PUV) ablated.

Retrograde urethral catheterization (RUC): Fetal endoscope is inserted into the amniotic cavity near fetal penis. Foreskin is grasped with 1 mm forceps. A 2 mm monopolar electrode is passed into the urethra under combined USG and endoscopic guidance. PUV is identified and ablation done.

Monitoring: The patient is monitored using external fetal monitor for 2 hours and uterine irritability treated with tocolysis and intravenous fluids. USG at 24–48 hours and then weekly for 4–6 weeks needs to be done to confirm proper catheter placement and function, amniotic fluid volume, and progressive resolution of bilateral hydronephrosis.

Prognostic Factors:

- Renal cystic dysplasia, renal cortical thinning, hyperechoic parenchyma and oligohydramnios are poor prognostic factors. If fetal urinary sodium, calcium, total protein, microalbulmin, phosphate, N-acetyl-beta-D-glucosaminidase, osmolality and β-2-microglobin are below the threshold of renal cystic dysplasia on vescicocentesis, fetal surgery can be offered
- Associated structural malformations may be present in 17–30%
- Chromosomal anomalies may range from 8% to 23% (trisomy 13, 18, 21).

As the bladder shrinks, dislocation and malfunction of the shunt may occur in 60% cases due to pull from skin into the fetal abdomen or shunt being pulled out of the fetus into the amniotic cavity. Antenatal treatment of obstructive uropathy, although widely performed, remains controversial. In one large study, 58 patients were followed up from 6 months to 6½ years (mean 3.9 years). Group 1 included 12 patients who had vesicoamniotic shunt placement and were confirmed postnatally to have PUV. Four fetuses died (33.3%); three out of the eight living had perinatal complications. Of the eight living neonates, three (37.5%) underwent valve ablation and five (62.5%) underwent urinary diversion (three vesicostomies and two cutaneous ureterostomies). Renal function returned to normal in only four (50%). Radiological abnormalities (hydronephrosis and/or reflux) resolved in three (37.5%), was downgraded in one (12.5%) and persisted in four cases (50%). Group 2 included 46 patients who were treated postnatally. Thirty-five (76%) underwent primary valve ablation, while 11 (24%) underwent urinary diversion (seven vesicostomies, four cutaneous ureterostomy and one pyelostomy). Renal function returned to normal in all babies who underwent valve ablation, except in three, while renal function returned to normal in only 3 of 11 patients who underwent urinary diversion. Radiological hydronephrosis and/or reflux resolved in 28 patients (60.9%), was downgraded in 6 patients (13%) and persisted in 12 patients (26.1%).

Thus, antenatal vesicoamniotic shunt placement appears to make no difference to the outcome and long-term results of patients with PUV and debate about its efficacy on renal outcome remains. Primary valve ablation is emerging as the keystone of treatment for patients with PUV that might achieve the primary goal of nephron preservation. The lowest creatinine concentration in the 1st year of life is the most appropriate predictor of future renal function.

LUNG DEFECTS

Congenital Cystic Adenomatoid Malformations

Congenital cystic adenomatoid malformation (CCAM) of the lung is a nonfunctioning benign lung tumor, hamartomatous or dysplastic in origin. They may be:

- Macrocystic—usually a single, 2-10 cm cyst within lungs
- Microcystic—appearing as solid, echogenic mass.

Hydrops fetalis and polyhydramnios warrant fetal intervention. Treatment by means of decompression can improve substantially the clinical results in these patients.

Fetal Surgery

Antenatal evaluation using USG, amniocentesis, percutaneous umbilical blood sampling (PUBS), cardiac echo should be carried out to look for the presence of other fetal anomalies and fetal prognostic markers. If fetal hydrops is not present, the mother should be followed by serial USG scans and arrangements made for appropriate postnatal care. An elective postnatal resection of lung mass at 4 weeks of age can be carried out. If the fetus has hydrops, or hydrops develops during follow-up, then management depends on the gestational age. For fetuses more than 32 weeks, delivery of the fetus and resection of the lesion ex utero in a center with extracorporeal membrane oxygenation (ECMO) facilities is appropriate.

For fetuses that develop hydrops before 32 weeks of gestation, treatment options are:

Microcystic CCAM

- Posterolateral thoracotomy with resection of involved lobe
- Percutaneous intrauterine laser therapy.

Macrocystic CCAM

Thoracoamniotic shunt placement carries a 70% success rate. Effect of prenatal pulmonary drainage (shunt, surgery or drainage) on perinatal survival was compared with no treatment, in fetuses with ultrasonic evidence of lung pathology. Sixteen controlled observational studies involving 608 fetuses showed that pulmonary drainage did not improve perinatal survival in cystic lung lesions compared with no drainage [odds ratio (OR) 0.56, 95% confidence interval (CI) 0.32-0.97, P=0.04] overall. However, there was a marked improvement with this therapy in a subgroup of fetuses with fetal hydrops fetalis (OR 19.28, 95% CI 3.67-101.27, P=0.0005) but not in the subgroup uncomplicated by fetal hydrops fetalis (OR 0.04, 95% CI 0.01-0.32, P=0.002).

Bronchopulmonary Sequestration

These are intralobar and extralobar lung masses of benign pulmonary tissue without tracheobronchial communication. They may be densely echogenic or with a cystic adenomatoid malformation component. Prenatal three-dimensional power Doppler USG may be useful in identifying the feeding vessel and thus establishing the diagnosis of pulmonary sequestration in the presence of a hyperechogenic pulmonary lesion, allowing its differentiation from CCAM. Fetal extralobar pulmonary sequestration (EPS) is sometimes complicated by massive pleural effusion (PE) leading to fetal hydrops. The underlying mechanisms as well as the origin of the fluid are not well understood, but venous obstruction may have a role to play.

Fetal Surgery

Pleuroamniotic shunting should be considered as a treatment option for fetal hydrothorax and hydrops associated with bronchopulmonary sequestration (BPS) (procedure same as vesicoamniotic shunt). Postnatally, of eight fetuses with hyperechogenic lung, there was isolated pulmonary sequestration (n=3), microcystic congenital adenomatoid malformation (n=4), and mixed (macrocystic and microcystic) congenital adenomatoid malformation (n=1). In three cases of fetal EPS complicated by fetal hydrothorax, thoracentesis and eventually thoracoamniotic shunt placement was performed. After birth, all three infants required mass resection for the control of PE. Twenty-two articles describing 308 cases of fetuses with CCAM, 25 cases of hydrothorax and 55 cases of BPS. Of the 388 cases, 250 fetuses were managed conservatively. Hydrops was identified as the worst prognostic factor—survival rate of 55.7%. The global survival was of 56.5% (155 cases) in the fetuses with CCAM, 98.1% (52 cases) in the fetuses with BPS and of 80% (20 cases) in the fetuses with hydrothorax. Initial reports were characterized by a high (about 30%) incidence of adverse features (e.g. hydrops). Sixty-seven fetuses had a cystic lung abnormality diagnosed from January 1995 to July 2001. The lesion was right sided in 29 (43%), left in 36 (54%), and bilateral in 2 (3%); it was characterized as dominantly macrocystic in 27 (40%), microcystic in 35 (52%), and mixed in 5 (8%). Mediastinal shift was present in 30 fetuses (45%). Fetal hydrops was present in five fetuses (7%). Antenatal intervention was performed in 4 fetuses [thoracoamniotic shunts (n=3) and percutaneous intrauterine laser therapy (n=1)]. Sixty-four (96%) of the fetuses were born alive. There was one TOP and two intrauterine deaths (all severe microcystic lesions). Forty-two infants (63%) underwent thoracotomy and appropriate excisional surgery at a median of 7.5 months (range, from 1 day to 34 months). Two infants (which included the fetus having intrauterine laser therapy) died early in the postnatal period. Both were large microcystic lesions and had antenatal features of hydrops. Twelve infants were investigated in the postnatal period but did not undergo surgery. Ten infants were not appropriately investigated or were lost to follow-up. Histologic examination showed definitive diagnostic features of CCAM (n=25) or PS (n=6). Other lesions with hybrid features of both were also seen (n=11). Surgical excision was required in 45% of lesions showing late-gestation "resolution". Thus, antenatally diagnosed "cystic lung disease" have an excellent prognosis in the absence of signs of hydrops.

Pleural Effusion

Fetal PEs may lead to lung compression and hypoplasia, and could be due to chylothorax.

Fetal Surgery: Thoracoamniotic Shunt

Evaluation of the efficacy of a thoracoamniotic shunt for the treatment of PE, by preload index (PLI) in the inferior vena cava (IVC), the maximal flow velocity of the descending aorta (VAomax), skin edema on the thorax and the ratio of lung to the thorax transverse area (L/T) as measured by USG in five fetuses with PE showed that the PLI and skin edema on the thorax decreased significantly after shunt placement compared to before shunt placement (PLI before: 0.488±0.036, after: 0.348±0.043, P <0.05; edema before: 15.3±2.06 mm, after: 9.00±0.63 mm, P <0.05). Furthermore, the L/T increased significantly after shunt placement compared to before (before: 0.220±0.013, after: 0.260±0.011, P <0.01). No significant difference in VAomax was seen between before and after shunt placement (before: 101.5±6.39 cm/s, after: 10.7.6±5.41 cm/s, P=0.16). Thus, shunt for PE improved PLI especially in the fetal hemodynamics significantly. Study of perinatal outcome following thoracoamniotic shunting for fetal PEs in hydropic fetuses with suspected chylothorax—performed immediately following diagnosis, on the basis of the rationale that mediastinal compression could lead to acute fetal distress showed that shunting was successful in all 60 cases attempted. There were 7 pregnancy terminations, 10 in utero deaths, and 43 live births, of which 7 children died in the neonatal period and 36 survived (33 without sequels). Among the liveborn, 26 were delivered preterm (72%), of which 7 (19%) had preterm premature rupture of membranes and 4 (11%) had chorioamnionitis. Perinatal death (24/60, 40%) was related to underlying anomalies (7cases), pulmonary hypoplasia (5cases), chorioamnionitis (2 cases), or treatment failure for unknown reasons (10 cases). All 36 survivors had chylothorax, 33 of which were primary, and 3 were secondary to right congenital diaphragmatic hernia, PS, or Noonan syndrome. PE with hydrops has survival rate more than 50% after shunting, but still have a high rate of morbidity and mortality.

SACROCOCCYGEAL TERATOMA

Sacrococcygeal teratomas (SCTs) are the most common neonatal tumors with an incidence of approximately 1:30,000. They can be entirely cystic, microcystic, mixed cystic and solid, or solid. The diagnosis of SCT is quite accurate using both magnetic resonance imaging (MRI) and sonography, though compared with sonography, MRI more accurately characterizes the intrapelvic and abdominal extent of the tumors and provides more information on compression of adjacent organs. The additional anatomic resolution provided by MRI results in more accurate prenatal counseling and improved preoperative planning for surgical resection.

Fetal Surgery

Fetal SCT necessitates frequent monitoring to ensure the detection of fetal or maternal complications by USG and Doppler ultrasound. The most important prognostic criteria are cardiomegaly, fetal hydrops, and increased preload indexes of the fetal venous system as sign of fetal heart failure. Many studies show that the occurrence of pulsations in the umbilical vein of a hydropic fetus correlates with a poor fetal outcome. The decision on the optimal time of delivery should therefore be made by a multidisciplinary team of specialists. Fetuses that develop hydrops before 32 weeks, need to be referred to tertiary care center for fetal surgery:

- Resection
- Laser vessel ablation
- Alcohol sclerosis
- Cyst drainage.

Open fetal surgery has been performed in hydropic fetuses or even before hydrops develops. One study of 27/41 SCTs managed antenatally, 6 underwent TOP, 12 underwent fetal intervention (laser vessel ablation: 4, alcohol sclerosis: 3, cyst drainage: 2, amniodrainage: 2, vescicoamniotic shunt: 1) for fetal hydrops of these, 3 died in utero, 9 born alive, median gestational age, 33 weeks (27–37 weeks) but 3 more died in the neonatal period. Six (50%) survived long-term. Without intervention, 17 infants were born alive at median 38 weeks (26–40 weeks), 16 had excision surgery at median 2 days (1–16 days) with no recurrences on follows up till median 39 months (8–86 months). Thus, overall survival was 77%, in utero intervention requirement being poor prognostic factor.

TWIN TO TWIN TRANSFUSION SYNDROME

This describes a continuum of complications that are seen in monozygotic, monochorionic diamniotic twins. In monozygotic twin pregnancies, there are placental vascular communications between the two fetuses. In 15% of such pregnancies there is an imbalance in net blood flow between the twins, resulting in the twin-twin transfusion syndrome (TTTS). The recipient twin may have severe hydramnios during the second trimester of pregnancy, and there is a high risk of perinatal death and cerebral palsy in survivors.

Fetal Surgery

- Serial amnioreduction: Under USG guidance, a needle is inserted into the amniotic cavity and amniotic fluid drained using suction drainage
- Laser ablation of arteriovenous anstomosis. Laser coagulation of placental vessels crossing the intertwin membrane on the chorionic surface under sonoendoscopic guidance, Endoscopic coagulation of the vascular anastomoses responsible for fetofetal transfusion with a neodymium:yttrium-aluminum-garnet (Nd:YAG) laser. With the use of local anesthesia and continuous USG visualization, a rigid fetoscope 2 mm in diameter, housed in a 2.7 mm cannula, was introduced transabdominally into the amniotic cavity of the recipient twin. A systematic search was made for all vessels approaching or crossing the membrane between the twins, and these were coagulated with an Nd:YAG laser by means of a fiber in the side arm of the cannula
- Umbilical cord ligation or occlusion
- Septostomy.

Intrauterine surgery was performed in 45 pregnant women carrying twins at 15–28 weeks of gestation (median, 21 weeks); in each case there was severe hydramnios in one fetus due to the TTTS. Coagulation of the communicating vessels was successful in all cases. The total number of fetuses who survived to delivery was 48 (53%), and the number of pregnancies with at least one survivor was 32 (71%). Among the liveborn infants, the median gestational age at delivery was 35 weeks (range, 25–40 weeks), and the median birth weight was 2098 g (range, 550–4, 252 g). The median interval between the endoscopic laser procedure and delivery was 14 weeks (range, 0–21 weeks). All the survivors were developing normally at a median age of 12 months (range, 2–24 months).

One hundred and thirty-two pregnancies complicated by severe TTTS, reflected by polyhydramnios and enlarged bladder of one twin and oligo- or anhydramnios and collapsed bladder of the other twin, presenting before 28 weeks of gestation. Endoscopic laser was carried out at a median gestation of 21 weeks. The total number of surviving infants were 144 (55%) and there was at least one survivor in 97 cases (73%). At a minimum age of 1 year neurological handicap was suspected in six survivors (4.2%). In comparison with serial amniodrainage, the survival rate may be similar, but the handicap rate in survivors appears much lower, stressing need for a prospective study comparing these two techniques.

CONGENITAL DIAPHRAGMATIC HERNIA

The risk to the neonate is death due to fetal lung hypoplasia, respiratory compromise and associated congenital or chromosomal anomalies.

Patient Selection

Degree of pulmonary hypoplasia—measurement of the lung-to-head ratio, greater than 1.4 have a good prognosis while those with a ratio less than 0.6 are not likely to survive without in utero therapy. The presence of liver herniation into the thorax is a poor sign.

Fetal Surgery

The operative goals are reduction of the viscera from the thoracic cavity, closure of the diaphragmatic defect, and elimination of potential duodenal obstruction due to nonrotation of the intestine.

Fetal Endoscopic Tracheal Occlusion (Clip or Balloon)

This procedure is performed at 23–27 weeks of gestation. Preoperative betamethasone is given to mother for fetal lung compliance. Under general anesthesia through low transverse maternal laparotomy, a 5 mm trocar is inserted into the uterus, and a 4 mm perfusion hysteroscope is guided through the fetal vocal cords under fetoscopic and USG guidance. A detachable silicone balloon (Target Therapeutics) is placed in the fetal trachea midway between the carina and vocal cords, and inflated with iso-osmotic contrast material so as to fill the fetal trachea (0.5 mm diameter) and for at least 2 cm length.

Tocolysis is maintained with preoperative indomethacin suppository (50 mg), intraoperative halogen and nitroglycerine and postoperative magnesium sulfate with indomethacin, followed by oral calcium-channel blocker till delivery.

At delivery, ex-utero intrapartum therapy (EXIT) procedure is done. At cesarean section, the fetal head is delivered, bronchoscopically the balloon is deflated and removed, the airway suctioned, endotracheal tube inserted, exogenous surfactant (3 mg/kg body weight) administered, and assisted ventilation begun before baby delivered and umbilical cord divided. The survival rate on day 90 was 73% (8/11), compared to those that received standard care 77% fetal surgery being associated with preterm delivery at approximately 31 weeks, brings to focus research studies on optimal timing and duration effect of short-term occlusion later in gestation, use of smaller (2 mm) fetoscopes and new techniques to seal the membranes.

Aqueductal Stenosis

Ultrasonographic examination should be done every 2 or 3 weeks to detect abrupt increase in ventriculomegaly. Spontaneous resolution of mild to moderate hydrocephalus has been reported in some cases. Progressive ventricular dilatation more than 1.5 cm can be offered open surgery in utero, but (Denver) shunts have not been very useful as they got dislodged or obstructed, with poor outcome, and the International Fetal Medicine and Surgery Society in 1985 agreed to a moratorium on the procedure.

Fetal Surgery

Through hysterotomy, as in standard neurosurgical procedures, a tube is placed in the lateral ventricle connected to a valve, and is placed subcutaneously downward into the peritoneal cavity.

Cesarean delivery is performed at term. In strictly selected cases, the prognosis for aqueductal stenosis is good. However, the complications with shunts requiring revision within 2 years of birth in 60% cases have to be realized.

Ovarian Cysts

These are the most frequent, prenatally diagnosed intra-abdominal cysts. Fetal or neonatal ovarian cyst may lead to complications such as torsion; and seems to be an indication for surgical intervention. In a total of 17 cases reported, postnatal surgery was performed in seven infants. Of these, four cases of ovarian cyst torsion were confirmed. In the remaining 10 fetuses, one case regressed completely during pregnancy, and the other nine cases including two complex cysts resolve spontaneously after birth. Postnatal symptomatic cysts or cysts with a diameter greater than 5 cm that do not regress or enlarge should be treated, but uncomplicated asymptomatic cysts less than 5 cm in diameter may only be observed and reassessed by serial ultrasonography. If they regress spontaneously, no surgical intervention is necessary independent of their sonographic findings. Though these cysts are usually benign corpus luteal cysts, they may enlarge to more than 5 cm size, undergo torsion leading to ultimate removal gangrenous ovaries at birth of female child.

Fetal intervention: USG guided ovarian cyst aspiration appears to be useful in large simple cysts in preventing torsion, with complete resolution. Smaller ones may undergo spontaneous resolution as seen on repeat scan monitoring.

Major concerns include the maintenance of uterine blood flow and uterine relaxation, as premature labor and delivery severely limit fetal benefits from surgery. When performing these procedures, physicians have a special responsibility to weigh maternal risks against fetal benefits and should not jeopardize the life of the mother for procedures with questionable fetal outcome. Less than 10% of the antenatal diagnostic workload reach operative repair. These babies are a highly selected group, which is a factor in the high postoperative survival. Like the open procedures, the efficacy of the fetoscopic procedures to improve fetal outcome over postnatal treatment strategies will have to be assessed in further studies under close supervision of committees for human research.

CONCLUSION

Fetal Endoscopic Surgery is the exciting new field of surgical expertise for limited but expanding indications, being practiced in few, select centers throughout the world. In India, it is still in its infancy. Slowly, progress is being achieved, and, there is wide potential for further development and research, though many obstacles need to be overcome.

The management of fetuses with treatable congenital malformation continues to be one of the most challenging subjects in Obstetric Surgery. The problems of establishing the correct differential diagnosis, accurately providing prognosis for subsequent organ function and the best mode of fetal therapy still requires further experience and refinement.

BIBLIOGRAPHY

1. Adzick NS, Harrison MR, Crombleholme TM, et al. Fetal lung lesions: management and outcome. Am J Obstet Gynecol. 1998;179:884-89.
2. Adzick NS, Harrison MR, Glick PI, et al. Diaphragmatic hernia in the fetus: Prenatal diagnosis and outcome in 94 cases. J Pediatr Surg. 1985;20:357-61.
3. Berris M, Shoham M. Febotics-a marriage of fetal surgery and robotics. Comput Aided Surg. 2006;11(4):175-80.
4. Cardoza JD, Filly RA, Podrasky AE. The dangling choroids plexus: a sonographic observation of value in excluding ventriculomegaly. Am J Roentgenol. 1988;151:767-70.
5. Crombleholme TM, Harrison MR, Golbus MS, et al. Fetal intervention in obstructive uropathy: prognostic indicators and efficacy of intervention. Am J Obstet Gynecol. 1990;162:1239-44.
6. Davenport M, Warne SA, Cacciaguerra S, et al. Current outcome of antenally diagnosed cystic lung disease. J Pediatr Surg. 2004;39(4):549-56.

7. Davis GH. Fetal hydrocephalus. Clin Perinatol. 2003;30:531-9.
8. Deka D, Malhotra N, Takkar D, et al. Prenatal diagnosis and assessment of fetal malformations by ultrasonography in India. Ind J Pediatrics. 1999;66:737-49.
9. Deka D. Role of Ultrasound in Invasive Prenatal Diagnosis. In: Shah PK, Pratap K, Malhotra N (Eds). Imaging in Obstetrics and Gynecology, 4th edition. New Delhi: Jaypee Brothers Medical Publishers (P) Ltd.;2002.
10. De Lia J, Cruiskshank D, Keye W. Fetoscopic Neodymium: YAG laser occlusion of placental vessels in twin-twin transfusion syndrome. Obstet Gynecol. 1990;75:1046-53.
11. Deprest J, Jani J, Lewi L, et al. Fetoscopic surgery: Encouraged by clinical experience and boosted by instrument innovation. Semin Fetal Neonatal Med. 2006;11(6):398-412.
12. Dicke JM, Blanco VM, Yan Y, et al. The type and frequency of fetal renal disorders and management of renal pelvis dilatation. J Ultrasound Med. 2006;25(8):973-7.
13. Flake AW. Open Surgery for Fetal Sacrococcygeal Teratomas. In: Evans MI, Platt LD, de la Cruz F (Eds). Fetal Therapy. New York, USA: Parthenon Publishing Group; 2001. pp. 63-6.
14. Gogarten W, Van Aken H, Marcus MA. Fetal surgery: general or regional anaesthesia? Curr Opin Anaesthesiol. 2000;13(3): 277-81.
15. Golombeck K, Ball RH, Lee H, et al. Maternal morbidity after maternal-fetal surgery. Am J Obstet Gynecol. 2006;194(3):834-9.
16. Harrison M. Surgically correctable fetal disease. In: Evans MI, Platt LD, de la Cruz F (Eds). Fetal Therapy. New York, USA: Parthenon Publishing Group; 2001. pp. 47-57.
17. Harrison MR, Adzick NS, Bullard KM, et al. Correction of congenital diaphragmatic hernia in utero VII: a prospective trial. J Pediatr Surg. 1997;32:1637-42.
18. Harrison MR, Adzick NS, Flake AW, et al. Correction of congenital diaphragmatic hernia in utero. VI. Hard-earned lessons. J Pediatr Surg. 1993;28:1411-7.
19. Harrison MR, Adzick NS, Longaker MT, et al. Successful repair in utero of a fetal diaphragmatic hernia after removal of herniated viscera from the left thorax. N Engl J Med. 1990;322:1582-4.
20. Harrison MR, Albanese CT, Hawgood SB, et al. Fetoscopic temporary tracheal occlusion by means of detachable balloon for congenital diaphragmatic hernia. Am J Obstet Gynecol. 2001;185:730-3.
21. Harrison MR, Filly RA, Paren JT, et al. Management of fetus with urinary tract malformation. JAMA. 1981;246:635-9.
22. Harrison MR, Langer JC, Adzick NS, et al. Correction of congenital diaphragmatic hernia in utero. V. Initial clinical experience. J Pediatr Surg. 1990;25:47-55.
23. Hedrick MH, Estes JM, Sullivan KM, et al. Plug the lung until it grows (PLUG): a new method to treat congenital diaphragmatic hernia in utero. J Pediatr Surg. 1994;29:612-7.
24. Johnson MP, Corsi P, Bradfield W, et al. Sequential fetal urine analysis provides greater precision in the evaluation of fetal obstructive uropathy. Am J Obstet Gynecol. 1995;173:59-65.
25. Kitano Y, Matsuoka K, Honna T, et al. Venous arterialization in extralobar pulmonary sequestration associated with fetal hydrops. J Pediatr Surg. 2006;41(3):490-4.
26. Knox EM, Kilby MD, Martin WL, et al. In-utero pulmonary drainage in the management of primary hydrothorax and congenital cystic lung lesion: a systematic review. Ultrasound Obstet Gynecol. 2006;28(5):726-34.
27. Kohl T. Fetoscopic surgery: where are we today? Curr Opin Anaesthesiol. 2004;17(4):315-21.
28. Kwak DW, Sohn YS, Kim SK, et al. Clinical experiences of fetal ovarian cyst: diagnosis and consequence. J Korean Med Sci. 2006;21(4):690-4.
29. Lakasing L, Cicero S, Davenport M, et al. Current outcome of antenatally diagnosed exomphalos: an 11 year review. J Pediatr Surg. 2006;41(8):1403-6.
30. Langer JC, Harrison MR, Schmidt KG, et al. Fetal hydrops and death from sacrococcygeal teratomas: rationale for fetal surgery. Am J Obstet Gynecol. 1989;160:1145-50.
31. Makin EC, Hyett J, Ade-Ajayi N, et al. Outcome of antenatally diagnosed sacrococcygeal teratomas: single-center experience (1993–2004). J Pediatr Surg. 2006;41(2):388-93.
32. Mari G, Roberts A, Detti L, et al. Perinatal morbidity and mortality rates in severe twin-twin transfusion syndrome: results of the international amnioreduction registry. Am J Obstet Gynecol. 2001;185:708-15.
33. Mychaliska GB, Bealer JF, Graf JL, et al. Operating on placental support: the ex utero intrapartum treatment procedure. J Pediatr Surg. 1997;32:227-30.
34. Nicolaides KH, Azar GB. Thoraco-amniotic shunting. Fetal Diagn Ther. 1990;5:153-64.
35. Phaloprakarn C, Bartsch EM, Harrison MR. Residual congenital cystic adenomatoid malformation and thoracic scar deformation after fetal surgery: a case report. J Pediatr Surg. 2006;41(2):e11-4.
36. Picone O, Benachi A, Mandelbrot L, et al. Emergency thoracoamniotic shunting in cases with compressive pleural effusion with hydrops: a retrospective study of 60 cases. J Gynecol Obstet Biol Reprod (Paris). 2006;35(7):652-7.
37. Quintero RA, Johnson MP, Romero R, et al. In-utero percutaneous cystoscopy in the management of fetal lower obstructive uropathy. Lancet. 1995;346(8974):537-40.
38. Ruano R, Benachi A, Aubry MC, et al. Prenatal diagnosis of pulmonary sequestration using three-dimensional power Doppler ultrasound. Ultrasound Obstet Gynecol. 2005;25(2):128-33.
39. Salam MA. Posterior urethral valve: outcome of antenatal intervention. Int J Urol. 2006;13(10):1317-22.
40. Teal LN, Angtuaco TL, Jiminez JF, et al. Fetal teratomas: antenatal diagnosis and clinical management. J Clin Ultrasound. 1988;16:329-36.
41. Vander Wall KJ, Skarsgard ED, Filly RA, et al. Fetendo-clip: a fetal endoscopic tracheal clip procedure in a human fetus. J Pediatr Surg. 1997;32:970-2.
42. Ville Y, Hecher K, Gagnon A, et al. Endoscopic laser coagulation in the management of severe twin-to-twin transfusion syndrome. Br J Obstet Gynaecol. 1998;105(4):446-53.
43. Ville Y, Hyett J, Hecher K, et al. Preliminary experience with endoscopic laser surgery for severe twin-twin transfusion syndrome. N Engl J Med. 1995;332:224-7.
44. Walsh DS, Johnson MP. Fetal intervention for obstructive urology. Semin Perinat. 1999;23:484-95.

Section 3

Gynecology

Section Outline

- Perioperative Measures and Positioning the Patient for Surgery
- Suture and Choice with Abdominal Wall Closures
- Hemostasis and Drains
- Abortions
- Vulva
- Vagina
- Cervix
- Tubes and Ovaries
- Uterus
- Laparoscopy
- Hysteroscopy
- Bladder, Urethra and Incontinent Surgery
- Small Bowel, Colon, Appendix in Gynecological Surgery
- Gynecologic Cancer Surgery
- Surgery for Ovarian Cancer
- Omentectomy, J-Flap, TRAM Flap
- Role of Colposcopy in Gynecology
- Overview of Assisted Reproductive Technologies Procedures
- Male Infertility Surgery
- Male Sterilization, Vasectomy
- Making of a Surgeon (A Practical Life and Guidance for Neosurgeons)
- Gynecological Surgery Instruments

CHAPTER

33 Perioperative Measures and Positioning the Patient for Surgery

Randhir Puri

INTRODUCTION

The success of an operation depends not only on careful clarification of the indications, selection of the right time for operating and technically neat operating techniques, but also on correct preoperative preparation and positioning of the patient. But this aspect in particular is frequently neglected, particularly by young surgeons, because technical details of the operation assume far greater attention, underestimating the contribution made by optimum positioning to a time-saving operation which runs as perfectly as possible. How easy is it for an operation to develop complications out of all proportion because the surgeon forgot certain "minor" matter during preparations! Anyone who has witnessed this themselves will appreciate just how important exact preoperative planning and preparation is, before an operation takes place.

PERIOPERATIVE HYGIENE

The causes of inadequate hygiene behavior are frequently psychological in nature, resulting on the one hand from the contradictions between hygiene standards. Wound infection is the most frequent nosocomial infection in surgery. Medical literature describes a large number of factors triggering and promoting infections. The starting point for infections can be patients, staff, equipment and instruments, materials, surfaces and the air. "The ten most important points for preventing infections are the ten fingers of every single person involved in the operation." This somewhat pithy statement does make it clear that personal hygiene measures must be given prime attention. The following descriptions refer to hygiene measures for preventing infections associated directly with the patient, the staff and the operation.

At the outset, a young surgeon experiences in the surgical department consists of all the instructions and warnings about sterility and asepsis. It is clear to anyone that surgical discipline creates possibilities for the penetration of germs or for the release and spreading of germs, so that there is an increased risk of infection. Consequently there is a logical demand for special measures over and beyond the general hygiene requirements in a hospital, with high priori acceptance of such surgical hygiene measures.

Most people working in operating suites today are relatively well informed about the most important aspects of perioperative behavior. But from time-to-time, drastic discrepancies emerge between required and actual behavior and recommendations and on the other hand from barriers to motivation.

Concrete Measures: Wound Infection

Wound infection is a treatment-specific risk of surgical operations. This risk must be minimized by methods corresponding to good medical practice and standards (hygiene status). In the event of any disputes, a medical expert decides whether avoidable hygiene violations were involved.

Clothing in the Operating Suite

Operating Suite Clothing

Everyone releases a large number of microorganisms all the time, particularly when walking. Normal hospital clothing (usually white healthcare work wear) is regularly affected by (facultative) pathogenic germs. This is joined by microorganisms released through the nose and throat when talking, coughing and sneezing. The hair of hospital staff has been proven to have a large number of germs, including in particular *Staphylococcus aureus*. It is advisable to reduce the contaminants and release of germs in the operating suite as far as possible. The guidelines for hospital hygiene and the prevention of infections therefore, require the staff to change their clothing completely in the staff sluice of an operating suite. The hospital clothing should be removed down to the underwear and replaced by germ-free surgical clothing (trousers, shirt, surgical shoes). The suite clothing must be disinfected and cleaned, and transported and stored with protection from contamination. Surgical clothing must not be worn outside the operating suite. This prohibition cannot be bypassed by wearing something else (e.g. white coat) on top. This strict rule makes it possible to monitor what goes into and out of the operating suite, underlining its special character.

Headgear and Face Mask

In the operating suite, everyone must wear hair covering which completely covers facial hair and hair on the head in order to prevent the exposure of the contaminated hair. The face mask fulfills two tasks: (1) it prevents the transport of pathogenic germs into the sterile operating suite and into the wound, and (2) protects the wearer from contamination with body fluids, e.g. sprays of blood. Protective goggles are also recommended as personal protection. Their meaningfulness or otherwise has been repeatedly discussed since the introduction of face masks. Already back in 1936, Rise achieved the lowest wound infection rates during so-called silent operations without a mask. It is a known fact that the release of germs during speaking can be significantly reduced by wearing a mask. Face masks should fit tightly over the mouth and nose. They should be worn in the operating theater and, for disciplinary reasons, in the immediately adjacent ancillary rooms as well. Multi-layer masks (MLMs) with fleece and polyester inlays are superior to single layer masks and gauze masks, because the latter are too permeable. As the mask becomes increasingly damp, the filter resistance is increased. The so-called edge leak rate increases, i.e. the passage of germs between the edge of the mask and the face. Damp masks must therefore be replaced (between two surgical procedures). If the face mask has been loosened (e.g. in the day room), it must be replaced. This should be followed by hygiene disinfection of the hands to eliminate contamination of the hands from the used mask.

Going to the Toilet

The guidelines for hospital hygiene and preventing infection recommend going through the complete operating suite sluice procedure after going to the toilet. Adam and Dasher do not find any scientific indication that the genital region of the surgeon or any other member of staff in the operating suite would constitute a special risk for postoperative wound infection. This presumes that the clothing is not soiled and that the operating staff wash their hands after going to the toilet and also disinfect them before every operation.

Sterile Surgical Clothing

The surgical team enters the actual operating theater through the scrub room where the surgical hand disinfection procedure takes place. On entering the operating theater, the sterile ankle-length operating gown is fitted. It is important that the gown fits closely around the neck and that the sleeves are long enough and also fit tightly around the wrists. The requirements for sterile surgical clothing depend essentially on the liquid levels. For high-moisture procedures, linen and cotton quickly lose their function as germ barrier.

In such cases, the surgical clothing must be impervious to liquid at least in the sleeves and front of the body. Sterile operating gloves are generally accepted as protection for patient and staff alike. It goes without saying that defective gloves must be replaced. The use of double gloves does not protect from punctures or cut injuries but does reduce the risk of contaminating the hands with blood. Everyone should be advised to use two pairs of gloves.

Cleaning and Disinfecting the Hands

Most infections in hospitals are transferred with the hands. Washing and disinfecting the hands are therefore the simplest, safest, most effective and cheapest means of controlling infection. Jewelry worn on the hands and lower arms make the measures less effective. Surgeons should ensure that their hands are not impaired by stubborn dirt and soiling from work performed in their free time, e.g. from oil, grease and lubricants.

Washing hands with detergents cleans the hands and reduces the germ count by a factor of 100.

One milliliter of pus contains about 10^7 germs, which can be reduced to about 10^5 germs by washing. The rule for washing hands is: first disinfect, then wash. This should prevent the spread of germs by the actual washing procedure. But no one can be expected to treat for example hands contaminated with sputum by rubbing with disinfectant first. In the case of coarse soiling, the hands can be cleaned first with a disposable wet-wipe soaked in disinfectant.

Disinfecting Hands

The word disinfection refers to the actual disinfection process, which always consists of the actual disinfectant, a reaction time and the means in which the disinfectant is applied. When disinfecting hands, it is necessary to distinguish between hygienic and surgical (preoperative) disinfection. Hygienic hand disinfection (3 mL alcoholic solution rubbed in for 30 sec) kills off the transient skin flora and reduces the germ count by a factor of 10,000 (i.e. in the example given above, reduction to approximately 10,000 germs). Surgical hand disinfection aims at achieving an essential reduction in skin flora to rule out the risk of the hands being a source of infection. Together with preoperative skin disinfection, surgical hand disinfection is the most important antiseptic measure for surgical procedures. The hands are washed initially to remove any coarse soiling. The former practice of washing the hands thoroughly with soap and a scrubbing brush is considered obsolete today. Dirt should always be removed immediately and not only in the scrub room before operations. When the skin is scrubbed with a brush, deeper skin layers are opened resulting in a higher germ count on the skin. Frequent handwashing also encourages eczematization. The pertinent guidelines for hospital hygiene and prevention of infection, still requires fingernails and the edges of the nails to be cleaned with a nailbrush. The washing procedure should not take more than 1 minute. After washing, any remaining soap is rinsed off thoroughly and the hands dried gently. Many hypersensitive reactions are caused by mixing remaining soap and disinfectants. Low-germ towels (textile) can be used to dry the hands. Paper towels are rejected by some authors because of possible spore contamination. It is very important for a suitable disinfectant to be applied to the dry skin. (This is easily explained: damp hands carry approximately 3 mL water; together with 3 mL 80% disinfectant, the water reduces the alcohol concentration to 40%, thus making it ineffective).

During the reaction time, the hands and lower arms should be coated with the disinfectant all the time. The disinfectant should be rubbed in, devoting particular attention to the nails and between the fingers. Approximately 12–15 mL disinfectant are required, depending on the reaction time and size of the hands. Experts fail to agree on the time that should be taken to disinfect the hands. Whereas Hingst et al. fundamentally demand 5 minutes, Adam and Daschner draw attention to the fact that surgeons abroad are already operating while their German colleagues are still disinfecting their hands in the scrub room. Generally, it is recommended 3 minutes before the first operation and another 1–2 minutes before further operations.

Preoperative Patient Preparation

Body flora in the patient's nose and throat, intestinal passage and skin can be the starting point for wound infection.

Day before the Operation

The length of stay in hospital before the operation is closely related to the wound infection rate. One reason could be contamination of the patient with opportunistic hospital germs. The aim should therefore be to reduce the length of stay in hospital before the operation. A multicenter study in various European countries has revealed that bathing in an antiseptic agent (chlorhexidine) on the evening before the operation has no influence on the infection rate.

But the procedure of shaving the site of the operation before surgery has a verified effect on the incidence of wound infections. Seropian and Reynolds showed that the use of a depilatory cream without mechanical hair removal resulted in a far lower infection rate than after shaving (0.6% compared to 5.7%). But depilatory agents frequently cause skin irritations. Studies by Cruse and Foord showed the wound infection rate to be 0.9% when no measures were taken, 1.7% when cutting the hair with scissors and 2.3% in shaved patients. The cause of the increased infection rate after shaving the patient on the evening before is presumed to come from germ settlement and infection of tiny skin injuries. Today the operating site is only shaved immediately before the operation (in the preparation room) if thick hair is expected to interfere with the operation and simply shortening the hair is not sufficient. A strip of approximately 2 cm along the incision should be sufficient. The skin should be shaved as gently as possible, i.e. with a disinfected, sharp razor blade and using shaving soap or cream to prevent any injuries to the skin as far as possible.

Skin Disinfection

The disinfectants used include alcohol, iodine preparations and more rarely, phenolic preparations. Alcohol disinfectants start to act very quickly and are ideal for wound infections caused by key germ types. Iodine preparations start to react more slowly and are used more for disinfection of the mucous membranes. The operating site must be intensively coated with disinfectant for the complete reaction time. Wiping disinfection is more effective than simply spraying. The disinfected area must extend well beyond the actual operating site. An area of 20 cm is recommended all around the operating site. In addition, all areas must be disinfected which are touched during the operation when changing the patient's position. For normal cases, Gundermann recommends a minimum of 2 minutes for alcoholic preparations and a minimum of 5 minutes for iodine preparations. Adam and Daschner stipulate 3 minutes.

POSITIONING THE PATIENT: LEGAL PRINCIPLES

A patient is to be positioned before, during and after an operation in such a way as to avoid any position-related injuries as far as possible. The doctors performing a surgical procedure and the nursing staff under their instruction share a legal obligation to ensure that the patient is positioned correctly. Interdisciplinary cooperation is required in positioning the patient.

In positioning a patient for an operation, doctors in various disciplines work together without being accountable to each other, in particular the surgeon and the anesthetist. This is the area of the so-called horizontal division of labor.

Operating Table (Fig. 1)

The centerpiece of every operating theater is the operating table. The operating table or the position in which it is erected is the basis for arranging all other high-tech devices, such as ceiling mounts for anesthesia systems and surgery, operating lights, possibly ceiling-mounted X-ray image intensifiers or surgical microscopes, together with air-conditioning ceilings and panels.

What exactly is an operating table? An attempt to explain this with the help of a dictionary is sure to fail. "Operating table" cannot be found in most dictionaries, although it is the central element of an operating theater.

The patient is positioned (in an anatomically correct fashion) for his operation on this table. In other words, an operating table has to satisfy the needs of the surgeon, the anesthetist and the patient. These needs are essentially those shown in Box 1.

In time, various special surgical disciplines have developed from so-called general surgery, so that special operating tables have been designed and produced to suit these requirements.

Patient Warming System (Fig. 2)

Before surgery, it is decided which parts of the body can be covered without impairing the surgical activities. Heat is supplied from above (conductive method).

The patient is covered outside the surgical or sterile area. Highly versatile, segmented and specially shaped blankets are ideal for individual use in every surgical discipline.

Box 1 Properties and requirements of an operating table

- Height adjustment to adapt to the surgeon's height to allow for ergonomic working
- Slanting (Trendelenburg or reverse Trendelenburg) to allow for immediate measures during crash or ileus intubation, risk of shock or embolism, and to control such measures during conduction anesthesia
- Tilting right or left to give a better insight into the body cavity and for organ positioning during minimally invasive procedures
- Adjusting the individual segments of the patient board to allow for the body to be bent in the anatomically correct positions and to position the extremities as required for the operation, e.g. bending, spreading, etc.
- Radiolucent patient board to work with the X-ray image intensifier without any problems
- Special foam core (SFC) padding, soft and radiolucent to avoid damage from pressure sores
- Mobility to bring the patient from the hospital bed or patient transfer board to the anesthetic preparation room and operating theater without having to transfer the patient

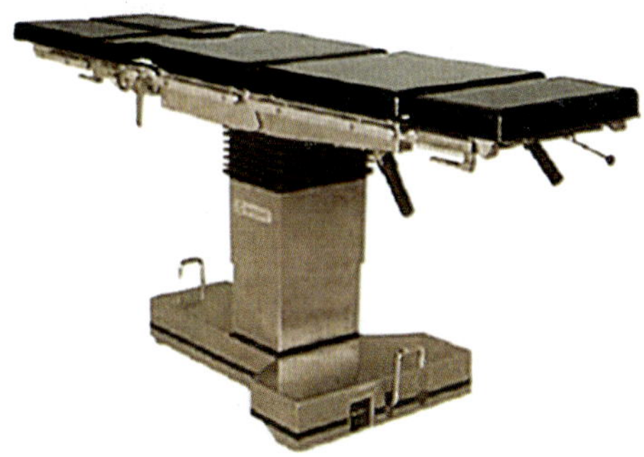

Fig. 1: Mobile universal operating table, Betastar® 1130

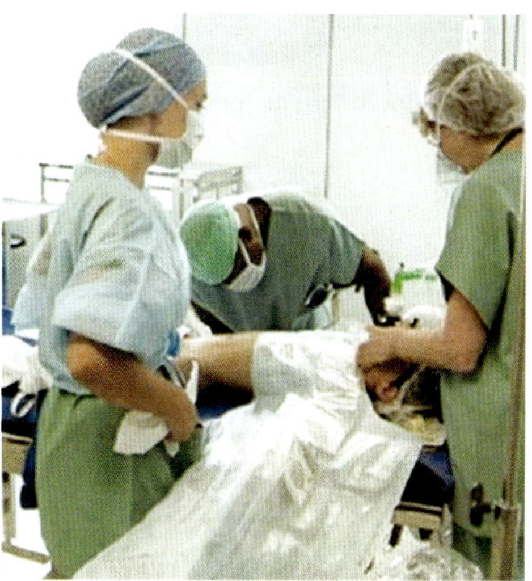

Fig. 2: Patient warming system

LITHOTOMY POSITION (FIGS 3 AND 4)

In the lithotomy position, shoulder supports are used in addition to position the head. Once again, the head should be held in the middle or neutral position.

The patient should be prevented from slipping if Trendelenburg positioning is required. It is also important to avoid a low position of the clavicle and to minimize pressure at the contact points, because not even well padded shoulder supports can always avoid damage to the plexus.

A short vacuum mat should always be used in this position as a procedure for longer operations or if required by the patient's size. This distributes the pressure across the back and relieves the pressure on the shoulders.

Back and Pelvis

Special attention and care is required when positioning the pelvis or sacrum. Excessive warmth from water mats and local loads on the sacrum will encourage the development of pressure sores. Here again, the vacuum mat can be used as a suitable precaution, because the mat molds itself to the whole back region, distributing the contact pressure which is thus also reduced at the exposed regions of the back. A dimpled gel mat with direct body contact can be beneficial for this kind of positioning because it distributes the contact pressure better. Furthermore, a drainage effect is achieved in case the drapes are inadequately adhered, so that the buttocks do not have to lie in disinfectants and body fluids.

Legs (Figs 5 and 6)

The legs are normally positioned in Goepel leg holders. Another possibility is to use modern pneumatic leg holders with well-padded calf boots. These leg holders are recommended for longer operations, because the pressure is on the soles of the feet and less on the calves. Another version is to position with feet in leg holders with removable heel loops. It is ideal if the leg holders are fitted at the level of the hip joint to prevent the patient from slipping on the operating table if the legs are moved. The

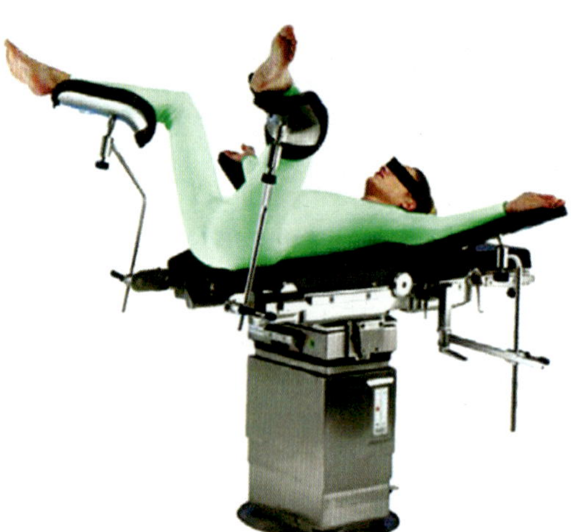

Fig. 3: The lithotomy position

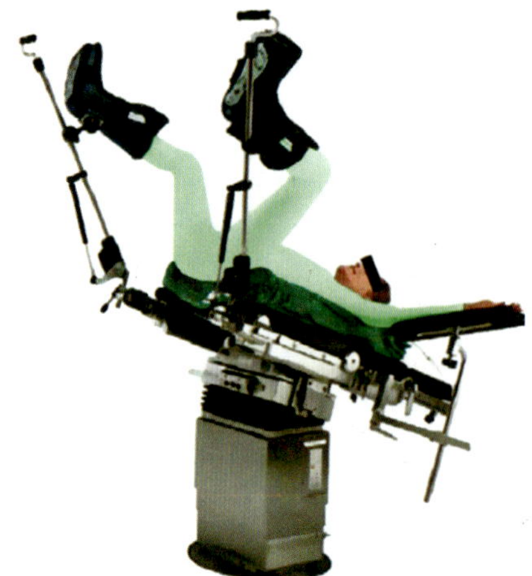

Fig. 4: Lithotomy position in Trendelenburg with vacuum mat and leg holders with one-hand operation, good decubitus and plexus prophylaxis

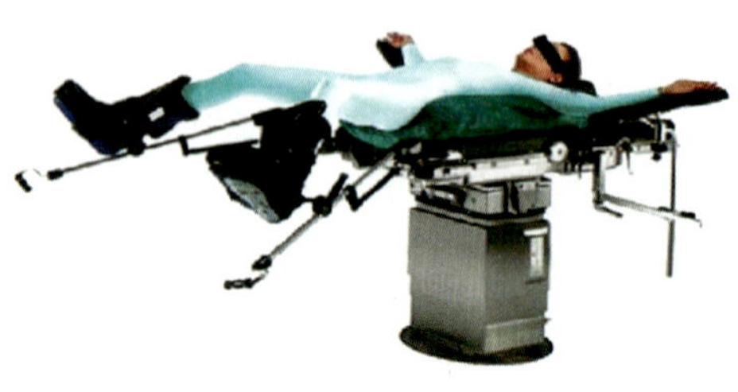

Fig. 5: Positioning the legs in special leg holders

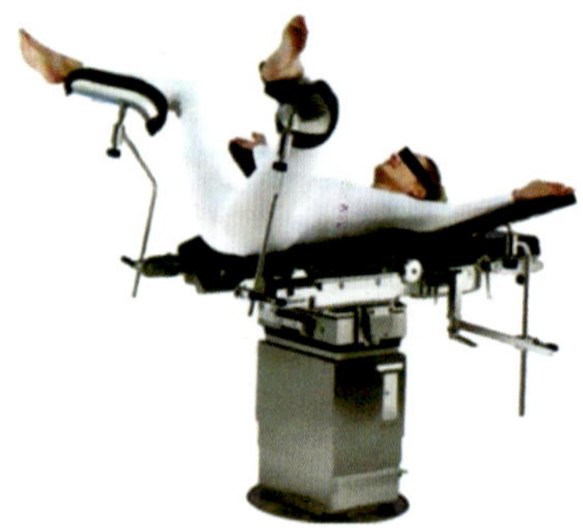

Fig. 6: Lithotomy position with Goepel leg holders

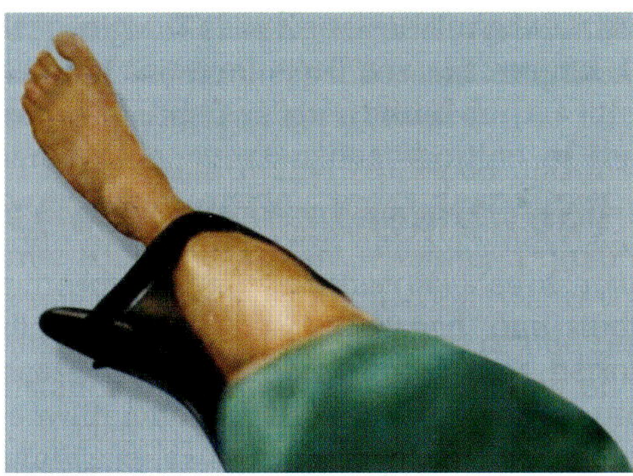

Fig. 7: Incorrect positioning of the leg in the holder, without padding and with pressure on the head of the fibula

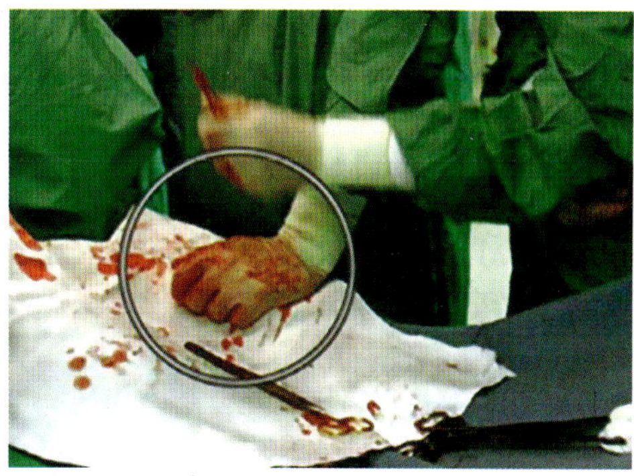

Fig. 8: Incorrect position of leaning hand on patient's leg and instruments placed wrongly

end of the foot and knee of a leg should form an axis with the opposite shoulder.

Unfortunately, compartment syndrome of the lower leg is not rare after an operation lasting several hours in the lithotomy position. Repeated, regular movement of the legs (not massage) during the operation by an assistant would help to prevent positioning complications and also reduce the risk of an embolism.

CONCLUSION

It is not only the standard positioning procedures, our positioning know-how and the positioning aids protect the patient from positioning injuries. The operating team must be disciplined in continuing to support the prophylaxis measures during the operation.

Frequently one of the team members will lean on the patient's knee without realizing it. The patient in Figure 7 has not been supported by a half roll under the knee. Here the left knee is straightened with increased pressure on the heels. Neither is it necessary for the instruments to lie on the legs (Fig. 8).

Our aim is for the patient to be satisfied after the operation, having been well-padded by the team during the operation, and kept in a dry, warm position.

CHAPTER

34

Suture and Choice with Abdominal Wall Closures

Kusum Gupta, Anupam Gupta

INTRODUCTION

The success of a gynecologic procedure performed through an abdominal incision depends on careful selection of the incision site and proper closure of the wound. The surgeon needs to consider multiple factors before making an abdominal incision. These factors include the disease process, operative exposure, simplicity, previous scars, cosmetic perspective and the need for quick entry into the abdominal cavity. The most important factor is adequate exposure to the operative field.

Complications during surgery can occur because of inadequate exposure, which is often due to the unwillingness of the surgeon to extend the incision. Incision location is particularly important when the patient has a gynecologic malignancy. These patients may need a colostomy, urinary diversion, or extraperitoneal lymph node dissection to satisfactorily treat the disease.

RELEVANT ANATOMY

A thorough understanding of abdominal wall anatomy is essential for choosing and making the proper surgical incision. The musculature of the abdominal wall is composed of two muscle groups. One group, consists of the external oblique, internal oblique and the transversus abdominis. The second group is composed of two muscles that run vertically, the rectus abdominis and the pyramidalis. The external oblique muscle is the largest and most superficial of the flat muscles of the abdominal wall. Arising from the lower eight ribs, the external oblique courses transversely to insert upon the iliac crests. The aponeurosis is a strong tendinous sheath that ends medially in the linea alba. The internal oblique muscle arises from the upper surface of the inguinal ligament, the iliac crest and the thoracolumbar fascia. This muscle courses at a right angle to the fibers of the external oblique muscle. The aponeurosis of the internal oblique splits at the edge of the rectus muscle to envelope the rectus. The anterior layer blends with the aponeurosis of the external oblique. Posterior to the rectus muscle, this aponeurosis blends with the aponeurosis of the transversus abdominis to form a portion of the posterior rectus sheath (Fig. 1).

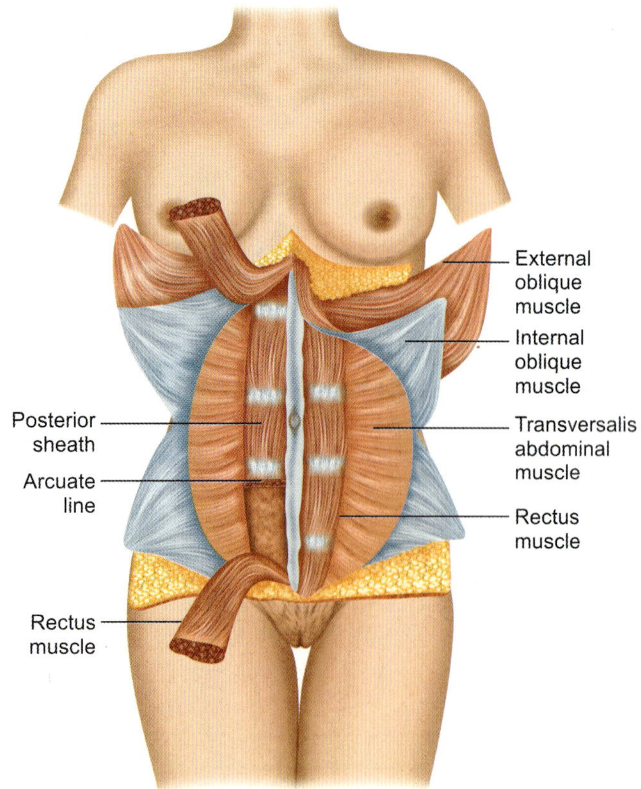

Fig. 1: Anatomy of abdominal wall

The innermost of the flat muscles is the transversus abdominis. This muscle arises from the inguinal ligament, the iliac crest, the thoracolumbar fascia and the lower costal cartilages. Coursing transversely to the midline, the upper three-fourths of the transversus aponeurosis lies behind the rectus muscle. The lower one-fourth of the aponeurosis passes in front of the rectus muscle. The aponeurosis of each flat muscle joins medial to the rectus muscle to form the linea alba.

Originating from the pubic crest, the rectus muscle runs vertically to insert into the xiphoid process, and the fifth, sixth and seventh costal cartilages. The muscle fibers contain three fibrous insertions known as the linea transversae. The rectus is surrounded by the rectus sheath, which consists of the aponeuroses of the oblique muscles and the transversus abdominis. A small, vestigial, triangular-shaped muscle, the pyramidalis, arises from the symphysis and inserts upon the linea alba. This muscle marks the midline and assists in the identification of the medial borders of the rectus muscle.

Two important surgical landmarks are formed by the aponeuroses of the abdominal wall muscles. The linea alba is in the midline between the two rectus muscles. Formed by the fusion of the aponeuroses of the external oblique, internal oblique and transversus abdominis, identifying this structure during a midline incision is important. A second surgical landmark is the arcuate line that is found below the rectus muscle, approximately halfway between the umbilicus and the symphysis pubis. Above the arcuate line, the aponeuroses of the internal oblique and transversus abdominis fuse to form the posterior rectus sheath. Below the arcuate line, the posterior rectus sheath is absent. This anatomic finding occurs as the aponeuroses of the oblique muscles and the transversus pass in front of the rectus muscle.

Blood Supply

The primary blood supply to the abdominal wall is from the superficial and deep vasculature. The superficial vasculature originates from branches of the femoral artery and includes the superficial epigastric, the superficial circumflex and the superficial external pudendal arteries. These vessels course through the tissues anterior to the rectus sheath.

The deep vasculature is composed of vessels from the external iliac artery and the internal thoracic artery. The inferior epigastric artery originates from the external iliac artery and courses posterior to the lateral one-third of the rectus muscle. Another branch of the external iliac is the deep circumflex artery which courses cephalad lateral to the inferior epigastric artery. The superior epigastric artery is the terminal branch of the internal thoracic artery. This artery has multiple branches leading to the rectus muscle and has an anastomosis with the inferior epigastric artery. The internal thoracic artery is the source of the musculophrenic artery which has an anastomosis with the deep circumflex artery. This large network of vascular anastomoses in the abdominal wall provides an excellent blood supply to all areas of the abdominal wall.

Nerve Supply

Innervation of the abdominal wall is by the thoraco-abdominal nerves, the ilioinguinal nerves and the iliohypogastric nerves. The thoracoabdominal nerves travel caudad between the transversus abdominis and the internal oblique. These nerves innervate the flat muscles of the abdominal wall and the rectus muscle.

Innervating the lower abdominal wall are the iliohypogastric nerves and the ilioinguinal nerves. Both of these nerves arise primarily from the first lumbar nerve root. Damage to these nerves results in sensory changes in the mons pubis and the labia majora.

TYPES OF ABDOMINAL INCISIONS

Vertical Incision (Figs 2A to D)

Several types of vertical abdominal incisions have been used in gynecologic surgery including midline, paramedian and wide paramedian incisions. The midline incision is the easiest and most versatile vertical incision for performing gynecologic surgery. This incision allows quick entry into the abdominal cavity with little blood loss and it is easily extended in length to accommodate the operative findings. The presumed disadvantages of a midline incision compared with a transverse incision include an increased risk of wound dehiscence and hernia formation. Most studies that support this idea are retrospective or lack proper statistical design. Recent studies have challenged this dictum and advocate that little difference exists in dehiscence rates between properly closed midline incisions and transverse incisions.

For a midline abdominal incision, the skin and subcutaneous fat are incised to the level of the fascia. The scalpel or electrocautery can be used to incise this tissue. Some surgeons believe the infection rate is higher with the use of electrocautery. However, recent prospective studies indicate no increased wound complications with electrocautery compared with a scalpel in midline abdominal incisions.

Using either instrument, the principle is to make long smooth strokes through the subcutaneous fat to the fascia. The subcutaneous fat should not be dissected from the fascia because this creates unnecessary dead space. Next,

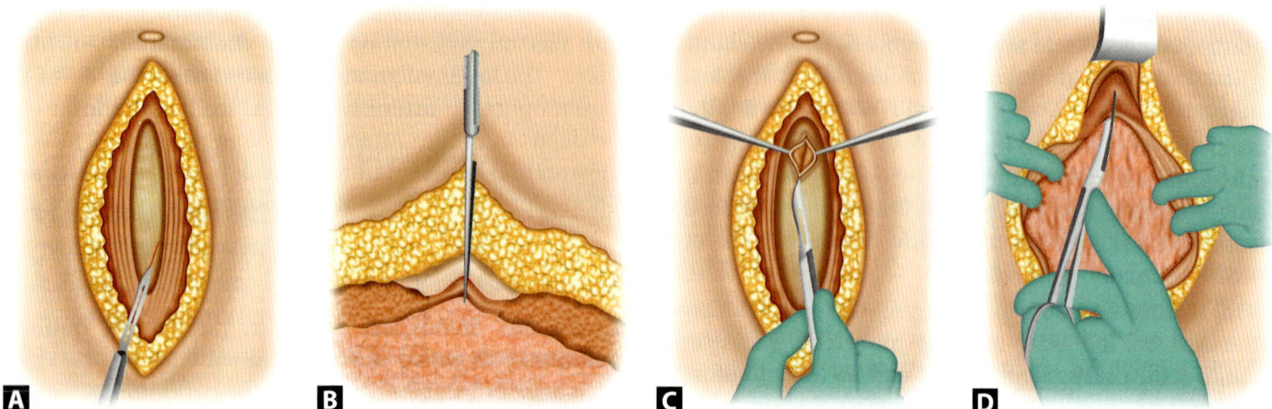

Figs 2A to D: Intraumbilical, vertical incision being made in layers. (A and B) Cutting of skin and subcutaneous tissue; (C) Incisioning the rectus sheath; (D) Extending rectus sheath incision

the fascia is incised, and the rectus muscles are separated vertically in the midline. The midline may not be evident in patients with previous abdominal surgery. Identifying where the rectus muscles diverge around the umbilicus or locating the pyramidalis muscles assists in identifying the midline. Once the rectus muscles are divided, the peritoneum is grasped between two hemostats opened with a scalpel and extended the length of the incision.

If the operative findings necessitate extending the incision above the umbilicus, avoid cutting through the umbilicus. Postoperative wound infections may be increased due to bacterial colonization of the umbilicus. Extension of the incision should pass to the left of the umbilicus to avoid cutting through the ligamentum teres.

Closure of the midline incision has evolved over the last 2 decades. Layered closure using interrupted sutures was previously the choice of many surgeons. Today, most surgeons prefer to close the abdominal wall with a continuous running suture using delayed absorbable sutures. The use of a continuous suture to close the fascia is faster with dehiscence rates comparable to those of interrupted closures. Two basic techniques are used to close the abdomen with continuous suture, the single-layer mass closure and the internal mass closure. The single-layer mass closure involves using a heavy monofilament delayed-absorbable or permanent suture. Fascial closure involves penetrating the fascia 1.5 cm from the edge with the suture. The suture should also include the underlying muscle and peritoneum.

Some surgeons close the wound using the internal mass closure technique advocated by Smead-Jones. This is a far-far, near-near suturing technique. The anterior fascia is included in the near-near bite. The initial stitch is similar to the single layer mass closure. The second bite only includes the anterior rectus fascia approximately 0.5 cm from the fascial edge. Either technique requires starting from each end of the incision. Securing the suture with 5 knots at each end is sufficient. In patients who are slender, burying the knot is helpful.

Transverse Incision

Several useful transverse abdominal incisions are available to the surgeon performing gynecologic surgery. Historically, the obstetrician-gynecologist had preferred this type of incision. Reported advantages include better cosmetic results, less pain and low incidence of hernia formation. The disadvantage is that transverse incisions limit exploration of the upper abdomen, they are associated with greater blood loss and they are more prone to hematoma formation when compared with a midline incision. Nerve injury, which can result in paresthesia of the overlying skin, is more frequent in a transverse incision compared with a midline incision.

Pfannenstiel Incision (Figs 3A and B)

The Pfannenstiel incision results in good exposure to the central pelvis but limits exposure to the lateral pelvis and upper abdomen. These factors limit the usefulness of this incision for gynecologic cancer surgery. If the patient is thin and has a gynecoid or platypelloid pelvis, this incision can be used. The incision is usually made 1–2 fingerbreadths above the pubic crest. Use of a marking pen is helpful to keep the incision symmetric. An incision length of 10–14 cm is sufficient. Increasing the length of the skin incision usually does not improve exposure due to the rectus muscles. The incision is made through the subcutaneous fat to the fascia. The superficial epigastric vessels are often near the lateral edges of the incision.

The anterior fascia is incised in the midline with a scalpel or electrocautery. Using curved scissors or electrocautery, the fascia is incised in a curvilinear fashion 1–2 cm lateral to the rectus muscle. The upper edge of the fascia is grasped with two Kocher clamps on either side of the midline. Using electrocautery, the rectus muscle is dissected free from the fascia. Electrocautery allows coagulation of multiple small vessels that perforate the rectus muscle to the fascia. The rectus muscles are mobilized off the fascia to the level of the umbilicus. Next, the lower fascial edge is grasped with Kocher clamps. Electrocautery is used again to dissect the rectus muscles and the pyramidalis muscle from the fascia. The rectus muscles are separated. The peritoneum is opened and incised vertically to complete a Pfannenstiel incision. Closure of the Pfannenstiel incision is straightforward. The peritoneum does not need to be closed separately as re-epithelization occurs within 48 hours. Closure of the peritoneum does not add to the strength of the incision. Regardless of whether the peritoneum is closed, the rectus muscles should be thoroughly irrigated with water or saline and any bleeding areas should be cauterized or ligated. Bleeding from small perforating vessels through the rectus muscle is the most common source of subfascial hematoma. The fascia is approximated with a delayed absorbable suture. Usually, a separate suture is started at each end of the fascial incision and all layers of the anterior rectus sheath are incorporated. Unless a large area of dead space exists between the fascia and the skin, closure of the Scarpa fascia is not needed. Placement of a closed drainage system, like a Jackson-Pratt drain, may be needed if a large amount of fluid collection is anticipated.

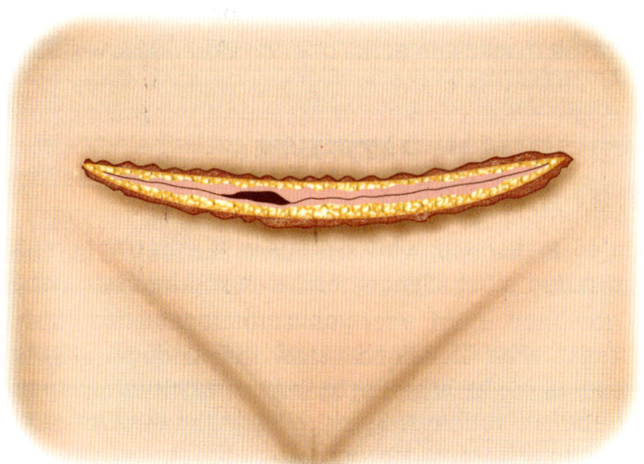

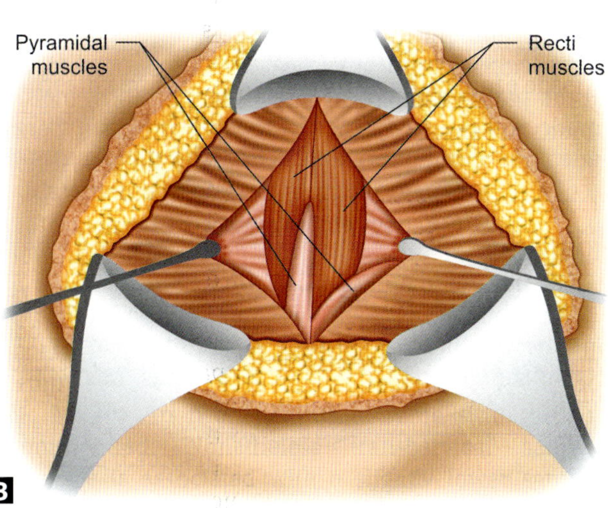

Figs 3A and B: Making of a Pfannenstiel incision

Transverse Incision (Figs 4 and 5)

Several useful transverse abdominal incisions are available to the surgeon performing gynecologic surgery. Historically, the obstetrician-gynecologist has preferred this type of incision. Reported advantages include better cosmetic results, less pain and low incidence of hernia formation. The disadvantage is that transverse

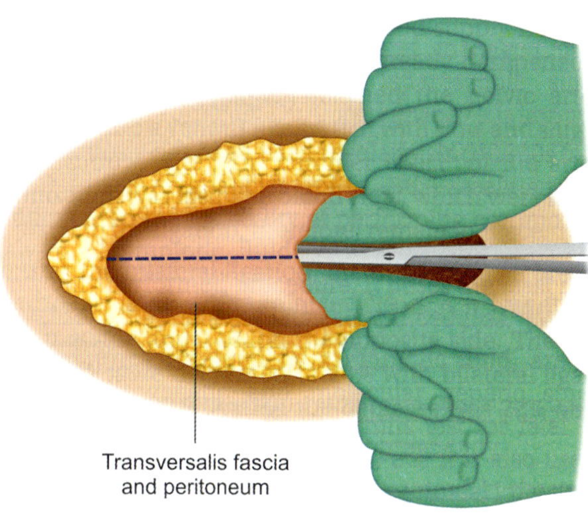

Fig. 4: Transverse layered incision

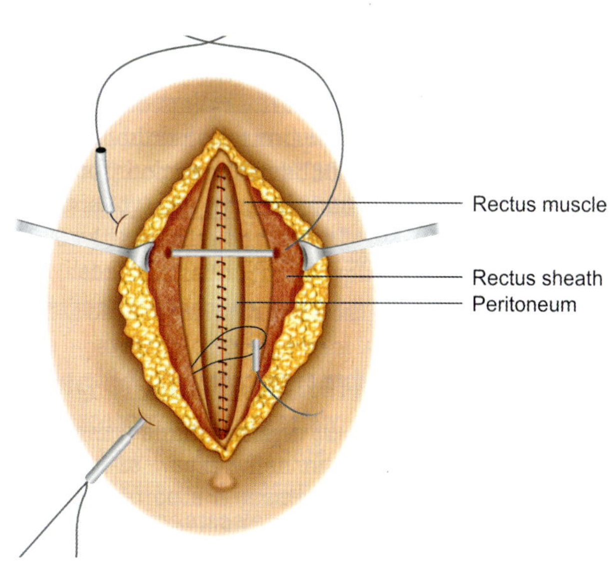

Fig. 5: Suturing and closure of abdomen in layers

incisions limit exploration of the upper abdomen, they are associated with greater blood loss and they are more prone to hematoma formation when compared with a midline incision. Nerve injury, which can result in paresthesia of the overlying skin, is more frequent in a transverse incision compared with a midline incision.

Maylard Incision

In an effort to improve surgical exposure to the lateral pelvic sidewall with a transverse incision, Maylard proposed a transverse muscle-splitting incision. This incision usually refers to a subumbilical transverse incision. For gynecologic surgery, the incision is made 3–8 cm superior to the pubis symphysis. The anterior rectus sheath is cut transversely. The inferior epigastric vessels are identified under the lateral edge of each rectus muscle and then are ligated. Patients with significant peripheral arterial disease may experience ischemia from ligation of the inferior epigastric vessels. These patients may have collateral flow from the epigastric vessels to the lower extremities. After ligation of the inferior epigastric vessels, electrocautery is used to transversely cut the rectus muscle. The peritoneum is opened and cut laterally.

To facilitate closure of a Maylard incision, flex the operating table. Close the peritoneum with an absorbable epigastric vessel and irrigate with water. Examine the cut edges of the rectus muscles for any bleeding areas. The fascia and underlying rectus muscle can be closed with a monofilament absorbable suture.

Cherney Incision

Cherney described a transverse incision that allows excellent surgical exposure to the space of Retzius and the pelvic sidewall. The skin and fascia are cut in a manner similar to a Maylard incision. The rectus muscles are separated to the pubis symphysis and separated from the pyramidalis muscles. A plane is developed between the fibrous tendons of the rectus muscle and the underlying transversalis fascia. Using electrocautery, the rectus tendons are cut from the pubic bone. The rectus muscles are retracted and the peritoneum opened. Closing a Cherney incision begins with closure of the peritoneum. Attach the cut ends of the rectus muscle to the distal end of the anterior rectus sheath with interrupted nonabsorbable sutures. Fixing the rectus muscle to the pubis symphysis can result in osteomyelitis. Next, the fascia is closed with two running, continuous, delayed-absorbable sutures.

Several types of incisions facilitate extraperitoneal para-aortic lymph node dissection. An upper abdominal transverse incision, which is a high Maylard incision, is made approximately 2 cm above the umbilicus. The incision is extended laterally and caudad to the anterior superior iliac spines. The fascia and rectus muscles are incised transversely, usually requiring ligation of the inferior and superior epigastric vessels. Next, the transversus abdominis muscle is cut exposing the peritoneum. Using blunt dissection, the peritoneal sac is dissected caudad to cephalad, to expose the psoas muscle, the aorta and the common iliac vessels. Often a drain needs to be placed in the area of the lymph node dissection.

Modified Gibson Incision

Some gynecologic oncologists perform an extraperitoneal lymph node dissection using a modification of the Gibson incision. This incision can be made on each side of the midline, but often, the skin is cut only on the left. The incision is started 3 cm superior and parallel to the inguinal ligament. Extension is made vertically 3 cm medial to the anterior superior iliac spine to the level of the umbilicus. The fascia is cut and the peritoneum bluntly dissected, as described above. The round ligament and the inferior epigastric vessels are ligated to facilitate surgical exposure. Care is needed when exposing the lymph nodes using only a left-sided incision. Too much traction on the peritoneum can result in avulsion of the inferior mesenteric vessels.

INCISIONS IN PATIENTS WHO ARE OBESE

Surgery in patients who are obese and morbidly obese represents a challenge for every surgeon. Wound complication rates are uniformly higher in patients who are obese, regardless of the type of incision. Obtaining adequate surgical exposure requires patience, understanding of changes in anatomical landmarks and proper surgical equipment.

The abdominal wall landmarks are distorted in patients who are obese, particularly in the presence of a large panniculus. The umbilicus is located caudad to its normal position. If a vertical incision is needed, first pull the panniculus downward. A periumbilical incision is made and the fascia incised to the symphysis. Care is needed not to buttonhole the skin under the panniculus. Use of a ring retractor, such as the Bookwalter, optimizes surgical exposure. The site of a transverse incision in patients who are obese should never be made under the fold of the panniculus. Wound complications are invariably higher compared with an incision made away from the panniculus. Ideally, a paraumbilical midline incision should be made. In some patients, this will not allow for adequate exposure to the pelvic organs. The surgeon may find the distance to the pelvic structures exceeds the length of the surgical instruments and the retractors. In this scenario, a panniculectomy should be performed. A panniculectomy allows the fascial incision to be within several centimeters of the pubic symphysis, allowing easier access to the pelvic organs. Large suction drains should be placed above the fascial closure with a panniculectomy and kept in place until the drainage is less than 30 mL in 24 hours.

SUTURES

A suture is any strand of material used to approximate tissue or ligate vessels. Various materials have been used for sutures throughout history. Materials incorporated into sutures include horsehair, linen, silk, animal intestines and wire. The ideal suture is yet to be created. Qualities important in a suture include uniform tensile strength, knot security, nonallergenic properties, and high tensile-strength retention during wound healing. Choosing the correct suture requires knowledge of the healing characteristics of tissues and understanding of the physical properties of various suture materials.

Absorbable Sutures

Today, sutures are classified based on their absorptive properties. Absorbable sutures are prepared from the collagen of animals or synthetic polymers. These sutures are removed from the body by enzymatic action or hydrolysis. The ability of the suture to retain tensile strength dictates where the suture should be used in wound closure. Do not confuse the loss of tensile strength with the rate of absorption. Sutures can maintain adequate tensile strength until wound healing is complete, followed by rapid absorption. Conversely, some sutures may loose tensile strength rapidly and undergo slow absorption. All absorbable sutures eventually completely dissolve.

Absorbable sutures have some limitations. For patients with fever, infection, or poor nutritional status, absorption of absorbable suture may accelerate and lead to premature diminution of tensile strength. If these sutures are exposed to significant moisture, such as ascites, absorption rates are accelerated. The common absorbable sutures used in gynecologic surgery are as follows:

- Surgical gut
  - Plain
  - Chromic
  - Fast absorbing
- Polyglactin 910 (Vicryl)
  - Uncoated
  - Coated
- Polyglycolic acid (Dexon)
- Poliglecaprone (Monocryl)
- Polydioxanone (PDS)
- Polyglyconate (Maxon).

Surgical gut sutures can be used to reapproximate mucosal surfaces or peritoneal edges, but they lack the tensile strength for use in fascial closure. Poliglecaprone 25 (Monocryl) is a newer absorbable suture that retains 50% of its tensile strength after 2 weeks but is not used to reapproximate the abdominal wall fascia.

Synthetic absorbable sutures are used extensively in many gynecologic surgeries. Polyglactin (Vicryl) and polyglycolic acid (Dexon) are frequently used to ligate pedicles during a hysterectomy. These sutures can be used to close a transverse incision in a healthy patient, although monofilament sutures are preferred by many surgeons for fascial closure of a transverse incision. Two monofilament delayed absorbable sutures useful in fascial closure are polyglyconate (Maxon) and polydioxanone (PDS). Both of these sutures invoke little tissue reaction and maintain 50% of their tensile strength at 4 weeks. These sutures are often used with midline incision closures in gynecologic surgeries.

Studies indicate that using a delayed absorbable suture in a mass closure of all layers of the abdominal wall is efficient and safe.

Nonabsorbable Sutures

Enzymatic activity or hydrolysis does not digest nonabsorbable sutures. These sutures are composed of multiple filaments of metal, synthetic fibers and organic fibers fashioned into a strand by twisting, braiding or spinning. The commonly used nonabsorbable sutures are as follows:

- Natural
  - Silk
  - Cotton
- Stainless-steel wire (Flexon)
- Nylon (Dermalon, Surgilon)
- Polypropylene (Prolene, Novafil)
- Braided synthetics (Dacron, Tevdek).

Some investigators recommend the use of nonabsorbable sutures, polypropylene (prolene) or polybutester (novafil) to close the fascia in a midline abdominal incision. A meta-analysis of 32 trials published in 2000 compared the closure techniques of the abdominal fascia. This study found a 32% decreased risk of incisional hernia when the fascia was approximated with nonabsorbable sutures compared with absorbable sutures. This study may have included patients with fascial closure using rapidly absorbed sutures such as vicryl or dexon. A study by van't Riet, in year 2002 found no difference in incisional hernia rates between delayed absorbable sutures and nonabsorbable sutures.

CHAPTER

35

Hemostasis and Drains

Randhir Puri, V Chandra

INTRODUCTION

Blood circulation is vital for our survival and any imbalance in the circulatory system or in hemostasis may either lead to death or severe debility. Thus, there is a great demand for therapeutic agents for blood loss.

Surgical procedures are inevitably associated with bleeding. The amount of blood loss may vary widely between different surgical procedures and depends on surgical as well as nonsurgical factors. Whereas adequate surgical hemostasis may suffice in most patients, prohemostatic pharmacological agents may be of additional benefit in patients with (diffuse) surgical bleeding or in patients with a specific underlying hemostatic defect. In general, surgical hemostasis and pharmacological therapies can be complementary in controlling blood loss.

PHARMACOLOGICAL THERAPIES

The use of pharmacological therapies to reduce blood loss and blood transfusions in surgery has historically been restricted to a few drugs. Antifibrinolytic agents (aprotinin, tranexamic acid and aminocaproic acid) have the best evidence supporting their use, especially in cardiac surgery, liver transplantation and some orthopedic, gynecological oncology surgical procedures. Meta-analyses of randomized controlled trials in cardiac patients have suggested a slight benefit of aprotinin compared with the other antifibrinolytics. Desmopressin is the treatment of choice in patients with mild hemophilia A and von Willebrand's disease. It has also been shown to be effective in patients undergoing surgery who received aspirin up to the time of operation. However, overall evidence does not support a beneficial effect of desmopressin in patients without pre-existing coagulopathy undergoing elective surgical procedures.

Topical agents, such as fibrin sealants have been successfully used in a variety of surgical procedures. However, only very few controlled clinical trials have been performed and scientific evidence supporting their use is still limited. Novel drugs, like recombinant factor VIIa (eptacog alfa) are currently under clinical investigation. Recombinant factor VIIa has been introduced for the treatment of hemophilia patients with inhibitors, either in surgical or nonsurgical situations. Preliminary data indicate that it may also be effective in surgical patients without pre-existing coagulation abnormalities. More clinical trials are warranted before definitive conclusions can be drawn about the safety and the exact role of this new drug in surgical patients. Future trials should also consider cost-effectiveness because of considerable differences in the costs of the available prohemostatic pharmacological agents.

HEMOSTASIS

Hemostasis refers to the physiologic process whereby bleeding is halted. Stopped bleeding is commonly referred to, however as coagulation, but coagulation is only one type of hemostatic process.

When a blood vessel is wounded several steps occur to staunch the flow of blood, namely:

- Vasoconstriction constricts the blood vessel, minimizing vessel diameter and slowing bleeding
- Primary hemostasis occurs, wherein platelets, one of the formed elements of the blood, bind to collagen in the exposed walls of the blood vessel to form a hemostatic plug within seconds after an injury
- Secondary hemostasis or coagulation occurs. This involves a complex cascade of coagulation factors, ultimately resulting in the transformation of fibrinogen, a blood protein, into polymerized fibrin, making a clot. This process takes several minutes

- The clot attracts and stimulates the growth of fibroblasts and smooth muscle cells within the vessel wall and begins the repair process which ultimately results in the dissolution of the clot (fibrinolysis).

Methods to Control Blood Loss During Surgery

During the course of nearly all types of surgery, blood vessels will be disrupted causing some bleeding. The practice of "meticulous hemostasis" refers to a surgical team's scrupulous attention to even the minutest areas of bleeding during the course of surgery. The theory is that by preventing the loss of even small amounts of blood, the surgical team is protecting the patient's red blood cell supply.

A variety of tools exist to quickly stop bleeding blood vessels. Specialized surgical equipment use heat to seal the ends of cut blood vessels (electrocautery) in order to prevent blood from leaking out. The "argon beam plasma coagulator" uses argon gas and high-frequency electrical current to keep bleeding under control.

Methods

Embolotherapy refers to various methods of blocking a bleeding blood vessel preventing further blood loss. Embolotherapy may employ:

- Chemical agents called sclerosants that scar the inside of the blood vessel allowing the resulting scar tissue to "dam up" the bleeding vessel
- Mechanical agents that block a bleeding vessel, including metal coils and latex or silicone balloons
- Particles or microspheres to shore up bleeding within a vessel, including gelatin foam
- Liquids that provide a barrier within a bleeding vessel, including injected liquid that quickly turns into a thicker gel-like or spongy mass to prevent bleeding from the vessel.

Fibrin glue is a substance made from human clotting factors. These clotting factors can be harvested from donor blood plasma or from a patient's own blood plasma. Fibrin glue can be applied to a bleeding vessel. It both blocks the vessel from bleeding and activates normal clotting/coagulation activity. Because fibrin glue is made from blood products, each individual will need to examine their own conscience to decide if its use is personally acceptable.

Platelet gel concentrates are made from a patient's own blood plasma, mixed with calcium and clotting compounds produced in cows. Platelet gel concentrates can be applied during the course of surgery to control bleeding. As with fibrin glue, platelet gel concentrates are produced from plasma, so their use by some individuals is a matter of conscience.

Biological hemostats are manufactured pads that are woven out of collagen (the kinds of fibers of which skin, tendons and bones are composed) and cellulose (plant fibers). These pads are placed on bleeding areas during surgery and appear to help stop bleeding more quickly.

Hemostasis by clamps may refer to the process of manually clamping a blood vessel, usually with hemostatic clamps in surgery or dissection, to prevent bleeding from that vessel. This also may be done when an abnormal blood vessel forms, as these vessels may have thin walls and be prone to rupturing.

New "Instruments" for Surgery

A variety of tools exist to quickly stop bleeding blood vessels. Specialized surgical equipment use heat to seal the ends of cut blood vessels (electrocautery) in order to prevent blood from leaking out. The "argon beam plasma coagulator" uses argon gas and high-frequency electrical current to keep bleeding under control.

When compared with the old traditional surgical scalpel, many of the newer instruments for performing surgery have the potential for causing far less blood loss. Such instruments include:

- High-tech scalpels that combine the ability to cut tissue and seal bleeding vessels, at the same time, such as the harmonic scalpel (Fig. 1) (which uses ultrasound waves) and the microwave-coagulating scalpel
- The gamma knife may be used for brain surgery. This technique utilizes a powerful and precise form of radiation that can destroy tumors or abnormal blood vessels.
- Laser surgery harnesses the energy from light to cut through tissues
- Cryosurgery destroys abnormal tissue through freezing.

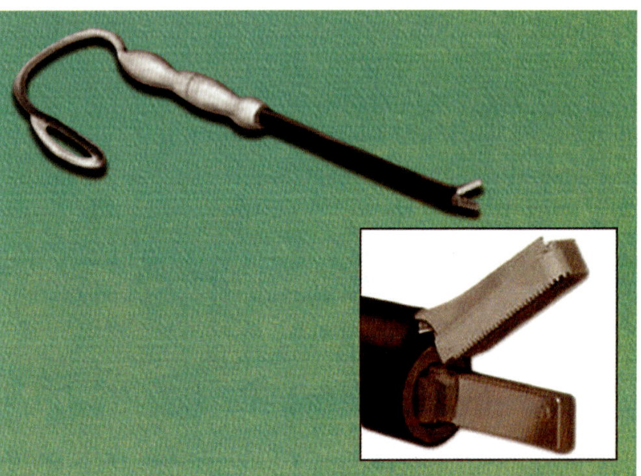

Fig. 1: The harmonic scalpel uses ultrasonic energy to both cut tissue and coagulate blood vessels

Laparoscopic Surgery

The increase in laparoscopic surgery has resulted in an increased need for a safe and reliable method of obtaining minimally invasive operative hemostasis. Because the traditional "open" methods of controlling bleeding (pressure, tying and suture ligating) are not as easily applied in the laparoscopic arena, a heavy reliance on forms of tissue and vessel coagulation is necessary. To better assess these forms we use monopolar, bipolar and ultrasound energy in addition to laser energy used in a novel application.

Although, each instrument has its place in the surgical armamentarium, the ultrasound technology appears to be the safest and most efficacious, commercially available device for obtaining hemostasis.

Lasers for hemostasis: The laser, as it is applied in minimally invasive surgeries, is also highly effective, but still a prototype device.

ADVANTAGES AND DISADVANTAGES OF LASERS

Advantages of Lasers

- Seals blood vessels while cutting any tissue
- No need to distend with high pressure fluids to stop bleeding—less swelling
- No need for repetitive diathermy to burn tissues to stop bleeding
- No need for drainage tubes to drain blood post-operatively (one cause of pain).

One Probe Does the Work of Many Instruments

- No need to keep changing instruments through the skin wounds
- Less damage to the portal tissues
- Less likelihood of breaking instruments
- Shorter operating and anesthetic times as ergonomically more efficient.

Small Diameter Instrument (2 mm)

- Less scuffing to adjacent joint surfaces
- Less damage to surrounding tissues which may be stretched to admit actions of conventional instruments, e.g. basket forceps
- Better access as it fits into very small spaces with gentle curve.

Cost Saving

- Once a hospital has a laser, the ongoing costs are less than conventional equipment, i.e. less disposable "single use" expensive equipment
- Reusable hand pieces.

Benefits, Especially for the Patient

- "Less subjective pain; less apparent bleeding and swelling"
  - The surgeon does not need to pump in fluid under pressure to stop the bleeding—this normally causes marked swelling and distention of tissues which is a cause of pain after the traditional laparoscopic/hysteroscopic operations
  - Tourniquets are not needed and they cause pain because of the period of ischemia and the pressure beneath
  - No drainage tubes which cause pain with movements
- Reduces surgical time
  - So less problems from the anesthesia, i.e. nausea and drowsiness
  - Patient gets over the operation more quickly
  - Less complications from the anesthesia—important if previously encountered medical problems
- No charring, therefore less irritation and inflammation
- Safety considerations
  - Surface ablation 0.4 mm per pulse
  - Surrounding tissue effect less than 1 mm and this seals the blood vessels
  - If beam does not come into contact with tissue within 4 mm, a harmless bubble forms as completely absorbed by the fluid—little likely damage to other tissues besides the one being targeted
- Precise surgery
  - Minimal damage/spread other tissues
  - Allows better sparing of adjacent tissues
  - Safe—danger zone only 3–4 mm in water
  - Very precise cutter, ablator, coagulator.

Disadvantages of Lasers

- Lasers are of high price and limited wavelength range
- Relatively few surgeons are trained in laser use
- Laser equipment is expensive and bulky compared with the usual surgical tools, such as scalpels
- Strict safety precautions must be observed in the operating room for example, the surgical team and the patient must use eye protection.

POSTPARTUM HEMORRHAGE

Postpartum hemorrhage (PPH) remains in the top five causes of maternal deaths in both developed and developing countries. Persistent blood loss of more than 1,000 mL should prompt predetermined measures to achieve resuscitation and hemostasis. A protocol including guidelines is given and volume replacement is discussed. The range of medical and surgical interventions that may be considered for the modern management of major hemorrhage unresponsive to oxytocin and ergometrine are discussed. The review discusses in depth the use of misoprostol, recombinant activated factor VII, the uterine tamponade procedures, artery ligation and uterine hemostatic suturing techniques. It also evaluates the place of interventional radiology and hysterectomy in modern obstetrics worldwide review of the uses of the uterine compression suture techniques as alternative to hysterectomy in the management of severe PPH.

Postpartum hemorrhage is a worldwide problem. The historical background dates back to William Smelley's in the 17th century in his famous treaty of the theory and practice of midwifery in 1752. Changes in clinical factors and surgical expertise compel the modern day midwife and obstetrician to be vigilant in identifying risk factors and apply appropriate solution early. The recent confidential enquiry into maternal death [why mothers die (2000–2002)] identifies areas of substandard care. The rising cesarean section rate adds to the rising incidence of PPH. The reduction in junior doctor's hours may limit the pool of experienced obstetric surgeons available to manage severe PPH competently. There can be major complications following radical surgery for PPH. These include loss of fertility, other morbidity and even maternal death. The invention of the B-Lynch surgical technique for the conservative management of PPH was first performed and reported by a consultant obstetrician and gynecological surgeon in Milton Keynes National Health Service (NHS) Trust publishing the first series of cases in BJOG, (an International Journal of Obstetrics and Gynaecology) 1997. This has made a significant impact on the conservative surgical management of massive PPH. There are now over 1,300 successful applications of this technique worldwide (CB-Lynch personal communication). Other similar or modified techniques such as Cho's square suture and Haymen's modification of the B-Lynch suture technique have been introduced adding to more available methods of conservative surgery. The current list of publications of successful application of the B-Lynch compression technique is encouraging and more outcome data can be reported by a letter or e-mail to enquiries@cblynch.com. Obstetricians and midwives both in developed and underdeveloped countries should seek training and attend fire drills in PPH control to avoid maternal morbidity and death. There should be special concentration on effective conservative surgery such as uterine compression techniques to avoid major morbidity and loss of fertility.

Parallel vertical compression sutures: A technique to control bleeding from placenta previa or accreta during cesarean section.

Fourteen women with placenta previa (including one who also had placenta accreta) undergoing cesarean section had massive bleeding after removal of the placenta. In order to preserve the uterus two parallel vertical compression sutures were placed in the lower segment to compress the anterior and posterior walls of the lower uterine segment. The hemorrhage from the lower segment stopped immediately after the knots were tightened. All women later resumed normal menstrual flow with no apparent complications. Two of the fourteen women had a spontaneous pregnancy 1–2 years after the operation. This parallel vertical compression suturing technique is simple, easy and effective for controlling bleeding in women with placenta previa or accreta. We suggest that this technique be tried first before other more complex procedures are undertaken.

SURGICAL DRAINS

Drains are put in by the surgeon to allow any fluid or air collecting at the operation site or in the wound to drain to the surface while allowing the main wound to heal. Fluids to be drained include blood, pus, urine, feces, bile or lymph.

Wound Drainage

1. Exudate—fluid, cells or other substances that have slowly exuded or discharged from cells or blood vessels through small pores or breaks in cell membrane.
2. Drainage—the removal of fluids from a body cavity, wound, or other source of discharge by one or more methods.
3. Types
   a. Serous
      i. Clear, watery fluid that has been separated from its solid elements (e.g. the exudate from a blister)
      ii. Serous fluid has characteristics of serum
      iii. Serum is clear, thin, sticky fluid portion of blood that remains after coagulation
   b. Sanguineous—Fluid contains blood
   c. Serosanguineous—Thin and red, described as pink.
4. Exudate/drainage greater than 300 mL in the first 24 hours should be treated as abnormal.

5. When patients first ambulate, a slight increase may occur.
6. If sanguineous drainage continues, small blood vessels may be oozing.
7. Not all surgical wounds drain.

   The following characteristics are important to note and chart:
   a. Color
   b. Amount
   c. Consistency (thick/thin)
   d. Odor.

TYPES OF DRAINS

Drains may be:
1. *Superficial,* i.e. in the wound
2. *Deep*
   a. Intraperitoneal, e.g. covering an intestinal anastomosis
   b. In a hollow organ or duct, e.g. a T-tube in the bile duct
   c. In an abnormal channel, e.g. a fistula
   d. To drain a deep cavity, e.g. an abscess or hematoma.

In addition drain may be:
1. *Open,* i.e. draining into a dressing or bag open to the air
2. *Closed,* i.e. draining into a sterilized air-tight tube and container. The drainage system may be:
   a. On tree drainage, e.g. drainage of ascites by gravity
   b. On suction, e.g. Redivac drains
   c. Controlled by a one-way valve, e.g. an underwater seal or chest drains.

TYPES OF DRAINS AND THEIR USES

Open Drains

Corrugated Rubber Drain

Rubber causes a tissue reaction and the drain track caused by this material persists longer than when inert materials are used. The drain is fixed by a suture at the end of the wound and a safety pin must be placed through the end to prevent the drain slipping inwards. Corrugated rubber drains can be used either for the wound or for deep drainage.

Yates' Drain

This is a corrugated drain made of a series of capillary tubes joined side to side. It is generally made of polyethylene which is less reactive than rubber. The drain site, therefore, tends to close more quickly once the drain has been removed. Its uses are similar to corrugated rubber drains and it is secured as described above.

Penrose Drain

This is a drain fashioned out of thin-walled rubber tubing and a gauze wick is threaded through the center of the tube. Fluid can then either drain down the track once the tube is removed or through the center whilst it is in place (Figs 2A to C).

Closed Drains

Redivac Drain

This is a fine tube with many holes at the end which is attached to an evacuated glass bottle providing suction. It is used to drain blood beneath the skin, e.g. after mastectomy or thyroidectomy, or from deep spaces, e.g. around a vascular anastomosis.

Jackson Pratt Drain (JP Drain or Bulb Drain)

It is a suction drainage device used to pull excess fluid from the body by constant suction. The device consists of a flexible plastic bulb—shaped something like a hand grenade—that connects to an internal plastic drainage tube. Removing the plug and squeezing the bulb removes air which creates a lower air pressure within the drainage tubing. The best way to accomplish this is to essentially fold the drain in half while it is uncapped, then while folded, recap the drain (Figs 3A and B). This action causes

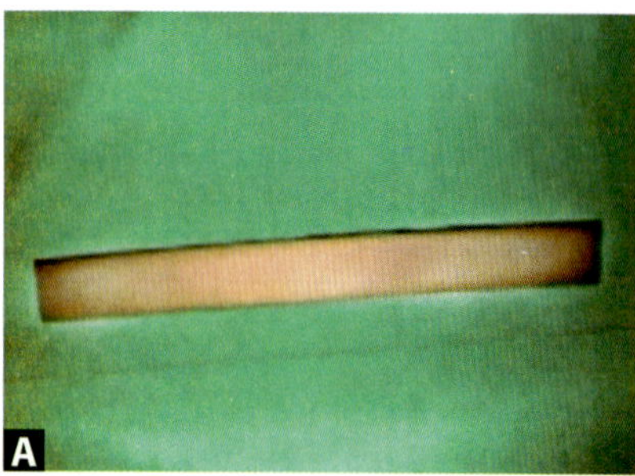

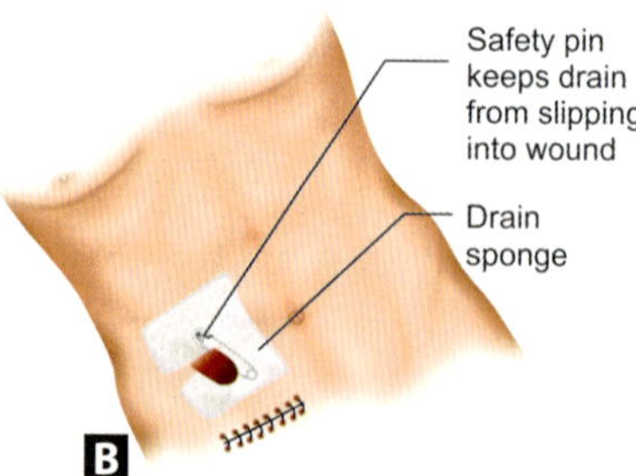

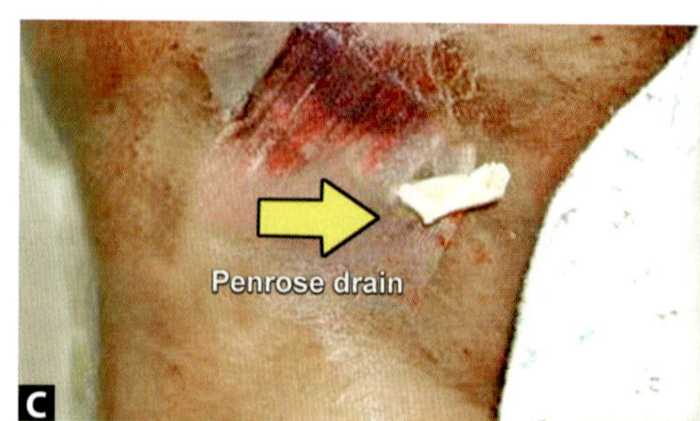

Figs 2A to C: Penrose drain and its placement

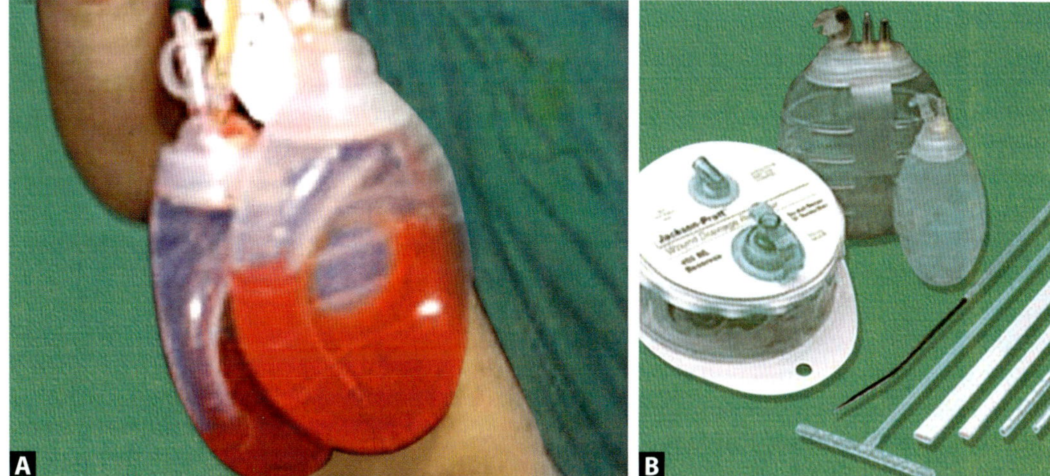

Figs 3A and B: (A) Jackson Pratt drain attached to a patient, (B) Complete set of JP drain

fluid to be gradually sucked of the body and into the bulb itself. The bulb may be repeatedly opened to remove the collected fluid and squeezed again to restore suction. It is best to empty drains before they are more than half full to avoid the discomfort of the weight of the drain pulling on the internal tubing.

'Shirlry' Wound Drainage

This is a suction drain with an intake tube supplying air to the bottom of the main tube. This allows continuous suction and the flow of air prevents the tube getting blocked.

Silastic Tube Drum

Silastic is a polymeric silicone and incites little tissue inflammation. Once this type of drain is removed, the track closes rapidly. A silastic tube drain can be used to provide closed drainage to deep pelvic cavity.

Red Rubber Tube Drain

This causes an intense tissue reaction and fibrosis. The track will, therefore, persist for some time after the drain is removed. This feature can be useful for drainage of chronic abscess cavities, such as an empyema or hepatic abscess.

Removal of Drains

A drain is removed as soon as it is no longer required. Hence, it is necessary to know the purpose for which it was inserted and you should ascertain this from the surgeon at the time of operation. The following are general guidelines:

1. Drains put in to cover perioperative bleeding and hematoma formation, can come out after 24–48 hours.
2. Drains put in to cover serous collections can come out after 3–5 days.
3. Where a drain has been put in because the wound may later become infected, it should be left for 1–5 days.
4. Drains put in to cover intestinal anastomoses should not be removed until after 5–7 days.

LOW VACUUM DRAINAGE: HANDYVAC

Introduction

Wound drains can be used when blood and lymphatic vessels are cut during surgery. Despite meticulous hemostasis performed by the surgeon, a wound may continue to ooze profusely necessitating placement of a wound drain. The usage as well as type of drainage system depends on the preference of the surgical team, procedure, patient and expected amount of fluid draining. If the wound is not drained, then a number of serious problems may occur including hematomas, infection, inflammation and pain. Such problems can increase the need for antibiotics as well as prolonging a patient's stay in hospital. A low vacuum drainage system is suitable for all procedures where gentle fluid removal is desired, especially when prolonged wound seroma production is foreseen. Low vacuum drainage may be used for several surgical procedures including breast, vascular, orthopedic, gynecology, general and some urological surgery. Besides skin irritation due to hard plastic drains, much of the discomfort for the patient is caused by the frequent need to replace the bottles which collect the drained fluids. The latter often necessitates a hospital visit where medical staff has to change bottles. Systems in which emptying of the fluid collector as well as reinstalment of vacuum pressure to the drainage system can be performed by the patient herself may, therefore, be preferred.

How to Use the HandyVac (Figs 4A and B)

The complete low vacuum drainage system comes in one sterilized package comprising of:

- Soft drain
- Compressible 125 mL vacuum chamber (initial vacuum 65 mm Hg)
- Drainage bag.

As shown in Figure 4B, the compressible low vacuum chamber (3) is at the top connected to a large soft plastic tube ending in a twist and lock connector (1) and at the bottom a short plastic tube which can be connected to the drainage bag (6) also by a twist and lock connector (5). Both tubes can be temporarily closed by blue clamps (2, 4). The drainage bag can contain 700 mL and can be emptied through a bottom outlet (7).

Step 1: Placement of the wound drain

The drain is placed into the wound and extruded through the skin using a trocar.

Separate the drain from the trocar using a large scissors. In order to properly fit the drain to the connector it should be cut at a right angle not oblique (Figs 5A and B).

Step 2: Connection to the compressible vacuum chamber (Figs 6 and 7)

It is of utmost importance that the twist and lock connector (1) is properly locked in order to prevent leakage and improper function of the low vacuum drainage system.

Once the connector is tightly screwed the patient drain can be connected to the tip of the plastic connector. In case of a slippery drain, use a gauze to hold the drain more easier (Fig. 8).

Step 3: Connection of the drainage bag (Fig. 8)

Connect the drainage bag to the bottom of the compressible vacuum chamber, i.e. the short tube with twist and lock connector (5). Make sure that the bottom outlet 7 of the drainage bag is closed.

Step 4: Installing low vacuum pressure (Figs 9A and B):

Both blue clamps (2, 4) on either side of the compressible vacuum chamber should be in the "open position". Compress the vacuum chamber (3). Repeat this maneuver until the vacuum chamber stays in a fully compressed form which corresponds with 65 mm Hg vacuum pressure.

Step 5: Reinstalment of low vacuum pressure

Due to persistent drainage the compressible vacuum chamber is filled up with fluid. Low vacuum pressure

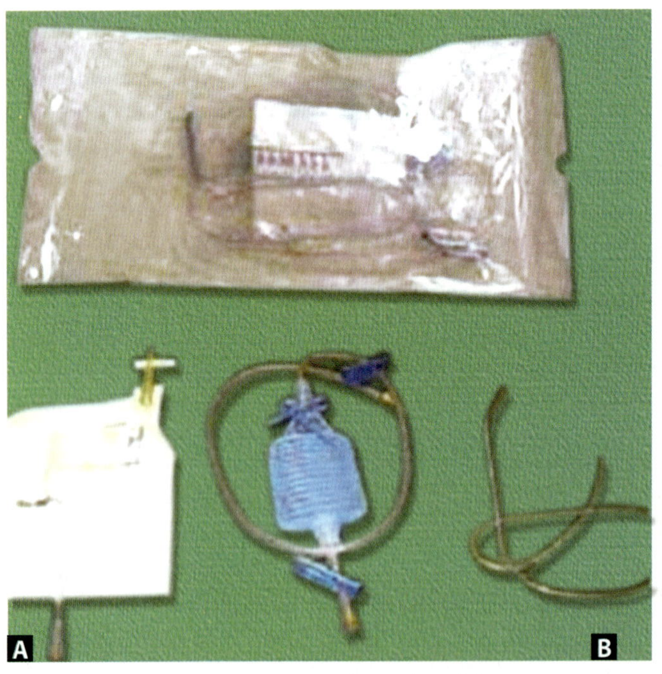

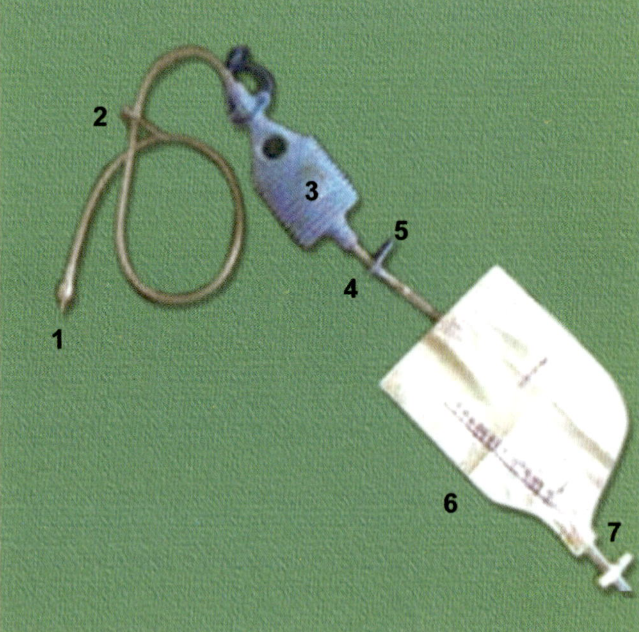

Figs 4A and B: Schematic overview of HandyVac drain with parts

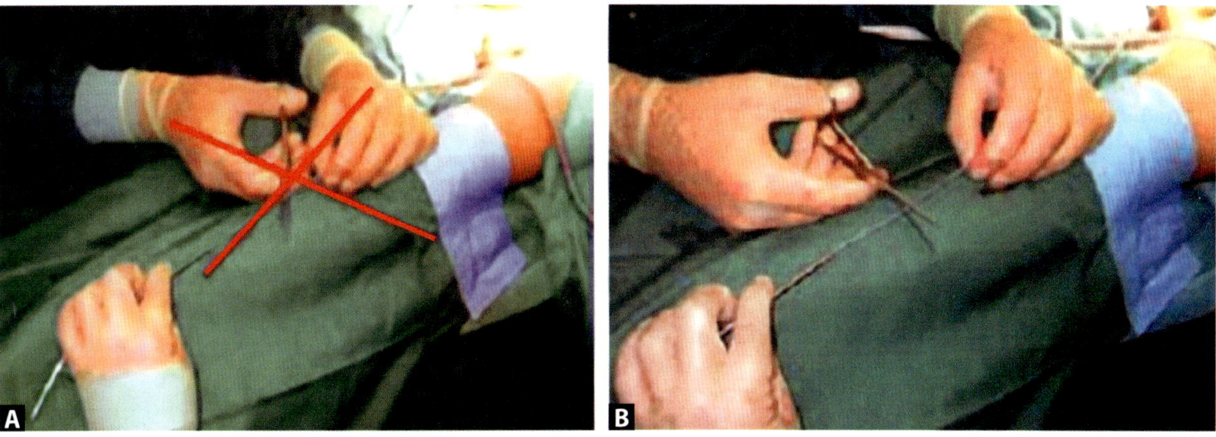

Figs 5A and B: Incorrect and correct method of cutting off the drain end after placement

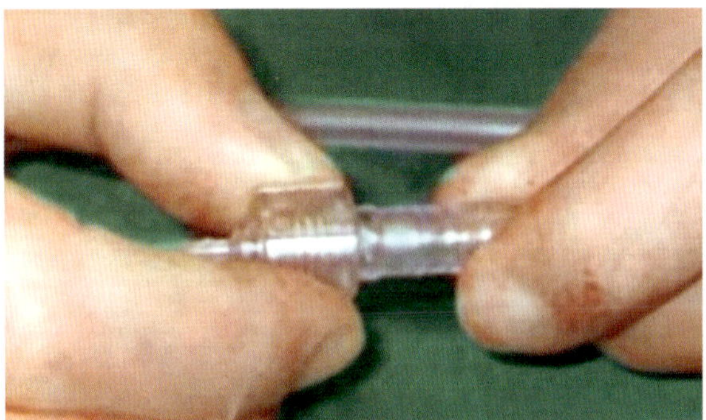

Fig. 6: How to correctly connect, the twist and lock connector

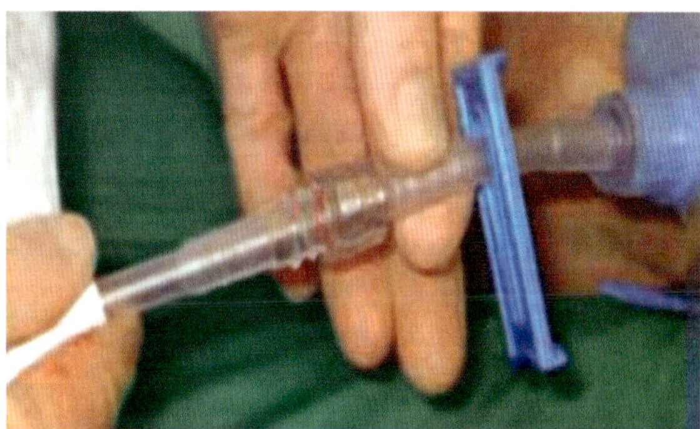

Fig. 7: How to correctly connect, the twist and lock connector

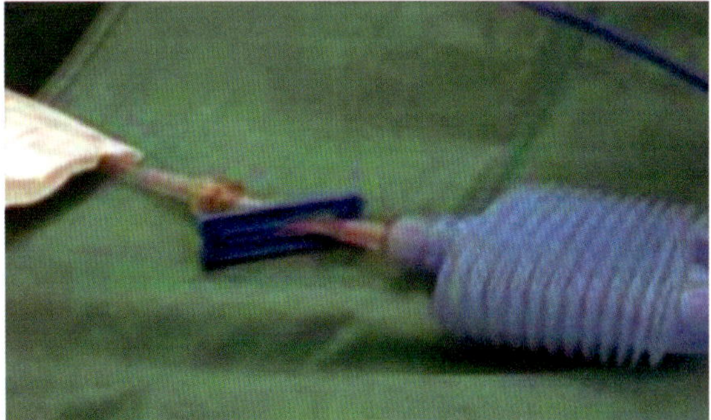

Fig. 8: Closure of lock connector

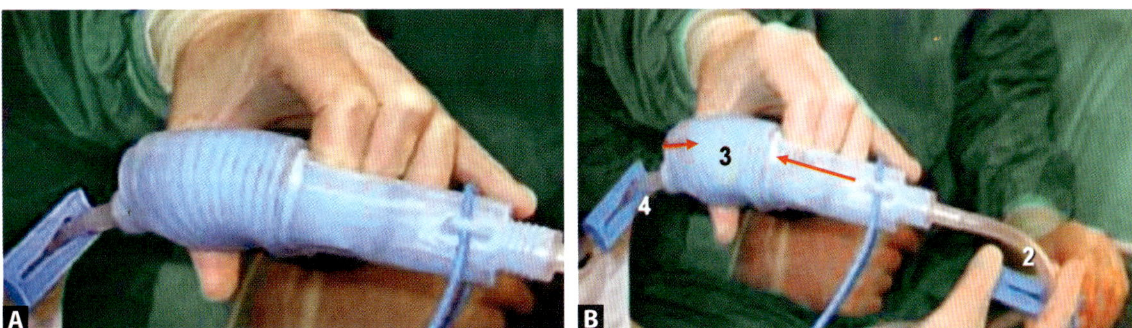

Figs 9A and B: Installing low pressure vacuum

decreases with filling of the chamber resulting in passive drainage instead of active vacuum drainage. To reinstall low vacuum pressure simple compress the compressible vacuum chamber thereby emptying the fluid in the large white collection bag. Clamps 2 and 4 must be left in the "open position".

Note:

- Due to non-return valves in the compressible vacuum chamber, fluids will not flow backwards.
- If it for some reason should be necessary to change the drainage bag, both clamps (2, 4) must be in closed position.

Step 6: Disconnection and/or emptying of the drainage bag

Before emptying the drainage bag, close the blue clamp (4) at the bottom of the compressible vacuum chamber. Clamp (2) can be left open (Fig. 10).

The drainage bag (6) can be emptied through a bottom outlet (7) (Fig. 11). Once the patient is mobilized on the ward or discharged from the hospital with the drainage system the drainage bag can be removed. Close the blue clamp (4) at the bottom of the compressible vacuum chamber. Unscrew the drainage bag from connector (5). The connector can be closed using a special cap (not shown).

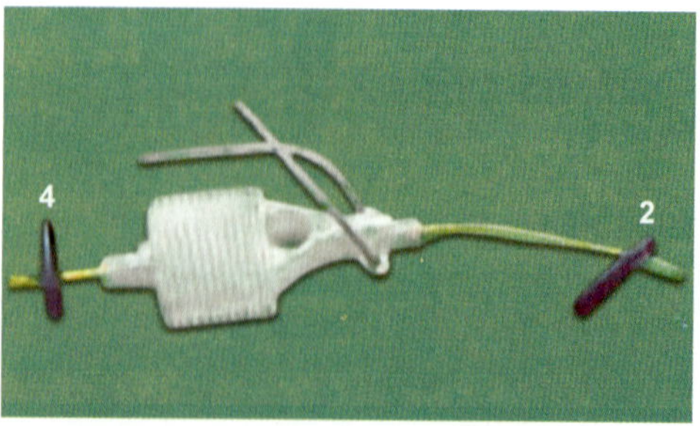

Fig. 10: Parts of vacuum installation set

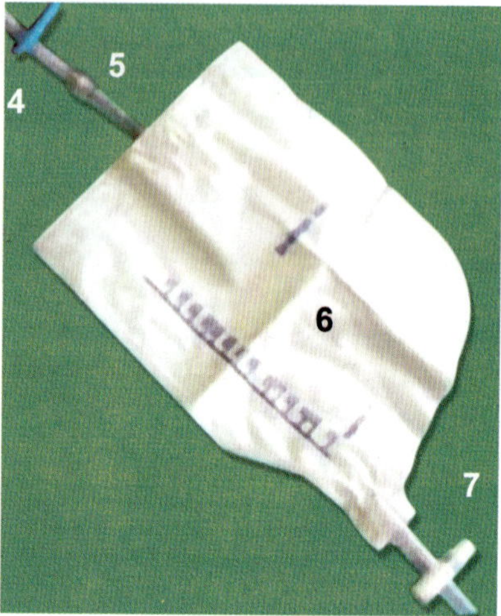

Fig. 11: Emptying of drainage bag

CHAPTER

36

Abortions

Ajita Mandlekar, Usha R Krishna

36.1 TERMINATION OF EARLY PREGNANCY BY MEDICAL METHODS

Ajita Mandlekar, Usha R Krishna

INTRODUCTION

The term "Medical Abortion" refers to pregnancy termination with medications. Termination of pregnancy was done by dilatation and curettage and later by electric suction evacuation. A lesser invasive method of manual vacuum aspiration is very acceptable. However, surgical methods do need perfect asepsis and training. A totally noninvasive method is the use of mifepristone (RU486), followed by prostaglandins (PGs) analog, misoprostol, which successfully terminates early pregnancy in about 95% of cases.

MECHANISM OF ACTION

Mifepristone (RU486) is the most widely used antiprogesterone compound. Mifepristone was invented in France at Roussel Uclaf by Dr E Baulieu in 1980. The chemical name of mifepristone is 11-[4-dimethylamino) phenyl]-17-hydroxy-17-(1-propynyl)-(11β,17β)-estra-4,9-dien-3-one. It is a derivative of norethindrone, and the 17α substitution is responsible for promoting higher binding affinity to the receptor. The 11β substitution is responsible for increasing antiprogesterone activity. It is the nature and position of substitutions in the steroid structure which appears to be critical for the progesterone antagonistic activity. The bioavailability of the drug after oral absorption is as high as 70% and the peak plasma concentration is reached within 1–2 hours. Although its half-life is about 20 hours, it is effective for several days and, therefore, it can be used as a single oral dose. The drug is extensively metabolized and there is no drug accumulation in the body. The drug has high affinity for progesterone receptors and also binds to glucocorticoid receptors and to a lesser extent to androgen receptors. Efforts are being made to prepare compounds with minimum antiglucocorticoid activity.

The antiprogesterones act on progesterone receptors in the myometrial, endometrial and decidual cells following which there is local withdrawal of progesterone. This causes the detachment of trophoblastic cells and the breakdown of endometrium, detachment of embryo followed by decline of human chorionic gonadotropin (hCG) and decline in progesterone. It initiates myometrial contractility, softening and dilatation of the cervix and even expulsion of the embryo. The method is successful in terminating early pregnancy in about 75% of cases. To make this method more successful, a small dose of PG is necessary, thus increasing the chance of successful expulsion in 95–98% cases. This was demonstrated by Bygdeman and Swahn in 1985. The side effects are minimal as the dose of the PG is very small but sets spontaneous contractions as the sensitivity to PGs has been increased by mifepristone. Different analogs have been used 36–48 hours after mifepristone administration. Tablet misoprostol given 48 hours after RU486, is the most practical and effective method as both RU486 as well as misoprostol can be given orally and do not require refrigeration.

Various analogs of PGs such as gemeprost vaginal suppository (16-dimethyl-trans 2PGE1), sulprostone, an injectable PG (16-phenoxy tetra non PGE2 sulfonylmide), carboprost [15(S)-15-methyl PGF2] as well as metenprost (9-deoxo-16,16-dimethyl-9) have been used. However, misoprostol (PGE1 analog) is the currently favored PG because of its safety, low cost, stability at room temperature, wide availability and easy oral administration. Misoprostol can also be administered by various other routes such as vaginal, buccal and sublingual. The mifepristone-misoprostol regimen in several dosage schedules have been found to be effective, feasible and acceptable method of induced abortion for women and providers of health care setting in various countries.

This antiprogestin mifepristone has many potential applications such as cervical softening and induction of labor besides termination of pregnancy. It is successfully used in cases of missed abortions. It has potential use as a contraceptive, and could be used for endometriosis, leiomyoma and even meningioma and breast cancer, and as an antiglucocorticoid.

PROTOCOLS

The standard drug administration protocol consisted of giving 3 tablets, i.e. 600 mg of mifepristone orally on day 1 followed by 400–800 μg of misoprostol on day 3. The World Health Organization (WHO) trial has proved the effectiveness of 200 mg same as 600 mg. A 17-center study was conducted by the WHO all over the world where two doses of mifepristone 200 mg and 600 mg followed by 400 μg of misoprostol for pregnancy termination up to 9 weeks gestation. The complete abortion rate was 91.5% in 200 mg group and 90.7% in 600 mg group, showing that both doses were equally effective.

The dose of mifepristone used now is 200 mg and misoprostol could be 400–800 μg orally or vaginally. Generally, misoprostol is given 48 hours after mifepristone. However, this time interval between the drugs had been reduced to as low as 6–24 hours and the patient could also be explained to administer misoprostol herself at home and come for follow-up to confirm pregnancy expulsion. Efforts are made to increase the efficacy, decrease the side effects and improve the acceptability. There are studies indicating better results if misoprostol is repeated 4 hours after the first dose. In a randomized study, women received one or two doses of 400 μg misoprostol orally. The repeat administration of misoprostol 400 μg improved the complete abortion rate from 87.4% to 92.6% and significantly reduced the rate of ongoing pregnancy from 7% to 0.7%.

Though sublingual administration of misoprostol has shown to be very effective and shows quick and higher rise of the drug, the success is more or less similar to vaginal administration.

The medical termination of pregnancy (MTP) is officially permitted till 49 days after last menstrual period. However, its acceptability and success has been shown even up to 56 days and even 63 days. The woman has to be counseled appropriately as it is the most essential part of the abortion program. When the client has chosen medical method, the drug schedule and importance of follow-up should be explained. It is necessary to inform her about the side effects and complications although they are rare. The patient could get nausea and vomiting, diarrhea and abdominal cramps. Occasionally, she can get fever. There is possibility of incomplete abortion or failure of the method. Profuse or prolonged bleeding needs medical attention and necessary treatment.

EFFICACY AND SAFETY

A successful medical abortion is defined as complete termination of pregnancy without the need for a surgical procedure. Failure is defined as recourse to a surgical procedure, which may be the result of continuation of pregnancy, incomplete expulsion or heavy bleeding. The majority of women expel the products of conception in 24 hours after misoprostol administration but the process may take up to 2 weeks to complete. Sonography is carried out if there is possibility of incomplete abortion.

Early medical abortions in controlled settings are extremely safe without long-term problems on women's health. Frequently cited safety concerns are excessive and prolonged bleeding, undiagnosed ectopic pregnancy and teratogenic effects. In cases of failure of abortion in spite of misoprostol treatment, it is necessary to carry out suction evacuation. The drug can cross the placenta and cause limb and skull deformities.

It is essential to do blood grouping, complete blood count and urine examination. Other laboratory investigations such as blood sugar, etc. are carried out when considered necessary. Pelvic sonography (trans-vaginal) is not routinely necessary unless there is a suspicion of ectopic pregnancy or the woman is not sure of her last menstrual period.

Rh-negative women should be protected by anti-D injection of 50 μg intramuscularly on the day of PG treatment to prevent Rh-immunization.

MEDICAL ABORTION MORTALITY

Seven deaths have been reported to the company responsible for the US distribution for mifepristone and to the Food and Drug Administration (FDA) since 2001, four of these are related to infection with a rare organism *Clostridium sordellii*. It may be necessary to consider giving antibiotics for 1 week with medical abortion. Metronidazole may be a good option. However, deaths from abortions by various methods are difficult to assess. It is certainly essential to understand that causes of abortion-related deaths, however, are rare.

CONCLUSION

Medical abortion is now freely available, but it is necessary that the provider is conscious of the contraindications such as chronic adrenal disease, hypertension, cardiac disease, concurrent long-term corticosteroid therapy, hemorrhagic disorders, anemia, undiagnosed adnexal mass, pregnancy with intrauterine device (IUD) and possibility of ectopic pregnancy. Allergy to misoprostol though rare should be enquired. Previous cesarean section or presence of leiomyoma is contraindication. Bronchial asthma is also not a contraindication for misoprostol as it is a weak bronchodilator. It is better to avoid medical abortion in women older than 35 years and who smoke more than 10 cigarettes per day. Counseling for proper follow-up, postabortal care as well as advice to follow contraception are essential. Contraception can be initiated as soon as termination of pregnancy is confirmed. There is a risk of repeat pregnancy as ovulation may occur by day 11 postabortion and 75% of women would have ovulated within 6 weeks postabortion. Condoms, combined oral contraceptive pills (COCPs), injectables, intrauterine contraceptive device (IUCD), male and female sterilizations can be offered. Studies indicate that COCPs and injectable can be started on day 3 after misoprostol has been used. Emergency backup services, transport facilities as well as blood transfusion facilities though rarely required should be available. The misuse of drugs in advanced pregnancy can cause mishaps and the proper dosage and systematic follow-up have to be emphasized.

By now there is a great deal of experience of medical method in India and most studies have shown a success rate from 90% to 95%. The initial trials by Indian Council of Medical Research (ICMR)used mifepristone (RU486) followed by 9-methylene PGE2 gel with a success rates in various centers ranging from 94.5% to 89.4%.

In the last 5 years, the authors have used 200 mg of mifepristone followed by 400 μg of misoprostol in more than 300 patients with a success rate of 95%. If the bleeding did not start after 4 hours, a second dose of 400 μg of misoprostol is given. Home administration of misoprostol is possible and successful with good counseling in majority of the cases.

Medical method is, therefore, very acceptable and has good impact on the program of safe abortion and safe motherhood.

BIBLIOGRAPHY

1. Baulieu EE. Contragestion and other clinical applications of RU 486, an antiprogesterone at the receptor. Science. 1989;245:1351-7.
2. Bygdeman M, Swahn ML. Progesterone receptor blockage. Effect on uterine contractility and early pregnancy. Contraception. 1985;32:45-51.
3. Coyaji K, Elul B, Krishna U, et al. Mifepristone abortion outside the urban research hospital setting in India. Lancet. 2001;357(9250):120-2.
4. Coyaji K, Krishna U, Ambardekar S, et al. Are two doses of misoprostol after mifepristone for early abortion better than one? BJOG. 2007;114(3):271-8.
5. Fischer M, Bhatnagar J, Guarner J, et al. Fetal toxic shock syndrome associated with Clostridium sordellii after medical abortion. N Engl J Med. 2005;353:2352-60.
6. Indian Council of Medical Research Task Force of Hormonal Contraception. A multicentre clinical trial with RU 486 followed by 9-methylene-PGE2 vaginal gel for termination of early pregnancy: a dose-finding study. Contraception. 1994;49:87-98.
7. Mittal S. Contraception after medical abortion. Contraception. 2006;74(1):56-60.
8. Winikoff B, Sivin I, Coyaji KJ, et al. Safety, efficacy, and acceptability of medical abortion in China, Cuba, and India: a comparative trial of mifepristone-misoprostol versus surgical abortion. Am J Obstet Gynecol. 1997;176:431-7.
9. World Health Organization Task Force on Post-ovulatory Methods of Fertility Regulation; Special Programme of Research, Development and Research Training. Comparison of two doses of mifepristone in combination with misoprostol for early medical abortion: a randomized trial. BJOG. 2000;107:524-30.

36.2 SECOND TRIMESTER—TERMINATION OF PREGNANCY

Usha R Krishna

INTRODUCTION

Although first trimester abortion can be performed by a registered medical practitioner, who has received MTP training certification, termination of pregnancy between 12 weeks and 20 weeks have to be approved by two doctors. Unsafe abortions are serious public health problem in India and about 15% of maternal deaths are due to unsafe abortions. This is a preventable mortality, if MTPs are carried out by safe and effective methods in well-equipped institutions. This specially applies to second trimester termination as it certainly has greater hazards and needs perfect asepsis and good expertise.

Even today, in spite of liberalization, illegal abortions are frequently performed by untrained persons. Singh R et al studied 48 cases of septic abortions over 6 years and found that untrained persons were responsible for septic abortions in 95.83% of cases. Septic abortions were more common in grand multiparas (62.5%) and there was maternal mortality in 16.6% of the cases. With awareness of the community and training of medical and paramedical staff, this tragedy could be avoided almost completely. The methods of doing terminations of pregnancy have improved tremendously. Aspirotomy and intra-amniotic use of hypertonic saline have been given up. Extra-amniotic ethacridine lactate is a widely used safe and successful method. PG analogs have been used by intra-amniotic, extra-amniotic, vaginal, cervical, intramuscular (IM) and oral routes.

ETHACRIDINE LACTATE

It is a lactoacridine, a yellow dye with antiseptic properties, and used as 0.1% solution. It is injected extra-amniotically via Foley catheter in the dose of 10 mL per gestation week for inducing abortion.

MECHANISM

Mechanical stimulation of the uterus by extensive detachment of the membranes and damage to decidual lysosomes leads to synthesis and release of PGs. This is followed by contractions of uterine muscle and rise in resting tension as well as cervical dilatation. The process can be accelerated by intravenous (IV) oxytocin or IM or extra-amniotic PG analog. It is necessary to monitor the patient meticulously and plan the drugs and dosage for acceleration to prevent problems like hypertonia or rupture of the uterus. Proper asepsis is essential to prevent pelvic infection. Postabortal hemorrhage can be prevented by timely action.

Chaudhuri et al compared intravaginal misoprostol with extra-amniotic ethacridine lactate for second trimester MTP in Kolkata to compare safety, efficacy, complications and cost effectiveness of each method. A randomized comparative study on 120 women between 13 weeks and 20 weeks showed that the success of abortion within 48 hours was 95% in each group. The interval of induction abortion was shorter in misoprostol group (15.5 hours compared to 31.3 hours) and the average cost of treatment was Rs. 57.95 for misoprostol as compared to Rs. 87.10 for ethacridine lactate. The side effects were rare in both the groups.

PROSTAGLANDINS

Intra-amniotic, extra-amniotic carboprost, IM sulprostone, vaginal gemeprost and PGE1 analog misoprostol can be used for second trimester termination. Misoprostol is most suitable as the cardiovascular effects and excessive motility of gastrointestinal tract are rare compared to other PG analogs. There is no bronchial constriction but mild bronchodilator effect.

PROTOCOL

Laboratory investigations such as blood grouping, complete blood count, blood sugar and urine examination are necessary. Other appropriate investigations are done according to the requirements. Sonography is done when the date of the gestational age is uncertain. It is also necessary in cases of twins, history of failed terminations, intrauterine fetal death, etc.

Misoprostol can be given orally or vaginally. The bioavailability is much higher with vaginal administration than oral. Two tablets of misoprostol (400 μg) should be introduced in the vagina. This can be followed by two to four additional doses 3 hourly. The dose can be delayed or decreased depending on the severity and frequency of the uterine contractions and the extent of cervical effacement and dilatation. Most often, three to five doses are sufficient to expel the product of conception. Proper monitoring is very essential to prevent hypertonia, rupture of the uterus or bucket handle tears of the cervix. The induction abortion period varies from 13 hours to 24 hours in various studies and the success rate is around 90%.

ADJUVANTS

Various modifications are made in the regimen depending on the uterine contractions and cervical dilatation as well as experience of the provider. At times, misoprostol is withheld after two or three doses and IV oxytocin is given to have better control over the frequency and intensity of uterine contraction. Occasionally, the process of abortion needs to be completed by IM injection of carboprost, especially when contractions have become weaker and infrequent. Mifepristone (RU486) 200 mg can be orally given 6–12 hours before initiating the process of second trimester abortion with misoprostol. This reduces the induction abortion period very substantially and increases the success rate. Baird, Thong and Tang have shown 98.8% success rate and induction abortion period of 7.8 hours. Randomized trials of mifepristone prior to PGs have shown significant reduction in the induction abortion interval and the dose of PG.

CERVICAL RIPENING

Cervical ripening is achieved through alterations in biochemical properties of the cervix, i.e. reduction in the collagen content, increase in water contents and change in the glycosaminoglycan. Endocervical or vaginal PGE2 gel can be used for cervical ripening prior to the process of second trimester termination. This softening, effacement and dilatation of the cervix certainly reduces the induction abortion interval. Cervical ripening can also be carried out by mifepristone as well as misoprostol and gemeprost vaginal suppositories. In cases requiring late first trimester or early second trimester terminations, suction evacuation can be done after cervical ripening. IV oxytocin or IM carboprost helps evacuation by contracting the uterus during suction evacuation. The possibility or perforation of the uterus and hemorrhage are significantly reduced. The methods used for second trimester terminations can be used for evacuation of vesicular mole. Cases with intrauterine death and fetal abnormalities can also be similarly treated.

SIDE EFFECTS AND COMPLICATIONS

The process of uterine contractions causes abdominal cramps similar to labor. Nausea and vomiting and at times diarrhea are side effects, which need to be looked after. Fever is not infrequent. This is more often due to misoprostol rather than infection.

Second trimester terminations certainly carry greater hazards and it is important that the women are made aware of the importance of approaching for medical help early in pregnancy. Delay in abortion from 8 weeks to 16 weeks increases the risk by more than 300% depending on the abortions techniques used.

Prostaglandins are the most effective abortifacients and, therefore, need caution because of its powerful action on the uterus and effect on other systems such as gastrointestinal, cardiovascular, etc. It is essential that the termination is carried out in an institution, where trained personnel, asepsis and emergency services including blood transfusions are available. Cases with previous cesarean section have to be carried out very meticulously with close monitoring. Cases with intrauterine death need thorough laboratory work-up including study of coagulation factors. When a case is referred from elsewhere after a failed termination or after some complications, it is very necessary to get detailed history and do a thorough examination as there is possibility of infection, perforation and anemia due to hemorrhage. Termination for female feticide is prevalent due to social reasons. Prevention of these tragedies needs awareness, education and implementation of law.

The risk of complications depends on the gestational age, parity, method of abortion and expertise of the provider. The immediate complications are hemorrhage often due to retention of the placenta. This needs immediate management. Severe hemorrhage can be associated with coagulopathy. Uterine and cervical trauma could be minimized by preoperative cervical ripening and controlled uterine contractions. Incomplete evacuation and infection are not infrequent. Women who harbor organisms such as *Neisseria gonorrhoeae, Chlamydia trachomatis* or anerobic organisms in lower genital tract are particularly vulnerable. Poor asepsis and prolonged procedures increase the possibility of infection. These pelvic infections can cause tubo-ovarian infection, peritonitis and toxic shock, which can be fatal. There is considerable morbidity such as chronic pelvic pain, secondary infertility due to tubal block and intrauterine synechia. Possibility of ectopic pregnancy and recurrent abortions should be considered. Prophylactic use of antibiotics is justified and cost effective. It is essential to give anti-D injection to Rh-negative women in the dose of 300 μg after second trimester termination to prevent Rh-immunization.

ULTRASONOGRAPHY

Sonography is useful when there is a doubt regarding gestational age. It is most useful when there is a failure of abortion or suspicion of incomplete abortion. The author was referred a case of failure of second trimester abortion where the products had moved between the two leaves of broad ligament through a lateral tear of the uterus causing a mass in left iliac fossa.

POSTABORTION COUNSELING

The second trimester termination cases need to be followed till the uterus is well involuted and the patient gets normal menstrual period. Family planning advice is essential.

The second trimester terminations should decrease over years with greater awareness about contraception, emergency contraceptives and easier access to facilities of first trimester abortion. This will substantially reduce the abortion-related complications and duration of hospital stay. The abortion-related maternal mortality would drastically fall and the long-term morbidity could be avoided.

A 17-year review of voluntary termination of pregnancy by Patel and Leuva in Ahmedabad indicated that there was no decline in the rate of induced abortion over the 17-year period. Most women (99.4%) were married and 72.5% had two or more living children. The rate of termination in multiparas has increased over the years and the rate of termination of pregnancy of 12 weeks has declined over the last 3 years.

There is certainly an unmet need of contraception. Is it a failure on the part of government, nongovernmental organizations (NGOs), community leaders or medical professionals? We all have a long way to go to prevent termination of pregnancy, especially second trimester. There has to be a sustained effort in the area of education, counseling and medical care to avoid the alarming maternal mortality and morbidity.

BIBLIOGRAPHY

1. Baird DT, Thong KJ, Tang OS. Second trimester medical abortion with mifepristone and gemeprost: a review of 956 cases. Contraception. 2001;64:29-32.
2. Chaudhuri S, Mitra SN, Chaudhuri N, et al. A comparison of intravaginal misoprostol with extraamniotic ethacridine lactate for second trimester MTP. Obstet Gynecol India. 2006;56:518-21.
3. El-Refaey H, Templeton A. Induction of abortion in the second trimester by a combination of misoprostol and mifepristone: a randomized comparison between two misoprostol regimens. Hum Reprod. 1995;10:475-8.
4. Gottlieb C, Bygdeman M. The use of antiprogestin (RU 486) for termination of second trimester pregnancy. Acta Obstet Gynecol Scand. 1991;70:199-203.
5. Grimes DA, Cates W. Complications from legally induced abortions: a review. Obst Gyn Survey. 1979;34:171-91.
6. Grimes DA, Schulz KF, Cates W. Prophylactic antibiotics for curettage abortion. Am J Obstet Gynecol. 1984;150:689-94.
7. Ho PC, Ma HK. Termination of second trimester pregnancy with sulprostone and mifepristone: a randomized double-blind placebo-controlled trial. Contraception. 1993;47:123-9.
8. Patel T, Leuva B. A 17-year review of voluntary termination of pregnancy (MTP). J Obstet Gynaecol India. 2006;56(6):522-8.
9. Singh R, Nagrath A, Taneja S. Evaluation of septic abortion over past 6 years in a teaching hospital. J Obstet Gynaecol India. 2007;57(1):61-3.
10. UK Multicenter Study Group. Oral mifepristone 600 mg and vaginal gemeprost for mid-trimester induction of abortion. An open multicenter study. Contraception. 1997;56:361-6.

CHAPTER

37

Vulva

Prabha Malhotra, Neharika Malhotra Bora, Narendra Malhotra, Neeta Singh, Randhir Puri, V Chandra, Malini KV, Ashwini Bhalerao-Gandhi Murad E Lala, Bimal Mody

Problems around the vulvar region are common and can lead to severe discomfort and embarrassment for women. They generally suffer in silence, ignore the problem until it gets very severe or use home remedies which worsen the situation. Conditions commonly seen are boils, abscesses, Bartholin's cysts, growths like warts, rashes like lichen simplex/psoriasis/lichen planus/lichen sclerosis as well as cancerous and precancer lesions.

37.1 LABIAL FUSION RELEASE/INCISION

Prabha Malhotra, Neharika Malhotra Bora

INTRODUCTION

Labial fusion (Fig. 1) is when the female's labia get attached and adhered to each other in the middle line, leaving a small opening or sometimes closing off the vagina. It is a rare event, especially in adults where it is an acquired lesion. It should not be confused with blue-domed membrane of imperforate vagina with hematocolpos within (Fig. 2).

In adults, it is mainly caused by poor hygiene, estrogen deficiency, lack of sexual activity, repeated urinary infections and inflammation that occurs secondary to various resultant scarring. Inflammation may cause the labia skin to peel off and during healing, the labia get fused together. But this usually happens after sexual abuse in a prepubertal child.

Very few adults require surgical correction and release of fusion. Local estrogen works even in patients who

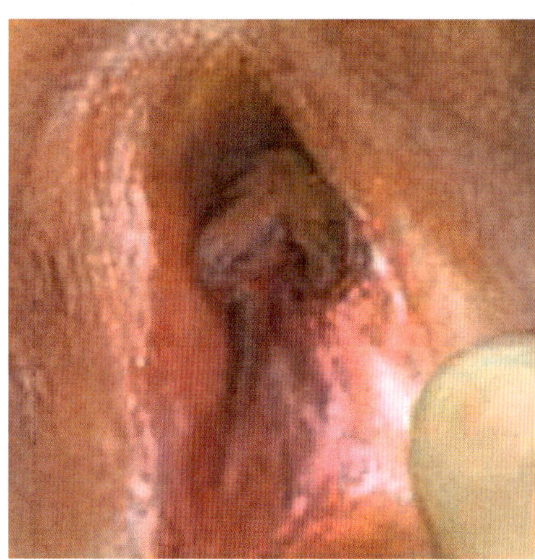

Fig. 1: Extensive labial adhesion

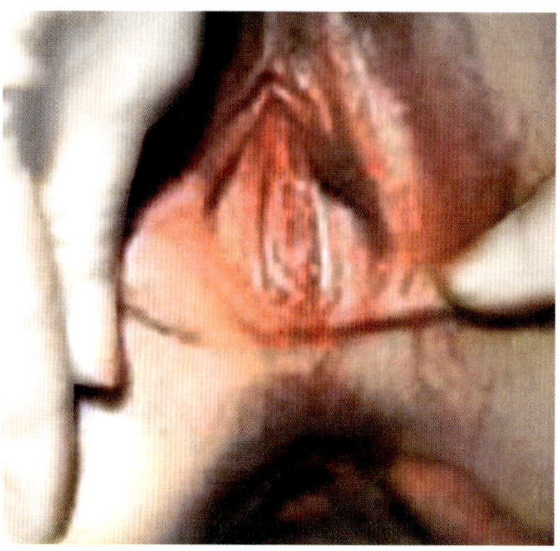

Fig. 2: Vaginal agenesis. Labial adhesion of Figure 1 is not to be confused with imperforate blue-domed translucent membrane

require surgery to prevent refusion and allay the patient's anxiety and emotional trauma.

In babies, it is congenital. In girls, 6 months to 6 years, it can be managed by a simple procedure of separating the fused labia or application of an estrogen cream.

Labial fusion is never seen in the reproductive ages but is more common in postmenopausal women.

Separating the fused labia using a blunt instrument is a simple office procedure.

If left untreated for long, it leads to repeated urinary tract infections, bladder distension and kidney problems due to urinary outflow obstruction.

Treatment may include simple reconstruction of the labia without any operation, or when the condition is caused by lack of estrogen, an estrogen cream can be prescribed. The cream is applied on the fused labia until when they separate.

Sometimes, the condition can also disappear without treatment when the adolescent girl attains menarche and gets her first periods. All patients require surgical lysis of labial adhesions under general anesthesia. Adhesions are incised sharply and the cut edges are reapproximated with 7-0 chromic suture.

LABIAL ADHESIONS

Labial adhesion, also referred to as labial agglutination, occurs in children when the inner vaginal lips (labia minora) fuse with each other. It often gives the appearance that the opening of the vagina has closed off. It may be noticed incidentally by a parent or by a physician during a medical examination, or the child may complain of irritation or difficulty urinating.

Because the adhesion sometimes creates a little pouch in front of the vagina where urine can collect, some children experience dribbling when they stand up after urinating. Occasionally, a child will get a bladder infection or will have difficulty passing urine due to the obstruction but most often labial adhesions are not significant enough to obstruct the flow of urine.

What Causes Labial Adhesion?

The most likely cause is that inflammation of the labia minora creates two raw surfaces at the edges of the lips, which eventually heal together in the middle, partly or fully covering the opening of the vagina.

Many factors can lead to inflammation and irritation of the vaginal lips. Exposure to irritants like fabric softener residue, perfumed soaps, or bits of stool; or a prolonged exposure to damp (as in wet diapers) all can cause irritation of the area. The lack of estrogen (which is normal before puberty) probably plays a role in this process.

When is Treatment Necessary?

Labial adhesions are commonly found in young girls between the ages of 3 months and 6 years. While experts used to think medical or surgical treatment was necessary, recent research has shown that cases involving adherence that is not obstructing the flow of urine usually resolve on their own over a period of 6–18 months.

However, even when treatment is used, the likelihood that the labial adhesions will recur is high. The best approach is to eliminate factors that lead to inflammation and then be patient. Active treatment may be most helpful if child is getting bladder infections, is extremely bothered by dribbling after urination, or has difficulty passing urine.

When treatment is necessary, a small amount of estrogen cream can be gently rubbed onto the area of fusion twice a day. Using a cotton-tipped applicator can assist you. Also put a bit of pressure along the fusion line. This therapy should be combined with careful avoidance of irritants and a daily bath in plain water. The labia usually will separate by 3–8 weeks. Parents should be aware that some girls, and even infants, will experience a small amount of breast development during treatment with topical estrogen cream because the hormone can be absorbed into the bloodstream. If estrogen treatment is not fully successful by 8 weeks, a topical anesthetic like xylocaine ointment cream can be used in the office and the practitioner can gently tease apart the lips.

Vulvar care measures, combined with estrogen treatment, when indicated is usually all that is needed. However, there have been reports of rare cases in which the labia totally heal together, forming a "skin bridge" that requires surgery.

Prevention of Recurrence

After the labia separate, daily bathing in a tub of plain water, avoiding irritants, and treating the area with petroleum jelly or ointment usually prevents recurrence. Good vulvar hygiene does not mean that you need to scrub the vaginal area. Rather, it means avoiding irritants and trying to expose the area to some air every day.

SURGICAL TECHNIQUE STEPS

1. Under general anesthesia, patient is cleaned and draped aseptically. At 30°, 5 mm laparoscope is introduced within the pocket formed by labial fusion. This is to define lower most edges of fourchette (Fig. 3A)
2. Incision is made with scissors in median raphe within the channel of metal probe inserted behind the labial fusion ridge (Fig. 3B)
3. Cut edges are reapproximated with 7-0 chronic sutures to enlarge the vulvar opening (Figs 3C and D).

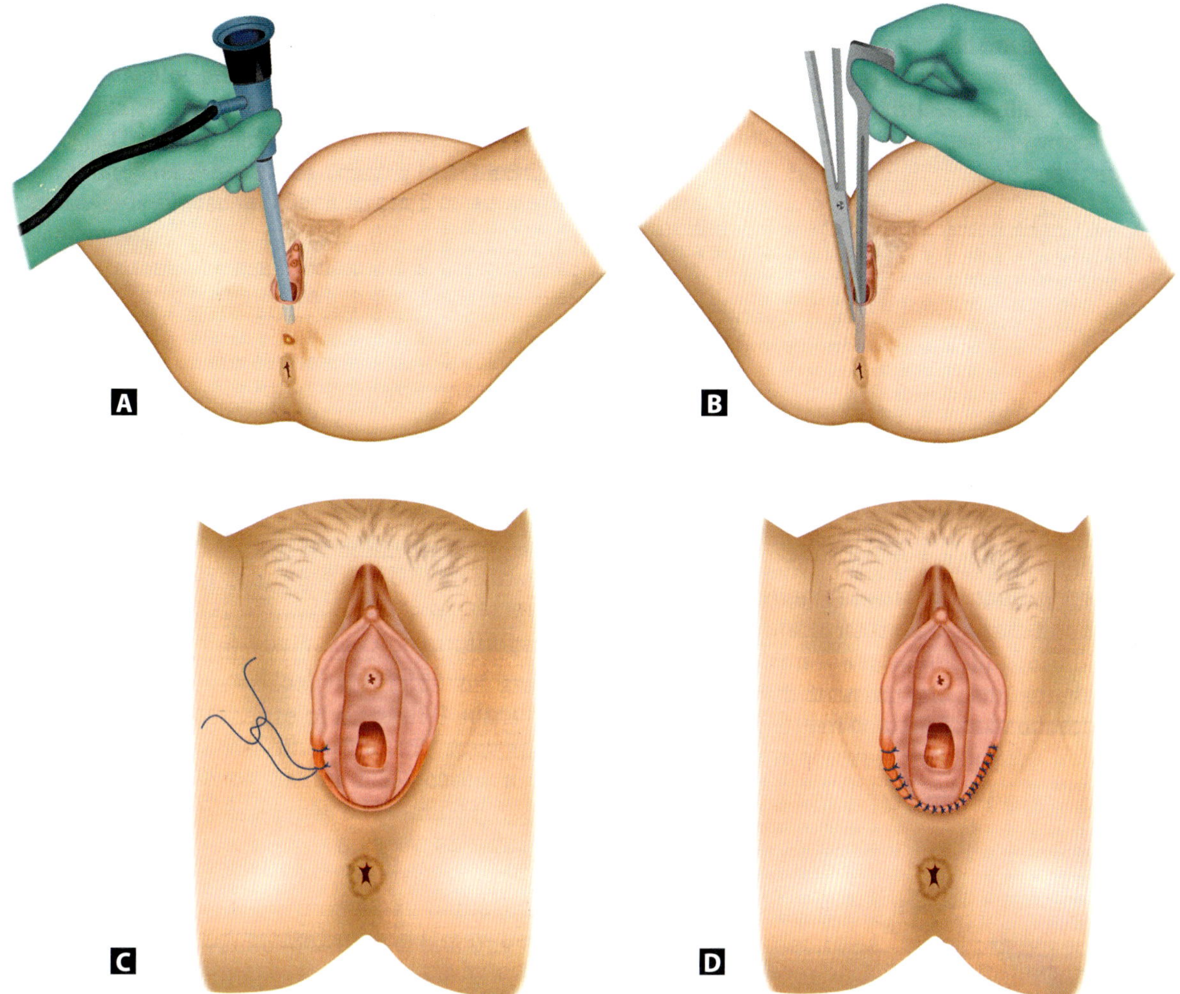

Figs 3A to D: Steps of labial fusion release. (A) Introduction of 5 mm laparoscope to know the extent of fusion and reach to fourchette for guidance of labial incision; (B) The incision with guard kept in vagina by a fenestrated metal probe; (C and D) Reconstruction by suturing of incised area to enlarge vulva opening after release of labial/incision/adhesion

37.2 HYMENORRHAPHY AND HYMENOPLASTY

Narendra Malhotra, Neharika Malhotra Bora

THE HYMEN

Hymen (HI-min): The hymen is a thin, delicate membrane (a membrane is like skin but much thinner). It partially covers the opening of the vagina in most girls.

- The hymen is simply the vestigial membranes of the vagina and urogenital sinus at their point of fusion (Fig. 1)
- An elastic and collagenous tissue
- In younger women, hymen is very vascular as opposed to menopausal women, which are very thin
- In adult virgin women, the hymen is of different thickness that surrounds the vaginal opening more or less completely
- The hymen is named after Hymenaeus, the Greek god of marriage and the wedding feast or song
- Hymenaeus, son of Aphrodite and Dionysus, is mentioned in the Illiad and the Aeneid and is typically depicted with the marriage torch held aloft

Function of the Hymen

- The biological function of the human hymen is still uncertain
- Scientists hypothesize that it protects the vagina from infection in infants
- The social function of the hymen, however, has been and still is a mythical symbol of virginity in many cultures
- Allows outflow of menstrual blood.

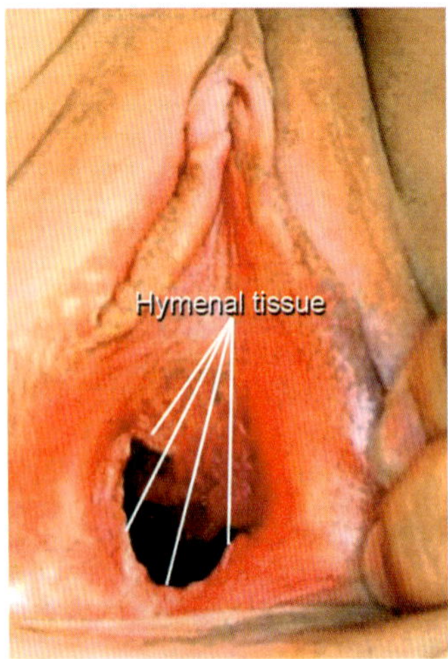

Fig. 1: Hymenal residual tissue

Types of Hymen (Figs 2A and B)

- Annular or circular—in which the hymen forms a ring around the vaginal opening
- Dentate fimbriated or denticular hymen—a hymen with an opening which has serrate edges
- Crescentric or lunar hymen, a moon-shaped hymen—anterior, posterior
- Hymen bifenestratus—a hymen with two openings side by side and a broad septum between them
- Septate—a hymen in which the opening is divided by a narrow septum
- Hymen subseptus—a hymen in which the opening is partially filled by a septum growing out of one wall, but not reaching the other
- Cribriform or fenestrated—full of holes
- Complete absence of hymen
- Microperforate—almost completely covers the opening but there is the opening which is very small
- Imperforate—completely covers the opening.

Causes for Tear

(Nonsexual or sexual)

Many girls and teens tear or otherwise dilate their hymen

- During first intercourse (coitus) or rape
- While participating in sports like bicycling, horseback riding, gymnastics
- Or inserting tampons
- Or while masturbating
- A girl may not even know this has occurred, since there may be little or no blood or pain involved when this happens.

Virgin

The term "virgin" typically means someone who has never had sexual intercourse (specifically the penis entering the vagina). For the most part, being a virgin is not about whether a woman's hymen is intact or broken. It used to be that on her wedding night if a woman's first sexual intercourse (losing her virginity) was painful and there was blood on the sheets, that is a proof that she was a virgin.

Surgeon Restores Hymens for

- For cultural reasons—very important situation for some women—and this operation quite honestly saves lives
- For tightening vagina walls for better sex

Hymenorrhaphy, Hymenoplasty, or Hymen Restoration or Hymen Replacement Surgery or Restoration of the Hymenal Ring

- It is a surgical procedure offered in western countries
- It is illegal in most Arab countries
- It is done on an outpatient basis and with or without anesthesia.

Types of Surgery

- If it is not too damaged (surgical repair)
  - Piecing together its remnants
- When the hymenal remnants are insufficient
  - Stitch across hymen
  - Cerclage around hymenal ring
  - Approximate undermined hymen remnants
  - Approximate a flap from the vaginal wall across the opening
  - Alloplant for hymenoplasty.

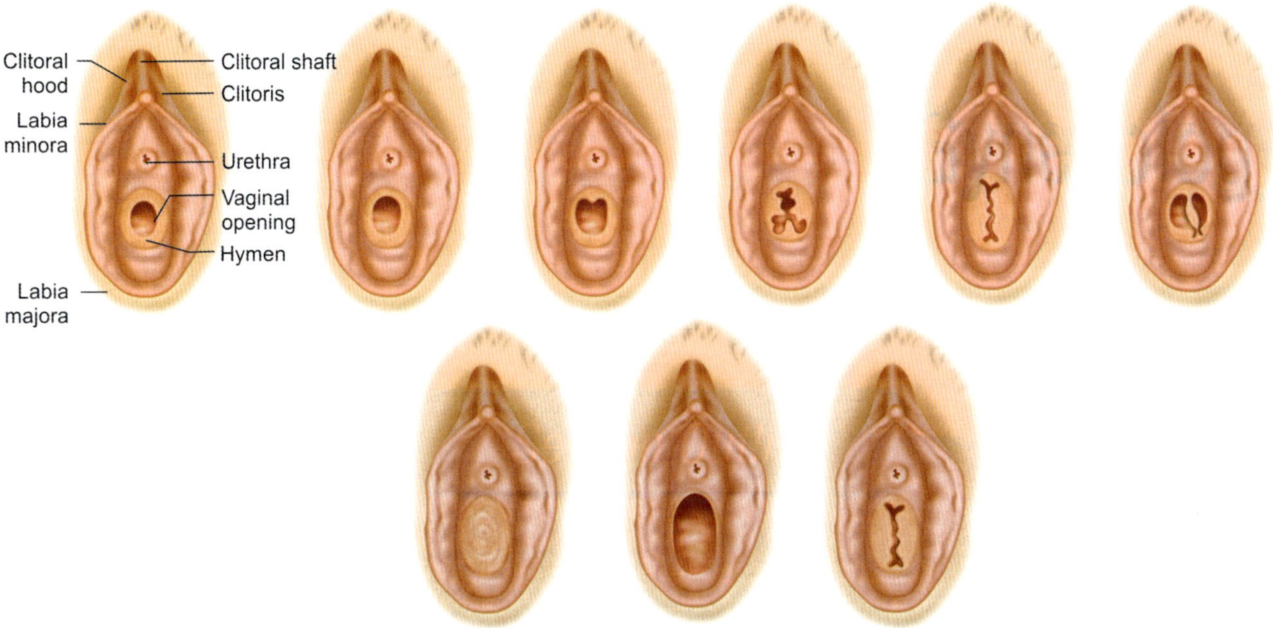

Fig. 2A: Types of hymen

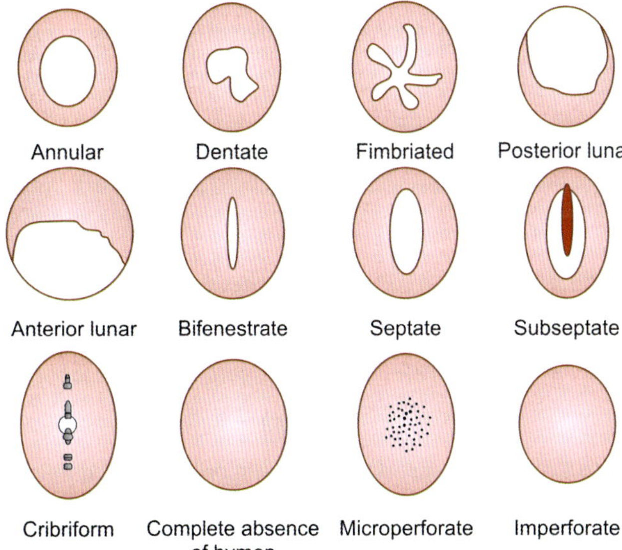

Fig. 2B: Diagrammatic representation of types of hymen

STEPS

The Simplest Technique of Hymenorrhaphy (Surgical Repair)

- Pain-killing medicine is taken 1 hour before the operation. The actual operation is performed under a general or local anesthetic with muscle relaxants
- The hymen is reconstructed, recreate the hymen by piecing together its remnants, if it is not too damaged, restoring its original appearance as a circular membrane with a central opening
- Surgery can also include inserting a gelatin capsule filled with a blood-like substance that will burst during intercourse, simulating bleeding
- Must be done 3–7 days before the wedding. Because the tissue is simply pulled together and the procedure does not last, catgut sutures are used to approximate hymen remnants
- Healing is rare because hymen is relatively avascular.

Stitch Across Hymen (Fig. 3)

By thread from underwear of wedding night tied inside and across. When the hymenal remnants are insufficient, cerclage around hymenal ring by thread from underwear of wedding-night, tied inside (Fig. 4).

A Gelatin Capsule

Inserting a gelatin capsule filled with a blood-like substance that will burst during intercourse, simulating bleeding

THE DEFINITIVE PROCEDURE

Hymen Replacement Surgery

- When the hymenal remnants are insufficient
  - Approximates undermined hymen remnants or a vaginal flap (Fig. 5)
  - Surgeon attaches a vaginal flap (a small section) from the vaginal wall across the opening, often producing vascular bands across the introitus (Figs 6A and B).

Alloplant for Hymenoplasty

The allografts with controllable extraction of glycosaminoglycans from collagen fibers having low antigenicity, nontoxic, not encapsulated, gradually reabsorbed and replaced mostly by natural recipient tissue, were named "alloplant".

Alloplant biomaterials can selectably stimulate the natural tissue regeneration. Therefore, alloplant biomaterials can be tried in surgery for selectable restoration of different tissues, as in hymenoplasty.

CONCLUSION

Hymenorrhaphy is justifiable in certain circumstances, when the woman would otherwise suffer disgrace or worse. More importantly, however, young women require appropriate sexual education and their families need to be educated about their adherence to the "bloody sheet" theory, to avoid mishaps.

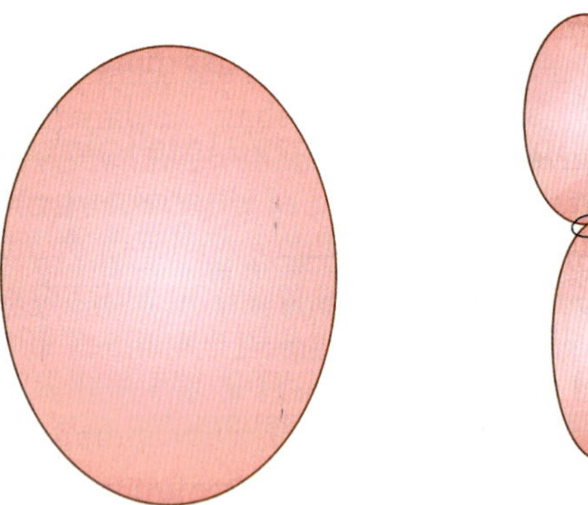

Fig. 3: Stitch across hymen

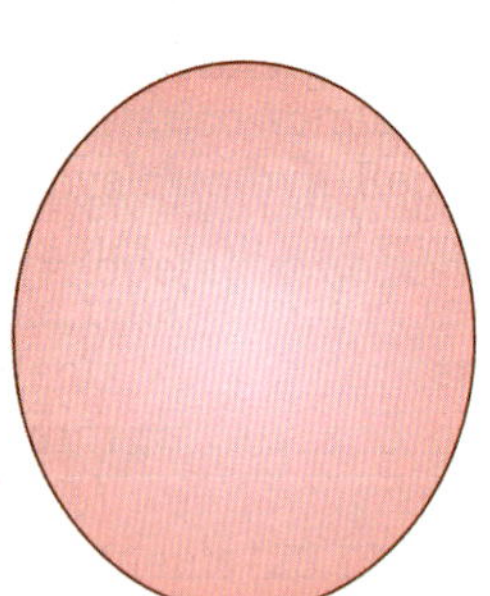

Fig. 4: Cerclage around hymen

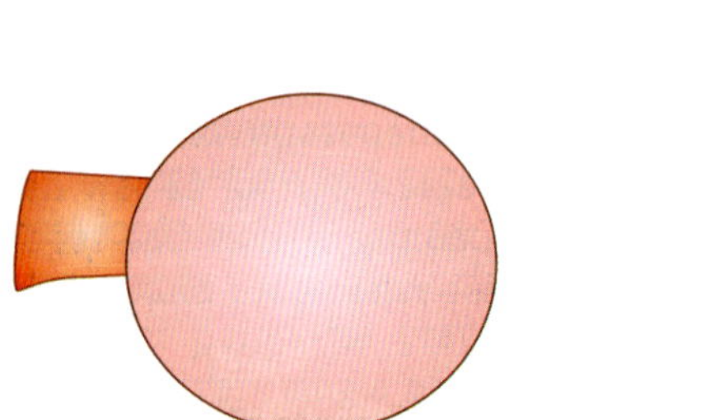

Fig. 5: Approximate undermined hymen remnants and they often produce vascular bands across the introitus, simulating hymen

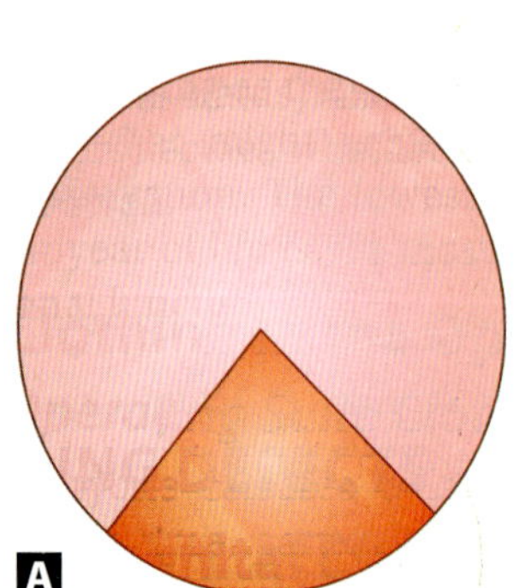

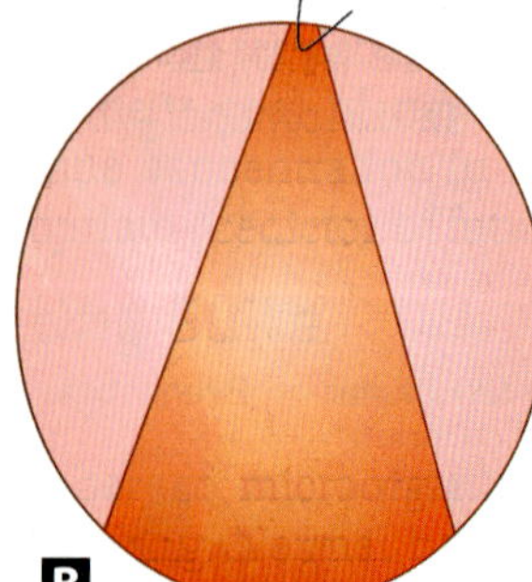

Figs 6A and B: (A) Vaginal flap from posterior vaginal wall freeing from upward leaving based attached; (B) Suture is attached to the upper end area at anterior vaginal wall

BIBLIOGRAPHY

1. Adler MW. Sexual health—a Health of the Nation failure. BMJ. 1997;314:1743-7.
2. De Cock KM, Low N. HIV and AIDS, other sexually transmitted diseases, and tuberculosis in ethnic minorities in United Kingdom: is surveillance serving its purpose? BMJ. 1997:314:1747-51.
3. Emans SJ, Wood ER, Allred EN, et al. Hymenal findings in adolescent women: impact of tampon use and consensual sexual activity. J Pediatr. 1994;125:153-60.
4. Fenton K, Johnson AM, Nicoll A. Race, ethnicity, and sexual health. BMJ. 1997;314:1703-4.
5. Kandela P. Egypt's trade in hymen repair. Lancet. 1996;347:1615.
6. Lacey CJ, Merrick DW, Bensley VC, Fairley I. Analysis of the sociodemography of gonorrhoea in Leeds, 1989-93. BMJ. 1997;314:1715-8.
7. Low N, Daker-White G, Barlow D, et al. Gonorrhoea in inner London: of a cross sectional study. BMJ. 1997;314:1719-23.
8. Underhill RA, Dewhurst J. The doctor cannot always tell: medical examination of the "intact" hymen. Lancet 1978;i:375-6.

37.3 BARTHOLIN'S GLAND—INCISION, DRAINAGE, MARSUPIALIZATION AND GLAND EXCISION

Neeta Singh

INTRODUCTION

Bartholin's duct cysts and gland abscesses are common problems in women of reproductive age. Bartholin's glands are located bilaterally at the posterior introitus and drain through ducts that empty into the vestibule at approximately 4 o'clock and 8 o'clock positions (Fig. 1A). These normally pea-sized glands are palpable only if the duct becomes cystic or a gland abscess develops. The goal of management is to preserve the gland and its function, if possible. Office-based procedures include insertion of a word catheter for a duct cyst or gland abscess and marsupialization of a cyst; excisional biopsy is reserved for use in ruling out adenocarcinoma in menopausal or perimenopausal women with an irregular, nodular Bartholin's gland mass.

SURGICAL ANATOMY

Bartholin's glands are bilateral vulvovaginal bodies located in the labia minora at approximately the 4 o'clock and 8 o'clock positions on the posterolateral aspect of the vestibule (Fig. 1B). The glands are normally about the size of a pea and are composed of cuboidal epithelium.

They drain into a duct approximately 2.5 cm long, which is composed mostly of transitional epithelium. The duct exits just external to the hymenal ring into a fold between the hymen and the labium where the duct lining becomes squamous epithelium. Therefore, either squamous carcinoma or adenocarcinoma can develop in a Bartholin's gland. The gland's secretions provide some moisture for the vulva but are not needed for sexual lubrication; thus, removal of a Bartholin's gland does not seem to compromise the vestibular epithelium or sexual function.

Epidemiology

- Bartholin's gland duct cysts and abscess incidence: 2%
- Most common in adult women under the age of 30 years.

Pathophysiology

- Bartholin's gland duct cyst
  - Results from distal duct obstruction
- Bartholin's gland abscess (more common than cysts)
  - May occur spontaneously or as infection of duct cyst.

MANAGEMENT OF BARTHOLIN'S GLAND CYSTS

Normally, the Bartholin's gland cannot be palpated. Bartholin's gland cysts develop from cystic dilation of

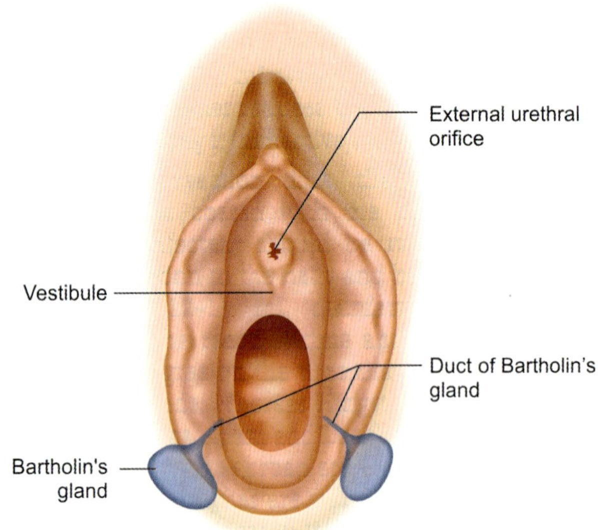

Fig. 1A: Anatomy of vulva depicting placement of Bartholin's glands bilaterally

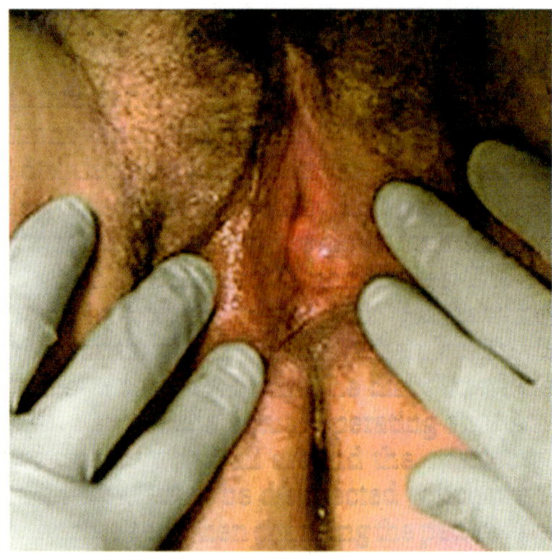

Fig. 1B: Swollen and infected Bartholin's gland

the duct following blockage of the duct orifice. They are generally 1–3 cm in size and are usually asymptomatic. The patient may notice a bulge in the labium majus or the cyst may be found during a routine gynecologic examination. When symptoms occur, the patient may report vulvar pain, dyspareunia, inability to engage in sports and pain during walking or sitting. Bartholin's gland cysts tend to grow slowly. Since noninfected cysts are usually sterile, routine antibiotic therapy is not necessary. Asymptomatic Bartholin's gland cysts in patients under age 40 years may not require treatment. As discussed below, some clinicians advocate excision of all Bartholin's gland cysts in patients over 40 years of age because of the possibility of malignancy. Various treatment options are available if a cyst causes cosmetic problems or bothersome symptoms. If a patient has a Bartholin's gland cyst that ruptures spontaneously, all she may need is hot sitz baths. Occasionally, use of broad-spectrum antibiotics is indicated if secondary infection develops. Definitive methods of treatment include placing a word catheter, marsupializing the cyst, performing a "window" procedure, using a carbon dioxide (CO_2) laser, applying silver nitrate to the cyst cavity or excising the entire cyst.

Anesthesia

Incision and drainage of a Bartholin's cyst or abscess requires anesthesia of the labial mucosa. Because infiltration of the labial mucosa with a local anesthetic may be painful, options such as intravenous narcotics and procedural sedation and analgesia can also be used.

Position, Draping

Place the patient in the lithotomy position and spread open the labia. An assistant may aid with traction of the labia during the procedure. Use the sterile skin preparatory solution to clean the labia and surrounding area. Infiltrate 2–3 mL of lidocaine 1% subcutaneously under the mucosa of the labia minora.

Excision

Although Bartholin's gland abscesses may rupture and drain spontaneously, recurrence is likely, and surgical excision may be necessary. Excision is not an office-based procedure. Cultures for *Neisseria gonorrhoeae* and *Chlamydia trachomatis* may be obtained. Excision of the Bartholin's gland should be considered in patients who do not respond to conservative attempts to create a drainage tract, but the procedure should be performed when there is no active infection. If multiple attempts have been made to drain a cyst or an abscess, adhesions may be present making excision difficult and resulting in postoperative scarring and chronic pain in the area.

Word Catheter Treatment (Figs 2 and 3)

It is a simple procedure to treat the Bartholin's gland cyst. After local anesthesia and sterile preparation, a stab incision is made 1 cm deep into the cyst just outside the hymenal ring, a hemostat is inserted to break up any loculations, now a word catheter is placed. Word catheter

Fig. 2: Medial stab incision of Bartholin's gland cyst, before placement catheter

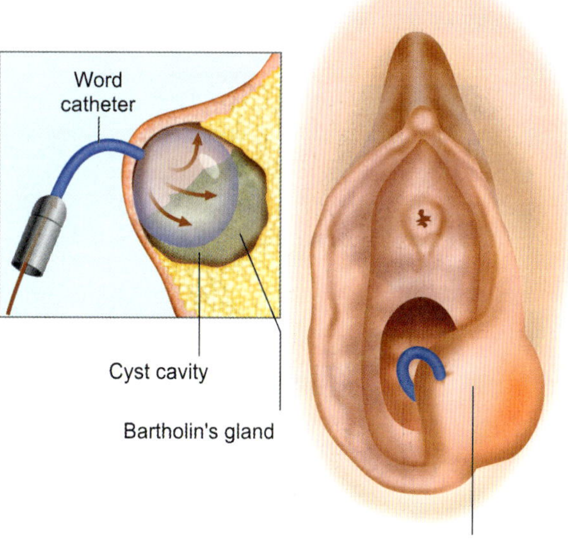

Fig. 3: Placement of Word catheter in a patient with a Bartholin's gland cyst

is a small rubber tube with inflatable balloon tip that is inserted with water or lubricating gel, free end is tucked up in vagina. The catheter is left in place for up to 4 weeks to permit complete epithelization of the new tract. Patient is advised pelvic rest and abstinence from intercourse until removal of catheter. The catheter is removed by deflating the balloon and over time the resulting orifice will decrease in size and become unnoticeable.

Marsupialization (Figs 4 and 5)

Marsupialization procedure can be performed if a cyst recurs despite treatment with a word catheter or if the physician prefers it as a first-line technique. After sterile preparation of the cyst and surrounding area, a no. 11 scalpel is used to make a vertical elliptic incision just inside or outside the hymenal ring but not on the outer labium majus. The incision should measure about 1.5 × 1.0 cm, cruciate and should be deep enough to include both the vestibular skin and the underlying cyst wall. An oval wedge of vulvar skin and underlying cyst wall should be removed. The cyst or abscess will drain. Loculations are broken if necessary; the cyst wall is sewn to the adjacent vestibular skin using interrupted 3-0 or 4-0 delayed-absorbable sutures on a small needle (Fig. 5). Silver nitrate sticks or direct pressure can be used for hemostasis of the skin edge. The new tract will slowly shrink over time and epithelialize forming a new duct orifice. The recurrence rate after marsupialization is about 10 %.

MANAGEMENT OF BARTHOLIN'S GLAND ABSCESSES

A Bartholin's gland abscess can be so painful that the patient is incapacitated. Common symptoms are severe dyspareunia, difficulty in walking or sitting, and vulvar pain. Signs in addition to a large, tender mass in the vestibular area are vulvar erythema and edema. Bartholin's gland abscesses usually develop over 2–4 days and can become larger than 8 cm. They tend to rupture and drain after 4–5 days. In the past, Bartholin's gland abscesses were thought to develop mainly from gonococcal or chlamydial infections.

Treatment of Bartholin's gland abscesses is similar to that of symptomatic cysts. If an abscess points and ruptures spontaneously, the patient may need only sitz's bath, antibiotics and pain medication. In fact, it is prudent to treat early abscesses with sitz baths until the abscess points, making incision and definitive treatment easier.

Bartholin's Gland Cyst in Pregnancy

Although none of the treatment methods discussed is contraindicated in pregnant women, the increase in blood flow to the pelvic area during pregnancy may lead to excessive bleeding when Bartholin's cysts or abscesses are treated. For this reason, surgical treatment for asymptomatic cysts should probably be withheld until after delivery. If treatment is necessary because a cyst

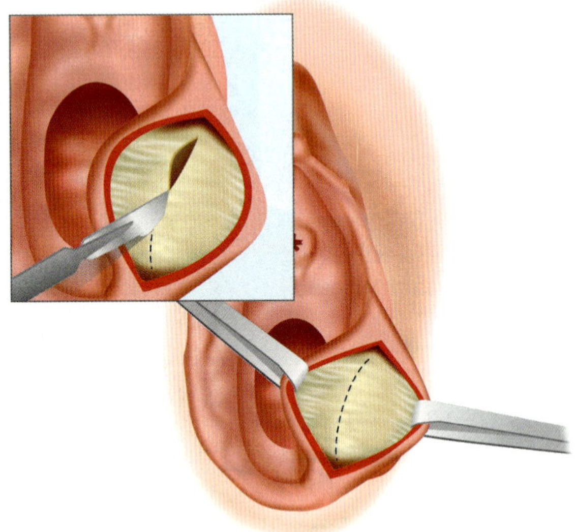

Fig. 4: Marsupialization of Bartholin's duct cyst. (Left) A vertical incision is made over the center of the cyst to dissect it free of mucosa

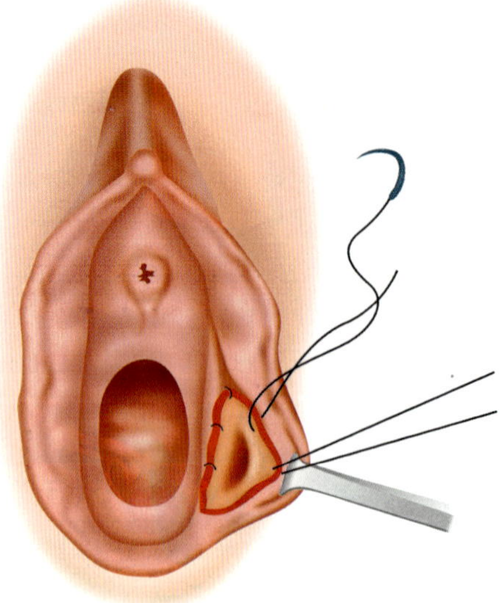

Fig. 5: (Right) The cyst wall is everted and approximated to the edge of the vestibular mucosa with interrupted sutures

becomes infected or the patient presents with an abscess, local anesthesia is not contraindicated, and most broad-spectrum antibiotics appear safe for use during pregnancy.

COMPLICATIONS

- Bleeding
- Progressive infection and sepsis.

Patients with compromised immune systems may exhibit these rare complications. Treat all immunocompromised patients with antibiotics. Closely monitor or even admit such patients in order to diagnose and treat progression to a deeper-seated infection.

Recurrence

Recurrence is the most common complication after incision and drainage. Premature dislodgement of the word catheter results in incision closure and high rates of recurrence.

BIBLIOGRAPHY

1. Apgar BS. Bartholin's cyst/abscess: word catheter insertion. In: Pfenninger JL, Fowler GC (eds). Procedures for primary care physicians. St. Louis: Mosby; 1994. pp. 596-600.
2. Azzan BB. Bartholin's cyst and abscess. A review of treatment of 53 cases. Br J Clin Pract. 1978;32(4):101-2.
3. Blakey DH, Dewhurst CJ, Tipton RH. The long term results after marsupialization of Bartholin's cysts and abscesses. J Obstet Gynaecol Br Commonw. 1966;73:1008-9.
4. Curtis JM. Marsupialisation technique for Bartholin's cyst. Aust Fam Physician. 1993;22:369.
5. Droegemueller W. Comprehensive gynecology, 2nd rev edition. St. Louis: Mosby; 1992. pp. 637-9.
6. Hill DA, Lense JJ. Office management of Bartholin gland cysts abscesses. Am Fam Physician. 1998;57:1611-6,1619-20.
7. Stenchever MA. Comprehensive gynecology, 4th edition. St. Louis: Mosby; 2001. pp. 482-6,645-6.
8. Wilkinson EJ, Stone IK. Atlas of vulvar disease, 5th ed. Baltimore: Williams and Wilkins; 1995. pp. 15.

37.4 NERVE DENERVATION—ALCOHOL AND CORTISONE INJECTION

Randhir Puri, V Chandra

INTRODUCTION

Basic considerations for using nerve blocks: The proper use of nerve blocks to treat pain requires a specially trained physician with a thorough understanding of pain and its syndromes. It is essential that a patient is selected for nerve block therapy only after an accurate diagnosis of the source of the pain is made. The examination may include a complete medical history, physical examination, laboratory studies, and a complete psychiatric and psychosomatic assessment. Nerve blocks relieve pain by interrupting pain sensory pathways and preventing them from reaching the brain. A local anesthetic is used to temporarily block the transmission of pain along these pathways. Two types of sensory pathways are sympathetic nerve plexus and somatosensory nerve.

Besides local anesthetics, various other drugs and methods are available:

Corticosteroids (triamcinolone, depomedrol) are used in conjunction with local anesthetics in nerve blocks when there is an area of inflammation, as in acute herniated disk syndrome, nerve entrapment syndrome or trigger point pain.

Opioids (morphine) are infused continuously into the area surrounding the spinal cord (called the epidural space) to control pain in a certain area of your body.

ALCOHOL INJECTION OF THE VULVA (FIG. 1)

In patients with chronic and severe pruritus of the vulva (Fig. 2) not amenable to steroid cream therapy, denervation of the vulva is often as needed to break the vicious cycle of itching, scratching, excoriation, microlacerations and irritation of cutaneous nerves. Alcohol injection of the vulva gives the patient a temporary period of denervation. Surgical denervation should be reserved for those patients in whom medical therapy and alcohol injection have failed and is based on cutaneous innervation areas of vulva nerve supply (Figs 3 and 4).

To prevent microulcerations and infection, care must be taken to inject the 95% alcohol into the subcutaneous space and not the intradermal space.

The purpose of this operation is to temporarily denervate the vulva by injecting alcohol in a systematic fashion that will denervate each of the cutaneous branches of the ilioinguinal, genitofemoral, posterior femoral and pudendal nerves. This denervation generally lasts 4–6 months.

Effects off: Denervation of the perineum blocks the awareness of itching, thereby eliminating the need for

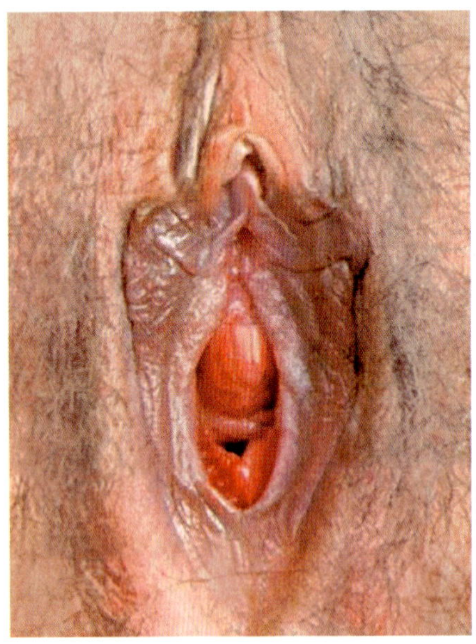

Fig.1: Normal anatomy, vulva

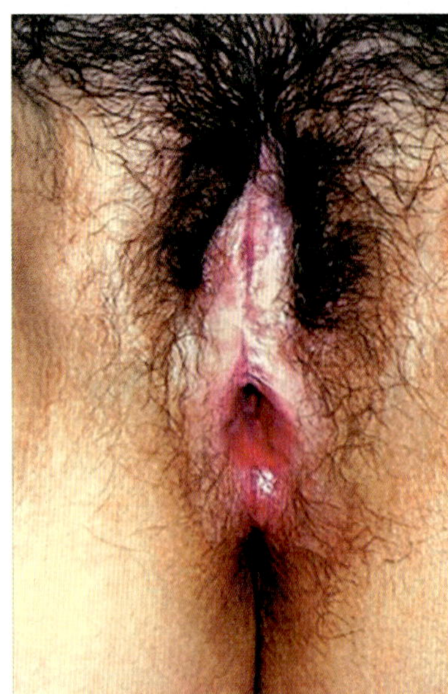

Fig. 2: Female genital lichen sclerosus (early). "Figure-of-eight" dystrophy with fusion of clitoral hood, and obliteration of labia minora

scratching. Scratching produces microlacerations that become infected, producing more itching, and thus the vicious cycle. By stopping the itching and eliminating the scratching, this procedure allows the perineum to heal during the 4–6 months of denervation.

Note: The alcohol must be injected subcutaneously, not subcuticularly, or sloughing of the epidermis will occur.

Technique

1. The patient is placed in the dorsal lithotomy position. The perineum is prepared and draped. The skin to be removed is carefully outlined with brilliant green solution (Fig. 5A)
2. An incision is made down to the dermis. An Allis clamp is placed on the skin and a scalpel is used to carefully dissect the skin off the dermis (Fig. 5B)
3. The dissection follows the outline of the incision around the external genitalia, removing the involved skin. Note that noninvolved structures may be left intact (Fig. 5C).

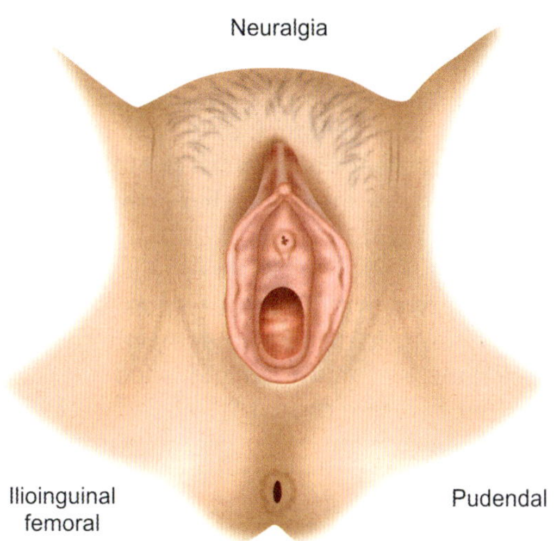

Fig. 3: Nerve supply, enervation of vulva

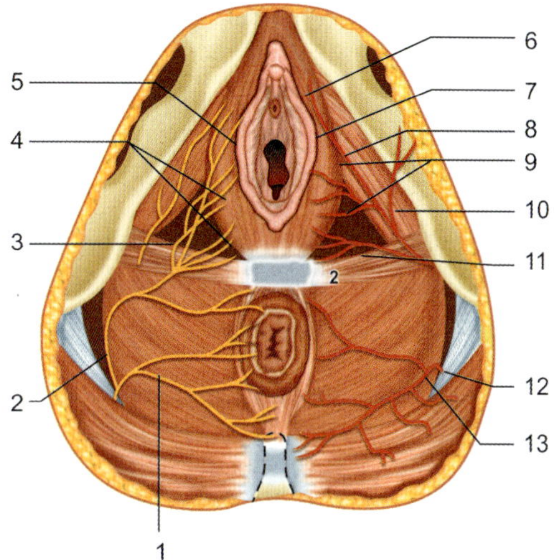

Arteries and nerves of pelvic floor as seen from below. Branching of internal pudendal artery and of pudendal nerve.

1. Anal nerve
2. Perineal nerve
3. Branch of pudendal nerve innvervating ischiocavernosus
4. Posterior labial nerves
5. Dorsal clitoral nerve
6. Dorsal clitoral artery
7. Deep clitoral artery
8. Ischiocavernosus muscle
9. Bulbocavernosus muscle and artery of vestibular bulb
10. Posterior labial artery
11. Perineal artery
12. Internal pudendal artery in Alcock's canal
13. Inferior rectal artery

Fig. 4: Rich nerve supply to the muscles of perineum

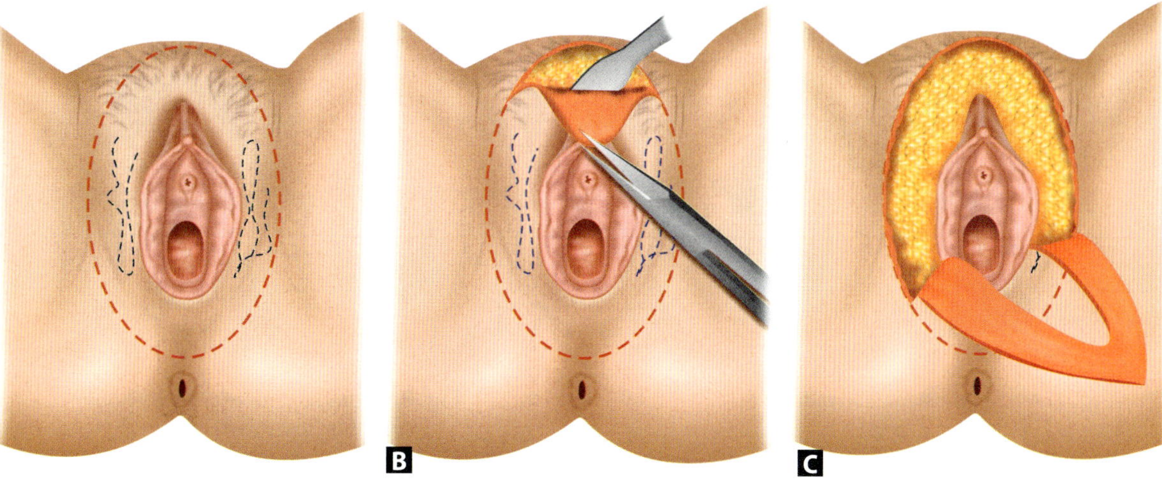

Figs 5A to C: Denervation, skinning-off vulva

CORTISONE INJECTION OF THE VULVA

In patients with chronic pruritus of the vulva (Fig. 6), subcutaneous injection of the vulva with a fluorinated cortisone preparation will often relieve the patient and break the vicious cycle of itching, scratching, excoriation, and irritation of cutaneous nerves.

Pruritus of the vulva is often associated with parakeratosis that does not allow steroid cream to penetrate the skin and reach the important subdermal area. The injection must cover the entire vulva. Particular attention must be given to those areas that the patient designates as especially troublesome with help of cotton swab test.

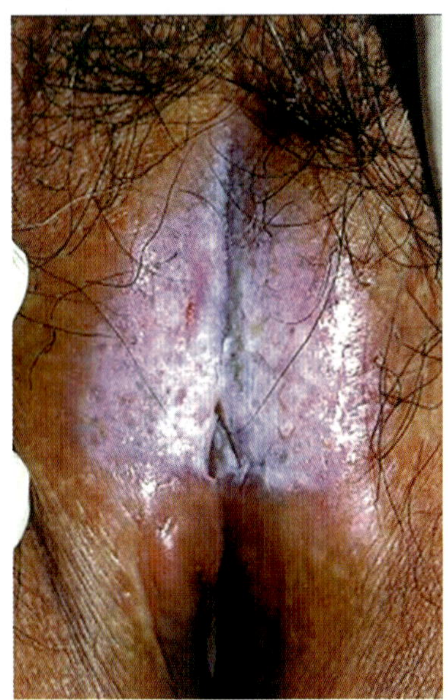

Fig. 6: Pruritis vulva with parakeratosis

Effects off: Pruritus of the vulva is eliminated. Cortisone reduces the inflammatory reaction and improves the vascular supply and thus improves the nutrition of the vulvar skin.

Note: Care must be exercised to inject the entire vulva and to avoid penetration of the perineal branches of the pudendal artery and nerve.

Technique

With the patient under general or local anesthesia in the lithotomy position, the surgeon outlines the inflamed areas of the vulva.

1. Innervation of the vulva including the ilioinguinal nerves, the genital branch of the genitofemoral nerve, the perineal branch of the posterior femoral cutaneous nerve and the perineal branches of the pudendal nerve is shown in Figure 4
2. 40 mg of a fluorinated steroid solution in a 20 mL syringe mixed with 1 mL of xylocaine are injected in a radial grid design underneath the squamous epithelium. The entire area affected is covered. The injection can be repeated 1–2 times/week for up to 4 weeks (Figs 7 and 8).

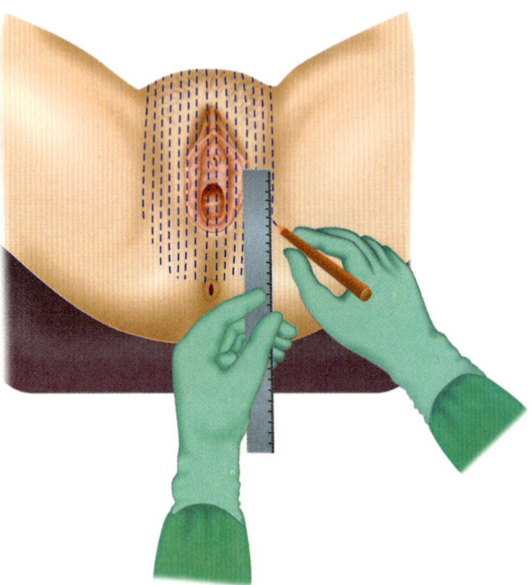

Fig. 7: Area of vulva marked radially

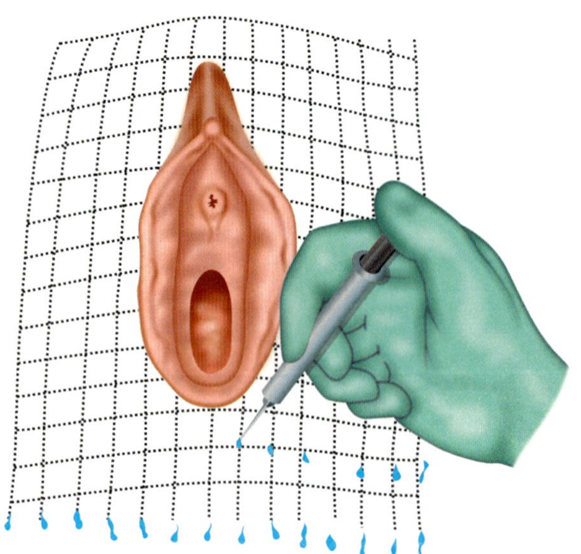

Fig. 8: Nerve, alcohol and/or cortisone injection, over marked grid

37.5 WIDE LOCAL EXCISION OF THE VULVA, Z-PLASTY FLAP

Randhir Puri, V Chandra

INTRODUCTION

A wide local excision is indicated for women with in situ or microinvasive carcinoma of the vulva. The goal of this operation is to remove the carcinoma and a 2 cm margin of normal skin surrounding the gross lesion (Fig. 1). It is imperative that prior to making the incision, the surgeon measure the margin with a centimeter rule and outline it with a marking pen to ensure that the specimen is adequate. If the 2 cm margin is not measured and the skin is not marked prior to the incision, all too often, the specimen sent to the pathologist will not have an adequate margin. In most cases, adjacent vulvar skin can be mobilized and used to affect a primary closure of the vulva. This is done in two layers after adequate hemostasis has been achieved. In cases where extensive lesions are removed and the defect is too large for primary closure, a Z-plasty flap may be used to cover the wound without resorting to a split-thickness skin graft.

Preoperative Considerations

Preoperative measurement and marking of the diseased areas are mandatory. The Z-plasty flap or primary closure should be completed as large defects should not be left in the vulvar area to simply granulate and epithelialize. If primary closure is to be performed, adjacent vulvar skin should be adequately mobilized so that the suture line enclosing the vulva is not under tension. If the excised defect is too large for primary closure, as demonstrated by tension on the suture line, the Z-plasty flap procedure should be performed.

In this case, care should be taken to ensure that (1) the distance from point A to point B on the Z-plasty flap is shorter than the distance from point B to the margin of excised defect and (2) there is an adequate blood supply entering the base of the flap (Fig. 2). It is essential that all tissues be adequately mobilized to avoid any tension on any suture line within the flap area.

Primary Closure Technique

1. Adequate mobilization of adjacent vulvar skin is made by sharp and blunt dissection. It is essential that the wound be closed without tension. Sutures should merely hold the tissue that has been adequately mobilized and approximated.
2. A continuous layer of 4-0 synthetic absorbable sutures stitched with an intestinal needle is used to close the subcutaneous space.

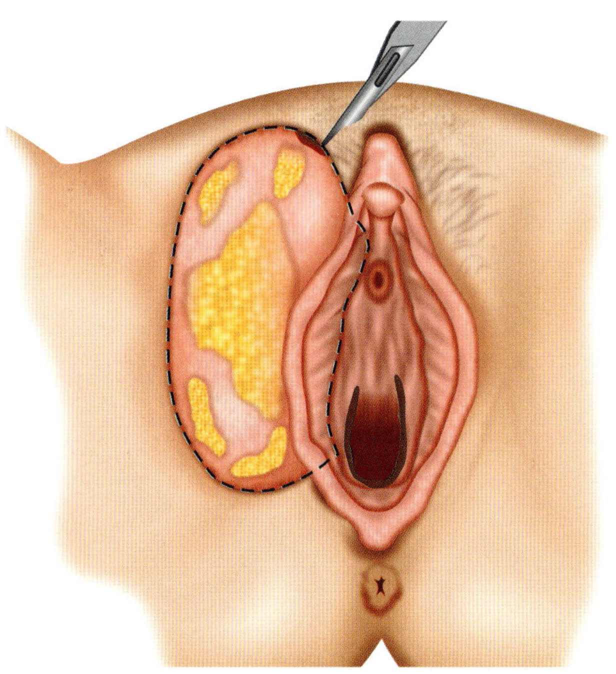

Fig. 1: 2 cm wide excision of tumor mark done

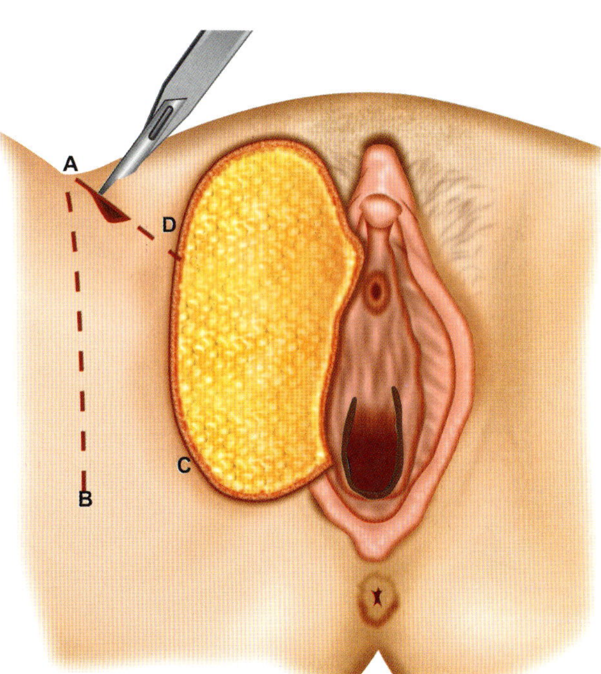

Fig. 2: Flap is marked

3. A subcuticular technique can be used to approximate the skin using 4-0 synthetic absorbable suture. Small stainless steel skin clips can also be used and can be removed on the 7th or 8th postoperative day. Fine nylon sutures can be used in either a mattress technique or the so-called flap stitch technique. These are removed on the 7th or 8th postoperative day.
4. If the lesion to be removed leaves an excessively large defect, primary closure may be impossible. In these cases, a Z-plasty flap may be the procedure of choice.
5. The defect is measured with a ruler. The medial margin usually extends from the clitoral area to the posterior fourchette of the vagina and is equal to the distance on the proposed flap by the line marked A-D. It is essential that the base of the flap from B to the lateral edge of the defect be wider than the length of the flap. The blood supply to the flap will enter through this area, and if the length of the flap is longer than the width of the base, the flap will have insufficient blood supply, and its tip may necrose. A scalpel is used to border off the flap through a full thickness of skin and subcutaneous fat. Meticulous hemostasis must be achieved at this point (Fig. 3).
6. The portion of the flap marked A should be stitched with fine synthetic absorbable suture to the ventral margin of the defect (Fig. 4). This suture should be in the form of a flap stitch that enters the full thickness of the skin of the margin of the defect and is brought through the flap with a subcuticular technique. The needle re-enters the full thickness of the margins of the defect from the subcutaneous layer and exits the cutaneous layer adjacent to the first suture. This flap stitch aids healing by less constricture of the blood supply in the flap.
   The second suture should be placed in the posterior fourchette of the vagina and be brought to the angle of the flap marked D with the same stitch described above. At this point, the part of the flap marked C should be sutured with the flap stitch to the angle (ABC) created by the entire Z-plasty (Figs 5A and B). After the margins of the flap have been sutured, the surgeon can make adjustments, if necessary. If undue tension is noted at any particular point, it can be released by greater mobilization of adjacent skin. Any dog-eared skin tags are removed.
7. Several techniques are acceptable for suturing the flap to the adjacent recipient skin and vaginal wall. The new stainless steel skin clips have the advantage of being inert and causing little tissue reaction. They can be left in for long periods of time to allow for complete closure and healing of the wound. Synthetic absorbable suture material can be utilized and, in general, gives improved cosmetic result. Sutures of fine nylon, in the flap stitch technique, can be used throughout the closure. These require removal after the margins of the wound have completely healed.

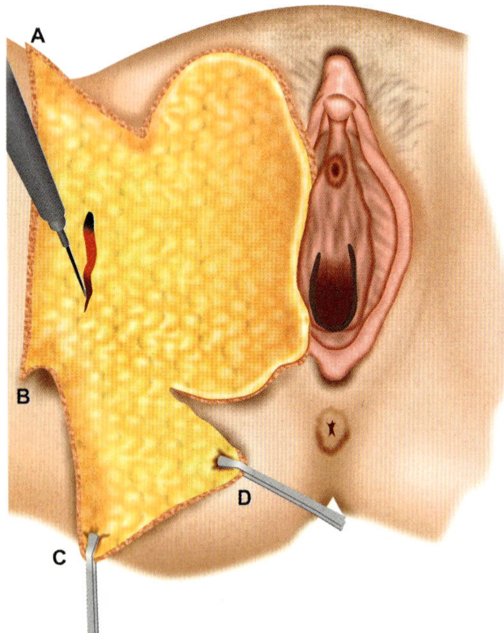

Fig. 3: Hemostasis ensured

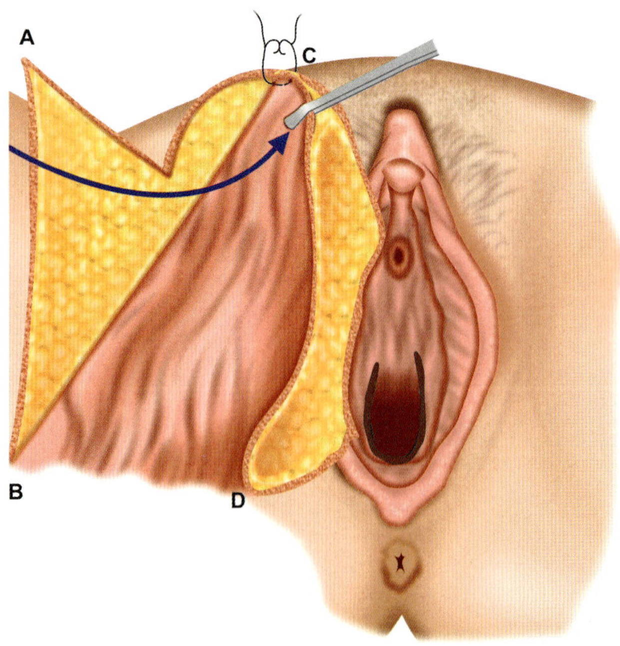

Fig. 4: Suturing of flap as per flap-stitch technique

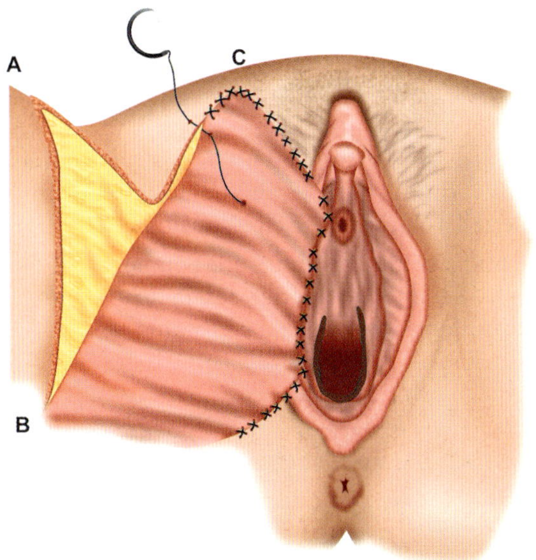

Fig. 5A: Suturing of vulvar flap

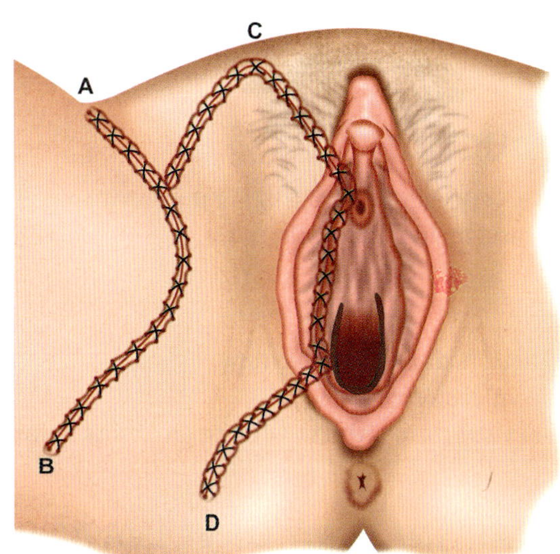

Fig. 5B: Flap in place by Z-plasty

Patients who have undergone large perineal Z-plasty flaps should remain in bed for a minimum of 6–7 days. Thromboembolic prophylaxis, utilizing the contemporary technique of intermittent pressure cuffs, is essential. Defecation should be delayed for 6–8 days until the margin of the flap has sealed. This is achieved by a low-residue diet and the administration of Lomotil tablets qid.

37.6 VULVECTOMY

Malini KV

INTRODUCTION

Vulvectomy is the surgical excision of the vulva employed for benign and malignant conditions.

Types

- Superficial (skinning) vulvectomy
- Simple vulvectomy
- Radical vulvectomy with or without groin dissection.

SURGICAL ANATOMY OF VULVA AND THE PERINEUM

Since surgery is the cornerstone in the management of vulvar cancer, knowledge of surgical anatomy of vulva and the perineum is very important (Fig. 1).

The female external genitalia are known as the vulva. They include:

- Mons pubis
- Labia majora
- Labia minora
- Clitoris
- Vestibule of the vagina
- Bulb of the vestibule.

Mons lies anterior and superior to the pubis symphysis. It is covered by pubic hair and with labia majora, is composed of fibro-fatty tissue. Labia majora extends from labiocrural skin folds laterally to labia minora medially. The overlying skin contains hair with sweat and sebaceous glands. Labia minora are skin folds devoid of hair. Anteriorly, they merge to form prepuce and the frenulum of the clitoris and posteriorly merge to form the fourchette. The area enclosed by labia minora is the vestibule into which the urethra and the vagina open. The clitoris is located anterior to the vestibule close to the symphysis.

Urogenital diaphragm is a fascial membrane bordered by the inferior pubic rami on each side and transverse perineal muscles posteriorly. The perineal muscles lie superficial to the inferior fascia of urogenital diaphragm. The two bulbocavernosus muscles, the transverse perineal muscles and external anal sphincter form the perineal body. The ischiocavernosus muscles arise from the inner surface of the ischial tuberosity and the ischial ramus and insert into the crus of clitoris. The gluteus maximus forms the floor of the posterior quadrant of vulva and the perineum (Fig. 2).

The Bartholin's glands lie underneath the lower end of bulbocavernosus muscles and opens by a duct into the vestibule at 4 o'clock and 8 o'clock positions.

The bulbs of the vestibule are composed of erectile tissue and lie on the inferior fascia of the urogenital diaphragm alongside the vaginal introitus.

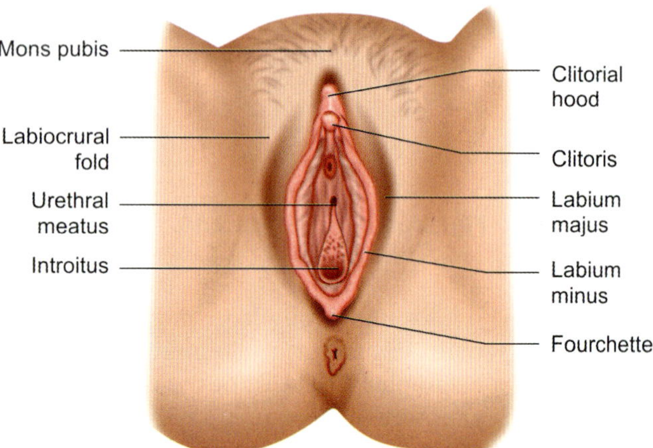

Fig. 1: The superficial structures of the vulva and perineum

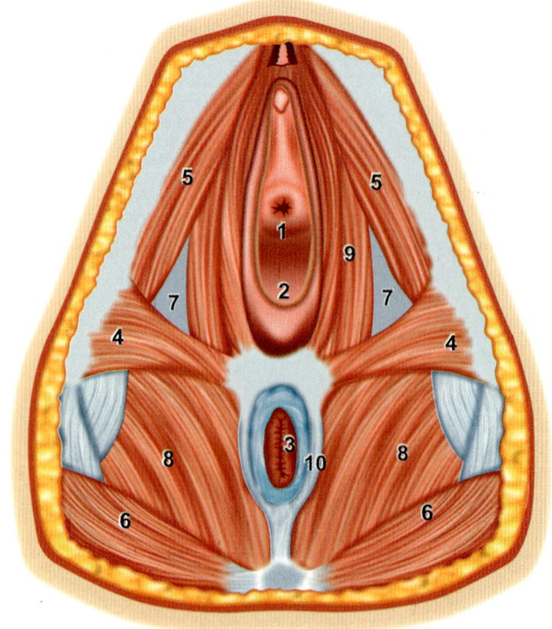

Fig. 2: Deeper structures of vulva and perineum. (1) Urethral orifice; (2) Vaginal introitus; (3) Anus; (4) Transverse perineal muscles; (5) Pubic ramus with ischiocavernosus muscle; (6) Gluteus maximus; (7) Urogenital diaphragm; (8) Levator ani muscle; (9) Bulbocavernosus muscle; (10) Sphincter ani

ARTERIAL SUPPLY TO VULVA AND PERINEUM

The main arterial supply is provided by internal pudendal artery, a branch of anterior trunk of internal iliac artery. It enters the perineum through lesser sciatic notch and pudendal canal where it lies lateral to the pudendal nerve.

In the posterior part of the pudendal canal, it gives off inferior rectal artery which runs medially to supply the anal canal and the sphincter. The perineal artery arises near the anterior end of the pudendal canal and gives off transverse perineal branches, posterior labial branches and the artery to the bulb as shown in Figure 3. The artery ends in dorsal and deep arteries of the clitoris.

External pudendal arteries arising from femoral artery contribute further blood supply. Deep external pudendal artery supplies the skin of labium and perineum. Superficial external pudendal artery supplies the skin of the lower abdomen and anterior labium majus.

NERVE SUPPLY OF VULVA AND PERINEUM

The vulva and the perineum have rich sensory nerve supply (Fig. 4).

The ilioinguinal nerve (L_1) and the genital branch of genitofemoral nerve (L_1, L_2) supply the anterior vulva and the mons. The pudendal nerve (S_2–S_4) gives off inferior rectal nerve and divides into perineal nerve and dorsal nerve of clitoris. Inferior rectal nerve passes medially and supplies external anal sphincter, the skin around the anus and the anal canal below the pectinate line. The perineal nerve gives off labial branches and also branches to the bulb of the vestibule and the urethra. The dorsal nerve of the clitoris is the terminal branch supplying the clitoris.

The perineal branch of the posterior cutaneous nerve of thigh (S1–S3) supplies the skin of the upper and medial thigh, the posterior vulva, the perianal area and the lateral perineum.

THE LYMPHATIC DRAINAGE OF THE VULVA

Understanding the lymphatic drainage of the vulva is critical for the proper management of vulvar cancer.

The principal lymphatic drainage is to the nodes in the groins. Lymph channels draining the vulva do not cross the labiocrural fold.

The groin lymph nodes consist of inguinal and the deep femoral group (Fig. 5).

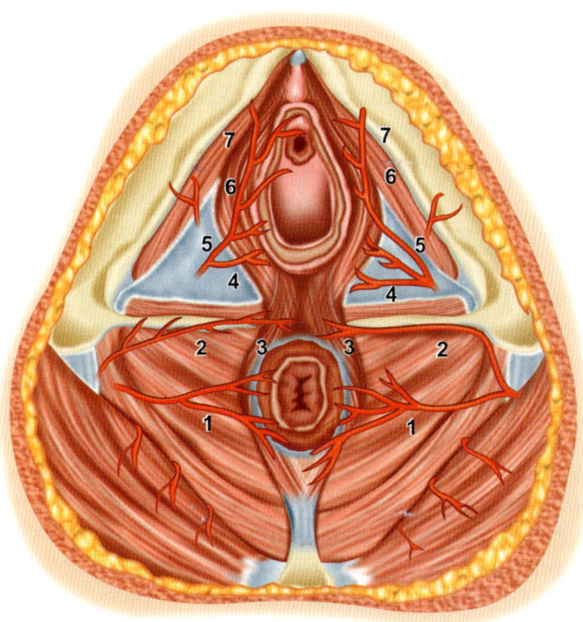

Fig. 3: Branches of internal pudendal artery. (1) Inferior rectal artery; (2) Perineal branch; (3) Transverse perineal branch; (4) Posterior labial branch; (5) Artery to the bulb of the vestibule; (6) Dorsal artery of the clitoris; (7) Deep artery of the clitoris

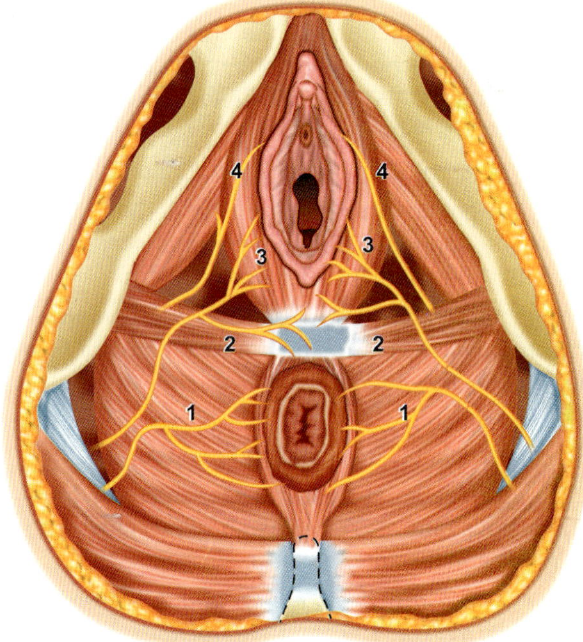

Fig. 4: Nerve supply of vulva and perineum. (1) Inferior rectal branch of pudendal nerve; (2) Perineal branches of pudendal nerve; (3) Nerve to bulb of the vestibule; (4) Dorsal nerve of clitoris

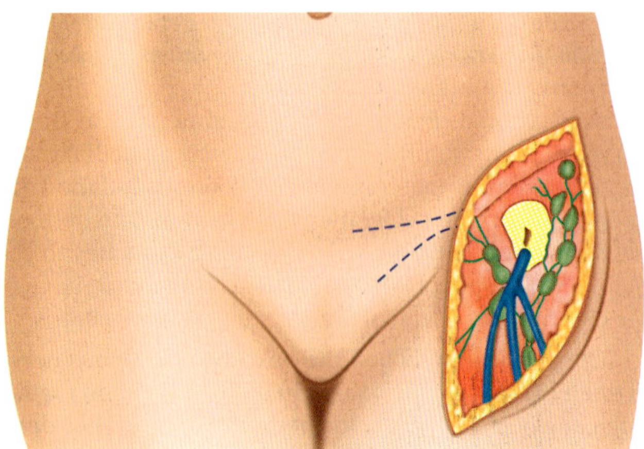
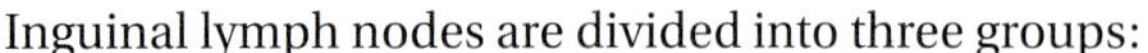

Fig. 5: Superficial inguinal lymph nodes

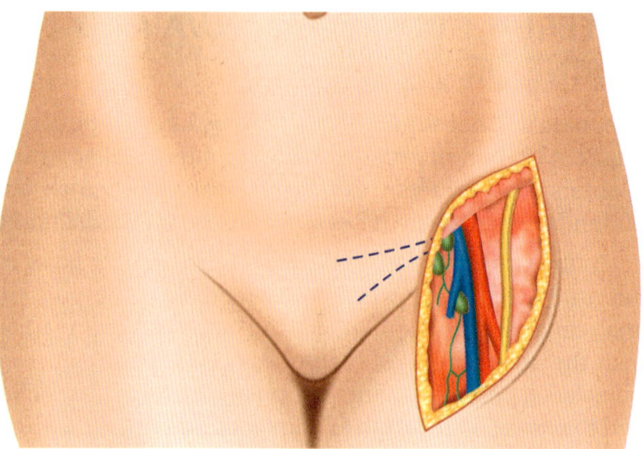

Fig. 6: Deep femoral lymph nodes

Inguinal lymph nodes are divided into three groups:

1. The lower vertical group placed along both sides of the terminal part of the great saphenous vein, contains 4–5 nodes
2. The upper lateral group placed below the lateral point of the inguinal ligament, contains 2–3 nodes
3. The upper medial group placed below the medial end of the inguinal ligament, contains 2–3 nodes.

All these drain into deep femoral nodes and thence to external iliac nodes, although the most lateral group may terminate directly in the external iliac nodes. Femoral nodes, 1–4 in number, lie medial to the femoral vein (Fig. 6). The most constant node lies just below the saphenofemoral junction and the next most constant lies just above the junction. The node of Cloquet is the most proximal node of this group, lies in the femoral canal and is absent in 50% of the cases.

Note: No nodes lie lateral to femoral vessels.

The lymphatic drainage from the perineum, clitoris and the anterior part of the labium minus is bilateral. Rest of the vulva drain into ipsilateral groin nodes.

Note: Ipsilateral groin dissection is appropriate for early stage vulvar cancer (T_1), provided it has not involved clitoris, perineum or labium minora.

The lymphatic vessels from the vulva course anteriorly and terminate in the inguinal lymph nodes.

The deep femoral nodes receive afferents from the inguinal nodes and also receive some direct channels from the clitoris and the anterior vulva.

Note: Groin dissection always should consist of the dissection of both inguinal and femoral nodes.

Lymphatic spread is by embolization and not by permeation.

Note: Radical local excision rather than radical vulvectomy is advocated for early tumors ($T_1N_0M_0$).

Preoperative Investigations and Preparation

The patient is admitted 2 days prior to surgery. Visual and colposcopic examination of the vulva, vagina and cervix is mandatory. Diagnostic biopsies are to be performed before planning treatment. Biopsy must include area of epithelium from normal and abnormal areas. It should be greater than 1 mm in depth to allow for proper staging and to be taken under local anesthesia.

Colposcopically directed biopsy, after application of either toluidine blue or 2–3% acetic acid in the absence of obvious lesions, is of value.

Further investigations are done to determine the disease extent and patient's fitness for surgery. They include:

- Complete blood count (CBC)
- Blood grouping and Rh typing
- Bleeding and clotting time
- Blood sugar
- VDRL (Venereal disease research laboratory), hepatitis B surface antigen (HbsAg), human immunodeficiency virus (HIV)
- Blood urea nitrogen (BUN) and creatinine
- Liver function test (LFT) (excludes liver metastases)
- Electrocardiogram
- Chest X-ray (excludes lung metastases)
- Cystoscopy, intravenous pyelogram (IVP) or proctoscopy is indicated if locally advanced cancer appears to involve bladder/rectum
- Lymphatic mapping is experimental, data is scanty and preliminary. Moreover, sentinel node is difficult to define in vulvar cancer
- Pelvic ultrasonography to detect associated pelvic pathology
- High resolution ultrasound (US) for diagnosis of lymph nodes may be of value.

Prophylactic antibiotic, antibiotic bowel preparation and enema to clear lower colon is advised the day before surgery, especially when radical surgery is planned.

Anesthesia and Position

Vulvectomy may be performed under general, epidural or spinal anesthesia. Patient is placed in dorsal lithotomy position with legs supported in stirrups. Slight Trendelenburg or elevation of buttocks in obese patients may facilitate access to perineum for radical vulvectomy.

Skinning vulvectomy: Removal of only skin up to dermis (Fig. 7).

Indication

- Vulvar intraepithelial neoplasia (VIN)
- Intractable benign lichen scleroses
- Vulvar atrophy
- Paget's disease.

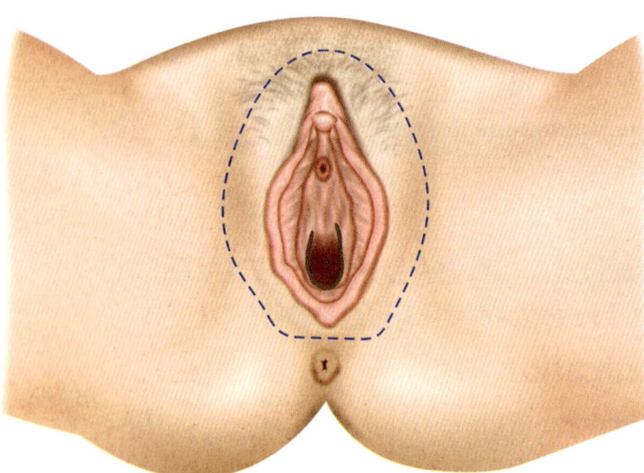

Fig. 7: Incision—skinning vulvectomy

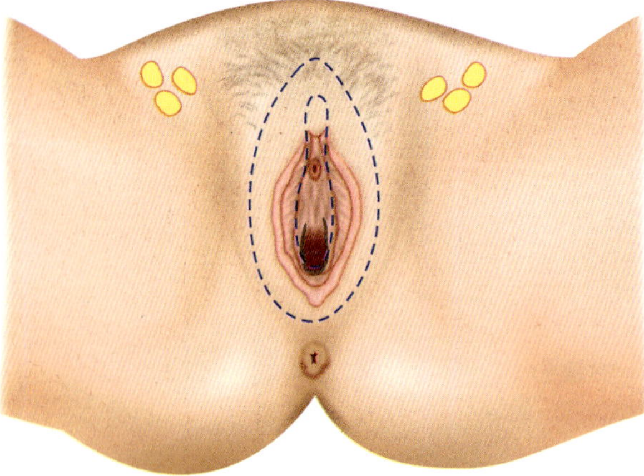

Fig. 8: Incision for simple vulvectomy

Procedure

The excision margins are selected after colposcopy and marked with pen. Skin is incised through the dermis and not deeper. Skin is dissected off the subcutaneous tissue. Clitoris is preserved if desired. Defect is closed by suturing the edges or by split thickness skin graft using 3-0 vicryl.

SIMPLE VULVECTOMY

Removal of whole of vulva down the fascia with perineal tissues as indicated.

Indication

- Widespread intraepithelial neoplasia
- Paget's disease
- Symptomatic vulvar dystrophy not responding to medical treatment

Procedure

Incision is placed as shown in Figure 8. Electrocautery (ESU) for cutting and coagulating is preferred. Outer incision is placed first and the dissection is carried through the skin and the labial fat pad. If shaft of the clitoris has to be removed, dissection is carried down to aponeurosis over the pubic symphysis.

Closure is affected by interrupted simple or mattress vertical sutures using 2-0 vicryl. Drains are unnecessary after simple vulvectomy (Fig. 9).

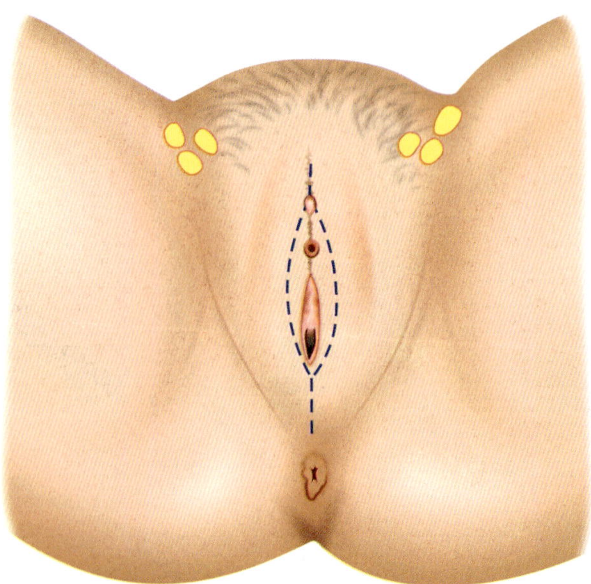

Fig. 9: Simple vulvectomy after closure

RADICAL VULVECTOMY

Wide radical excision of the whole of the vulva together with adjacent tissues to a "minimum" of "10 mm" of surgical margins around the lesion.

Indication

It is the primary treatment for vulvar cancer.

The type of incision is individualized depending on the site and size of the tumor and often is performed with or without unilateral or bilateral groin dissection.

Type of surgery when lesion is confined to the vulva:

- Radical local excision
- Radical hemivulvectomy
- Modified radical vulvectomy (anterior, posterior or total)

When Lesion is Beyond the Vulva

Radical vulvectomy with additional procedures like:

- Excision of lower urethra
- Partial/total vaginectomy
- Excision of anus and/or distal rectum
- Anterior/posterior/total exenteration

WIDE LOCAL EXCISION WITHOUT GROIN DISSECTION (FIG. 10)

Indication

Lesion less than 2 cm and stromal invasion less than 1 mm (FIGO stage IA)

WIDE LOCAL EXCISION WITH GROIN DISSECTION

Indication

- Stromal invasion greater than1 mm (FIGO stage IB)
- Tumor greater than 2 cm (FIGO stage II)

MODIFIED RADICAL HEMIVULVECTOMY WITH IPSILATERAL GROIN DISSECTION

Indication

Lateral tumor with wide margin, at least 1 cm beyond the tumor, where edge would not involve midline structures like clitoris, urethra, vagina, perineal body or anus.

Incision: As shown in Figure 11

If ipsilateral nodes are positive, contralateral nodes are also removed.

ANTERIOR RADICAL VULVECTOMY WITH BILATERAL GROIN DISSECTION

Indication

Anterior midline lesions

Incision: As shown in Figure 12

POSTERIOR RADICAL VULVECTOMY WITH BILATERAL GROIN DISSECTION

Indication

Posterior midline lesion

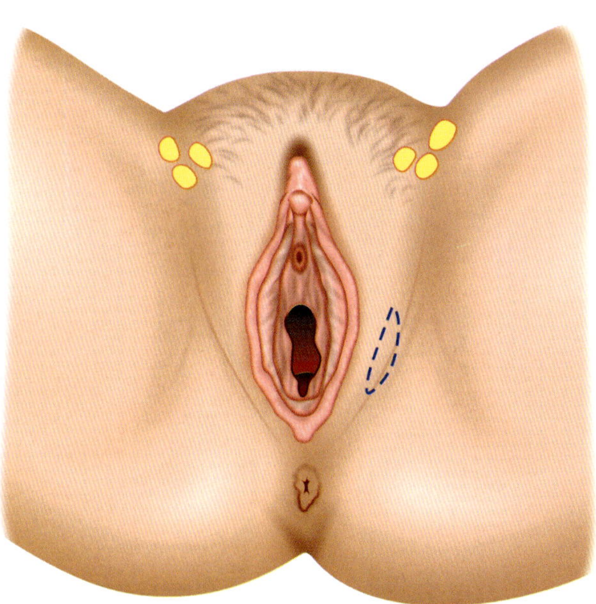

Fig. 10: Incision for wide local excision

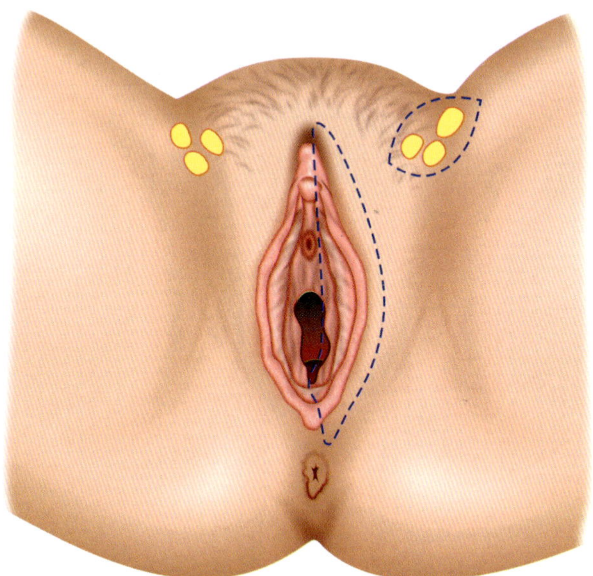

Fig. 11: Incision for modified radical hemivulvectomy

Incision: As shown in Figure 13.

TOTAL RADICAL VULVECTOMY WITH BILATERAL GROIN DISSECTION

Indication

Patients with T_2 and T_3 tumors and N_{0-1} nodes.

Preoperative preparation: Same as mentioned earlier, but good bowel preparation and thorough skin preparation are required.

Patient is carefully explained and counseled with regard to sequelae of the procedure.

Incision

a. Modified butterfly incision for en bloc dissection as shown in Figure 14, or
b. Triple incision as shown in Figure 15

TECHNIQUE OF EN BLOC RADICAL VULVECTOMY

Patient is placed in low lithotomy position with legs supported. A crescent-shaped incision is made, starting from 2 cm medial and caudal to the anterior superior iliac spine. The in cision is extended about 1 cm above the inguinal ligament, arching above the pubic bone to the other side.

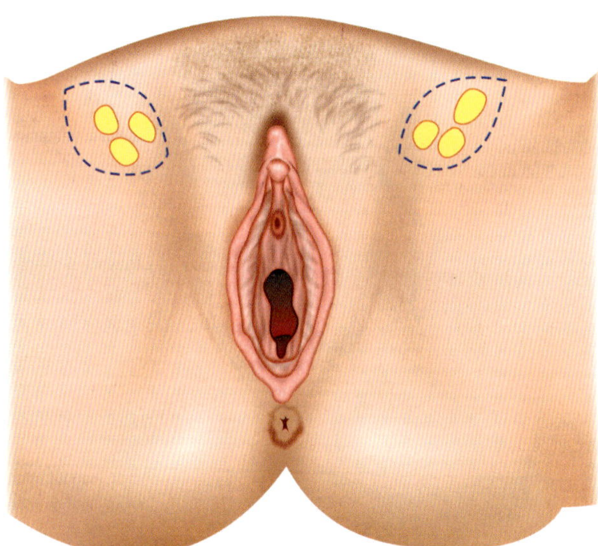

Fig. 12: Incision for anterior radical vulvectomy

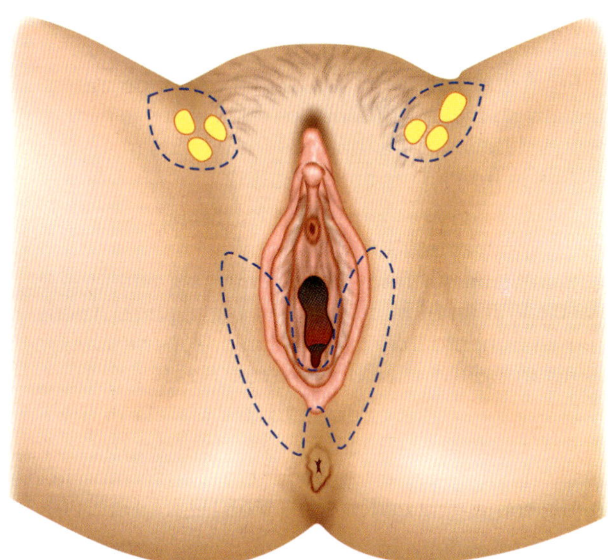

Fig. 13: Incision for posterior radical vulvectomy

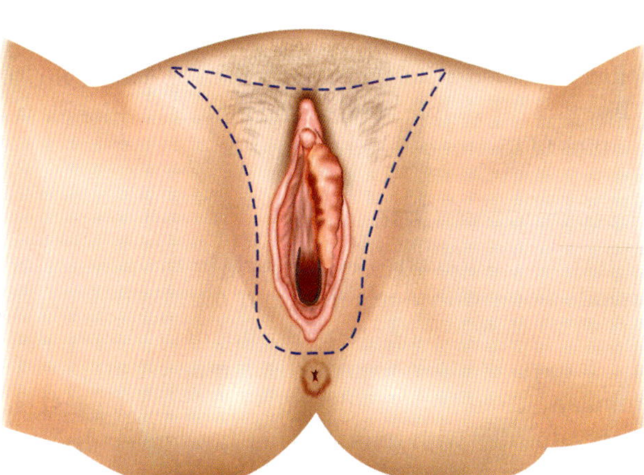

Fig. 14: Modified butterfly incision

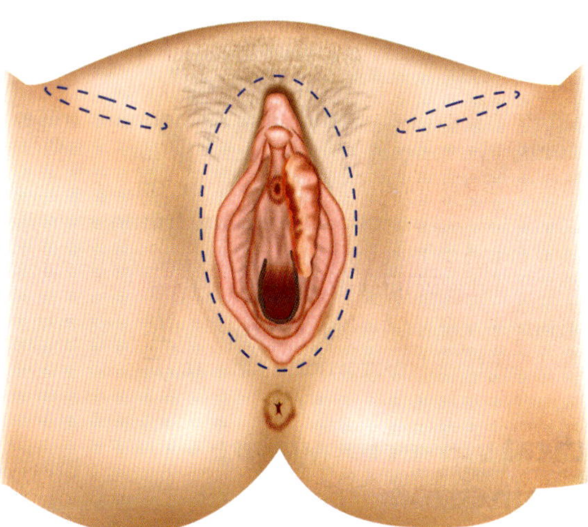

Fig. 15: Triple incision

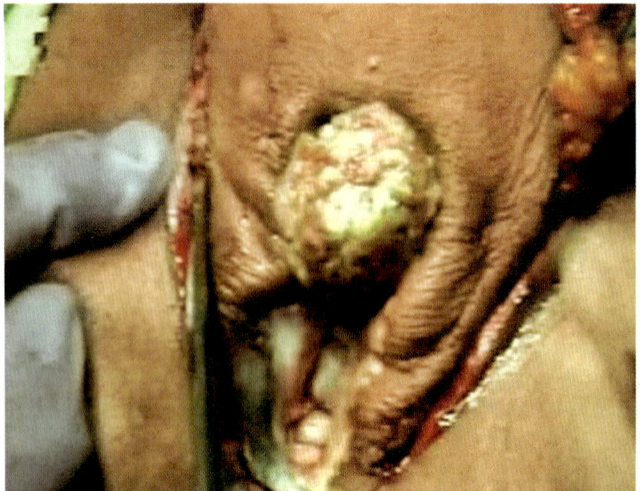

Fig. 16: Incision along the labiocrural folds

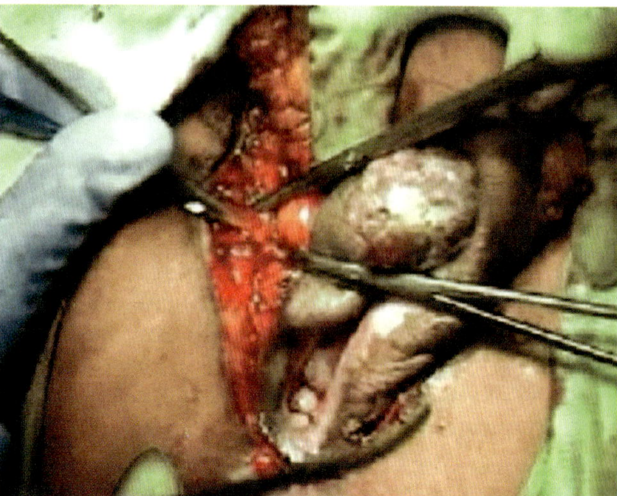

Fig.17: Dissection through subcutaneous fat

From the lateral point, caudal incisions are carried medially so that a width of 2 cm skin strips is included. It is carried down along the labiocrural folds to meet in the midline in front of the anus (Fig. 16).

The dissection is carried down through subcutaneous fat up to aponeurosis of external oblique muscle 3 cm above inguinal ligament. Fatty tissue containing lymph nodes is dissected off and lower margin of the inguinal ligament is exposed. Superficial circumflex iliac and superficial epigastric vessels are ligated when encountered (Figs 17 and 8).

Dissection is taken down to deep fascia of the thigh, about 6 cm from the inguinal ligament over the sartorius muscle, femoral vessels and adductor longus muscle. Fatty bundle containing nodes is taken off (Figs 19 and 20).

Anteromedially, long saphenous vein is identified and is followed down to saphenofemoral junction. Femoral artery pulsation can be taken as a landmark to identify the femoral vein. Femoral nodes lying medial to femoral vein are removed. Any fatty tissue in femoral canal is removed (Fig. 21).

Long saphenous vein is "preserved" to prevent postoperative groin wound and subsequent lower limb problems. Sartorious muscle which forms the lateral boundary of femoral triangle may be transpositioned to protect femoral vessels. Skin flaps are trimmed and closed with 1-0 vicryl or black silk, using vertical mattress sutures. Suction drain is kept at the groin.

If defect is too large, it is closed with a skin flap. Light dressing is placed after wound closure (Fig. 23).

Radical Vulvectomy with Triple Incision

More recently, radical vulvectomy is performed with separate incisions placed over the groin and the vulva.

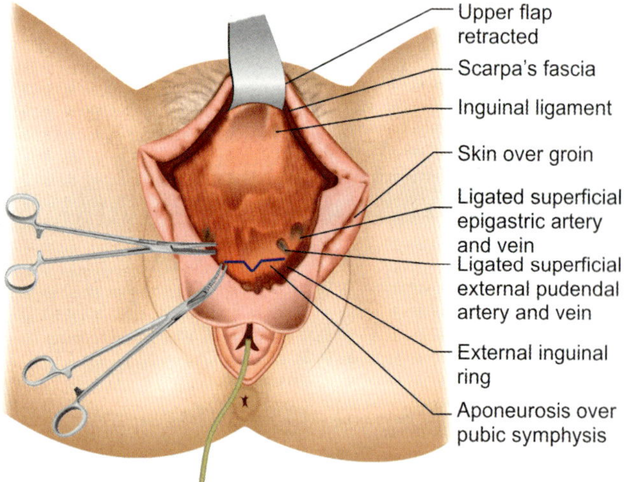

Fig.18: Exposure of external oblique aponeurosis

The technique is same as described earlier. But the groin incisions are elliptical in shape and end medially, 2 cm below and medial to the pubic tubercle. Vulval incision is like that for simple vulvectomy but with wider excision margins of 15 mm beyond the tumor.

Postoperative Care

Prophylactic antibiotic is continued in the postoperative period, along with analgesics and intravenous fluids. If wound is closed under tension, ambulation is restricted to 3–5 days. Bladder drainage is continued till patient is ambulant. Liquid diet is advised on the next day and later, low residue diet with stool softener. Low molecular weight (LMW) heparin is given intraoperatively and continued for 5 days in the postoperative period. Drains are kept till the drainage fluid is less than 50 mL.

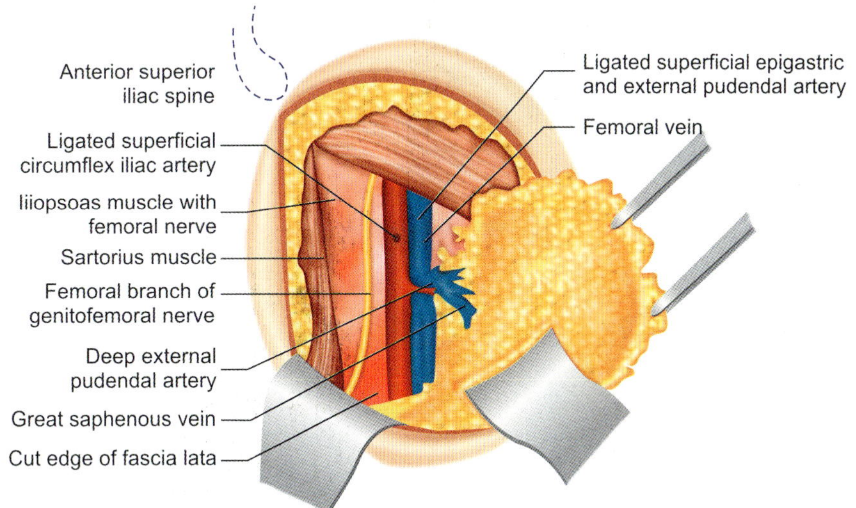

Fig.19: Inguinal lymphadenectomy

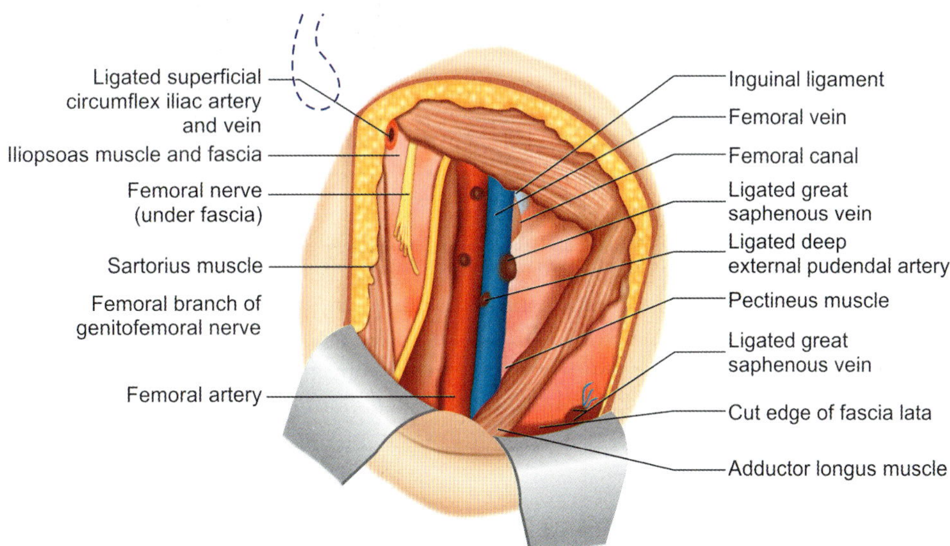

Fig. 20: Structures of femoral triangle after inguinal lymphadenectomy

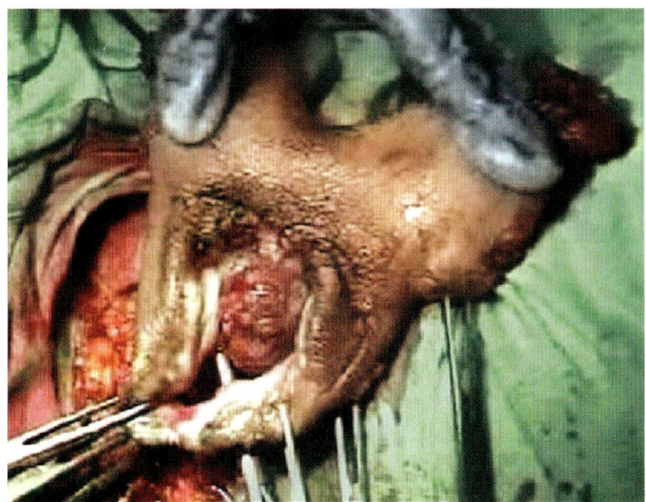

Fig. 21: Specimen after dissection

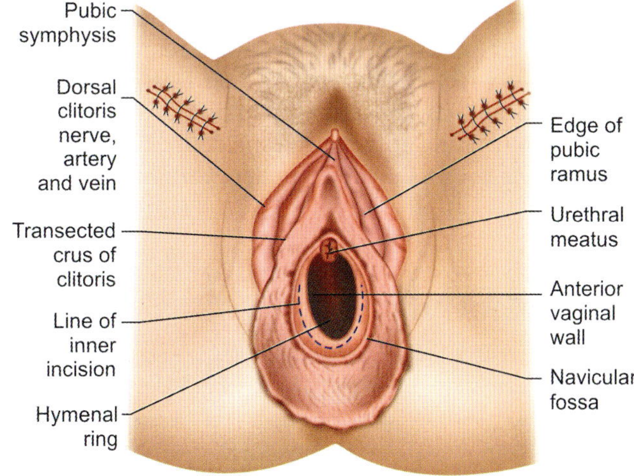

Fig. 22: Dissected anterior portion of the specimen

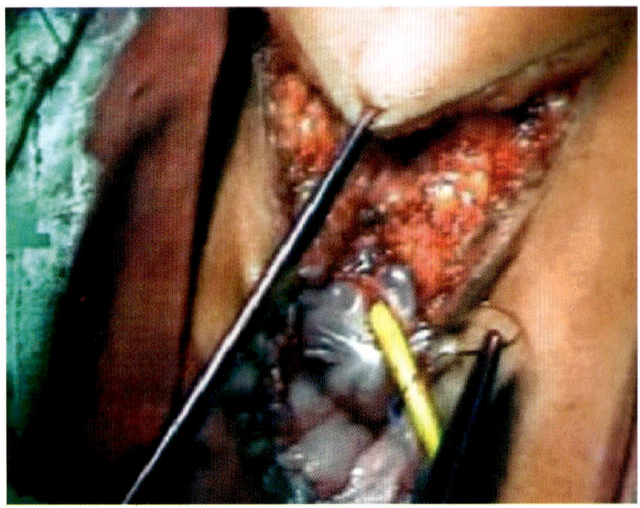

Fig. 23: Closure of wound

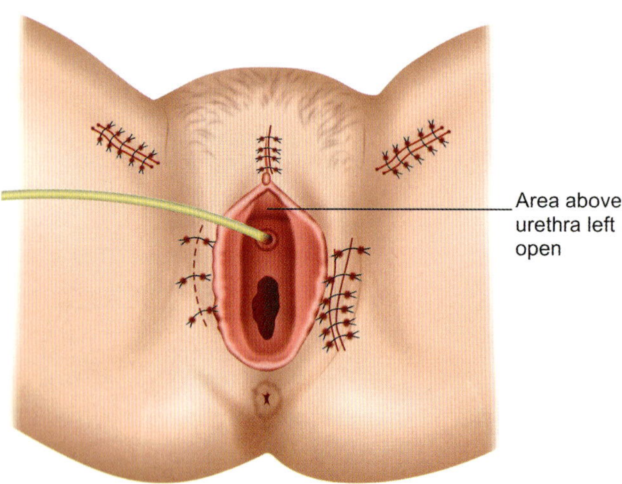

Fig. 24: Triple incision after closure

Postoperative Complications and Management

The immediate morbidity includes wound infection and wound breakdown. With triple incision, incidence of wound breakdown is reduced by 50%. Local dressings and wound debridement, if necrosis is present, will help in healing. Other complications are deep vein thrombosis (DVT), pulmonary embolism and hemorrhage. Use of LMW heparin will avoid thromboembolic complications. About 10–20% may develop lymphocysts which can be aspirated. Temporary numbness and paresthesia of anterior thigh is common and will improve slowly (Fig. 24).

Late Complications

Common late complication is chronic leg edema. Preservation of saphenous vein has reduced this problem.

Compressor stockings and intermittent elevation of leg may help. Rarely, femoral hernia may develop. Closure of femoral canal by suturing the Cooper's ligament to inguinal ligament may prevent this. Urinary and fecal incontinence may develop which can be repaired later. Dyspareunia due to scarring and psychosexual complications can occur. With vulval sparing surgery, the incidence is less likely. Preoperative counseling of the patient with husband may be of value.

CONCLUSION

- Type of vulvectomy should be individualized depending on the site and size of vulvar lesion
- Preoperative confirmation by biopsy is a must
- Vulvar sparing surgery is appropriate for early vulvar cancer
- A minimum margin of 15 mm of disease free tissue is optimum
- Triple incision technique reduces morbidity and recurrence, in early stage disease
- Groin node dissection is not needed in stage IA carcinoma
- In lateral tumor, only ipsilateral groin node dissection is appropriate
- Groin dissection should include removal of both inguinal and femoral nodes to prevent recurrence
- Preservation of long saphenous vein may decrease both groin wound and lower limb problems.

ACKNOWLEDGMENTS

- Dr Dhananjaya, Professor and HOD (Retd), Dept of OBG, BMC, Bangalore
- Dr Uma, Professor, KMIO, Bangalore
- Dr Rajesh and Ms Anusha, BMC, Bangalore.

BIBLIOGRAPHY

1. Borgono G, Micheletti L, Barbero M, et al. Topographic distribution of groin lymph nodes. J Reprod Med. 1990;35:1127-9.
2. Burrell MO, Franklin EW, Campion MJ, et al. The modified radical vulvcetomy with groin dissection: an eight-year experience. Am J Ostet Gynecol. 1988;159:715-22.
3. Ghurani GB, Penalver MA. An update on vulvar cancer. Am J Obstet Gynecol. 2001;185:294-9.
4. Hacker NF, Berek JS, Lagasse LD, et al. Individualization of treatment for stage I squamous cell vulvar carcinoma. Obstet Gynecol. 1984;63:155.

5. Hacker NF, Berek JS. Practical Gynaec Oncology, 2nd edition. William Wilkin's publications; 1994.
6. Hacker NF, Leuchter RS, Berek JS, et al. Radical vulvectomy and bilateral inguinal lymphadenectomy through separate groin incisions. Obstet Gynecol. 1981;58:574-9.
7. Hacker NF. Current management of early vulvar cancer. Ann Acad Med Singapore. 1998;27:688-92.
8. Iverson T, Abeler V, Aalders J. Individualized treatment of stage I carcinoma of the vulva. Obstet Gynecol. 1981;57:85.
9. Lees DH, Singer A. A color atlas of gynecologic surgery. Wolfe Medical Publications Ltd; 1980.
10. Leusley DD. 'Future of Surgery in Gynecological Oncology'. In: Studd J (ed.). Progress in obstetrics and gynaecology, 14th edition. Churchill Livingston; 2000.
11. Mann WJ, Stovall TG. Gynaecologic Surgery. Churchill Livingstone; 1996.
12. Monaghan JM, Lopes T, Naik R. Bonney's Gynaecological Surgery, 10th edition. Blackwell Science; 2005.
13. Morrow CP, Curtin JP. Gynaecologic Cancer Surgery. Churchill Livingston Inc; 1996.
14. Moskovic EC, Shepherd JH, Barton DP, et al. The role of high resolution ultrasound with guided cytology of groin lymph nodes in the management of squamous cell carcinoma of the vulva: a pilot study. Br J Obstet Gynaecol. 1999;106:863-7.
15. Stehman FB, Bundy BN, Dvoretsky PM, et al. Early stage I carcinoma of the vulva treated with ipsilateral superficial inguinal lymphadenectomy and modified radical hemivulvetomy: a prospective study of the Gynecologic Oncology Group. Obstet Gynecol. 1992;79:490-7.
16. Stehman FB, Bundy BN, Dvoretsky PM, et al. Early stage I carcinoma of the vulva treated with ipsilateral superficial inguinal lymphadenectomy and modified radical hemivulvectomy. Obstet Gynecol. 1992;79:490-7.
17. Te Linde RWRock JA, Thompson JD. Te Linde's Operative Gynecology, 9th edition. Lippincott-Raven Publications; 2003.
18. Zhang SH, Sood AK, Sorosky JI, et al. Preservation of the saphenous vein during inguinal lymphedenectomy decreases morbidity in patients with carcinoma of the vulva. Cancer. 2000;89:1520-5.

37.7 SURGICAL MANAGEMENT OF SOLID VULVAR TUMORS

Ashwini Bhalerao-Gandhi, Murad E Lala, Bimal Mody

SOLID BENIGN TUMORS OF VULVA

The incidence of solid benign tumors in the vulva is low; but a variety of benign tumors including fibromas, fibromyomas, lipomas, hemangiomas, neurofibromas and endometriomas have all been reported. These tumors can originate from any of the three germinal layers that constitute the anogenital area. Most solid tumors should be excised, both to ascertain the diagnosis and to relieve the patient's discomfort.

CONDYLOMA ACUMINATUM

This is one type of morphologic manifestation of human papillomavirus (HPV) infection in the lower genital tract. They are frequently associated with cervical, vaginal and anal HPV infection.

Careful clinical evaluation, PAP smear (Papanicolaou test) and colposcopy are essential in patients presenting with vulvar warts. This is necessary not only to exclude cervical and vaginal dysplasia but also to define the extent of condylomatous involvement. The most common approach to vulvar condylomata is the local application of 25% podophyllum resin. Multiple applications may be necessary. Use is restricted to the vulva in nonpregnant patients. Vaginal application may lead to undesirable absorption and neurotoxicity. Surgical excision/cautery/laser ablation are indicated in (1) extensive lesions; (2) multicentric HPV infections, particularly with involvement of the vagina, urethra or anus; (3) failure of topical chemical agents; (4) additional presence of significant intraepithelial neoplasia.

HIDRADENOMA OF VULVA

These are small, firm to soft tumors of vulva. Most are found in the interlabial folds, in the labia majora or in the perineum. Because these tumors are apocrine in origin, the labia minora location is unusual. Hidradenomas are classically asymptomatic and most lesions are discovered during a routine pelvic examination. Curative treatment consists of local excision.

VULVAR INTRAEPITHELIAL NEOPLASM

The first two cases were described by Bowen, in 1912. The vulvar intraepithelial lesions are subdivided into VIN I corresponding to mild dysplasia, VIN II similar to moderate dysplasia and VIN III which corresponds to severe dysplasia or carcinoma in situ (CIS). VIN in young women is commonly associated with HPV. However, HPV is less frequently identified in VIN lesions of older women suggesting some other etiology. Itching is the primary symptom in 50% of patients with in situ cancer. Other presenting complaints are the presence of a lump, bleeding and pain. Careful inspection of the external genitalia including perianal areas, thighs and buttocks under a bright light and magnification is always helpful. Colposcopy is preferred modality.

Although surgical excision of VIN is favored, patients typically do not require total vulvectomy. Wide local excision is usually successful but an attempt should be made to obtain clear margins. The CO_2 laser has also been successfully used. It is used particularly in areas where excision hampers presentation of anatomy such as in the clitoral/perianal region. Simple vulvectomy is recommended in patients with extensive Paget's disease of the vulva or widespread VIN where it is difficult to rule out invasive cancer, even with multiple biopsies. Procedures performed for extensive VIN 3 or Paget's disease include total or partial vulvectomy, skinning vulvectomy and multiple wide excisions. These may result in large denuded areas requiring vulvar reconstruction.

CANCER OF THE VULVA

Most often it affects the inner edges of the labia majora or the labia minora. Less often cancer occurs on the clitoris or in Bartholin's glands. In the United States, vulvar cancer accounts for about 4% of cancers in the female reproductive organs and 0.6% of all cancers in women. Over 90% of cancers of the vulva are squamous cell carcinomas. The second most common type of vulvar cancer (about 2–4%) is melanoma. A small percentage of vulvar cancers develop from glands and are called adenocarcinomas. Adenocarcinomas can also form in the sweat glands of the vulvar skin. Paget disease of the vulva is a condition in which adenocarcinoma cells are found in the vulvar skin. Between 20% and 25% of patients with vulvar Paget's disease also have an invasive adenocarcinoma of a Bartholin's gland or sweat gland. In the remaining 75–80%, the malignant cells are found only in the skin's top layer. Less than 2% of vulvar cancers are sarcomas, tumors of the connective tissues under the skin that tend to grow rapidly. Unlike other cancers of the vulva, vulvar sarcomas can occur at any age, including childhood.

Almost 85% of women with vulvar cancer are over 50 years of age and half are over 70 years of age at the time their cancer is first diagnosed. However, 15% of new patients are under the age of 40 years. The average age of women diagnosed with invasive cancer is 70 years, whereas women diagnosed with noninvasive vulvar cancer averages about 20 years younger. In general, vulvar cancer in younger women tends to be associated with infection with the high-risk HPV types. In elderly women, HPV is less likely to be a risk factor. Women who are infected with a high risk HPV have a much higher risk of developing vulvar cancer if they smoke. The risk of vulvar cancer appears to be slightly increased by Lichen sclerosus et atrophicus (LSA) with about 4% of women with LSA later developing vulvar cancer. Women with a family history of melanoma or dysplastic nevi (atypical moles) elsewhere on the body are at risk for developing a melanoma on the vulva.

Recent studies suggest that squamous cell vulvar cancer (the most common type) can develop in at least two ways. In about one-third to half of the cases, HPV infection appears to have an important role. Vulvar cancers associated with HPV infection seem to have certain distinctive features. In addition to being younger, women with these cancers often have multiple areas of VIN elsewhere on their vulvas and are usually smokers.

The second process by which vulvar cancers develop does not involve HPV infection. Vulvar cancers not linked to HPV infection usually are diagnosed in older women (age 55–85 years) who rarely have VIN, but often have LSA. DNA tests from vulvar cancers in older women not infected by HPV often show mutations of the p53 tumor suppressor gene.

The most common symptom of VIN is persistent itching that does not improve. However, many patients do not have symptoms. Areas of VIN are usually thicker and lighter in color than the surrounding skin. However, some cases of VIN can appear red, pink, or darker than the surrounding skin. The signs and symptoms of early invasive vulvar cancer are similar to those of symptomatic VIN. As invasion and growth progress, a distinct tumor is more likely to be recognized. The most common symptoms are a red, pink, or white bump or bumps with a wart-like or raw surface. An area of the vulva may appear white and feel rough. About half of the women with vulvar cancer complain of persistent itching and a growth. Some also complain of pain, burning, painful urination, bleeding and discharge not associated with the normal menstrual period. An ulcer that persists for more than a month is another sign.

TNM CATEGORY/FIGO STAGE

Primary Tumor (T)

- TX: Primary tumor cannot be assessed
- T0: No evidence of primary tumor
- Tis/0: Carcinoma in situ (preinvasive carcinoma)
- T1/I: Tumor confined to the vulva or vulva and perineum, 2 cm or less in greatest dimension
  - T1a/IA: Tumor confined to the vulva or vulva and perineum, 2 cm or less in greatest dimension, and with stromal invasion no greater than 1 mm
  - T1b/IB: Tumor confined to the vulva or vulva and perineum, 2 cm or less in greatest dimension, and with stromal invasion greater than 1 mm
- T2/II: Tumor confined to the vulva or vulva and perineum, more than 2 cm in greatest dimension
- T3/III: Tumor of any size with contiguous spread to the lower urethra and/or vagina or anus
- T4/IVA: Tumor invades any of the following: Upper urethra, bladder mucosa, rectal mucosa, or is fixed to the pubic bone.

Regional Lymph Nodes (N)

- NX: Regional lymph nodes cannot be assessed
- N0: No regional lymph node metastasis
- N1/III: Unilateral regional lymph node metastasis
- N2/IVA: Bilateral regional lymph node metastasis.

Distant Metastasis (M)

- MX: Distant metastasis cannot be assessed
- M0: No distant metastasis
- M1/IVB: Distant metastasis (including pelvic lymph node metastasis).

Survival (Table 1)

A recent report from the Mayo clinic divided patients into 2 groups—those with or without lymph node spread of the cancer. Women who had no lymph node spread had a 5 year survival of 96%. Those with spread to the lymph nodes had a 5 year survival of 64%.

Standard treatment in vulvar cancer is surgery with or without adjuvant radiation therapy. Because of the psycho-sexual consequences and significant morbidity associated with standard radical vulvectomy, there is a definite trend toward vulvar conservation and individualized management of patients with early vulvar cancer.

Table 1: Survival rates at every stage

Stage	Relative 5-Year Survival Rate
I	93%
II	87%
III/IVA	43%

PRINCIPLES OF MANAGEMENT

Stage 0 (Carcinoma In Situ)

Vulvar intraepithelial neoplasia occupying nonhairy areas can be considered an epithelial disease; however, VIN occupying hairy sites usually involves the pilosebaceous apparatus and requires a greater depth of destruction or excision.

Standard treatment options:

- Wide local excision or laser beam therapy or a combination of both
- Skinning vulvectomy with or without grafting
- Use of 5% fluorouracil cream (response rate of 50–60%). The use of topical fluorouracil is not a reliable first choice for treatment.

Stage I

Treatment options depend on the size and depth of the cancer and whether the patient also has VIN. For microinvasive lesions (< 1 mm invasion) with no associated severe vulvar dystrophy, a wide (5–10 mm) excision is indicated. For all other stage I lesions, if well lateralized, without diffuse severe dystrophy, and with clinically negative nodes, a radical local excision with complete unilateral lymphadenectomy should be performed, Candidates for this procedure should have lesions 2 cm or less in diameter with 5 mm or less invasion, no capillary lymphatic space invasion, and clinically uninvolved nodes. A literature review suggests that the local recurrence rate is 7.2% after radical local excision compared with 6.3% after radical vulvectomy.

If the cancer is larger and quite extensive, another option is a radical vulvectomy with bilateral inguinal node dissection. The definition of radical vulvectomy is being extended with the realization that the effect of radical surgery is limited by the closest resection margin rather than the achievement of total organ ablation. One study suggested that the margin of clearance of the tumor is the best predictor of local recurrence. All of the recurrences were with surgically free margins less than 8 mm.

Stage II

The treatment for most stage II vulvar cancers is partial radical vulvectomy and bilateral inguinal node dissection. Adjuvant local radiation therapy may be indicated for surgical margins less than 8 mm, capillary-lymphatic space invasion, and thickness greater than 5 mm, particularly if the patient also has positive nodes.

Stage III

Some of these bulky cancers can be cured by radical operations—modified radical vulvectomy with inguinal and femoral node dissection. Radiation therapy of 45–50 Gy to the pelvis and groin is indicated when there is capillary-lymphatic space invasion and a thickness of greater than 5 mm, particularly if the nodes are involved.

For those patients unable to tolerate radical vulvectomy or who are deemed unsuitable for surgery because of site or extent of disease, radical radiation therapy may result in long-term survival. Where radiation therapy is being tested for primary definitive treatment of vulvar cancer, some prefer to add concurrent 5-fluorouracil or 5-FU and cisplatin, as chemotherapy adjuvant.

Stage IV

1. Radical vulvectomy and pelvic exenteration
2. Surgery followed by radiation therapy to the vulva for large resected lesions with narrow margins. Localized adjuvant radiation therapy consisting of 45–50 Gy may also be indicated when there is capillary-lymphatic space invasion and thickness greater than 5 mm, particularly if the nodes are involved. Radiation therapy to the pelvis and groin should be performed if two or more groin nodes are involved
3. Radiation therapy of large primary lesions to improve operability followed by radical surgery. A radiation dose of up to 55 Gy with concomitant 5-FU has been suggested.

Recurrent Vulvar Cancer

Treatment options will depend on how soon the cancer comes back and whether it is local, regional, or distant.

If the recurrence is local, it may still be possible to remove the cancer by surgery or by using combinations of chemotherapy, radiation therapy and surgery. When local recurrence occurs, more than 2 years after the initial treatment, the prognosis is better than if the cancer had recurred sooner.

When the cancer is unresectable, chemotherapy and/or radiation therapy may be used to help relieve symptoms such as pain caused by the cancer, or to shrink the tumor so that surgery may become an option.

Case 1

Sixty two year postmenopausal multiparous female patient came with a large ulcer in vulvar region since few months. On examination, an ulcerative growth involving bilateral labia majora in lower two-third was seen. Upper one-third of labia majora had hypopigmented patches with thickening. Foul-smelling discharge was present. Biopsy confirmed the diagnosis of invasive squamous cell carcinoma of vulva. Sonography of abdomen and pelvis was normal and magnetic resonance imaging (MRI) pelvis revealed mass arising from labia majora bilaterally extending into lower ome-third of vagina. Bilateral inguinal and external iliac lymph nodes were enlarged. Total vulvectomy with partial vaginectomy, and perineal reconstruction and diversion colostomy was done on 3.12.04 (Margins sent for histopathology were found free of tumor on frozen section. Left iliac fossa sigmoid loop colostomy was done. Perineum was reconstructed with bilateral rotation flaps taken from medial side of thighs). Histopathology revealed invasive squamous cell carcinoma of vulva. The patient received radiotherapy (teletherapy 37 sitting and brachytherapy 3 sittings) till May, 2005. Computed tomography (CT) of abdomen and pelvis done in August, 2005 revealed multiple enlarged lymph nodes along right external iliac and both obturator vessels.

The woman received three cycles of chemotherapy cisplatin-phosphatidyl-choline-lipiodol (CPL), 5-FU, and taxol]. Patient developed vulvar ulcers and swelling of right lower limb in October, 2005 and died after 6 months. (Figs 1A to E).

Case 2

A 57-year-old postmenopausal lady presented with a fungating mass in the vulvar region of 3 months duration. The lady was operated for vulvar cancer 2 years prior in a hospital outside. After investigations she underwent a radical vulvectomy with bilateral groin dissection. The urethra was spared since on frozen section it was found to be uninvolved by tumor. Postoperatively she received radiation treatment. Eighteen months later the patient had a second recurrence in the perineal region. After counseling she was taken up for an anterior exenteration with ileal conduit with wide local resection of vulva (Figs 2A to F).

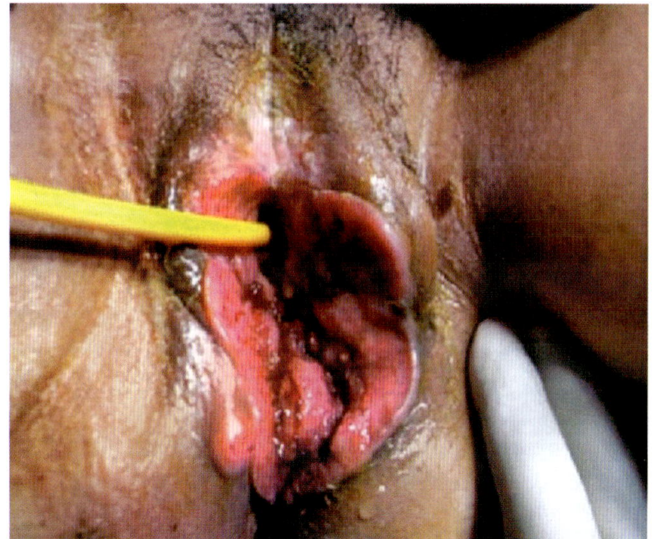

Fig. 1A: Carcinoma of vulva—extensive lesions (Case 1–A)

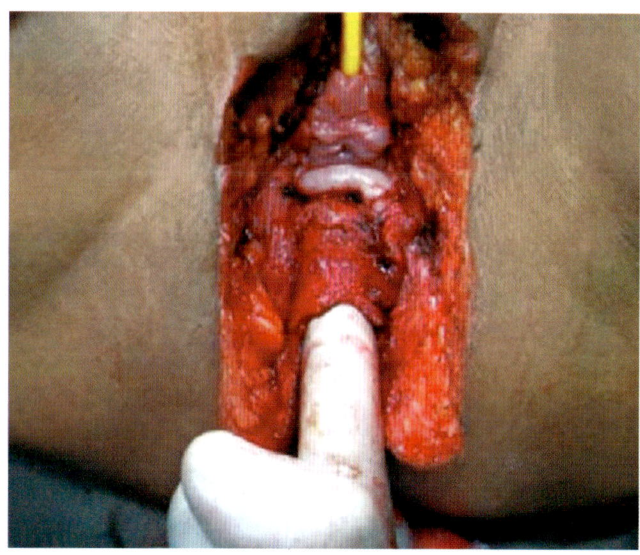

Fig. 1B: Wide excision of vulva with partial vaginectomy (Case 1–B)

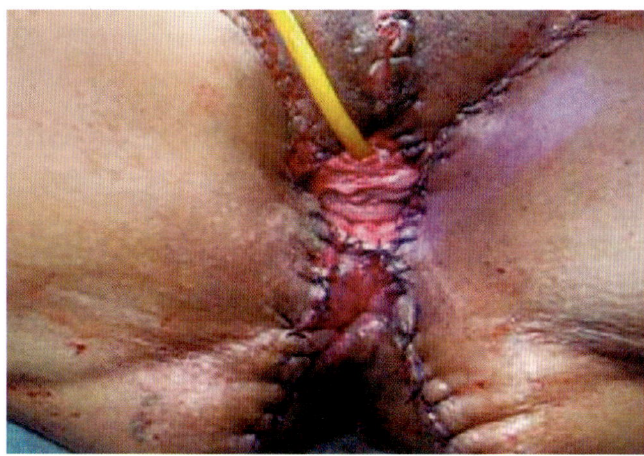

Fig. 1C: Perineal reconstruction with bilateral rotation flaps from medial side of thighs (Case 1–C)

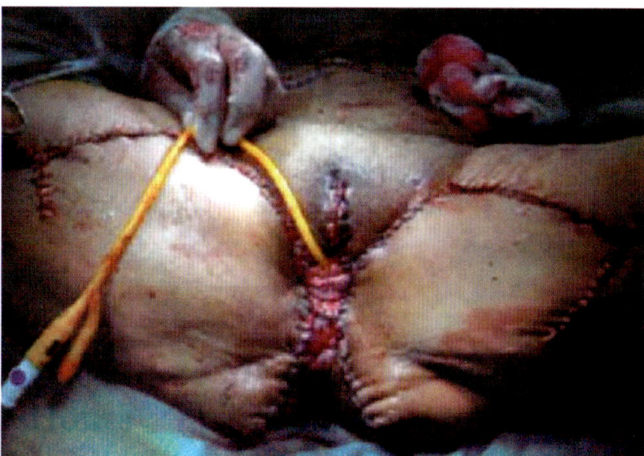

Fig. 1D: End result after surgery (Case 1–D)

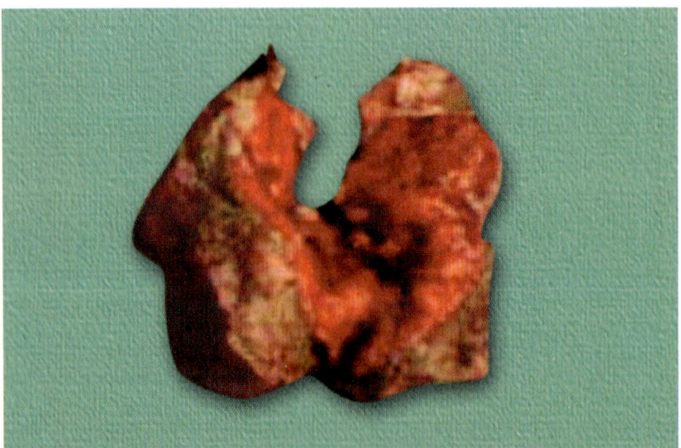

Fig. 1E: Excised specimen from vulva, perineum and lower vagina (Case 1–E)

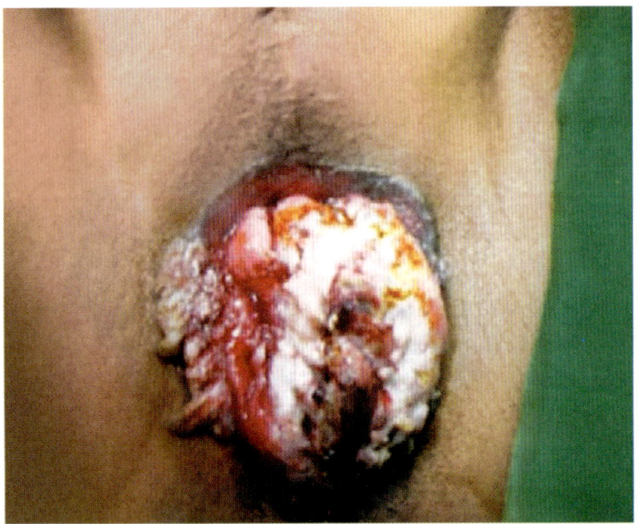

Fig. 2A: Fungating recurrent mass (Case 2–A second surgery)

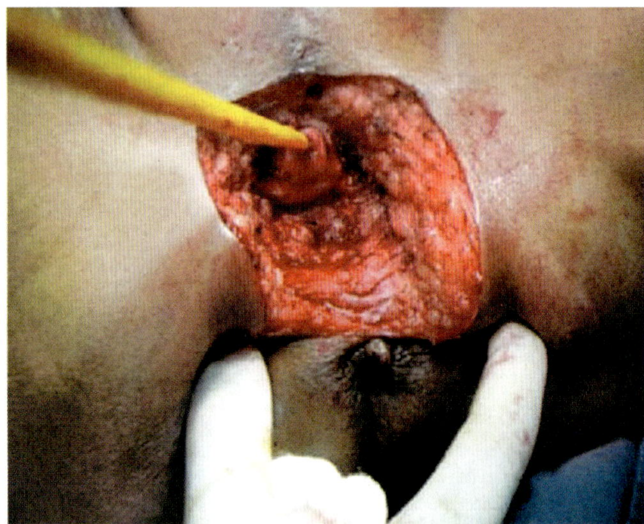

Fig. 2B: After wide excision, urethra intact (Confirmed to be free of tumor on frozen section (Case 2–B second surgery)

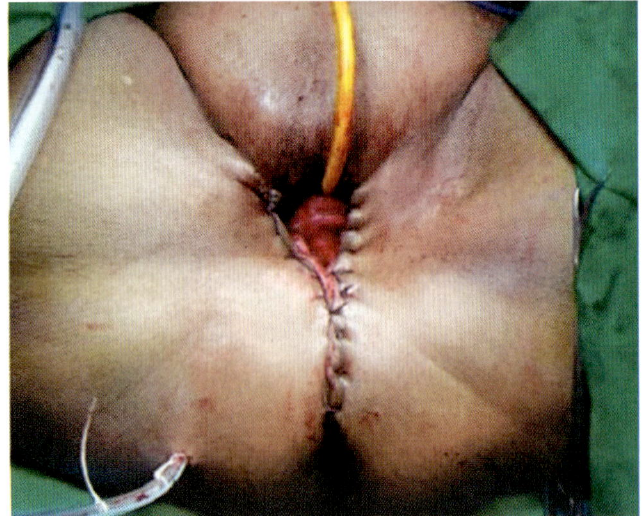

Fig. 2C: Perineal closure (Case 2–C second surgery)

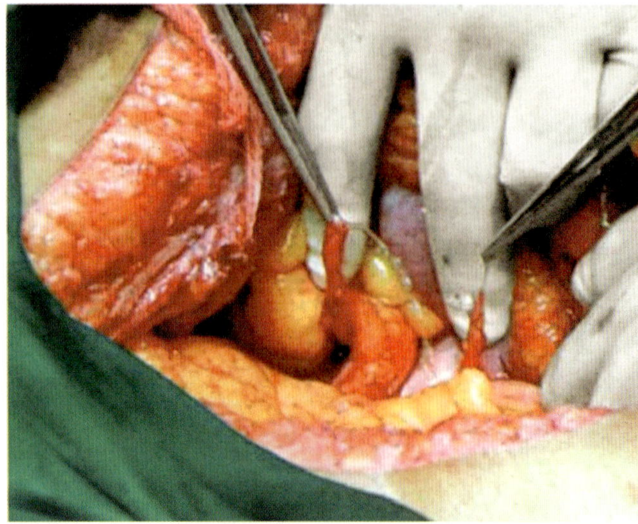

Fig. 2D: Ureters ready to be implanted into ileal conduit—anterior exenteration for second recurrence (Case 2–D third surgery)

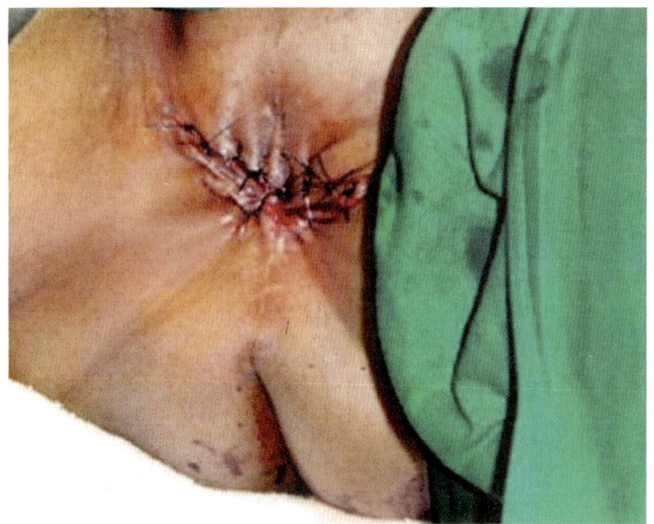

Fig. 2E: Closed perineal wound

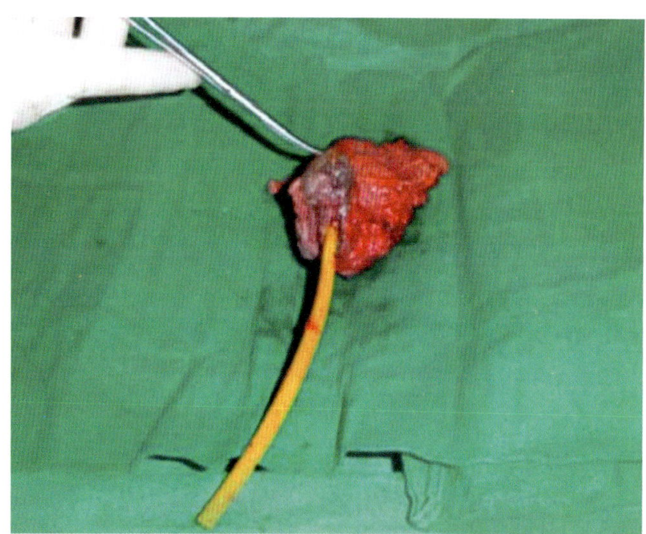

Fig. 2F: Resected specimen of urethra and bladder (Case–2 F, third surgery)

BIBLIOGRAPHY

1. Hacker NF, Van der Velden J. Conservative management of early vulvar cancer. Cancer. 71 1993;(4 Suppl):1673-7.
2. Heaps JM, Fu YS, Montz FJ, et al. Surgical-pathologic variables predictive of local recurrence in squamous cell carcinoma of the vulva. Gynecol Oncol. 1990; 38(3): 309-14.
3. Malfetano JH, Piver MS, Tsukada Y, et al. Univariate and multivariate analyses of 5-year survival, recurrence, and inguinal node metastases in stage I and II vulvar carcinoma. J Surg Oncol. 1985;30(2):124-31.
4. Stehman FB, Bundy BN, Dvoretsky PM, et al. Early stage I carcinoma of the vulva treated with ipsilateral superficial inguinal lymphadenectomy and modified radical hemivulvectomy: a prospective study of the Gynecologic Oncology Group. Obstet Gynecol. 1992;79(4):490-7.
5. Thomas GM, Dembo AJ, Bryson SC, et al. Changing concepts in the management of vulvar cancer. Gynecol Oncol. 1991;42(1): 9-21.
6. Woodruff JD, Julian C, Puray T, et al. The contemporary challenge of carcinoma in situ of the vulva. Am J Obstet Gynecol. 1973;115(5): 677-86.

CHAPTER

38

Vagina

MS Urala, SS Trivedi, Suchitra Pandit, Barun Sarkar, Swaraj Batra,
S Singh, Lakhbir Dhaliwal, SK Rath, Phool Chandra, Jasleen

38.1 EXCISION OF TRANSVERSE VAGINAL SEPTUM

MS Urala

EMBRYOLOGY OF VAGINA

In the embryologic language, the human female is a default state of development due to lack of Y chromosome. Y chromosome contains a DNA sequence on its short arm [sex determining region of Y (SRY)] that leads to production of testicular determining factor which in turn controls the development of testes from the undifferentiated gonad. Lack of this Y chromosome makes the undifferentiated gonad to develop into ovary. As ovaries do not produce Müllerian inhibiting factor, the Müllerian ducts persist to develop into uterus and vagina.

Around 60 mm crown rump (CR) length embryo following events occur in stages for development of vagina (Figs 1 to 5).

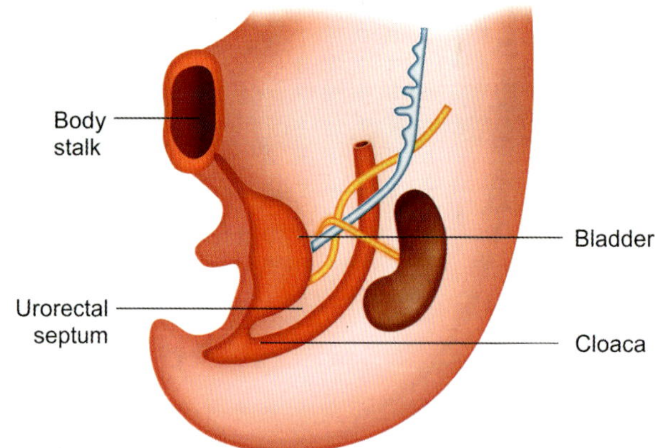

Fig. 2: The urogenital sinus forming as urorectal septum of mesoderm divides the cloaca and hindgut

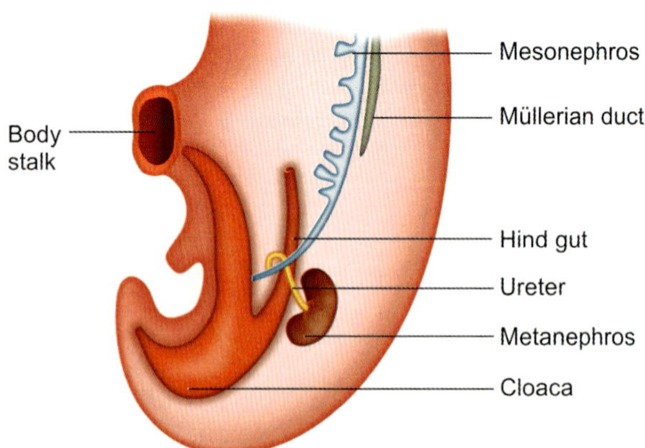

Fig. 1: Development of hindgut and cloaca from endoderm

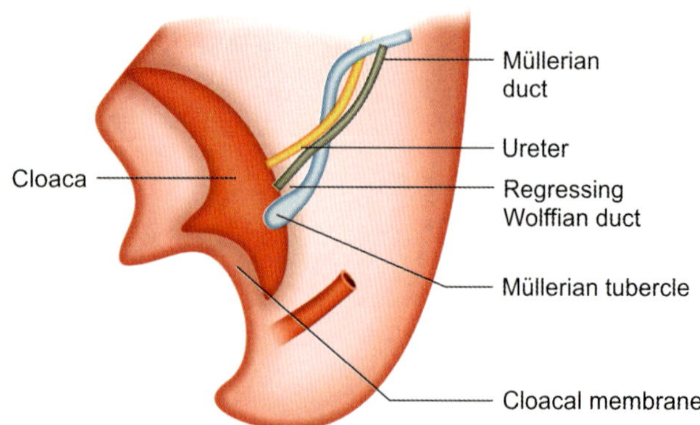

Fig. 3: Müllerian ducts impinge on urogenital sinus to form Müllerian tubercle; the sinovaginal bulb develops at this site

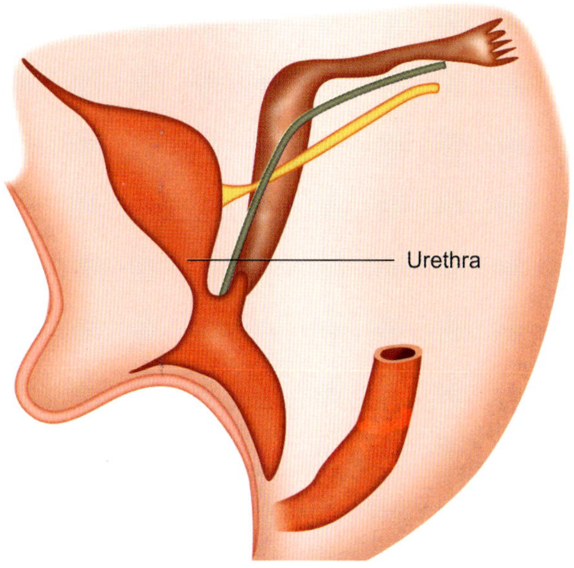

Fig. 4: Urogenital sinus above the Müllerian tubercle narrows to form the urethra

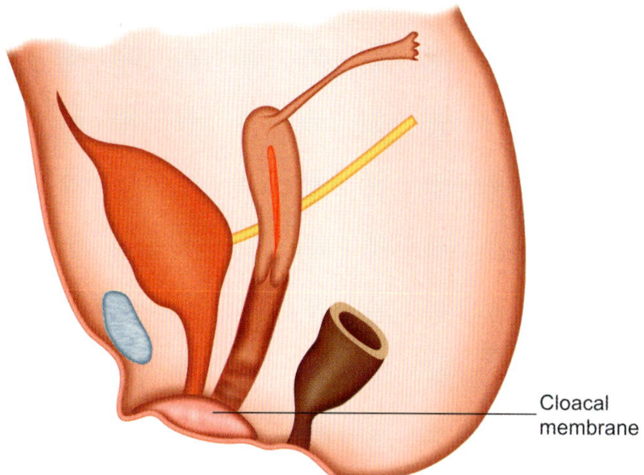

Fig. 5: Cloacal membrane breaks to expose the opened up lower part of the urogenital sinus—vulva. Posterior part opens up to form the anus

Stage I

Starts with beginning of fusion of two Müllerian ducts in caudal to cranial direction. An epithelial proliferation (sinovaginal bulb) arises from dorsal wall of urogenital sinus in the region of the sinus tubercle and its origin marks the site of future hymeneal orifice. This proliferation gradually extends as a solid anteroposteriorly flat-ended plate, inside the mesodermal condensation of uterovaginal primordium that will eventually become the fibromuscular wall of vagina.

Stage 2

Formation of uterovaginal canal: By 3rd month, the anlage of the vagina cervix and uterus are formed as the fusing Müllerian ducts merge with paired outpouching (sinovaginal bulb) that develop from posterior wall of urogenital sinus making contact with an area termed the Müllerian tubercle.

Stage 3

Growth of primordial vagina: This occurs due to proliferation of a solid mass of stratified squamous epithelium—The vaginal plate which appears between and separates the lumina of the uterovaginal canal and the urogenital sinus may be mesonephric or cloacal in origin.

Stage 4

Mesodermal proliferation: The mesoderm surrounding the vaginal plate proliferates to form the muscle of uterus and vagina.

Stage 5

Canalization of vagina: Commencing from lower end, the solid vaginal plate enlarges into a cylindrical structure with the central cells desquamate to form the vaginal lumen. At the upper end, it enlarges and grows up into the mesoderm around cervix to form the fornices. The lower end also enlarges, it invaginates the dorsal wall of urogenital sinus around the hymeneal orifice trapping a thin layer of mesoderm around the orifice to form the hymen. Thus, the hymen is lined by vaginal epithelium at the upper end and sinus epithelium at the lower part. In the later stages, lower surface of hymen and large part of vestibule become lined by the common vaginal epithelium. The urogenital sinus undergoes relative shortening in the craniocaudal direction to form the vestibule that opens on the surface through the cleft between the genital folds.

During the later months, vaginal epithelium enormously hypertrophies under the influence of maternal/placental hormones.

Classification of Müllerian Anomalies

The American Fertility Society (AFS) classification of Müllerian anomalies has been given in Table 1.

Transverse Vaginal Septum

It is the rarest of the anomalies of female genital tract. Delanmae in 1877 first discussed this condition. But it is the most common problem of the vagina. Incidence varies from 1:2,100 (Lodi et al.) to 1:84,000 (New York Medical

Table 1: American Fertility Society classification of Müllerian anomalies

Class	Anomaly
Class I	Segmental Müllerian agenesis hypoplasia A. Vagina B. Cervix C. Fundus D. Tube E. Combined anomalies
Class II	Unicornuate A. Communicating B. Noncommunicating C. No cavity D. No horn
Class III	Didelphys
Class IV	Bicornuate A. Complete division down to internal os B. Partial
Class V	Septate A. Complete (septum up to internal os) B. Partial
Class VI	Arcuate uterus
Class VII	Diethylstilbestrol raised

(***Source***: Adapted from the American Fertility Society classification of Müllerian anomalies. Fertil Steril. 1988;49:944)

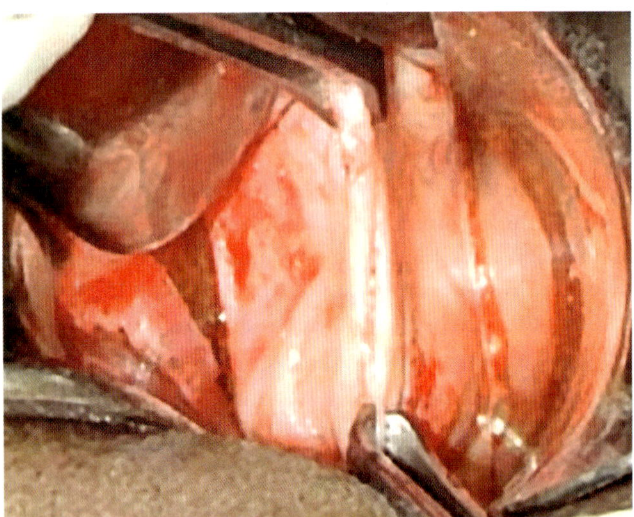

Fig. 6: Transverse vaginal septum in a cut specimen of uterus

College). Davidson (1939) described septum recognized during late pregnancy.

Transverse vaginal septum usually means a high vaginal septum (Fig. 6). The septa of upper vagina are more than 1 cm thick and that of lower vagina are thinner. However, they block free menstrual flow leading to retrograde menses and formation of endometriomas or may carry a small opening to excrete part of menstrual blood.

Etiology

Exact cause is still uncertain but may be due to:

- Failure of complete canalization of vagina by 20 weeks of gestation
- Vertical fusion defect between Müllerian ducts and urogenital sinus
- McKusick has noted the possibility of a sex-linked recessive gene
- Dungy et al. have explained an association of a hereditary transverse vaginal septums and polydactyly
- Bowman and Scott observed the occurrence of secondary vaginal septa following trauma of severe inflammations and fibrosis after a forgotten foreign body
- Brenner et al. noted the possibility of an iatrogenic substance swallowed by the present mother before 20 weeks for inducing abortion. They can be associated with other body deformities like coarctation of aorta, defects of atrial septae and lumbar spines.

Clinical Presentation

Depends upon whether the septum is perforate or imperforate. Twenty five percent of patients may be asymptomatic (Brerch and Lanfel, 1999).

Imperforate septum may first be noted in a newborn or early infancy as a case of hydrometrocolpos or mucocolpos because of entrapped cervical and uterine glandular secretions due to influence of maternal estrogens. The septa may be in the upper, mid and lower vaginal septa in 46:40:40 (Lodi, 1951).

Complete transvaginal septum may present in prepubertal girls with accumulation of fluid from endocervical and Müllerian glands. These collections can be large enough to compress ureters, vena cava and rectum and lymphatics of lower limbs and vulva.

Postpubertal patients may represent with cyclic pain, vaginal discharge, pelvic mass amenorrhea with inability to use a tampon or have sexual intercourse.

Other symptoms could be dysmenorrhea, infertility, menstrual irregularities, dyspareunia and soft tissue dystocia during labor.

Investigations

- Transabdominoperineal sonography can help to diagnose conditions like transverse vaginal septum, imperforate hymen and vaginal agenesis. This is particularly true when other conventional approaches prove inadequate. Transperineal scanning clearly images lower uterine segment, cervix bladder, urethra, vagina and moreover it helps to determine the anatomic relationships between these structures better than the abdominal scan (Fig. 7)

- Other investigations include colpohysterography cystogram, plain X-ray abdomen, intravenous (IV) pyelography, barium enema. A diagnostic laparoscopy is also of immense help to look for problems of internal genitalia
- Magnetic resonance imaging (MRI) to know the pelvic anatomy before surgery.

Treatment

1. *No treatment*: In 10 out of 42 cases (Lodi et al.), no treatment was given as they were mostly asymptomatic. This approach is unwise if future pregnancy is contemplated or problem of soft tissue dystocia during delivery expected. Delay final surgery till the girl is 22 years (mature enough to understand the problem and keep the prosthesis inside) or married and regular coitus prevents stenosis of the repair site.
2. Simple incision of the septum for drainage of mucocolpos in a compromised newborn. But subsequent exploration including laparotomy may be mandatory or recurrence of septum or vaginal stenosis is common.
3. Dilatation of a large perforated transverse septum is useful to provide a functional vagina. Bowman and Scott explain a case of vaginal dilatation after cesarean section by frank procedure. Teach patient how to dilate for 3–4 days in the hospital using graduated glass dilators. Patient goes home and dilates the vagina for 15–20 minutes three or four times a day for 8–10 weeks.
4. Acute decompression of hematocolpos (Figs 8 to 10) to relieve pain, endometrial suppression and preoperative passive vaginal dilatation to facilitate resection of septum and vaginal anastomosis. The hematocolpos can be aspirated to relieve the acute pain and delay surgery. Further recurrence of hematocolpos can be delayed by continuous use of oral contraceptive pills. Vaginal dilatation for 6–8 months helps to lengthen lower vaginal segment to facilitate resection and anastomosis effective. This can increase the length of lower vagina from 1 cm to 5 cm. If coitus assumed at earliest, 85% girls achieve a functional vagina without requirement of further surgery.
5. Excision of septum with an electric knife—the procedure is useful if the septum is perforated. If the septum is complete where upper vagina cannot be identified laparotomy and hysterotomy is done to push a Duncan's dilator from above through cervix to appreciate the thickness of septum, which can be excised from the vaginal route.
6. *End-to-end anastomosis*: A transverse incision is made on the lower septal wall and the body of septum excised. Now excise the upper vaginal wall transversely resulting into formation of four mucosal flaps a, b, A, B. The corresponding upper and lower flaps are sutured by interrupted 3-0 chromic catgut (Fig. 11).
7. Z-plasty (Figs 12A to F) of transverse vaginal septum using Garcia's procedure and Grunberger's modification. Oblique crossed incisions are made through vault of short vagina and four triangular vaginal mucosal flaps (anterior portion of the barrier) are separated by sharp and blunt dissection. The obliquity of the crossed incision provides horizontal baselines of the superior and inferior triangular flaps so that the bladder and rectum can be saved during

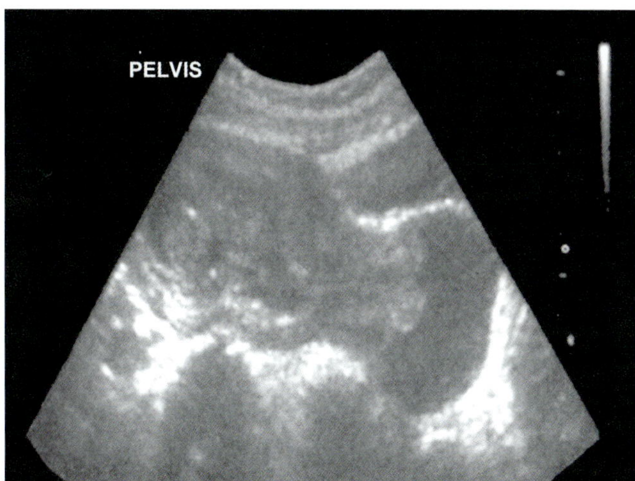

Fig. 7: Transvaginal ultrasound with intrauterine pregnancy and transverse vaginal septum

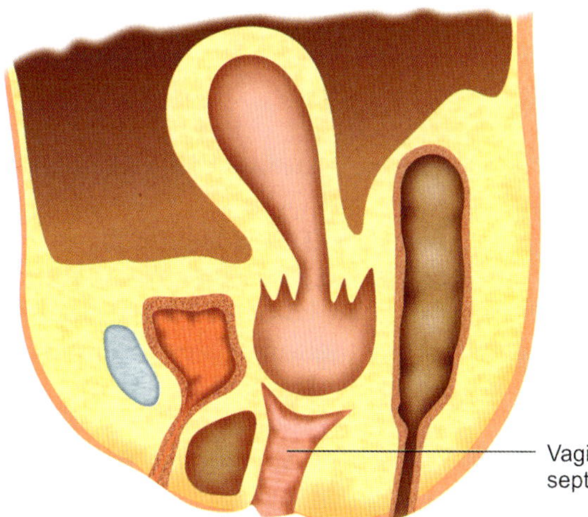

Fig. 8: Hematocolpos, hematometra above the vaginal septum

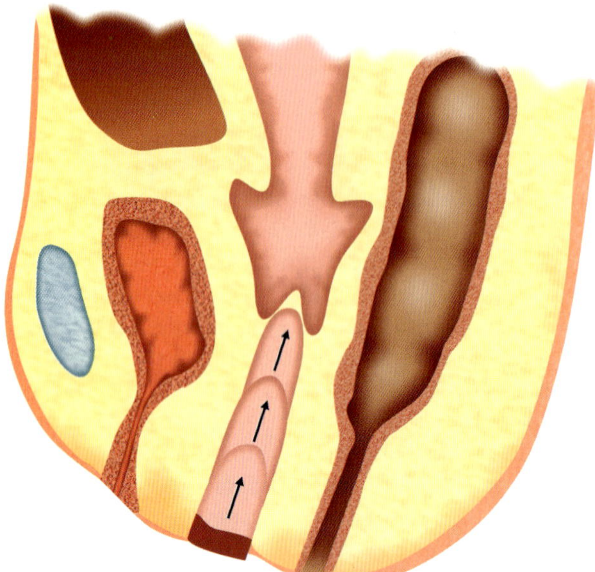

Fig. 9: Passive dilatation of vagina using progressively larger dilators to increase the depth of the vagina

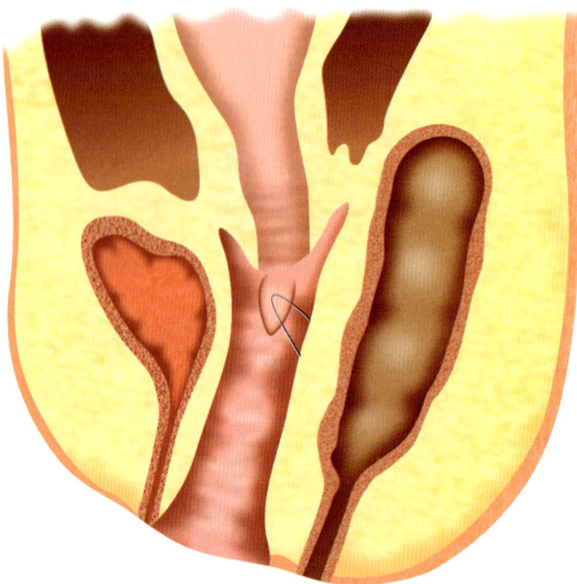

Fig. 10: Upper and lower vaginal anastomosis can be performed after excising the septum

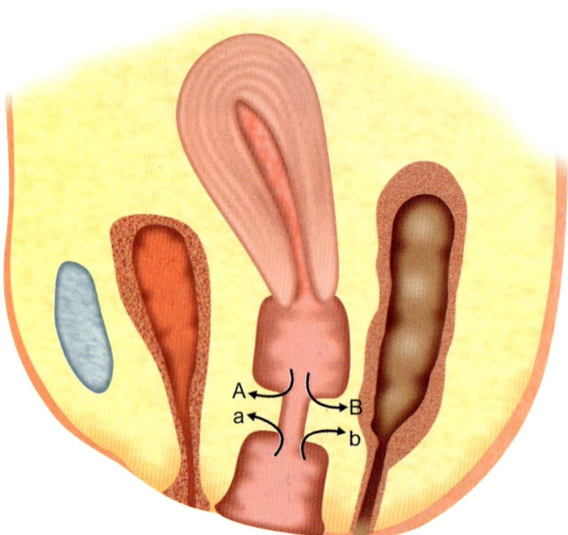

Fig. 11: Excision of the septum and end-to-end anastomoses

the blind procedure. Depending on the diameter of the sinus tract opening in some cases tissue portions of different sizes are to be cut of the lower vaginal mucosa between triangular flaps to ensure optimal flaps, meticulous marking and stabilization of vaginal mucosa flaps by stay sutures are to be done. Abundant areolar tissue between anterior and posterior vaginal mucosa must be carefully resected and kept by local sharp knife dissection and electrocautery. Urethral catheter in site and frequent per rectal (PR) examination done to protect bladder and rectum. Four more triangular vaginal mucosa flaps are prepared by two crossed incisions through upper vaginal mucosa of the vaginal pocket (posterior portion of the barrier). Lower and upper incisions are rotated 45° against each other. If preparation and resections of midseptum and dissection of upper vaginal mucosa are difficult because for thick septa, a balloon catheter is passed through the central opening into upper vaginal pocket, careful traction of catheter simplifies surgery and allows sharp knife dissection of areolar tissue. Avoid destruction of upper vaginal mucosa. Any areolar tissue remnants beneath upper vaginal mucosal flap can still be dissected before joining upper and lower flaps. In case of obstructed transvaginal septa, it is better to inject same fluid into the upper vaginal pocket through an ultrasound-guided needle or balloon catheter in the very beginning of the surgery (Figs 12A to F).

The edges of the upper and lower vaginal mucosal flaps are joined in the form of a continuous and Z-plasty anastomosis using interrupted single layer delayed absorbable suture.

A rigid plastic vaginal mold (Figs 13A and B) is inserted after smearing it with estriol cream to be taken out, cleared and reinserted everyday till discharge. Patient is discharged with an elastic mold for next 6–8 weeks after which sexual relation can be advised. If patient is unmarried, she may use the mold for next 6 months during night time.

In summary, the Grunberger's method of vaginoplasty using upper and lower mucosal flaps of the septum can keep the vagina adequately enlarged for the subsequent sexual function.

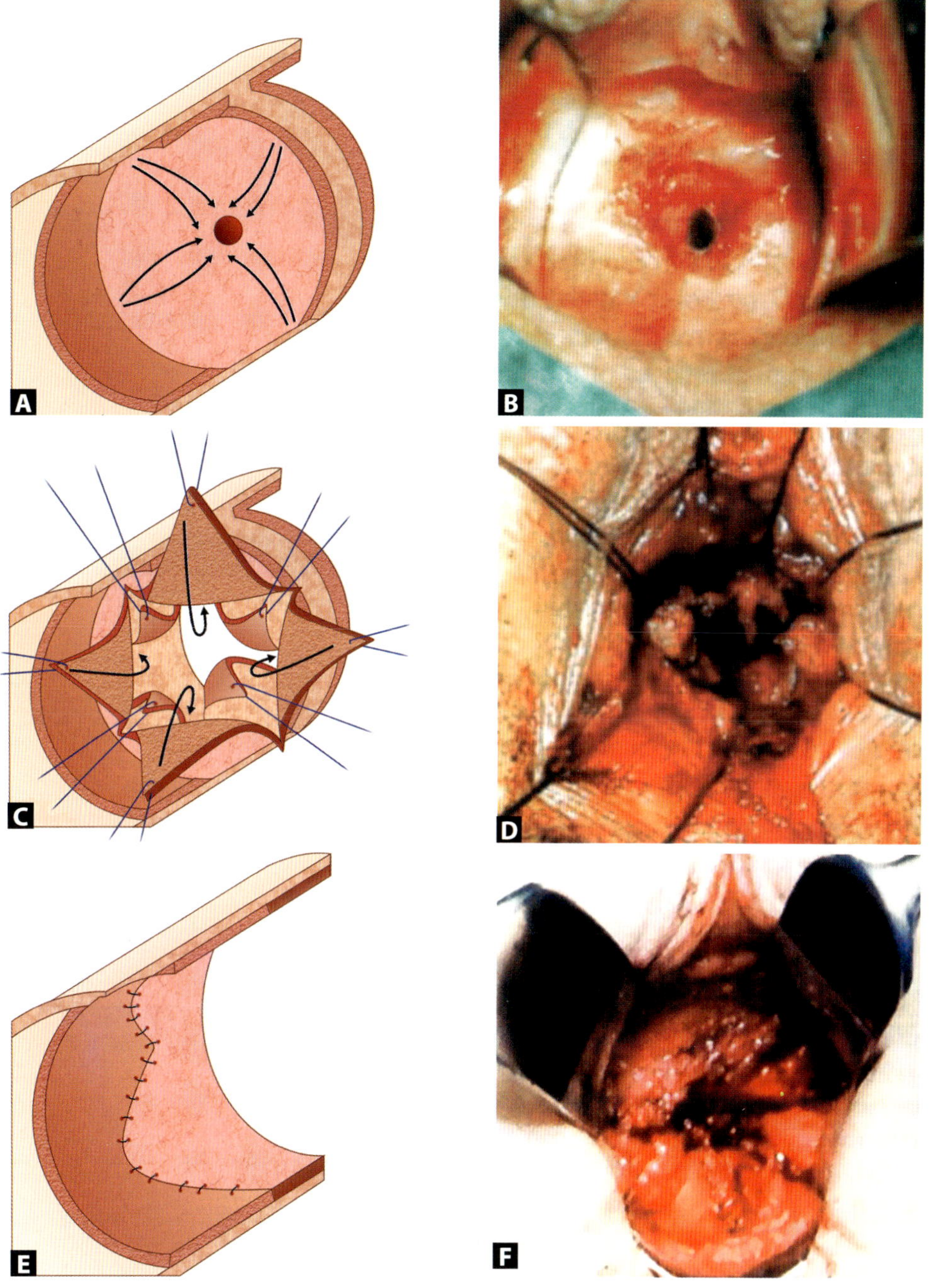

Figs 12A to F: Z-plasty

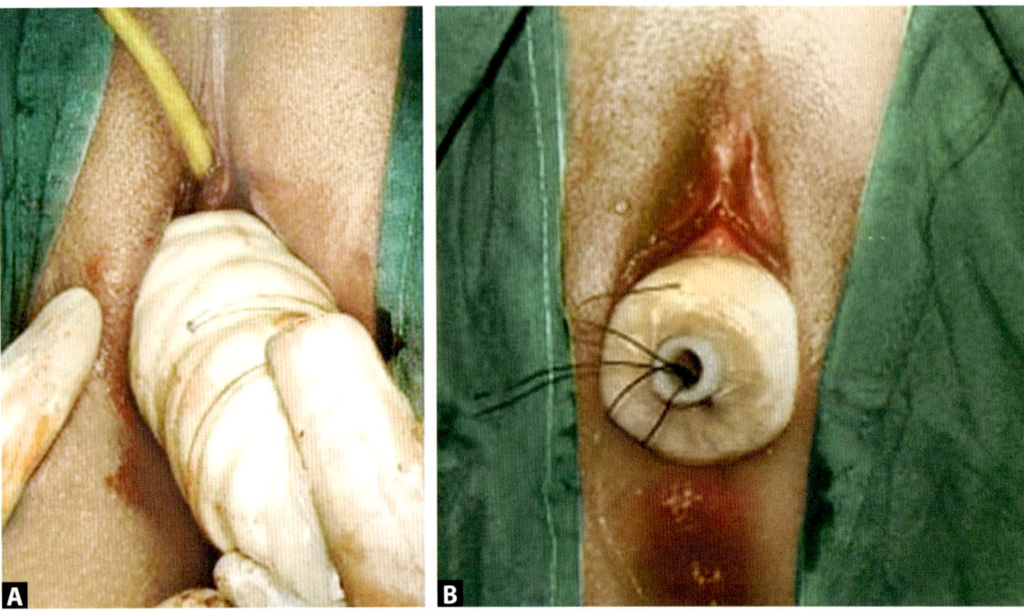

Figs 13A and B: Vaginal mold after surgery

BIBLIOGRAPHY

1. Blanton EN, Rouse DJ. Trial of labor in women with transverse vaginal septa. Obstet Gynecol. 2003;101:1110-2.
2. Edmonds DK. Congenital malformations of the genital tract. Obstet Gynecol Clin North Am. 2000;27(1):49-62.
3. Gibson ED. Transverse upper vaginal septum presenting in pregnancy: a case report and review of the literature. Aust N Z J Obstet Gynaecol. 2003;43:381-3.
4. Hurst BS, Rock JA. Preoperative dilatation to facilitate repair of high transverse vaginal septum. Fertil Steril. 1992;57(6):1351-3.
5. Jeffcoate N. Jeffcoate's Principles of Gynaecology. London: Butterworths; 1987.
6. Meyer WR, McCoy MC, Fritz MA. Combined abdominal-perineal sonography to assist in diagnosis of transverse vaginal septum. Obstet Gynecol. 1995;85:882-4.
7. Rock JA, Zacur HA, Dlugi AM, et al. Pregnancy success following surgical correction of imperforate hymen and complete transverse vaginal septum. Obstet Gynecol. 1982;59(4):448-51.
8. Weirrani F, Bodner K, Spängler B, et al. "Z" plasty of the transverse vaginal septum using Garcia's procedure and the Grünberger modification. Fertil Steril. 2003;79(3):608-12.
9. Wenof M, Reyniak JV, Novendstern J, et al. Transverse vaginal septum. Obstet Gynecol. 1979;54(1):60-8.

38.2 VAGINECTOMY AND EPISIOTOMY OR STENOTIC RELEASE SURGERY OR STRICTURE RELEASE

SS Trivedi

INTRODUCTION

Vaginectomy or colpectomy is the partial or total excision of the vagina. This surgery is not commonly performed except with radical hysterectomy for carcinoma cervix. Other indications for vaginectomy include vaginal intraepithelial neoplasia (VAIN) III, vaginal cancer stage I and selected cases of severe genital prolapse. Residual VAIN, following hysterectomy for cervical intraepithelial neoplasia (CIN) is the commonest indication for vaginectomy. Therefore, it is imperative that extension of cervical premalignant lesion on to the vagina should be identified preoperatively by colposcopy and excised completely.

Vaginectomy has a limited role in treatment of vaginal cancer. Women with stage I disease involving the upper posterior vagina can be treated by radical vaginectomy and pelvic lymphadenectomy with hysterectomy (if uterus is present). However, it is not an appropriate and adequate procedure for invasive carcinoma of vagina and majority of tumors are treated by radiation therapy. Rarely chronic benign conditions like severe lichen planus may warrant vaginectomy.

SURGICAL ANATOMY OF VAGINA (FIG. 1)

Vagina is an elastic fibromuscular canal. Inferiorly it is related to vulva. From vulva, it extends upward and backward at an angle of 60–70° to the horizontal. Superiorly cervix projects into it dividing the vaginal vault into four fornices. Ureter and uterine vessels lie in the base of broad ligament, over the lateral fornix and only 1–2 cm away from the cervix.

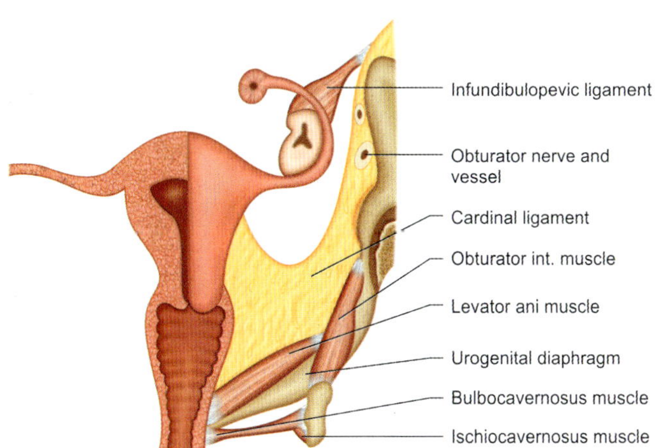

Fig. 1: Surgical anatomy of vagina

The anterior and posterior vaginal walls lie in apposition, thus obliterating the lumen of the vagina. Anteriorly, the vagina is related to the bladder above and urethra below. Posteriorly, from above downward, vaginal wall is related to peritoneum of pouch of Douglas (POD), ampulla of rectum and perineal body. Laterally from above downward, the vagina is related to lower part of cardinal ligaments, levator ani with the paracolpos, ischiorectal fossa, urogenital diaphragm and bulbospongiosus muscle.

VAGINECTOMY

Preoperative Preparation

Bowel preparation is done. Preoperative colposcopic evaluation is done to identify the margins of lesion. If vaginectomy is being performed abdominally a stitch may be put at the inferior border of vaginal lesion. Identification of this stitch during surgery ensures adequate excision.

Anesthesia

Surgery can be performed under general, epidural or spinal anesthesia. Use of epidural/spinal anesthesia reduces blood loss during surgery.

VAGINAL VAGINECTOMY

Vaginectomy is usually performed vaginally. It has been suggested that ideally hysterectomy for CIN and associated VAIN should also be performed vaginally. Vaginal route is appropriate if the entire lesion margins can be visualized.

The procedure is done in lithotomy position. Bladder is catheterized. Examination under anesthesia is indicated if the procedure is done in a posthysterectomy case to exclude the presence of any invasive lesion above the vaginal vault. Saline can be infiltrated in subepithelial tissues. This helps in defining tissue planes during surgery. A large Sims speculum is used to retract posterior vaginal wall and a smaller vaginal retractor is placed in anterior vagina to achieve good access and visualization of vault. Lesion is identified. Colposcopy or Lugol's iodine is used to demarcate the area. Incision is given below the margin of lesion (Fig. 2). Using Allis forceps, appropriate traction is applied to the skin flap. Using blunt scissors, subepithelial plane is developed laterally and superiorly toward vaginal vault (Fig. 3). As the tissue planes get developed, the skin edges are incised around the circumference of the mapped lesion. The incision is completed all around the entire lesion and the dissection continues till the vaginal vault is reached (Fig. 4). Firm traction is now applied to the vaginal skin and the attachment to vaginal vault is cut from right and left, thereby releasing the vaginal specimen. While dissecting in vaginal fornices, care should be taken not to damage the ureters.

If the peritoneal cavity is opened, it can be left open or closed using continuous stitch. Hemostasis is secured and the raw vault is left unsutured and allowed to heal by granulation. Split thickness skin graft can be used to cover denuded vagina, if substantial areas of vagina are excised.

Alternatively peritoneal edges may be sutured to vaginal mucosa by interlocking sutures. Peritoneal defect is sutured high up by purse string suture (Fig. 5).

Vaginal pack and self-retaining catheter is left for 24 hours. Routine postoperative care is given and patient can be discharged next day.

Complications

- *Bleeding*: Vagina is a highly vascular structure and brisk bleeding can occur from sinusoidal or cavernous structures. These should, therefore, be sutured as they are encountered
- *Damage to surrounding viscera*: Damage to surrounding structures including ureter, rectum and anus can occur. While dissecting in vaginal fornices, care should be taken not to damage the ureters

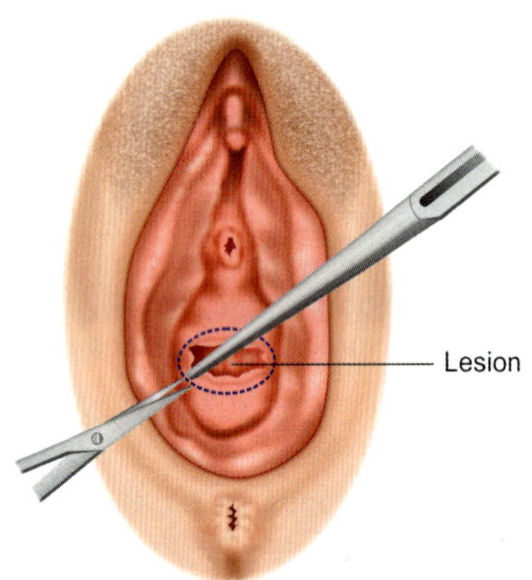

Fig. 2: Vaginal incision

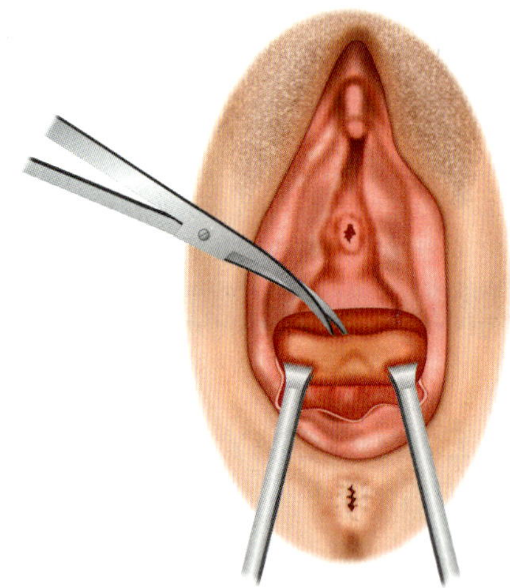

Fig. 3: Dissection of vagina

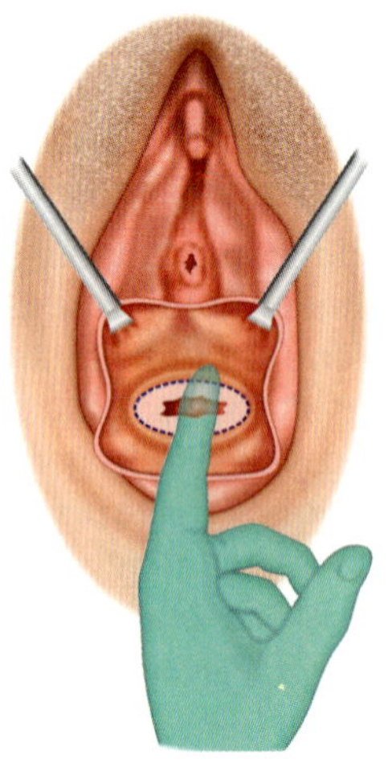

Fig. 4: Raising vaginal flaps

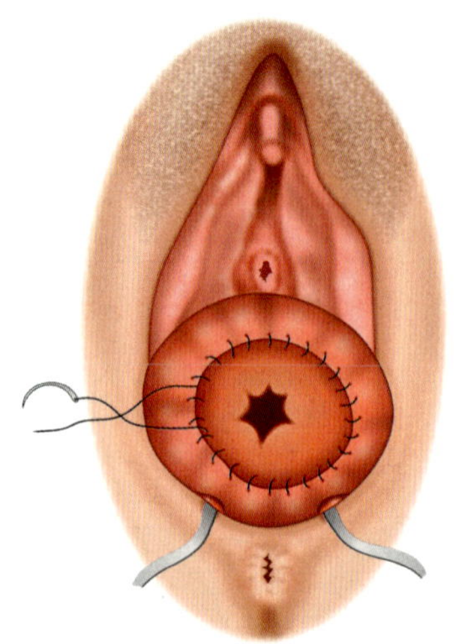

Fig. 5: Peritoneal edge sutured to vaginal mucosa

- Postoperative vaginal stenosis and sexual function morbidity can occur following vaginectomy.

VAGINECTOMY WITH UTERUS IN SITU

It is an integral part of hysterectomy when the surgery is done vaginally for CIN or stage I carcinoma cervix. Operative procedure starts in similar fashion as for vaginectomy. Incision is given posteriorly and is continued anteriorly around the entire circumference of the vagina. Anteriorly, bladder is dissected free of vagina and cervix. Blunt dissection is continued superiorly in submucosal space till the anterior and posterior cul-de-sacs are entered. The vaginal cuff margins are then clamped together below the cervix. Lateral traction is given using these clamps and paravaginal tissue is clamped close to the lateral vaginal wall. Extent of paravaginal tissue removed depends on the type of radical hysterectomy being performed. Hysterectomy is continued as per the indication.

ABDOMINAL VAGINECTOMY

Although vaginectomy is usually performed vaginally, abdominal approach may be appropriate if the lesion can not be fully visualized vaginally or there are extensions with dog ears at the vaginal vault angles in a hysterectomized woman.

Abdomen is opened by vertical incision to gain adequate access. The adhesions from previous surgery, if any, are cleared and the ureters are identified. Peritoneum between the remnant of the round ligament and the infundibulopelvic ligament is incised and retroperitoneal space is entered taking care of the ureters. Uterine artery is identified and divided as lateral as possible and drawn medially thereby exposing the ureteric tunnel. Now transverse incision is given in the peritoneum anteriorly and bladder is separated from the anterior surface of the vagina and pushed down. The insertion of the ureter into bladder is identified, and ureter is traced back to its passage through ureteric tunnel. The roof of the ureteric tunnel is incised thus freeing the ureter, which is now displaced laterally. Transverse incision is made in the peritoneum at the upper posterior part of vagina and is extended laterally on both sides over the uterosacral ligaments. Vagina is separated from the rectum by blunt dissection (Fig. 6). Thus, vagina is released laterally from ureters, anteriorly from bladder and posteriorly from rectum. Uterosacrals and the paracolpos are now held and clamped and the preoperatively decided length of vagina is removed (Fig. 7). The original marker stitch, if placed, is identified to confirm adequate excision of the vagina. If total vaginectomy is required, then the patient is put in lithotomy position and lower vagina is dissected, proceeding upward to meet the abdominal dissection and the entire vagina is removed. Vaginal vault may be left open to drain. A pelvic drain may be put if extensive dissection has been done.

Complications

- Hemorrhage
- Damage to surrounding structures and formation of ureterovaginal and vesicovaginal fistula (VVF)
- Febrile morbidity
- *Bladder dysfunction*: The incidence of significant bladder dysfunction is reported to be high. Disruption

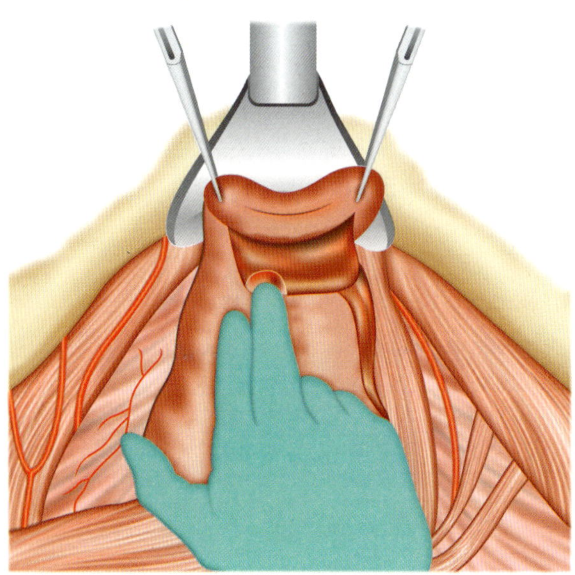

Fig. 6: Dissection of rectovaginal space

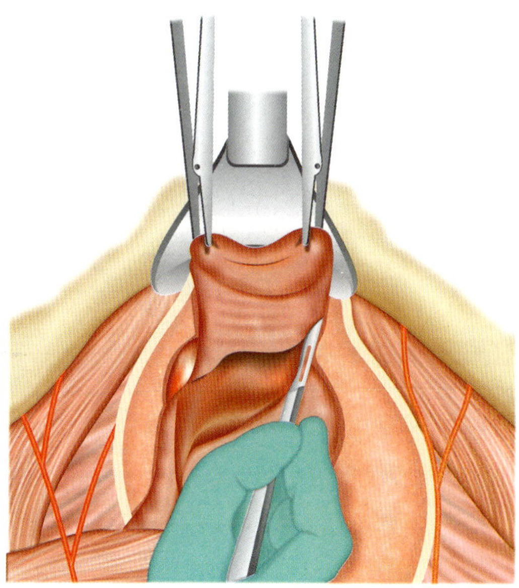

Fig. 7: Removal of vagina

of parasympathetic and sympathetic nerve fibers to bladder and urethra is the main identifiable cause. Preventing over distention and maintaining adequate bladder drainage during postoperative period is important.
- Vaginal stenosis.

VAGINAL STENOTIC RELEASE SURGERY

Congenital stenosis of vagina is rare, more often it occurs as a result of scarring from previous surgery in vagina. Episiotomy, lacerations at the time of delivery, posterior colporrhaphy and anterior colporrhaphy can lead to vaginal scarring and stenosis. Radical surgery or radiation for advanced pelvic malignancies can lead to extensive scarring and nonfunctional vagina. In these cases, specialized reconstructive surgery using different types of musculofascial grafts is required for satisfactory results. Some of the commonly performed surgeries for vaginal strictures for benign conditions are described below.

Perineotomy

Midline perineotomy or episiotomy is performed for release of introital stenosis. A small vertical incision is given at the fourchette (Fig. 8). The vaginal mucosa is sutured transversely to the skin of perineum with 2-0 or 3-0 delayed absorbable suture (Fig. 9). For selected cases of idiopathic vaginismus, division of the bulbospongiosus muscle has been advocated (Fenton's repair).

Incision of the Ring or Ridge

Constriction ring or ridge in the vagina can be incised to relieve the stricture. Vertical incision is given over the ring or ridge which is then closed transversely with 3-0 delayed absorbable suture after achieving hemostasis. More than one incision may be required. Incision at 4 and 8 o' clock avoid damage to urethra, bladder and rectum. It is important to excise the fibrous bands till loose connective tissue is reached. Vaginal incisions may not be stitched and left to heal by granulation.

"Z"-Plasty

For well-circumscribed stricture or stenosis of vagina with not too much of scarring, a Z-plasty operation can be done with good results. A vertical or a transverse Z-plasty can be performed depending on the site of stricture in vagina. A Z-shaped incision with about 2 cm arms and 60° angle between the arms is made (Fig. 10). Length and angle can be varied depending on the size of stricture and requirement of the flaps. Flaps are raised and transposed as shown in Figure 11. Suturing is done with fine absorbable suture after obtaining complete hemostasis (Fig. 12). Vaginal pack and indwelling urinary catheter are left for 24 hours.

A labial cutaneous flap may also be used to cover the defect in the vagina if the constriction is near the introitus. An incision is given at introitus and extended into the vaginal wall. Scar tissue is excised. Incision from introitus is extended anteriorly and laterally to labia minora and then posteriorly over the labia majora in a Z-shaped fashion. The flaps are mobilized. The apex of the labial flap

Fig. 8: Perineotomy incision

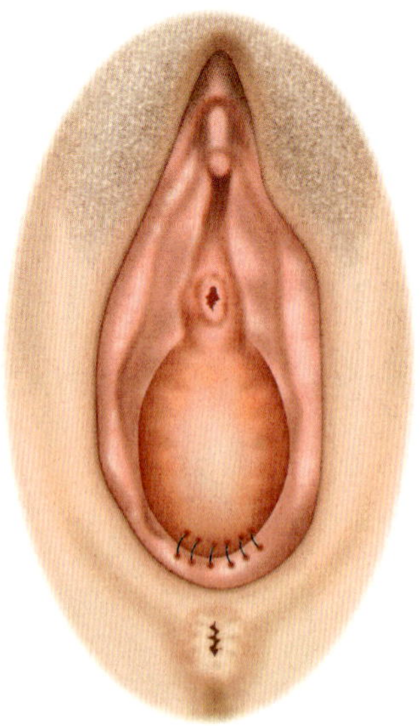

Fig. 9: Transverse suturing of incision

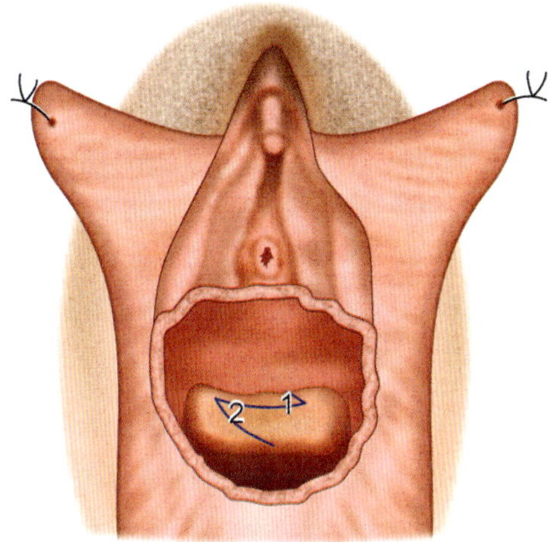

Fig. 10: Z-plasty incision

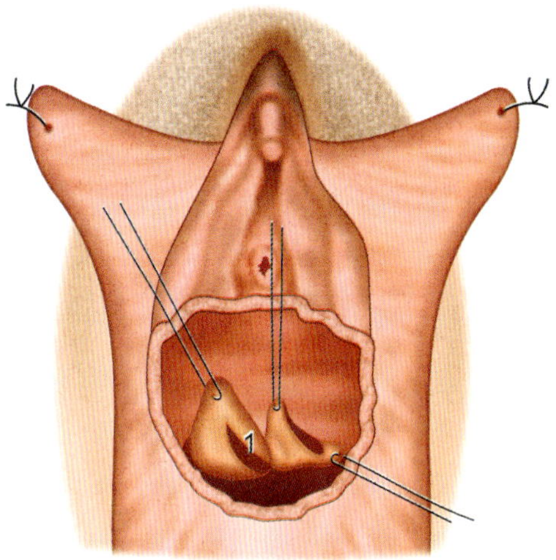

Fig. 11: Z-plasty transposition of flaps

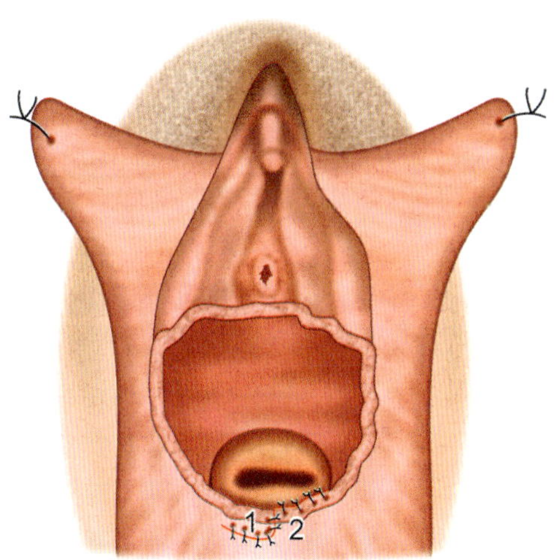

Fig. 12: Suturing of Z-plasty incision

is then stitched to apex of vaginal incision with 3-0 delayed absorbable suture. Rest of the incision is then stitched.

Advantage of Z-plasty operation is that it does not reduce the length or caliber of vagina. Healthy vaginal mucosa, however, is a prerequisite as healthy vaginal flaps are required to cover the defect in vagina.

Vaginal Flap Advancement

In this operation, an incision is made through the vaginal scar and scar tissue is excised. Surrounding healthy vaginal mucosa is mobilized to cover the incision.

It is important to achieve complete hemostasis before suturing is done. Vaginal packing is done. Vaginal shortening may occur with this procedure.

Free Skin Graft

In cases of extensive vaginal scarring, it may not be possible to perform the above mentioned procedures and skin graft may be required. Full thickness graft with epidermis and dermis is preferred as chances of contracture are less as compared to those with split thickness graft. Elliptical graft can be taken from the donor site, e.g. iliac crest and sewn over the vaginal defect formed as the result of excision of large area of scar tissue. The advantage of the free skin graft is that it can be used in any part of the vagina including the proximal areas because the graft is not on the pedicle.

Depending on the extent and location of the stricture, the most suitable procedure among the ones described above can be used to relieve the vaginal stenosis. Success rate of 85% has been reported. As there is high risk of restenosis, vaginal dilatation is recommended after all above procedures.

BIBLIOGRAPHY

1. Baggish MS, Karram MM. Vaginectomy. Atlas of Pelvic Anatomy and Gynecologic Surgery. WB Saunders and Company; 2001. pp. 520-3.
2. Bidus MA, Elkas JC. Cervical and vaginal cancer. Berek and Novak's Gynecology, 14th edition. Lippincott Williams and Wilkins; 2007. pp. 1448.
3. Cardosi RJ, Bomalaski JJ, Hoffman MS. Diagnosis and management of vulvar and vaginal intraepithelial neoplasia. Obstet Gynecol Clin North Am. 2001;28(4): 685-702.
4. Hudson CN, Setchell ME. Surgery of vulva and vestibule. Shaw's Textbook of Operative Gynaecology, 6th edition. BI Churchill Livingstone Pvt Ltd.; 2001. pp. 293.
5. Hurst BS, Rock JA. Iatrogenic and congenital vaginal abnormalities. Atlas of Pelvic Anatomy and Gynecologic Surgery. WB Saunders and Company; 2001. pp. 508.
6. Monaghan JM, Lopes T, Naik R. Operations on the vagina. Bonney's Gynaecological Surgery, 10th edition. Oxford: Blackwell publishing; 2004. pp. 146-61.
7. Vassallo BJ, Karram MM. Management of iatrogenic vaginal constriction. Obstet Gynecol. 2003;102:512-20.

38.3 ANTERIOR COLPORRHAPHY/CYSTOCELE REPAIR

Suchitra Pandit

INTRODUCTION

Anterior vaginal wall prolapse occurs commonly and may coexist with disorders of micturition. Mild anterior vaginal wall prolapse often occurs in parous women but usually presents few problems. As prolapse progresses, symptoms may develop and worsen, and treatment becomes indicated. Following proceeding reviews the anatomy and pathology of anterior vaginal wall prolapse and describes traditional and innovative methods of vaginal prolapse repair.

ANATOMY AND PATHOLOGY

Anterior vaginal wall prolapse (cystocele) is defined as pathologic descent of the anterior vaginal wall and overlying bladder base. According to the International Continence Society standardized terminology for prolapse grading, the term *anterior vaginal wall prolapse* is preferred over *cystocele* (Fig. 1). The pubocervical fascia is trapezoid which is described by Bonney. The fascia or the fibromuscular tissue of the anterior vagina fuses with the perineal membrane distally. It is attached to the pubic ramus and anterior to the ischial spines bilaterally. It is also attached to the cervix or to the vaginal cuff base of the broad ligament and cardinal-uterosacral ligaments. There are four clinically identifiable defects:

1. Laterally, where the pubocervial fascia attaches to the pelvic side wall (paravaginal defect)

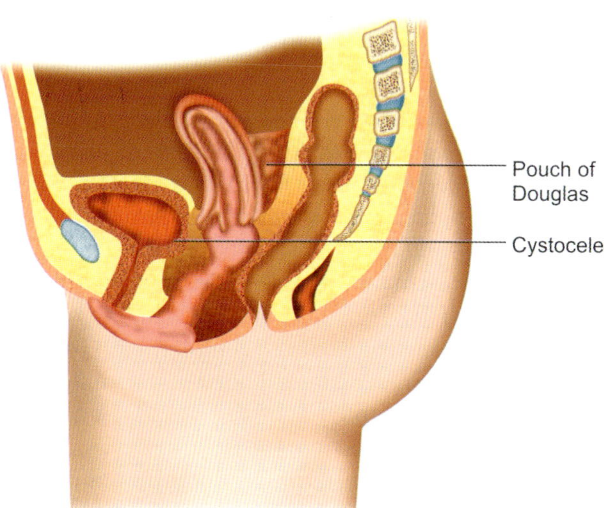

Fig. 1: Cystocele and its anatomy

2. Transversely, in front of the cervix, where the pubocervical fascia blends in the paracervical ring of fibromuscular tissue
3. Centrally, in the area immediately above the vaginal mucosa in between the lateral margins of the vagina (midline defect)
4. Distally, where the urethra perforates the urogenital diaphragm.

THEORIES OF ANTERIOR VAGINAL WALL PROLAPSE

Nichols and Randall described two types of anterior vaginal wall prolapse: (1) distention and (2) displacement. Distention was thought to result from overstretching and attenuation of the anterior vaginal wall, caused by overdistention of the vagina associated with delivery or atrophic changes associated with aging and menopause. The distinguishing physical feature of this type was described as diminished or absent rugal folds. The other type, displacement, was attributed to pathologic detachment or elongation of the anterolateral vaginal supports to the arcus tendineus fasciae pelvis, resulting in descent of the anterior segment with the rugae intact.

Evidence Till Date

In a study of 71 women with anterior vaginal wall prolapse and stress incontinence who underwent retropubic operations, DeLancey described paravaginal defects on the left in 87% of patients and on the right in 89%. The arcus tendineus fasciae pelvis was usually attached to the pubic bone but detached from the ischial spine for a variable distance. The pubococcygeal muscle was visibly abnormal with localized or generalized atrophy in more than half of the women.

DIAGNOSTIC TESTS

- A urinalysis should be performed to evaluate for urinary tract infection if the patient reports any lower urinary tract dysfunction
- If urinary incontinence is present, further diagnostic testing is indicated to determine its cause
- Urodynamic (simple or complex), assessments of filling and voiding function are generally indicated only when symptoms of incontinence or voiding dysfunction are present

- In women with severe prolapse, it is important to check urethral function after the prolapse is repositioned
- Detects residual urine, which involves a timed, measured void followed by urethral catheterization or bladder ultrasonography to measure residual urine volume.

Recent Advances in Pelvic Imaging

Magnetic resonance imaging easily identifies various measurements such as the urethrovesical angle, the descent of the bladder base, the quality of the levator muscles and the relationship between the vagina and its lateral connective tissue attachments. Aronson et al. used an endoluminal surface coil placed in the vagina to image pelvic anatomy with MRI.

PREOPERATIVE PREPARATION

- The patient needs a daily vaginal douche and an antiseptic vaginal pack for a few days prior to surgery. If there is edema then glycerin with acriflavine packs can be used for a couple of days till such time that the edema is cleared
- Estrogen cream applied locally for senile vaginitis should be stopped a few days prior to surgery as increased bleeding during surgery will be undesirable
- The patient should receive a course of antibiotics if urinary infection is present
- Blood should be arranged for the operation
- A vaginal 0.5% betadine douche should be given in the morning of the operation about an hour before the patient leaves the ward. This should be a cleansing douche and should not contain any very strong antiseptic
- Immediately before the patient leaves the room, i.e. her ward bed, the bladder should be emptied completely.

INDICATIONS

- Cystocele grade II and III
- As a combined procedure with vaginal hysterectomy, Fothergill's surgery where cystocele is associated
- In cases where stress urinary incontinence (SUI) is present, appropriate procedures have to be combined.

POSITION, DRAPINGS AND INCISION

- The operation can be done under general, regional or local anesthesia
- The patient is put in lithotomy position with proper padding under the popliteal fossa to prevent undue pressure over the nerves
- Bladder is catheterized
- Crepe bandage over both the legs is preferred in all patients where anterior repair is associated with other major procedures.

Special drapes with leggings are available for vaginal procedures. Or instead one large towel is used to cover the legs and the lower abdomen, while a rectangular towel is used to cover the lower portion of the perineum on one side and the other end is attached to the surgeon.

STEPS OF OPERATION

- Grasp the cervix with a traction forceps and draw it well down until the anterior vaginal wall is practically a level even surface. Liberal infiltration around 80–90 mL with saline adrenaline 1 in 300,000 is done at the portio vaginalis (in cases with hypertension, plain saline infiltration is sufficient)
- When this is determined, an inverted T-shaped incision (Fig. 2A) is made as far from the cervix as possible, keeping in mind always the location of the lower edge of the bladder. The incision must be so placed such that its horizontal part should cover the cervix from 11 o' clock to 2 o' clock position and the vertical incision is carried to within a short distance of the urethral opening
- The anterior vaginal wall is then separated (Fig. 2B), using dissecting scissors, being careful to raise it from the bladder wall without doing any damage. An Allis forceps is placed at this point. Two other Allis forceps are then placed on the margin of the flaps at the base so as to assist in retracting.
- The flaps, which consist of the anterior vaginal wall, are then dissected from the bladder and the dissection is carried well out toward the pubic rami. This is done with a piece of wet gauze over the finger. Great care being exercised so that the wall is not perforated.
- The redundant portion of the vagina is then excised. Allis forceps are reapplied on the lateral margins of the vagina.

"The objective of anterior colporrhaphy is to plicate the layers of vaginal muscularis and adventitia overlying the bladder (pubocervical fascia) or to plicate and reattach the paravaginal tissue in such a way as to reduce the protrusion of the bladder and vagina."

- If SUI is present then simple Kelly's stitch with number 1-0 vicryl (Fig. 3)
- The pubovesicocervical fascia underneath the base of the flaps laterally is approximated in the midline by no. 1/0 vicryl interrupted sutures (Fig. 4). Reducing the cystocele above this repair
- The edges of the vaginal mucosa are approximated with no. 1-0 vicryl, continuous interlocking sutures (Fig. 5). Each suture also takes a thin bite through the fascia over the underlying urinary bladder so as to occlude

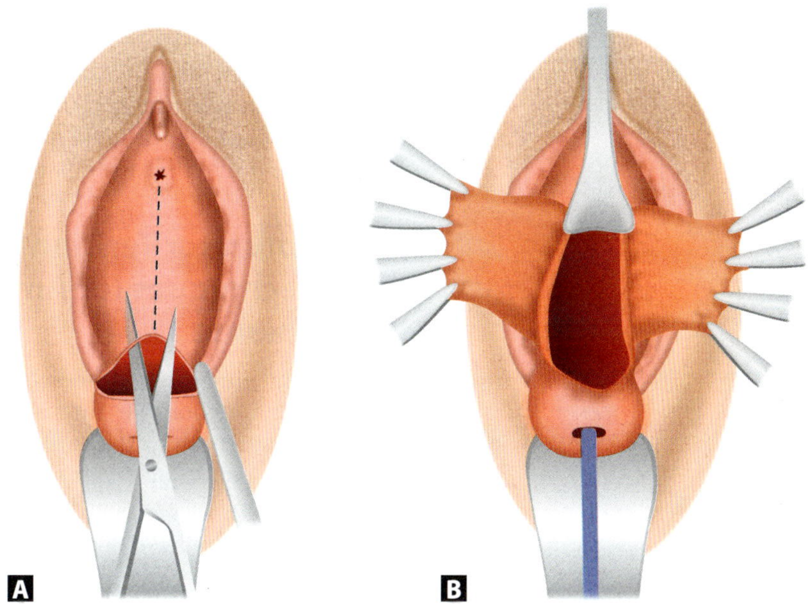

Figs 2A and B: (A) Anterior colporrhaphy excising the pubocervicovaginal fascia; (B) Creating the plane of dissection

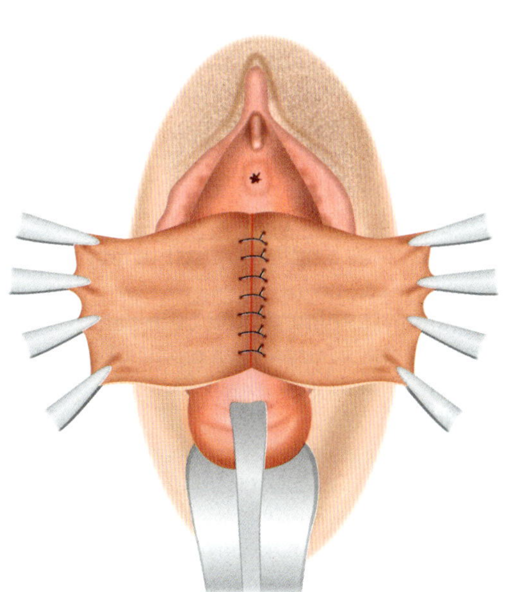

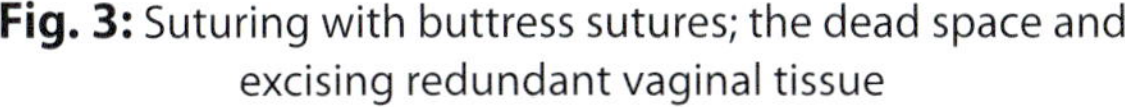

Fig. 3: Suturing with buttress sutures; the dead space and excising redundant vaginal tissue

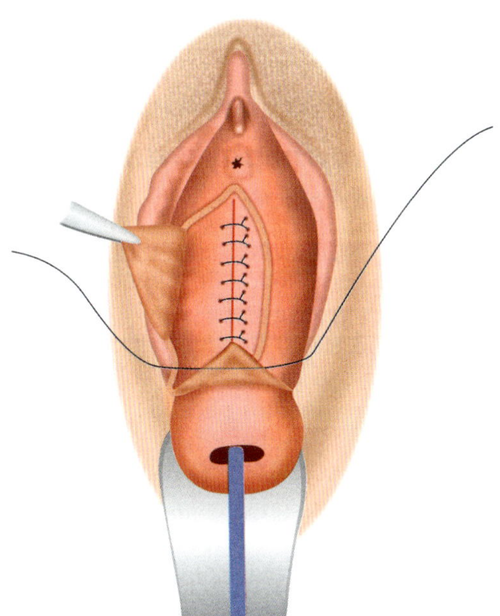

Fig. 4: Longitudinal sutures

the dead space in between. Finally, the transverse incision in the vaginal mucosa is similarly sutured.

POSTOPERATIVE MANAGEMENT

- Appropriate antibiotics, analgesics and IV fluids to be given
- Continuous bladder drainage till 48 hours and in cases where surgery for a large cystocele with SUI is done, then drainage for 5 days is preferable
- If the residual urine volume after removal of the catheter is more than 50 mL, the catheter is passed again and bladder drill taught
- Abstinence from sexual relation for 4 weeks.

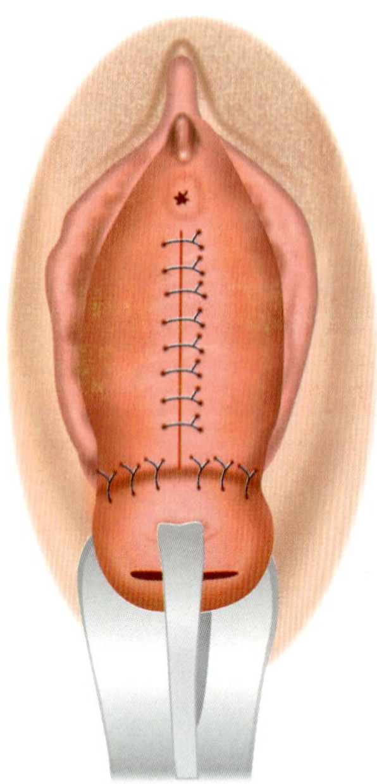

Fig. 5: Longitudinally and transversely suturing the vagina

OTHER INNOVATIVE PROCEDURES

Anterior Colporrhaphy with Graft Augmentation

One modification of anterior colporrhaphy involves use of a prosthetic material to aid in support of the anterior vagina. Other is to place a piece of polyglactin 910 mesh into the fold of imbricated bladder wall below the trigone and apical portion of the anterior colporrhaphy. In a second modification, after the plication sutures have been placed and tied, the prosthetic layer is placed over the stitches and anchored in place at the lateral limit of the previous dissection, using interrupted stitches of no. 2-0 absorbable or nonabsorbable suture. The anchor points are usually at or near the arcus tendineus fasciae pelvis or obturator fascia bilaterally, anti-incontinence operations are often performed at the same time.

Vaginal Paravaginal Repair with and without Graft Augmentation (Figs 6A to D)

The objective of paravaginal defect repair for anterior vaginal wall prolapse is to reattach the detached lateral vagina to its normal place of attachment at the level of the white line or "arcus tendineus fasciae pelvis". This can be done using a vaginal or retropubic approach.

This repair is a three-point closure involving the vaginal epithelium, the vaginal muscularis and endopelvic fascia (pubocervical fascia), and the lateral pelvic side wall at the level of the arcus tendineus fasciae pelvis. Vaginal tissue should not be trimmed until all the stitches are tied. The vaginal flaps are trimmed and closed with a running subcuticular or interlocking delayed absorbable suture.

Transobturator Tension-free Vaginal Mesh Techniques for Anterior Vaginal Wall Prolapse

More recent innovative approaches for anterior vaginal wall repair anchor is an allograft, xenograft, or polypropylene mesh without tension via strips placed through the obturator foramen with a special device (Perigee, American Medical Systems, Minnetonka, MN; and Anterior Prolift, Gynecare, Somerville, NJ). These techniques await safety and efficacy studies but are increasing in use.

INTRAOPERATIVE COMPLICATIONS

- Excessive bleeding may occur, requiring blood transfusion, or a hematoma may develop in the anterior vagina; this is probably more common after vaginal or paravaginal repair than after anterior colporrhaphy. In such cases, a good compression with a roller gauze is preferred postsurgery and vigilant monitoring for hemodynamic instability
- The lumen of the bladder or urethra may be entered in the course of dissection
- Accidental cystotomy should be repaired in layers at the time of the injury. After repair of cystotomy, the bladder is generally drained for 7–14 days to allow adequate healing
- Ureteral damage or obstruction occurs rarely (0–2% incidence) usually with very large cystoceles or with apical prolapse. Ureteric catheterization with repair of bladder in liaison with the urosurgeon is necessary
- Other rare complications include intravesical or urethral suture placement (and associated urologic problems) and fistula, either urethrovaginal or vesicovaginal
- If permanent sutures or mesh material are used in the repair, erosion, draining sinuses, or chronic areas of vaginal granulation tissue can result. The incidence of these complications is unknown but may be as high as 13%
- Urinary tract infections occur commonly, especially with prolonged concurrent catheter use, but other infections (e.g. pelvic or vaginal abscesses) are less common

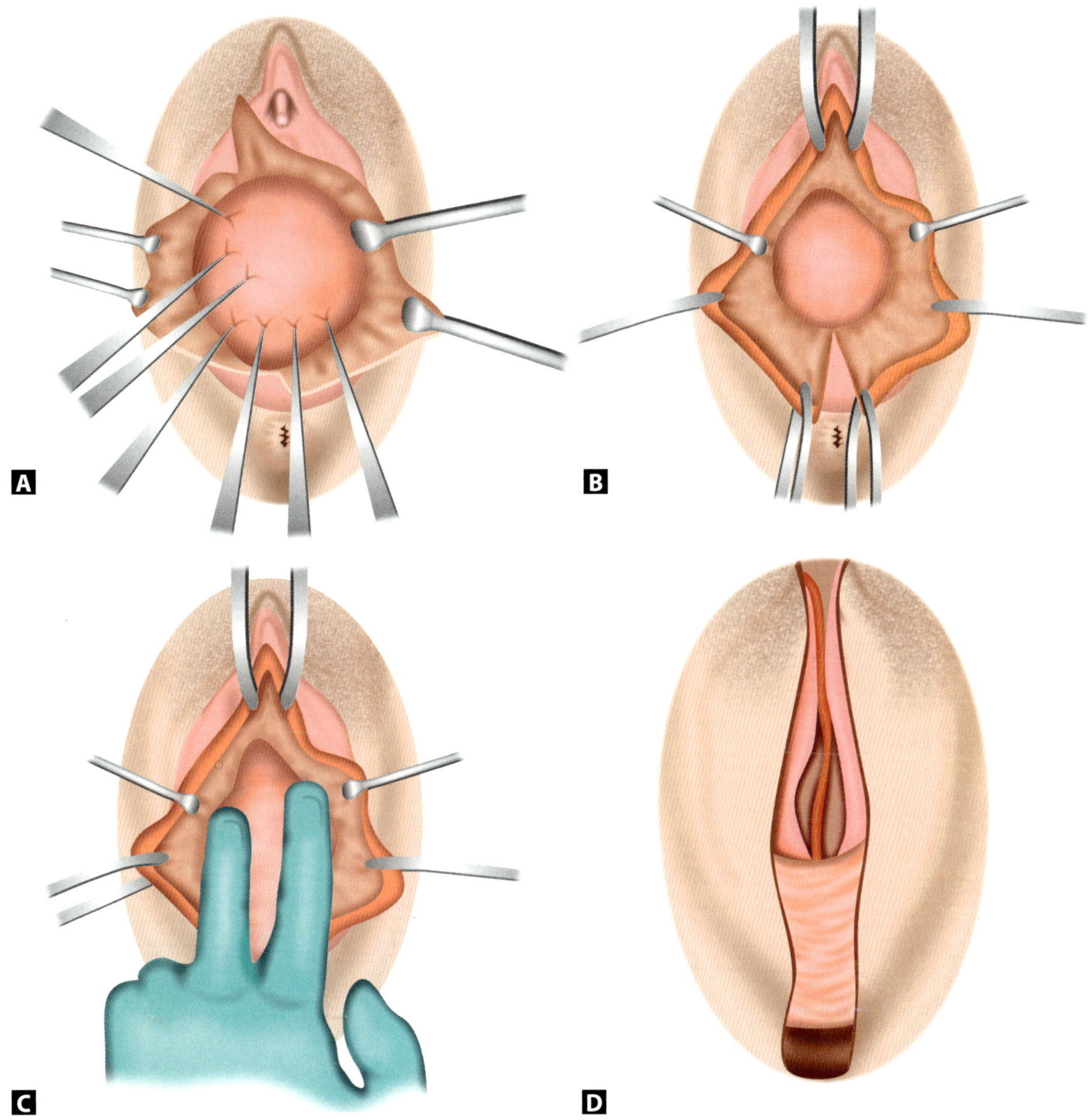

Figs 6A to D: Steps of cystocele repair: (A) Paravaginal sutures on right side to close the paravaginal defect; (B) After tying of sutures restoration of pubocervical septum; (C) Completed anterior vaginal reconstruction and polyester fiber graft; (D) Excessive vaginal tissue has been trimmed

- Voiding difficulty can occur after anterior vaginal wall prolapse repair. The average time to adequate voiding after cystocele repair with suburethral plication is 9 days. This problem may occur more often in women with subclinical preoperative voiding dysfunction. The treatment is bladder drainage or intermittent self-catheterization until spontaneous voiding resumes, usually within 6 weeks
- Sexual function may be positively or negatively affected by vaginal operations for anterior vaginal wall prolapse.

BIBLIOGRAPHY

1. Aronson MP, Bates SM, Jacoby AF, et al. Periurethral and paravaginal anatomy: an endovaginal magnetic resonance imaging study. Am J Obstet Gynecol. 1995;173:1702-8.
2. Baden WF, Walker T. Evaluation of uterovaginal support. In: Baden WF, Walker T (Eds). Surgical Repair of Vaginal Defects. Philadelphia: JB Lippincott; 1992. pp. 51.
3. Bonney V. On diurnal incontinence of urine in women. J Obstet Gynaecol Br Emp. 1923;30:358-65.
4. Bump RC, Mattiasson A, Bo K, et al. The standardization of terminology of female pelvic organ prolapse and pelvic floor dysfunction. Am J Obstet Gynecol. 1996;175:10-7.
5. DeLancey JO. Fascial and muscular abnormalities in women with urethral hypermobility and anterior vaginal wall prolapse. Am J Obstet Gynecol. 2002;187:93-8.
6. Flood CG, Drutz HP, Waja L. Anterior colporrhaphy reinforced with Marlex mesh of the treatment of cystoceles. Int Urogynecol J Pelvic Floor Dysfunct. 1998;9:200-4.
7. Kobak WH, Walters MD, Piedmonte MR. Determinants of voiding after three types of incontinence surgery: a multivariable analysis. Obstet Gynecol. 2001;97:86-91.
8. Kwon CH, Goldberg RP, Koduri S, et al. The use of intraoperative cystoscopy in major vaginal and urogynecologic surgeries. Am J Obstet Gynecol. 2002;187:1466-72.
9. Nichols DH, Randall CL. Vaginal Surgery, 4th edition. Baltimore: Williams and Wilkins; 1996.
10. Richardson AC, Lyon JB, Williams NL. A new look at pelvic relaxation. Am J Obstet Gynecol. 1976;126:568-73.
11. Shull BL, Benn SJ, Kuehl TJ. Surgical management of prolapse of the anterior vaginal segment: an analysis of support defects, operative morbidity, and anatomic outcome. Am J Obstet Gynecol. 1994;171:1429-39.
12. Weber AM, Walters MD. Anterior vaginal prolapse: review of anatomy and techniques of surgical repair. Obstet Gynecol. 1997;89:311-8.
13. White GR. An anatomical operation for the cure of cystocele. Am J Obstet Dis Women Child. 1912;65:286-90.
14. White GR. Cystocele--a radical cure by suturing lateral sulci of vagina to white line of pelvic fascia. 1909. Int Urogynecol J Pelvic Floor Dysfunct. 1997;8(5):288-92.
15. Young SB, Daman JJ, Bony LG. Vaginal paravaginal repair: one-year outcomes. Am J Obstet Gynecol. 2001;185:1360-6.

38.4 LE FORT SURGERY (CLOSURE OF OUTLET)

Barun Sarkar

INTRODUCTION

- This is one of the historical procedures for the surgical treatment of prolapse
- Its relevance in current surgical practice is limited
- The operation was first described by Neugebauer and subsequently perfected by Le Fort.

SURGICAL ANATOMY

In third degree prolapse and procidentia, there is a complete distortion of the anatomy particularly in long-standing cases which are not very rare in our rural population.

It is, therefore, imperative that a thorough preoperative assessment is carried out not only to rule out medical complications associated with this geriatric age group but assess the urinary tract as kinking of the ureters along with hydroureter and hydronephrosis may be associated.

Preoperative Assessment

Vaginal smear, endometrial curettage—both these investigations are mandatory before venturing on the surgical procedure to rule out any pathology, particularly malignancy. Intravenous pyelograms (IVP)—in long-standing cases, because of kinking of the ureter, there is a tendency towards, associated hydroureter and hydronephrosis. Cystoscopy and renal function tests are also essential in longstanding cases to rule out concomitant renal pathology. Routine investigations like hemogram, blood sugar, bleeding time (BT), clotting time (CT) are part of the work-up.

Preoperative Treatment

Treatment of any existing medical conditions like respiratory disease, cardiac disease, hypertension, diabetes or associated local infection goes a long way in enhancing the success of the operation.

Initial wrapping and packing of uterus and of the prolapsed organ with glycerin and acriflavine to reduce the edema thus facilitating reposition of the prolapsed uterus. Moreover, there is invariably associated decubitus ulcer which only heals after reposition of the uterus for 2–3 weeks.

The surgery should be carried out only after the decubitus ulcer has healed.

Indications

The indications for the procedure are limited in current surgical practice. It is indicated in elderly widows, elderly couples not interested in sexual intercourse or patients who are extremely debilitated and therefore, unable to tolerate any type of general anesthesia and prolonged surgery. Regardless of the age, vaginal closure should be done only after counseling the patient regarding total cessation of sexual life.

Anesthesia

- Spinal is preferred
- Local can be used in selected cases.

SURGICAL STEPS

Principle: The basic idea is to create two rectangular areas on the anterior and posterior vaginal walls and approximating them to effect vaginal closure thus preventing descent of the cervix.

- Position the patient in lithotomy
- Part is painted and draped
- The anterior lip of the cervix is held with a vulsellum
- The area to be denuded anteriorly is delineated by a knife (Fig. 1A)
- The upper limit of the incision is 5 cm below the uretheral meatus, while the lower limit is 2 cm from the tip of the cervix
- By a combination of sharp and blunt dissection, the mucosal strip is removed (Fig. 1B)
- A similar procedure to remove a rectangular piece of the same size is carried out on the posterior vaginal mucosa (Fig. 1C)
- The mucosal edges are approximated transversely with interrupted sutures using 1-0 vicryl on a round body eyeless needle (Fig. 1D)
- The denuded areas of the anterior and posterior vaginal mucosa are approximated with interrupted sutures of 1-0 vicryl. The suturing starts at the top (Figs 1E to G)
- In the end, the mucosal edges are approximated using interrupted sutures of 1-0 vicryl (Fig. 1H)

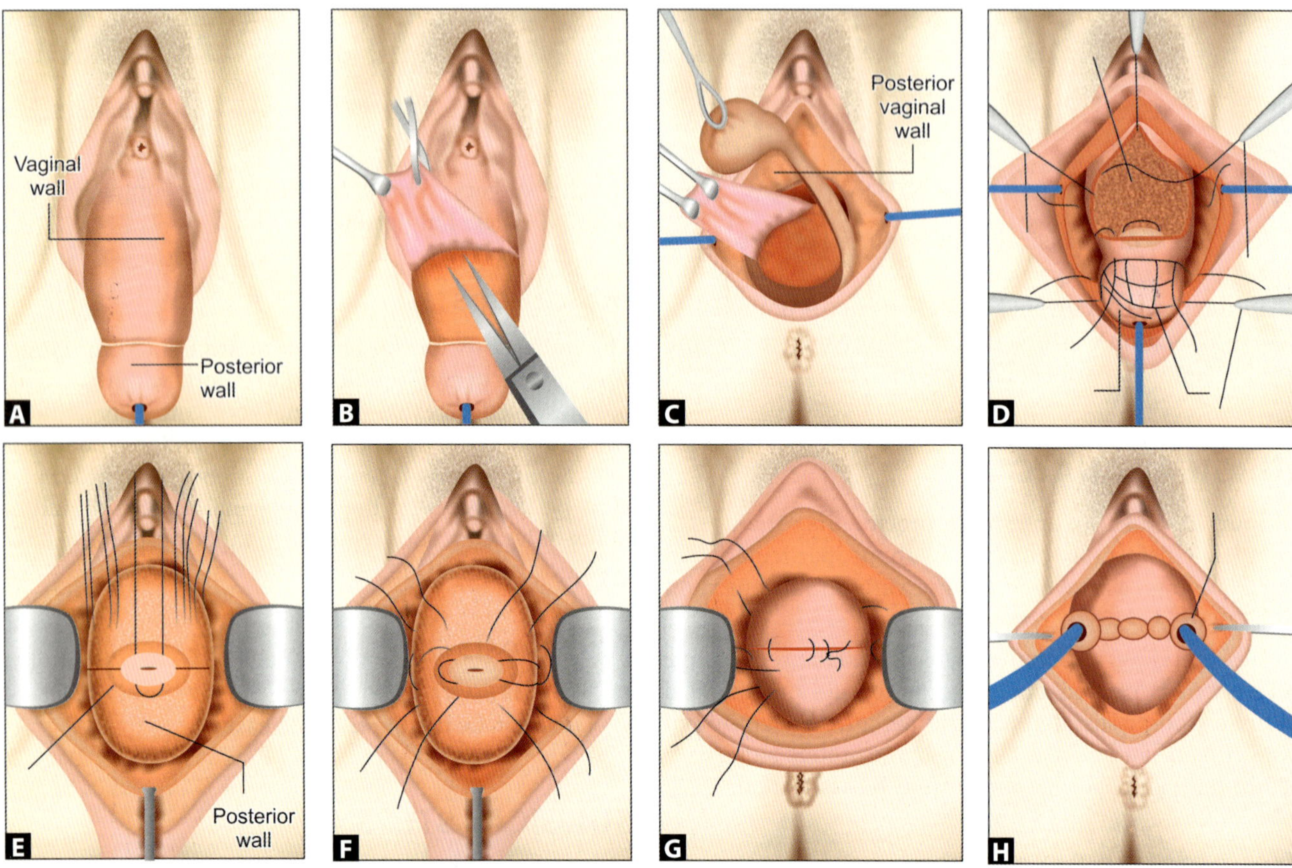

Figs 1A to H: Steps of Le Fort operations

- Care is taken to leave two lateral mucosa lined tunnels as shown by artery forceps (Fig. 1H).

COMPLICATIONS

- Bladder, uretheral injury
- Rectal injury
- Urinary incontinence—it may result due to pull of the posterior vaginal wall on the anterior vaginal wall which is intimately attached to the trigone and urethra. Ridley has reported an incidence of 24% partial urinary incontinence after this procedure
- Mucocolpos—secretions may collect in the upper part of the vagina if the drainage is inadequate
- Vaginal or cervical carcinoma, if it occurs would be detected late.

GOODALL-POWER MODIFICATION OF LE FORT OPERATION

Goodall and Power created two triangular denuded areas on the anterior and posterior vaginal walls in the upper part. The base of the triangles was above and the apices below. This resulted in partial vaginal closure thus allowing sexual intercourse.

CONCLUSION

In the third world countries where patients may present with long-standing neglected procidentia, there exists a small though definite need for this procedure.

BIBLIOGRAPHY

1 Baldy JM. The treatment of uterine displacements. Surg Gynecol Obstet. 1908;8:421.

2 Emge LA, Durfee RB. Pelvic organ prolapse: four thousand years of treatment. Clin Obstet Gynecol. 1966;9:997-1032.

3 Goodall JR, Power RMH. A modification of the Le Fort operation for increasing its scope. Am J Obstet Gynecol. 1937;34:968-76.

38.5 RECTOVAGINAL/URETHROVAGINAL FISTULA REPAIR

Swaraj Batra, S Singh

INTRODUCTION

The passage of flatus and stool per vagina are symptoms of a rectovaginal fistula and can be extremely distressing, painful and socially awkward for the patient. It is difficult to determine the true incidence but obstetrics trauma accounts for majority of them. There are numerous surgical techniques described but the anatomic location and size of fistula, as well as presence of infection, inflammation and history of radiation is important factor in choosing treatment modality.

SURGICAL ANATOMY

The anorectal region is composed of both visceral and somatic components. The visceral components include the rectum, internal anal sphincter and lining of upper part of the anal canal.

Voluntary or somatic components are the epithelium of the lower part of the anal canal as well as the striated muscles of the pelvic floor and the external anal sphincter. The rectal mucosa consists of mucous secretory columnar goblet cells which invaginate to form tubular glands. The mucosa is surrounded by a muscularis mucosa and inner layer of circular smooth muscle. This circular muscle layer thickens distally to become internal anal sphincter. The outer longitudinal layer of smooth muscle transitions distally into fibrous fascicles that travel between the internal and external anal sphincter and insert into perianal skin anchoring the sphincter complex and creating the puckering effect (Figs 1 and 2). The anal canal in female is 2.5-4 cm in length. The main blood supply to the rectum and anal canal is from the branches of superior and inferior hemorrhoidal arteries, inferior rectal branches of the pudendal nerve (S2 to S4) supply the external sphincter; they also provide the sensory supply to the area which extends 1-2 cm above pectinate line.

ETIOLOGY

- Congenital
- Acquired
  - Obstetric injury: Fourth degree tear; breakdown/infection of repair of episiotomy, forceps injury
  - Trauma: Operative—hysterectomy, vaginoplasty, molds, low anterior resection, anorectal instrumentation, coital injury. Penetrating/blunt accidents— rectal/vaginal lacerations, fecal impaction
  - Inflammation and infection: Inflammatory bowel disease, ulcerative colitis, Crohn's disease, endometriosis, drug reaction, chemical burns, crypoglandular abscess, Bartholin's gland infection, diverticulitis, tuberculosis, amebiasis, schistosomiasis, lymphogranuloma venereum
  - Radiation and malignancy: Pelvic—Rectum, anus, vagina, perineum, metastatic deposits, leukemia.

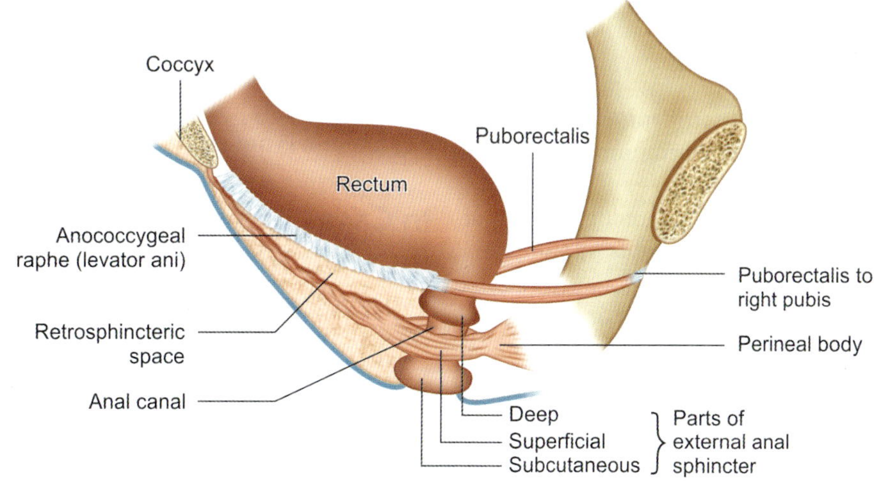

Fig. 1: Puborectalis and the external anal sphincter from the right. The three traditional parts of the sphincter are shown, but they merge with one another and the deep part is continuous with the puborectalis part of levator ani

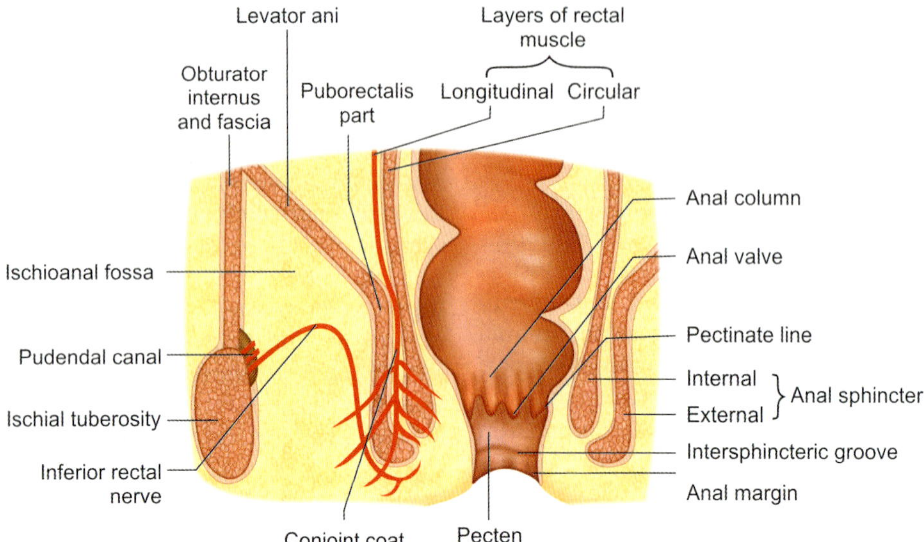

Fig. 2: Coronal section of the anal canal and the right ischioanal (ischiorectal) fossa. The inferior rectal nerve is shown leaving the pudendal nerve in the pudendal canal; the corresponding vessels pursue a similar course across the fossa

CLASSIFICATION

There are various classifications.

1. Location:
   a. *Low*: Vaginal opening near posterior fourchette.
   b. *Mid*: From the level of the cervix to just superior to the posterior fourchette.
   c. *High*: Fistula in the area of posterior fornix, it is above the level of puborectalis.
2. Complexity:
   a. Simple
   b. Complex

Obstetric fistula and following cryptogenic abscess are often low, simple and small.

Crohn's disease, radiation or diverticulitis cause typically high and complex fistulas.

Symptoms

Rectovaginal fistula caused by obstetric trauma can occur immediately after delivery but more commonly appears 7–10 days postpartum.

- Most women complaint of foul-smelling vaginal drainage or passage of involuntary flatus or stool per-vaginum
- It may be associated with perineal sepsis or proctitis in women with inflammatory bowel disease
- More serious fecal incontinence may be present in cases of sphincteric tears and defects.

Preoperative Assessment and Preparation

- A complete and detailed history should be elicited from the patient
- *Physical examination*: The location and size of the fistula and number of openings can be identified. The route of fistula may be outlined by the passage of thin probe from the vagina through the fistulous tract into the anal or rectal canal, examining finger should also be placed in the rectum. The contraction of the puborectalis and external anal sphincter should be evaluated for competency. The perineal body and sphincteric defects can be palpated as thin, with minimal or no motion during squeeze efforts
- Fistula caused by radiation or patient with history of carcinoma should have a biopsy performed to rule out carcinoma
- Proctosigmoidoscopy and anoscopy can be used to assess the underlying pathology
- *High rectovaginal fistula*: A proctoscopic and possibly a flexible sigmoidoscopic examination will be needed to plan treatment.

Occasionally a water soluble contrast enema or vaginogram is necessary (Fig. 3).

In Cases of Suspected Fistula (but Not Identified)

- Methylene blue enema may be given to the patient after insertion of a vaginal tampon. Removal of tampon after 10–15 minutes of waiting period may show evidence of blue dye at the tip of tampon, thus confirming the diagnosis
- With a patient in slight Trendelenburg position with a size 20 Foley urinary catheter, a 5 mL balloon is placed in anal canal and air is instilled through the catheter while the water-filled or soap-covered vagina is observed for any escape of air bubbles.

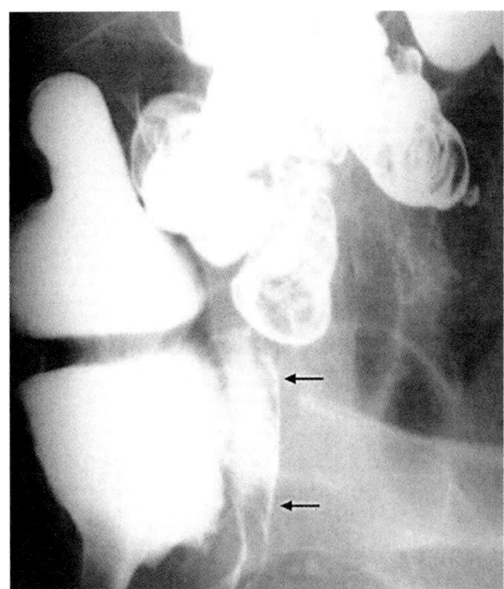

Fig. 3: Photograph of Barium enema showing spill into vagina suggestive of rectovaginal fistula

Management

Various factors determine the route, timing and approach of repair:

- Number and cause of fistula
- Location and accessibility
- Status of the anal sphincter
- Condition of vaginal and anal tissues.

Approach

- Transvaginal—performed by gynecologist
- Transanal—performed by rectal surgeons
- Transabdominal—performed for complex and high fistulas.

Timing

- *Early repair*: The practice has been abandoned as there are high chances of failure due to tissue edema and infection. So it is better to wait at least 8 weeks before any surgical intervention is done to allow surrounding inflammation to resolve. Venkatesh et al. report 50% of small fistulas may heal without operative intervention during the first 6–8 weeks postpartum
- *Delayed repair*: This is the preferred timing for repair especially in cancer cases after completing the treatment and excluding the local disease by biopsy.

Preparation of the Patient

1. General condition of the patient should be improved with correction of anemia, nutritional status. Perineal infection and proctitis should be treated with antibiotics and steroids.
2. A good mechanical bowel preparation is essential and it should be preceded by a short period of residue reduction by starting low residue diet with bowel wash for 3 days prior to surgery, in some cases parenteral nutrition may be indicated.
3. Fecal diversion may be indicated for high, difficult or recurrent fistula but bowel preparation is still required.

Routes of Repair

Abdominal repair: It is carried out under general anesthesia or regional block.

It is done in two conditions:

1. High rectovaginal fistula
2. High rectovaginal fistula with distal circumferential rectal loss.

Vaginal repairs: It is carried out under general anesthesia regional block with patient in lithotomy position.

High Fistula

It can be repaired vaginally if:

- It is nonadherent to the bone
- Reasonable access is possible from below.

Dissection should be done between the posterior vaginal wall and rectum till POD is reached. Peritoneum covered rectum is mobilized, fistula is closed. POD is closed by stitching peritoneum anterior to rectum to posterior of the cervix. Vagina may not be closed as squamous metaplasia later occurs.

Midvaginal Fistula

1. Fistula margin is incised until clear of scar tissue preserving as much as possible of adjacent visceral wall. Vaginal wall is separated from rectum.
2. Rectum may be elevated by a finger in the rectum. A rectum is closed in two layers by starting above the apex using vicryl 3-0 on atraumatic needle. In first layer submucosa and muscularis is taken and second layer is taken including the perirectal fascia and muscularis in continuous/interrupted Lembert sutures
3. Vagina is closed with similar vicryl 3-0 sutures in continuous/interrupted sutures. Puborectalis if exposed in lower fistula should be stitched in center.

In these cases, flap repair is done (Figs 4 to 9).

Low Fistula

It is usually associated with incomplete healing of perineal laceration and with sphincter damage. Under

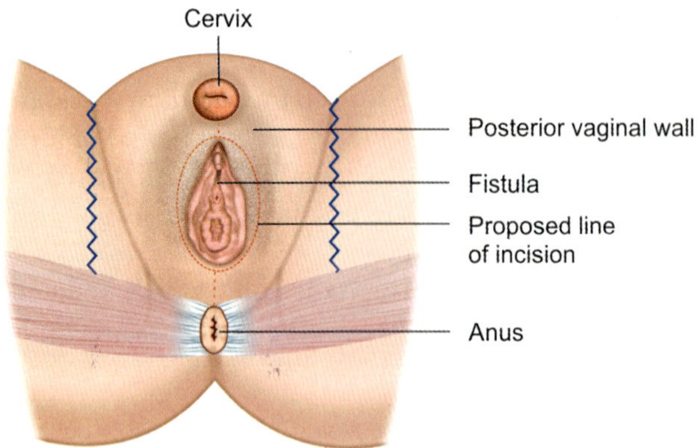

Fig. 4: Incision is given around the fistulous tract and extended upward and downward

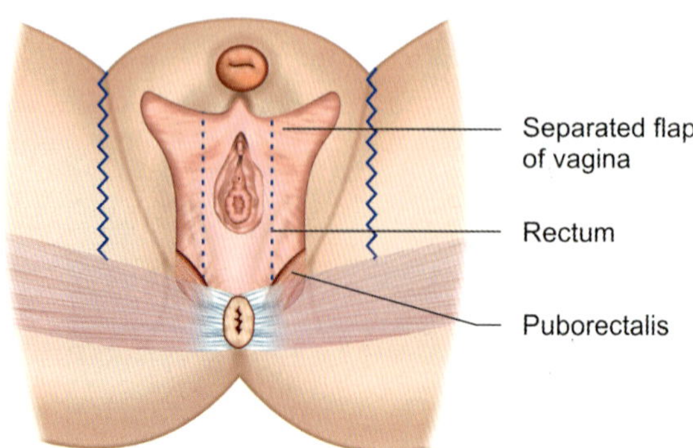

Fig. 5: Mobilization of posterior vaginal wall from anterior wall of rectum. Puborectalis visualized

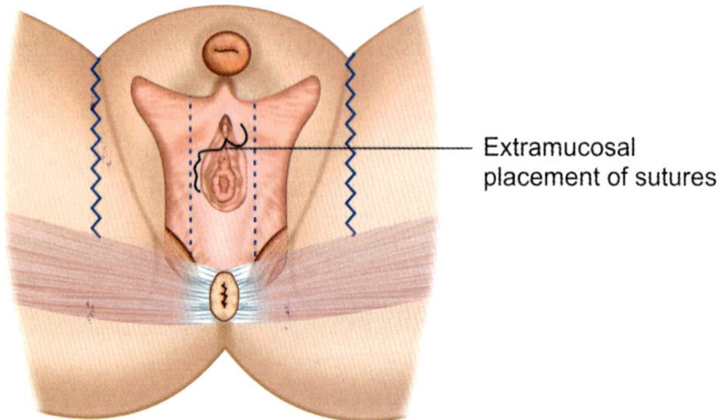

Fig. 6: First layer suture including muscularis and submucosa

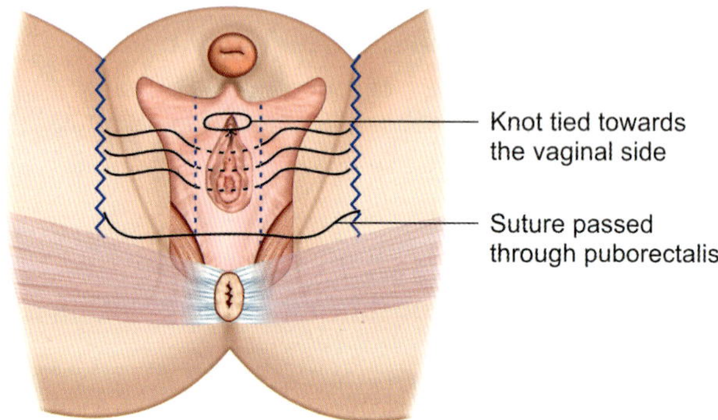

Fig. 7: First layer continued

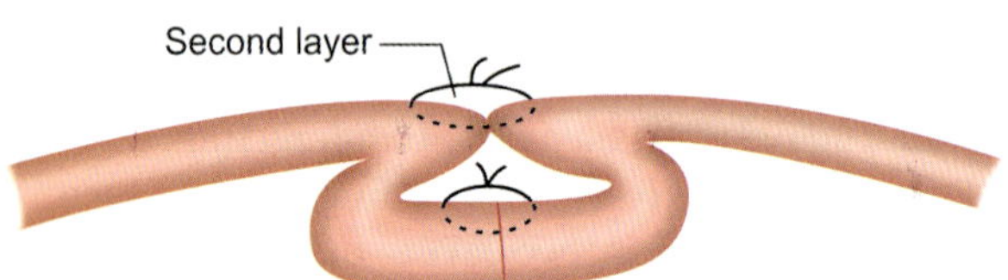

Fig. 8: Second layer in muscularis and prerectal fascia inverting first layer

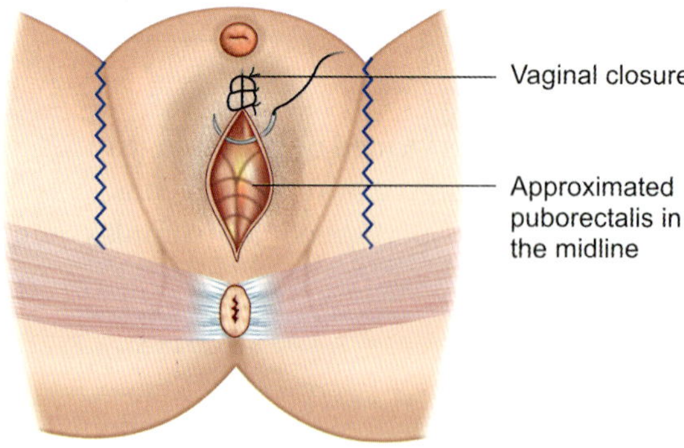

Fig. 9: Converting low fistula into fourth degree perineal tear

such circumstances, the bridge of scar tissue should be incised and cut back to healthy tissue on either side to form complete perineal tear and repair is done as for complete perineal tear. In this type of deficiency, rectum and anus are separated from vagina, and anal sphincter is exposed by taking incision posteriorly over it. After closure of rectum and anus, external sphincter and levator ani are stitched (Figs 10 and 11).

Radiation Fistula

The fistula must be reachable by a finger inserted per rectum. If this is not so, fecal loss is at the apex of sigmoid loop and colpocleisis should not carried out.

Colpocleisis with interposition graft (gracilis or bulbospongiosis) is the treatment of choice for irradiated rectovaginal fistula.

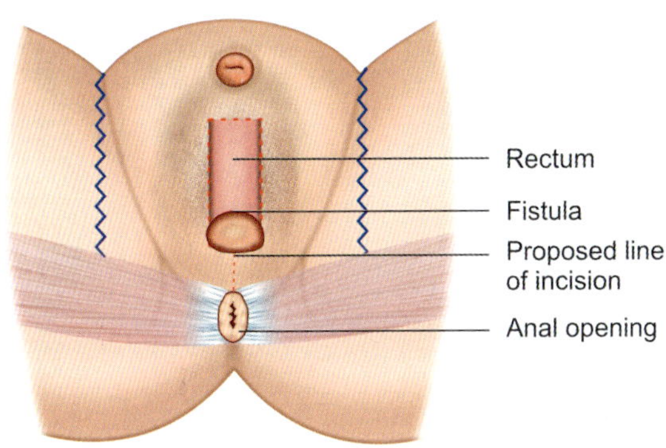

Fig. 10: Approximation of puborectalis followed by vaginal closure

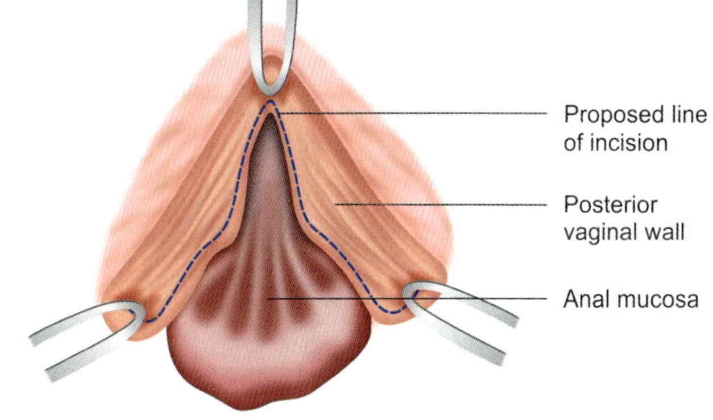

Fig. 11: Complete perineal tear

Gracilis muscle transposition has been used with good results for complicated fisulas.

Postoperative Care

- Any anesthesia related complication should be monitored
- Adequate pain relief should be provided otherwise pain increases intraluminal tension and may strain sutures
- For complete perineal tear repair cases sterile pad should be provided for first 3 days and perineal care should be done for 1 week
- Patient is kept nil per orally for first day followed by clear fluids on second day with stools softener from second night onward for 1 week. Soft diet is started from 3rd day for 1 week
- Constipation and early purging should be avoided.

Complications

Immediate

- *Infection*: Febrile morbidity which can further progress to gram-negative septicemia, and mortality
- *Inadvertent fistula enlargement/formation of false passage*: This can occur during separation of vaginal mucosa from rectum, when fresh injury can be caused to rectal mucosa
- *Hemorrhage*: It arises, if dissection is carried out in the wrong tissue plane or in case where early repair has been under taken, mostly due to unresolved tissue edema and inflammation.

Delayed

- *Vaginal stricture*: Can result after repair of large fistula with considerable reduction in vaginal bore with subsequent impact on coital ability
- *Failed repair*: Usually occurs in large fistula, radiation fistula or nonrecognition of intrinsic pathology (Crohn's disease).

URETHROVAGINAL FISTULA

Surgical Anatomy

The female urethra is 4 cm long and 6 mm in diameter. It begins at the internal urethral orifice at the neck of the urinary bladder roughly 5 cm behind the middle of the pubic symphysis. It runs downward and forward embedded in the anterior wall of the vagina, traverses the urogenital diaphragm and ends at the external urethral orifice in the vestibule. The urethra normally is supported by the endopelvic fascia, which attaches to the pelvic side walls along the arcus tendineus fascia; it permits the urethra to be compressed closed during episodes of increased intra-abdominal pressure. Levator ani provides muscular component to urethral support (Fig. 12). When these are damaged, urethral hypermobility results which presents as stress incontinence. Automatic (sympathetic) innervation of the urethra is mediated by alpha-adrenergic receptor in urethra and bladder neck, proximal part is supplied by the inferior vesical artery and distal part by branch of internal pudendal artery.

They are uncommon and unusually occur:

- After prolonged or obstructed labor
- Postsurgery for:
  - Urethral diverticulum
  - Anterior vaginal wall prolapse or urinary incontinence, e.g. vaginal slings and suspension procedures
- Following radiotherapy
- Difficult operative vaginal delivery
- Prolonged indwelling transurethral catheter or vaginal mold after vaginoplasty.

Fistula results due to tissue ischemia, radiation necrosis and pressure necrosis.

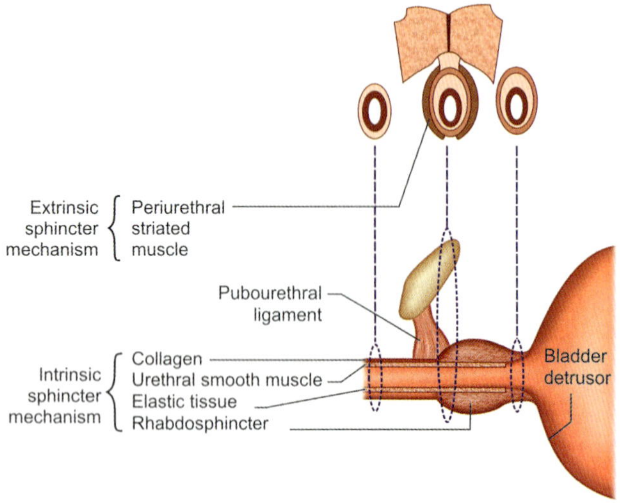

Fig. 12: The bladder neck and urethra showing the components of the urethral sphincter mechanism

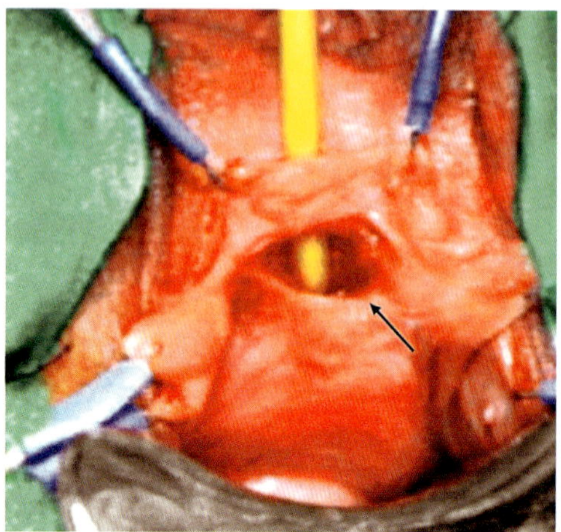

Fig. 13: Urethrovaginal fistula

Symptoms

Depending on the location of fistula patient may present with variety of complaints.

Distal Fistula

- May be asymptomatic
- Spraying of urine/abnormal urinary stream.

Midurethral Fistula

- Asymptomatic
- Stress incontinence
- Recurrent cystitis.

Proximal Urethra/Bladder Neck

- Continuous dribbling of urine similar to VVF.

Examination

It should be performed with good light, adequate exposure. A malleable probe per urethra is inserted and it can be directly observed coming through vagina in per speculum examination (Fig. 13).

Investigations

Routine investigations including renal function test, routine urine and culture should be done in all cases prior to surgery.

Dye Test

It is done to exclude the associated ureteric and bladder fistula.

Inference

- If dye stains highest swab near the vaginal apex, small VVF is present. If it is wet with urine with no blue dye then leakage from ureterovaginal fistula is suspected
- If distal swab near the vaginal introitus is blue, urethral incontinence is present. Stress incontinence should be excluded.

Urethrocystoscopy

It should be done in all cases to rule out associated bladder fistula and its relation to the ureteric orifice, bladder calculi, location and size of fistula.

Ultrasonography of Kidney, Ureter and Bladder

It demonstrates calyceal dilatation or any back pressure changes if associated.

Cystourethrogram

It can identify the site and number (Fig. 14).

Preoperative Preparation

Once investigations have confirmed both the diagnosis and location of fistula, the following factors should be taken into consideration:

- *Tissue condition*: Tissue healing and successful repair is affected by prior irradiation, concomitant malignant disease, infection, and gross scarring (due to previous surgery). Biopsy may be necessary
- *Tissue loss*: Partial or complete urethral loss will affect the closure without tension

- *Presence of double fistula*: It may be associated with vesicovaginal, urethrovaginal and intestinal fistula, repair may be taken up simultaneously or one by one
- *Scar formation*: Previous route of surgery and previous type of surgery will affect the present successful repair
- *Intercurrent infections*: They include vulval urinary excoriation and urinary tract infection. These must be identified and treated.

Therapeutic Options

No treatment: If the patient is asymptomatic or it is a small fistula, it may heal on its own.

Surgical Intervention

Timing of intervention:

- A clean traumatic fistula may be repaired almost at once, if recognized within 48 hours
- Delay of preferably 3–6 months should be done in:
  - Postpartum—due to tissue necrosis and edema
  - Prior radiation
  - Infection
  - Previous failed repair.

Repair is carried out under general/regional anesthesia.

Low Fistula

It can only be treated by vaginal approach as it is hidden from the view of an abdominal operator by the arch of the inferior pubic rami.

Symmonds Technique (Figs 15 to 18)

- The anterior vaginal wall is incised and extending around the margins of the urethral defect
- Scar tissue is excised
- The urethral margin is a mobilized enough to provide a tension-free closure over a 12 Foley catheter with interrupted delayed absorbable sutures with 3-0, 4-0 vicryl
- Mobilized paraurethral fascia is sutured on each side of total length of the urethra with no. 4-0 vicryl
- Vaginal mucosa is closed without tension with interrupted or continuous vicryl 3-0.

Repair of Segmental Loss of Urethra (Figs 19 to 21)

In case of segmental loss of urethra, the lower urethral opening towards the fistula may get obliterated. It should be checked by passing sound through the external meatus and incision is given on the tip of the sound to open it.

Urethra is separated from vaginal wall by giving longitudinal incision in vagina and separating the vaginal flaps.

The upper and lower segment of urethra should be mobilized. Posterior wall with posterior wall of urethra and anterior wall with anterior wall are stitched with no. 3-0 vicryl.

Paraurethral fascia is stitched over it before closing the vagina (Figs 17 and 18).

Invariably sphincter loss is always present so bladder buttressing sutures should always be taken.

Total/Partial Urethral Loss

In these cases, urethral reconstruction is carried out (Figs 22 to 28).

Fig. 14: Cystourethrogram showing urethrovaginal fistula

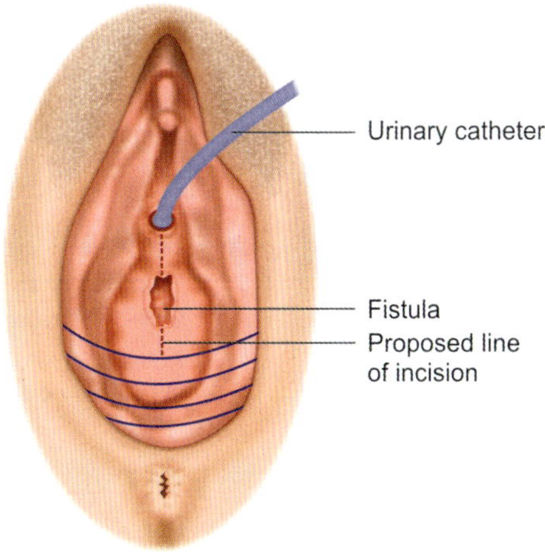

Fig. 15: Fistulous tract mobilized from vagina

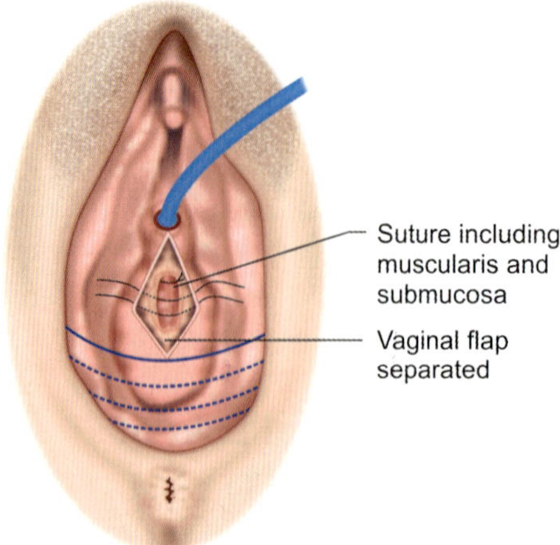

Fig. 16: First layer of fistula closure

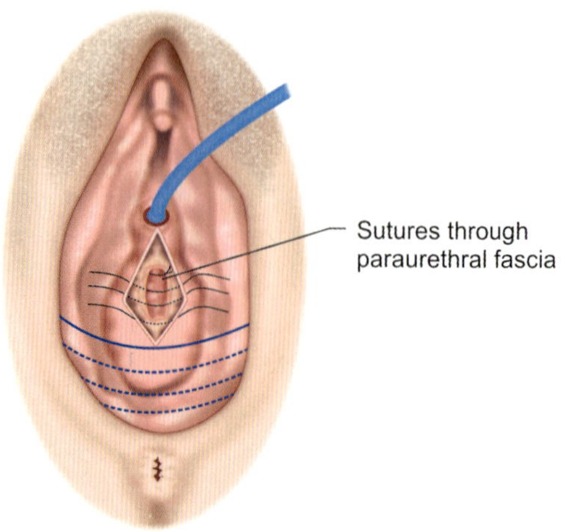

Fig. 17: Second layer of fistula closure

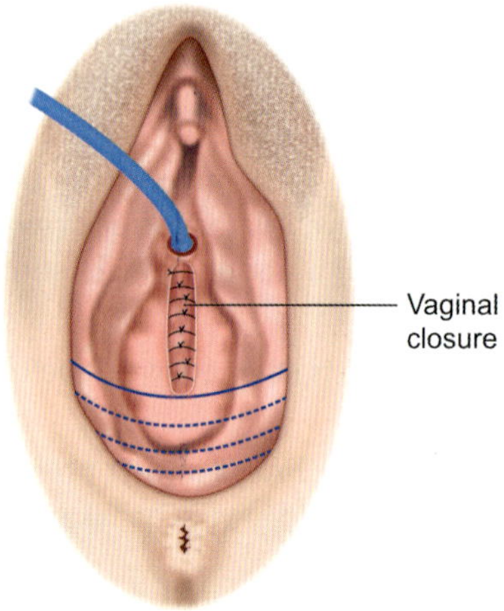

Fig. 18: Repair completed with vaginal closure and bladder neck plication

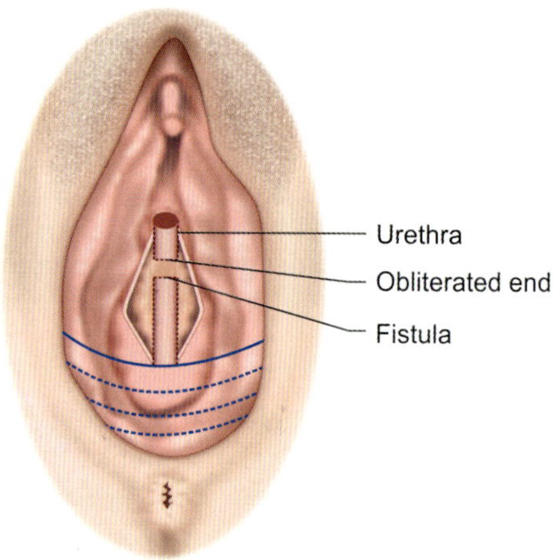

Fig. 19: Segmental loss of urethra with distal segment obliterated. Sutures for plication of bladder neck, scalpel, bladder sound, proposed line of incision

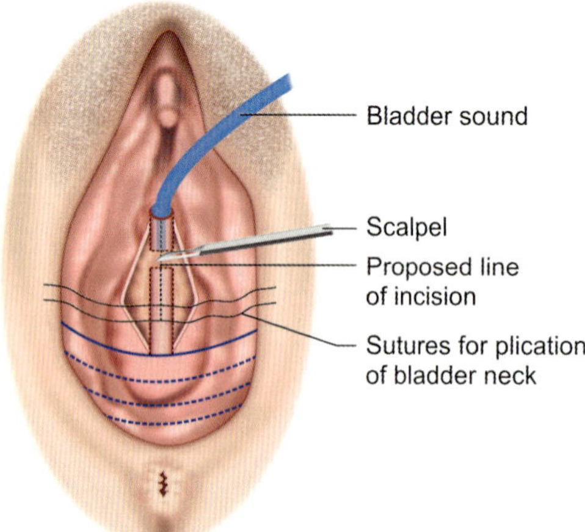

Fig. 20: Obliterated end made prominent by bladder sound and incision given on it. Anterior vaginal wall separated, reconstructed urethra, urinary catheter

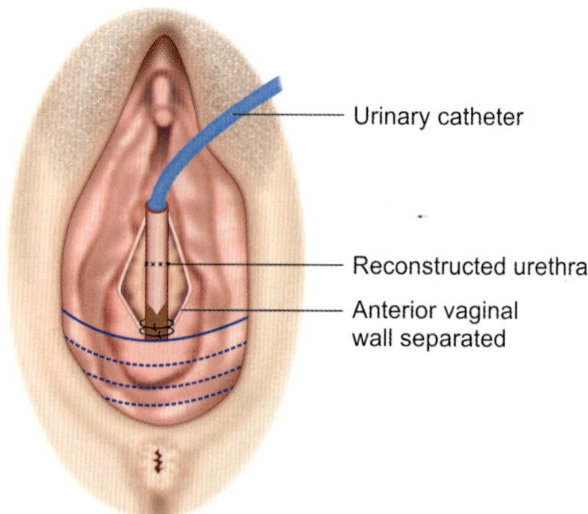

Fig. 21: Urethral segments reunited. Bladder plication sutures taken

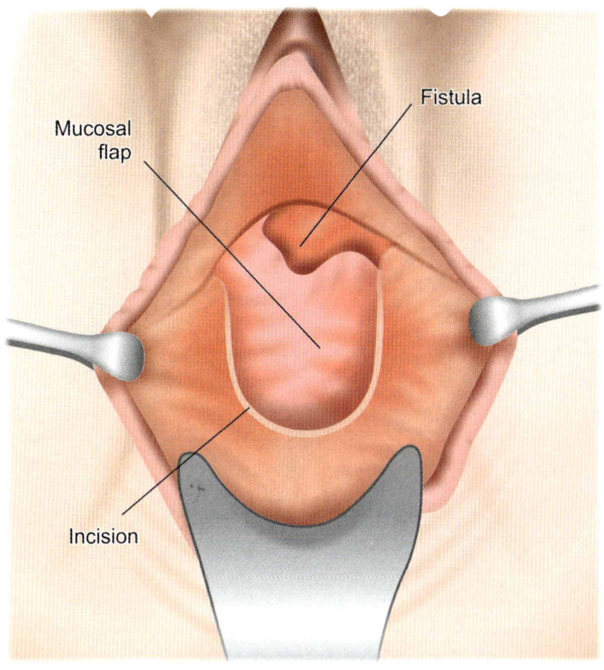

Fig. 22: A U-shaped incision is made through the vaginal epithelium

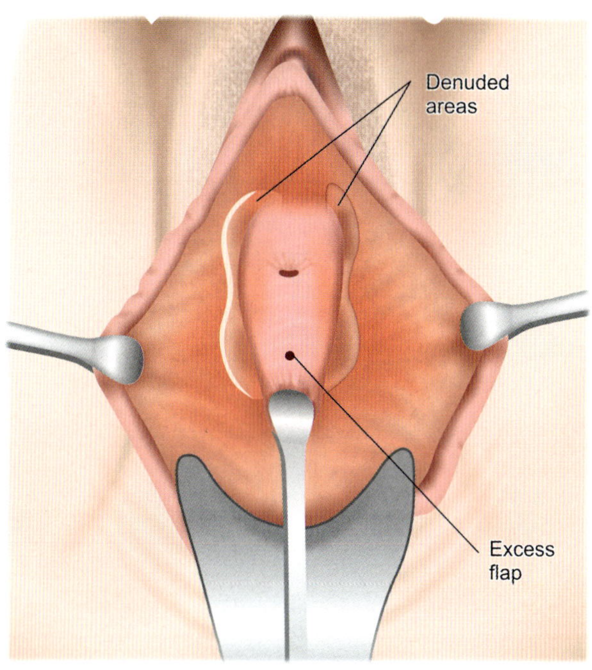

Fig. 23: The incision is extended on both sides

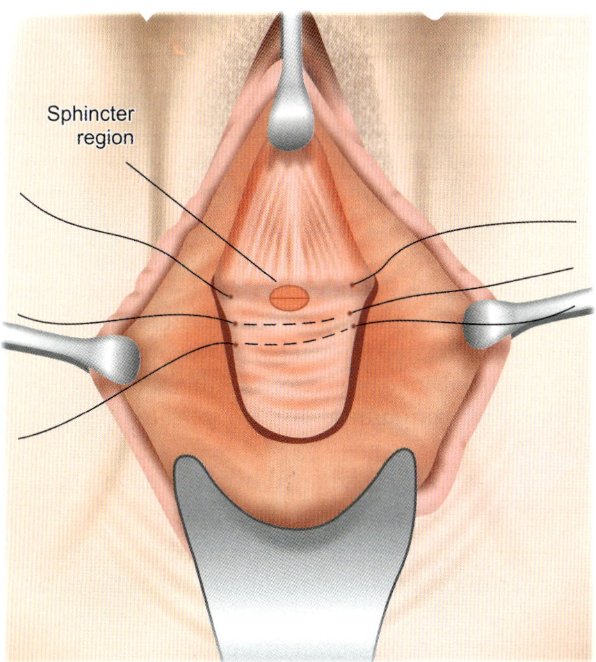

Fig. 24: The flap is mobilized and rotated over the fistula

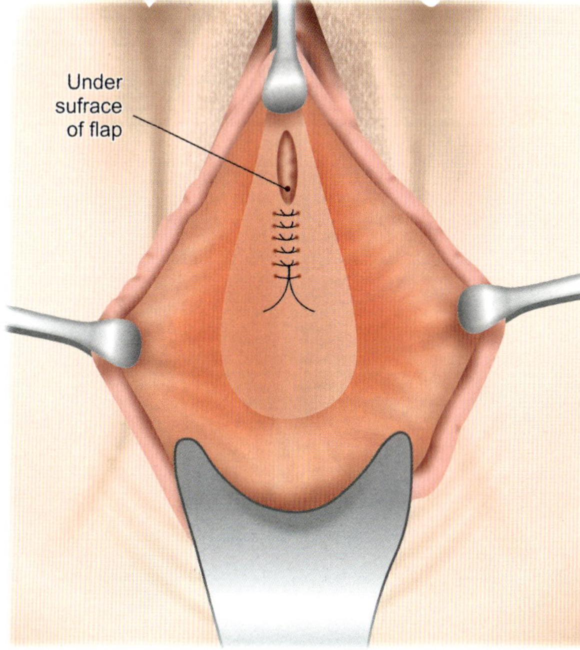

Fig. 25: Three interrupted delayed absorbable sutures are placed in the sphincter region

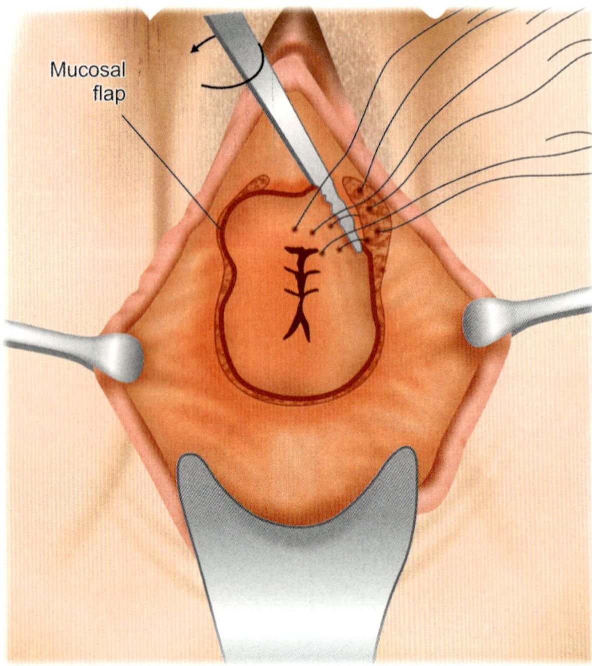

Fig. 26: The incision edge approximated to form a tube

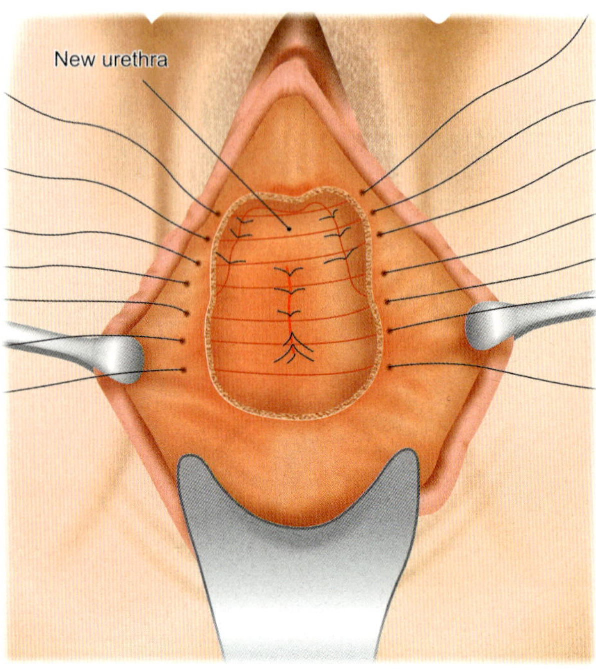

Fig. 27: A layer of paraurethral fascia is plicated beneath the urethra. The vagina is approximated over the neourethra with interrupted delayed absorbable sutures

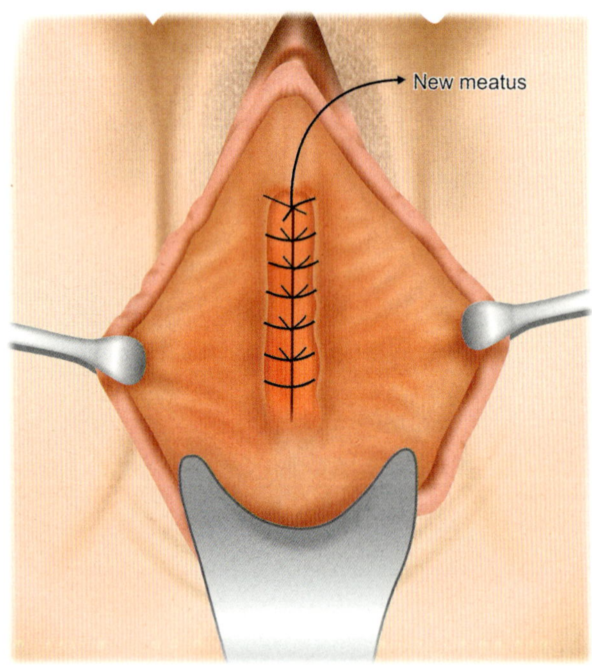

Fig. 28: Completion of the reconstruction, showing interrupted suture closure of suburethral mucosa

Dennis Browne (Modified by Chassar Moir 1964)

1. A U-shaped vaginal mucosal flap is made exposing the underside of trigone and sphincter
2. Flap is rotated forward, two to three deep sutures are placed in the region of sphincter and when tied will tighten the internal orifice
3. The flap of mucosa is drawn downward and an area of 6–7 mm wide is denuded forward for a distance equal to length of flap and flap is stitched back to the denuded margins. This step is repeated on the opposite side and an epithelial lined tube is formed that serves as urethra. A layer of paraurethral fascia is plicated beneath the urethra
4. The vagina is approximated over the neourethra with interrupted delayed absorbable sutures.

Interposition graft (modified Martius graft)may be used for either vaginal technique of urethral reconstruction, this helps to reduce postoperative incidence of stress incontinence and breakdown of repair.

Abdominal Approach

- Bladder wall advancement technique
- Bladder spout technique.

Postoperative Care

- A suprapubic catheter is placed to allow continuous drainage for 14–21 days. In repair of segmental loss of urethra, a fine silicon catheter should be left in situ for 2 weeks to maintain the patency of the urethra
- Good bladder irrigation should be maintained so that catheter is not blocked by blood clot resulting in retention which might disrupt the suture line. A strict 1 hourly input output chart is maintained
- Early ambulation is possible if adequate bladder drainage is obtained
- Urine routine and cultures should be obtained every 48 hours to detect early onset of urinary tract infection
- An antibiotic prophylaxis should be given for 10–14 days
- Patient should be given adequate balanced diet.

Subsequent Care

- Before discharging the patient she should be advised frequent voiding of urine and residual postvoid urine should be measured
- Sexual intercourse should be resumed only after complete wound healing, i.e. after 3 months
- If the patient conceives again, she should be advised elective cesarean section whenever indicated.

Complications

Intraoperative

- *Hemorrhage*: It can occur when mobilizing urethral mucosa from vagina. It is mostly venous bleeding and should be controlled with pressure
- Inadvertent enlargement of fistula.

Postoperative

- Acute urinary retention
- Urinary tract infection
- *Failure of repair*: More likely in large and radiation fistulas
- *Appearance of stress incontinence*: The patient should be counseled preoperatively regarding this complication. It occurs in 13% of patients where there was sphincter involvement and 16% where there is both sphincter involvement and tissue loss.

CONCLUSION

Correct diagnosis and selection of proper technique and adequate postoperative care will help in achieving good results. Obstetric fistulas are mostly preventable and good intranatal care will help in preventing these fistulas. Operative trauma should be identified and repaired immediately. The fistulas following mold insertion after vaginoplasty can be prevented by using foam molds.

BIBLIOGRAPHY

1. Anatomy of pelvis: Lasts textbook of anatomy, chapter 19, 10th edition. 2001. pp. 305-6.
2. Baskin D, Tatlidede S, Karsidag SH. Martius repair in urethrovaginal defects. J Pediatr Surg. 2005;40:1489-91.
3. BD Chaurasia. Urinary bladder and urethra. Human Anatomy Regional and Applied, 3rd edition. pp. 310.
4. Cardozo L. Anatomy and embryology. Textbook of Urogynecology. 1997. pp. 34-5.
5. Hudson CN, Setchell ME, Howkins J. Genital fistula. Shaw's Textbook of Operative Gynecology. 6th edition. New Delhi: Elsevier; 2001. pp. 237-70.
6. Rock JA, Jones HW. Anal incontinence and rectovaginal fistula. Te Linde's Operative Gynecology, 9th edition. Philadelphia: Lippincott Williams and Wilkins; 2003. pp. 1121-51.
7. Rock JA, Jones HW. Vesicovaginal urethrovaginal fistulas. Te Linde's Operative Gynecology, 9th edition. Philadelphia: Lippincott Williams and Wilkins; 2003. pp. 1099-119.
8. Venkatesh KS, Ramanujam PS, Larson DM, et al. Anorectal complications of vaginal delivery. Dis Colon Rectum. 1989;32:1039-41.
9. Zmora O, Tulchinsky H, Gur E, et al. Gracilis muscle transposition for fistulas between the rectum and urethra or vagina. Dis Colon Rectum. 2006;49(9):1316-21.

38.6 VAGINOPLASTY

Lakhbir Dhaliwal

INTRODUCTION

Vaginoplasty is a major surgical procedure, wherein, an artificial vaginal cavity is created either in cases of congenital absence of vagina due to vaginal agenesis or in the case of male-to-female sexual or gender reassignment surgery (SRS or GRS) where a vaginal cavity did not exist before. As this surgery is most often done for vaginal agenesis (Fig. 1) consequent to a variety of maldevelopment of Müllerian ducts, a comprehensive and distinctive preoperative evaluation of form of anomaly of each patient with suspected malformation of Müllerian ducts is essential. Müllerian dysgenesis occurs in approximately 1 in 5,000 live born females. Despite clear understanding of anomaly of Müllerian agenesis in a particular patient, a correct form of defect may not be established until the time of surgical correction. A sound knowledge of surgical anatomy of this region is of paramount importance to have successful outcome of this procedure. The physician can help patient to allay her anxieties by making a prompt evaluation and giving a full and accurate description of the reproductive implications of her uterovaginal anomaly and correction thereof. A thorough counseling of the patient along with parents regarding her modified marital prospects concerning sexuality, getting married to a person not keen to have children out of the married relation, social and financial self-sufficiency, etc. are of utmost importance.

SURGICAL ANATOMY

The reproductive system in the female consists of external genitalia, gonads and an internal duct system.

Embryologically, these components originate from different primordia and in close association with the urinary system and hindgut (Fig. 2). The Müllerian duct system is stimulated to develop preferably over the Wolffian duct system, which regresses in early female fetal life. The Müllerian ducts persist and attain complete development to form the Fallopian tubes, the uterine corpus and cervix and a portion of the vagina. Vagina is formed partly from Müllerian ducts and partly from urogenital sinus (Figs 3A to D). A solid vaginal cord results from proliferation of cells at the caudal tip of the fused Müllerian ducts. The cord gradually elongates to meet bilateral sinovaginal bulb developing from the urogenital sinus below. Subsequent canalization of vagina and epithelialization with cells mostly derived from urogenital sinus leads to complete formation of vagina. Hymen is the embryologic septum between the sinovaginal bulbs above and urogenital sinus proper below which is not derived from the Müllerian ducts. Failure in the development of Müllerian duct at any time between their origins from coelomic epithelium to fusion with urogenital sinus is the underlying basis of different forms of vaginal agenesis. Failure of development of a Müllerian duct may also be associated with failure of development of ureteric bud from the caudal end of the

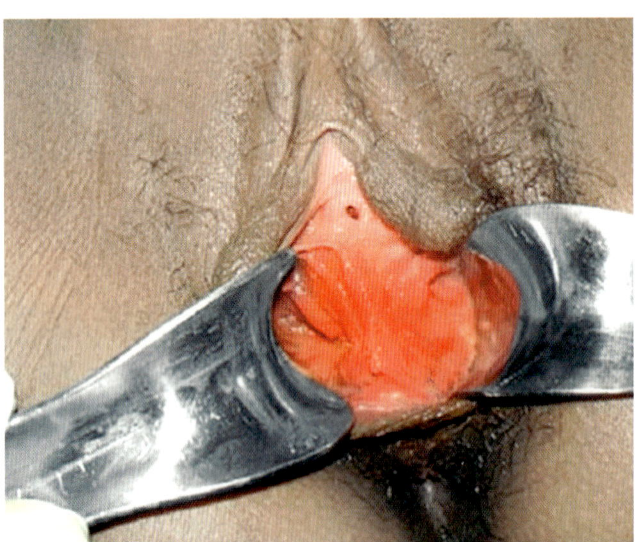

Fig. 1: Fibrotic bands and closure of neovagina

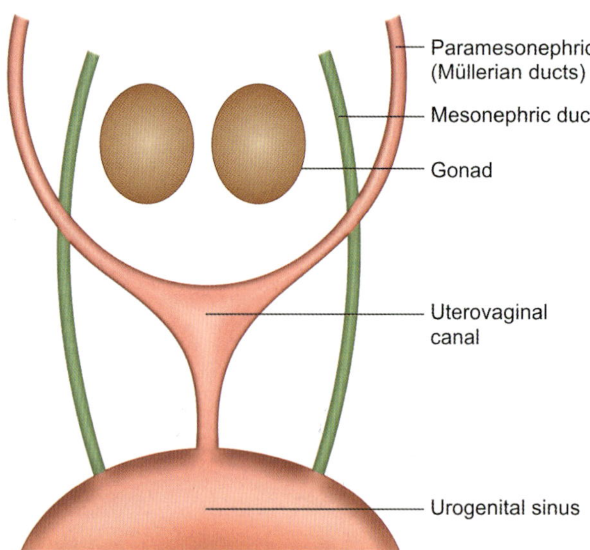

Fig. 2: Embryological development of female genital tract

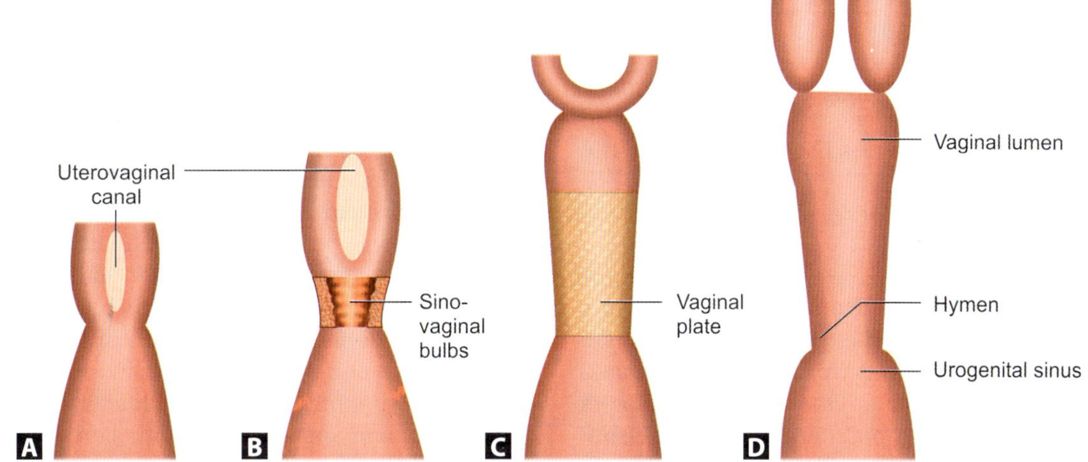

Figs 3A to D: Embryological development of vagina

Wolffian duct leading to congenital absence of kidney on the side of ipsilateral to the agenesis of a Müllerian duct. A significant percentage of these female patients with congenital absence of the kidney may be found to have associated genital anomalies.

INDICATIONS OF SURGERY

- *Congenital absence of uterus and vagina,* commonly known as Mayer-Rokitansky-Küster-Hauser syndrome is the most common indication of vaginoplasty
- However, an incomplete form with *a transverse vaginal septum* or partially atretic vagina with intact uterus also requires vaginoplasty
- In *testicular feminization syndrome or androgen insensitivity syndrome,* the vagina may be incompletely developed because of the existing male gonadal suppression of the development of the Müllerian ducts. These genetically male patients with female phenotype, without a completely formed vagina should be surgically corrected, in order to have a satisfactory sexual function in their female gender role
- Similarly, an *ineffective suppression of Müllerian ducts* may lead to ambiguous genitalia associated with small rudimentary uterus or a partially developed vagina requiring vaginoplasty in *congenital adrenal hyperplasia*
- *Male-to-female SRS or GRS* in collaboration with psychologist with laid standard guidelines for care of such individuals by Harry Benjamin International Gender Dysphoria Association.

PREOPERATIVE EVALUATION

A thoroughly motivated patient is the cornerstone of a successful vaginoplasty surgery. The management of an adolescent girl with congenital absence of vagina needs a gentle sympathetic approach in which the problem is explained to her in simple terms and is made to understand what can be done for her. The realization that, suitably treated, she can live a normal sexual life, can transform a depressed, withdrawn teenager into an optimistic, cooperative young lady. Time spent with such a patient is invaluable to the ultimate result, as she gives wholehearted cooperation. The timing of start of treatment must be carefully decided after an assessment of the patient attitude and emotional maturity. More recently, it has become usual to perform the procedure when patients are 17–20 years old and emotionally mature and intellectually reliable enough to manage without difficulty, the vaginal mold that will be used to maintain the neovaginal space. Alternatively, vaginoplasty may be planned a few months prior to marriage in order to initiate regular sexual activity for maintenance of vaginal cavity. The most difficult point to manage is the inevitable infertility of the affected patient. To help her accept this, very gentle, sympathetic handling indeed is necessary.

INVESTIGATIONS

- *Abdominal ultrasonography* helps in revealing an absent uterus and may differentiate between hematocolpos, hematometra, endometrial and other ovarian cysts, and pelvic kidney. Scan for other renal anomalies should also be done
- *Intravenous pyelogram* to delineate the renal anomalies
- *Magnetic resonance imaging* may be diagnostic for both uterine, vaginal and renal findings
- *Chromosomal analysis,* if there is suspicion of ovarian dysgenesis or androgen insensitivity syndrome.

DIFFERENT APPROACHES TO CONSTRUCT VAGINA

There is no consensus regarding the correct approach to the problem of vaginal agenesis. Both surgical and nonsurgical methods of correction have their benefits and limitations.

Nonsurgical Methods

Various nonsurgical methods like intermittent pressure on the perineum have shown the functional success rate up to 80%. The basis of this approach is the graduated dilatation of vaginal dimple at the introitus. Dilators (Fig. 4) are placed against the fourchette and firm pressure is kept up for 15 minutes twice a day or more often. The dilatation will go further slowly till a full length vagina can be achieved. Recently graduated dilators that can be worn inside a panty belt are available, continuous dilatation will be achieved by girl sitting on bicycle seat; the ridge of the seat will give a firm upward thrust to the dilators. The patient's enthusiasm must be reinforced by the attendant supervising her case.

Surgical Methods

The surgical techniques include:

1. *McIndoe procedure*: This procedure was first described by Abbe, further modified by McIndoe and Banester, and a number of researchers. In this operation, a space is created between rectum and bladder, largely by blunt dissection through a 0.5 cm incision made across the region of fourchette. Blunt finger dissection is then carried out to achieve optimum vaginal length of 10–12 cm. The finger pressure must be exerted laterally and posteriorly to prevent entry into rectum. Gauze pressure is sufficient to achieve hemostasis. Sheares used Hegar dilators to stretch up the region of paramesonephric duct on each side of a midline septum between them, which is then divided by scissors. The space is then lined by split skin graft taken from the buttock, thigh, or suprapubic region/or amnion graft (Figs 5 to 9). The graft is then sewn over a suitable mold with deep surface of the graft facing outward so that it will be in contact with the newly created vaginal wall. The molds may be rigid over of dental stent or malleable made from rubber foam packed into rubber condoms. It should be of sufficient length and width to fit snugly into new cavity, without causing extra pressure onto rectum, bladder and urethra. The labia are then approximated with skin suture to hold the mold in place. McIndoe originally left the mold in

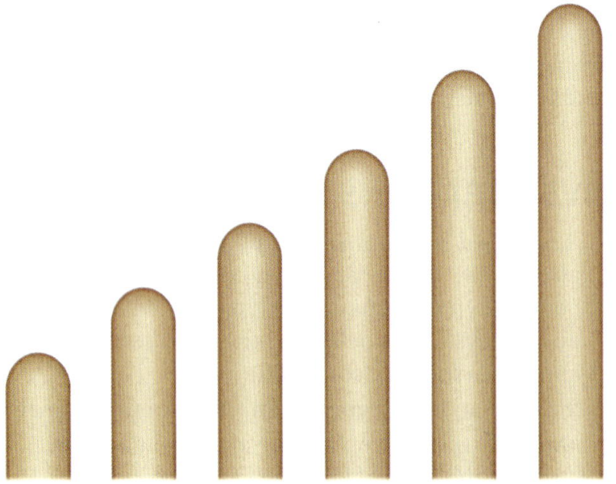

Fig. 4: Variable sized vaginal dilators

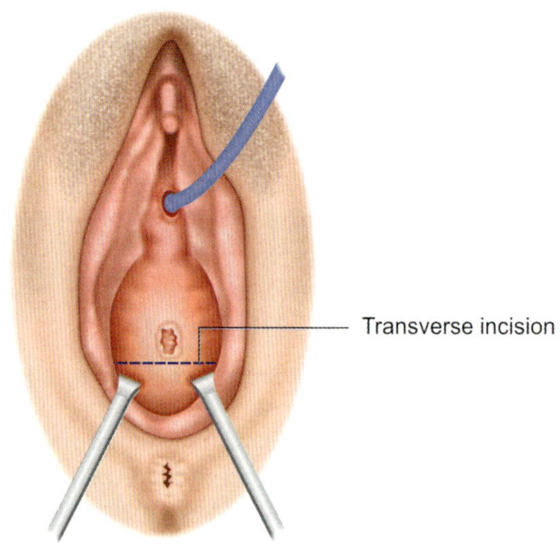

Fig. 5: Transverse incision across the apex of vaginal dimple

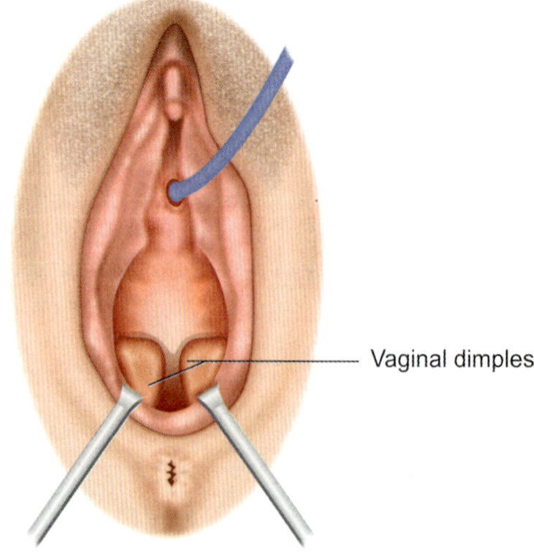

Fig. 6: Vaginal dimple on either side of median raphe

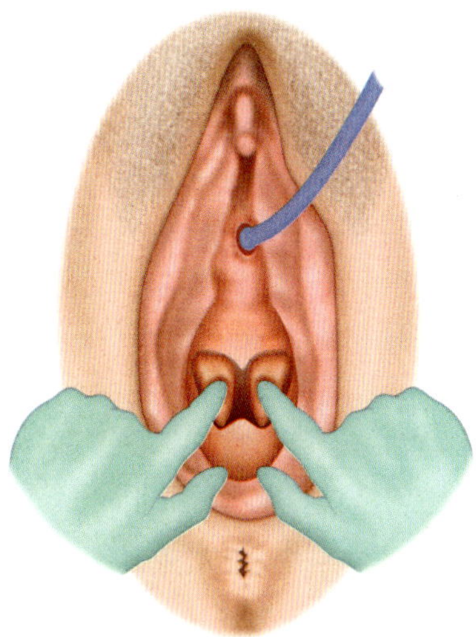

Fig. 7: Blunt dissection with fingers on either of median raphe

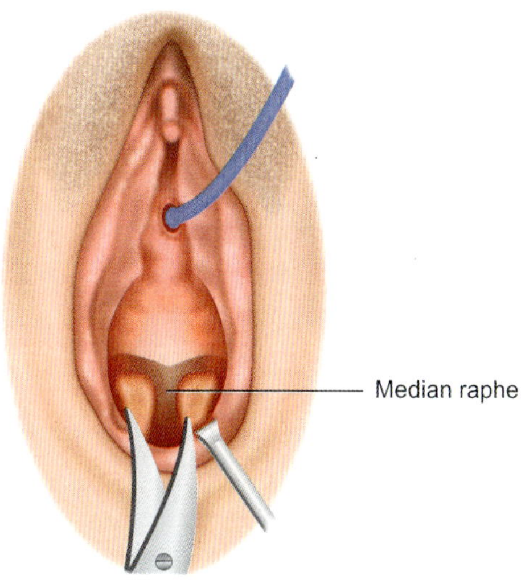

Fig. 8: Excision of median raphe

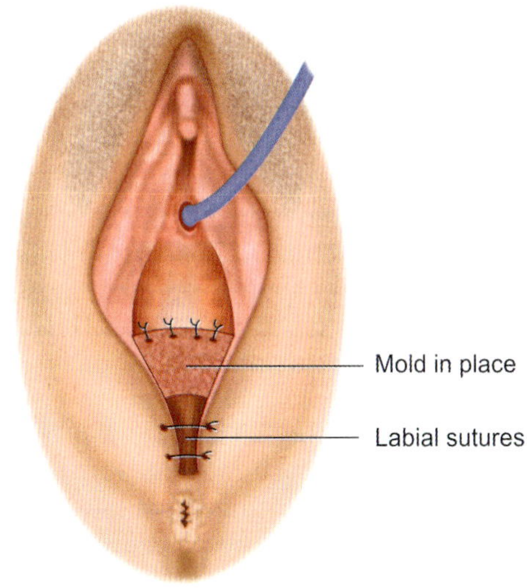

Fig. 9: Vaginal mold in place with labial sutures

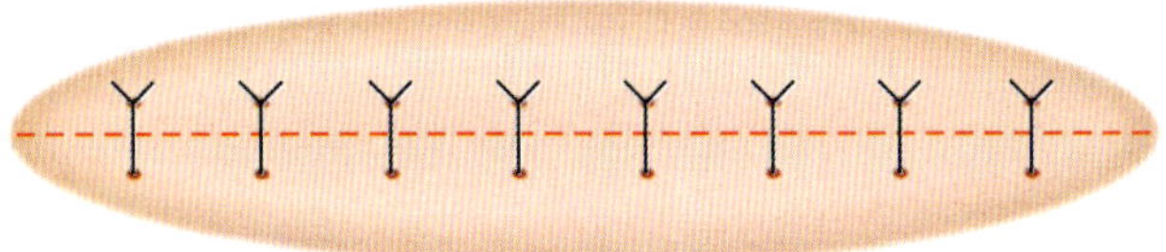

Fig. 10: Mold with amnion stitched in situ (chorionic surface facing outward)

place for 3 months to avoid contraction of new vagina. Undoubtedly, the prolonged suturing together of the labia is uncomfortable and distressing so that removal of mold after 1 week followed by repeated insertion whenever possible by wearing it at night appears more than sufficient

The amniotic membrane can be harvested a day or two prior to the vaginal procedure, from the placenta of clean vaginal or cesarean delivery tested negative for hepatitis B, C and human immunodeficiency virus (HIV). It should be washed in sterile saline and stored in refrigerator in sterile saline-containing antibiotic and hydrogen peroxide. The amnion is draped around the mold with its deep or mesothelial surface facing outward before insertion (Fig. 10). The mold is removed and cavity cleaned after 1 week to reveal a new vaginal cavity lined with glistering white membrane. Vaginal epithelialization may be superior with amnion but risk of contraction of new vagina is same as when skin is used, and efforts to prevent this are mandatory until regular coitus is practiced. The main advantage of amnion over skin is that there is no painful or unsightly donor site on the patient's leg or buttock.

2. *Penile inversion vaginoplasty*: This procedure is done in males seeking a sex or gender reassignment. The penile skin and scrotal skin is used to make a vaginal tube which is inverted to construct a neovagina. After catheterization of the bladder, the penile structures are pruned while skin along with its nerve supply is salvaged in order to construct vagina. Some portion

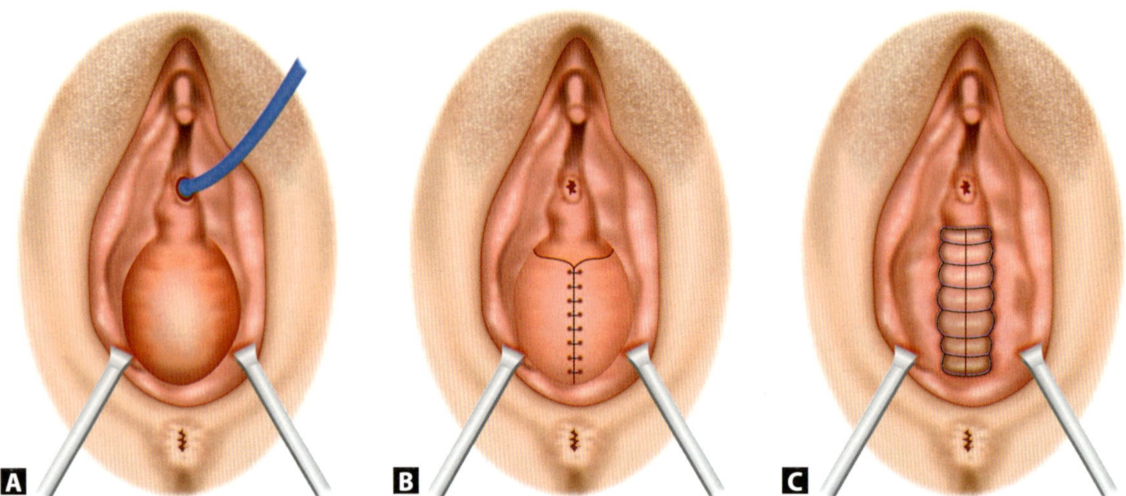

Figs 11A to C: Williams vulvovaginoplasty: (A) Making incision; (B) Making of vaginal pouch; (C) Completed layered closure

of the glans is also preserved to mimic as clitoris as an important component of vulval reconstruction. A vaginal cavity is then prepared in the same manner as McIndoe procedure and the mold is covered with vaginal tube formed out of penile and scrotal skin. A bilateral orchidectomy is also performed at the same occasion and the redundant scrotal skin is used to reconstruct labia majora and minora

3. *Colon vaginoplasty*: This procedure uses a segment of rectosigmoid colon as a covering structure in place of split thickness graft after creating a vaginal space in a similar manner as in McIndoe procedure. This is often done when McIndoe procedure or penile inversion vaginoplasty fails to achieve satisfactory results.
4. *Williams vulvovaginoplasty*: Williams described the construction of a perineal bridge which can be used as vaginal canal. An advantage of this technique is its technical simplicity where no mold is needed, and hence, the new vagina has no tendency to contract even though it is neither dilated nor used for natural coitus for some time after the operation.

   In this operation, a horseshoe-shaped incision is made in the vulva lateral to the midline and passing superior to the urethral orifice for similar distance after insertion of an indwelling catheter in the bladder. The base of incision thus passes across the region of fourchette in a gentle curve. Edges are freed by gentler undercutting and the internal edges on each side and stitched together in the midline with knots inside the vaginal lumen. Finally, the internal skin margins are approximated with interrupted sutures (Figs 11A to C). It should be possible to insert two fingers into the pouch to a depth of 3 cm. Catheter should stay in place for 5–6 days and should be strapped into the abdomen. Good result can be achieved with procedure with regard to coital orgasm, because the angle of the new vagina formed allows maximum clitoral stimulation during penile insertion. However, an unusual angle of vagina may result in minor urinary difficulties requiring manual squeezing out of last few drops of urine from this neovagina at the end of urination.
5. *Laparoscopic neovaginoplasty (Vecchietti procedure)*: Vecchietti operation originally described in 1965 can be considered as surgical version of Frank's method of vaginal graduated dilatation. Constant pressure is exerted on vesicorectal space from above to an acrylic olive, which is pulled upward, causing a deep invagination in this space in 7–8 days. The constructed neovagina must be maintained by daily application of artificial dilators. In 1994, a laparoscopic version of above was described. The criterion for anatomic success was a neovagina more than 6 cm long, allowing easy introduction of two fingers, within 6 months after corrective surgery. Hundred percent of anatomic and approximately 98% of functional success have been achieved so far in various studies.

POSTOPERATIVE CARE

All the techniques of vaginoplasty need a meticulous postoperative care and follow-up for neovagina to maintain its desirable shape and size. After 1 week of surgery, labial sutures are removed and the cavity is inspected for healing and progress of epithelialization. The mold is washed and patient is demonstrated a reinsertion so as to continue self-dilatation of the neovaginal cavity. The patient is instructed to continue dilatation of neovagina four to six times a day to a total period of 45 minutes per day. Initially, this dilatation appears cumbersome and painful, however, with time, it becomes less frequently required and thus less unpleasant. A natural sexual intercourse may be attempted as early as 6–8 weeks, although 10–12 weeks abstinence is usually more rewarding in terms of long-term outcome of the procedure. The neovagina has a strong tendency to shrink at any stage of life in absence of regular sexual intercourse or alternative artificial dilatation of the neovagina. Hence, a neovagina requires a lifelong maintenance in order to retain its benefits.

COMPLICATIONS

Vaginal stenosis is by far the most common and the most significant complication of vaginoplasty. Indeed a long period of not dilating can result in shrinkage of neovagina, in terms of both diameter and length. With careful perseverance and a little discomfort this loss can usually be recovered. Failure of primary surgery usually results in infection and formation of fibrotic vaginal bands. Repeat surgery in such patients carries the greatest risk of fistula formation because the dissection through tough fibrous tissue is quite difficult as compared to loose soft tissues at the first operation. Fistula formation is the most serious complication, if it occurs during operation, the original procedure should be abandoned and treatment to close the fistula should be instituted first. Pulmonary embolism from deep vein thrombosis is another complication that can be avoided with intermittent leg compression and anticoagulant therapy. It is not unusual to notice some spraying of urine during micturition; this usually resolves itself as genital swelling subsides. Particularly for GRS, patient's urine stream points more forward than normal female. Patient should be reassured regarding natural consequences of new vaginal geography and tendency to get used to with time.

CONCLUSION

Initial approach to Müllerian agenesis using vaginal dilator therapy can successfully create a functionally useful vagina in 85–90% of cases, with sexual function equivalent to normal controls. In segmental vaginal agenesis, a primary corrective surgery, however, has great benefits and is supported by the clinical guidelines published by The Australian Society of Pediatrics and Adolescent Gynecology (TASPAG). Rarity of the disease and availability of vast number of procedures have led to limited number of follow-up studies available; comparing various outcomes. Primary surgery should be definitive and performed by well-trained experts.

BIBLIOGRAPHY

1. Abbe R. New method of creating a vagina in a case of congenital absence. Med Rec. 1898;54:836.
2. Ashworth MF, Morton KE, Dewhurst J, et al. Vaginoplasty using amnion. Obstet Gynecol. 1986;67:443-6.
3. Atkinson E, Bennett MJ, Dudley J, et al. Consensus statement: the management of congenital tract anomalies in women. Aust N Z J Obstet Gynaecol. 2003;43:107-8
4. Bürger RA, Riedmiller H, Knapstein PG, et al. Ileocecal vaginal construction. AM J Obstet Gynecol. 1989;161:162-7.
5. Farber M, Mitchell GW. Surgery for congenital absence of the vagina. Obstet Gynecol. 1978;51:364-7.
6. Fedele L, Bianchi S, Zanconato G, et al. Laparoscopic creation of a neovagina in patients with Rokitansky syndrome: analysis of 52 cases. Fertil Steril. 2000;74:384-9.
7. Feroze RM, Dewhurst CJ, Welply G. Vaginoplasty at the Chelsea hospital for women: a comparison of two techniques. Br J Obstet Gynaecol. 1975;82:536-40.
8. Fliegner JR. Congenital atresia of the vagina. Surg Gynecol Obstet. 1987;165:387-91.
9. Frank RT. The formation of an artificial vagina without operation. Am J obstet Gynecol. 1938;35:1053-7.
10. Hensle TW, Reiley EA, Vaginal replacement in children and young adults. J Urol. 1998;159:1035-8.
11. Hurwitz RS, Fitzpatrick TJ. Vaginal urethra, clitoral hypertrophy and accessory phallic urethra: a rare syndrome of female pseudohermaphroditism. J Urol. 1982;127:1165-8.
12. Ingram JM. The bicycle seat stool in the treatment of vaginal agenesis and stenosis: a preliminary report. Am J Obstet Gynecol. 1981;140:867-73.
13. Kaloo P, Cooper M. Laparoscopic-assisted Vecchietti procedure for creation of a neovagina: an analysis of five cases. Aust N Z J Obstet Gynaecol. 2002;42:307-10.
14. McIndoe AH, Banister JB. An operation for the care of congenital absence of the vagina. J Obstet Gynaecol Br Emp. 1938;45:490-4.
15. McIndoe AH. The treatment of congenital absence and obliterative conditions of the vagina. Br J Plast Surg. 1950;2:254-67.
16. Morton K, Dewhurst CJ. The use of bowel to create a vagina: a follow up study. Ped Adol Gynaecol. 1984;2:51.
17. Morton KE, Dewhurst CJ. Human amnion in the treatment of vaginal malformations. Br J Obstet Gynaecol. 1986;93:50-4.
18. Nadarajah S, Quek J, Rose GL, et al. Sexual function in women treated with dilators for vaginal agenesis. J Pediatr Adolesc Gynecol. 2005;18:39-42.
19. Roberts CP, Haber MJ, Rock JA. Vaginal creation for Müllerian agenesis. Am J Obstet Gynecol. 2001;185:1349-53.
20. Rock JA, Jones HW. Construction of a neovagina for patients with a flat perineum. Am J Obstet Gynecol. 1989;160:845-51.
21. Sheares BH. Congenital atresia of the vagina: a new technique for tunneling the space between bladder and rectum and construction of a new vagina by a modified Wharton technique. J Obstet Gynaecol Br Emp. 1960;67:24-31.
22. Williams EA. Congenital absence of the vagina: a simple operation for its relief. J Obstet Gynaecol Br Commonw. 1964;71: 511-2.

38.7 SACROPEXY AND COLPOPEXY

SK Rath

INTRODUCTION/PREOPERATIVE CONSIDERATIONS

The main goal of any procedure aimed at suspending the vaginal vault should be to suspend as near as possible to its normal anatomic position. This should reapproximate the upper vagina in the midline over the levator plate. Distortion of the vaginal vault, whether in an anterior or posterior direction, can lead to a recurrent prolapse.

The ultimate goal of pelvic reconstructive surgery is to restore anatomy, restore visceral function, and maintain or restore normal sexual function. Hence, it is extremely important to determine preoperatively whether lower urinary tract dysfunction, sexual dysfunction and defecator dysfunction exist. Urinary dysfunction may be masked in patients with advanced pelvic organ prolapse by obstructing or kinking of the urethra. Thus, reductive maneuvers aimed at simulating what surgery will accomplish should be employed in the hope of identifying those patients who will require a continence procedure in conjunction with their pelvic reconstructive surgery. Local estrogen therapy may be required preoperatively in patients who have urogenital atrophy.

Many operations have been described for suspending the prolapsed vaginal vault. There is no general consensus on what is the best procedure. The procedure that the surgeon ultimately chooses is influenced by many factors, including the comfort and skill of the surgeon, whether prolapse is primary or recurrent, the patient's age, state of health, anticipated outcome, sexual activity and overall state of the tissues. Most cases can be approached transvaginally, reserving abdominal colpopexy for patients who have a failed previous vaginal approach, have a foreshortened vagina, or in whom a compensatory procedure with the insertion of mesh is necessary to obtain a long-term durable repair. The vaginal approach to pelvic prolapse has the advantage of decreased operative time, decreased incidence of adhesion formation and quicker recovery time. Obliterative procedures, including partial Le Fort colpocleisis and colpectomy, and colpocleisis can be used in elderly fragile patients who are no longer sexually active.

VAGINAL PROCEDURE TO SUSPEND THE VAGINAL APEX

Sacrospinous Ligament Fixation

Surgical Anatomy

The sacrospinous ligament is a cord-like structure that exists within the body of the coccygeus muscle. The complex is collectively called the coccygeus-sacrospinous ligament (CSSL) complex. It attaches medially to the sacrum and coccyx. Laterally, it is attached to the ischial spine. Following important structures lie in immediate vicinity. Pudendal nerve and vessels pass directly posterior to the ischial spine. The sciatic nerve lies superior and lateral to the sacrospinous ligament. The inferior gluteal vessels and the hypogastric venous plexus lie superior to the ligament. To avoid trauma to these structures, it is important to place the fixation sutures 3 cm medial to the ischial spine.

Steps of Operation (Figs 1 to 11)

- The apex of the vagina is grasped with two Allis clamps so the extent of the prolapse can be assessed
- The vagina is than reduced to the sacrospinous ligament. Most surgeons prefer to use the sacrospinous ligament opposite their dominant hand; i.e. the right-handed surgeon uses the right sacrospinous ligament, although some surgeons perform a bilateral fixation
- Marking sutures can be used to identify the intended vaginal apex throughout the operation. It may be necessary to choose a different fixation point than the original vaginal cuff scar. This is best illustrated in a patient with a foreshortened anterior segment and a large enterocele. In this case, the new fixation point would be moved to an area over the enterocele. If the patient requires an anterior vagina wall repair or an anti-incontinence procedure, this should be performed in conjunction with the sacrospinous fixation

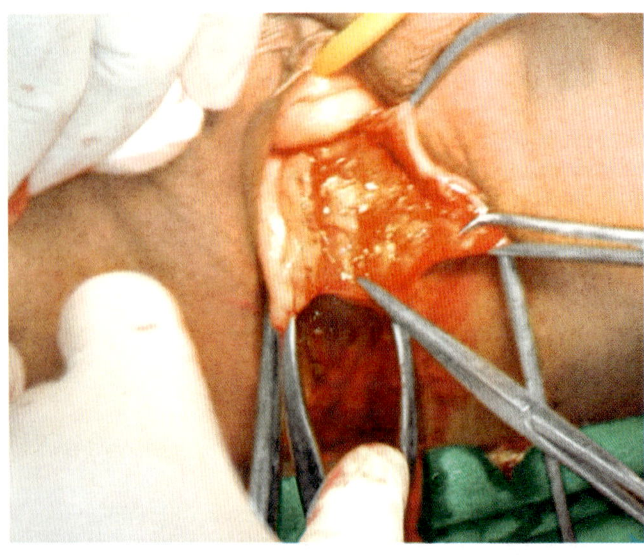

Fig. 1: Opening of vault

- A posterior vaginal incision is made. Almost always an enterocele sac is present. It should be mobilized off the posterior vaginal wall up to its neck; the sac is then opened and the peritoneum excised. The defect is closed with purse string sutures
- The next step is entry into the perirectal space. The rectal pillar separates the rectovaginal space from the perirectal space. A window is created, which is best accomplished by blunt dissection just lateral to the enterocele sac over the ischial spine. The window can also be created with the tips of scissors or a hemostat. The window should be gently enlarged to accommodate the vagina
- The sacrospinous ligament can then be palpated next to the spine and moving the fingers dorsal and medial. Once the window has been created and the ligament is identified, a retractor is used to displace the rectum medially. Care must be taken to avoid raking the retractor over the anterior surface of the sacrum and causing damage to presacral nerves and vessels
- When doing ischial right sacrospinous ligament fixation, the middle and index finger of the left hand are placed on the medial surface of the ischial spine
- Then, under direct vision, the tip of the long-handled ligature carrier penetrates the sacrospinous ligament two fingers medial to the ischial spine. There should

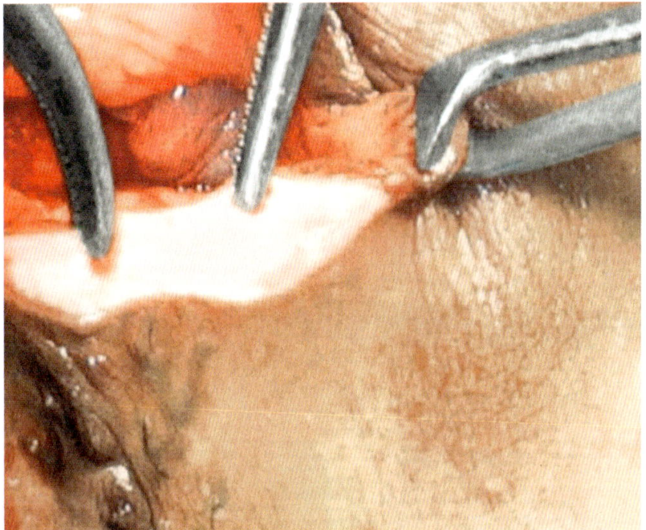

Fig. 2: Posterior colpotomy incision is given and extended to do colporrhaphy

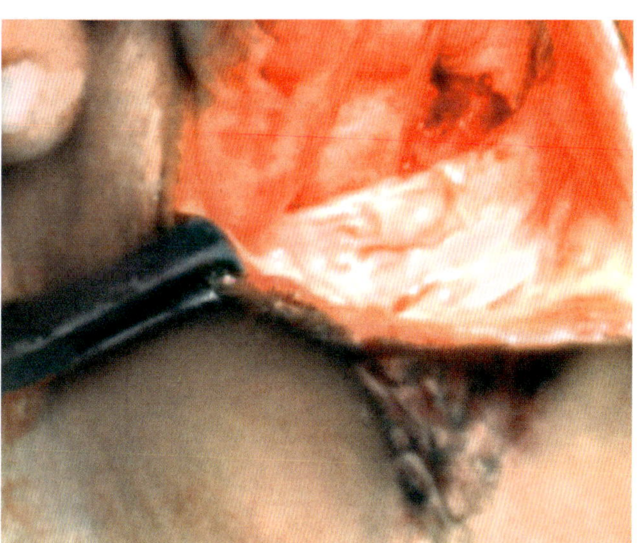

Fig. 3: Visualization of peritoneum

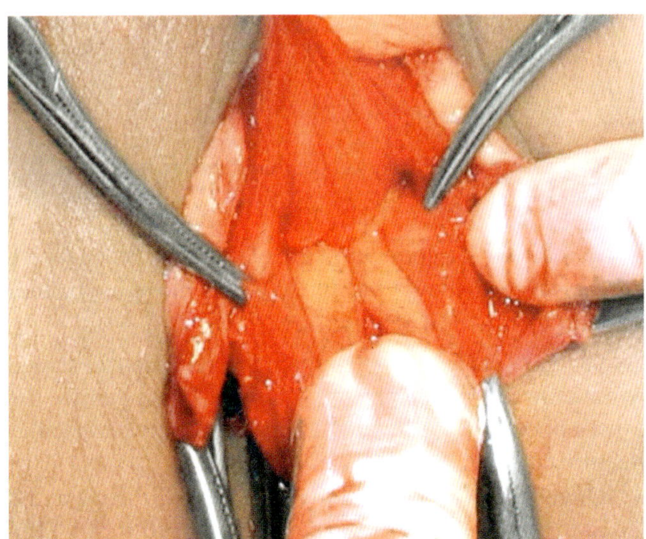

Fig. 4: Reduction of enterocele

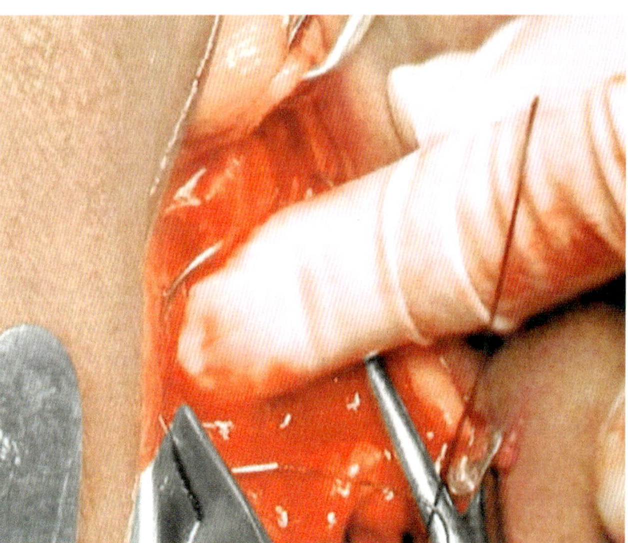

Fig. 5: Developing presacral space to define sacrospinous ligament

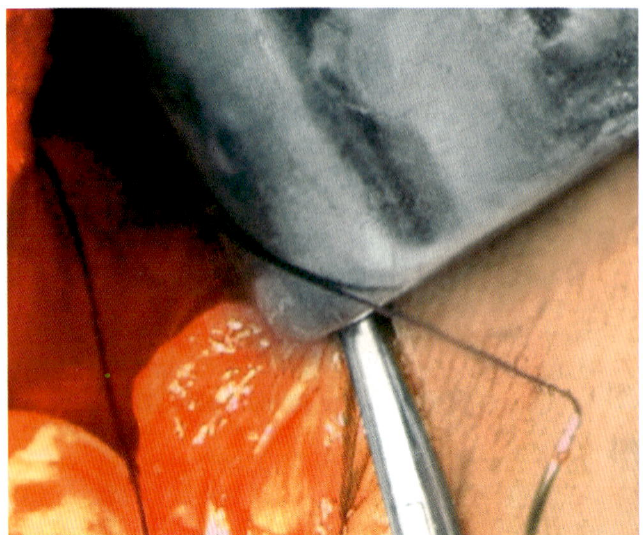

Fig. 6: Placement of sacrospinous 1-0 prolene suture

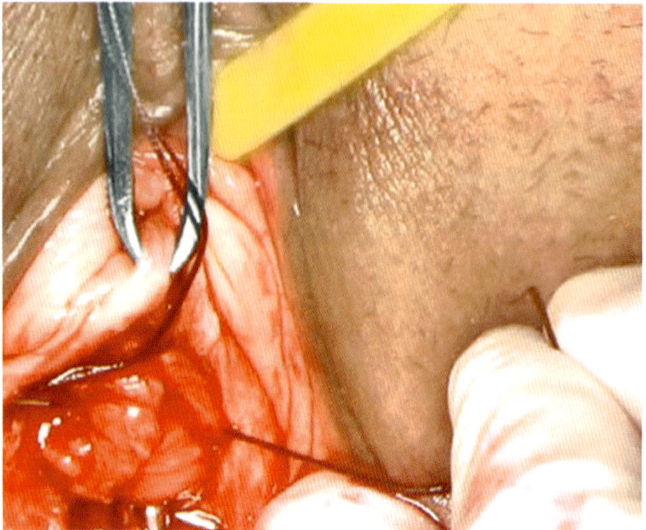

Fig. 7: Fixation of vault to sacrospinous ligament

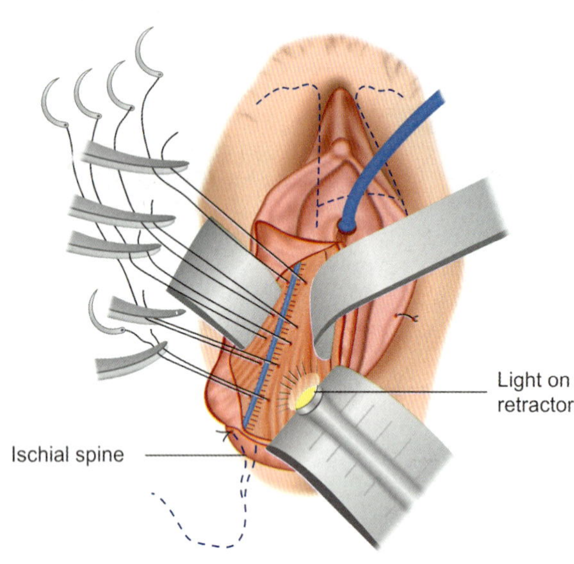

Fig. 8: Visualization of sacrospinous ligament

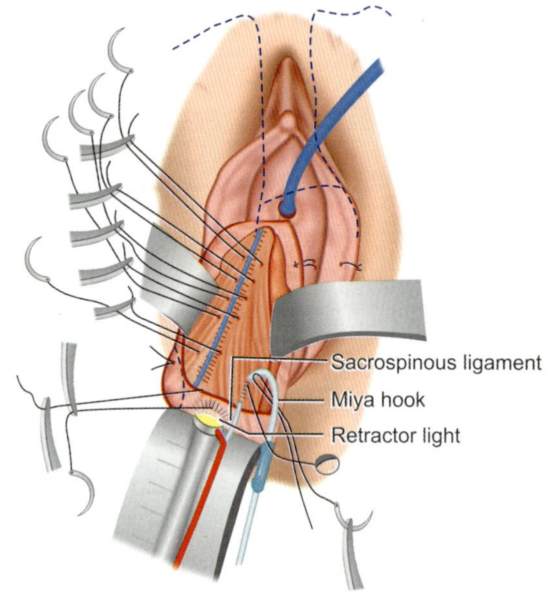

Fig. 9: Placement of suture at CSSL complex using Miya hook

be considerable resistance as the carrier is pushed through the body of the ligament. If no resistance is felt, then the carrier is either passed in front of or around the ligament. The ligament can be grasped with an Allis clamp or babcook in order to isolate the tissue away from the vessels and nerves. After the suture has been passed, the fingers of the left hand are withdrawn. The suture is then grasped with a hook. A second suture is placed in similar fashion approximately 1 cm medial to the first. If the surgeon does not desire a second passage, the suture can be cut in the midline and each end of the cut loop can be paired with its respective free suture. If a good purchase of tissue has been taken, the surgeon should be able to gently move the patient with the traction of the suture

Several specialized instruments have been designed to pass the suture through the ligament. These include the Miya's hook, Laurus needle driver and Nichols-Veronikis ligature carrier.

- Once the surgeon has two sutures through the sacrospinous ligament, the vaginal vault can then be suspended. There are two ways for the surgeon to attach the sutures to the vagina. The first is to use a pulley stitch. Here the free end of the suture is threaded

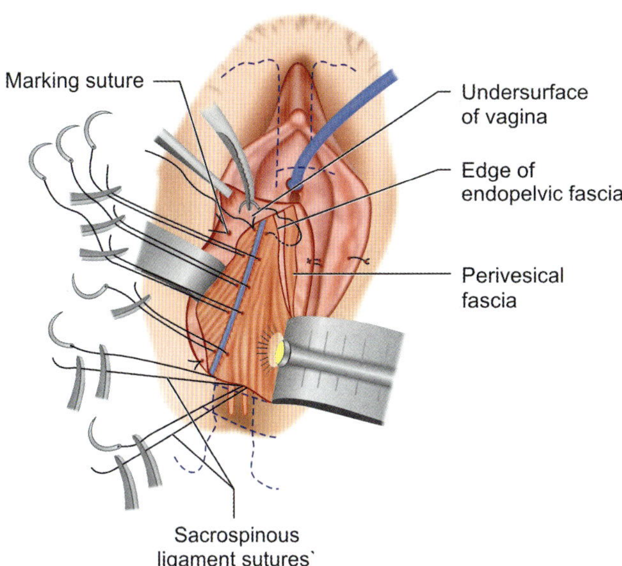

Fig. 10: Placement of another set of sutures through CSSL

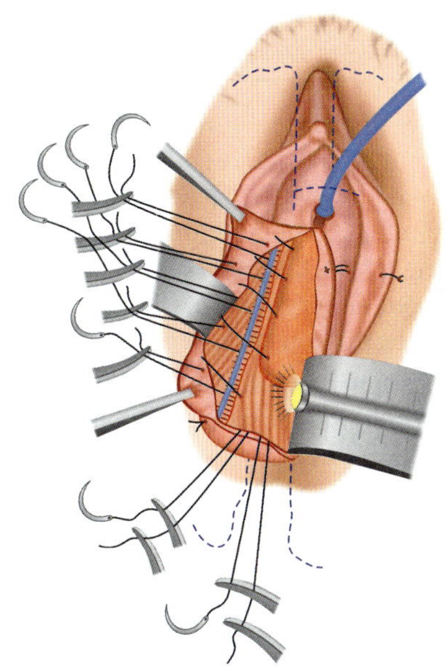

Fig. 11: Repair of presacral sac to obliterate the space opened during dissection

through a free needle, sewn into the full thickness of the fibromuscular layer on the undersurface of the vagina (excluding the epithelium), and then tied by a half hitch. Traction on the free end of the suture pulls the vagina directly onto the ligament. A square knot is then used to fix the suture in place. Generally, when using this technique, permanent suture should be used.

- The second technique can be used if the vagina is thin or if greater vaginal length is desired. This technique involves each end of the sutures through the full thickness of the vagina using 1-0 or 2-0 absorbable suture. The upper portion of the posterior vaginal wall should be closed with interrupted or running 3-0 absorbable sutures before tying the colpopexy sutures. If the colpopexy sutures are tied before the posterior wall is closed, the visibility of the vault is reduced and the colporrhaphy sutures are difficult to place. The vagina should come into contact with the sacrospinous ligament, especially if absorbable sutures are used. A suture bridge can predispose to recurrent prolapse because a strong scar will not form before suture absorption.
- After the colpopexy sutures are tied, a posterior colporrhaphy and perineorrhaphy is done. The vagina is then packed with moist gauze for 24 hours.

RESULTS

The overall results from sacrospinous fixation have been good. In 1997, Karram reviewed the literature on sacrospinous suspension and of the 1,137 patients available for follow-up, 36 (3.6%) had recurrent vault prolapse. Ninety-six (8%) had anterior wall prolapse and 25 (2%) had posterior wall prolapse. Some authors (Shull, 1992) have reported a high incidence of anterior wall prolapse following sacrospinous fixation, others have not. Smilen and colleagues in 1998 compared patients with anterior vaginal wall defects undergoing anterior colporrhaphy with and without sacrospinous fixation to patients with a well-supported anterior vaginal wall who undergoing pelvic reconstructive procedures with and without sacrospinous fixation. They found no difference between the groups for subsequent anterior wall prolapse during the follow-up period.

Complications

Complications can occur and the some common complications are discussed here. It is important to do frequent rectal examinations during this procedure to make sure that no inadvertent proctotomy has occurred if evidence of suture penetration is evident. The offending suture should be removed and replaced. Lacerations should be closed in a standard two-layer fashion.

Hemorrhage can result from injury to the hypogastric venous plexus, which can occur from overzealous dissection or inappropriate needle passage through the sacrospinous ligament. If bleeding does occur initially, pressure should be applied to the bleeding area. Continued bleeding should be addressed with suture ligation and hemoclips. Because this area is difficult to approach transabdominally, every effort should be made to control bleeding transvaginally. An improperly placed retractor or inattentive assistance can cause damage to the presacral vessels by taking the tip over the bony sacrum.

A patient who complains of severe postoperative gluteal pain that runs down the posterior surface of the affecting leg, most likely has a pudendal nerve injury. Sutures that are placed too close to the ischial spine risk injury to the pudendal nerves and the sciatic nerve. If the patients have evidence of nerve injury, she should immediately undergo reoperation with removal of those sutures impinging on the nerve. New colpopexy sutures should be placed either more medial on the same side or the opposite sacrospinous ligament can be used.

In our experience, approximately 10–15% of patients have transient moderate to severe buttock pain on the side of the sacrospinous suspension. It is usually self-limiting and resolves by 6 weeks postoperatively. Reassurance and anti-inflammatory agents are all that are necessary.

Vaginal stenosis can occur if too much vaginal tissue is removed before closing the vaginal incision. An aggressive posterior repair can also cause a constriction ring. If a constriction ring is present while the patient is still under anesthesia, it should be addressed at that time.

ILIOCOCCYGEUS FASCIA SUSPENSION

In 1993, Shull and colleagues reported this technique to treat 42 women. Their approach was to identify all fascial defects preoperatively. Before iliococcygeus suspension, any anterior compartment defects are fixed. A cul-de-sac repair may be undertaken to shorten and approximate the uterosacral ligaments.

Steps

- Cuff suspension and posterior colporrhaphy are approached by excising a diamond-shaped section of tissue from the perineum and introitus
- The vaginal epithelium is then freed from the rectum rectovaginal fascia, and the dissection is carried laterally to the levators and cephalad to the cuff
- The iliococcygeus muscle is identified lateral to the rectum and anterior to the ischial spine. The surgeon then uses the nondominant hand to press rectum medially
- A suture is placed just anterior to the ischial spine
- Both ends of the suture are then passed through the ipsilateral vaginal apex. The same procedure is repeated on the patient's opposite side
- If delayed absorbable suture is used, it should be passed through the full thickness of the vagina
- If nonabsorbable suture is used, a pulley stitch similar to that described sacrospinous fixation should be used
- The sutures are then held to be tied after posterior colporrhaphy is finished.

A total of 152 patients were treated with this technique by Shull and colleagues and by Merks and colleagues. A total of 13 patients (8%) developed recurrent prolapse at various sites. Two developed vault prolapse, eight developed anterior vaginal wall relaxation, and three developed posterior wall defects. They reported one rectal and one bladder laceration and two cases of hemorrhage requiring transfusion. Postoperative follow-up ranged from 6 weeks to 5 years.

ABDOMINAL SACRAL COLPOPEXY

Suspension of the vagina to the sacral promontory or into the hollow of sacrum with an intervening mesh has been shown to be an effective treatment for vault prolapse.

Position of Patient

The patient is placed in Allen stirrups and is prepared and draped. Alternatively, the patient could be placed in the frog-leg position. Either position allows access to the vagina during operation. A way Foley catheter is used to drain the bladder.

Steps

- A laparotomy incision is made via a low transverse or vertical midline approach
- Moist laparotomy sponges are then used to pack the bowl into upper abdomen. Any adhesions should be carefully taken down
- The course of the ureters and the cul-de-sac should be inspected and palpated
- If the patient has uterus, a hysterectomy should be done first and cuff closed
- The vagina is elevated and peritoneum is then dissected off the anterior vaginal wall. The peritoneum on the posterior aspect of the vagina is incised in the midline and carried down into the cul-de-sac. The peritoneum is dissected free laterally
- Three to five pairs of 0 nonabsorbable sutures are placed on the posterior aspect of the vagina about 1.5–2 cm apart. The suture should incorporate the full thickness of the vagina without entering the vaginal lumen
- The sutures are then placed through the mesh and tied down. In 1997, Cundiff recommended extending the mesh to the perineum. We generally extend the mesh approximately halfway down the posterior wall. We also place two to four pairs of 0 nonabsorbable sutures in the anterior aspect of the vagina and attach a separate piece of mesh
- This anterior mesh is sewn to the posterior mesh just proximal to the vaginal apex. Other potential configurations have been described

- A Moschowitz procedure is done to obliterate the cul-de-sac
- To expose the presacral area, the rectosigmoid is then reflected to the left
- The bifurcation of the aorta is palpated and again the right ureter is identified and retracted laterally
- The peritoneum over the sacral promontory is opened and carried down over the anterior surface of the sacrum. With the peritoneum reflected, the middle sacral artery and vein are identified
- A subperitoneal tunnel can be created into the cul-de-sac by blunt and sharp dissection
- The graft can then be placed retroperitoneally. Alternatively, the graft can be placed over previous culdoplasty and can then be extraperitonealized by sewing the serosa of the sigmoid to the lateral peritoneum of the cul-de-sac
- The sacral promontory and the anterior longitudinal ligament are then exposed by blunt and delicate dissection
- Two to four sutures of 0 nonabsorbable are placed through the longitudinal ligament over sacral promontory
- The appropriate amount of graft material is cut and sutures are placed through the graft and tied. There should be no tension on the graft material
- The peritoneum over sacrum is then closed with a 2-0 absorbable suture. The peritoneum over the anterior vaginal wall is closed, thereby covering mesh. The abdomen is then closed
- The vagina is inspected and evaluated for any remaining defects. Usually a posterior colporrhaphy is required.

It has been shown by multiple investigators that abdominal sacral colpopexy is durable and strong surgical correction of vaginal vault prolapse. Benson and colleagues randomized patient's with prolapse to abdominal sacral colpopexy versus bilateral sacrospinous ligament fixation. They found superior result with abdominal sacral colpopexy. The reoperation rate in the vaginal group was 33% and in the abdominal group 16%, optimal results were obtained in only 29% of the vaginal group and 58% of the abdominal group. Although the exact indication for abdominal sacral colpopexy is controversial, many surgeons use it as their primary surgery for all cases of posthysterectomy vault prolapse.

Complications

Intraoperative complications are unusual, through injury to bowel, bladder and infection, as with all abdominal surgery, have been described. Hemorrhage, especially from presacral vessels, can be life-threatening. Hemostasis can be difficult because damaged presacral vessels tend to retract beneath the bony surface.

HIGH UTEROSACRAL LIGAMENT SUSPENSION

After the abdomen has been opened and the bowel has been packed away, the remnants of the uterosacral ligaments are identified and tagged with suture near the ischial spine. The ureters are identified bilaterally. The enterocele is then addressed by obliteration of cul-de-sac. The peritoneum over the vaginal apex is opened and the endopelvic fascia is reapproximated to form a continuous covering of endopelvic fascia over the vaginal epithelium. Nonabsorbable sutures are then used to suspend the vagina with the now intact endopelvic fascia to the uterosacral ligaments.

Results for the abdominal approach to high uterosacral suspension should be similar to those for the vaginal approach. There are, however, no long-term studies available. Complications are similar to those for the vaginal approach.

Laparoscopic Approach

The techniques and concepts described earlier can also be approached via laparoscopy. The laparoscopic approach to the patient for positioning, port placement, and equipment is outside the scope of this chapter. These procedures require patience, attention to detail, and the realization that there is a steep learning curve. It is our belief that the operation and subsequent outcomes should not be compromised for the purpose of having achieved the operation by this approach. Therefore, the surgical measures taken to achieve the underlying concepts should not be significantly altered or changed.

OBLITERATIVE PROCEDURES

Le Fort Partial Colpocleisis

At times a patient may be sufficiently bothered by uterovaginal or vault prolapse but they are medically unable to undergo major reconstructive surgery. An obliterative procedure may then be undertaken. A Le Fort procedure is an option if the patient has her uterus and is no longer sexually active. The rate of postoperative urinary stress incontinence has been reported to be as high as 30% after this procedure, and, because the uterus is retained, it will be difficult to evaluate any future uterine bleeding or cervical pathology. Therefore, endometrial biopsy and Papanicolaou must be done before surgery.

Steps

This procedure has been described in detail elsewhere in this book.

38.8 UTEROVAGINAL PROLAPSE: ETIOLOGY, MANAGEMENT WITH ANTERIOR ABDOMINAL SLING SURGERY

Phool Chandra, Jasleen

DEFINITION

What is Prolapse?

Pelvic organ prolapse is a very common condition particularly among elderly women with normal vaginal deliveries. These women experience prolapse of any part of organ, at later period of life.

Prolapse is also called as uterine prolapse, uterovaginal prolapse, pelvic relaxation, pelvic floor dysfunction, urogenital prolapse or vaginal wall prolapse.

Types of Prolapse

Pelvic organ prolapse occurs when the pelvic muscles, fascia and ligaments become weak and damaged and are no longer able to support the pelvic organs like cervix, uterus and vagina. These organs are displaced from their place.

Pelvic organ prolapse is divided according to the site in pelvic area such as front wall, back wall and top of the vagina. Patient may have more than one type of pelvic organ prolapse.

Anterior Vaginal Wall Prolapse

Cystocele: When urinary bladder prolapses, it falls toward the vagina and creates large bulge in front wall of vaginal wall, it is called cystocele (Fig. 1). If it remains outside without treatment for a longer period there can be keratinization of vaginal epithelium.

When anterior one-third of vaginal wall, where urethra is situated falls forward, it is called urethrocele, usually there is combination of two called cystourethrocele.

Postvaginal Wall Prolapse

Lower two-thirds of vagina when fall down and bulge into vaginal canal, it is called rectocele because the postvaginal wall is associated with rectum (Fig. 2).

When upper one-third of vagina falls down, it is called POD prolapse, which is having small bowel in it and is called enterocele (Fig. 3).

Uterine Prolapse

Degree I (Type I, Stage I): When along with cervix, uterus descends down and reaches up to the level of ischial spines, it is called type I or stage I prolapse.

Degree II (Type II, Stage II): When cervix and uterus descend down but cervix reaches up to the vaginal opening, it is called type II, or stage II prolapse (Fig. 4).

This prolapse can further be differentiated into two types. First type when uterus remains at its own level but it is the cervix only which descends down up to the introitus, because the supravaginal portion of cervix elongates due to good upper ligamentary support which pulls the uterus up and poor lower ligamentary support hangs cervix down. Second type is when uterus along with cervix descends down into the pelvis and cervix reaches up to the introitus. This is due to total deficient ligamentary support in the pelvis.

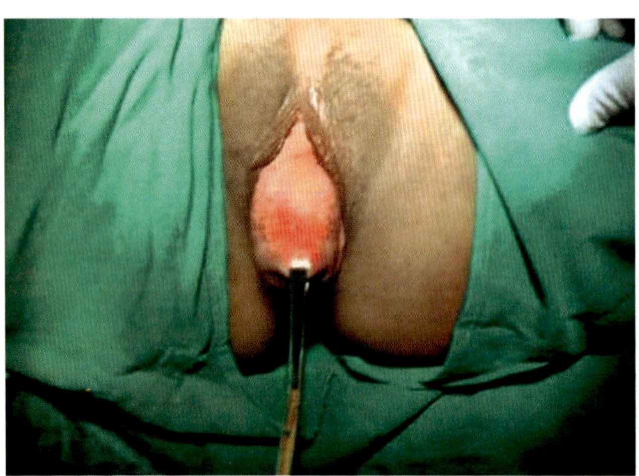

Fig. 1: Cystocele

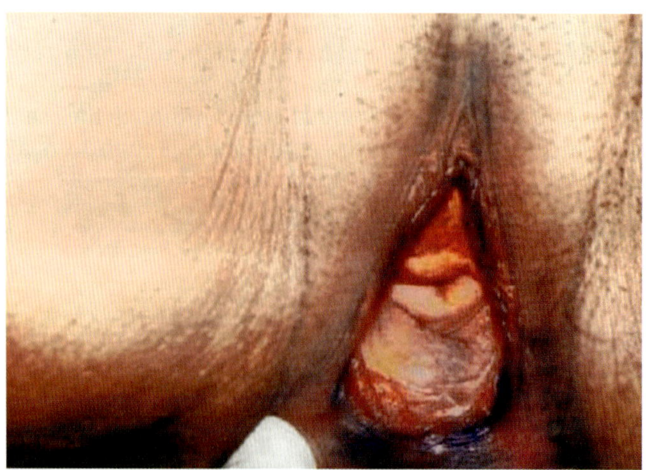

Fig. 2: Rectocele

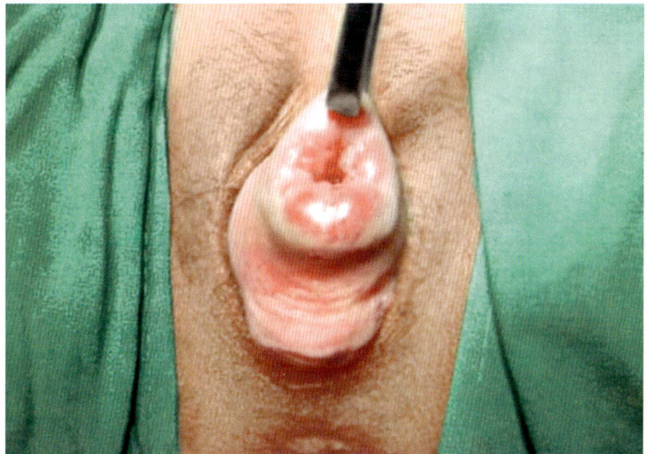

Fig. 3: Enterocele

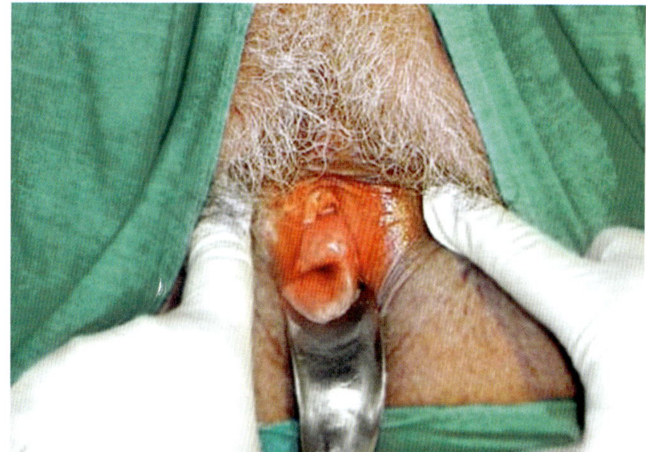

Fig. 4: Second degree uterovaginal (UV) prolapse

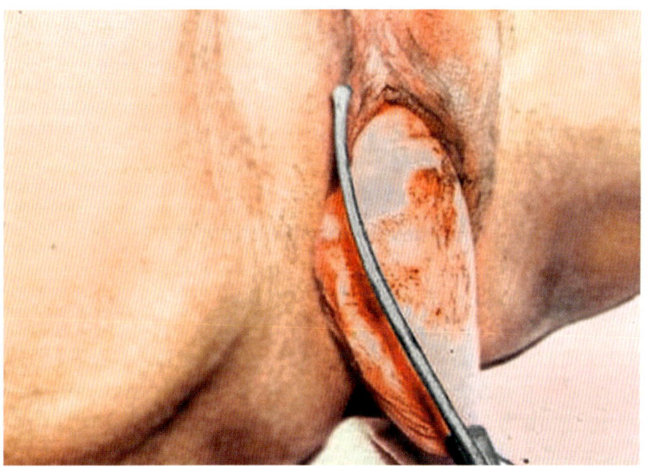

Fig. 5: Third degree uterovaginal (UV) prolapse

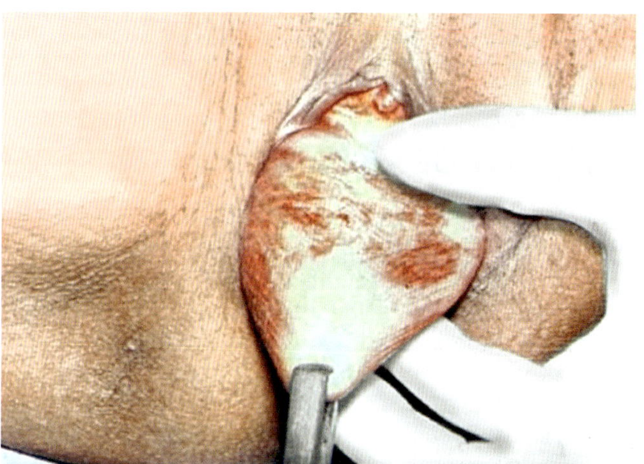

Fig. 6: Procidentia

Degree III (Type III, Stage III): When cervix comes out of the introitus and uterus is still in the pelvis, it is called stage III or type III prolapse (Fig. 5).

Degree IV (Stage IV): When uterus and cervix along with its appendages descend down out of the pelvis, it is called procidentia (Fig. 6). There is formation of decubitus ulcer in long-standing cases.

Vault Prolapse

It is defined as total vaginal prolapse after hysterectomy which may be abdominal or vaginal. Incidence is on rise due to increase in life span of women, and more hysterectomies performed nowadays. It may be after abdominal or vaginal hysterectomy, but it is more after vaginal hysterectomy, due to lack of surgical skill. Nowadays, elderly women seek remedy to vault prolapse due to inconvenience created by vault prolapse and for sexual satisfaction (Figs 7 and 8).

SUPPORTS OF UTERUS

Uterus is bent forward on itself at the level of internal os and is called anteflexion. It is maintained in the position of anteflexion, anteversion by its own weight and round ligaments which holds the fundus forward. Uterosacral ligament keeps the supravaginal cervix back in the pelvis.

Uterus is supported by transverse cervical ligament (Mackenrodt's ligament) at the level of supravaginal cervix, upper part of vagina and uterosacral ligaments. Broad ligaments and round ligaments also have a steadying effect on uterus. They do not, however, have any significant action in preventing descent of the uterus.

Vagina is supported in its upper part by transverse cervical ligaments which are fused with fascial sheaths of lateral pelvic wall, vesicovaginal fascia, pubocervical fascia and rectovaginal septum. Middle part of vagina is supported by levator ani, pelvic fascia and urogenital diaphragm. Lower part of vagina is supported by perineal

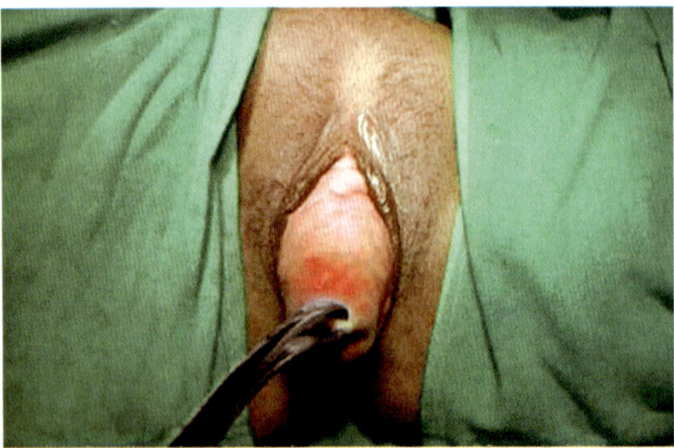

Fig. 7: Vault prolapse

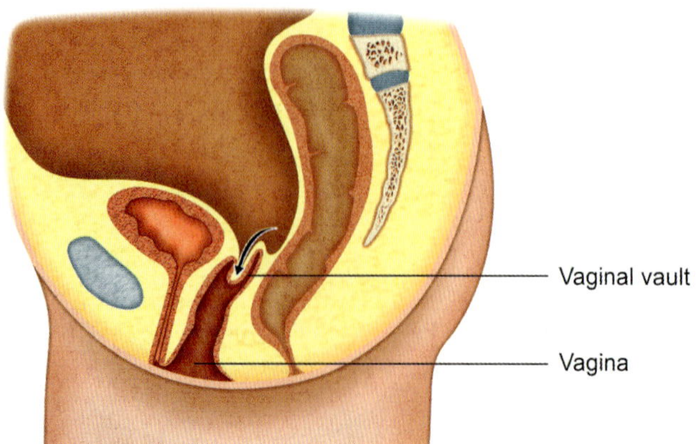

Fig. 8: Vaginal vault prolapse

muscles, perineal body and pelvic diaphragm. However, support given by perineal muscles, perineal body and pelvic diaphragm are minimal.

ETIOLOGY OF VAULT PROLAPSE

Causes of vault prolapse may be wrongly chosen case for surgery and faulty executed cases.

During hysterectomy, the cardinal uterosacrals and round ligaments if not identified and stitched over the vault can later lead to vault prolapse. This is more so after vaginal than abdominal hysterectomy. In long-standing cases of prolapse, the cardinal and uterosacral ligaments are already stretched and damaged and if proper preoperative assessment is not done, and during surgery not properly identified and stitched over the vault will lead to vault prolapse.

Immediate Postsurgery

If enterocele is not repaired during hysterectomy and absent ligamentary support to vault of vagina can lead to vault prolapse later.

Delayed Causes

Delayed causes are age-related weakness of tissue supporting vagina, menopausal tissue atrophy due to estrogen deficiency, increase in intra-abdominal pressure due to pulmonary ailments, chronic cough, chronic constipation and obesity.

Predisposing Factors of Uterovaginal Prolapse and Vault Prolapse

Predisposing factors of uterovaginal prolapse leading to postsurgical vault prolapse are congenital weakness or developmental weakness of supports of uterus, easy deliveries causing precipitate labor, familial incidence, birth trauma due to instrumental delivery, prolonged labor, repeated childbearing, premature bearing down, pulling down after coming head in partially dilated cervix, pressure on the fundus (Crede's method), surgical injury more after subtotal than total hysterectomy, faulty hysterectomy of uterovaginal prolapse lead to vault prolapse.

Activating Factors

Activating factors of uterovaginal prolapse later on leading to vault prolapse are increased intra-abdominal pressure which can be because of chronic cough, ascites, intra-abdominal tumor, heavy weight lifting; increased weight of uterus like in subinvoluted uterus, myohyperplasia of uterus, multiple fibroid in uterus and traction of uterus due to large cervical fibroid.

Identification of Apex of Vagina in Vault Prolapse

While performing the surgery for prolapse uterus, identification of lack of support to apex of vagina is important. If it is not identified and only anterior vaginal wall and posterior vaginal wall are repaired, it leads to vault prolapse.

PREVENTION OF UTEROVAGINAL PROLAPSE

To prevent uterovaginal prolapse, which can lead to vault prolapse later, during labor one must avoid premature attempt of delivery, prolonged second stage, wrong application of forceps and vacuum extraction. All layers of episiotomy should be repaired properly. Liberal episiotomy in pelvic organ prolapses (POPs) and malpresentations and proper management of third stage of labor should be done to prolapse and vault prolapse after hysterectomy. During puerperium, perineal exercises by the mother are helpful in preventing prolapse. Puerperal constipation should be properly treated and weight lifting be avoided. During menopause, women should be given hormonal therapy and advised pelvic floor exercises. During hysterectomy, cardinal ligaments, uterosacral ligaments and round ligaments should be identified properly and stitched over the vault to prevent vault prolapse later.

CLINICAL MANIFESTATIONS OF VAULT PROLAPSE

Women with prolapse into the vagina often complain of sensation of pelvic pressure, bearing down sensation, inguinal discomfort, dyspareunia or low back pain. These symptoms become gradually worse due to gradual increase in size of the prolapse. With repetitive increase in intra-abdominal pressure, the prolapsed vault may protrude from the vagina on standing, leading to chronic discharge and bleeding from chronic ulceration. The danger of vaginal evisceration is always there. Vaginal vault prolapse is frequently accompanied by cystocele, rectocele, enterocele or combination of these disorders.

MANAGEMENT OF VAULT PROLAPSE

Management of vault prolapse may be:
- Surgical or hormonal.

Surgical

Abdominal Sling Operation: Rectus Sheath Sling

Preoperative Management

- Routine investigations as per surgical norms to ensure her fitness for major surgery
- Ultrasound examination of lower abdomen
- Intravenous pyelogram if required.

Preoperative Preparation

Bowel preparation for 2-3 as advised by anesthesia:
- Premedication
- Reduction of vault by betadine-soaked vaginal packing (Fig. 9)
- Catheterization with Foley catheter (Fig. 10)
- *Anesthesia*: Depends upon medical examination. General anesthesia/spinal anesthesia can be decided depending upon the condition of the patient (Fig. 11)
- Cleaning and draping for suprapubic transverse incision (Fig. 12).

Operations

Rectus sheath sling steps of operations:
- Suprapubic transverse incision is given in the skin and fat (Fig. 13)
- Rectus sheath is identified and exposed by dissecting the fat (Figs 14 and 15)
- Transverse incision is given in the sheath, a flap/sling is made, which is cut in the middle, divided into two

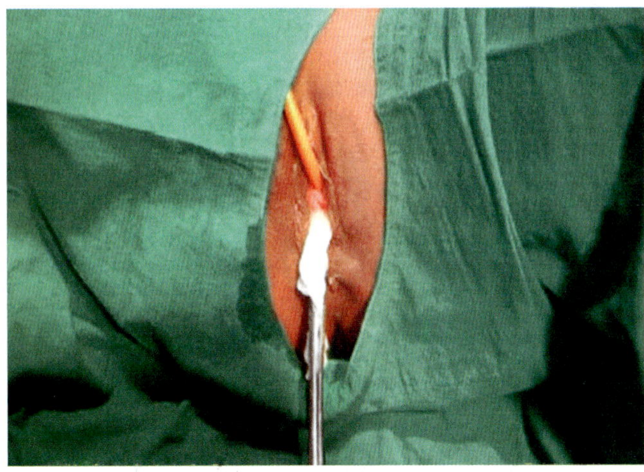

Fig. 9: Vaginal packing removal prior to surgery

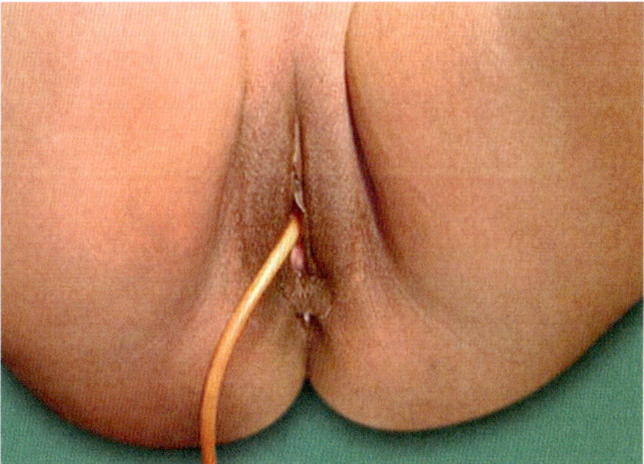

Fig. 10: Catheterization of urinary bladder after reducing the prolapse

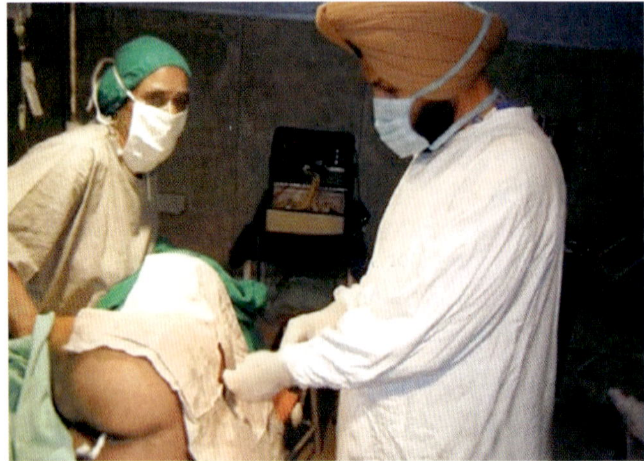

Fig. 11: Giving spinal anesthesia

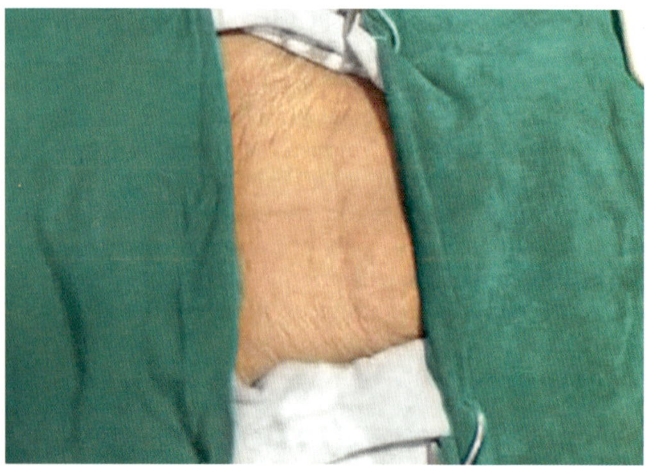

Fig. 12: Cleaning and draping of abdomen

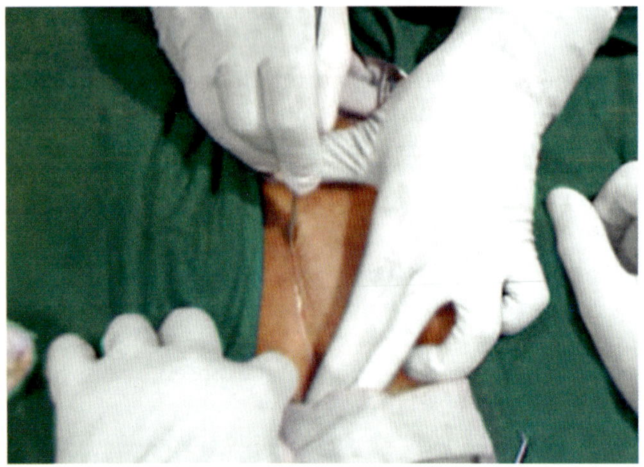

Fig. 13: Transverse incision in the lower abdomen

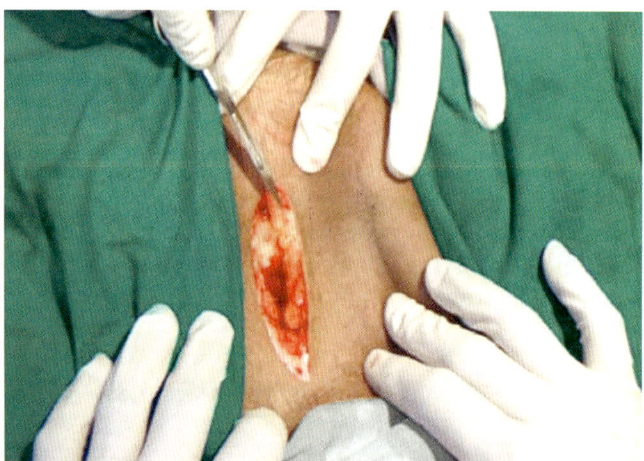

Fig. 14: Opening of abdomen up to rectus sheath

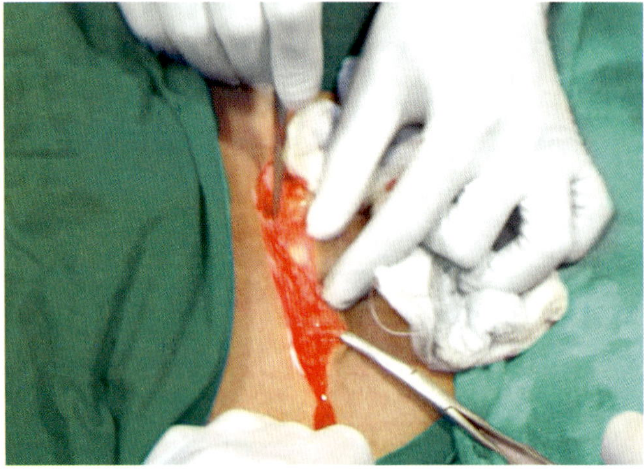

Fig. 15: Identifying of rectus sheath

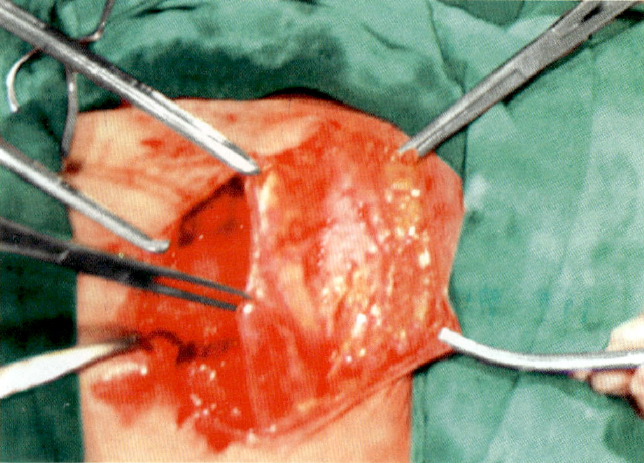

Fig. 16: Separation of rectus sheath

parts, kept attached to the lateral side of the sheath (Figs 16 and 17)

- Abdomen is opened and packs placed into displace the gut
- Vault, anterior and upper margins of urinary bladder are identified (Fig. 18)
- Rectus sheath sling is brought in the abdomen through lateral abdominal wall on both sides by a false opening away from the rectus muscle (Figs 19 and 20)
- Sling is passed through the two leaves of peritoneal folds, up to the vault as vault is kept upright by the vaginal packing
- Vaginal packing is removed from below
- Both slings are attached over the vault posteriorly with nonabsorbable suture (Figs 21 and 22)
- Sling keeps vault suspended in the pelvic cavity (Fig. 23)
- Abdominal packs are removed and rectus sheath gap stitched by prolene (Fig. 24)
- Abdomen is closed in layers after maintaining hemostasis
- Rectocele repair is done from below (Fig. 25).

Complications

- Anesthetic complications
- Injury to bladder, if upper margin not identified properly.

Other Methods

Artificial Supports

Artificial support can also be used in the form of Mersilene/nylon tapes. These are stitched over to the top of the vault and brought laterally and retroperitoneally out and stitched to lateral border of aponeurosis of external oblique muscle. Recent review by Nygaard et al. shows that success rate with this support management ranges from 78% to 100%.

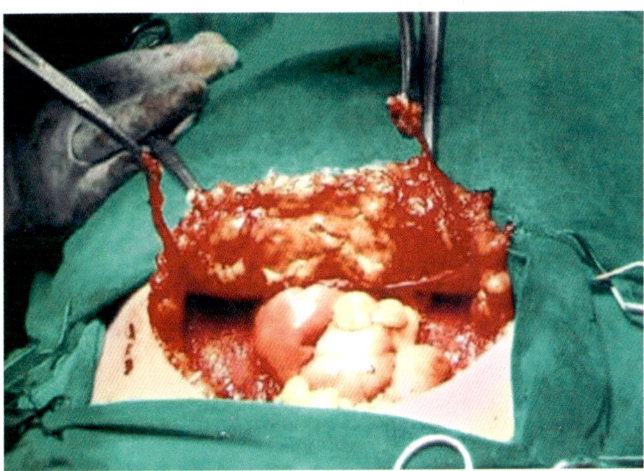

Fig. 17: Rectus sheath sling

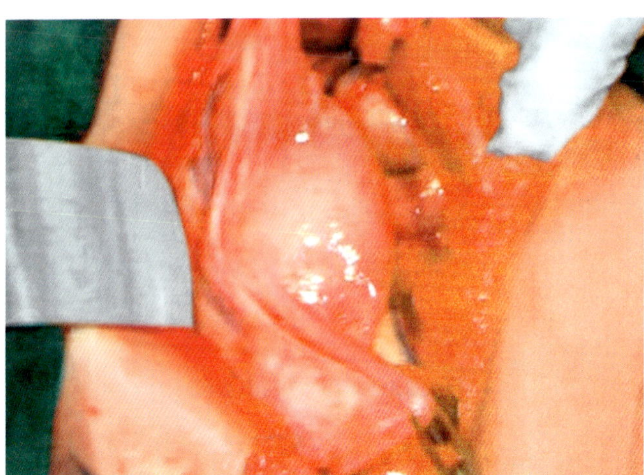

Fig. 18: Identification of vault and urinary bladder

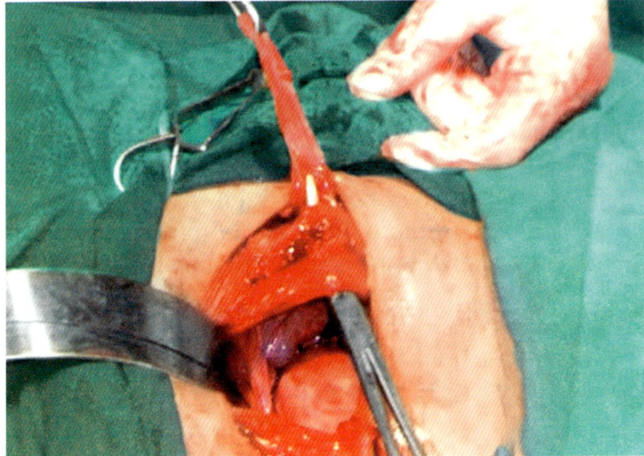

Fig. 19: Introducing sling in the abdomen through false opening away from rectus muscle

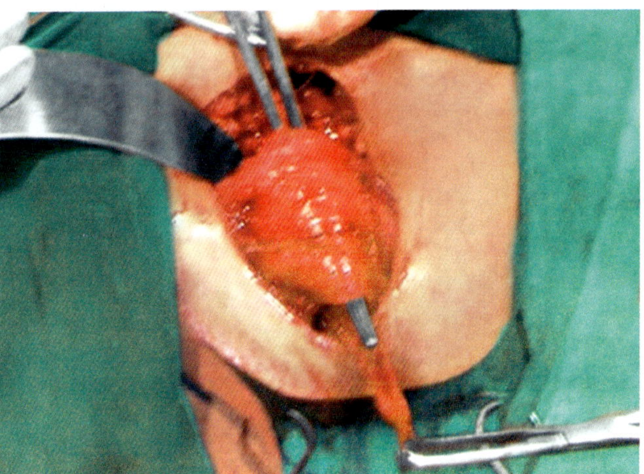

Fig. 20: Introducing sling in the abdomen through false opening away from rectus muscle on ipsilateral side

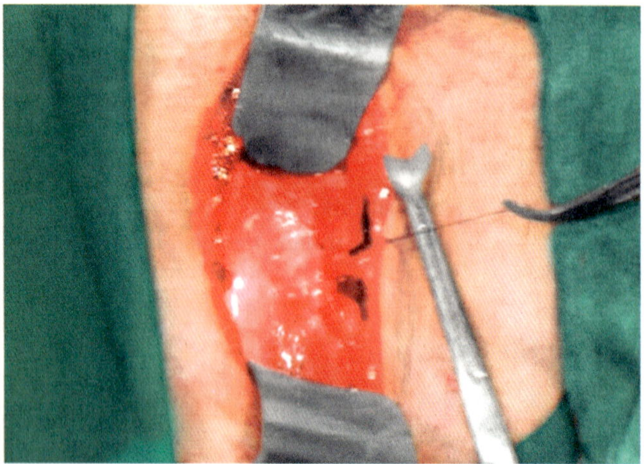

Fig. 21: Stitching of rectus sheath sling on the posterior side of vault

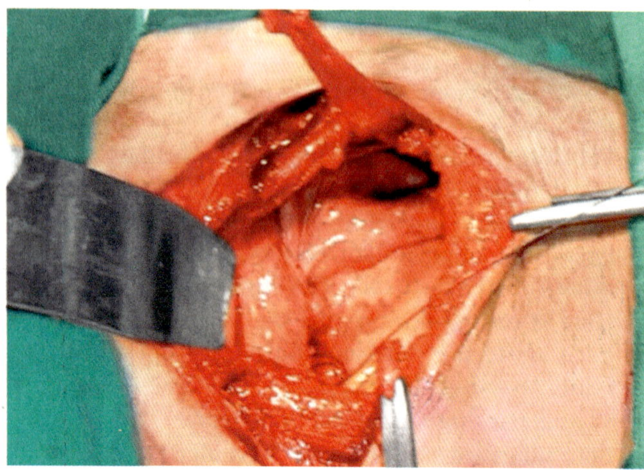

Fig. 22: Stitching of rectus sheath sling on the posterior side of vault on their side

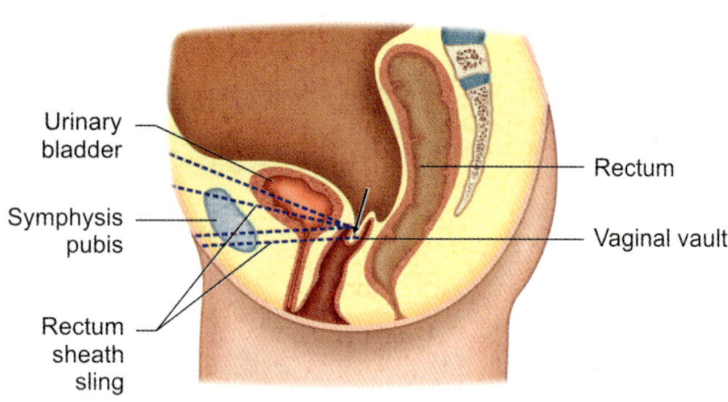

Fig. 23: Rectus sheath sling

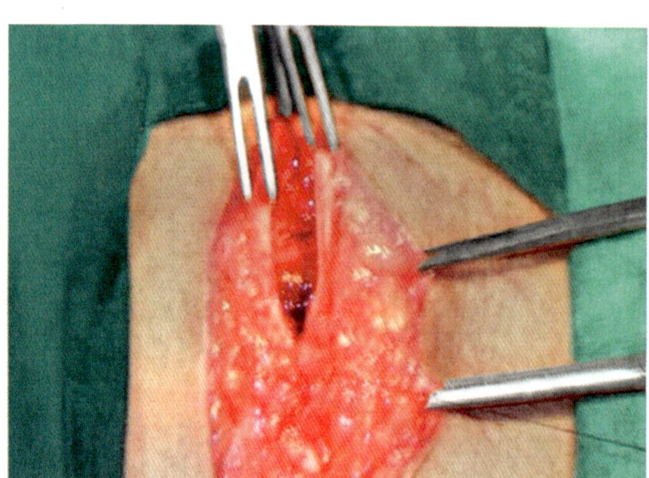

Fig. 24: Closure of rectus sheath

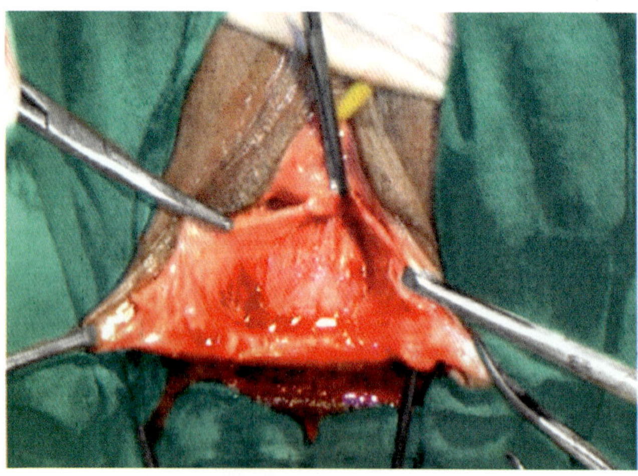

Fig. 25: Rectocele repair

Moschcowitz's Repair

It is done to obliterate the POD and enterocele. Purse string sutures are applied between the posterior surface of cervix and vagina near the POD and presacral peritoneum to obliterate the POD.

Shirodkar's Sling

Shirodkar's procedure, uterosacral ligaments to be identified and stitched over the vault. It is more useful in nulliparous women, because in old women the uterosacrals ligaments are already atrophied.

Transabdominal Sacral Colpopexy

Transabdominal sacral colpopexy comprises suspending the vault to the sacral promontory using Mersilene tape. It can be done extraperitoneally or can be put in the hollow of sacrum.

Laparoscopic Colpopexy

Laparoscopic colpopexy is a very useful and skillful technique as shown by Cossom et al. Here Mersilene or nylon tape is used which is stitched to fundus of the vault and brought to the anterior superior iliac spine or sacral promontory.

Infracoccygeal Sacropexy

Infracoccygeal sacropexy with a tension-free tape has been tried on day care basis. It has a failure rate of 6% and is a bit difficult procedure requiring skill. One may injure rectal and sacral vessels. Attempts directed solely at repairing the anterior and posterior vaginal walls will not solve the problem of apical support loss.

Khanna's sling Operation

In Khanna's sling operation, Mersilene tape is fixed to the fundus of uterus and the two free ends are brought out through lateral abdominal wall and stitched over the anterior superior iliac spine on either side.

Pelvic Floor Repair

Pelvic floor repair will not be successful as there will not be any support to the apex of the vault.

Colpocleisis

Colpocleisis is rarely performed.

Le Fort's Repair

Le Fort's repair is also obsolete nowadays.

Pessary Treatment

Cases unfit for surgery, ring pessary can be used but it needs repair of deficient perineum to retain the ring pessary.

Hormonal Therapy

All the posthysterectomy cases should be given oral and local hormonal therapy (LHT) as per guidelines.

CONCLUSION

Vaginal vault prolapse is due to faulty surgical procedure at the level of apex during vaginal or abdominal hysterectomy. To prevent vault prolapse, uterovaginal prolapse should be preoperatively assessed for decision of abdominal/vaginal hysterectomy and all the procedures of prevention of vault prolapse should be taken during surgery.

Mackenrodt's uterosacral and round ligaments should be identified and stitched over the vault in abdominal hysterectomies, wherever vagina is lax and cervical elongation is present. Enterocele should be identified and buttressing of two uterosacral ligaments and peritoneum over it should be done.

Vault prolapse can be repaired by abdominal route with suspension operation to prevent recurrence. Various suspension operations have been enumerated in the literature. Rectus sheath sling is stitched by abdominal route over the apex of the vault after identifying urinary bladder. It keeps uterine vault suspended in the pelvic cavity. The vagina does not get narrowed and shortened as seen in surgery by vaginal route. Deficient perineum and rectocele is repaired from below. Additional hormonal therapy for local application for short duration should be prescribed after the surgery.

BIBLIOGRAPHY

1. Addison WA, Livengood CH, Sutton GP, et al. Abdominal sacral colpopexy with Mersilene mesh in the retroperitoneal position in the management of posthysterectomy vaginal vault prolapse and enterocele. Am J Obstet Gynecol. 1985;153:140-6.
2. Barrington JW, Edwards G. Posthysterectomy vault prolapse. Int Urogynecol J Pelvic Floor Dysfunct. 2000;11:241-5.
3. Birnbaum SJ. Rational therapy for the prolapsed vagina. Am J Obstet Gynecol. 1973;115:411-9.
4. Cosson M, Rajabally R, Bogaert E, et al. Laparoscopic sacrocolpopexy, hysterectomy, and burch colposuspension: feasibility and short-term complications of 77 procedures. JSLS. 2002;6:115-9.
5. Cruikshank SH. Sacrospinous fixation—should this be performed at the time of vaginal hysterectomy? Am J Obstet Gynecol. 1991;164:1072-6.
6. Davila GW. Introduction and review of current approaches to vault prolapse. [online] Available from www.ivstunneller.com/content/USS interviews Aug 2003 intro.htm.
7. Farnsworth BN. Posterior intravaginal slingplasty (infracoccygeal sacropexy) for severe posthysterectomy vaginal vault prolapse—a preliminary report on efficacy and safety. Int Urogynecol J Pelvic Floor Dysfunct. 2002;13:4-8.
8. Morley GW, DeLancey JO. Sacrospinous ligament fixation for eversion of the vagina. Am J Obstet Gynecol. 1988;158: 872-81.
9. Nygaard IE. McCreery R, Brubaker L, et al. Abdominal sacrocolpopexy: a comprehensive review. Obstet Gynecol. 2004;104:805-23.
10. Parikh M. Editorial. J Obstet Gynecol India. 2005;55(1):20-1.
11. Petros PE. Vault prolapse II: restoration of dynamic vaginal supports by infracoccygeal sacropexy, an axial day-case vaginal procedure. Int Urogynecol J Pelvic Floor Dysfunct. 2001;12:296-303.

CHAPTER

39

Cervix

Surveen Ghumman, Sonia Kamboj, Jaideep Malhotra, Narendra Malhotra, Chandrawati, Priti Kumar, Mala Arora, Vandana Walvekar, Geetha D Balsarkar, Nidhi Gupta, Kamal Gupta, VL Lahiri, Manashi Ray

39.1 CERVICAL BIOPSY AND ENDOCERVICAL CURETTAGE

Surveen Ghumman

INTRODUCTION

Cervical biopsy forms an important diagnostic follow-up in cases with abnormal cytology or colposcopic finding in premalignant and malignant conditions of the cervix. Cervical cancer is one of the most common malignant diseases in women. Results of cervical biopsy determine further management of the lesion. Cone biopsy could also be therapeutic if it is excisional. Since these specimens are often very small, careful handling and work-up is required.

If there is suspect or evident dysplasia in cytology, but not in the biopsy, there is a possibility that the dysplastic lesions might be rather small and difficult to reach, and therefore might not have been targeted by a biopsy. For that reason histology and cytology should be closely correlated in such cases, and if the changes found in the biopsy do not explain the cytological changes, a repeat biopsy should be considered.

ANATOMY

The cervix consists of the ectocervix which is part of the cervix exposed to the vagina. It is a convex round surface with a slit-like or circular opening (external os) into the endocervical canal. The endocervical canal is 2–3 cm in length and opens into the endometrial cavity at the internal os. The cervical mucosa contains both stratified squamous epithelium, characteristic of exocervix and mucus secreting columnar epithelium characteristic of endocervical canal. The intersection of these epithelia is the squamocolumnar junction or the transformation zone which is the vulnerable site for development of neoplasia. The transformation zone changes location with age in response to hormonal stimulation.

Squamous epithelium: It consists of four layers:

1. *Basal layer:* Single layer of immature cells with large nuclei.
2. *Parabasal cells:* 2–4 rows of immature cells.
3. *Intermediate layer:* 4–6 layers of cells with large amounts of cytoplasm in a polyhedral shape.
4. *Superficial layers:* 5–8 rows of flattened cells with small uniform nuclei and cytoplasm. These cells form the basis for Pap smear (Papanicolaou test).

Columnar epithelium: It has a single layer of columnar cells with mucus at the top and round nucleus at the base.

Metaplastic epithelium: It begins at the columnar reserve cell. Under stimulation of lower vaginal acidity the reserve cells proliferate lifting the columnar epithelium. The immature metaplastic cells have large nuclei and small amount of cytoplasm. As the metaplasia replaces the columnar epithelium, the central capillary of the villus regresses and the epithelium flattens out, leaving the epithelium with its typical vascular network. Metaplasia replaces the cervical cleft incompletely leading to entrapment of mucus secreting cells and formation of nabothian follicles.

PREOPERATIVE PREPARATION

Preoperative evaluation by Pap smear and colposcopy should have been done. Although punch biopsy is done under local anesthesia, fasting for 6–8 hours is recommended in case of any complication where the need to give general anesthesia, may arise. An informed consent must be taken.

Indications

1. Positive cytology.
2. Suspect cytology.
3. Suspect colposcopy (leukoplacia, condyloma, polyps).
4. Persistent symptoms.
5. Suspicious lesion or growth.

Anesthesia

It is done under local anesthesia. Cone biopsy may be done under regional or general anesthesia.

Position

Patient is placed in lithotomy position.

Types of Cervical Biopsy

- Punch biopsy
- Wedge biopsy
- Cone biopsy
- LEEP (loop electrosurgical excision procedure).

The punch biopsy and the wedge biopsy may be colposcopically directed. Single or multiple punch biopsies may be taken according to the colposcopic findings.

Choice of Biopsy

If neoplasm is visible punch biopsy will suffice. As a rule cervical biopsy should contain tissues from squamo-columnar junction and border between normal and suspicious area. If cytology is positive and no lesion visible on gross or colposcopic examination, an endocervical currettage or conization will be necessary in order to survey the entire squamocolumnar junction.

Technique

Defining lesions for biopsy: The first step is to identify the area requiring biopsy.

Intraepithelial neoplasms rarely produce changes in the cervix which are visible to the naked eye. Thus speculum examination of the cervix may not reveal the source of abnormal cells and there may be difficulty in deciding where to target the biopsy. For this reason several techniques have been developed which can be used to identify the site of the biopsy:

1. *Schiller's iodine:* The test is defined by the reaction iodine has when painted on the portio vaginalis of cervix and vaginal mucosa. Normal squamous epithelium, which is glycogen rich, stains brown; whereas, cancerous area which does not contain glycogen will not take up the stain. Surgery can be directed to iodine negative areas
   Fallacy: There is a false positive reaction in areas of immature metaplasia, atrophic and glandular epithelium which does not take up the stain. A few cancers may be rich in glycogen and may take up the stain.
   Precaution: Either Schiller's or Lugol's iodine may be used. Alcoholic solution of iodine should not be used as it spoils the tissue for histopathology.
2. *Colposcopy:* It consists of stereoscopic binocular microscope with central illuminating device of high intensity which is used to inspect the cervix at a magnification of 4–40 times. Abnormal epithelium can be biopsied under direct vision.

Abnormal findings on colposcopy which need to be biopsied are:

1. Atypical transformation zone
   i. Whiteness of epithelium after application of acetic acid
   ii. Changes in angioarchitecture
   iii. Keratosis
   iv. Slight surface irregularity.
2. Changes suggestive of invasive carcinoma
   These findings are then graded.

PUNCH BIOPSY

The cervix is exposed after the patient has been positioned. The area of biopsy is marked out. The biopsy is taken by a punch biopsy forceps (Figs 1A and B). The area marked is exposed and the punch biopsy forceps is introduced (Fig. 2). Adequate bite of the tissue must be obtained. A biopsy should contain sufficient subepithelial connective tissue so that the possibilty of microinvasion can be ruled out. The punch biopsy forceps is sharp and will provide a depth of 3–5 mm of stroma in addition to surface epithelium which helps to identify microinvasion (Fig. 1B). Specimens are usually small, difficult to orient and easily crushable. Oblique sectioning causes false impression that invasion is present. This can be minimized if mucosal surface of the biopsy is identified and aligned correctly so that it is at right angles to the plane of section.

WEDGE BIOPSY

Punch biopsy has largely replaced wedge biopsy with use of colposcope for directing the biopsy. It still has a place in pregnant patients where biopsy should be avoided unless suspecting invasion or microinvasion. In such cases, a wedge is preferred to punch as it is easier to control bleeding by suturing the raw edges of biopsied area. Since, it is a wider and deeper biopsy it is used when punch biopsy

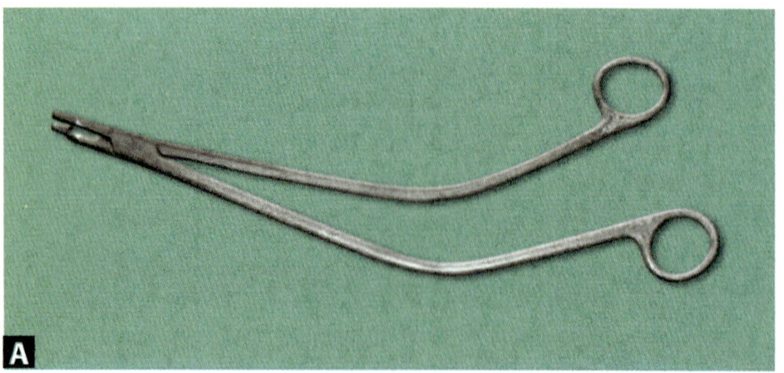

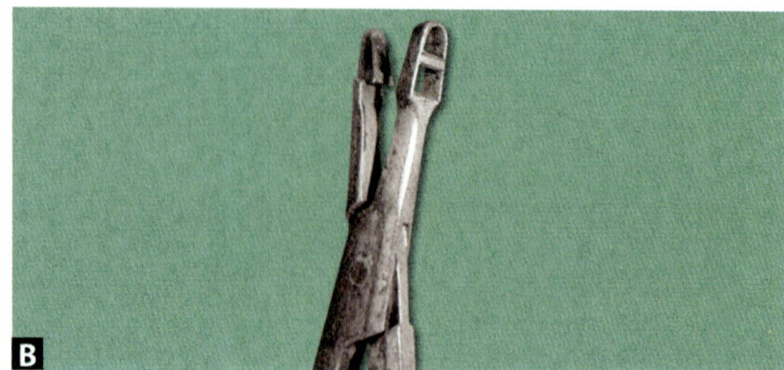

Figs 1A and B: Punch biopsy forceps

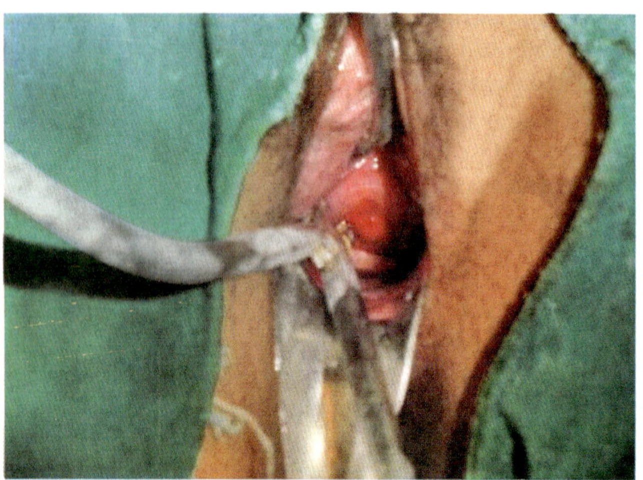

Fig. 2: Punch biopsy forceps being used for taking a biopsy at 9 o'clock position on cervix

is inconclusive or micro invasion or invasion is suspected. A wedge is cut with a knife taking care to include both endocervix and ectocervix. The raw edges may be sutured with interuppted stitches.

CONE BIOPSY

A cone biopsy is a procedure to obtain a larger sample than that obtained by cervical punch biopsy or colposcopically directed biopsy. It could be diagnostic or therapeutic. A small cone-shaped sample of tissue is removed from the cervix which includes the cervical canal. A cone biopsy removes abnormal tissue that is high in the cervical canal. A sample of tissue can be removed for a cone biopsy using:

1. Surgical Knife.
2. Carbon dioxide (CO_2) laser.
3. LEEP.

INDICATIONS

1. Diagnostic evaluation and clarification where there is lack of correlation between cytology, biopsy and colposcopy.
2. If previous punch biopsy specimen of grossly suspicious lesion shows noninvasive precancerous lesion not completely excised.
3. Lesion extending into endocervix beyond the limits of colposcopy.
4. Endocervical histology positive for high-grade squamous intraepithelial lesion (HSIL).
5. Cytology persistently positive for low-grade squamous intraepithelial lesion (LSIL).
6. Colposcopy reveals that endocervix is involved.

The cone should contain the entire squamocolumnar junction Depending on age of the patient, the junction may be located on ectocervix as in reproductive age requiring a shallow cone or the endocervix as in older patients requiring a clongated cone (Figs 3 and 4) Colposcopy can help decide location of squamocolumnar junction.

COLD KNIFE EXCISION

Technique: Cervix is grasped with a single toothed tenaculum laterally at 3 o' clock and 9 o' clock position outside the lesion and pulled down. One can apply sutures of absorbable material laterally in the region of descending branch of uterine artery. Lugol's iodine is applied to dilineate extent and a 5 mm margin is left. As the incision is deepened, it is angled towards the canal in the shape of a cone. Bleeding points are electrocoagulated. If raw area is large then Strumdorff suture may be applied to cover the cervix.

The disadvantage of cold knife excision is that it is impossible to monitor the endocervical canal margin of excision to ensure that full length of the lesion has been removed. Also there is significant morbidity related to obstetric and reproductive sequelae. Today this technique has been mostly replaced by large loop excision of the transformation zone (LLETZ)-conization as there is increased incidence of postoperative bleeding.

LASER CONIZATION

Laser is used in cutting mode at highest power. A 3 mm margin is taken from lesion site. The disadvantage of

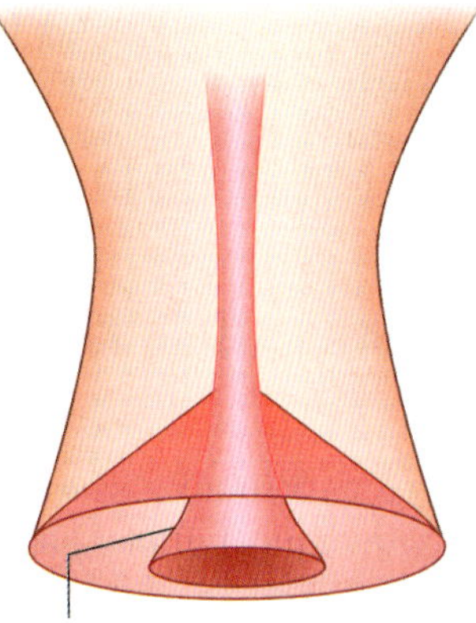

Fig. 3: Shallow cone is taken when squamocolumnar junction is located on ectocervix

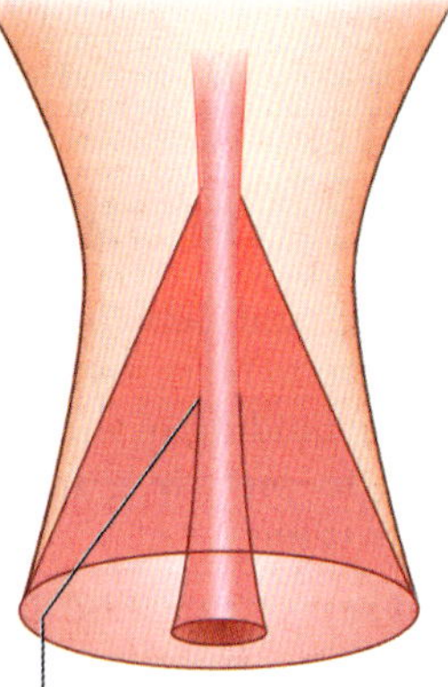

Fig. 4: Deep cone is taken when squamocolumnar junction is located on endocervix

laser conization is that resection margins are in most cases damaged by the heat and a large wound is left. This technique is performed rarely today and has been mostly replaced by LLETZ-conization.

Equipment: It consists of a set of stainless steel wire loops of various sizes attached to an insulated handle.

Technique: As cutting current is passed, it is essential to follow rather than push the loop through the cervix. If looped is dragged, a shallow cut is made. The loop is placed over the lesion with enough pressure to bend wire slightly. For this technique, the specimen is sent to the pathological laboratory, mostly in two portions, one ectocervical and a second endocervical one. The surgeon should try to retrieve the ectocervical specimen intact as it enables the pathologist to determine if a lesion (dysplasia) has been resected totally.

Handling and labeling of cone specimen: The specimens are quite large and can be orientated easily. The cone should be marked such that the pathologist can understand its anatomical location. A suture can be put at the 12 o'clock position. The surgeon should not attempt to open the cone or remove the mucus or blood from the raw surface as abnormal epithelium is very delicate and may detach. It should not be cut till it is fixed as epithelium is very fragile. It should be fixed for 24 hours. The edges of the cone must be free of abnormal cells otherwise further intervention is required.

POSTOPERATIVE COMPLICATIONS

- *Hemorrhage:* It occurs in 6% of cases, usually on the eighth to tenth postoperative day. Treatment consists of packing, antibiotics, diathermy coagulation or sutures
- *Infection:* Seen in 0.2% cases
- *Perforation:* Perforation is a rare complication occurring in 0.005%
- *Cervical Stenosis:* It occurs in 0.7% of cases
- *Cervical incompetence:* Cervical incompetence may occur if a large specimen is removed
- Infertility
- *Persistence of disease:* Postcone endocervical curettage was found to be the most statistically significant factor for predicting persistent disease.

COLD KNIFE VS LLETZ VS LASER

Loop removes less healthy tissue without reducing chances of complete excision. The chances of postoperative bleeding are less. If amount of tissue removed is related to occurrence of cervical incompetence at a later date, it may be preferred in women who have not completed a family. LLETZ is easier and less time consuming. The disadvantage is that there are electrocautery artifacts, so evaluation of margin is not possible. Laser has the disadvantage of high cost, time consumption and significant alteration of tissue. The cold knife excision biopsy provided a cervical specimen that had less fragmentation and less thermal damage with margins that were less likely to be indeterminate than those obtained with the large loop electrosurgical procedure. The status of margins is a better predictor of abnormal follow-up in cold knife conization than in LLETZ specimens. 77% of cases with LLETZ had artifacts which interfered in interpretation compared to cold knife conization where they were present in 38%.

POSTOPERATIVE CARE AND COUNSELING

After the procedure, there may be some cramping or discomfort for a week or so. Patient should avoid sexual intercourse, douching and use of tampons for about 4-6 weeks. For 2-3 weeks after the procedure, there may be heavy, bloody, or a yellow-colored discharge. Some vaginal bleeding is normal for up to 1 week.

COLLECTION AND FIXING

The collection, fixing and labeling is to be done by gynecologist. It is extremely important for the clinicians to have a clear understanding of the requirements of the pathologist in order to provide a specimen which is of maximum diagnostic value.

Care must be taken to immerse the tissue fully in a fixative. Small specimens from punch biopsy or wedge biopsy require fixation for 6 hours, whereas larger tissues like cone biopsy specimen require fixation for 24 hours. All specimens must be labeled correctly.

SECTIONS

Punch Biopsy/Wedge Biopsy

Small specimens should be worked up in toto in serial sections. For paraffin embedding, it should be considered that the cutting plane level should be at a normal angle to the surface of the specimen. Larger specimens should be divided in half and should also be worked up in serial sections.

Cone Biopsy

Macroscopic description: Anteroposterior diameter, height of the specimen, location of the cervical channel (central, paracentral, at the margin) and any macroscopically visible lesion should be noted.

Serial sectioning: It can be done as step sectioning or radial slicing after dividing the specimen into half

1. Step sectioning (Fig. 5).
2. Radial slicing (Fig. 6).

It is recommended to make all the sections at 0.1–0.2 mm. This method, resulting in 100–200 sections/specimen, enables the pathologist to assess possible microinvasion and vasular involvement more reliably. Each tenth section is placed on a silanized slide, thus allowing immunohistochemistry.

The histopathological diagnosis should include:

- Histological type
- Grade of the lesion (LSIL, HSIL)
- Circumference of the lesion
- Uni/multifocal
- Human papilloma virus (HPV)-typical changes
- Margins
- Stroma reaction
- Invasion: Uni/multifocal, depth of invasion, circumference of invasion, stroma reaction, lymphovascular invasions.

Immunohistochemistry to support diagnosis of microinvasion or vascular involvement

Immunohistochemical markers (antibodies directed to extracellular matrix components of the basal lamina) could be used in selected cases for the assessment of microinvasion and vascular invasion.

ENDOCERVICAL CURETTAGE

Indications

- May be included as a routine in colposcopy of older women when squamocolumnar junction recedes as neoplastic changes can be missed by cytology and colposcopy
- Suspect glandular cells in cervical smear
- When cone suggests incomplete removal and hysterectomy is contraindicated.

Endocervical curettings (ECC) are usually scanty. If bulky specimen is received endocervical polyp or adenocarcinoma is suspected.

Technique

Patient is placed in lithotomy position. Posterior vaginal wall is retracted by a Sims speculum. Anterior lip of cervix

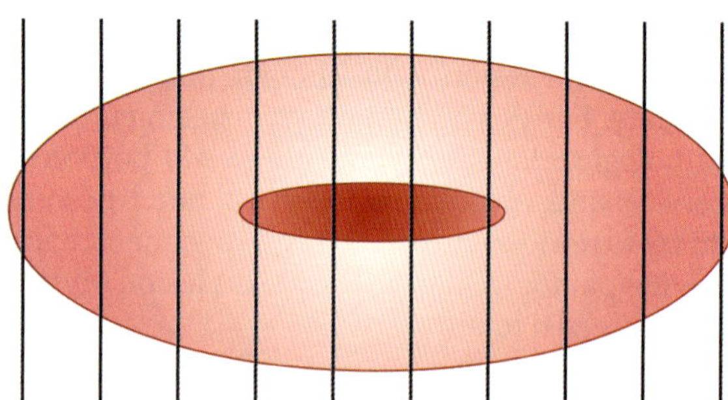

Fig. 5: Step sectioning of cone biopsy specimen

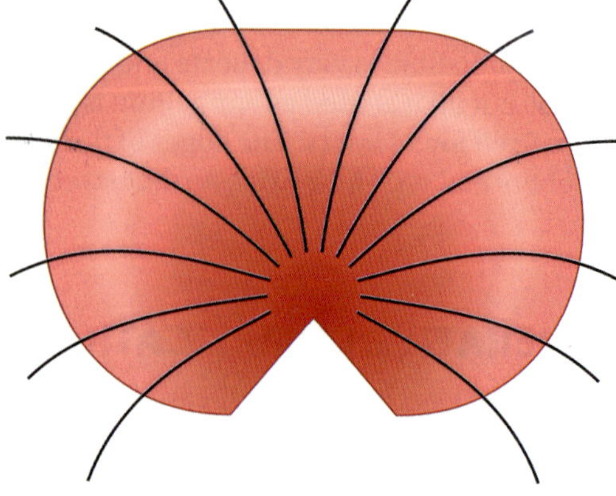

Fig. 6: Radial slicing of cone biopsy specimen

is held by a vulsellum. Endocervical curettage is usually done by means of an endocervical curette. The specimens may be very small. There should be several sections of the specimen. Endocervical cytology can also be taken by the endocervical brush (ECB).

Our findings suggest that the colposcopic study is optimized when it is performed in conjunction with ECB as opposed to ECC, and that intensive ECB may be superior to ECC. There is good agreement between grade of dysplasia on preoperative ECC and on subsequent conization specimen. Colposcopic examination was not a good predictor of pathology in the endocervical canal. Routine ECC should be part of the preoperative assessment of an abnormal Pap smear.

Important information to be communicated by the pathologist to the gynecologist report should include a clear diagnosis of the primary lesion and if the resection margins are clear. Since microinvasion has a severe impact on clincial managment of patients, complete work-up of specimens in serial sections is recommended. Additional immunohistochemistry could support a diagnosis of possible microinvasion or vessel involvement.

CONCLUSION

Cervical biopsy though a minor procedure is an important step for deciding management of cervical intraepithelial neoplasia (CIN) and invasive cancer of cervix. The clinician's role is vital in taking the specimen from the right site with an adequate depth, proper handling and fixing of these small specimens, and marking anatomical location on the specimen for the pathologist.

BIBLIOGRAPHY

1. Birner P, Obermair A, Schindl M, et al. Selective immuno-histochemical staining of blood and lymphatic vessels reveals independent prognos-tic influence of blood and lymphatic vessel invasion in early-stage cervical cancer. Clin Cancer Res. 2001;7(1):93-7.
2. Fine BA, Feinstein GI, Sabella V. The pre- and postoperative value of endocervical curettage in the detection of cervical intraepithelial neoplasia and invasive cervical cancer. Gynecol Oncol. 1998;71(1):46-9.
3. Fischer NR, Alexandarian D, Gagliardi S, et al. Evaluation of the cone biopsy excisor compared with the large loop for electrosurgical excision of cervical lesions. Prim Care Update Ob Gyns. 1998;5(4):161-2.
4. Girardi F, Hegdarfadai M, Koroschetz F, et al. Cold knife cone vs loop excision: Histopath and clinical results of randomised trial. Gynecol Oncol. 1994;55:368-70.
5. Ioffe OB, Brooks SE, De Rezende RB, et al. Artifact in cervical LLETZ specimens: correlation with follow-up. Int J Gynecol Pathol. 1999;18(2):115-21.
6. Lu CH, Liu FS, Kuo CJ, et al. Prediction of persistence or recurrence after conization for cervical intraepithelial neoplasia III. Obstet Gynecol. 2006;107(4):830-5.
7. Maksem JA. Endocervical curetting vs. endocervical brushing as case finding methods. Diagn Cytopathol. 2006;34(5): 313-6.

39.2 CERVICAL CONIZATION

Sonia Kamboj

INTRODUCTION

Cervical conization may be used to diagnose possible cancer or to excise CIN or other abnormal (on colposcopy) tissue extending beyond the field of vision up the cervical canal (10–15% of cervical cancers develop in the upper cervical canal).

A biopsy of malignant tumors can never give information about the depth of invasion. If the clinical signs fail to reveal how deeply a tumor has invaded, e.g. a crater is seen, a conization must always be performed. This is the only method on which to base the decision of whether further treatment should consist of simple surgical procedures (enlarged cone or simple hysterectomy) or involve more extensive methods (radical surgery or irradiation). A conization should always contain the entire squamocolumnar junction. Depending upon the age of the patient, that junction may be localized on the ectocervix, as during the reproductive age, requiring a flat conus, or be up in the endocervical canal, as in old age, requiring an elongated conus (Fig. 1). Since, however, neoplastic transformation of the endocervical reserve cells may extend into or even start in the endocervical canal, a large and elongated conus is often advisable in young patients, too. The cone should be marked so that the pathologist understands how it was located anatomically; the same marking procedure should be used in all cases. For example, a suture mark at "12 o'clock" will help the pathologist orient the specimen and pinpoint the site of a lesion on either the anterior or posterior lip, or both. Especially, when a precancerous lesion reaches the excisional margins of the cone, correct localization of the lesion will help the gynecologist in his follow up treatment of the patient. The lateral margins of a cone may contain cervical glands that project deep into the tissue, possibly with precancerous lesions. Therefore, these parts of the tissue must also be carefully examined. To avoid the possibility of leaving the bottoms of glands behind, many surgeons prefer excising a more cylindrically shaped piece of cervical tissue. In most instances, precancerous lesions are totally excised by conization and no further surgery will be necessary. Accordingly, diagnostic conization serves also serves as a therapeutic measure. Occasionally cervical conization may be required as a means of treatment, e.g. in patients with resistant vaginal discharge. Here, careful histological examination of the squamocolumnar junction is advisable to ensure that possible precancerous changes are not overlooked.

Most cervical conizations are performed as outpatient surgical procedures. Paracervical or general anesthesia may be required. Antiseptic solutions may be used, but care is taken not to touch the external cervical os. Suspicious areas that should be biopsied have generally previously been mapped by colposcopy. Conization is most commonly accomplished by LEEP, scalpel (cold conization), or laser and involves removing a thin circular portion of the cervix exterior to the squamocolumnar junction and extending variably up the endocervical canal. Rarely should the excision extend to the level of the internal os.

COLD KNIFE CONIZATION

Traditional cold knife conization has been used successfully for generations to excise lesions that extend into the endocervical canal to rule out invasive cancer. The cone is generally planned to be both diagnostic and therapeutic, and the technique is widely understood and practiced. The cone usually is performed in an operating room under anesthesia and, thus it is expensive. Because of the size of the specimen excised, bleeding and other sequelae such as cervical stenosis and infection are more common.

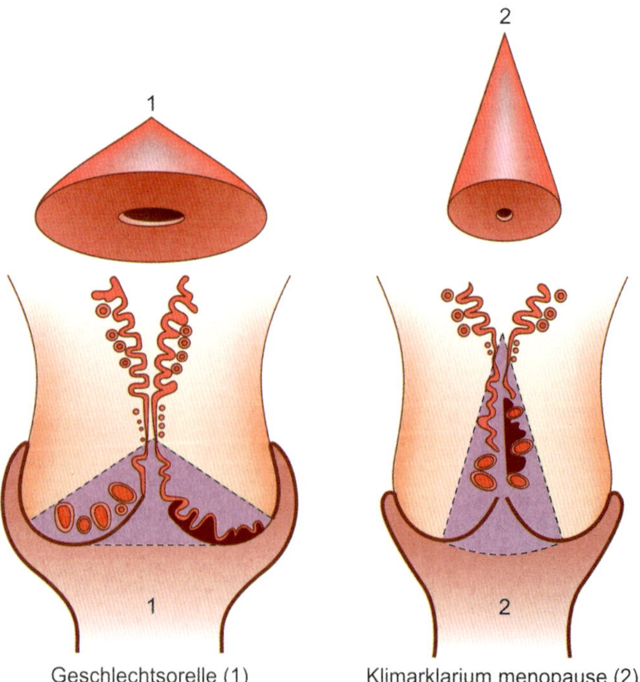

Fig. 1: Location of the squamocolumnar junction indicating zone of possible neoplastic transformation and shape of the conus usually recommended in (1) reproductive age and (2) in old age

A cold knife conization is clearly indicated when:

- The lesion extends into the endocervix
- A previous biopsy indicated a microinvasive carcinoma
- An adenocarcinoma in situ (ACIS) has been suspected in cytology
- A discrepancy exists between cytology, colposcopy and histology of a previous punch biopsy.

Scalpel cervical conization may be facilitated by introduction of a uterine sound to or just beyond the internal os so the tip of the blade approximates the sound. (Figs 2A to C). Generally, the tissue removed exceeds 0.3 cm in thickness. A suture usually is inserted at the top of the cone to aid the pathologist in tissue orientation for histology. A major problem of conization is damage to the internal cervical os. Moreover, the majority of lesions occur at the squamocolumnar junction and during the reproductive years the squamocolumnar junction is located on the portio of the cervix. Therefore, to avoid the potential of internal os injury many authorities currently recommend taking the specimen in a "doughnut" configuration without an extended endocervical portion. The endocervix is then curetted and the tissue submitted for analysis. If the cervix is deeply lacerated, segmental excision of tissue may be required to constitute a complete sample. Each fragment must be identified and a diagram to aid the pathologist facilitates accurate analysis.

LOOP ELECTROSURGICAL EXCISION

Loop electrosurgical excision procedure waas introduced in the United Kingdom as LLETZ after the modification of techniques originally developed in France. LEEP was introduced in the North America in the early 1990s, and as in Europe, rapidly became the procedure of choice for the management of CIN.

Loop electrosurgical excision procedure (LEEP) takes advantage of the properties of modern, solid-state, electrosurgical generators coupled with loop electrodes, made with a thin stainless steel or tungsten wire, to excise areas of CIN. It is also possible to electrocoagulate tissue with a 5 mm ball electrode. LEEP is used under colposcopic control and has the advantage of being a diagnostic and therapeutic procedure at the same time. The fact that a tissue specimen is provided makes the procedure particularly useful in ruling out early invasive cancer and in identifying unsuspected ACIS. Many authors have reported that 4–6 per 1,000 cases diagnosed by colposcopy, punch biopsies and endocervical curettage as having CIN in fact have invasive cancer or AIS in the specimen removed by LEEP. Because LEEP is easy to learn, easy to teach and easy to apply, it can be used to treat patients with high-grade CIN without the disadvantages and great cost of cold knife conization. The major advantage of LEEP over conventional cold knife conization is that the procedure can be performed under colposcopic control and the margins can be examined colposcopically after the initial excisions are completed. This gives the operator the opportunity to re-excise additional tissue if it is found colposcopically that residual CIN remains. For LEEP to be used effectively, the extent of excision and the choice of electrodes must be tailored to the size and distribution of the lesion. When disease extends into the canal, however a loop endocervical excision procedure can be performed with use of a 1×1 cm loop electrode. If the lesion is present on both the portio and the canal, a "reverse cowboy hat" combined endocervical-portio excision is appropriate.

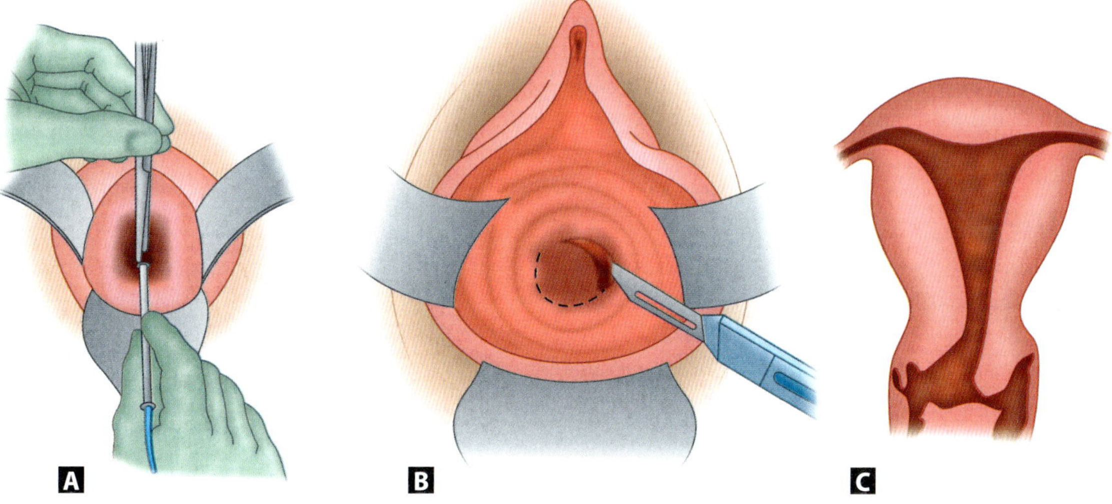

Figs 2A to C: Scalpel conization

The preferred electrode for the portio excision should not exceed 2.5 cm in width and 7 mm in depth. The use of extremely large electrodes may lead to inadvertent cervical amputations and significant reproductive and obstetric morbidity. The side effects and complications of LEEP are almost identical to those of the CO_2 laser.

Although low-grade lesions can readily be treated with cryotherapy, many gynecologists choose LEEP excision instead because of its ease of use, its limited morbidity and the fact that it provides a specimen. Caution is advised in choosing LEEP for small lesions in women who have only small areas of CIN in a small, nulliparous cervix because it is possible to produce irreversible cervical damage. With few exceptions, all high-grade lesions should be removed with use of an excisional, rather than an ablative procedure.

"See-and-treat"

Because LEEP is a simple procedure that can be used for both diagnosis and treatment during a single office visit, its use has been recommended in the so-called "see-and-treat" mode. With this application, patients who are detected as having an abnormal Pap smear are seen for colposcopy and when a clear-cut colposcopically visible lesion is present, the lesion is removed in its entirely with use of the loop electrode (Fig. 3). The patient does not first have to undergo cervical biopsies and an endocervical curettage.

The advantages to this approach are that the procedure is done in one office visit, thus reducing patient anxiety by eliminating the need to wait for a diagnosis to be rendered and to then return for additional treatment, and if used appropriately, it may save time and money. The disadvantage to this approach is that the colposcopic appearance of squamous metaplasia, repair, or other non-HPV-related changes may mimic CIN, and some patients who do not have a CIN lesion may have benign epithelium excised inappropriately. For see-and-treat to be used effectively and appropriately, the colposcopist must be certain that the colposcopic changes that are seen

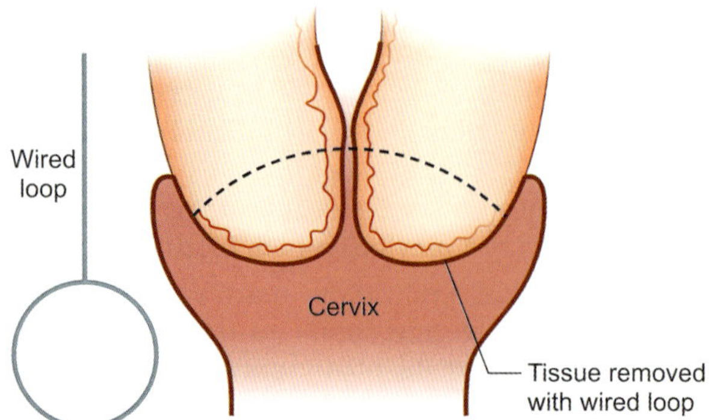

Fig. 3: Loop electrosurgical excision

are sufficiently characteristic for the diagnosis of an HPV-related lesion can be assured. Under these circumstances, see-and-treat may be the procedure of choice. It has been shown that the LEEP see-and-treat approach is highly beneficial and provides the opportunity to treat patients with significant lesions who might otherwise not return for their scheduled therapeutic follow-up visits.

MORBIDITY

The influence of previous cone biopsy on the morbidity of radical hysterectomy is controversial. Mikuta et al. reported an increased risk of postoperative complications, including febrile morbidity and urinary fistulas, although the interval between conization and radical hysterectomy was less than 3 weeks. Velden et al. reported no significant difference in morbidity but the conizationradical hysterectomy interval in their study was 6 weeks. They believed that delaying the definitive surgery may allow the tissue reaction to subside, thereby decreasing morbidity. Others have found the interval between the conization and radical hysterectomy to have no influence on morbidity and recommend proceeding without delay. Our policy is to proceed immediately with radical hysterectomy if the surgical margins of the cone biopsy are involved, but to postpone surgery for 6 weeks if the cone margins are clear.

BIBLIOGRAPHY

1. Dallenbach-Hellweg G. On the origin and histological structure of adenocarcinoma of the endocervix in women under 50 years of age. Pathol Res Pract. 1984;179(1):38-50.
2. Hamperl H, Kaufmann C. The cervix uteri at different ages. Obstet Gynecol. 1959;14:621-31.
3. Mikuta JJ, Giuntoli RL, Rubin EL, et al. The 'problem' radical hysterectomy. Am J Obstet Gynecol. 1977;128(2):119-27.
4. Murta EF, Silva AO, Silva EA. Clinical significance of a negative loop electrosurgical excision procedure, conization and hysterectomy for cervical intraepithelial neoplasia. Eur J Gynaecol Oncol. 2006;27(1):50-2.
5. Phongnarisorn C, Srisomboon J. Surgical morbidity associated with total laparoscopic hysterectomy in women with prior diagnostic excision of the cervix. J Obstet Gynaecol Res. 2007;33(4):519-23.
6. van der Velden J, Samlal R, Schilthuis MS, et al. A limited role for adjuvant radiotherapy after the Wertheim/Okabayashi radical hysterectomy for cervical cancer confined to the cervix. Gynecol Oncol. 1999;75(2):233-7.

39.3 CERVICAL INCOMPETENCE—McDONALD'S SUTURE

Jaideep Malhotra, Narendra Malhotra

INTRODUCTION

Fetal loss is a painful experience. A history of second or early third trimester fetal loss, after painless dilatation of the cervix, prolapse or rupture of the membranes and expulsion of a live fetus despite minimal uterine activity, is characteristic for cervical insufficiency.

Cervical incompetence was described by Palmer and LaComme in 1948 as a condition in which the cervix fails to retain the conceptus during pregnancy, with cervix length less than 25 mm. Cervical incompetence is defined "classically" as painless dilation of the cervix leading to delivery between 16 weeks and 28 weeks gestation. Unfortunately, this diagnosis is made retrospectively and attempts to make the diagnosis prospectively have been fraught with unknown validity. Treatment options include bed rest or serial assessment of the cervix digitally or by ultrasound and surgical procedures such as Shirodkar, McDonald, or abdominal cerclage.

INCIDENCE

Although it has been estimated to complicate as many as 1% of all pregnancies, the prevalence of cervical incompetence is likely to be in the range of 0.05–0.2%.

DIAGNOSIS

Attempts to make the diagnosis prospectively by passage of a # 8 Hegar dilator or a # 16 Foley catheter remain unproven. The diagnosis is routinely made based on a mid-trimester loss in which the patient presents with complaints of pelvic pressure and/or vaginal discharge, without regular contractions, and on digital examination is found to be significantly effaced and/or dilated, and delivers within a short interval.

INDICATION/TIMING FOR CERCLAGE PLACEMENT

If in the previous pregnancy, there was painless dilation of the cervix culminating in painless and rapid labor in the mid-trimester, most clinicians would place a cerclage in the next pregnancy. Previously, cerclage was delayed until early in the second trimester of a subsequent pregnancy, rather than placing the cerclage in the first trimester in order to lessen the chance that the surgery would be followed by a spontaneous abortion. However, the identification of the fetal heart motion by ultrasound allows early intervention, if desired, since the odds of miscarriage decrease markedly once fetal viability is documented.

ROLE OF ULTRASONOGRAPHY

Recently, ultrasonography has become gold standard and being utilized more frequently to make diagnosis of incompetent cervix in individuals without a "classic" history as well as to study patients during pregnancy that have had a prior premature birth.

The ultrasound criteria for the diagnosis of incompetence cervix vary and there is no uniform consensus. One research group defined cervical incompetence as progressive shortening of the cervical canal length to less than 2 cm, either spontaneously or after application of transfundal pressure (Fig. 1). Cervical incompetence was also assumed if a single endocervical canal measurement of less than 2 cm was recorded. Using this definition to determine the need for cerclage placement, more patients requiring cerclage had a prior mid-trimester pregnancy loss. In one of the studies by Iams JD et al. noted that the worse the obstetrical history (i.e., the more premature the prior birth), the greater the frequency of an ultrasound diagnosis of cervical incompetence. Of 36 cases of ultrasound diagnosed cervical incompetence, 91.7% occurred in woman who had a prior birth less than 27 weeks gestation at delivery.

Funneling of the cervix with the changes in forms TYVU (correlation between the length of the cervix and the changes in the cervical internal os).

The TYVU (Trust Your Vaginal Ultrasound) stages and the bulging membranes (Figs 2A to D).

INDICATIONS FOR CERCLAGE

A history of a cervical cone biopsy is often considered a risk factor for cervical incompetence. If a large portion of the cervix is surgically removed, this may weaken the structure, particularly if the internal cervical os is incorporated in the biopsy. Unfortunately, reviews of studies include patients with differing depth and width of cone biopsy. Thus, it is impossible to conclude that cone biopsy carries no risk for cervical incompetence. It is reasonable to follow patients with prior cone biopsy and no intervening term pregnancy expectantly with weekly or biweekly cervical exams or ultrasound measurement of cervical length from 16 weeks gestation.

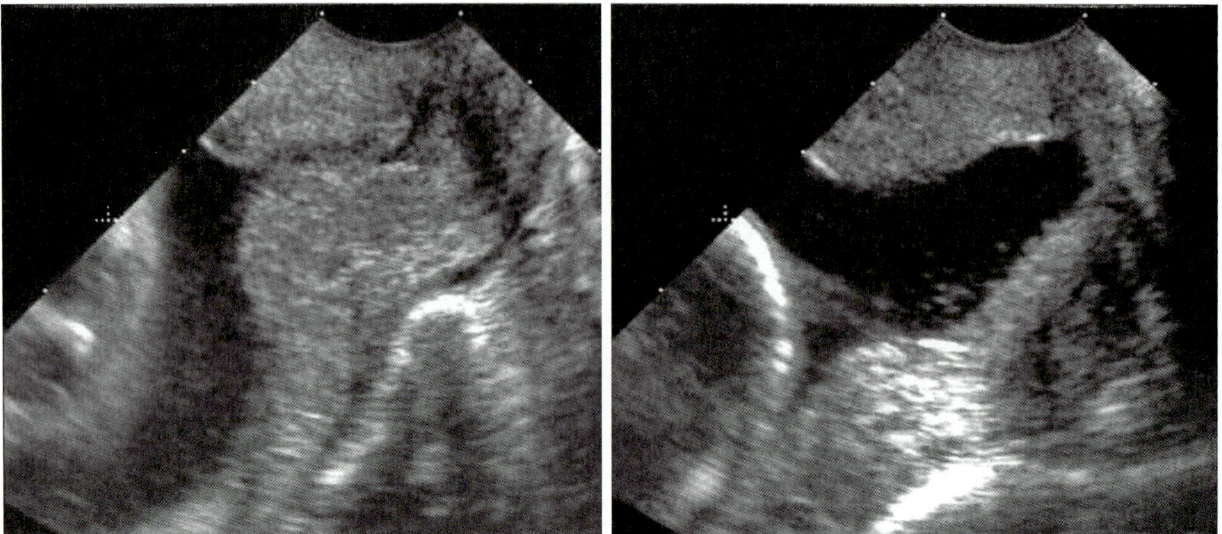

Fig. 1: Ultrasonographic image of same cervix 20 seconds apart, without and with fundal pressure

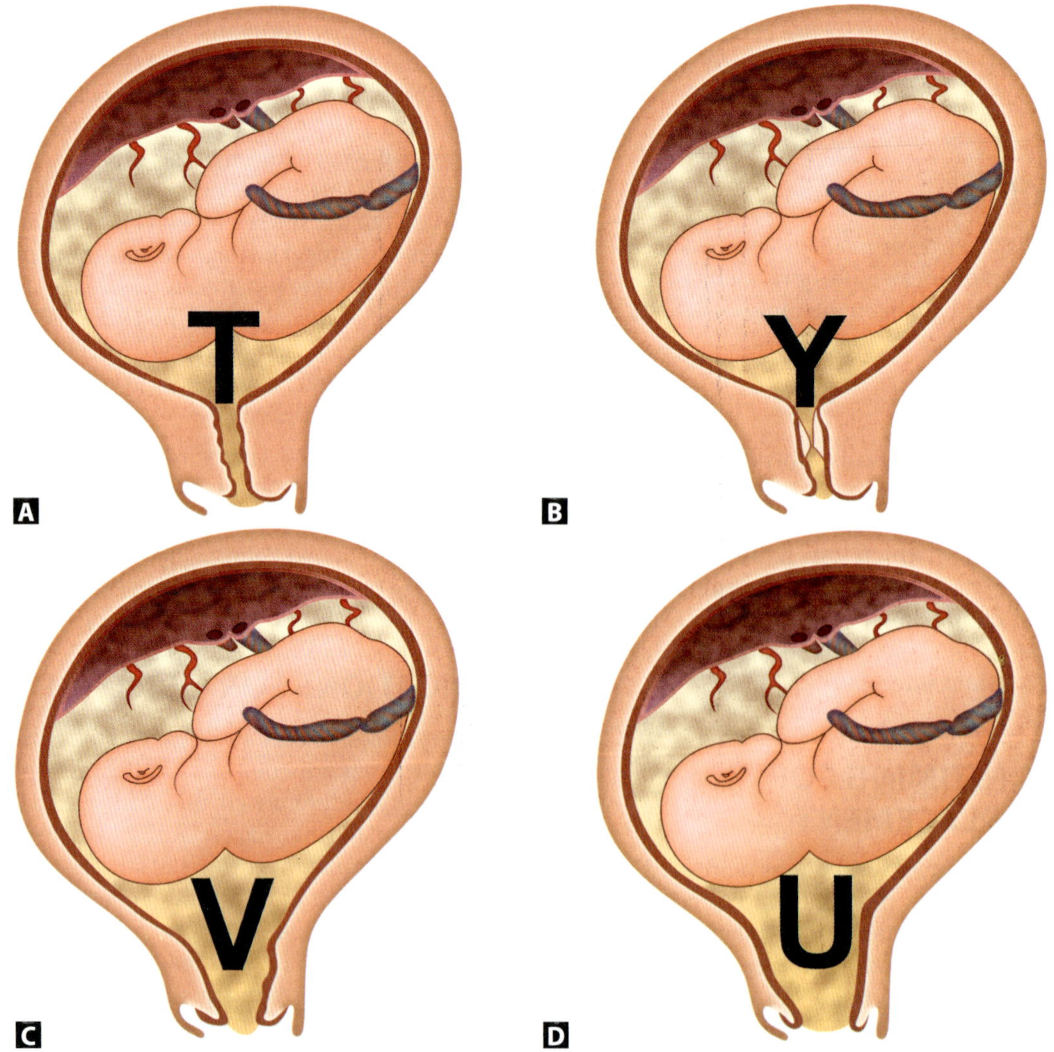

Figs 2A to D: Trust your vaginal ultrasound (TYVU) type of cervical canal defects

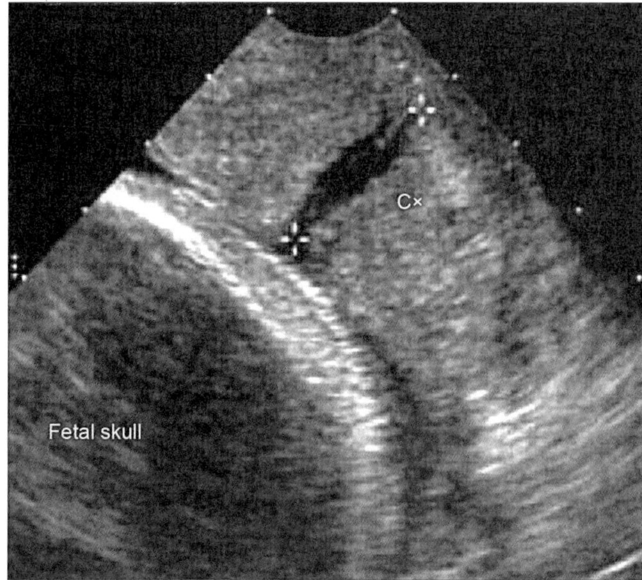

Fig. 3: Cervix length less than 25 mm

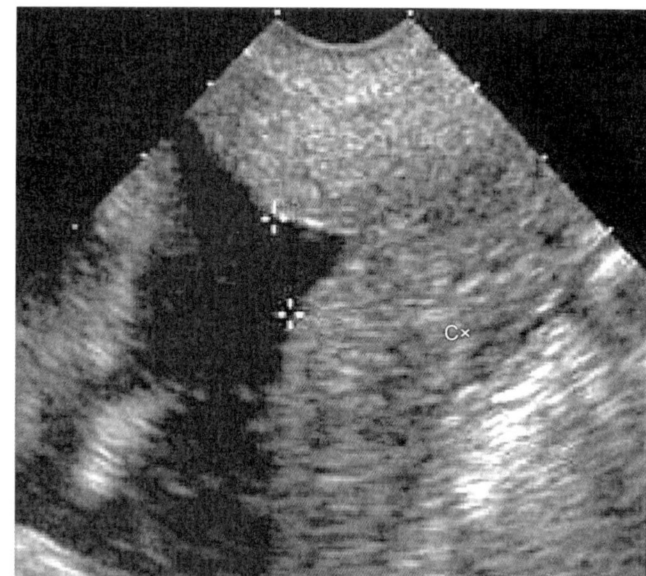

Fig. 4: V sign

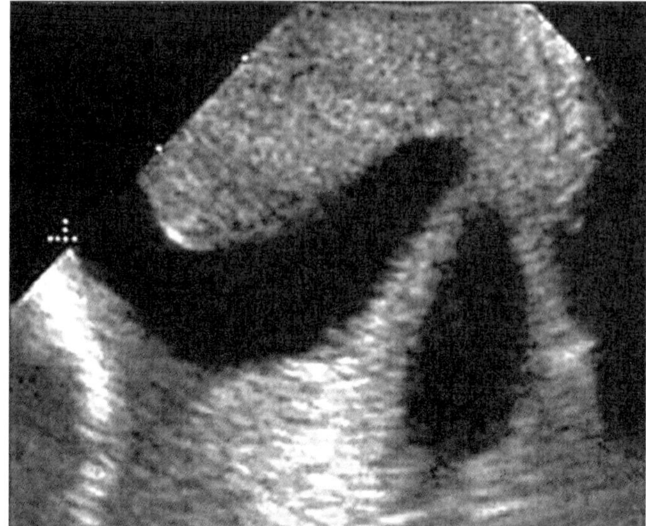
Fig. 5A: Dilated cervical canal

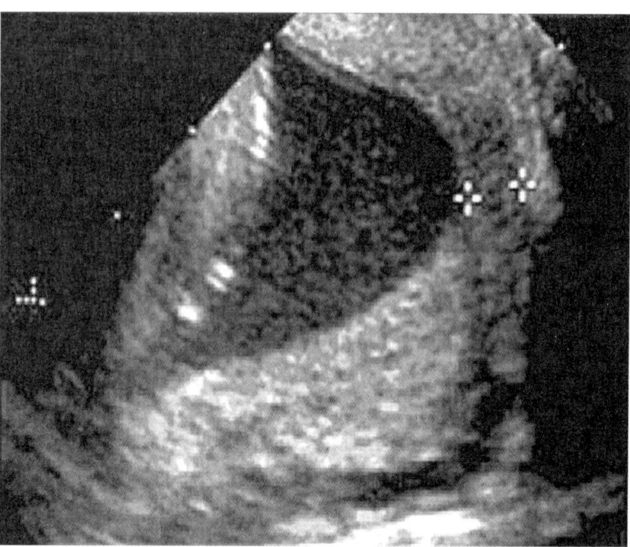
Fig. 5B: Protrusion of the membranes with short cervix

The trauma associated with abortion by dilation and curettage carries a higher risk for subsequent pregnancy loss than abortion by suction aspiration. Harlap found a relative risk of 3.27 for mid-trimester loss among the nulliparous women who had an induced abortion by dilation and cerclage, a risk that disappeared after cervical dilation by lamanaria was introduced.

Finally, there is no evidence to support prophylactic cerclage in women with two or more induced abortions, women with congenital uterine anomalies, women with symptomatic placenta previa, and women with multiple gestations (Figs 2. to 5).

CONTRAINDICATIONS

Absolute contraindications to cervical cerclage include:

- Uterine contractions or labor
- Unexplained vaginal bleeding
- Intrauterine or vaginal infection
- Rupture of fetal membranes
- Intrauterine fetal demise
- Major fetal anomaly, and
- A gestational age beyond 28 weeks.

Factors, such as placenta previa, a mucopurulent cervical discharge with membrane opacification, fetal

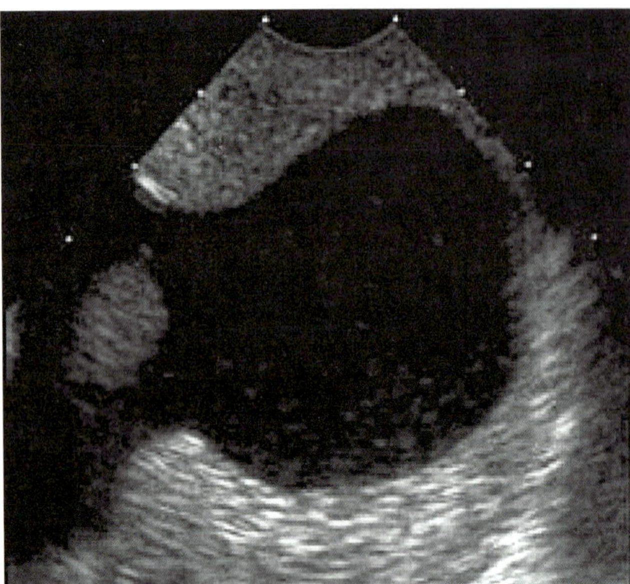

Fig. 6: Presence of fetal parts in the cervix or vagina

membranes prolapsing through the cervical os, and intrauterine fetal growth restriction may be regarded as relative contraindications to emergent cerclage.

Cerclage is an appropriate intervention when the clinical history for cervical incompetence is "classic". In circumstances such as diethylstilbestrol exposure, prior preterm birth without a "classic" history, multiple prior pregnancy terminations, or multiple gestations, frequent cervical exams or ultrasound assessment of the cervix should be instituted. A cerclage should be reserved for those patients demonstrating cervical change (Fig. 6).

RISKS OF CERCLAGE

- Premature rupture of membranes (1–9%)
- Chorioamnionitis (Infection of the amniotic sac, 1–7%) (This risk increases as the pregnancy progresses and is at 30% for a cervix that is dilated more than 3 cm).
- Preterm labor
- Cervical laceration or amputation (This can be at the procedure or at the delivery, from scar tissue that forms on the cervix)
- Bladder injury (rare)
- Maternal hemorrhage
- Cervical dystocia
- Uterine rupture

PROCEDURES/OPERATIVE TECHNIQUE

Three Types of Suturing (Fig. 7)

Based on timing, one may differentiate between:

- Prophylactic cerclage prior to conception

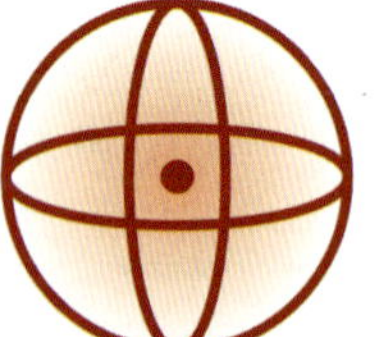
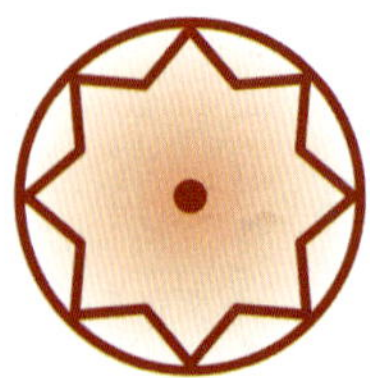
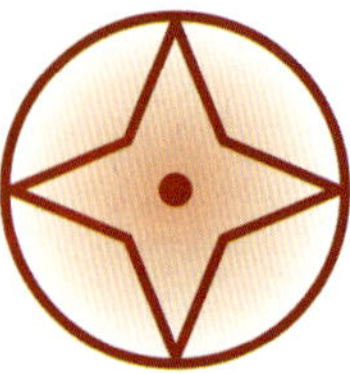

Fig. 7: Types of suturing

- Prophylactic cerclage in pregnancy
- Urgent cerclage after shortening of the cervix, and
- Emergency cerclage after exposure of the membranes.

The choice of McDonald's cerclage versus the Shirodkar procedure should be based on operator experience, since at present there are no "head-to-head" comparison studies. Retrospective studies have confirmed similar outcomes with either procedure (Fig. 8).

McDONALD'S PROCEDURE

McDonald's originally reported in 1957 on 70 cases in which a cerclage was placed at an advanced state of dilation, with a 43% neonatal survival. Subsequently, he reported an 80% success rate, an improvement he had attributed to prophylactic suturing at 14 weeks gestation. Advantages of the McDonald's procedure include its relative simplicity and less blood loss. The McDonald's procedure may be more practical when the cervix is markedly effaced (Fig. 9).

The following are steps of the Mcdonald's procedure:

1. Regional anesthesia is performed, although general anesthesia or recent reports using only paracervical block have been published.
2. After vaginal preparation, a sterile speculum is placed in the vagina and Sims retractor anteriorly is utilized for visualization.
3. The anterior cervical lip at 12 o'clock and the cervical lip at 9 o'clock are grasped with long Allis clamps (Fig. 10A). A 5 mm mersilene tape, swedged onto a medium size curved needle, is coated with sterile surgilube. Use of alternative suture materials includes gortex or silk.
4. The first bite of tissue is at 12 o'clock, at the cervicovaginal junction identified by a change in the rugae pattern. The needle exits at 9:30, re-enters at 9:00, exists at 6:30, re-enters at 6:00, exists at 3:30, re-enters at 3:00, and exists at 12:00, the site of the original insertion (Figs 10B and C).
5. Once the needle has been removed from the end of the suture, the purse-string suture is drawn closed over an assistant's finger (Fig. 10D). The operator places a surgeon's knot into the stitch and slides it down on the anterior aspect of the cervix. After 4–5 throws are

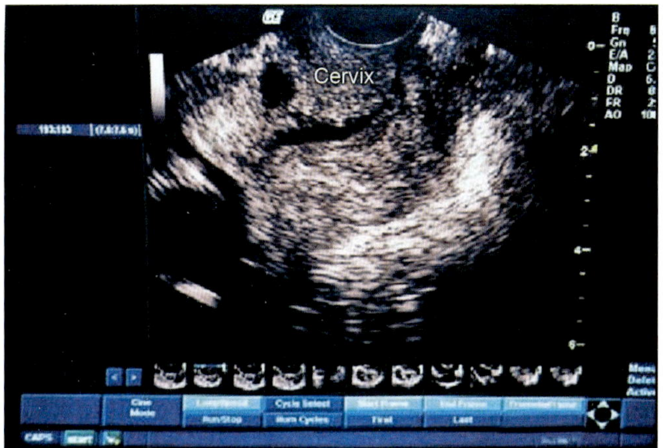

Fig. 8: Cervical canal dilatation

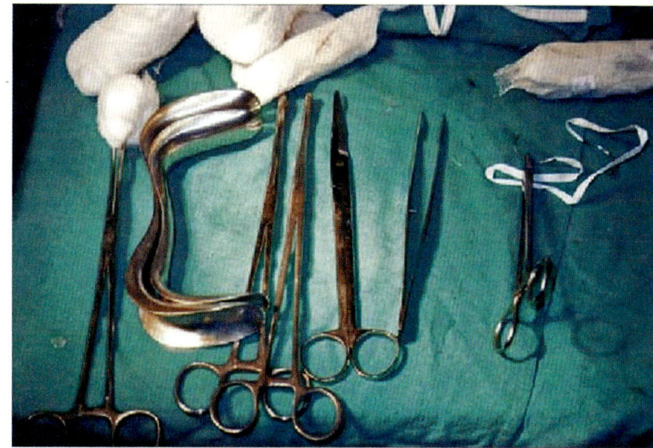

Fig. 9: Tray for McDonald's suture

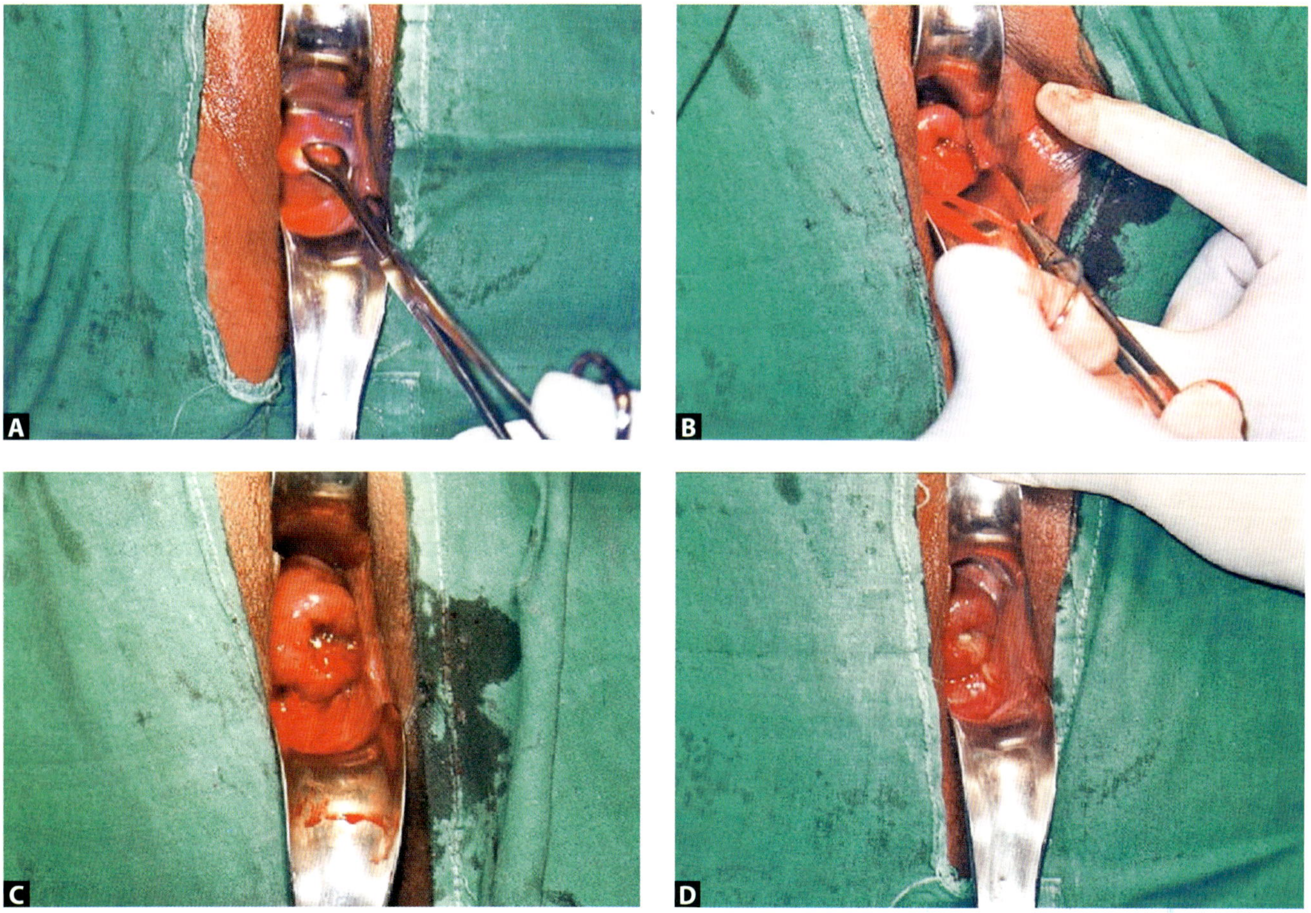

Figs 10A to D: Steps of placing McDonald's cervical encerclage

placed in the knot, the ends are trimmed to 2–3 cm to allow easy identification and manipulation at the time of removal.

SHIRODKAR PROCEDURE (FIGS 11A TO E)

Originally Shirodkar procedure was described in 1955. Later, refinements and additional modifications to the

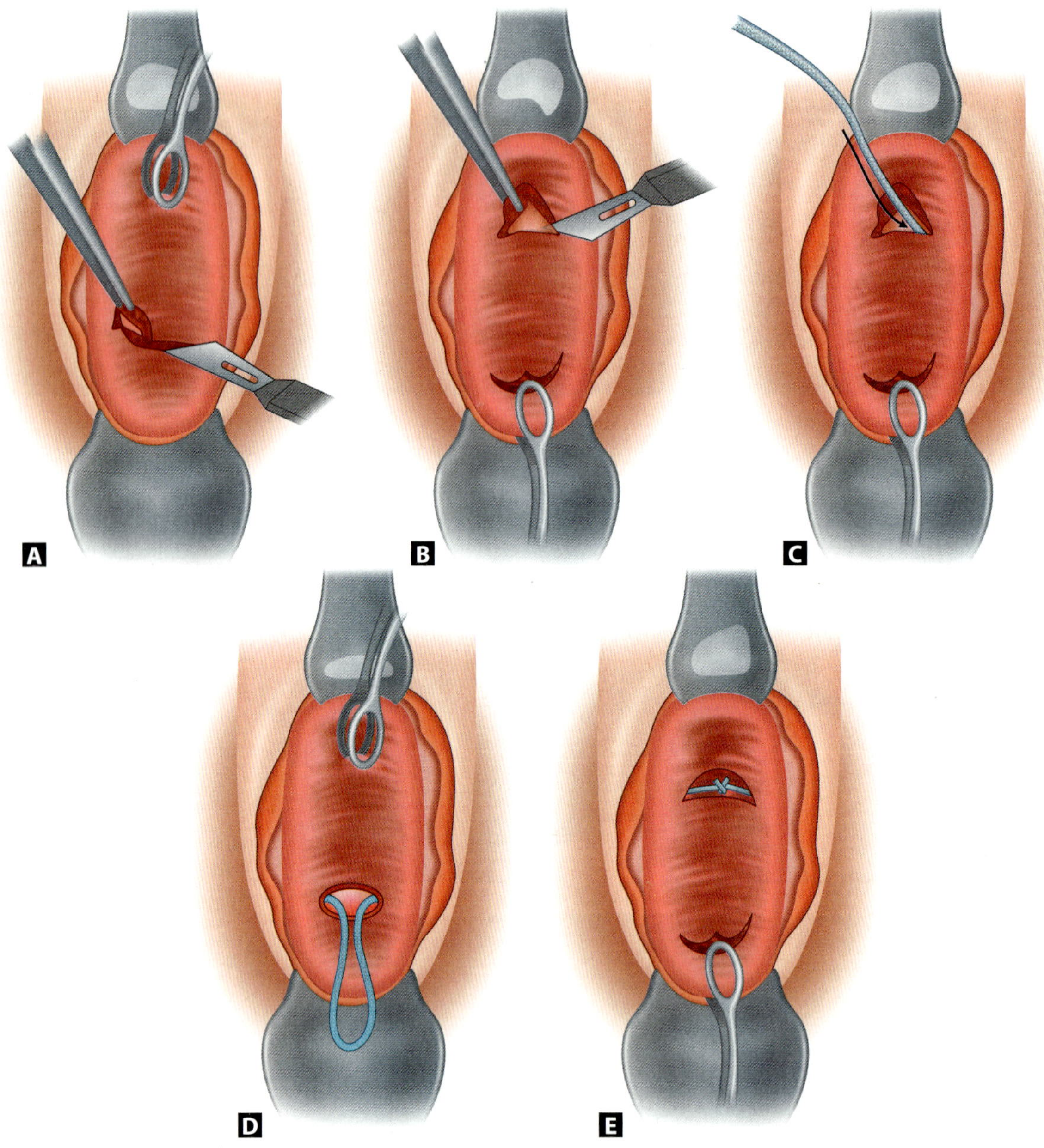

Figs 11A to E: Shirodkar's procedure

original operation have been suggested. The advantages of this procedure center around the fact that the anterior mucosal incision and the reflection of the bladder upward allow the stitch to be placed high on the cervix, near the location of the internal os. Also, the suture is buried under the vaginal mucosal, thus reducing the risk of infection. Disadvantages include greater technical difficulty placing the suture, as well as difficulty removing the suture at term.

The following are steps of the Shirodkar procedure:

1. Regional anesthesia is preferred.
2. The vagina is prepared with betadine.
3. A long weighted speculum and Sims retractor are placed in the vagina. The anterior and posterior lips of the cervix are grasped with Allis clamps/sponge holders.
4. A 2 cm transverse incision is made 2.5 cm proximal to the external os posteriorly and blunt section is utilized to develop a plane between the cervical mucosa and cervical stroma.
5. The cervicovesical reflection is identified anteriorly by moving the cervix, allowing visualization of the slight ballooning of the bladder. The anterior mucosal

incision is made transversely, approximately 2 cm long, at this reflection. A 5 mm mersilene tape, swedged onto a medium-sized atraumatic needle is utilized.

6. The first bite of tissue is taken from posterior to anterior. The needle is drawn directly upward through the paracervical tissue, emerging into the anterior mucosal incision.
7. The process repeated on the right side of the cervix, except that the needle is driven from anterior to posterior, emerging in the posterior mucosal incision.
8. The mersilene band is anchored to the anterior cervical substance with absorbable suture.
9. The knot is tied posteriorly as the assistant removes a finger inserted into the endocervical canal.
10. The edges of the anterior and posterior mucosal incisions are reapproximated with dissolvable suture.
11. The cerclage ends are trimmed to 3 cm long.

ABDOMINAL CERCLAGE

The indications for an abdominal cerclage, as described by Novy, include extensive cervical conization, cervico-vaginal laceration following abortion, or previous failed vaginal cerclage. Novy reported the results of 20 abdominal cerclage procedures performed since 1982, with a perinatal survival rate of 90%. The advantage to an abdominal cerclage is that it is performed in patients who can not be treated adequately with a vaginal cerclage. The main disadvantage of abdominal cerclage is that the patient must undergo two laparotomies, since most authors advocate delivery by cesarean section. This procedure must be reserved for highly selected cases and performed by experienced surgeons.

LAPAROSCOPIC CERVICOISTHEMIC CERCLAGE

Wurm Procedure

1. The Hefner cerclage, also known as the Wurm procedure, is used for later diagnosis of the incompetent cervix.
2. It is usually done with a U or mattress suture, and is of benefit when there is minimal amount of cervix left.

Emergency Cerclage

McDonald, Shirodkar and abdominal cerclages are best performed prior to cervical dilation; however, patients without a "classic" history of incompetent cervix may present in the second trimester with dilation/effacement requiring emergency cerclage. Retrospective reviews comparing prophylactic versus emergency cerclage have demonstrated a lower overall success rate with emergency cerclage. With emergency cerclage, 65% of patients delivered greater than 28 weeks, with only 49% of patients delivering greater than 34 weeks. Prior to proceeding with cerclage, premature labor, placental abruption and premature rupture of membranes must be excluded. If, in the absence of abruption, uterine contractions can be suppressed with tocolytic therapy and the clinician is convinced premature labor was a result of cervical dilation rather than the cause of it, emergency cerclage should be considered.

Prophylactic antibiotics are recommended when emergency cerclage is performed, based on a 2.6-fold increase chorioamnionitis when cerclage is performed after, compared to before, 18 weeks gestation. Broad-spectrum antibiotics should be initiated prior to the procedure, and may be continued orally for 1–3 days post surgery.

Cerclage Removal

It is practice to remove a cerclage at 37 weeks gestation, at a point in pregnancy when the risk of prematurity is minimal. If the patient has significant uterine activity, possibly leading to rupture of the uterus and avulsion of the cervix, then the cerclage must be removed after 35 weeks gestation, or in patients refractory to therapy that suppresses uterine activity at any gestational age.

- Should a cerclage be removed in a patient with preterm premature rupture of membranes and no evidence of labor?

There are no prospective studies randomizing patients with preterm premature rupture of membranes to removal versus allowing the cerclage to remain in situ. One group reported on 32 patients managed expectantly with preterm premature rupture of membranes and a cerclage in place. The cerclage was removed immediately in each case. The patients were compared to 32 matched-controls with premature rupture of membranes without a cerclage in place. The latency period and infectious complications were similar in both groups, suggesting that the presence of a pre-existing cerclage in the face of preterm premature rupture of membranes is not a contraindication to expectant management as long as the cerclage is removed. When the cerclage was left in situ following premature rupture of membranes, another retrospective comparative study demonstrated prolongation of pregnancy but increased maternal and perinatal mortality. The optimal management of preterm premature rupture of membranes in the presence of a cerclage has yet to be determined.

CONCLUSION AND RECOMMENDATIONS

That following are based on available published data supplemented by consensus and an expert opinion with the caution that the recommendations may not apply uniformly to patients at the extremes of gestational age.

The following recommendations are based on good and consistent scientific evidence (Level B):

- A patient with "classic" history of mid-trimester painless dilation with rapid labor and delivery may benefit from a cerclage after viability is determined in a subsequent pregnancy
- There is no indication for prophylactic cerclage in patients with diethylstilbestrol exposure, multiple abortions, uterine anomalies, multiple gestations, and patients with symptomatic placenta previa
- Use of an emergency cerclage in patients with advanced dilation/effacement in the second trimester results in a poorer outcome as compared to procedures done prophylactically. Cerclage procedures are contra-indicated in patients with active labor, premature rupture of membranes and unexplained vaginal bleeding.

The following recommendations are based primarily on consensus or expert opinion (Level C):

- The utilization of either serial digital exams or serial ultrasounds after 16 weeks gestation in patients without a "classic" history of incompetence cervix may decrease the requirement for cerclage placement in these patients
- The type of cerclage utilized should be dependent on operator experience
- Prophylactic broad-spectrum antibiotics should be utilized in any patient undergoing a mid-second trimester cerclage procedure
- Cerclages should be removed in patients with preterm premature rupture of membranes at the time of membrane rupture. There is no contraindication to conservative management in these patients, as the latency period for infectious complications seems to be similar to patients with preterm premature rupture of membranes without prior prophylactic cerclage placement.

BIBLIOGRAPHY

1. Aarts JM, Brons JT, Bruinse HW. Emergency cerclage: a review. Obstet Gynecol Surv. 1995;50(6):459-69.
2. Althuisius SM, Dekker GA, van Geijn HP, et al. Cervical incompetence prevention randomized cerclage trial (CIPRACT): Study design and preliminary results. Am J Obstet Gynecol. 2000;183:823-9.
3. Bengtsson LP, Acta Gynecol Scand, suppl. 1968;47:9.
4. Benson RC, Durfee RB. Transabdominal cervicouterine cerclage during pregnancy for the treatment of cervical incompetency. Obstet Gynecol. 1965;25:145-55.
5. Berghella V, Daly SF, Tolosa JE, et al. Prediction of preterm delivery with transvaginal ultrasonography of the cervix in patients with high-risk pregnancies: Does cerclage prevent prematurity? Am J Obstet Gynecol. 1999;181:809-15.
6. Cammarano CL, Herron MA, Parer JT. Validity of indications for trans-abdominal cervicoisthmic cerclage for cervical incompetence. Am J Obstet Gynecol. 1995;172:1871-75.
7. Charles D, Edwards WR. Infectious complications of cervical cerclage. Am J Obstet Gynecol. 1981;141:1065.
8. Chasen ST, Sliverman NS. Mid-trimester emergent cerclage: a ten year single institution review. J Perinatol. 1998;18(5):338-42.
9. Dor J, Shalev J, Machiach S, et al. Elective cervical suture of twin pregnancies diagnosed ultrasonically in the first trimester following induced ovulation. Gynecol Obstet Invest. 1982;13: 55-60.
10. Goldenberg RL, Mercer BM, Meis PJ, et al. The preterm prediction study: Fetal fibronectin testing and spontaneous preterm birth. Obstet Gynecol. 1996;87:643-48.
11. Guzman ER, Mellon C, Vintzileos AM, et al. Longitudinal assessment of endocervical canal length between 15 and 24 weeks gestation in women at risk for pregnancy loss or preterm birth. Obstet Gynecol. 1998;92:31-7.
12. Guzman ER, Mellon R, Vintzeleos AM, et al. Relationship between endocervical canal length between 15-24 weeks gestation and obstetric history. J Matern Fetal Med. 1998;7(6):269-72.
13. Haney AF. Prenatal DES exposure: The continuing effects. OBG Management. 2001;13(10):33-44.
14. Harger JH. Comparison of success and morbidity in cervical cerclage procedures. Obstet Gynecol. 1980;56(5):543-8.
15. Harlap S, Shiono PH, Ramcharan S, et al. A prospective study of spontaneous fetal losses after induced abortions. NEJM. 1979;301(13):677-81.
16. Hassan SS, Romero R, Maymon E, et al. Does cervical cerclage prevent preterm delivery in patients with a short cervix? Am J Obstet Gynecol. 2001;184:1325-9.
17. Heath VC, Souka AP, Erasmus I, et al. Cervical length at 23 weeks of gestation: The value of Shirodkar suture for the short cervix. Ultrasound Obstet Gynecol. 1998;12:318-22.
18. Heath VC, Southall TR, Souka AP, et al. Cervical length at 23 weeks of gestation: Prediction of spontaneous preterm delivery. Ultrasound Obstet Gynaecol. 1998;12:312-17.
19. Hibbard JU, Snow J, Moawad AH. Short cervical length by ultrasound and cerclage. J Perinatol. 2000;3:161-5.
20. Iams JD, Goldenberg RL, Meis PJ, et al. The length of the cervix and the risk of spontaneous premature delivery. N Engl J Med. 1996;334:567-72.

21. Iams JD, Johnson FF, Sonek J, et al. Cervical competence as a continuum: a study of ultrasonographic cervical length and obstetric performance. Am J Obstet Gynecol. 1995;172: 1097-106.

22. Lazar P, Gueguen S, Dreyfus J, et al. Multicentred controlled trial of cervical cerclage in women at moderate risk of preterm delivery. Br J Obstet Gynaecol. 1984;91:731-5.

23. Lazar P, Gueguen S, Dreyfus J, et al. Multicentred controlled trial of cervical cerclage in women at moderate risk of preterm delivery. Br J Obstet Gynecol. 1984;91(8):731-5.

24. Lockwood CJ, Senyei AE, Dische MR, et al. Fetal fibronectin in cervical and vaginal secretions as a predictor of preterm delivery. N Engl J Med. 1991;325:669-74.

25. Ludmir J, Bader T, Chen, L, et al. Obstet Gynecol. 1994;84:823-6.

26. Ludmir J, Bader T, Chen L, Lindenbaum C, Wong G. Poor perinatal outcome associated with retained cerclage in patients with premature rupture of membranes. Obstet Gynecol. 1994;84:823-6.

27. McDonald IA. Incompetent cervix as a cause of recurrent abortion. J Obstet Gynaecol Br Commonw. 1963;70(1):105-9.

28. McDonald IA. Suture of the cervix for inevitable miscarriage. J Obstet Gynaecol Br Emp. 1957;64:346-50.

29. McElrath TF, Norwitz ER, Lieberman ES, Heffner LJ. Management of cervical cerclage and preterm premature rupture of the membranes: Should the stitch be removed? Am J Obstet Gynecol. 2000;183:840-6.

30. McGregor JA, Jackson GM, Lachlin GC, et al. Salivary estriol as risk assessment for preterm labor: A prospective trial. Am J Obstet Gynecol. 1995;173:1337-42.

31. Mordel N, Zajicek G, Benshushan A, et al. Elective suture of uterine cervix in triplets. Am J Perinatol. 1993;10:14-6.

32. MRC/RCOG Working Party on Cervical Cerclage. Final report of the medical research council/royal college of obstetricians and gynaecologists multicentre randomised trial of cervical cerclage. Br J Obstet gynecol 1993;100:516-23.

33. Nichols DH. Gynecologic and Obstetric Surgery. Chapter 63, 1031, Mosby-Year Book, Inc., St. Louis, MO, 1993.

34. Norwitz ER, Goldstein DP. Transabdominal cervicoisthmic cerclage: Learning to tie the knot. J Gynecol Tech. 1996;2:49-54.

35. Novy MJ. Contemporary Ob/Gyn. 1977;10:17.

36. Novy MJ. Transabdominal cervicoisthmic cerclage: a reappraisal 25 years after its introduction. Am J Obstet Gynecol. 1991;164:1635-41.

37. Novy MJ. Transabdominal cervicoisthmic cerclage: A reappraisal 25 years after its introduction. Am J Obstet Gynecol. 1991;164:1635-41.

38. Palmer R, LaComme M. Gynecol Obstet (Paris). 1948;47:905.

39. Rush RW, Isaacs S, McPherson K, et al. A randomized controlled trial of cervical cerclage in women at high risk of spontaneous preterm delivery. Br J Obstet Gynaecol. 1984;91:724-30.

40. Rush RW, Isaacs S, McPherson K, et al. A randomized controlled trial of cervical cerclage in women at high risk of spontaneous preterm delivery. Br J Obstet Gynecol. 1984;91:724-30.

41. Shirodkar VN. The Antiseptic. 1955;52:299.

42. Yeast JD, Garite TR. The role of cervical cerclage in the management of preterm premature rupture of the membranes. Am J Obstet Gynecol. 1988;158:106.

39.4 FOTHERGILL'S REPAIR

Chandrawati, Priti Kumar

INTRODUCTION

Pelvic organ prolapse, along with urinary incontinence, fecal incontinence, voiding dysfunction and defecatory dysfunction, make up an interrelated group of conditions known collectively as disorders of the pelvic floor. These disorders share many common risk factors and often coexist with one another. Pelvic organ prolapse, like other pelvic floor disorders, rarely results in severe morbidity or mortality; rather, it causes symptoms that can impact a woman's daily activities and negatively affect her quality of life.

Some sort of surgical procedure is nearly always the best treatment for established prolapse but is only necessary if the condition is causing symptoms or is interfering with the women's normal activities. Youth and intention to have more children in the future are not contraindication to operation and require a modified surgical technique called Fothergill's repair. Besides surgical treatment, conservative forms of therapy such as pessaries and pelvic floor therapy can be successfully used in selective patients with prolapse.

FOTHERGILL'S REPAIR

In 1888, Donald, of Manchester, England, began treating prolapse of the uterus by anterior and posterior colporrhaphy combined with amputation of the cervix. This operation continues to be performed in Manchester and other areas of England by many gynecologists.

Before Fothergill modified the operation, the procedure included amputation of the cervix, followed by an anterior colporrhaphy. Fothergill made the incision for the anterior repair triangular in shape with the base at the cervix, and then carried the incision around the cervix to perform the amputation. This exposed the base of the broad ligaments to better advantage than did the method previously used and facilitated the approximation of these supporting structures in front of the remainder of the cervix. This operation, with slight variation, has been performed by different members of the Manchester Clinic staff since 1888. Manchester operation has a limited place in modern gynecology but may be appropriate when there is a cytostocele associated with only a first or second-degree prolapse, when childbearing no longer needs to be considered, and when the uterus is not in marked retro position, or when the retrodisplaced uterus is a small atrophic structure not contributing to the patient's symptoms. The operation is particularly satisfactory under the preceeding condition when much of the apparent prolapse is due to cervical elongation.

We believe that there is a definite objection to the operation when future pregnancy is likely because of the amputation of the cervix. Leonard found that after cervical amputation, the incidence of sterility was abnormally high, premature delivery between the sixth and eighth months increased, and cervical dystocia was common. Shaw's results also seem to condemn the operation during the childbearing period because few of his patients subsequently had children. It is a subject of controversy to perform such conservative's surgeries if further child bearing is needed. The modern management and advances in treatment of prolapse has an edge over such surgeries. Thus Fothergill's repair is best indicated in young females with I or II degree prolapse desiring or not desiring conception in future.

Preoperative Steps

- Proper selection of patients for the Fothergill's repair is very important. The patient should be properly examined by senior gynecologist
- Proper counseling of patient regarding postoperative problems, both recent and remote, should be done before surgery
- Correct general health of the patient
- Treat urinary tract infection, if present
- Assess renal system
- Treat vaginal infection and cervical lesions
- Treat for any existing medical problem-precipitating prolapse
- Vaginal toileting with weak betadine solution (0.5%) for 2 days prior to surgery
- Light diet is preferred 2 days prior to surgery
- Bowel should be evacuated prior to surgery
- If family is complete, consent for ligation should be taken
- Complete preoperative hematological investigations to be performed.

Main Objectives

The objectives of this procedure are:

- To amputate the vaginal portion of the cervix, particularly when there is supravaginal elongation

- Approximation of the cardinal ligaments in front of the cervical stump. This shortens these ligaments and thus elevates and displaces the cervix posteriorly. This backward displacement encourages anteversion of uterus and helps to prevent prolapse in future.

The operation should always be combined with anterior repair and should always search for an enterocele. Posterior repair is common but not obligatory. Thus proper preoperative evaluation of the patient is very important as to decide the additional corrective surgeries needed.

Operative Steps

- The patient is laid in the lithotomy position and a Sims' speculum introduced into the vagina. The lateral vaginal walls are retracted away by assistant using vaginal retractors. The cervix is pulled down with the Vulsellum forceps in the middle.
- The repair of the cervix can be carried out more easily after the cervical canal has been dilated. Some surgeons like to use a dilute adrenalin infiltration (1;400000). Check for uterocervical length by putting the uterine sound. These are the crucial steps in assessing the length of the cervix to be amputated. The length of cervix to be amputed is such that the effective uterocervical length is three and a half inches. The cervical canal is dilated properly up to Hegar 8, so that the formation of cervical lip later on is easy. There should not be too vigorous or more dilatation of the cervix as it may lead to cervical incompetence in future. The uterine cavity is preferably curetted before the surgery to rule out any endometrial pathology. The endometrial tissue should be sent for histopathological examination.
- *Selection of Fothergill's four points:* (Fig. 1) Fothergill's four points are now selected and the vaginal skin is grasped in small-toothed Allis forceps as follows: The first point is just below the urethral orifice, the second behind the cervix in the posterior fornix and in the midline about the lower level of the uterine isthmus, or roughly 2.5 cm from the external os. Two lateral points are so placed that when approximated to each other in front of the cervix, the vaginal vault is of the right caliber. If the prolapse is severe, naturally these lateral points will be placed farther laterally. When considering surgical correction for anterior wall defects, the surgeon should remember to evaluate for masked stress urinary incontinence. Significant anterior wall descent may lead to a urethral "kinking" effect that masks the symptom of stress urinary incontinence. Resupporting the anterior vaginal wall and straightening the urethra may reveal previously hidden incontinence. An easy way to test this preoperatively is to simply support the anterior wall defect with a pessary or speculum to straighten the urethra. The patient is then asked to cough and bear down with a comfortably full bladder. If urinary leakage is elicited, then the patient is likely to demonstrate stress urinary incontinence with surgical correction of her anterior vaginal wall defect and a concomitant incontinence procedure should be planned. After checking for this, empty the urinary bladder by putting K-90 catheter.
- Either an inverted T incision or an inverted V incision is given in anterior vaginal wall and extended round the cervix. The vaginal flaps are carefully dissected and elevated. Hemostasis is secured.
- *Dissection of urinary bladder:* The bladder must now be freed and advanced to a higher plane. The vesicocervical ligament and the lateral bladder pillars are therefore cut with scissors and all vessels secured. It is necessary to free the bladder from the lateral vaginal skin flaps before it can be adequately pushed up by blunt finger and gauze dissection. The bladder should now be elevated as high as the uterovesical peritoneal pouch, which can always be recognized if the surgeon is in the proper plane. If the plane of dissection is not proper, the dissection will be always very difficult and there are high chances of damaging the bladder. It is a checkpoint for the operating surgeon (Fig. 2).
- The cervix is now pulled upwards and forwards to expose the posterior fornix and the vaginal skin mobilized by sharp and blunt dissection from the region of pouch of Douglas. The peritoneum of which is soon apparent. If there is any tendency to a hernial sac in this region, this sac or enterocele should be freed from the cervix in front, and the vagina behind right up to the level of the rectum. It is recognizable by its fat and longitudinal muscle fibers and blood vessels.
- *Shortening of Mackenrodts or cardinal ligaments:* The cardinal ligaments on either side of the cervix can now be clearly seen (Fig. 2) and they are grasped in strong forceps or clamp, such as McCullough's and cut

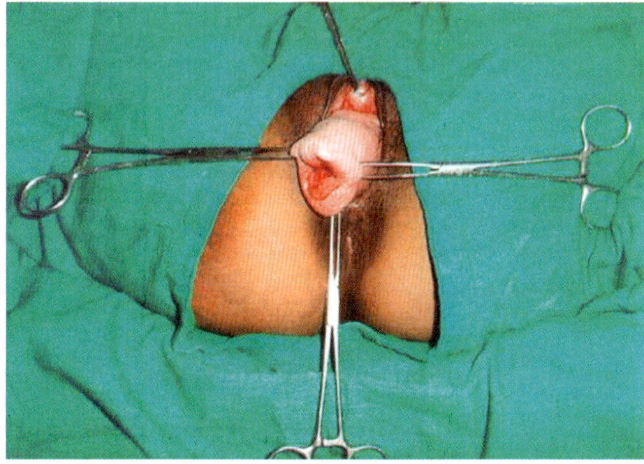

Fig. 1: Fothergill's repair—Fothergill's 4 points

through up to the level of the internal os. They are then transfixed and tied with a preferably vicryl 1/0 suture. A second suture ligature is similarly placed and left long as a tractor (Fig. 3).

- *Amputation of the cervix:* The cervix is now amputated; at whatever level the surgeon deems necessary. The decision of how much the cervix to be ampulated is vital. The effective uterocervical length should be three and a half inch; after the amputation of cervix.
- *Repair of enterocele and suture of uterosacral ligaments over it:* The enterocele sac is then opened and transfixed at its highest point after the opening has been drawn down as low as possible. The neck is tied preferably by vicryl 1/0 and excised, and the two uterosacral ligaments approximated in the midline by two or three transfixing sutures so that the fascial hiatus is effectively bridged.
- *Suture of posterior vaginal skin over the amputated cervical stump:* The next step is the covering of the amputation site with vaginal skin. The surgeon should start posteriorly at 6 o'clock and anchor Fothergill's posterior point with a Bonney-Sturmdorf suture so that the vaginal mucosa is snugly enfolded into the cervical canal. A series of radial sutures is passed through the cervix and the vaginal mucosa on both the sides in such a way that the new posterior lip of the cervix is fashioned and completely covered with vaginal mucosa shown in Figures 4 and 5.
- *Formation of anterior cervical lip by Fothergill's key suture (Fig. 6)*: The redundant vaginal tissue is excised. The quantity of vaginal mucosa trimmed is at the surgeon's discretion. Because the vagina is structurally a tube, excising too much mucosa can result in narrowing the vaginal diameter with resultant dyspareunia later

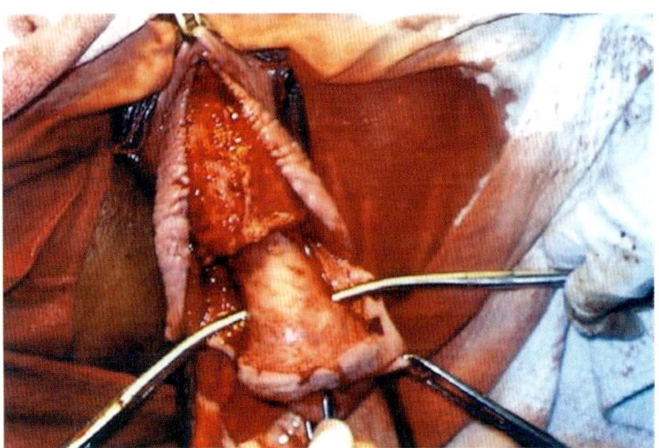

Fig. 2: Vaginal flaps dissected, urinary bladder pushed up and Mackenrodt's ligament held by the clamp

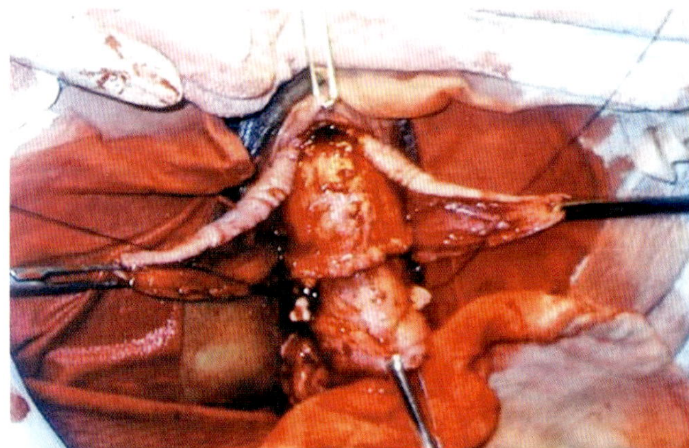

Fig. 3: Mackenrodt's ligaments are cut and ligated and one suture is held long

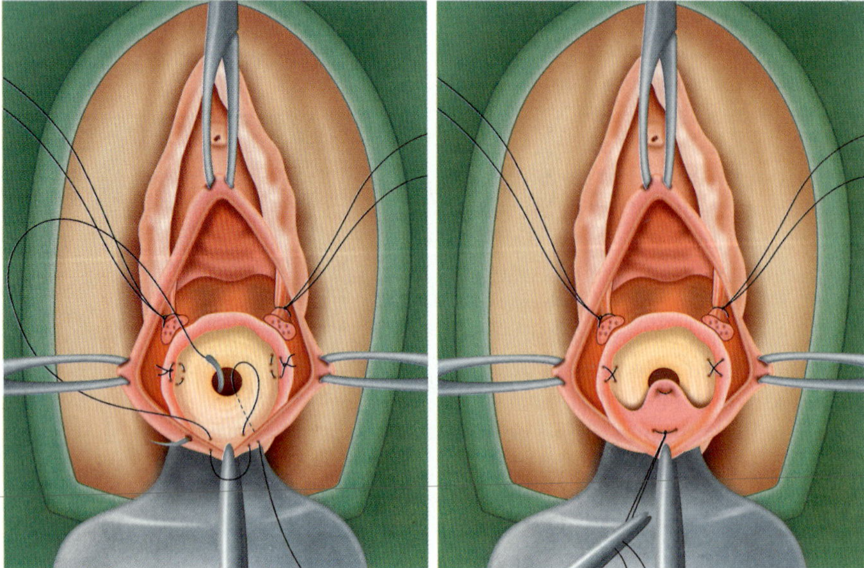

Figs 4 and 5: The posterior lip of cervix is re-epithelized by using Sturmdorf suture (Diagrammatic representation)

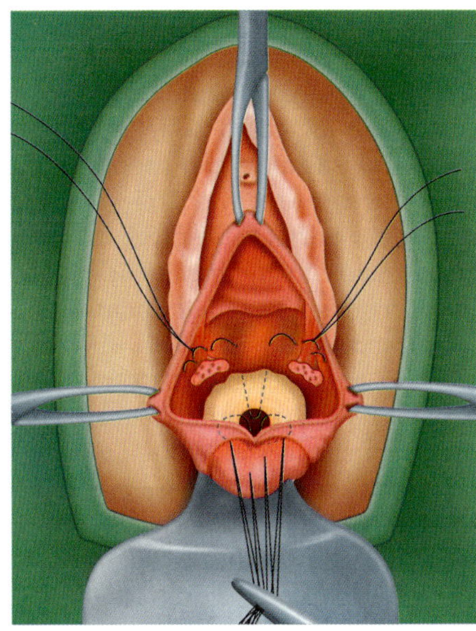

Fig. 6: Fothergill's suture to form the anterior cervical lip (Diagrammatic representation)

on. When removing vaginal epithelium during any of the repairs described in this chapter, it is generally wise to take the attitude that "you can always cut out more, but you cannot put it back once it is gone."

This is particularly a concern when concomitant posterior colporrhaphy is performed or if the patient has undergone a previous anterior repair with resection of vaginal mucosa. Now vaginal skin is folded inside to form anterior lip of cervix. The inferior lip of cervix is formed by passing Forthergill's suture (Fig. 6).

This enters the vaginal skin at the level of Fothergill's lateral point and transfixes a good bite of the cut cardinal ligament pedicles. The needle is now repassed from with outwards and through the cardinal ligament pedicle of the other side and finally out at Fothergill's other lateral point. A second, somewhat similar suture, at a slightly higher level may be used, or alternatively, the previously inserted cardinal lingament ligatures may be tied together in the anterior midline in front of cervix. When tied with the fingers in the vagina, this suture advances the new cervix upward, backwards and effectively anteverts the uterus. Bladder buttressing is done with 2-0 chromic catgut to support the bladder in its place. It is important to see that there is not a significant gap left between the cervical stump and the buttressing of the bladder.

Closure

After excising the redundant vaginal tissue, the vaginal wall is best closed with delayed absorbable sutures like vicryl 2/0. The hemostasis is obtained and any collection at the stichline should be specifically checked for. Posterior perineal relaxation should be assessed, if needed, perineorrhaphy can be done.

Although spontaneous micturition may occur after anterior colporrhaphy and associated operations, it is prudent to insert an indwelling Foley's catheter for 48–72 hours. This avoids difficulties with over-distension and reduces the risk of infection from repeated catheterization. It is necessary to look for clear urine in the bladder. It is essential to perform a gentle per rectal examination after surgery.

Postoperative Care

- Light diet for 2 days and if enterocele repair done, liquid diet is given for 3 days
- Laxatives given to avoid constipation for 2–3 days
- Perineal cleaning and care
- Any collection or infection at stitch line to be checked
- Cathetor removed after 48–72 hours of surgery
- Avoid any straining in perineal area.

Remote Complications

- Avoid frequent future pregnancies and vaginal delivery that may cause recurrence
- Pregnancy related complications are sterility, premature labor and cervical dystocia
- Difficult labor should be avoided. The patient should be planned for elective lower segment cesarian section (LSCS) for mode of delivery in cases where prolonged or difficult labor is anticipated
- Dyspareunia
- Maintaining tissue strength in postmenopausal period is also necessary as it can precipitate recurrence of prolapse.

Outcome Measures

Long-term follow-up of patients is important. Tipton and Atkin presented a long-term follow-up (6–12 years) of 82 patients between the age of 29 years and 52 years treated for prolapse with the Manchester operation. After the operation, thirty four patients (41%) had uterine disease or unwanted pregnancy. Two patients developed uterine carcinoma, and one of these patients died. Seventeen patients (21%) required uterine operations, including eight hysterectomies. Contraception and fear of pregnancy were problems in many cases.

Outcome measures are the tools used to determine the efficacy, safety and side effects of a treatment. For an individual patient, the most important outcome of a surgical procedure is the relief of her symptoms and improvement in her quality of life, yet until recently, these areas have largely been ignored. As for as our personal experience is concerned, sterility and obstetric complications were relatively more and other pelvic symptoms like urinary symptoms, bowel symptoms and heaviness were relieved to a great extent. Elective and emergency cesarean rates were higher due to cervical factors.

Place of Fothergill's Repair in Modern Management of Prolapse

Much is still unknown regarding the etiology of pelvic organ prolapse. Current theories do not adequately explain why a nullipara can develop pelvic organ prolapse, whereas a gravida nine may have excellent pelvic organ support. Similarly, we cannot always explain why one patient develops recurrence after repair of all support defects, whereas another patient with the same repair has permanent cure.

Basic science research in pelvic floor dysfunction is increasing and is required to meet the needs created by increased numbers of patients with pelvic organ prolapse, incontinence and other pelvic floor conditions. Surgical innovation is increasing in the direction of minimally invasive surgery. Future surgeons will use materials that have increased benefits to patients as a result of their sophistication and specialization through tissue engineering. Future physicians will complete their management with pharmacologic agents specific to the patient's genetic makeup and metabolism with advanced laxity of tissue. Fothergill's repair could not be ideal in some patient's because firstly, often, the causes of the patient's prolapse are multifactorial, secondly the anterior colporrhaphy corrects the central bladder prolapse only and there are high chances of lateral prolapse of urinary bladder. Among the many etiologies are neuromuscular damage or dysfunction of the pelvis, environmental factors placing a strain on the pelvic floor and perhaps genetic differences in connective tissue. Reusing the same connective tissue that has already failed once without addressing the risk factors responsible for prolapse in a particular patient makes little sense. Thus future place of Fothergill's repair in management of prolapse in young females would pose controversial issues.

BIBLIOGRAPHY

1. Barber M, Walters M, Bump R. Association of the magnitude of pelvic organ prolapse and presence and severity of symptoms. J pelvic Med and Surg. 2003;9:208.
2. Burrows LJ, Meyn LA, Walters MD, et al. Pelvic symptoms in women with pelvic organ prolapse. Obstet Gynecol. 2004; 104:982-88.
3. Ellerkmann MR, Cundiff GW, Melick CF, et al. Correlation of symptoms with location and severity of pelvic organ prolapse. Am J obstet Gynecol. 2001;185:1332-38.
4. Jackson SL, Weber AM, Hull TL, et al. Fecal incontinence in women with urinary incontinence and pelvic organ prolapse. Obset Gynecol. 1997;89:423-27.
5. Luber KM, Boero S, Choe JY. The demographics of pelvic floor disorders:current observations and future projections. AM J Obstet. Gynecon. 2001;184:1496-503.
6. Luber KM, Boero S, Choe JY. The demographics of pelvic floor disorders: current observations and future projections. AM J Obstet Gynecol. 2001;184:1496,1501; discussion 1501-3.
7. Nichols NM, Gill EJ, Nguyen T et al. Anal sphincter injury in women with pelvic floor disorders. Obstet Gynecol. 2004; 104:690-96.
8. Samuelsson EC, Victor FTA, Tibblin G, et al. Signs of genital prolapse in a Swedish population of women 20 to 59 years. of age and possible related factors. AM J Obstet Gynecol. 1999;180: 299-305.
9. Swift SE, Tate SB, Nicholas J. Correlation of symptoms with degree of pelvic organ support in a general population of women: What is pelvic organ prolapse. Am J Obstet Gynecol. 2003; 189:372-79.
10. Swift SE, Tate SB, Nicholas J. Correlation of symptoms with degree of pelvic organ support in a general population of women: what is pelvic organ prolapse. Am J Obstet Gynecol 2003;189:372-79.

39.5 TRACHELORRHAPHY (OLD CERVICAL TEAR REPAIR)

Mala Arora

INTRODUCTION

Cervical tears are often produced during descent of the fetal head in the second stage of labor. They result in traumatic post partum hemorrhage and they are best repaired soon after delivery to control hemorrhage. However, if the blood loss is not excessive, they may go unnoticed, at that time and are either picked up at an interval pelvic examination or during the next pregnancy when they will present with cervical incompetence and may result in a mid-trimester pregnancy loss. Therefore, repairing the tears in the nonpregnant state will reduce the incidence of cervical incompetence.

Increased risk of cervical tears is seen with:

- Fetal macrosomia
- Rapid descent of fetal head through a partially dilated cervix as in precipitate labor
- Vaginal manipulations like manual rotation of fetal head in deep transverse arrest
- Forceps application both rotational and non-rotational
- Ventouse extraction if the cervical rim gets caught in the ventouse cup
- Vaginal destructive procedures
- Duhrssens incision over cervix to release the after coming head in a breech delivery.

Hence, in above cases, it is recommended to explore the cervix after delivery and repair the cervical tear. The technique of cervical exploration requires adequate light, the use of three sponge forceps and a Sims' retractor for the anterior and posterior walls. The sponge forceps are applied at 12 o'clock, 2 o'clock and 4 o'clock postions, the cervix inspected and the 2 o'clock forceps moved to 6 o'clock. The forceps are advanced clockwise till a tear is found, at which point the apex of the tear is visualized and an absorbable suture of chromic catgut is applied, continuously to approximate the tear (Fig. 1). If the apex is not visualized, the suture is placed at the highest point, held with an artery forceps and pulled downwards to bring the apex into view. Alternatively, the ring forceps or an artery forceps can be applied to the bleeding point and left in situ for 4 hours. It can then be slowly released and removed if no bleeding is observed. Repair of the tear in this case is done as an interval procedure.

In case of bleeding from a ragged cervical edge is encountered, it can be under run with locking by an absorbable chromic catgut suture much like the edging of a button hole. If the tear is involving the lower uterine segment, it is best repaired at laparotomy, for if left unattended may result in a broad ligament hematoma or hemoperitoneum, both of which can lead to postpartum collapse, hypovolemia and death.

ADVERSE EFFECTS OF CERVICAL TEARS

- Subfertility may result due to destruction of cervical glands that act as reservoir for spermatozoa
- Chronic cervicitis due to ascending infection with vaginal bacteria
- Chronic endometritis due to loss of protective cervical mucous
- Cervical incompetence which may result in mid-trimester pregnancy loss or premature delivery
- Preterm premature rupture of membranes secondary to ascending infection due to loss of cervical mucous plug.

The above factors obviate the need for trachelorrhaphy, as the obstetric outcome is improved after the procedure.

DIAGNOSIS

Per speculum visualization of the cervix will clearly show the extent and location of the cervical tear. Using a Sims speculum with an anterior vaginal wall retractor and grasping the anterior and posterior cervical lips with tenaculums will give better information of the upper extent of the tear.

If a digital examination alone is performed, the tear may be easily missed, although it may sometimes be palpable digitally as well.

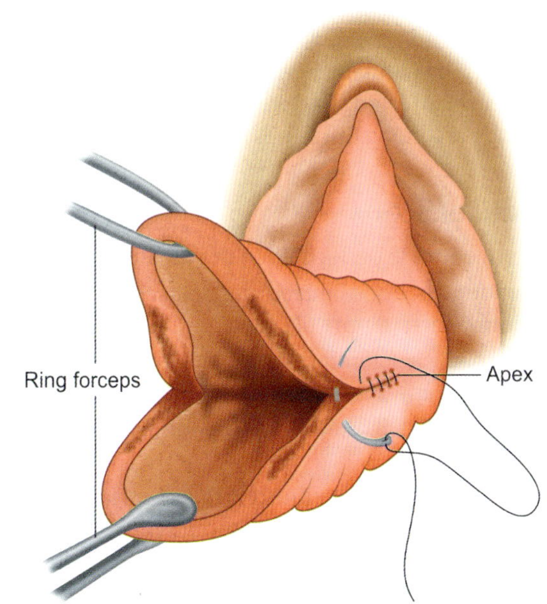

Fig.1 : Repair of old cervical tear

Transvaginal ultrasound scan that shows a wide cervical canal greater than 6 mm in width should raise the possibility of the presence of a cervical tear, which should be confirmed by a speculum examination.

TIMING OF AN OLD CERVICAL TEAR REPAIR

The procedure is best done soon after the cessation of a menstrual period as it ensures that the patient is not pregnant and allows time for cervical healing prior to the onset of the next period. Blood being a good culture medium may predispose to infection of a raw site on the cervix.

PROCEDURE

Anesthesia

The procedure is best done under general or spinal anesthesia. This gives good pelvic relaxation that is required for adequate visualization of the apex in deep cervical tears.

However, in superficial lacerations, local infiltration anesthesia can be used in the cervix. Plain 2% xylocaine in a 10 cc syringe and a 24 gauge needle is used to inject local at the edges of the cervical tear. Alternatively the cervix is injected at 4 o'clock and 8 o'clock position where the nerves enter the cervix. Care should be taken to avoid the 3 o'clock and 9 o'clock positions as the blood vessels are more likely to be hit.

A pudendal block is also effective and is given with a special pudendal block needle which is 15 cm long and of 24 gauge. It has a ring guard through which the index finger is passed. The ischial spine is palpated on the left side with the right hand and the needle inserted just beneath it for a distance of 0.5 cm under the vaginal mucosa. 5 cc of plain 1% xylocaine is injected. The procedure is repeated on the other side by reversing the hands.

Procedure/Steps

- The procedure is performed in the theater
- The patient is anesthetized and placed in lithotomy position with an empty bladder
- Alternatively, a self retaining Foley's catheter size 16 is inserted under anesthesia
- The vagina is cleaned with betadine solution and draped
- The operating light is adjusted to fall into the vagina from behind the surgeon's left shoulder
- The assistant retracts the posterior vaginal wall with a Sims speculum and if the need be the anterior vaginal wall is also retracted with another Sims speculum
- The two ends of the cervical tear are held by two long Allis forceps or single tooth tenaculums. The edges need to be freshened by superficial shaving with a knife till they appear raw and start bleeding, as described by Emmet. This is best done by gently stroking the knife blade up and down the cut, superficially on either side
- Alternatively, the tissue on the cut surface may be held with a toothed dissecting forceps and cut with a sharp scissors to freshen the edges. This is an important step as the healing is much quicker if the edges are fresh.

Suture

- The repair can be done in a single layer of interrupted absorbable sutures like chromic catgut number 1 or vicryl number 1 either plain or rapide on a reverse cutting needle
- The first suture is applied to the apex or the highest visible point, if the apex is not in view. The suture is tied securely and the ends are kept long and held on an artery forceps for traction and visualization of the apex
- This technique will allow the visualization of the apex in the majority of cases. Interrupted sutures provide better approximation. If the cervix is thick, the repair can be done in two layers. These are the inner and outer layers. It is important to do the inner layer first and then the outer layer.

Alternative Techniques

If conventional repair is not possible due to a high tear, alternative methods described are occlusion of the uterine isthmus with Shirodhkar's stitch in early pregnancy. Traditionally, the knot is placed anterior and buried under the vaginal mucosa. The suture may be removed after 38 weeks or left in situ, if a cesarean section is planned. The suture may then serve future pregnancies as well. A combination of repair and cerclage can be done at the same sitting under anesthesia in the non-pregnant state, if so desired.

Another technique of repairing the isthmus, less commonly employed, is that of Lash and Palmer. Occlusive trachelorrhaphy is rarely performed these days in the reproductive age group. It was described in 1956 and has been currently replaced by Shirodhkar or McDonald sutures. It involves interrupted sutures to obliterate the cervical canal with nonabsorbable sutures to prevent preterm labor. It may be of use in selected cases where the cervix is extremely short to permit cerclage, e.g. post Fothergill's surgery.

Postoperative Care

Since the vagina is an ecosystem comprising of many low virulent anaerobic and micro-aerophilic organisms, the wound should be smeared with metronidazole or betadine ointment. The same should be applied daily intravaginally at night. Intercourse and intravaginal tampons should be avoided for 2 weeks to allow healing.

Oral antibiotics may be administered which need to cover gram negative and anaerobic bacteria. A good combination will be a quinolone like ciprofloxacin or ofloxacin with metronidazole, secnidazole or ornidazole.

Complications

- Reaction to local anesthetic, especially if inadvertantly injected in a blood vessel can cause cardiac dysrhythmia, seizures
- Nonunion of the tear is encountered if the edges are not freshened or if infection occurs
- Partial union may occur if the sutures are placed at a distance from each other
- Cervico vaginal fistula is a complication of induced mid-trimester abortion. Cervical cerclage is preferred to trachelorrhaphy in these cases. In case vaginal cerclage is not feasible, transabdominal cerclage can be performed
- Tear during subsequent pregnancy and childbirth may be encountered and requires resuturing
- Hemorrhage may be encountered during freshening the edges which may be brisk but will settle as the sutures are applied
- Inability to visualize the apex vaginally may lead to incomplete healing of the tear.

BIBLIOGRAPHY

1. Benson RC, Durfee RB. Transabdominal cervicouterine cerclage during pregnancy for the treatment of cervical incompetency. Obstet Gynecol. 1965;25:145-55.
2. Cammrano CL, Herron MA, Parer JT. Validity of indications for trans-abdominal cervicoisthmic cerclage for cervical incompetence. Am J Obstet Gynecol. 1995;172:1871-5.
3. Gordon RT Cervicovaginal fistula as a result of saline abortion. Am J Obstet Gynecol. 1972;112(4);578-9.
4. Hall HH. Occlusive trachelorrhaphy for repeated abortion due to cervical incompetence. Am J Obstet Gynecol. 1956;71(1): 225-6.
5. Ilobachie GC, Onah HE. Cervical-vaginal fistula from induced abortions causing subsequent spontaneous midtrimester abortions in Nigerians: case report. Niger Postgrad Med J. 2002;9(2):99-101.
6. Lippi UG, Modda A, Ogata AJ, et al. Cerclage of the cervix uteri via a trans abdominal route: report of 2 cases. Rev Paul Med. 1989;107(3):189-90.
7. Lischke JH, Gordon HR. Cervicovaginal fistula complicating induced mid trimester abortion despite laminaria tent insertion. Am J Obstet Gynecol. 1974;120(6):852-3.
8. Machado LM. Conservative surgery of the uterine cervix; current concept of Emmet's trachelorrhaphy. Rev Gynecol Obstet. 1954;48(4):630-6.
9. Musset R, Poitout P, Truc JB, et al. An original and effective technic for trachelorrhaphy. J Gynecol Obstet Biol Reprod (Paris). 1976;5(1):105-11.
10. Novy MJ. Transabdominal cervicoisthmic cerclage: a reappraisal 25 years after its introduction. Am J Obstet Gynecol. 1991;164:1635-41.
11. Novy MJ. Transabdominal cervicoisthmic cerclage for the management of repetitive abortion and premature delivery. Am J Obstet Gynecol. 1982;143-4.
12. R, Goldstein DP. Transabdominal cervicoisthmic cerclage: Learning to tie the knot. J Gynecol Tech. 1996;2:49-54.
13. Wallenberg HC, Lotgering FK. Transabdominal cerclage for closure of the incompetent cervix. Eu J Obs. Gynecol Reprod Biol. 1987;25:121.

39.6 CRYOSURGERY

Vandana Walvekar, Geetha D Balsarkar

INTRODUCTION

Cryosurgery is a form of treatment of dysplasia of the cervix by destroying the abnormal tissue by freezing it to extremely cold temperatures using probes.

CRYOGEN

A substance with a very low boiling point, such as liquid nitrogen called cryogen, is used in cryotherapy treatment. Liquid nitrogen is cooled and liquefied at a temperature of -321°F. Such liquefied nitrogen can easily pass through the probes.

PHYSICS OF CRYOTHERAPY

The cold temperature required for cryotherapy is introduced through a probe which has liquid nitrogen or CO_2 circulating through it. To destroy dysplastic cervical cells, the tissue is cooled suddenly to below 20°C. The tissue frozen may be allowed to thaw and then be refrozen for another 2–3 minutes. A single freeze treatment for 5 minutes may also be used. Other procedures that control pain or bleeding for which liquid nitrogen is used are cooled to a lesser degree to prevent tissue damage.

INDICATIONS

Cryosurgery is used for treatment options of cervical dysplasia that can lead to cancer of the cervix, warts, including genital warts from HPV in gynecology.

OTHER USES

Cryotherapy has been tested mainly in various other specialities of medicine. Hence, it is widely used for the folllowing conditions:

- Tumors or cancer, especially those of the skin, cervix, eye and brain.
- This treatment is also being used for other cancers, such as prostate cancer and liver cancer.
- Actinic keratosis, a skin condition caused by sun exposure, can be treated with cryotherapy.
- Acne
- Hemorrhoids, which are enlarged veins in the rectum
- Certain types of chronic pain or nerve irritation, such as a condition called trigeminal neuralgia
- Other common skin lesions, such as skin tags, hemangiomas, or seborrheic keratoses
- A retinal tear or retinal detachment
- Bleeding during standard surgery.

PROCEDURE OF CRYOSURGERY

Cryosurgery, in gynecology, is performed as an office procedure. During the procedure a speculum is inserted to visualize the cervix. The cryoprobe is inserted into the vagina and placed firmly on the surface of the cervix (Fig. 1), covering the abnormal tissue. Compressed gaseous nitrogen (temperature approximately 50°C) flows through the instrument which can be identified by a hissing noise, making the metal cold enough to freeze and destroy the tissue. Cryosurgery is painless and produces little scarring. An iceball forms on the cervix killing the superficial abnormal cells. For optimal treatment, the freezing is done for 3 minutes. The cervix is allowed to thaw, then the freezing is repeated for an additional 3 minutes (Fig. 2).

PATHOPHYSIOLOGY

Liquid nitrogen causes a stinging and burning pain while the growth is being frozen and this burning continues while it thaws. Some time after liquid nitrogen treatment, the frozen tissue will become inflamed causing a blister.

A scab (crust) will form. The crust will fall off by itself in 2–4 weeks. The dysplastic cells will come off with the scab, leaving behind healthy tissue. Liquid nitrogen treatment causes a permanent white flat scar.

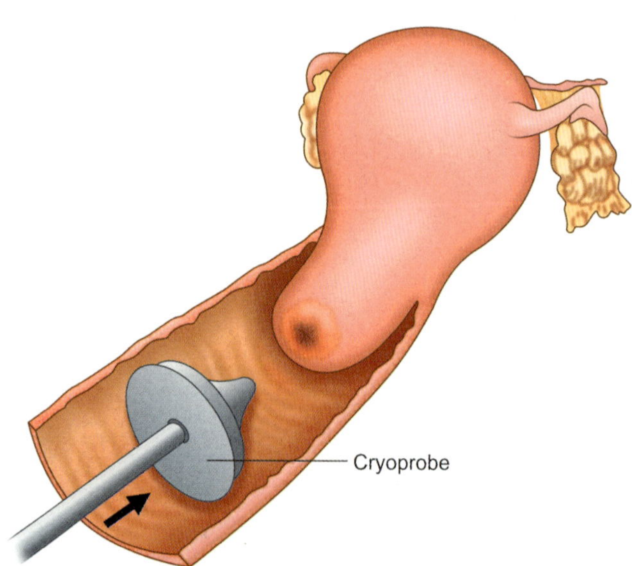

Fig. 1: Cryoprobe being applied at cervix

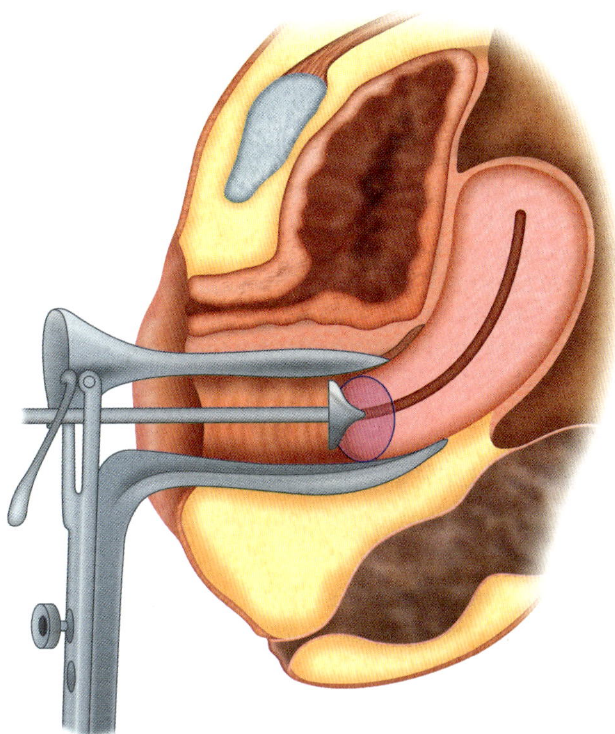

Fig. 2: Formation of iceball at cervix during cryofreezing

FOLLOW-UP OF CRYOSURGERY

A repeat Pap smear or biopsy as required depending on the primary pathology is recommended after 3 months to ensure that the procedure was successful in killing abnormal tissue. Patients may report with fever, moderate to heavy bleeding during periods, cramping pelvic pain, bad-smelling or yellowish vaginal discharge due to an infection.

AFTER CARE INSTRUCTIONS

Regular follow-up pelvic examinations are mandatory after cryotherapy of the cervix. Pap smear will be usually repeated in 3 months. If this first Pap smear is normal, then they will be repeated every 3 months for 1 year and every 6 months the second year, if each Pap smear test is normal. After this 2 year schedule, yearly pap smears are again recommended.

Almost all normal activities can be allowed immediately after surgery. Avoidance of sexual intercourse, as well as douching, may be recommended for several weeks till complete healing has taken place. For 2–3 weeks after the surgery, patients should be counselled that there will be a lot of watery discharge caused by the shedding of the dead cervical tissue.

COMPLICATIONS

- Bleeding from cervical tissue
- Infection of the dead cells causing yellowish vaginal discharge
- Cervical stenosis due to scarring, which may lead to secondary infertility, or cause secondary amenorrhea
- Incomplete procedure causing continuing growth of abnormal tissues, necessitating radical treatment.

ADVANTAGES

Cryotherapy offers some advantages over other methods of treatment like conization, cauterization and laser excision.

- It is less invasive than regular surgery
- It may eliminate the need for cuts in the tissue and subsequent bleeding
- Pain, bleeding and other risks of surgery are reduced
- It is often less expensive than other forms of surgery
- The person often has a shorter recovery time.

For individuals with CIN and vulval intraepithelial neoplasm (VIN), cryotherapy can be added to other standard treatments.

DISADVANTAGES

Cryotherapy, like almost all treatments, has side effects. However, they may be less severe than the side effects of regular surgery. The main risk is damage to surrounding healthy tissue. This can be quite serious, such as in brain surgery, when the healthy tissue is very important but not so in cervix.

PLACE OF CRYOTHERAPY TODAY

Cryotherapy is an effective method for destroying abnormal cervical tissue, depending on the size, depth, and type of abnormal tissue. Cryotherapy destroys all of the abnormal tissue in more than 85–90% of cases.

BIBLIOGRAPHY

1. Avasthi KK, Midha U, Kang B. Cryo Surgery in benign cervical epithelial lesion following up with cervical culture. Ind J Obstet and Gynaecol. 1990;40(3):436-40.
2. Hilgarth M, Hillemanns HG, Roll H. The special case: squamous epithelial carcinoma of the cervix after cryotherapy in a 23 year old patient. Fortschr Med. 1979;97(46):2145-9.
3. Mitchell MF, Tortolero-Luna G, Cook E, et al. A randomized clinical trial of cryotherapy, laser vaporization, and loop electrosurgical excision for treatment of squamous intraepithelial lesions of the cervix. Obstet Gynecol. 1998;92:737-44.

39.7 DILATATION OF CERVIX

Nidhi Gupta, Kamal Gupta

INTRODUCTION

It is the most frequently performed surgical procedure in gynecology. It should, therefore, be carefully learnt and practiced.

INDICATIONS

Dilatation of cervix is an important, preliminary to many gynecological procedures:

- Uterine curettage
- Early termination of pregnancy
- Cervical cautery
- Insertion of intrauterine contraceptive device (IUCD) in nulliparous patient (stenosed cervix)
- Intracavitary radiotherapeutic procedures
- Removal of intrauterine polyp
- Insertion of hysteroscope
- Suction evacuation procedure
- Manchester repair, Fothergill's surgery
- Conization of cervix
- Post-traumatic/atrophic stenosis
- Post-radiotherapy pyometra
- Post-surgical hematometra.

ANESTHESIA

Any procedure which includes dilatation of cervix is very painful, and therefore, the patient should have proper anesthetic backup prior to the procedure. Following are the options:

- Regional anesthesia—paracervical block
- Sedation
- General anesthesia
- Spinal/epidural anesthesia.

The choice of anesthesia depends on the procedure planned. General anesthesia is preferable, whenever available. Regional anesthesia (paracervical block), when correctly done, provides the advantage of early discharge after the procedure which is desirable since most of these cases are done on an outpatient basis.

Paracervical Block

It is an easy and better alternative to other types of anesthesia options, wherever indicated. The autonomic fibers, which supply uterus and vagina, form a plexus in parametrium; anesthetizing them will minimize the pain of cervical dilatation. This is achieved by performing a paracervical block wherein local anesthetic is injected submucosally into the lateral fornices of vagina to block the nerve transmission through the paracervical ganglion. About 10–15 mL of 1% lignocaine or 0.125% or 0.25% bupivacaine with or without adrenaline is used to block at the 3 o'clock and 9 o'clock position.

TYPES OF CERVICAL DILATATION

- Fast dilatation
- Slow dilatation.

Fast dilatation is dilatation of cervix immediately before the planned procedure which includes dilatation with Hegar's dilators.

Slow dilatation includes dilatation with drugs like prostaglandins, mechanical objects like laminaria tents.

PATIENT PREPARATION AND OPERATIVE PROCEDURE

- No need to shave the patient prior to the procedure
- Patient must be asked to empty her bladder
- She should preferably be empty stomach
- Lithotomy position is made and patient is brought to the edge of the table
- Prior use of misoprostol (oral or vaginal) 200–400 μm helps in easy accomplishment of the procedure, especially in cases of nulliparity and primary infertility.

After the preparation for the procedure is over, the following steps are to be followed:

- Clean the vulva and vagina with local antiseptic solutions like povidone-iodine (betadine) or cetrimide (savlon) or chloroxy-lenol or cetrimide (dettol)
- Drape the parts
- Prior knowledge of position of uterus with a sound is important so as to avoid inadvertent injury to the cervix, do pelvic examination
- A Sims' speculum is inserted in the vagina and posterior vaginal wall is retracted (Fig. 1)
- The cervix and the upper vagina are once again cleansed with antiseptic
- Anesthesia of choice is administered if not already given
- Anterior lip of the cervix is caught with a vulsellum. Sometimes it is better to use two Allis forceps.

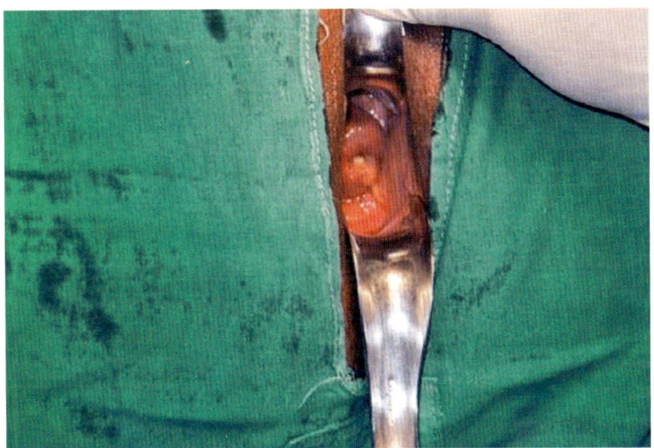

Fig. 1: Cervix visualized with Sims' speculum in situ

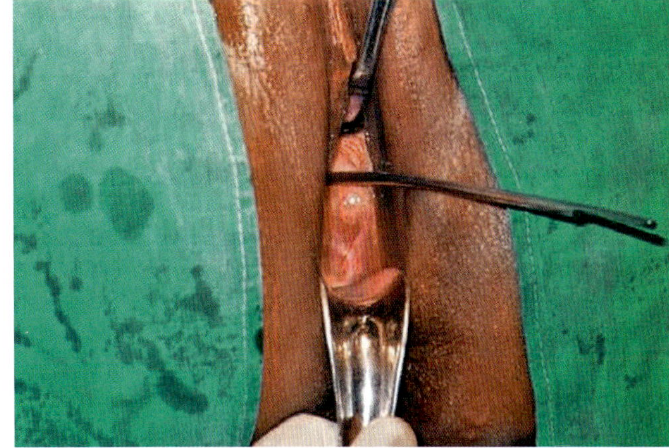

Fig. 2: Hager's dilator left in situ for some time, instead of frequent to and fro movements

DIFFICULTIES IN PERFORMING THE DILATATION

Inability to Pass a Sound or Dilator

Alternatively, a single tooth tenaculum can be used.

- Traction is applied on the cervix to straighten the uterocervical canal
- A uterine sound is gently passed till the fundus of the uterus to find out the direction of the uterocervical canal and the lengths of the cervix and the uterine cavity. Normal length of the cervical canal is 2.5 cm and that of the uterine cavity 4 cm
- The cervix is now dilated with lowest gauge of dilators first and then gradually ascending up. Hegar's dilators serially graduated in 0.5 mm thickness are the best. Cervix should essentially not be dilated beyond number 8 Hegar's dilator as doing this will damage the fibrous tissue and may result in repeated miscarriages later on due to incompetent os
- Dilator should be grasped between the thumb and the index and middle fingers while the ring and little fingers are fully extended (like a pencil). The last two fingers act like a guard to prevent application of unnecessary force which might otherwise injure the cervix
- The dilator should not be repeatedly slided in and out of the os, rather it should be left with its tip just beyond the internal os for a few seconds and then next thicker dilator is used (Fig. 2). Dilator should never be pushed beyond the sounded length of the uterine cavity

  After this process is over, next steps are to be taken for whatever the cervix is dilated
- Sometimes when a smaller dilator fails to enter the internal os, a thicker dilator might do the trick as it easily rides over the small cul-de-sacs in the canal
- Straightening the cervical canal with a slight traction on the cervix helps
- If there is total inability to pass the dilator, then this should be accepted as a stenosed/scarred cervix and the procedure to be performed should be modified likewise.

Point of Caution

Excessive force should never be applied as it can injure the cervix or it might go tearing the cervix into a false passage. If this is not noticed, the end result may be rupture of the cervix or uterus. This problem is obviated if the surgeon meticulously follows the axis of the uterus as defined at bimanual examination.

COMPLICATIONS OF DILATATION

1. *Tearing and laceration of the cervix:* Laceration is most likely to happen if excessive force is used or the cervix is dilated too widely or if spasm of the cervix is not allowed to relax before proceeding. A sudden give way sensation is suspicious of the tear. The tear might even extend from the cervix into the uterus followed by broad ligament. If the surgeon suspects that a tear may have occurred, dilatation should be stopped immediately. If the laceration is visible and bleeding, suture of the damaged area is mandatory. Even when there is no bleeding, suturing will restore the anatomy and obviate further bleeding developing later, but will probably not restore the functional integrity of the cervix if the internal os is damaged.
2. *Early bleeding:* Sometimes due to injury to the cervix during dilatation, it might bleed; in such a case, putting a pressure tampon is sufficient. In case, there is hemorrhage due to cervical tear, then offending vessel is sought for and sutured. If the bleeding point is not visible then there is a controversy regarding simple pressure packing or laparotomy. In case pressure

packing has been done then patient's vitals are to be monitored carefully.

If the bleeding is considerable and coming from an invisible site in the upper cervix, packing should not be considered. The cervix should either be split to demonstrate the bleeding point, or if the site cannot be identified, the uterine artery on that side should be exposed as in for vaginal hysterectomy and separately ligated.

3. *Perforation of the uterus:* If injudicious, excessive force is used, then it might perforate the uterus. The position of the dilator should be noted and the procedure terminated. The exception to this will be when evacuation of the uterus is imperative, such as in termination of a pregnancy, in which circumstances the remainder of the procedure should be performed with extreme gentleness and care; preferably under ultrasound guidance. When the suspected perforation has occurred during a clean procedure, such as curettage for menorrhagia or for endometrial sampling, observation of the patient by half hourly pulse and blood pressure is all that is necessary. If there is suspected infection, the same observation should be accompanied by antibiotic cover for at least 7 days.
4. *Cervical incompetence:* As already discussed above, injudicious excessive dilatation of cervix beyond number 8 hegar's dilator might result in cervical incompetence.

CONCLUSION

It is a very common procedure done in field of gynecology. The nuance of learning correct method of dilation will go long way in avoiding complications in a common procedure of daily use.

ENDOCERVICAL CURETTAGE

Curettage of the endocervical canal before cervical dilatation is done is called endocervical curettage.

Indications

- Carcinoma cervix
- Carcinoma endometrium
- Abnormal pap smear
- Unsatisfactory colposcopy.

Procedure

- A specialized endocervical curette or a uterine curette is introduced into the endocervical canal to the level of cervicoisthemic junction. Using firm linear strokes the entire surface is curetted, allowing the mucous laden specimen to at the external os
- The removal of the specimen can be difficult and is most easily accomplished by twirling the curette at the external os and allowing the specimen to wrap around the end of the curette A cotton swab applicator stick is then used to put pressure on the specimen against the curette. The specimen can then be withdrawn and placed in a bottle of 10% formalin for histopathologic evaluation.

BIBLIOGRAPHY

1. Ayim E, Bewes PC, Bion JF, et al. Nerve blocks. In: King MH (ed). Primary Anaesthesia. Oxford University Press; 1986. pp 40.
2. Currie JL. Malignant tumors of the uterine corpus. In: Rock JA, Thompson JD (eds). Te Linde's Operative Gynaecology. 8th edition. Lippincott Williams and Wilkins; 1997. pp. 1511-2.
3. Dutta DC. Operative obstetrics. In: Textbook of Obstetrics, 4th edition. New Central Book Agency Publishers; 1998. pp. 599-601.
4. Monaghan JM, Lopes AB, Naik R. Operations on the cervix. In: Bonney's Gynaecological surgery, 10th edition. Blackwell Publishing; 2004. pp. 27-32.
5. Ostergard DR, Berman ML, Yee B. Cervical biopsy and Endocervical curettage. In: Atlas on gynaecological surgery. WB Saunders Company; 2000. pp. 298-9.
6. Parikh MN. Dilatation of cervix and uterine curettage. Ind J Obstet Gynaecol. 1998; 48(6):181-84.

39.8 APPLICATION OF CYTOLOGY IN OBSTETRICS AND GYNECOLOGY

VL Lahiri, Manashi Ray

INTRODUCTION

The Pap smear is named after Dr George Papanicolaou, who with Dr Herbert Truta, a pathologist, perfected the technique. It had a tremendous impact on reducing the number of deaths from cervical cancer worldwide. At first it was hoped that the technique will catch cervical cancer in the early stages, but it has come to a point when precancerous lesions are detected and then eliminated reducing the morbidity and mortality of cervical cancer.

The technique has extended to other uses and other sites. Here professor Wahi should be remembered, who introduced cytopathology as a routine diagostic tool in the country.

Traditionally, cervical vaginal cytology has usually been considered a screening test and the reports considered requiring biopsy confirmation. However, with the involvement of trained pathologists cytology has evolved to a diagnostic discipline.

From numeric class I to V, the report have moved through to histologic terminology with a definitive confidence that the cytologic diagnosis is as good as histopathology. This trend is for fine needle aspiration cytology (FNAC) as well as in exfoliative cytology, and the reports will always lead to treatment and prognostication. This has been aided by the accuracy of sampling of deep seated lesions under imaging.

In comparison to biopsy, cytologic diagnosis has the advantage of more clarity on cell and nuclear morphology but lacks in orientation of cells and intertissue relationship like invasion. For dependable diagnosis and quality of report, the cytopathologist should not only have a qualification in cytology but have a good background of clinical/imaging data, histopathology and available information on cytodiagnostic features, cytochemistry and immunohistology.

The clinican should provide requisite information and keep up communication with the cytopathologist.

The accuracy is dependent on the direct involvement and supervision at every step of the procedure.

PAP SMEAR

Technique

Collection and transport of samples of Pap smear:

- The patient should avoid intercourse douches, intra-vaginal tablets, ointments, etc. for at least 24 hours.
- Select the collection procedure in light of the clinical data/findings
- Visualize the cervix and os
- Ayres spatula and ECB and endometrial aspirate canula are sufficient
- The material should be spread uniformly and fixed (without any drying) in liquid fixative or by fixative spray. Thick smears, blood or exudates may obscure the findings
- Stains such as Papanicolaous stain, H&E, May-Grünwald are used
- Giemsa and additional stains are used as indicated.

If there is suspicion of infective process, separate requisition for such tests as hanging drop, aflatoxin biomarker (AFB), Gram's, fluorescent antibody test, culture and sensitivity, fungal stains should be made.

APPLICATION OF PAP SMEAR

Screening for Cervical Cancer

In the USA, 50 million women are screened for changes in the morphology of the cells from cervix, vagina or endometrium and receive treatment accordingly.

However, the prohibitive costs and ignorance about usefulness have not made this possible as a general program in our country. It is, however, necessary to motivate women to undergo the test on a regular basis.

It has been established that mass screening effectively reduces mortality from cervical cancer by earlier diagnosis of invasive disease, by Adami, in 1994.

A strong correlation has been reported between screening intensity in a population and cervical cancer mortality. In the USA, in unscreened women, the invasive cancer rate is 310/1,00,000, while in screened women only 50/1,00,000.

Our figures are similar for the unscreened women with the added fact of high morbidity and mortality due to nonavailability of adequate medical support, especially for the economically weaker segment and rural population.

The Pap smear is almost painless procedure requiring very little time and is quite efficient.

The additional information which can be given regarding inflammatory and infective or infestations may help in the management of symptomatic cases.

Even if definite, screening protocol cannot be followed, a woman in reproductive/postmenopausal phase having irregularity of cycle, discharge or other relevant symptoms must have a Pap smear.

Table 1: American Cancer Society Guideline Screening (2002)

Criteria	Screening Program
Age to initiate screening	Three years after the onset of sexual activity; no later than 21 years, every year
Screening frequency	Annually with conventional cytology
Screening after hysterectomy	No cytologic screening required after hysterectomy for benign condition

It is difficult to decide the actual time to start screening. The following is a useful guide adopted from the American Cancer Society, Guideline Screening (2002) (Table 1).

- Women with three consecutive normal tests may be screened every 2-3 years or if they develop any symptoms
- Pregnancy should not be a cause for avoiding screening.

The efficacy for screening in preventing invasive cancers is about 3 out of 4 possible cases. The correct detection of invasive cancer is between 97% and 99% and of invasive carcinoma is between 88% and 94%.

Diagnostic Cytology—(Cervix, Uterus, Vagina and Vulva)

Samples

a. Cervix—ectocervical scrape smear with Ayres spatula Endocervix—brush smear/aspirate from endocervix, a combination of Ayres spatula and brush is ideal.
b. Vagina, vulva—scrape/brush smear.
c. Endometrium
   i. From posterior vaginal fornix
   ii. Aspirate from endocervical canal
   iii. Aspirates from the uterine cavity using a canula and syringe with/without sterile saline injection or a brush smear.

Fix without drying if Paps stain is used.

Stains - (Pap stain, H& E, May-Grunwald, Giemsa)

The Pap smear, specially with other stains can also give positive information about many infective lesions like:

Trichomonas: fungus, *Chlamydia: Amoeba,* herpes simplex: HPV, etc. It is important to realize that the positive report is important but the absence of it does not exclude the infections.

A judicious use of hanging drop preparation/Grams stain/cytochemical and immunofluorescent stains can provide helpful information.

Reporting Pap Smear

Terminology for reporting the Pap smear has been a difficult problem The Bethesda System (2001, revised) is being given.

The 2001 (revised) Bethesda System for Pap smear, reports:

As per the recommendations, the:

- Pap smear is considered a medical consultation
- Pathologist is responsible for diagnosis
- Referring physician is to provide clinical data
- Recommendations regarding follow-up should be made by the cytopathologist.

Report should contain comments on:

- The adequacy of Pap sample
- Incidental findings such, as evidence of infection, type of infection and cause if possible
- Evidence of lesions like dysplasia or carcinoma or other
- Presence of endometrial cells.

New Bethesda System—Classification of Smears (2002)

These refer mainly to epithelial cell changes:

1. LSIL
   a. Cellular changes associated with HPV
   b. Mild (slight) dysplasia/CIN I.
2. HSIL
   a. Moderate dysplasia/CIN II
   b. Severe dysplasia/CIN III
   c. Carcinoma in situ/CIN III.
3. Atypical squamous cells (ASC)
   a. Unspecified ASC (ASCUS)—includes unspecified and favor benign/inflammation
   b. Cannot exclude HSIL (ASCH).
4. Atypical glandular cells of uncertain significance (AGCUS): Endocervical, endometrial, or not otherwise specified origin or endocervical ACIS.
   a. Atypical glandular cells of unspecified significance (AGS-US)
   b. Atypical glandular cells, favor neoplastic (AGC-H) category are always to be closely followed up.

The various terms used:

- Normal (euplasia)—no abnormal cells are detected. No treatment or testing is required till next Pap smear and pelvic examination is due
- Atypical squamous cells of undertermined significance: The Pap smear reveals slightly abnormal squamous cells, but the changes do not clearly suggest SIL dysplasia. A test for HPV should be carried out and patient should be kept under follow up by Pap's smear.

- *Squamous intraepithelial lesion (SIL)/dysplasia:* This indicates that the cells may be precancerous. If the changes are low-grade, that if a precancerous lesion is present, it's likely to progress to cancer in some cases. If the changes are high-grade, there's a greater chance that the lesion may develop into cancer early. A close follow up by cytology colposcopy biopsy and tests for HPV may be indicated
- *Atypical glandular cells:* Atypical glandular cells may appear to be slightly abnormal, but it's unclear whether they're cancerous.

  Further testing is needed to determine the source of the abnormal cells. A repeat smear and colposcopy and biopsy are required
- *Squamous cancer or adenocarcinoma cells:* The cells collected for the Pap smear are so abnormal that the pathologist is almost certain a cancer is present in the vagina, cervix or, occasionally, the uterus. Squamous cavernoma refers to cancers arising in the flat surface cells of the cervix or metaplastic cells in endocervix or uterus. Adenocarcinoma refers to cancer of glandular cells of endocervix or endometrium. These categories in Bethesda system or other terminology such as SIL/ dysplasia are helpful in deciding basis of follow-up and procedures, however, these are not water tight compartments, especially because a large proportion of women in our population suffer from pelvic inflammatory disease and cervical infections of various etiologies, i.e. chlamydia, tuberculosis, etc., which may be causing epithelial changes similar to mild dysplasia or LSIL or the actual SIL lesion may be accompanied by infection.

Further there is always difficulty in categorizing changes when there is overlap of epithelial growth processes like retroplasia, proplasia and dysplasia/SIL.

In such circumstances a follow-up with smear, colposcopy or biopsy/cone biopsy is indicated.

Basis of Cytologic Reports

Cytologic reports are based on cellular morphology and the milieu which reflects biologic activity. It reflects the response of the host tissue end response at cellular level. It shows genetic and molecular response of cells to the various endogenous and exogenous agents.

Generally, proliferative activity is reflected best in structure of the nucleus and functional activity in the morphology of cytoplasm differentiation. The variations are recognized by morphology nucleus. The nuclear size, nucleus to cytoplasm (N/C) ratio, chromatin, parachromatin, chromatin rim, chromatin net, nuclear membrance, nucleoli which are all examined and changes considered.

Growth Patterns

i. *Euplasia:* Normal pattern of tissue is noted as euplasia. It is dominated by round or smooth nuclear character, i.e. rounded (nucleus, nucleolus, chromocenter) uniform or regular pattern of chromatin, predictable from one nucleus to another in a group or giant cells and normal N/C ratio.

ii. *Proplasia:* Innumerable processes are capable of causing progressive change—stimulation, replication, repair all cause proplasia, has characteristics of roundedness of nucleus, nucleoli, regular chromatin-parachromatin and predictability of structure remains, hyperchromasia binucleation, nucleolar enlargement occur. Mitosis is few and bipolar.

iii. *Retroplasia* (regressive process or decreased activity): loss of control over water content—hydropic degeneration, altered cytoplasmic staining, nuclear membrane wrinkling, blurring of chromation-parachromatin interface, chromatin clumping, karyorrhexis, pyknosis karyolysis, etc.

iv. *Mixed and changing growth process*: This is common slippery ground for the cytopathologist. Overlapping changes of euplasia, proplasia, retroplasia and sometimes neoplasia cause diagnostic difficulties, e.g. in chronic cervicitis, the endocervical cells show metaplastic changes with an active zone of transformation which exults cells showing changes of reaction to injury, features of repair and altered metabolic cell reaction. These may be mistaken for preneoplastic changes. Retroplasia, as in menopause, healed lesions, postradiation changes can be mistaken for neoplasia/dysplasia.

v. *Dysplasia* [CIN, systemic lupus erythematosus (SLE] is disordered form (disordered proliferation and differentiation). In cervix, the term dyslasia is applied to a spectrum of hetroplastic reactions of squamous or metaplastic epithelium characterized by abnormal/ irregular maturation or absence of it. Highest degrees of morphological changes to reported.

Dysplastic reactions occur more frequently on the anterior lip than the posterior lip and frequently in the transformation zone. Most lesions including cancer are thought to arise in area of squamous metaplasia in the endocervical canal or the transformation zone. It represents a reaction to various injurious agents. It has variable biologic behavior.

The concept of dysplasia, carcinoma in situ and squamous carcinoma are considered to form a continuous spectrum of morphological changes.

However, the degree of morphologic abnormality, grade of dysplasia does not necessarily correlate with biologic potential of the epithelial changes and all dysplastic lesions will not progress—some will regress, some persist and some will progress.

Table 2: Abnormal Pap smear—Natural progression and regression

Abnormal class	Regression to normal (%)	Progression to higher grade over 24 months (%)	Progression to invasive cancer over 24 months (%)
ASCUS	68	7	0.25
LSIL	47	21	0.15
HSIL	35	23	1.44

Abbreviation: ASCUS, atypical squamous cells unspecified; LSIL, low-grade squamous intraepithelial lesion; HSIL, high-grade squamous intraepithelial lesion

Table 2 shows abnormal Pap smear natural progression and regression

It is also important to realize that only 5-10% dysplasias reported on cytology can be confirmed by biopsy because of topography, size and depth of lesion. Moreover, sometimes a punch biopsy may remove an entire lesion of dysplasia or even intraepithelial carcinoma.

Cytologic smear gives a comprehensive idea of the epithelial lining of cervix, uterus and vagina. Grading of dysplastic change may not relate to accurate prognosis, it may give more insight into the morphologically different types of dysplasia as well as help in comparing potential of these lesions and relate to possible cause.

It is important to realize that the mean age at which cervical intraepithelial lesions/dysplasia are diagnosed is decreasing. This might be related to earlier sexual activity and number of partners as well as awareness of cytological tests.

vi. *Malignant neoplasia* (intraepithelial carcinoma and invasive carcinoma): There is no perfect or absolute feature of malignancy. The malignant diathysis includes nuclear and cytoplasmic changes as well as intercellular relationship.
   - *Nucleus:* Irregular shape, irregular chromatin rim; nuclear membrane irregularity and thickening; nucleolus-enlarged, irregular, multiple; chromatin—shows irregular lumps and staining. Anisonucleosis, variable morphology and non predictable in cell groups (anisonucleosis and anisochromasia); abnormal mitosis is tripolar or resette, etc.
   - Nuclear/cytoplasmic ratio is increased. Changes of degeneration are frequent but a degenerating cell should never form basis of diagnosis
   - Human papilloma virus (Koilocytotic) type 6, 11, 16, 18 and 31 are considered to be causatively linked to dysplasia and squamous cancer of cervix
   - Glandular neoplasms of cervix are increasingly seen
   - Adenocarcinomas accounting for 14–34% of cervical cancers. Epidemiological factors like age at starting sexual activity, member of partners or pregnancies do not seem to be related
   - However, wart virus infections, oral contraceptive use, HPV may be related. Precursor lesions involve the squamocolumnar junction and the canal. Various histologic variants have also been recognized.

Adenocarcinoma in Situ

The lesion shows all features of adenocarcinoma, except invasion. Similar lesions are found adjacent to invasive cancers also. The exfoliated cells also resemble those from adenocarcinoma. This lesion can be detected in smears, but not by colposcopy.

Adenocarcinoma in situ: The main types are—

i. Pure adenocarcinoma
ii. A combined adenosquamous carcinoma
iii. Adenoma maligmum or minimal deviation adenocarcinoma
iv. Clear cell carcinoma
v. Adenoid cystic carcinoma, basaloid adenoid carcinoma.

In smears, glandular carcinomas are associated with inflammatory exudates and necrosis, which makes identification of malignant cells difficult. While tumor diathesis in cells is the sole criteria of diagnosis, nuclear abnormality and deoxyribonucleic acid (DNA) content have been found to be important in prognostication.

Endometrial Cancer

The frequency of endometrial cancer has risen. In 1965, in the USA and some other countries, the incidence surpassed that of cervical cancer. This is mainly due to increase of older population, change in social milieu, use of unopposed estrogens and lack of screening program for endometrial cancer.

Cytological examinations can contribute to the detection of endometrial cancer and its precursors.

However, the sampling technique has to be appropriate. In the vaginal pool and endocervical aspirate, nearly 2% cases show endometrial cells-1.8% being normal. Hyperplasitc endometrial cells in 0.2% and carcinoma cells in 0.04%. While endometrial aspirates are ideal, the Pap smear (including the endocervical aspirate) provides information in most cases.

The morphology of spontaneously desquamated endometrial cells differs from forcibly aspirated cells from endometrium.

These may be glandular, stromal or both.

These cells are most frequently seen in menstrual phase and for few days in first half of cycle these are considered normal, but when seen in second half of cycle or postmenopausal period, they indicate abnormal shedding. This is seen in impending abortion, postpartum period, dysfunctional uterine bleeding, contraceptive device, anovulatory changes, endometritis, pyometra or endometrial polyp, submucous myoma and endometriosis of cervix and vagina. Their presence in post-menopausal women may indicate neoplastic pathology. Often it is not possible/advisable to differentiate between benign/malignant lesion on smear alone.

However, hyperplasia (without atypia) is usually benign. In vaginal/endocervical aspirate the morphology of endometrial hyperplasia with atypia is indistinguishable from adenocarcinoma in situ or differentiated adenocarcinoma. The accuracy of diagnosis is 90–95%. The accuracy is best in samples obtained from uterine cavity. Morphological variants are easy to diagnose, including mucinous carcinoma, papillary adenocarcinoma, undifferenciated carcinoma and adenosquamous carcinoma, malignant mixed mullerian tumor, etc.

Extra-uterine Tumors

Pap smear can have cells from all cancers of vagina, ovary, fallopian tube, colon, urinary bladder; melanomas, lymphomas, etc. can be detected. These reach the smears pool by the path of ovum or direct invasion of the uterus, cervix, etc., or through blood stream invasion. Other malignant tumors of uterine body like sarcomas, choriocarcinoma, can also be diagnosed.

Lesions of Vagina and Vulva

Cytology can provide adequate and useful information on lesions of vulva, vagina. Variety of inflammatory lesions like herpes simplex, molluscum, cytomegalo virus tuberculosis, leukoplasia, HPV, kraurosis, lichen sclerosis leukoplakia, fungal infections condyloma, etc. can be detected on smears.

Vulva intraepithelial neoplasm can also be detected. Squamous cell cancers, squamous cell carcinoma in situ, Pagets disease, melanoma, Bartholin cancer, metastatic tumors can be diagnosed if proper sample is collected. Basal cell carcinoma and verrucous carcinoma are difficult to diagnose.

Vaginal Vault Smear

After hysterectomy, the vaginal vault smears are examined and may give useful information about (Fig. 1 to 4):

i. Infection and formation of granulomas from stitch or other foreign body, parasite, etc.
ii. Cytohormonal status
iii. Presence of vault intraepithelial lesion (VAIN) has been reported and needs management.
iv. Squamous carcinoma and other malignant lesions of vault can occur and be diagnosed on smear.
v. Stump carcinoma, is still encountered in our country and can be detected.

Iatrogenic Changes

There are many physician induced morphological changes which are seen after curettage, cryosurgery, biopsy, IUCDs, laser ablation, loop electrical excision procedure (LEEP), hormonal therapy, chemotherapy and radiotherapy, even for other sites. In absence of information on the type of treatment, etc., these changes can be interpreted as dysplasia or even malignancy.

HORMONAL CYTOLOGY

It is based on the assumption that the degree of cellular maturity or contextual morphology of cell patterns is quantitatively proportional to the sex steroid levels, i.e. estrogens, progesterone, testosterone, etc. and also reflects the end organ response.

Collection of sample is important. The smear should be obtained from lateral wall of upper one-third of vagina without forceful scraping.

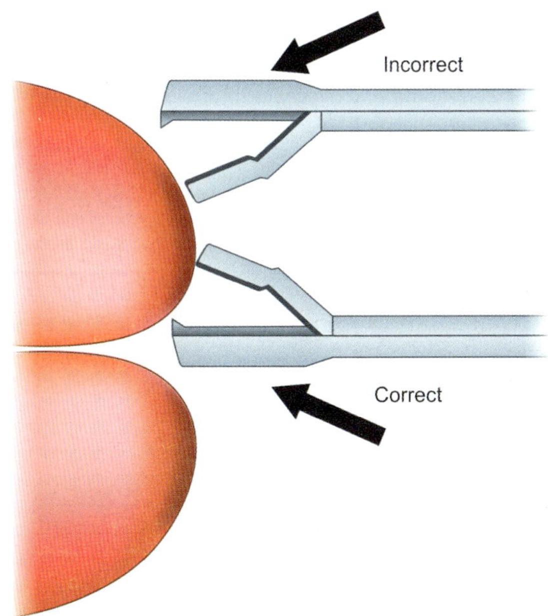

Fig. 1: Taking cervical biopsy including outer margin of lesion

However, it is only conditionally correct because as the hormones may act as synergists or antagonists and depends on end organ response which may vary due to many intrinsic and extrinsic factors.

However, if done in a proper clinical context it provides a cheaper adjunct to clinical and chemical assessments.

The various indices used are:

a. Maturation index and value
b. Navicular cell index
c. Eosinophilic index
d. Folded cell index
e. Crowed cell index

It is important in postmenopausal women, after pan-hysterectomy, cases of amenorrhea, threatened abortions, sexual disorders, etc.

SEX CHROMATIN (BARR BODY)

Nuclear sex dimorphism is a feature easily seen in leukocytes and vesicular nuclei of eukaryotic cells. Oral and vaginal epithelial cells are easy to sample. 1.8% leukocytes show drumstick appearance. In oral and vaginal epithelial cells, the sex chromatin is found.

Barr body is a biconvex chromatin mass of inactivated X chromosome. As only one X chromosome can be active, the number of Barr bodies is number of X chromosomes—1. They are seen in 8–61% nuclei in the females and less than 1% cells in normal males. These are important in diagnosis of genetic sex organ disorders and in management of sex organ abnormalities.

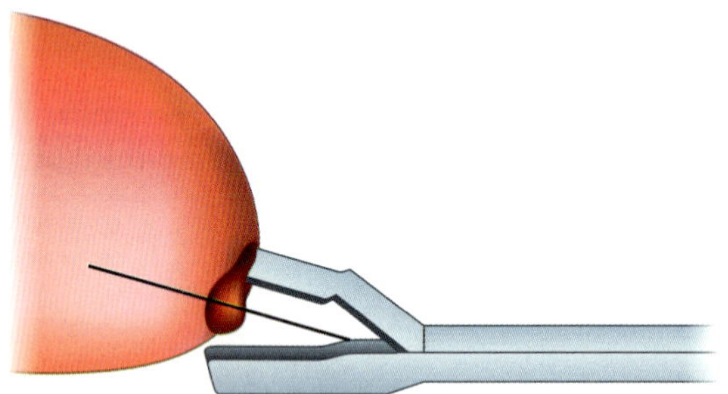

Fig. 2: Incorrect method of cervical biopsy excluding the margin

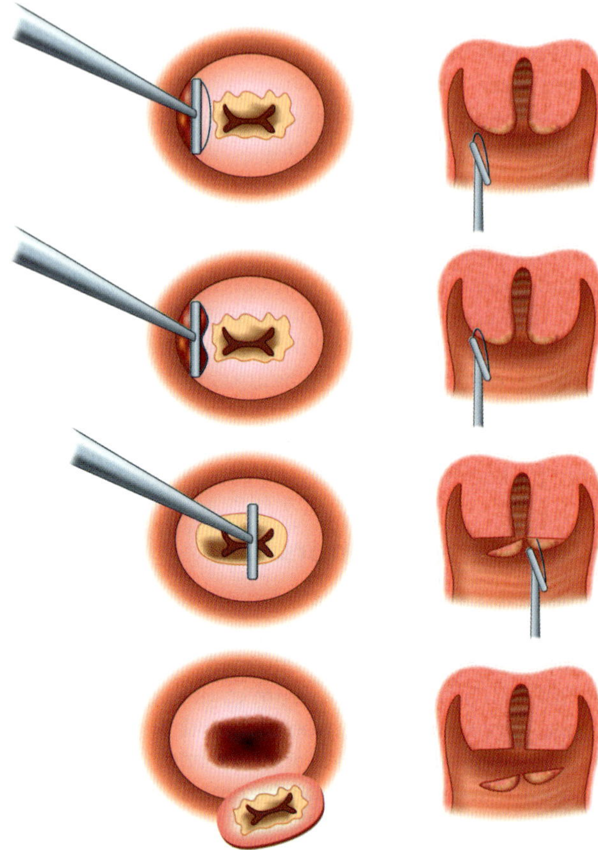

Fig. 3: Taking a loop biopsy of squamocolumnar junction

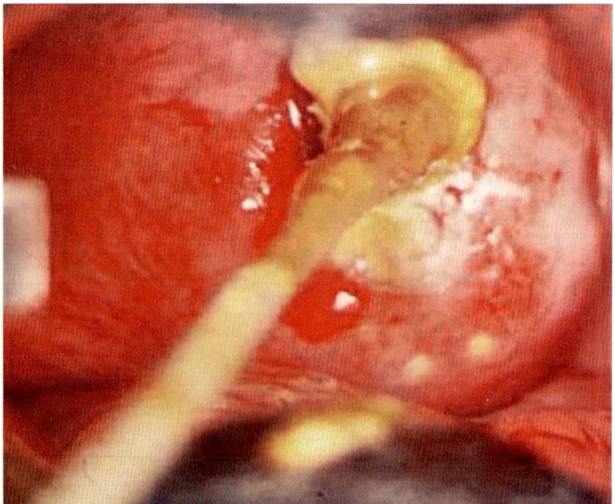

Fig. 4: Taking a surface smear

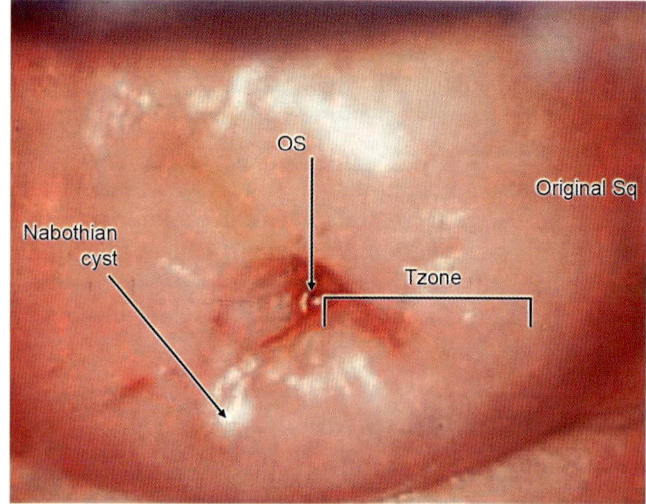

Fig. 5: Normal colposcopic appearance of cervix

The assessment of Barr body provides useful information in diagnosis and deciding course of treatment in congenital/genetic disorders of genital tract, i.e. Turner's syndrome, Klinefelter's syndrome, ambiguous genitalia, etc.

VARIOUS COLPOSCOPIC FINDINGS AND PATTERNS (FIGS 5 TO 14)

Fluid Aspiration Cytology

Peritoneal fluid and fluid from cul-de-sac can provide valuable information on the inflammatory or neoplastic nature and in a large proportion the possible sites of primary mitotic lesion.

The cytology is important in management of ovarian malignancy.

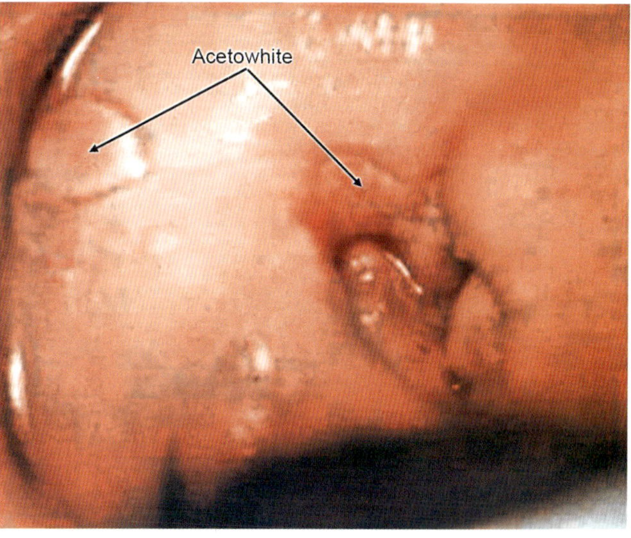

Fig. 6: Acetowhite lesion with small endocervical polyp

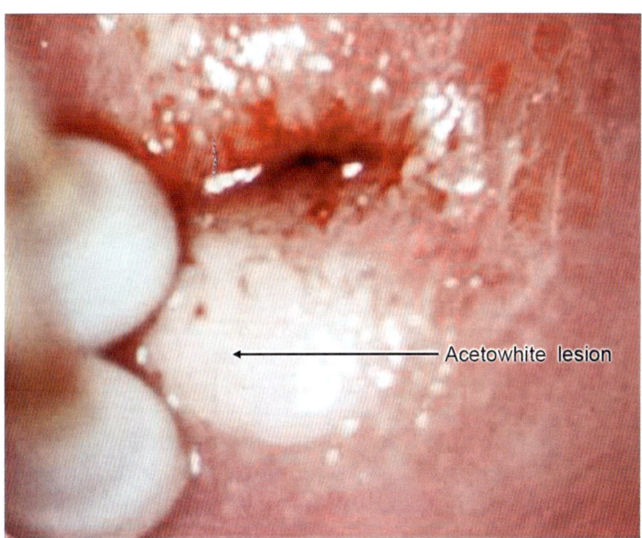

Fig. 7: Acetowhite lesion

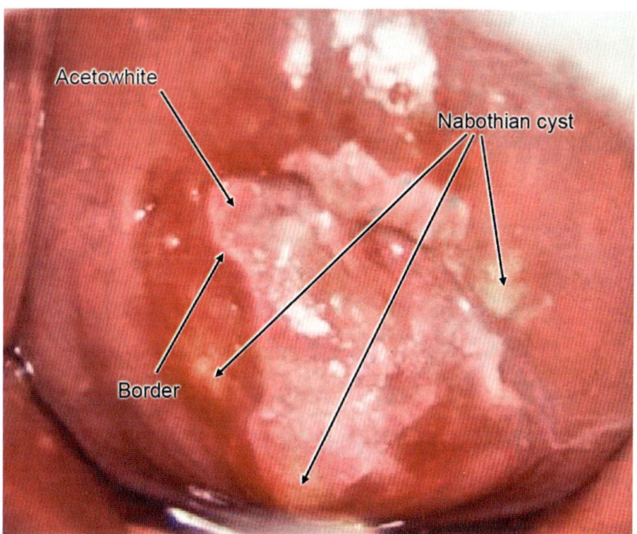

Fig. 8: Nabothian cyst with acetowhite lesion

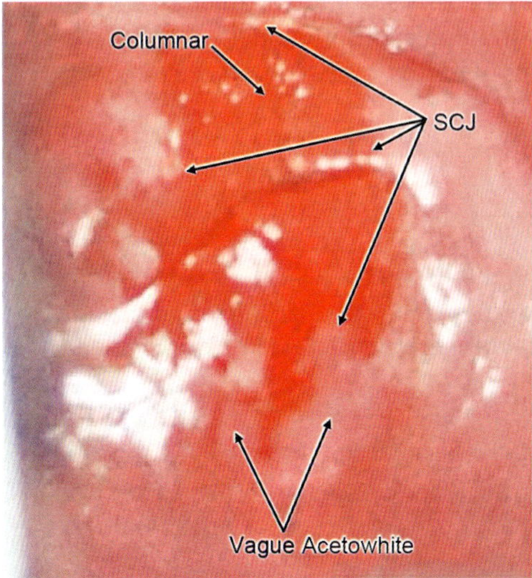

Fig. 9: Squamocolumnar epithelium junction

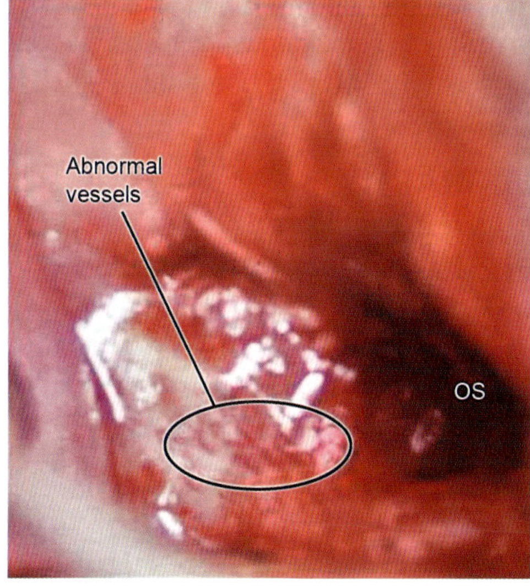

Fig. 10: Abnormal vascular pattern on colposcopy

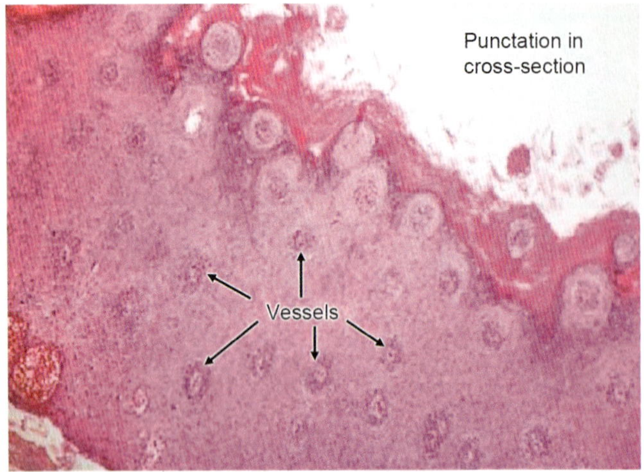

Fig. 11: Abnormal vasculature

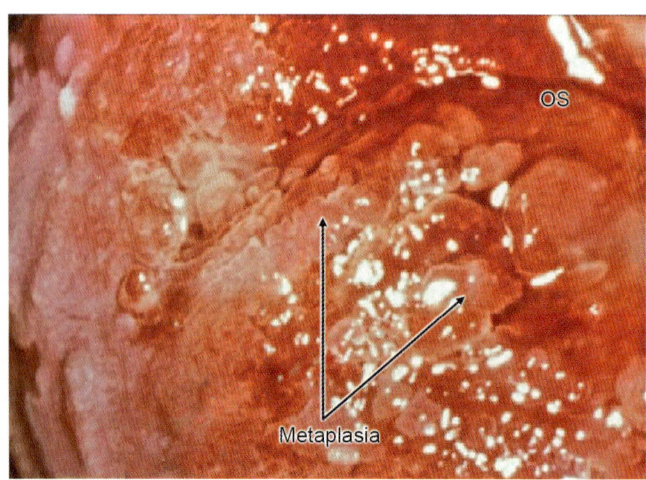

Fig. 12: Colposcopic metaplastic changes

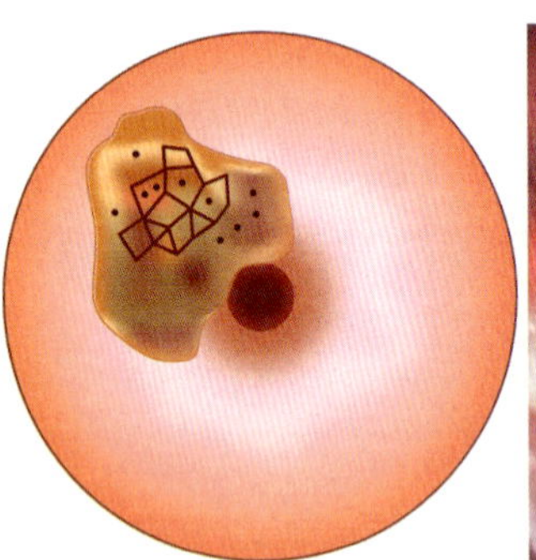

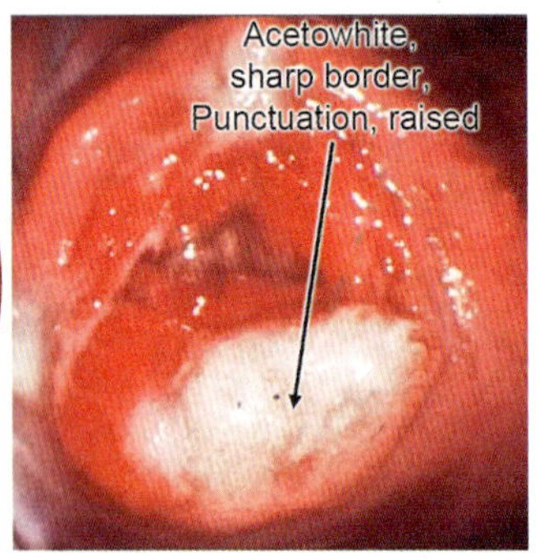

Fig. 13: Raised acetowhite lesion with punctation

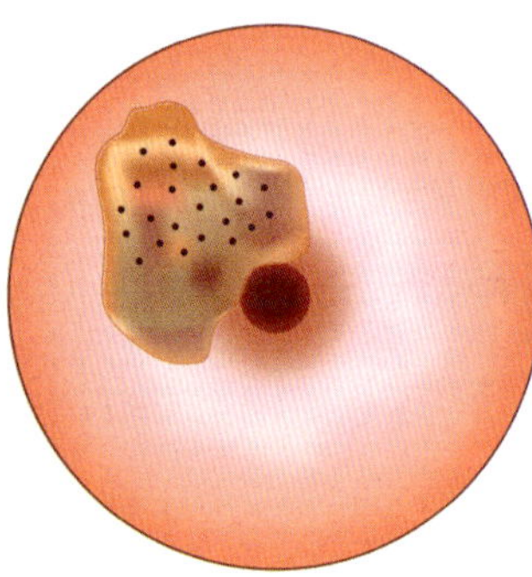

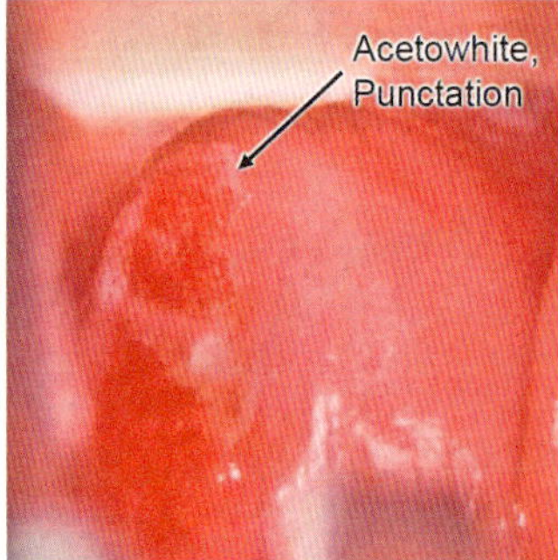

Fig. 14: Punctate lesion

FINE NEEDLE ASPIRATION CYTOLOGY

Ovary

This is a very important addition to the diagnostic facilities for ovarian lumps.

Using ultrasound guided aspiration or direct aspiration in a mass palpable per abdomen, benign cysts like simple cyst, follicular and luteal cysts, endometriosis, dermoid and serous or mucinous cyst adenomas can be diagnosed. In malignant lesions like serous cyst adenocarcinoma and mucinous cyst adenocarcinoma, the aspirates must be obtained from solid areas.

Fine needle aspiration cytology of lesions of vulva, vagina, inguinal, lymph nodes, etc. are very useful in diagnosis of lumps, cysts, tumors, etc.

BIBLIOGRAPHY

1. Adami N, Pontén J, Sparén P, et al. Cytologic screening reduces cancer cervix by early diagnosis. Cancer. 1994;73:140-7.
2. Kingholm SA, Micks DA. Inplications of inflammatory changes in cervical cytology. BMJ. 1990:300:638-40.
3. Lindau ST, McCarville MA, Bannetc L. Bethesda System 2001. JAMA. 2002;287:2120-8.
4. Lindau ST, Timoric, McCanrlle MA, Renet CL. University of Chicago clinical scholars programme, 2005.
5. Papanicolaou GN, Trant HF. The diagnostic value of vaginal smears in carcinoma of uterus. Am J Obst Gynecol. 1941;42:193.
6. Papanicolaou GN. New Cancer diag. In proceedings 3rd Race Betterment Conference. Race Betterment Foundation, 1928;528-30.
7. Saslow D, Runowicz CD, Solomon D, et al. ACS recommendations for detection of cervical cancer. JAMA. 2002;287:2120-9.
8. Wild GL, Bilbo M. Evaluation of endocrinologic condition by exfoliative cytology. In: Gold JJ (ed.) Gynaecology, 2nd edition. Hgerstown Harper and Row; 1975.

CHAPTER

40

Tubes and Ovaries

MB Bellad, Kavita N Singh, Monica S Chauhan, Tamkeen Rabbani, Usha Sharma, Mandakini Parihar, Shilpa Mangal, Atul Munshi, Sujal Munshi, Parimala Devi

40.1 ECTOPIC PREGNANCY—SURGICAL ASPECTS

MB Bellad

INTRODUCTION

Ectopic pregnancy (Fig. 1) is the outcome of an abnormal implantation of the blastocyst outside the normal endometrial cavity of the uterus. Fallopian tube is the commonest site for this (95–98%), the remaining once occur in the cornua of the uterus, oristrimus cervix or abdominal cavity. Since none of these sites can accommodate a growing embryo with placenta, hence, there is always a potential for rupture and hemorrhage.

In spite of advances in all the fields of medicine, ectopic pregnancy is a fertility and life-threatening condition, which continues to be responsible for maternal morbidity and mortality both in developing and developed world, and more so in the developing world due to delay in diagnosis, delay in transfer and delay in necessary intervention. Ten to fifteen percent of all maternal deaths are due to ectopic pregnancy.

The incidence of ectopic pregnancy has greatly increased in the last 3–4 decades, i.e. 4.5/1000 pregnancies in 1970 to an estimated 19.7 per 1000 in 1992. The rise in the incidence is partly due to increase in risk factors but mainly due to improved diagnostic facilities. However, in spite of rise in incidence the case fatality has declined from 3.55 maternal deaths/1000 ectopic pregnancies in 1970 to 0.38/1000 ectopic pregnancies in 1989.

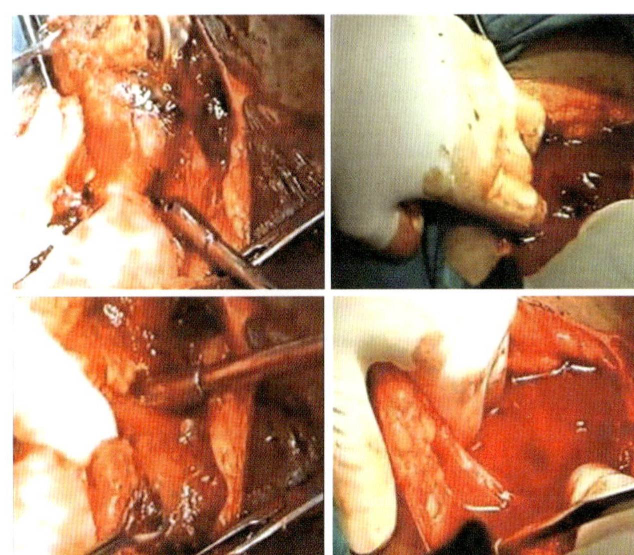

Fig. 1: Ectopic pregnancy at laparotomy

CLINICAL PRESENTATION

Usually menstrual aberration precedes the symptoms of ectopic pregnancy this may be the amenorrhea in majority but it may vary from premenstrual spotting to irregular bleeding or intermenstrual bleeding. The actual period of amenorrhea depends upon site of implantation within the tube. It is shorter for isthmic, up to 12 weeks for ampulla and still more in cases with interstitial and rudimentary born ectopic pregnancies (up to 16 weeks or more).

SITES OF ECTOPIC PREGNANCIES (FIG. 2)

Risk Factors

Strong evidence for association with followings:

- Pelvic inflammatory disease (PID)

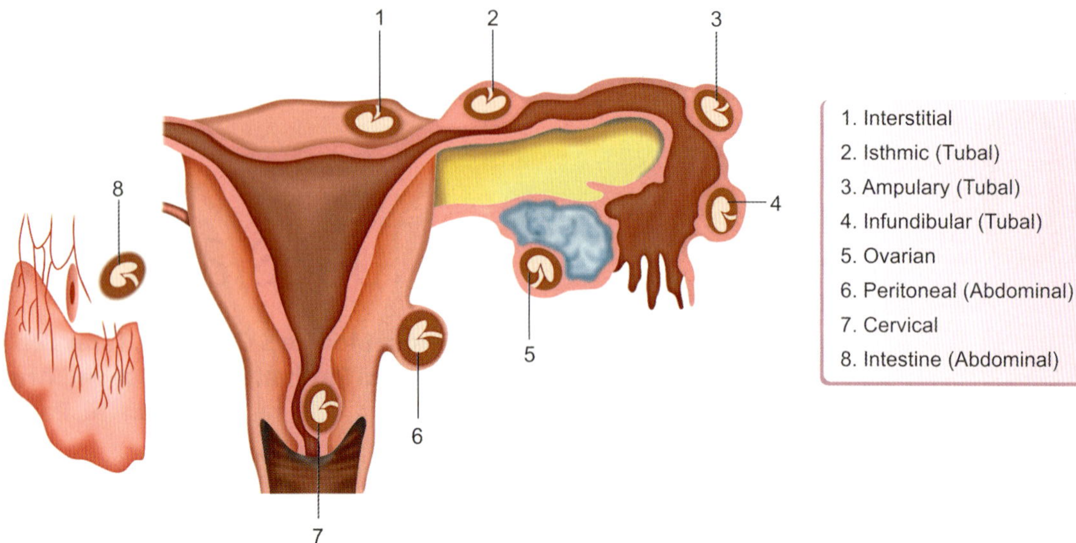

Fig. 2: Sites of ectopic pregnancies

- Previous ectopic pregnancy
- Endometriosis
- Previous tubal surgery
- Previous pelvic surgery
- Infertility and infertility treatments
- Utero-tubal anomalies
- In utero exposure to diethylstilbestrol
- Cigarette smoking.

Weaker evidence for association:
- Multiple sexual partners
- Early age at first intercourse
- Vaginal douching.

Any factor which interferes with normal fallopian tubal function increases the risk of ectopic pregnancy. Normally, an egg that is fertilized in the fallopian tube travels down the tube to the uterine cavity. This may be anatomical (scarring, partial block) or functional (impaired motility).

Pelvic inflammatory disease (PID) is the most common and important risk factor for ectopic pregnancy. *Neisseria gonorrhoeae, Chlamydia trachomatis* and mixed aerobes and anaerobes are the common organisms that afflict the fallopian tube. The important feature of *N. gonorrhoeae* and *C. trachomatis* is that they can produce silent infections unlike mixed aerobes and anaerobes. Even early treatment may not prevent the tubal damage in such infections. Intrauterine devices (IUDs) per se do not increase the risk for ectopic pregnancy [as there is no evidence to suggest currently available that IUDs) cause PID]. The explanation for the mistaken association with ectopic with IUDs may be that in presence of an IUD, ectopic pregnancy occurs more often than intrauterine pregnancy, as IUDs are effective in prevention of intrauterine pregnancies.

Previous ectopic pregnancy is a significant risk factor with each consecutive occurrence. The recurrence rate ranges from 15–20% with one previous ectopic to 32% with two previous ectopic pregnancies. However, an intervening intrauterine pregnancy reduces the recurrence rate.

Tubal and pelvic adhesions result from endometriosis, tubal and pelvic surgery. These adhesions lead to abnormal tubal function and thus increase the risk for ectopic. The drugs/hormones administered to improve fertility and ovulation affect the tubal function (the mechanism is not clearly understood).

Uterotubal anomalies with or without diethylstilbestrol (DES) exposure increase the risk for the occurrence of an ectopic pregnancy.

The ciliary function of respiratory tract is affected by smoking, the similar mechanism in cilia of fallopian tubes may be responsible for increase in the risk of ectopic pregnancy with smoking. Early age, at first intercourse, multiple sexual partners and vaginal douching increase the risk of ectopic pregnancy indirectly by increasing the occurrence of sexually transmitted infections, leading to ascending infection, thus damaging the normal tubal function.

DIAGNOSIS

High index of suspicion is the essential factor for the diagnosis of ectopic pregnancy. Proper history and physical examination remain the foundation for accurate and timely diagnosis of ectopic pregnancy. Careful attention to risk factors with subtle symptoms helps in the diagnosis. Scoring systems to facilitate earlier diagnosis of ectopic pregnancy have been proposed.

The early diagnosis (unruptured) of ectopic pregnancy is possible due to the advancement in technologies. This has, to a large extent, reduced the occurrence of life-threatening surgical emergency. The classical triad of presentation of pain and uterine bleeding with an adnexal mass has been the clinical hallmark of ectopic pregnancy. This still remains the commonest mode of presentation of symptomatic ectopic pregnancy. Vaginal bleeding, syncope, radiating pain to shoulder are other symptoms noted less commonly in ectopic pregnancy. The hypovolemic shock is usually seen with ruptured ectopic pregnancy presenting as acute abdomen.

Physical findings include slightly enlarged/normal uterus with tender cervical movements and palpable adnexal mass. Hypotension, tender abdomen with guarding and rebound tenderness suggests ruptured/leaking ectopic pregnancy. Rarely viable abdominal ectopic pregnancies have been discovered.

Tests to Help Diagnosis

Urine pregnancy test—qualitative assessment of human chorionic gonadotropin (hCG): The standard test has a sensitivity and specificity of 99% for pregnancy with ability to detect the beta-hCG level of 25 mIU/mL.

Some clinicians continue to use serum progesterone determinations. The viable intrauterine pregnancies are observed with a sensitivities of 91% and 97.5% at 11 ng/mL (35 nmol/L) and 25 ng/mL (80 nmol/L) respectively. It is difficult to differentiate an ectopic from failing intrauterine pregnancy when serum progesterone levels are less than 11 ng/mL. Additionally, ectopic pregnancies are known to occur even when serum progesterone levels are more than 25 ng/mL.

Serum quantitative beta-hCG with ultrasonography (USG) are more commonly used to diagnose ectopic pregnancy.

Creatine kinase and fibrogen levels, though investigated, but are not accepted due to inadequate diagnostic sensitivity.

Ultrasonography

A gestational sac must be visualized when the serum beta-hCG level of greater than 6500 mIU/mL with transabdominal sonography (TAS) whereas 1500 mIU with transvaginal sonography (TVS) (Figs 3A and B). This is called as discriminatory zone. An ectopic pregnancy should be suspected when ultrasound examination cannot visualize the gestational sac with the above discriminatory levels of beta-hCG.

The sensitivity and specificity to detect ectopic pregnancy by TVS ranges from 69–99% and 84–99.6% respectively.[19-21]

Unclear (uncertainty) at the first (initial) evaluation: If the initial evaluation is not conclusive of the diagnosis and the woman has signs and symptoms suggestive of ectopic pregnancy a laparoscopy will assist in both diagnosis and management. If the woman is hemodynamically unstable laparotomy is the other option.

If the woman is asymptomatic and hemodynamically stable, serial evaluation with serum beta-hCG will assist in the diagnosis. Lack of 48 hour beta-hCG doubling will assist in the diagnosis, but does not identify the location of abnormal pregnancy. Absence of chorionic villi on uterine curettage (nonviable intrauterine pregnancy is suspected) and or failure of decline in beta-hCG at least by 15% is suggestive of ectopic pregnancy.

Other Modalities

Culdocentesis is rarely done these days and is used where USG is not readily available. As ultrasound usually reveal the presence of free fluid in the peritoneal cavity. The presence of nonclotting bloody fluid strongly suggests ruptured/bleeding ectopic pregnancy. Immediate surgery (laparotomy/laparoscopy) is essential.

MANAGEMENT

The primary objective of accurate and early diagnosis of ectopic pregnancy is to reduce morbidity and eliminate mortality resulting from this condition. With the early diagnosis in a clinically stable state, ectopic pregnancy can be managed either by medical therapy or by laparoscopy with the potential benefit of conservation of fallopian tube. However, laparotomy is still the main stay of therapy in a patient who is hemodynamically unstable with suspected tubal rupture.

With advent of newer diagnostic and hormone evaluation facilities, following options are available for the management of ectopic pregnancy:

1. Expectant management
2. Medical management
3. Surgical management.

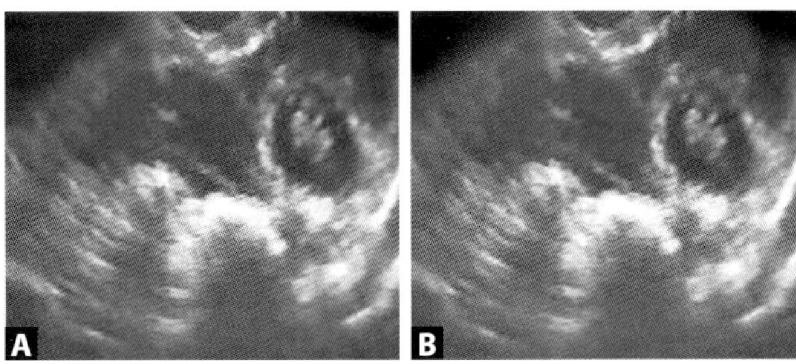

Figs 3A and B: Transvaginal ultrasonographic pictures of ectopic pregnancy

However, any of the options may be useful when the criteria for its use are strictly adhered to. Expectant and medical management warrant close monitoring. Moreover, re-evaluation of the woman (after the diagnosis of ectopic pregnancy) is essential before the management.

Expectant management may be attempted in a woman with ectopic pregnancy with a smaller mass size (less than 3.5 cm in greatest dimension) whose beta-hCG levels are either low, declining. It is also noted in studies that almost up to 75% (68–77%) of ectopic pregnancies resolve spontaneously without any intervention. Till date there are neither scoring systems nor the predictable factors are available to accurately identify which subset of ectopic pregnancies resolve or rupture. However, close monitoring of the women for any signs and symptoms of deterioration of the condition is essential. This is done usually with daily monitoring of beta-hCG and ultrasound.

Medical management is one of the options for the management of ectopic pregnancy. This is possible mainly due to early diagnosis of ectopic pregnancy. Avoidance of surgery, its associated complications, conservation of tubal function and low cost are the potential advantages with the medical management.

Direct injections of agents like hyperosmolar glucose, urea and prostaglandins have been investigated. Administrations of methotrexate (MTX) and mifeprostone have been used. The most studied of these agents is MTX, a folic acid antagonist acts by inactivating the enzyme dihydrofolate reductase (DHFR), leading to depletion of cofactors required for deoxyribonucleic acid (DNA) and ribonucleic acid (RNA) synthesis (folinic acid is used as a rescue medication to prevent some of the otherwise adverse effects of methotrexate).

Methotrexate can be administered orally, intramuscularly (IM), intrathecally and by continuous infusion. However, for the treatment of ectopic, it is usually administered by intramuscular route though oral administration is also successful. The two regimes commonly used are the single dose and the multidose with folinic acid. A single dose, i.e. 50 mg/m^2 body surface area is administered by intramuscular injection after calculation of woman's body surface area. Folinic acid is not given with this regimen. Although, it is called single dose, a repeat dose may be administered after 7 days if the beta-hCG levels do not adequately decline (at least 15% between fourth day to seventh day after the treatment). 20% of the women require more than one treatment cycle. However, it is difficult to predict which woman with ectopic pregnancy may need more than single MTX dose. The multidose intramuscular regimen, i.e. 1 mg/kg/day on days 1, 3, 5 and 7 of a week with folinic acid administered on 2, 4, 6 and 8 day of a week. A second course may be given after 1 week if there is plateau or increase in atleast two consecutive beta-hCG values. Women after the MTX therapy (irrespective of regimen used) must be followed with beta-hCG until it is undetectable in the serum; the only way to ensure complete resolution of ectopic pregnancy. Careful attention is a must in ectopic pregnancies which had rise of more than 66% in 48 hours before the treatment, as these ectopic pregnancies may cause tubal rupture even when the MTX regimen is on and beta-hCG levels are declining. The risk of tubal rupture may be as high as 20% in ectopic pregnancies with increasing beta-hCG even after MTX administration.

SURGICAL MANAGEMENT

Operative laparoscopy has changed the scenario of the surgical field and especially in the management of ectopic in particular. Earlier laparotomy and salpingectomy was the gold standard treatment option for ectopic pregnancy. It is still an option where the woman is hemodynamically unstable or facilities to perform laparoscopy are not available. The main principle of laparotomy is "quick in and quick out". Adequate replacement of blood volume is essential to avert the woman's death due to hypovolumic shock. This is one of few surgical conditions where dictum of concurrent resuscitation with fluids and blood is undertaken as patient is being prepared for laparotomy.

Laparoscopy

The advantages of laparoscopy need not be over emphasized as it clearly outscores the laparotomy in a woman with ectopic pregnancy who is hemodynamically stable.

Laparoscopically following procedures are done for ectopic pregnancy:

1. Salpingectomy and partial salpingectomy (Segmental excision)
2. Salpingostomy
3. Salpingotomy.

Salpingectomy: This is preferred in patients with uncontrolled bleeding, recurrent ectopic and with extensive tubal damage. This is also the procedure of choice in a woman who wants sterilization.

Partial Salpingectomy (Segmental resection): This is the conservative procedure for isthmic ectopic pregnancy. Here, the segment with ectopic is removed and end-to-end anastomosis is performed at a later date.

Salpingostomy

This is the most preferred conservative surgery, especially for ampullary ectopic. The disadvantages associated with this procedure are the increased recurrence risk and persistence of trophoblastic activity. A single dose of postoperative MTX may be an additional useful option in high-risk cases.

Salpingotomy

This is less preferred over salpingostomy and the disadvantages associated with this procedure are same as that of salpingostomy.

Almost all conservative surgeries warrant the beta hCG follow-up till it reaches the nonpregnant level.

Role of Anti-D Prophylaxis

Women who Rh negative and not sensitized with confirmed/suspected ectopic pregnancy should receive anti-D prophylaxis with 50 μg dosage.

Special Conditions

Broad Ligament Ectopic Pregnancy

Rupture and hematoma into broad ligament or intraligament of a tubal ectopic gives rise to tumor like situation with or without shock. Uterus is usually displaced to one of the sides and if the bleeding is extensive it leads to shock. Rarely, late pregnancies have been documented. If it continues to be viable, it may grow as secondary broad ligament or retroperitoneal ectopic pregnancy.

Chronic Ectopic Pregnancy

A steady and large bloody leak from tubal ectopic may present like a big pelvic tumor occupying the whole of the pelvis. This gives rise to what is known as chronic ectopic pregnancy. This is usually confused with other conditions like fibroid and ovarian tumors due to the solidification of clot. At times this may cause bowel obstruction, if intestines are adherent, otherwise it may cause retention of urine. This is usually diagnosed at laparoscopy/laparotomy.

Interstitial Intrauterine Pregnancy (Fig. 4)

The ectopic pregnancy occurs at the interstitial portion of tube in normal uterus. Since uterotubal myometrium provides a stouter and more resistant capsule to trophoblast, the rupture is usually delayed up to sometimes 16 weeks. This is highly vascular area, hence bleeding following the rupture can be dangerous.

Rudimentary Horn (Cornual Extrauterine Pregnancy) Ectopic Pregnancy

When one-half of the uterus is imperfectly developed, it is called rudimentary horn of the uterus. When the implantation occurs in this rudimentary horn of the uterus is called rudimentary horn ectopic pregnancy. The pregnancy in this type of ectopic may reach up to 16 weeks or more, the duration depends upon the development of rudimentary horn myometrium. If well developed, the duration before rupture may be more than 16 weeks. Careful TVS is essential to look for other pelvic masses in early pregnancies, other wise at times it is diagnosed as normal intrauterine pregnancy. The bleeding following rupture may be dangerous.

Ovarian Pregnancy

Primary ovarian pregnancy is the rarest of all extra uterine pregnancies. To diagnose primary ovarian pregnancy, following features must be fulfilled:

1. The tube on the side of the ovarian pregnancy must be normal anatomically and histologically (if removed).
2. Tube must be free and separate from the gestational sac.
3. The wall of the gestational sac must contain histologically demonstrable ovarian tissues.
4. The gestational sac attachment to the uterus must be with ovarian ligament.

Most of the ovarian ectopic pregnancies rupture early with profuse bleeding.

Abdominal Pregnancy

Secondary: Partially extruded ruptured tubal ectopic with sufficient attachment continue to remain alive and the extruded trophoblast invades sometimes into any of adjacent intra-abdominal viscera, including parietal peritoneum, and forms a secondary placenta thus leading to formation of secondary abdominal ectopic pregnancy.

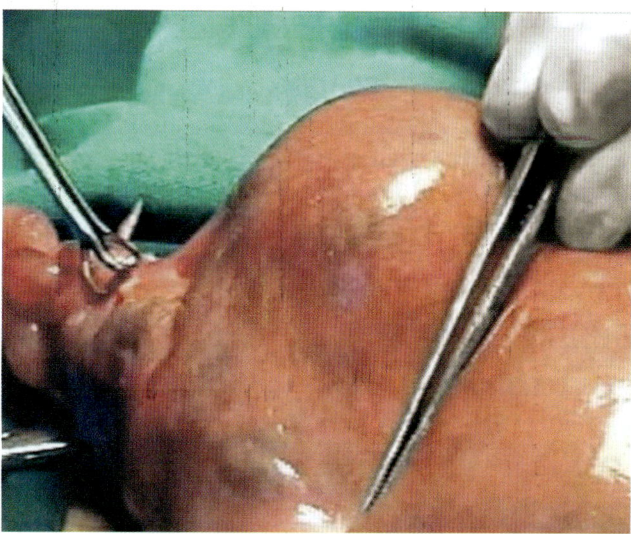

Fig. 4: Interstitial intrauterine pregnancy

This type of placenta may involve any intraperitoneal organ or peritoneum. There is no plane of cleavage between placenta and the structure to which it is attached. Heavy hemorrhage is associated with attempts to separate during the operation, at times it may not be possible to separate.

Primary: When the ectopic pregnancy is noted anywhere in the peritoneal cavity (on viscera or structures including peritoneum) fulfilling the following criteria is called primary abdominal pregnancy:

- Both tubes and ovaries are normal and without any evidence of recent or remote injury
- Without any uteroperitoneal fistula
- Exclusively, pregnancy on the peritoneum without any evident implantation in tube.

The most common primary abdominal pregnancies noted are on the posterior wall of the uterus and broad ligaments.

Bilateral Ectopic Pregnancy

This is extremely rare but has been described. This also is the other reason to look and examine the other side tube in case of ectopic pregnancy. At times associated with hematosalpinx is confused with this condition.

Heterotropic Pregnancy (Combined Intra- and Extrauterine Pregnancies)

It is a type of twin pregnancy with one developing within the uterus and other one ectopically. Diagnosis is usually by ultrasound or following surgery. This is more commonly seen with assisted reproductive technique. The treatment is laparoscopy in early pregnancy and laparotomy for late pregnancy with salpingectomy living the intrauterine pregnancy undisturbed.

Cervical Ectopic Pregnancy

This is one of the rare ectopics [incidence 1 in 1000 (Japan) to 1 in 16000 (Mayo clinic)]. Rubins following criteria must be fulfilled:

1. Cervical glands must be opposite the placental attachment
2. Placental attachment of the uterine vessels or below the peritoneal reflection of the anterior and posterior surfaces of the uterus
3. Fetal elements must be absent from the corpus uteri.

Paalman and McElin proposed five more practical criteria for the diagnosis of cervical ectopics:

1. Uterine bleeding without cramping pain following a period of amenorrhea
2. A soft, enlarged cervix equal to, or larger than the fundus (the " hourglass" uterus)
3. Products of conception entirely confined within and firmly attached to the endocervix
4. A closed internal cervical os
5. A partially opened external os.

This condition is usually confused with neoplasm of the cervix (because of marked vascularity and friability and inevitable/incomplete spontaneous abortion. Treatment is usually surgical, often requires hysterectomy. Other conservative approaches are use of Foley catheter with 30 mL balloon, use of MTX and misoprostol.

CONCLUSION

Ectopic pregnancy is one of the common and serious problem with significant morbidity rate and a potential for maternal death. Though the incidence of ectopic pregnancy is on the rise, the mortality, due to it, is declining.

Many a times the risk factors and classical clinical features (symptoms and signs) of ectopic may not be present. USG and beta-hCG measurement (single or serial) play an important role not only in diagnosis but also in the management.

Strict adherence to criteria for particular mode of management ensures increased success rate.

Surgical treatment is particularly an important option for women who are hemodynamically not stable or not likely to comply with post-treatment monitoring or who do not have facilities for immediate medical care. However, in others, the choice of treatment should be guided by proper counseling after a detailed discussion about monitoring, outcome, risks, benefits and the cost.

BIBLIOGRAPHY

1. ACOG practice bulletin no. 3. Medical management of tubal pregnancy. Clinical management guidelines for obstetrician-gynecologists. Washington DC: American College of Obstetricians and Gynecologists; 1998.
2. Ankum WM, Van der Veen F, Hamerlynck JV, et al. Suspected ectopic pregnancy. What to do when human chorionic gonadotropin levels are below the discriminatory zone. J Reprod Med. 1995;40:525-8.
3. Braffman BH, Coleman BG, Ramchandani P, et al. Emergency department screening for ectopic pregnancy: a prospective US study. Radiology. 1994;190:797-802.
4. Cates W, Rolfs RT, Aral SO. Sexually transmitted diseases, pelvic inflammatory disease, and infertility: An epidemiologic update. Epidemiol Rev. 1990;12:199-220.
5. Centers for Disease Control and Prevention. Ectopic pregnancy-United States, 1990-1992. MMWR Morb Mortal Wkly Rep. 1995;44:46-8.

6. Clausen I. Conservative versus radical surgery for tubal pregnancy: a review. Acta Obstet Gynecol Scand. 1996;75:8-12.
7. Darai E, Vlastos G, Benifla JL, et al. Is maternal serum creatinine kinase actually a marker for early diagnosis of ectopic pregnancy? Eur J Obstet Gynecol Reprod Biol. 1996;68:25-7.
8. Dorfman SF. Ectopic pregnancy surveillance. MMWR Morb Mortal Wkly Rep. 1983;32(SS01):19-21.
9. Dudley PS, Heard MJ, Sangi-Haghpeykar H, Carson SA, Buster JE. Characterizing ectopic pregnancies that rupture despite treatment with methotrexate. 2004;82:1374-8.
10. Falcone T, Mascha EJ, Goldberg JM, et al. A study of risk factors for ruptured tubal ectopic pregnancy. J Womens Health. 1998;7:459-63.
11. Franks AL, Beral V, Cates W, Hogue CJ. Contraception and ectopic pregnancy risk. Am J Obstet Gynecol. 1990;163(4 pt 1):1120-3.
12. Goldner TE, Lawson HW, Xia Z, et al. Surveillance for ectopic pregnancy-United States, 1970-1989. MMWR CDC Surveill Summ. 1993;42:73-85.
13. Hankins GD, Clark SL, Cunningham FG, et al. Ectopic pregnancy. In: Operative obstetrics. Norwalk: Appleton & Lange. 1995. pp. 437-56.
14. Hankins GV, Clark SL, Cunningham FG, et al. Abdominal pregnancy. In: Operative obstetrics. Norwalk: Appleton & Lange; 1995. pp. 425-36.
15. Kaplan BC, Dart RG, Moskos M, et al. Ectopic pregnancy: prospective study with improved diagnostic accuracy. Ann Emerg Med. 1996;28:10-7.
16. Lipscomb GH, Bran D, McCord ML, et al. Analysis of three hundred fifteen ectopic pregnancies treated with single-dose methotrexate. Am J Obstet. Gynecol. 1998;178:1354-8.
17. Lipscomb GH, Meyer NL, Flynn DE, et al. Oral methotrexate for treatment of ectopic pregnancy. Am J Obstet Gynecol. 2002;186: 1192-5.
18. Lundorff P, Thorburn J, Lindblom B. Diagnosis and treatment of tubal pregnancy as related to risk determinants. Eur J Obstet Gynecol Reprod Biol. 1991;40:191-6.
19. McCord ML, Muram D, Buster JE, et al. Single serum progesterone as a screen for ectopic pregnancy: Exchanging specificity and sensitivity to obtain optimal test performance. Fertil Steril. 1996;66:513-6.
20. Montgomery Irvine L, Padwick ML, Serial serum hCG measurements in a patient with an ectopic pregnancy: a case for caution. Hum Reprod. 2000;15:1646-7.
21. Nederlof KP, Lawson HW, Saftlas AF, et al. Ectopic pregnancy surveillance, United States, 1970-1987. MMWR CDC Surveill Summ. 1990; 39(4):9-17.
22. Phillips RS, Tuomala RE, Feldblum PJ,. The effect of cigarette smoking, Chlamydia trachomatis infection, and vaginal douching on ectopic pregnancy. Obstet Gynecol. 1992;79:85-90.
23. Pisarska MD, Carson SA, Buster JE. Ectopic pregnancy. Lancet. 1998;351:1115-20.
24. Sadek AL, Schiotz HA. Transvaginal sonography in the management of ectopic pregnancy. Acta Obstet Gynecol Scand. 1995;74:293-6.
25. Saraiya M, Berg CJ, Kendrick JS, et al. Cigarette smoking as a risk factor for ectopic pregnancy. Am J Obstet Gynecol. 1998;178:493-8.
26. Stovall TG,Ling FW. Buster JE. Outpatient chemotherapy of unruptured ectopic pregnancy. Fertil Steril. 1989;51:435-8.
27. Tulandi T, Hemmings R, Khalifa F. Rupture of ectopic pregnancy in women with los and declining serum beta human chorionic gonadotropin concentrations. Fertil Steril. 1991;56:786-7.
28. Valley VT, Mateer JR, Aiman EJ, et al. Serum progesterone and endovaginal sonography by emergency physicians in the evaluation of ectopic pregnancy. Acad Emerg Med. 1998;5:309-13.
29. Vitoratos N, Gregoriou O, Papadias C, et al. Clinical value of creatinine kinase in the diagnosis of ectopic pregnancy. Gynecol Obstet Invest. 1998;46:80.

40.2 SALPINGECTOMY/SALPINGOSTOMY

Kavita N Singh, Monica S Chauhan

INTRODUCTION AND SURGICAL ANATOMY

The fallopian tubes, also known as oviducts, uterine tubes and salpinges are very fine tubes leading from the ovaries of female mammals into the uterus (Fig. 1). There are two fallopian tubes, attached to either side of the cornual end of the uterus, and each terminating near ovary forming a structure called the fimbria.

In humans the fallopian tubes are about 7–14 cm long. There are four regions of the fallopian tube from the ovary to the uterus, infundibulum contains fimbria and is 1.25 cm long, Ampulla is the usual site of fertilization is about 5 cm, isthumus is about 2.5 cm and intramural oviduct which is inside the wall of uterus is 1.25 cm long. The fallopian tube is supplied by ovarian and uterine artery and venous drainage is through the pampiniform plexus into ovarian veins. Lymphatic drainage is into lumbar lymph nodes.

SALPINGECTOMY

Definition

Salpingectomy is the removal of one or both of a woman's fallopian tubes. The procedure was first described by Lawson Tait in patients with bleeding tubal pregnancy.

Indications

Salpingectomy can be unilateral/bilateral, partial/total.

- Unilateral salpingectomy-removal of one tube usually perfomed, if the tube has become grossly infected (chronic salpingitis) and to treat an ectopic pregnancy.

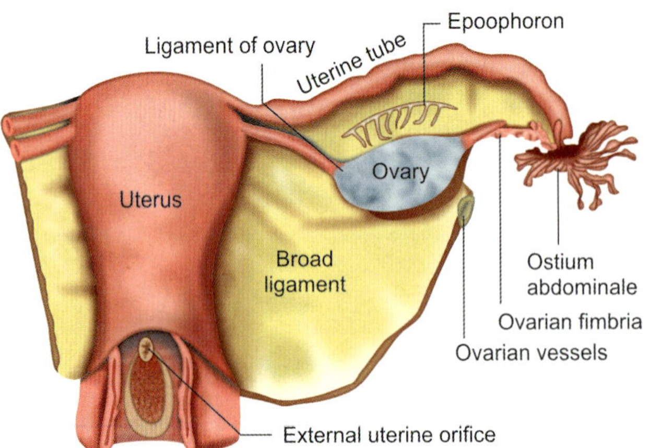

Fig. 1: Uterus. Right broad ligament, seen from behind

- *Bilateral salpingectomy*—removal of both the tubes is usually done if the ovaries and the uterus are also going to be removed. If the fallopian tubes and the ovaries are both removed at the same time, this is called a salpingo-oophorectomy.
- *Partial salpingectomy*—the conservative procedure of choice for isthmic and interstitial pregnancies. The procedure removes the tubal segment containing ectopic pregnancy.
- *Total salpingectomy*—whole of the fallopian tube is removed. Procedure is the treatment of choice when the preservation of fertility is not an issue, when the tube has been markedly destroyed by rupture or in the presence of large hydrosalpinx.

Diagnosis

Diagnosing ectopic pregnancy is mainly based on presentation of symptom, a positive pregnancy test and detection of a pregnancy outside of the uterus by means of USG (Figs 2A and B) and/or laparoscopy (Fig. 3).

Diagnosis of hydrosalpinx or other defects of the fallopian tubes by hysterosalpingogram or using a laparoscope (Fig. 4).

Anesthesia

Regional or general anesthesia (GA) may be used. The procedure has been traditionally done via opening the abdomen (laparotomy), more recently, however, laparoscopically which has become more common as a part of minimal invasive surgery.

Procedure (Laparotomy)

A suprapubic Pfannenstiel/vertical incision is used, and the distended tube is elevated. The mesosalpinx is clamped with a succession of Kelly clamps as close to the tube as possible to preserve ovarian vasculature.

Transfix and tie the divided mesosalpinx with 2-0 chromic catgut suture before releasing clamps (Figs 5A to C).

Laparoscopic Salpingectomy

In this procedure, the surgeon makes a small incision just beneath the navel and two accessory ports are made. The tubal segment to be removed is coagulated (Figs 6A and B) and cut off with bipolar forceps. The mesovarium is also coagulated and cut off as close to tube. The tube was subsequently removed with polyp forceps through one of the suprapubic punctures.

Complications

Immediate complication:

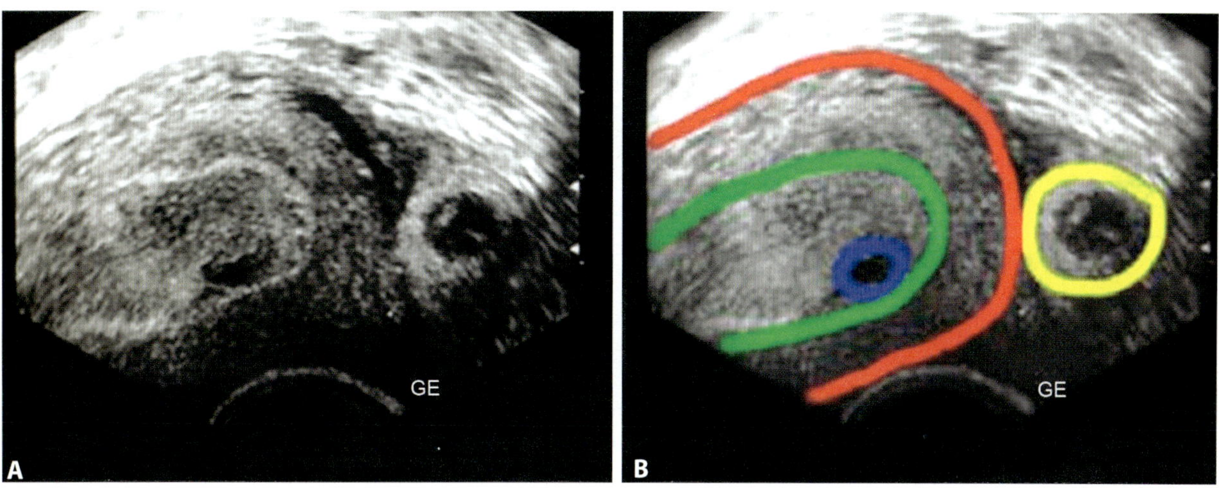

Figs 2A and B: (A) Ultrasonography showing uterus and tubal pregnancy; (B) Same image—uterus outline in red, uterine lining green, ectopic pregnancy yellow. Fluid in uterus at blue circle called a "pseudosac"

***Source*:** Ultrasonography images from causes and treatment of ectopic pregnancy and tubal infertility issues. http://www.advanced fertility.com/ectopic.htm.

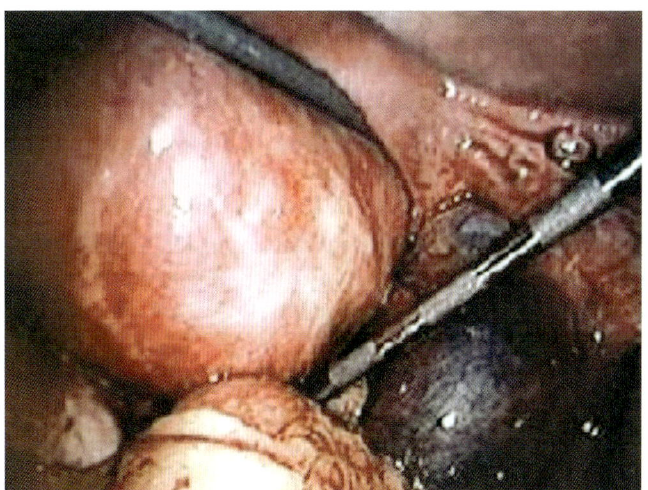

Fig. 3: Laparoscopic view of unruptured ectopic pregnancy

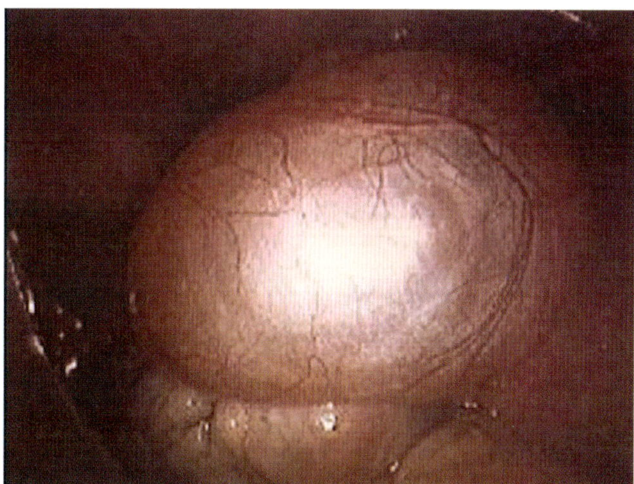

Fig. 4: Hydrosalpinx view during laparoscopy, ovary is seen behind the dilated tube

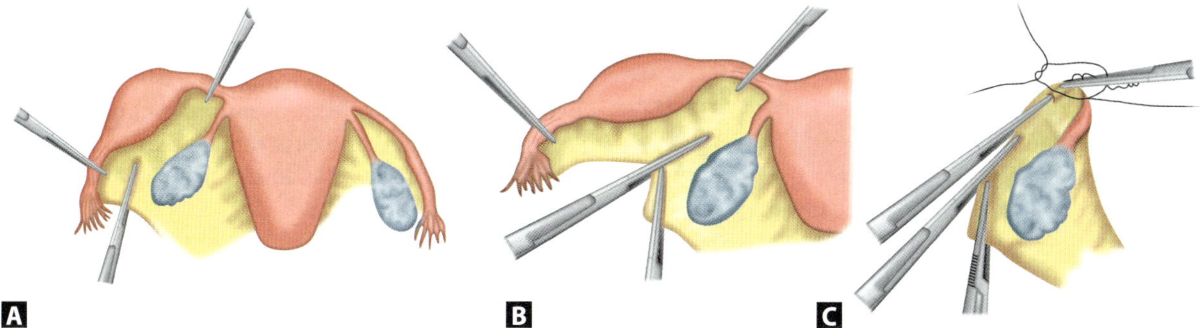

Figs 5A to C: Salpingectomy for ectopic pregnancy

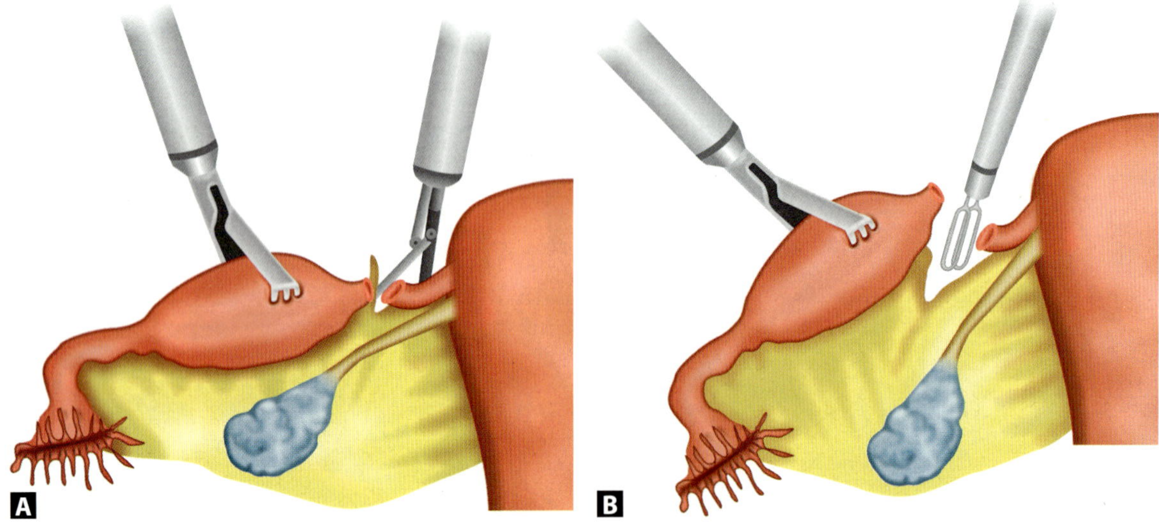

Figs 6A and B: (A) Cutting of the proximal segment after coagulation; (B) Coagulation repeated on the mesovarian

- Hemorrhage, due to slippage of ligature
- Bowel/bladder injury
- Anesthetic complications.

Late complication:

- Infection
- Pelvic adhesion
- Chronic pelvic pain.

A modified surgical technique—one trocar salpingectomy for the treatment of tubal pregnancy: A "marionette-like" technique has been reported by Fabio Ghezzi, et al. Laparoscopic salpingectomy for the treatment of tubal pregnancy has traditionally been performed with two ancillary trocars. A single-port technique requiring only an umbilical operative laparoscope and a percutaneous midline suture, inserted with a straight needle, to retract the affected fallopian tube. A total of 10 ectopic pregnancies have been successfully treated with no complications.

LINEAR SALPINGOSTOMY

Rarely, when there is little damage to the tube, the gestational sac can be removed and the tube conserved. This should be done only in cases where the conservation of fertility is very important to the woman, since she is at risk for another ectopic pregnancy.

Salpingostomy may be performed via laparotomy or laparoscopy, under general or regional anesthesia.

STEPS OF OPERATION

Open the abdomen and expose the appropriate ovary and fallopian tube. Apply traction forceps (e.g., Babcock) on either side of the unruptured tubal pregnancy and lift to view. Use a scalpel to make a linear incision through the serosa on the side opposite to the mesentery and along the axis of the tube, but do not cut the gestational sac (Figs 7A to D). Use the scalpel handle to slide the gestational sac out of the tube. Ligate bleeding points. Return the ovary and fallopian tube to the pelvic cavity.

Procedure can be done laparoscopically. An advantage of laparoscopic salpingostomy is that the operation is less invasive, thus the recovery time is quicker and less painful.

Risks

Complications associated with the surgical procedure include reaction to anesthesia, excessive bleeding, injury to other organs, infection, persistent tubal ectopic gestation and the risks of future ectopic pregnancy.

Alternatives

Some ectopic pregnancies may be managed expectantly up to 25% of ectopic pregnancies will resolve on its own. Treatment with MTX is gaining popularity and has been shown to have success rate similar to laparoscopic salpingostomy, if multiple doses are given and the patient is in stable condition.

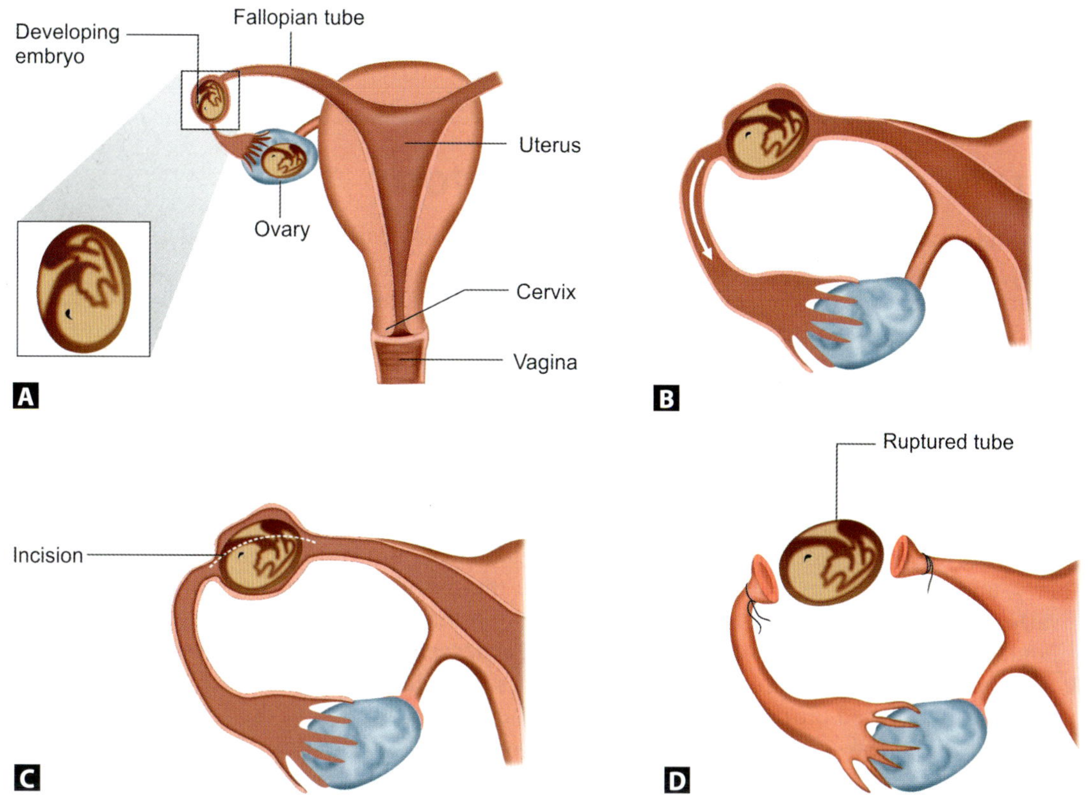

Figs 7A to D: Salpingostomy/salpingectomy

Dilemmas in Approach and Choice of Surgery

Laparotomy vs Laparoscopic Approach

Even with rising trends in endoscopic sugery, laparotomy still remains the majority treatment for ectopic pregnancy. Certainly there are factors that dictate whether laparotomy/ laparoscopy should be performed and certain factors are looked at in order to make a decision, they are: (a) size of ectopic pregnancy (b) amount of hemoperitoneum (c) stability of the patient. Moreover, surgical skills and availability of equipment are important while considering the approach.

Salpingectomy/Salpingostomy

The primary choice is based on future child-bearing, desires of the patient, and anatomical destruction both prior to and incurred by the presence of the ectopic pregnancy. On balance, if one does salpingostomy, the patient has function in that fallopian tube where as if one does salpingectomy the chances are that persistance of an ectopic pregnancy syndrome is diminished. As far as future child bearing, a salpingostomy carries a good chance of success for functionality of the tube that was operated on.

BIBLIOGRAPHY

1. Daniel BR. Surgical management of ectopic pregnancy," emedicine, Jan. 13, 2003 [online]. Available from www.emedcine.com/med/ topic3316.htm. [Accessed November, 2013].
2. DeCherney AH. Ectopic pregnancy: laparoscopic salpingectomy vs salpingostomy. In: The first world congress on controversies in obstetrics. Prague:Gynecology and Infertility; 1999.
3. Dubisson JB, Morice P, Chapron C, et al. Salpingectomy - the laparoscopic surgical choice for ectopic preg. Hum Reprod. 1996;11:1199-203.
4. Ghezzi F, Cromi A, Fasola M, et al. One-trocar salpingectomy for the treatment of tubal pregnancy: A 'marionette-like' technique. BJOG. 2005:112(10):1417-19.
5. Rulin MC. Is salpingostomy the surgical treatment of choice for unruptured tubal pregnancy Obstet. Gynecol. 1995;86:1010-13.
6. Salpingectomy for ectopic pregnancy. http://www.who.int/ reproductive-health/impac/procedures/salpingectomy-p109-p111.html.
7. Seifer DB, Gutmann JN, Doyle MB, et al. Persistent ectopic linear salpingostomy. Obstet. Gynecol. 1990;76:1121-5.

40.3 SALPINGO-OOPHORECTOMY

Tamkeen Rabbani

INTRODUCTION

The human ovary has many important role in a woman's life cycle, starting from puberty to menopause, and even later. It has a striking propensity to develop a wide variety of problems and enlargements, which may be physiological or pathological. The management of ovarian tumors, whether functional, benign or malignant, involves difficult decisions. This may have devastating consequences that may affect a woman's hormonal status, her fertility or increased future risk of malignancy and medical disorders. Thus, the importance of the ovaries in a woman's life cannot be debated and the organ should be well preserved prior to puberty and during a woman's reproductive career. The ovaries may be removed due to potential for developing neoplastic growth, once a woman is in the menopausal age group. Salpingo-oophorectomy is the commonest operation performed during total abdominal hysterectomy because of this risk.

DEFINITIONS

Cystectomy

Removal of a benign tumor by shelling out the cyst from the capsule in order to preserve endocrine and reproductive functions.

Ovariotomy

It is a misnomer. It involves removal of the whole ovary along with the tumor when there is any doubt about the nature of the tumor, especially when the patient is in the perimenopausal or postmenopausal age group. Maybe combined with opposite salpingo-oophorectomy to prevent future problems.

Salpingo-oophorectomy

It is the removal of a normal ovary along with the tube to pre-empt later problems in a peri- or postmenopausal woman who is undergoing pelvic surgery.

Radical Oophorectomy

Removal of the ovary after high ligation of the ovarian artery at its origin, along with underlying peritoneum, and combined with retrograde hysterectomy for malignant ovarian tumors.

ANATOMY

The ovaries are oval flattened structures about 3.5 × 2 × 2 cm in size and weighing 4–8 g, the right ovary being slightly larger. The size, however, is slightly variable depending on the woman's age and her phase of menstrual cycle. The surface is corrugated and pale and it is the only organ in the abdomen not covered by the peritoneum. The ovaries are attached to the posterior leaf of the broad ligament with their mesentries and are suspended with the help of the ovarian ligament to the uterus and to the lateral pelvic wall by the infundibulopelvic ligament (Fig. 1). The ovarian ligament is the vestigial gaburnaculum which continues as the round ligament. Developmentally the ovaries are abdominal organs and later descend down to the pelvis. The descent is arrested at the ovarian fossa or Waldeyer's fossa present as a shallow depression in the bony pelvis. They lie just anterior to the ureter and hypogastric vessels covered by peritoneum. Thus in cases of endometriosis, oophoritis or malignancy, they may be adherent to the underlying peritoneum and the ureter which may be damaged during surgery. Unlike the testes, the serosal covering and tunica albugenia of the ovaries is quite thin making the graffian follicles and the corpus luteum visible to the naked eye and also this causes no pain during these physiological enlargements. The part of the ovaries where the mesovarium is attached and through which all vessels and nerves pass into the ovaries is called the hilum.

RELATIONS

The tubes, ovaries and their mesentries are so closely related that together they are known as the *adnexa*. The

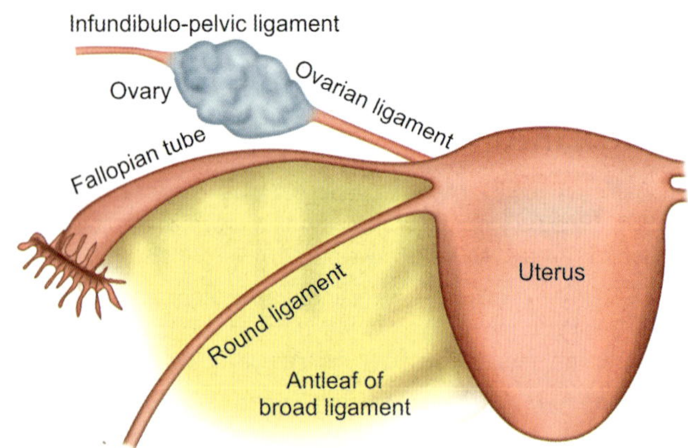

Fig. 1: Anterior view of relations of ovary

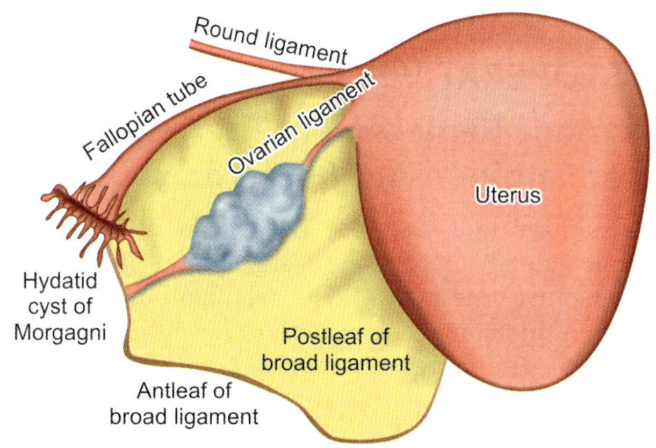

Fig. 2: Postview of relations of the ovary/free surface of ovary

exact position of the ovaries varies considerably in the pelvis from being near the pelvic brim to uterorectal pouch or may be in front of the uterus. The mobility and position depends on absence or presence of adhesions or associated pathology. However, it usually lies in the ovarian fossa bounded above by external iliac vessels and internal iliac vessels and ureter behind. The obturator nerve crosses the floor of the fossa (Fig. 2).

CHANGES WITH AGE

Infancy and Childhood

Tiny elongated structure, with a smooth surface situated near the pelvic brim, packed with primary oocytes, with few small follicles just after birth due to maternal hCG stimulation, but later has only primordial follicles.

Menopause

It becomes smaller in size and shriveled in appearance due to atrophy of the medulla and later still surface becomes smooth as in childhood. There are no follicles in old age.

BLOOD SUPPLY

Ovarian arteries arise directly from the abdominal aorta just below the origin of the renal arteries as developmentally ovaries are abdominal structures. They course downwards and cross laterally over the ureters at the level of the pelvic brim giving off branches to the ureter and the fallopian tubes, and end into giving an anastomosing branch to the uterus. The uterine arteries also give off branches to the ovaries.

Ovarian veins are two in number and form the pampiniform plexus in the mesovarium and form a single large ovarian vein to terminate into the inferior vena cava on the right side and the renal vein on the left side.

LYMPHATIC DRAINAGE

Lymphatics from the ovaries pass via the infudibulopelvic ligament to the pelvic and aortic lymph nodes. Some lymphatics drain directly into the inguinal lymph nodes along the round ligament while some crossover to the opposite ovary along the fundus of the uterus, so tumors are commonly bilateral.

NERVE SUPPLY

The ovaries and the fallopian tubes are supplied by both sensory and motor nerves of the sympathetic and parasympathetic nervous system arising from the preaortic plexus. These accompany the ovarian vessels entering the ovary along the infudibulopelvic ligament and ending at the hilum. They are derived from T10 or T11 for the ovary and T11–12 for the fallopian tubes.

Pain from adnexa is usually referred to the lower abdomen on the sides but can be central also. The ovaries are insensitive to all sensations except squeezing and pressure resulting in dyspareunia or pain during bimanual examination. The fallopian tubes, however, are very sensitive to sensations and cutting, cautery, pressure, pulling, etc. are all painful to the patient.

SALPINGO-OOPHORECTOMY

Salpingo-oophorectomy is the most common surgical procedure performed concurrently with hysterectomy—abdominal, vaginal or laparoscopic. Prophylactic oophorectomy is done to prevent development of benign or malignant ovarian tumors in peri- and postmenopausal women undergoing hysterectomy. Patients need hormone replacement therapy (HRT) after this so prior counseling should be done explaining the risks and benefits of removal of normal ovaries. The risk of development of carcinoma of the ovary is lesser in previous hysterectomized women than in the normal population. It is 0.14 % as opposed to 1.4% in the general population, probably due to the fact that it is a selected population, i.e. only normal ovaries are preserved at hysterectomy. The risk of developing a benign tumor is 5% or less. In those with family history of ovarian malignancy, risk increases to 3–50%.

PROCEDURE

The infundibulopelvic ligament is identified and doubly clamped and a third clamp is applied to control back bleeding (Fig. 3). Identification of the ureter should be done to prevent injury before cutting and ligation of infundibulopelvic ligament. The uterine end of the tube

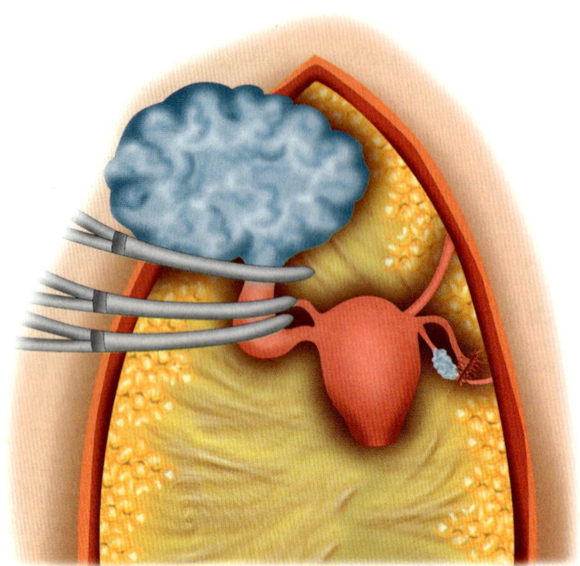

Fig. 3: Clamping the pedicle of a large ovarian cyst with double clamps

and ovarian ligament are excised from the uterus in a wedge shaped manner. The ascending uterine arteries are ligated just below the cornu and the cornual wound is closed with 2.0 figure of eight suture. The infundibulopelvic ligament is doubly ligated with 2.0 or 3.0 vicryl and cornual wound is peritonized. It is preferable to antevert the uterus by round ligament suspension.

SALPINGO-OOPHORECTOMY FOR CHRONIC SALPINGITIS

The chronically inflamed tubo-ovarian mass is dissected free of the underlying peritoneum and course of ureter should be identified to prevent injury to it in such cases.

PARADOXICAL OOPHORECTOMY

It is the removal of the severely pathologic adnexa to improve fertility in patients with strictly unilateral tubal disease. The approach involves removal of contralateral ovary when there is single tubal patency so that ovulation occurs each time in the same ovary which is present on the side of the patent fallopian tube, increasing the chances of conception. This was historically advocated by Jeffcoate and found to be beneficial in some recent studies by Scott and workers. But with the advent of assisted reproduction technology (ART) and the concept of superovulation for better results in ART this approach needs to be reassessed by proper controlled trials.

COMPLICATIONS AND POSTOPERATIVE CONSIDERATIONS

Hormone Replacement Therapy After Salpingo-oophorectomy

Few subjects in gynecology have been more debated and generated more controversy than HRT. In the postoperative period, after salpingo-oophorectomy, important metabolic changes occur because of estrogen deficiency. The more important of these are vasomotor symptoms, genitourinary atrophy, osteoporosis, cardiovascular diseases and cognitive disturbances. Hence, the importance of counseling prior to removal should be remembered. The long-term complaince with HRT is low and only 20–40% women continue HRT beyond 5 years. Also, those who develop breast cancer cannot be given estrogen.

However, prophylactic oophorectomy is beneficial in women greater than 45–50 years of age because cancer ovary is an important cause of death in this age group and cure rate is poor, moreover in developing countries patient follow-up is poor.

Ovarian Remnant Syndrome

Ovarian remnant syndrome occurs in patients who have undergone previous oophorectomy. They present with chronic pelvic pain with or without a pelvic mass. Histological examination confirms the presence of ovarian tissue. Studies have demonstrated that devascularized ovarian tissue can reimplant on abraded or intact surfaces and regenerate and retain ovarian function. Therefore, great care should be exercised to remove all ovarian tissue, particularly when doing laparoscopic surgery. Difficulty may arise in conditions where there is increased pelvic vascularity leading to difficulty in hemostasis, in the presence of adhesions as in endometriosis, pelvic inflammatory disease or when neoplasms distort the anatomy.

Residual Ovary Syndrome

Residual ovary syndrome is characterized by recurrent pelvic pain or persistent pelvic mass or dyspareunia in patients where ovaries have been preserved. Before surgery, the surgeon should discuss the various risks and benefits of castration and should encourage the patient to participate in any decision concerning the fate of her ovaries. The incidence of residual ovary syndrome is between 1–2%, so they should be counseled accordingly for risk of residual ovary syndrome when they decide to conserve the ovaries.

BIBLIOGRAPHY

1. Minke T, Depond W, Winkelmann T, et al. Ovarian remnant syndrome: Study in laboratory rats. Am J Obstet Gynecol. 1994;171:1440.
2. Randall CL, Hall DW, Armenia CS. Pathology in the preserved ovary after unilateral oophorectomy. Am J Obstet Gynecol. 1962;84(9):1233-41.
3. Ryan PJ, Harrison R, Blake GM, et al. Complaince with hormone replacement therapy (HRT) after screening for postmenopausal osteoporosis. Br J Obstet Gynaecol. 1992;99:13225-8.
4. Scheppe KE, Beller FK. Prophylactic oophorectomy. Geburtshilfe Frauunheilkd. 1979;98:662-6.
5. Scott JS, Lynch EM, Anderson JA. Surgical treatment of female infertility: value of paradoxical oophorctomy. Br Med J. 1976;1:631-4.
6. Stovall TG. Hysterectomy. In: Berek JS, Novak E (eds). Berek and Novak's Gynecology, 12th edition; pp. 767.
7. Symmonds RE, Petit P. Ovarian remnant syndrome. Obstet Gynecol. 1979;54:175.
8. Thompson JD, Warshaw J. Hysterectomy. In: Rock JA, Thompson JD. Telinde's Operative Gynecology, 8th edition. Lippincott-Raven Publishers; 1997. pp. 840-1.

40.4 TUBAL STERILIZATION PROCEDURES

Usha Sharma

Occlusion of fallopian tubes in some form is the most popular method of female sterilization all over the world. About 190 million couples throughout the world rely on female sterilization for birth control. Tubal ligation was first performed by Dr J Blindell of London in 1823. Initially, it was used for therapeutic reasons only and was not widely used for voluntary sterilization of women till 1930s. Since 1970, tubal ligation as a contraceptive measure has grown rapidly in India due to several factors such as relaxation of age and parity requirements, greater interest of doctors and sterilization providers, development of newer techniques such as minilaparotomy and laparoscopy and most importantly government on going family planning services in our country.

COUNSELING

Counseling of cases prior to tubal sterilization is essential. Myths and misinformation about sterilization procedure should be removed. The couple should be explained that though reversibility is possible, the procedure should be largely considered as a permanent method. Possible failure of the operation and risk of ectopic pregnancy should be explained. Alternative temporary methods of contraception should be told and a cafeteria approach should be provided. Complications like infection and bleeding should be explained and the patient should be told that menstrual disturbances, if they occur post-ligation, are not due to the procedure. Women may get obese after the procedure, but this is due to the fact that they get more rest and nourishment when they stop having frequent child births due to sterilization.

SELECTION OF CASES

World Health Organization's (WHO) medical eligibility criteria for female sterilization are:

Contraindication (Table 1)

No permanent contraindications.

Table 1: Conditions listing relative contraindications for sterilization

*Delay the procedure**	*Following pregnancy conditions*
Known or suspected pregnancy	Puerperal sepsis
Active pelvic infection, peritonitis	Prolonged rupture of membranes (24 hours or more)
Acute systemic infection	Pregnancy with persistent hypertension
Active liver disease	Antepartum or postpartum hemorrhage
Skin infection at operative area	Severe trauma to genital tract
STD infection	Postpartum psychosis
Severe anemia	Unhealthy newborn/stillbirth
Acute respiratory disease	Recent septic abortion
Current cerebrovascular or CAD	Severe postabortal hemorrhage (delay should be for at least 6 weeks after delivery or abortion)
Complicated valvular heart disease malignant trophoblastic disease	
Any other temporary operative risk	
Any psychiatric condition	
Special precautions/Refer client†	
Conditions that increase anesthetic risk:	*Conditions that increase surgical difficulties and risk:*
Past cardiovascular disease	Endometriosis
Chronic respiratory problems	Past pelvic infection
Hypertension (BP > 160/100 mm Hg)	Past complicated abdominal or pelvic surgery
Hyperthyroidism	Marked obesity
Diabetes with vascular disease	Umblical hernia
Moderate anemia (Hb 7–10 gm/dL)	Coagulation disorders
Severe chronic liver disease	

*conditions must be treated and pt recovers before operation

†refer to center with facilities for general anesthesia and other medical supports, where an equipped surgeon or staff can perform the procedure

Abbreviations: STD, sexually transmitted disease; CAD, coronary artery disease; BP, blood pressure; Hb, hemoglobin.

TIMING OF TUBAL LIGATION

Nowadays, tubal ligation can be done at any time according to suitability of the patient. The operation can be performed as:

- *Puerperal ligation:* The operation can be done 24–48 hours after delivery. The optimum time is after 6 hours and within 48 hours. Its chief advantage is that it is technically simple. Postoperative and postpartum convalescence period coincide, so hospitalization is minimally increased.
- *Interval ligation:* The operation can be done beyond 6 weeks following delivery or abortion. Ideal time is postmenstrual, in the proliferative phase.
- *Postabortal ligation:* Sterilization can be performed along with termination of pregnancy.
- *Cesarean ligation:* When there are indications for a cesarean section and the patient needs tubal ligation, the two procedures can be combined.

METHODS OF TUBAL STERILIZATION

- Tubal sterilization is a surgical procedure which involves occlusion of the fallopian tubes.
- Tubal occlusion can be done by resection of a segment (tubectomy) or blocking of the fallopian tubes by use of rings or clips.
- Female sterilization can be done by any of the three methods/routes:
  - Abdominal tubectomy
  - Vaginal tubectomy
  - Laparoscopic sterilization.

ABDOMINAL TUBECTOMY

It is a simple and safe procedure requiring only a minimal amount of equipment and dressings but sterilization of the material must be perfect and proper aseptic precautions should be taken. This approach is usually used in health centers, remote villages and camps for mass sterilization with safety and good results in developing countries like India.

Preoperative procedures: Written and informed consent of the women is necessary in most countries. In these matters, national rules and norms should be followed.

Besides a counseling session, the preoperative work-up consists of history taking, physical examination, urine analysis, blood counts and hemoglobin (Hb) estimation.

Methods of Abdominal Tubectomy

- Conventional laparotomy
- Minilaparotomy.

Conventional Laparotomy

Anesthesia: Operation is performed under general or spinal or local anesthesia. In mass camps, local anesthesia is preferable. In case of local anesthesia, premedication with injection Pentazocin 30 mg with Phenargan 50 mg IM is to be given at least 20 minutes prior to surgery and the incisional area is infiltrated with 1% lignocaine.

Incision: In puerperal cases, where uterus is felt per abdomen, the incision is made two fingers breadth (1") below the fundal height. In interval ligations, incision is made two fingers breadth above the pubic symphysis.

The incision is made either midline, paramedian or transverse. The abdomen is opened by usual steps.

Delivery of Tubes: The index finger is introduced through incision and is passed across the posterior surface of uterus and then to posterior leaf of the broad ligament from where the tube is hooked out. The tube is identified by fimbrial end and mesosalpinx containing utero-ovarian anastomosing vessels.

Tubal Ligation is Performed by one of the Following Techniques

A. Pomeroy's
B. Modified pomeroy's
C. Parkland
D. Uchida
E. Fimbriectomy
F. Madlener.

Pomeroy's Technique (Figs 1A and B)

In this method, the tube is grasped in its mid-portion, usually with a small atraumatic forceps such as Babcock and loop of tube is elevated. The base of tube is ligated with number 1 plain catgut or number 0 chromic catgut. About 1.2–1.5 cm of the segment of the loop distal to the ligature is excised. Segment of loop removed is to be inspected to be sure that the wall has not been partially resected. The same procedure is repeated on the other side. The cut ends become independently sealed off and retract widely from each other.

The Pomeroy's technique has several advantages, like it is easy, safe and highly effective in spite of the simplicity of technique. It has a low failure rate of 0.1–0.5%.

Modified Pomeroy's Technique

A silk suture of moderate thickness is put near and medial to the stump ligature, following Pomeroy's technique with a view to cause necrosis of intervening portion of the tube to lessen the chances of failure.

The abdominal parieties are closed in layers following usual technique. Skin is closed and stitches removed on fifth day and patient is discharged.

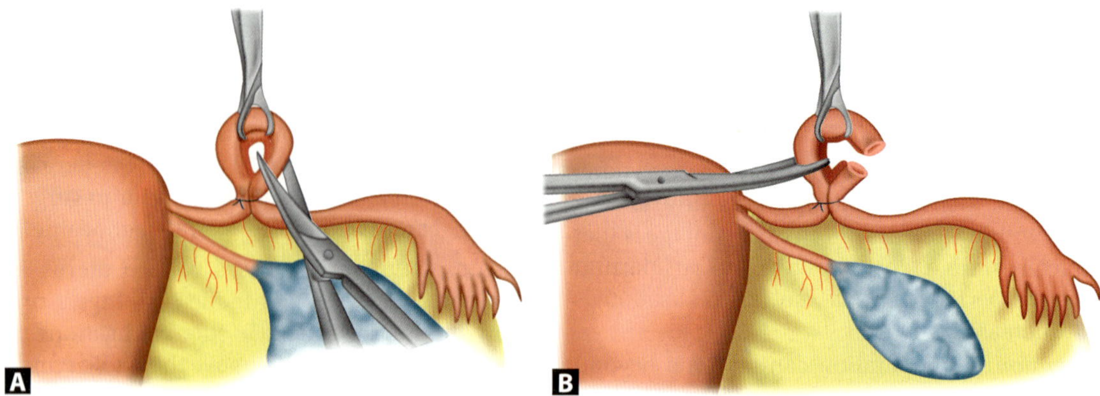

Figs 1A and B: Pomeroy's technique for tubal ligation: **(A)** A loop of the isthmic portion of the tube is elevated and ligated at its base with one or two ties of number 1 plain catgut suture. If performed through a minilaparotomy incision, these ties should be held long to prevent premature retraction of the tubal stumps into the abdomen when the loop of the tube is transected; (B) A fenestration is bluntly created through the mesentery within the tubal loop, and each limb of the tube on either side of this fenestration is individually cut. The cut ends of the tube are inspected for hemostasis and allowed to retract into the abdomen

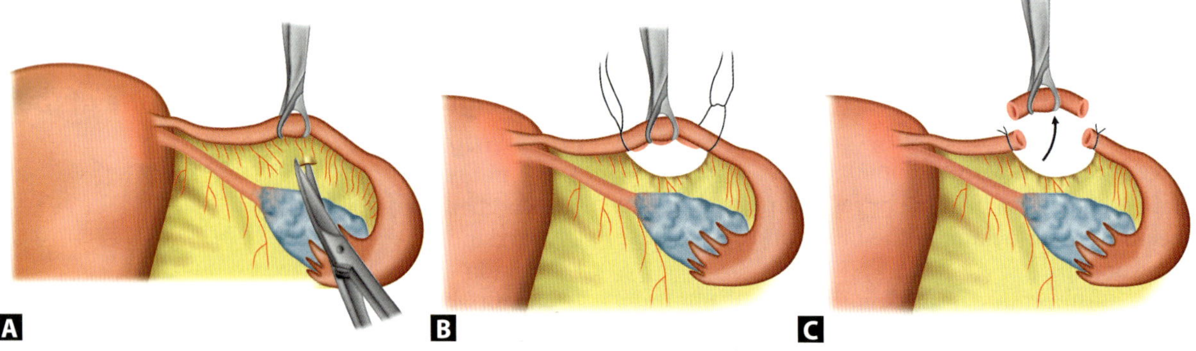

Figs 2A to C: Parkland technique: (A) A 2–3 cm fenestration is made beneath the isthmic portion of tube either with scissors or bluntly with a hemostat; (B) Ligation of the tube. Pulling up on the suture during ligation or during transection of the tube can shear the tube off the underlying mesentery, resulting in troublesome bleeding; (C) Portion of tube removed

Parkland Technique (Figs 2A to C)

After bringing out one of the fallopian tubes, an avascular site in mesosalpinx adjacent to the tube is perforated with a small artery forceps and the jaws are opened to separate the tube from adjacent mesosalpinx for about 2.5 cm. The freed tube is ligated proximally and distally with number 0 chromic catgut and intervening segment of about 2 cm is excised with scissors.

After inspecting for hemostasis, the two portions of ligated tube are pushed inside the two leaves of broad ligament and procedure is repeated on the other side.

Failure rate with this technique is about 1 in 400 procedures.

Uchida Technique (Figs 3A to D)

Saline with epinephrine is injected into mesosalpinx, which is then cut upon. The muscular tube is pulled out.

After removing a portion of tube two ends are ligated and medial stump is buried in mesosalpinx.

This technique is practically not followed nowadays.

Fimbriectomy (Kroener's Technique)

The fimbrial end of tube is doubly ligated with silk/catgut sutures and then removed. Although, this technique is a simple one, but it has high failure rate of 2–3% and chances of success of recanalization are very low, hence it is not popular.

Madlener's Technique

It is the easiest method. A loop of the tube is crushed with an artery forceps and the crushed area is tied. The loop is not excised.

Failure rate is very high to the extent of 3%, so its use has been practically abandoned.

Minilaparotomy

When tubectomy is done through a small abdominal incision along with some device to elevate the uterus then the procedure is called minilaparotomy. It was first described in Bangkok, in 1974.

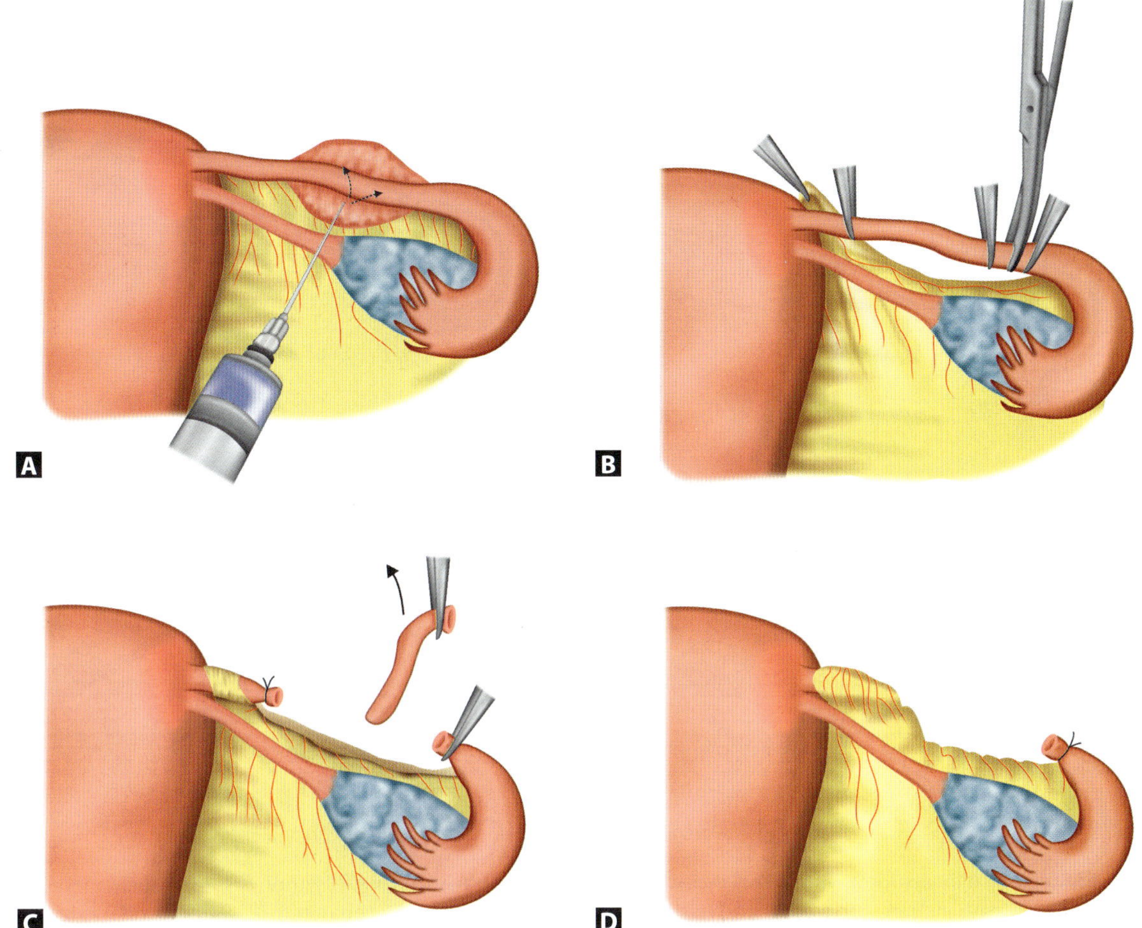

Figs 3A to D: Uchida technique for tubal ligation: (A) Injection of vasoconstricting solution beneath the serosa of the tube about 6 cm from the uterotubal junction. The serosa is then incised (dashed line); (B) The antimesenteric edge of the mesosalpinx is pulled back toward the uterus, exposing about 5 cm of the tube; (C) The tube is ligated proximally and cut, and the tied stump is allowed to retract into the mesosalpinx. The hemostat on the distal stump remains attached to facilitate exteriorization of this portion of the tube; (D) The mesosalpinx is closed. A purse string stitch of the mesosalpinx around the exteriorized tubal stump secures it in a position open to the abdomen, whereas the ligated proximal stump is buried within the mesosalpinx. Once the purse-string suture is tied, the hemostat can be removed

Preoperative checkup: Patients with fatty abdomen and/or rectroverted uterus with restricted mobility are unsuitable for minilaparotomy and are usually not selected for the procedure.

Anesthesia: Local anesthesia is preferable.

Incision: Incision should be half inche to three-fourth of an inch length, and the site selected is as in conventional method.

Steps (Figs 4A to E)

- Abdomen is opened areas
- Uterus is elevated or pushed to one side or other by the elevator which is already introduced transvaginally into uterine cavity. This helps in bringing the tube close to incision site
- The appropriate technique is performed for tubectomy. Tubal ligation is usually performed by Pomeroy's technique, alternatively Parkland technique may also be used
- Peritoneum is closed by purse string suture
- The patient is usually discharged within 24–48 hours
- Major complications such as uterine perforation and bladder trauma occur in less than 2% of cases.

Advantages of Minilaparotomy

- It is a safe and effective method
- It can be used in camps and primary healthcare centers (PHCs) and also as an outpatient procedure
- It can be performed even by residents and trainers
- No special equipment is required

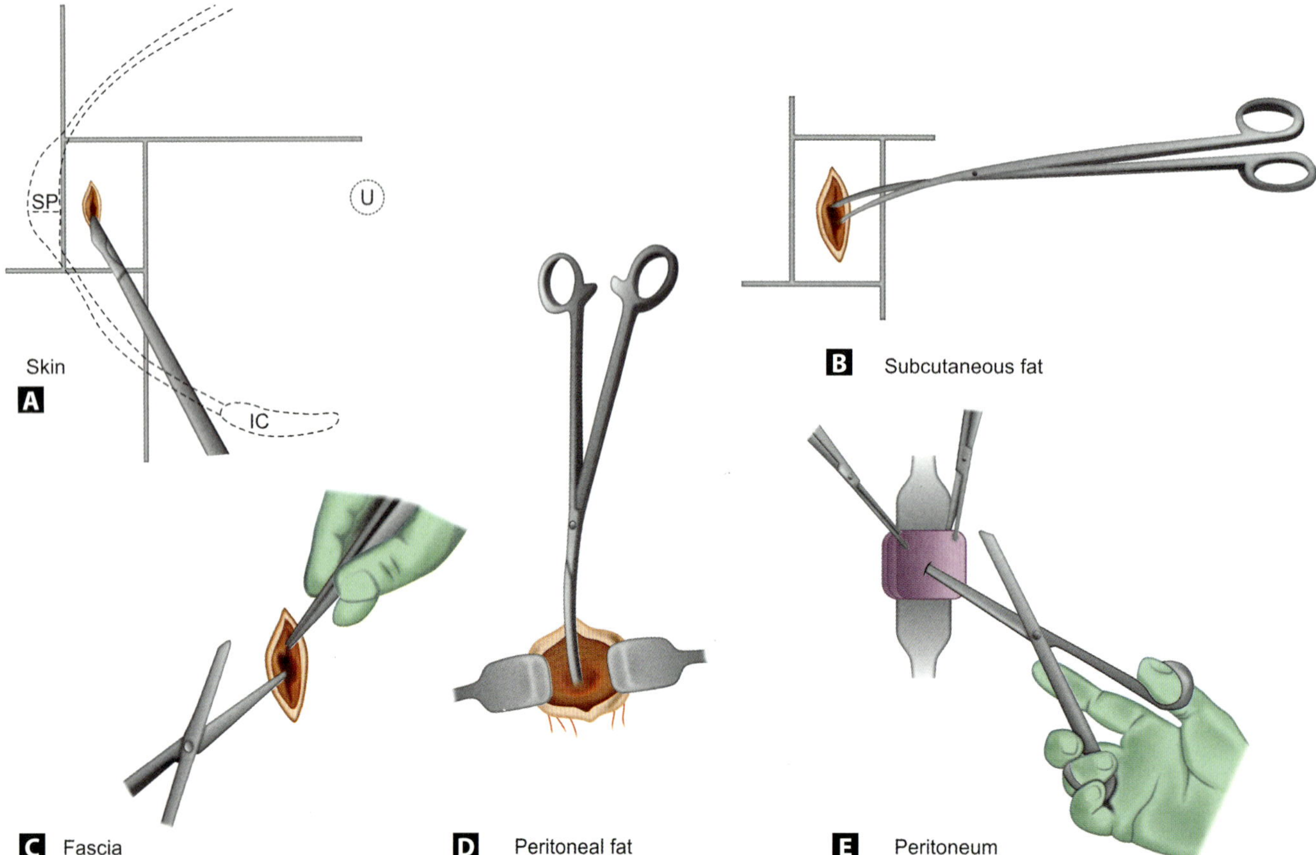

Figs 4A to E: Steps of minilaparotomy: (A) Skin incision made 2.5 cm above the pubic symphysis; (B) Subcutaneous fat bluntly dissected; (C) Rectus sheath incised with scalpel and scissors and rectus muscle bluntly separated; (D) Peritoneal fat bluntly dissected; (E) Peritoneum incised taking care to injure bladder and bowel

Abbreviations: SP, symphysis pubis; U, umbilicus; IC, iliac crest

- Complications are usually minimal
- It can be performed at any time.

Drawbacks of Minilaparotomy

- Wound and pelvic infection is more
- Postoperative pain is more
- Convalescence period is longer than laparoscopic ligation.

VAGINAL TUBECTOMY (FIGS 5A TO D)

It is a safe, effective and useful method. However, it is technically more difficult and needs special training. It is also not suitable for mass sterilization in camps and ill equipped operating places.

Vaginal tubectomy is usually done along with vaginal plastic operation by surgeon. When performed in isolation, approach is through posterior colpotomy. It can be done only in interval cases or following delivery when uterus is smaller than 12 weeks. Complications in the form of hemorrhage, broad ligament hematoma, injury to the rectum and infection are observed. Failure rate is more, so it is not very popular.

Contraindications for this procedure include vaginal infections, restricted uterine mobility due to operation or endometriosis obesity and recent second trimester abortion.

Advantages of Vaginal Tubectomy

- Abdominal scar is not present
- Postoperative pain is minimal
- Special equipment are not needed.

Drawbacks of Vaginal Tubectomy

- It is more difficult, so proper training is needed
- Failure rate is higher
- Usually GA is needed
- Intraperitoneal infection is more common
- Has to be converted to laparotomy in up to 2–3% cases

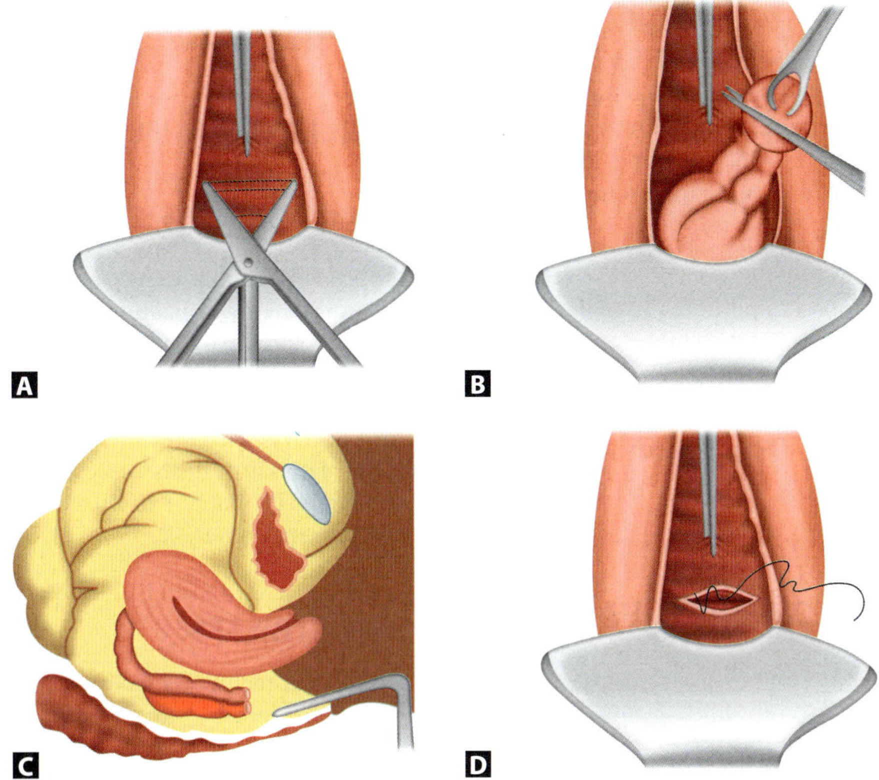

Figs 5A to D: Steps of vaginal tubectomy: (A) Posterior vaginal fornix is being opened; (B) The tube is brought out, ligated and cut; (C) The cut and ligated tube is pushed in; (D) The vagina is closed

- Sexual intercourse is delayed
- Vaginal tubectomy is not commonly used currently.

Complications of Tubectomy

- Complications following abdominal or vaginal tubectomy depend on several factors, which include method of sterilization, type of anesthesia, route of ligation, timing of ligation, place of operation, age of the patient, selection of the patient and skills of the operator. It has been observed that complications are more frequent with vaginal ligations and following cesarean and postabortal ligations.
- Major complications occur in 1.8% cases and minor in 14% cases of minilaparotomy.
- Following conventional laparotomy, minor complications occur in 8% of cases.
- Operative complications include anesthetic hazards, bowel and bladder injury, injuries to tubes and ovaries, broad ligament hematoma, and uterine perforation in minilaparotomy.
- Postoperative complications include wound infection, wound hematoma, pelvic infection, peritonitis, urinary infection, hemorrhage, bladder and bowel fistulae.

LAPAROSCOPIC STERILIZATION

Laparoscopy for female sterilization has been widely practiced since 1970. It is the most popular method of tubal ligation, especially in camps. This is because it is safe, simple, effective and can be performed through a very abdominal incision under sedation and local anesthesia.

POST LIGATION SYNDROME

This includes pelvic pain, menorrhagia along with cystic ovaries. However, these menstrual disturbances are more likely due to aging or development of a fresh gynecological disorder.

It has been reported that except for menstrual pain, there is no increased in adverse menstrual function, however, high serum estradiol and low serum progesterone have been found in some cases following tubal sterilization. This is more following techniques which cause obstruction of utero-ovarian flow. Therefore, it is considered desirable to preserve blood flow through the mesosalpinx to minimize the possibility of post-tubal ligation syndrome, if any. Cumulative evidence provides little support to the existence of post ligation syndrome. In addition there is alteration in libido in some patients.

FAILURE RATE

The overall failure rate following female sterilization by tubal ligation is about 0.7%. In India, the reported failure rate is 0.2–1.3%. Failure rates with different techniques are 0.1–0.5%, Pomeroy's; 1.5–3%, Madlener's; 0.5–0.6%, laparoscopy and 0.1–0.3% with minilaparotomy.

The major causes of failure are:

- Fistula formation or spontaneous reanastomosis
- Faulty selection of tubes, sometimes round ligament or broad ligament are confused with tube
- Failure rate is also increased when done through vaginal route or during cesarean section
- Luteal phase pregnancy—occurs when the patient was already pregnant and the time of surgery in cases of interval ligation.

MORTALITY FOLLOWING TUBAL STERILIZATION

Mortality following tubal sterilization is rare and in the developed countries, it is around 1.5/100,000 procedures performed, much lower than that from child birth. Mortality following ligation in India is higher, up to 72/100,000 procedures for all methods. Following puerperal ligation, mortality is 7/100,000 procedure and for laparoscopic ligation mortality is 5–10/100,000 procedure.

TUBAL LIGATION VERSUS LAPAROSCOPIC STERILIZATION

1. Both tubal ligation and laparoscopic sterilization are highly effective procedures with comparable failure rates. Both can be performed safely under local or GA, on inpatient or outpatient basis.
2. Tubal ligation is a simple procedure which can be performed by junior doctors or even health workers after a basic training with standard surgical equipment. Laparoscopic sterilization on the other hand needs expensive, high maintenance equipment, trained gynecologists, anesthetists and a fully equipped operating room.
3. Tubal ligation requires a large incision associated with more chances of wound infection, postoperative pain and long convalescence as compared to laparoscopic sterilization.
4. Though complications are less with laparoscopy, they are of a more serious nature and may even be life-threatening.
5. Therefore, it is almost globally accepted that tubal ligation is the safer and most practical method of female sterilization, especially in developing countries like India.

STERILIZATION IN A CAMP SET-UP

Camps are designed to meet the sterilization demands of women in rural areas. They are organized at PHCs or district hospitals. An expert team visits the center with its specialized equipment on predecided days and a large number of sterilization operations are performed. Nowadays, laparoscopic sterilization is the method employed in camps because of its efficacy, safety and acceptability. Patients are motivated for several weeks prior to the camps. A full physical examination and essential laboratory tests are carried out preoperatively. Postoperatively, patient is observed for 4-6 hours and thereafter sent home.

REVERSIBILITY

Microsurgical technique gives excellent results following tubal reanastomosis. However, it is costly, difficult and the ectopic pregnancy rate is high. The chances of success are best with clips and worst with electrocoagulation. Pregnancy rate after reversal are high, approximately 80% following clips or rings. So, informed consent must be obtained after adequate counseling prior to sterilization and the couple must understand the permanency of the procedure.

AUTHOR'S EXPERIENCE AND OPINIONS

Indeed, even vaginal ligation is a very good method and was widely accepted by the public when family welfare camps were organized during intensive drive period between 1974 and 1976 but later on it went into disrepute to the extent that no one is coming forward to accept this method today. Can we hold the method responsible for this? Certainly not. The method still remains very good but the acceptance has completely vanished due to over-enthusiastic use, which may happen with laparoscopic sterilization also. In my opinion laparoscopic sterilization is a very good method provided we are able to take care of the quality of the service available at every level and do not allow every doctor to perform these operations without taking care of their proper training. In few places, this method has gone into little disrepute; at other places, it is still widely acceptable and large number of cases are being operated by this technique which clearly indicates that it is due to some local deficiency in the services provided for laparoscopic sterilization. We still have enough time to review the acceptability in places where it is going into disrepute. The policy of the government should be such that we could provide all techniques of family planning, i.e. minilaparotomy, laparoscopic sterilization or vaginal ligation, at every level, ensuring the expertise of such methods. Let the public have the option to select whatever method they like according to their own suitability. Let us not impose on them the method to be opted by them, but let them be the choosers so as to have the maximum acceptability of every method. We must identify the places for laparoscopic sterilization and minilaparotomy with great caution. If we are able to maintain prolonged acceptability of these methods then only it will be possible for us to achieve our targets, rather than to criticize a method without considering the factors responsible for the method failure.

In my opinion laparoscopic sterilization is one of the best methods suited for our society due to minimum complications and least hospitalization. At few places, the failures were more because doctors were allowed to conduct camps without adequate training and capability of treating complications. If such things are not allowed to recur, we can be sure of prolonged and wide acceptability of this method. Once again I emphasize that all the methods of sterilization are equally good or bad provided we ensure the quality of service. We must popularize both the techniques. Let laparoscopic sterilization be performed by few experts in the institutions and camps conducted by them at peripheral hospitals to provide door-step service and minilaparotomy by all the doctors in routine at PHC level, that too after proper training. The skilled persons should only be given responsibility of performing laparoscopic sterilization if we want family planning program to succeed.

I have performed more than 1000 camps of laparoscopic sterilization since 1981 and with my own experience I can say that it is very difficult to refuse cases if they have come in large numbers during camps, because once refused, not only that they do not come again for operation but will also loose faith in the organizers of the camps resulting in negative impact on family planning programs. To avoid such circumstances, comparatively large number of cases can only be tackled by laparoscopy and not by minilaparotomy. No method can be chosen or condemned; we must educate the public regarding all methods of contraception. Let the public be a customer and we the providers of all methods and selection can be made by them, which will be finally provided by us considering the suitability of the method for the individual.

Our policy should be to work hard to find the reasons, why at places laparoscopic technique is going into disrepute rather than to discard it and to promote any other technique because the other technique will also have the same fate as vaginal ligation had, and laparoscopic ligations are being foreseen to have.

We must understand that every technique is perfect and good with experts having all possible facilities and the same may be discarded totally if used by inexperienced surgeons or with little facilities.

BIBLIOGRAPHY

1. Allyn DP, Leton DA, Westcott LA, et al. Presterilization counselling and women's regret about having been sterilized. J Reprod. Med. 1986;31:1027-32.
2. Bhiwandi Wala PP, Mumford SD, Feldblun PJ. A comparison of different laparoscopic sterilization occlusion techniques in 24,439 procedures. Am J Obstet Gynecol. 1982;70:319-31.
3. Bhiwandi Wala PP, Mumford SD, Kennedy KI. Comparison of the safety of open and conventional laparoscopic sterilization. Obstet Gynecol. 1985;66:391-4.
4. Bordahl PE, Raeder JC, Nordentoft I, et al. Laparoscopic sterilization under local or general anesthesia? A randomized study. Obstet Gynecol. 1993;81:137-41.
5. Brenner WE, Edelman DA. Permanent sterilization through a posterior colpotomy. Int J Gynecol Obstet. 1979;14(1):46-52.
6. Brian J, El-Toukhy T, Chandakas S, et al. Laparoscopic laser sterilisation: an alternative option. J Obstet Gynaecol. 2005;25(7): 681-4.
7. Dede FS, Dilbaz B, Akyuz O, et al. Changes in menstrual pattern and ovarian function following bipolar electrocauterization of the fallopian tubes for voluntary surgical contraception. Contraception. 2006;73(l):88-91.
8. Department of Reproductive Health, World Health Organization (1996). Medical Eligibility Criteria for Contraceptive use. [online]. Geneva: WHO; 1996.
9. Destefano F, Perlman JA, Peterson HB, et al. Long-term risks of menstrual disturbances after tubal sterilization. Am J Obstet Gynecol. 1985;152:835-41.
10. Emens JM, Olive JE. Timing of female sterilization. BMJ. 1978;2:1 126.
11. EsKobedo LG, Peterson HB, Grubb GS, et al. Case-fatality rates for tubal sterilization in U.S. hospitals, 1979 to 1980. Am J Obstet Gynecol. 1989;160:147-50.
12. Gentile GP, Helbig DW, Zacur H, et al. Hormone levels before and after tubal sterilization. Contraception. 2006; 73(5):507-11.
13. Gentile GP, Kaufman SC, Helbig DW. Is there any evidence for a post-tubal sterilization syndrome? Fertil Steril, 1998;69: 179-86.
14. Greenberg JA. Long-acting methods of contraception. N Engl J Med. 2006;354(6):645-6.

15. Grubb GS, Peterson HB. Luteal phase pregnancy and tubal sterilization. Obstet Gynecol. 1985;66:784-8.
16. Handa VL, Berlin M, Washington AE. A comparison of local and general anesthesia for laparoscopic tubal sterilization. J Women's Health. 1994;3:135-41.
17. Hillis SD, Marchbanks PA, Tylor LR, et al. Poststerilization regret: Findings from the United States Collaborative Review of Sterilization. Obstet Gynecol. 1999;93:889-95.
18. Hillis SD, Marchbanks PA, Tylor LR, et al. Tubal sterilization and the long-term risk of hysterectomy: Findings from the United States Collaborative Review of Sterilization. Obstet Gynecol. 1997;89:609-14.
19. Huber AW, Mueller MD, Ghezzi F, et al. Tubal sterilization: complications of laparoscopy and minilaparotomy. Eur J Obstet Gynecol Reprod Biol. 2006;134:105-9.
20. Indian Council of Medical Research. Collaborative study on sequalae of tubal sterilization. New Delhi: Indian Council of Medical Research; 1982. pp. 1-88.
21. International Planned Parenthood Federation. Med Bull 1999 33(4): 3.
22. Jamieson DJ, Hillis SD, Duerr A, et al. Complications of interval laparoscopic sterilization: findings from the United States Collaborative Review of Sterilization. Obstet Gynecol. 2000;96: 997-1002.
23. Kelekci S, Erdemoglu E, Kutluk S, et al. Risk factors for tubal ligation: Regret and psychological effects impact of Beck Depression Inventory. Contraception. 2005;71(6):417-20.
24. Kelekci S, Yilmaz B, Yakut Y, et al. Hormonal and ovarian stromal blood supply changes after laparoscopic tubal sterilization: a prospective controlled study. Contraception. 2006;73(3):279-83.
25. Koetsawang S, Gates DS, Suwanichati S, et al. Long-term follow up of laparoscopic sterilizations by electrocoagulation, the Hulka clip, and the tubal ring. Contraception. 1990;41:9-18.
26. Kovacs GT, Krins AJ. Female sterilisations with Filshie clips: What is the risk failure? A retrospective survey of 30,000 applications. J Fam Plann Reprod Health Care. 2002;28(l):34-5.
27. Levie MD, Chudnoff SG. Office hysteroscopic sterilization compared with laparoscopic sterilization: a critical cost analysis. Minim Invasive Gynecol. 2005;12(4):318-22.
28. Liskin L, Rinehart W, Blackburn R, et al. Minilaparotomy and laparoscopy: safe, effective, and widely used. Pop Rep C. 1985;9:C-125-67.
29. Litta P, Cosmi E, Sacco G, et al. Hysteroscopic permanent tubal sterilization using a nitinol-dacron intratubal device without anaesthesia in the outpatient setting: Procedure feasibility and effectiveness. Hum Reprod. 2005;20(12):3419-22.
30. Machado KM, Ludermir AB, da Costa AM. Changes in family structure following tubal sterilization. CadSaude Publica. 2005;21(6):1768-77.
31. Makar AP, Vanderheyden JS, Schatteman EA, et al. Female Sterilization failure after bipolar electrocoagulation: a six-year retrospective study. Eur J Obstet Gynecol Reprod Biol. 1990;37:237-46.
32. Moore CL, Vasquez NF, Lin H, et al. Major vascular injury after laparoscopic tubal ligation. J Emerg Med. 2005;29(l):67-71.
33. Mumford SD, Bhiwandiwala PP, Chi IC. Laparoscopic and minilaparotomy female sterilisation compared in 15,167 cases. Lancet. 1980;2:1066-70.
34. Nisanian A. Outpatient minilaparotomy sterilization with local anesthesia. J Reprod Med 1990;35:380-3.
35. Padhye S, Karki C. Voluntary surgical contraception: A study on level of satisfaction. Nepal Med Coll J. 2003;5(l):18-21.
36. Penava D, Daskalopoulos R, Nisker J, et al. Lack of timely access to tubal ligation increases risks of unintended pregnancy. Women Health Issues. 2006;16(1):1-3.
37. Penfield AJ. The Filshie clip for female sterilization: a review of world experience. Am J Obstet Gynecol. 2000;182:485-9.
38. Peterson HB, Jeng G, Folger SG, et al. The risk of menstrual abnormalities after tubal sterilization. N Engl J Med. 2000;343: 1681-7.
39. Peterson HB, Xia Z, Hughes JM, et al. The risk of ectopic pregnancy after tubal sterilization. N Engl J Med. 1997;336:762-7.
40. Peterson HB, Xia Z, Hughes JM, et al. The risk of pregnancy after tubal sterilization: Findings from the U.S. Collaborative Review of Sterilization. Am J Obstet Gynecol. 1996; 174:1161-8.
41. Rulin MC, Turner JH, Dunworth R, et al. Post-tubal sterilization syndrome-a misnomer. Am J Obstet Gynecol. 1985;151:13-9.
42. Schwartz D, Wingo PA, Antarsh L, et al. Female sterilizations in the United States, 1987. Fam Plann Perspect. 1989;21:209.
43. Sciara JJ. In: Sciara JJ, Aztuchni GI, Speidel JJ, (eds). Proceedings of a workshop on reversal of sterilization. PARFR Series. Hageerstown: Harper and Row; 1978.
44. Shobeiri MJ, Atashkhoii S. The risk of menstrual abnormalities after tubal sterilization: a case control study. BMC Womens Health. 2005;5(1):5.
45. Siegler AM, Grunebaum A. A short history of tubal sterilization. In: Phillips JM (ed). Endoscopic female sterilization: a comparison of methods. Downey: American Association of Gynecologic Laparoscopists, 1983:3.
46. Stuart GS, Castano PM, Sheffield JS, et al. Postpartum sterilization choices made by HIV-infected women. Infect Dis Obstet Gynecol. 2005;13(4):217-22.
47. Trussell J, Hatcher RA, Gates W, et al. A guide to interpreting contraceptive efficacy studies. Obstet Gynecol. 1990;76:558.
48. Uchida H. Uchida tubal sterilization. Am J Obstet Gynecol. 1975;121:153-8.
49. WHO. Progress in human reproduction research. Geneva: WHO; 1996.
50. World Health Organization Task Force on Female Sterilization, Special Programme of Research, Development and Research Training in Human Reproduction. Minilaparotomy or laparoscopy for sterilization: a multicenter, multinational, randomized study. Am J Obstet Gynecol. 1982;143:645-52.
51. Zite N, Wuellner S, Gilliam M. Barriers to obtaining a desired postpartum tubal sterilization. Contraception. 2006;73(4):404-7.
52. Zite N, Wuellner S, Gilliam M. Failure to obtain desired postpartum sterilization: risk and predictors. Obstet Gynecol. 2005;105(4):794-9.

40.5 OVARIAN WEDGE RESECTION

Mandakini Parihar, Shilpa Mangal

"An enigma wrapped in riddle and surrounded by mystery."
—**Sir Winston Churchill**

INTRODUCTION

Polycystic ovarian syndrome or PCOS, as it is called today, was first diagnosed and called as Stein Leventhal syndrome. However, even before that Hippocrates had described women, who showed evidence of male sprouting, would face difficulty to procreate.

Polycystic ovarian syndrome is a common and heterogeneous disorder of women of reproductive age, characterized by chronic anovulation and hyperandrogenism. One problem in understanding the etiology has been the wide variability in clinical manifestations. Features of PCOS may manifest at any age, ranging from childhood (premature puberty), teenage years (hirsuitism, menstrual abnormalities), early adulthood and middle life (infertility, glucose intolerance) to later life (diabetes mellitus and cardiovascular disease). Hyperinsulinemia has proved to be a key link in the enigmatic generation of the symptoms of PCOS, i.e. anovulatory infertility and the skin stigmata induced by hyperandrogenism. As obesity exaggerates the expression of the symptoms induced by hyperinsulinemia, a low calorie diet and lifestyle change resulting in loss of weight for obese women with PCOS is capable of reversing these symptoms. For this endocrine disorder, there is an emerging picture of a strong familial component. Hence now, PCOS is a recognized as a multiorgan endocrine disorder with certain long-term potential health risks, e.g. type II diabetes and endometrial cancer.

Rotterdam Consensus Meeting on PCOS, in 2003, now defines the syndrome of PCOS as presence of any two of the following three criteria:

1. Ultrasound appearance of polycystic ovaries
2. Menstrual disturbances
3. Evidence of hyperandrogenism, acne, hirsuitism, etc. after other causes of hyperandrogenism have been ruled out, especially congenital adrenal hyperplasia.

Since, hyperandrogenia has been postulated as the main cause of symptoms of PCOS, techniques to decrease the androgen circulation have been popularized since its initial description in 1935.

Ovarian wedge resection was first described in 1935 by Stein and Leventhal, and it was a path-breaking discovery and helped us understand the endocrinopathy of PCOS. The procedure helped in decreasing the androgens associated with PCOS and hence achieved ovulation and pregnancy in infertile anovulatory patients.

With the advent of minimally invasive surgery, there has been renewed interest in offering some procedure for decreasing androgen levels in women with PCOS. This renewed interest came as many patients in the original series had become pregnant after wedge resection and hence the hypothesis that decreasing androgen levels will help in achieving pregnancy gained momentum. The second important discovery was application of minimally invasive techniques to achieve this decrease in the androgen levels by Gjonasses, in 1984. The newer modalities of decreasing the androgen microenvironment in PCOS with ovarian drilling are discussed in this chapter and its merits and demerits are highlighted.

Historical Perspective

In 1935, the only way to confirm presence of ovulation was by doing an ovarian biopsy. Two enterprising medical health providers identified a subset of women who they suspected being anovulatory. They went ahead and did an ovarian biopsy on these women to confirm their diagnosis of anovulation. To their surprise, 80% of these women started getting regular cycles and become pregnant too. Thus was born the therapeutic technique of ovarian wedge resection/biopsy. This was the only method of management of patients suspected as having ovulatory infertility prior to the availability of clomiphene citrate (CC) in 1961.

Ovarian wedge resection was described by Irving Stein and Michael Leventhal (Fig. 1) for management of obese, hirsute anovulatory women. That time PCOS was diagnosed during laparotomy. It was found that ovarian biopsies taken to make the diagnosis subsequently led to ovulation. This surgical procedure was then developed for the treatment of PCOS based on a simple premise. If the ovary is producing too much of androgens, then removing part of the ovarian tissue should decrease the amount of androgens produced. Although, this premise is not completely accurate, the procedure has been successful and remained a viable option. Though there are many hypothesis stating the mechanism by which wedge resection of polycystic ovary resolves anovulation, but the most accepted theory is based on the fact that removal of androgen secreting stroma and theca reduces the amount of abnormal steroid production. It has been proved that after wedge resection, the mean level of

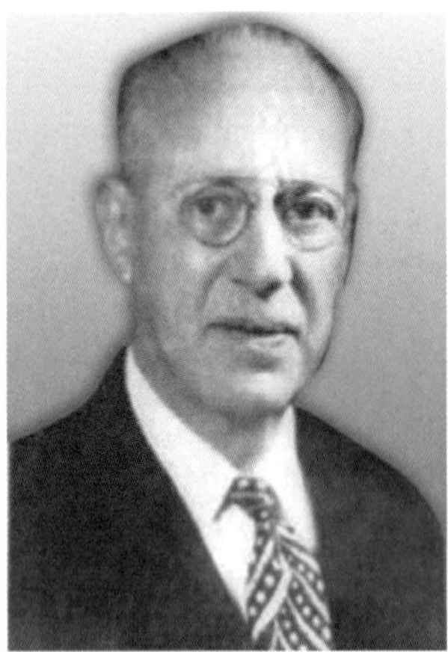
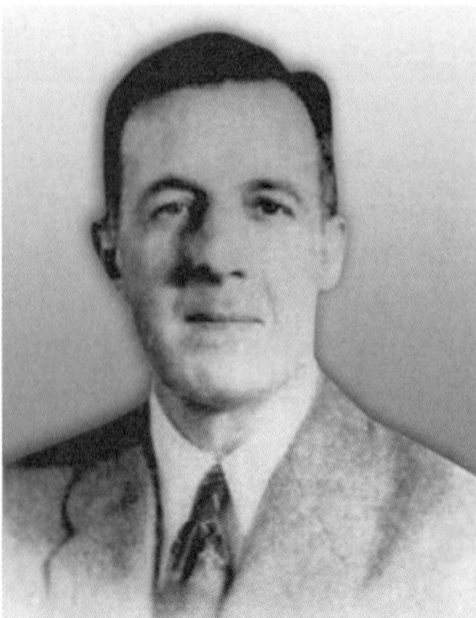

Fig. 1: Prof Stein and Prof Leventhal

17-hydroxyprogesterone, dehydroepiandrosterone, testosterone as well as transient decrease in estradiol occurs. This reduction in the steroidogenesis of androgens allows normalization of luteinizing hormone-follicle stimulating hormone (LH-FSH) ratio, thus establishes ovulation.

Stein reported experience of 108 cases and found that 95% of patients resumed normal cycles and 87% of those wishing to conceive did so, on at least one occasion. Furthermore he stated that surgery cured the condition such that the ovarian pathology did not recur.

A large review of 187 reports summarized data on 1079 ovarian wedge resection, with an overall rate of ovulation of 80% and pregnancy of 62.5%.

Another controversial point was the amount of ovarian tissue that is to be removed during wedge resection. Halbe and coworkers had done a study taking 38 patients who wanted to conceive, divided them in three groups and resected one-fifth, one-third and half to three-fourth part of ovarian tissue, respectively and found that best pregnancy rate and best ovulation rate were achieved after removal of at least half of the ovarian medulla. However, size of ovary may vary with the spectrum of PCOS, this has no bearing on selection of patient for wedge resection.

Until the introduction of CC therapy in 1961, wedge resection was the only treatment for anovulatory PCOS. Kistner and Patton recommended wedge resection for patients who did not conceive after seven or eight cycles of treatment with CC. However, most appropriate indication is the patient who is unresponsive to CC with maximum permissible dose when combined with hCG and have subsequently failed a trial of pure FSH ovulation induction. Some patients who can not afford costly gonadotropins, or who may not want to take the risk of multiple pregnancy or hyperstimulation were offered wedge resection, but with the advent of newer reproductive technologies and laparoscopy this procedure is now abandoned. The main disadvantage of the procedure was that surgical intervention by laparotomy converted anovulation as cause of infertility to mechanical cause by causing adhesions and tubal damage. Hence, in the years following availability of CC this procedure was abandoned for favor of ovulation induction.

Beside the routine preoperative investigation, baseline serum LH, FSH, thyroid-stimulating hormone (TSH) and prolactin levels should be checked. Husband's semen analysis in patients who wish to conceive should also be done.

Operative Procedure (Historical) (Figs 2A to E)

Abdomen was opened by a midline infraumbilical incision. Keeping in mind that approximately half of the ovarian tissue is to be removed, 2–3 cm elliptical incision was given over the thickened capsule. Incision was made on the convexity of the ovary along the antimesenteric border in such a manner that a sickle shaped segment of ovarian tissue can be created. While giving the incision, due care was taken to avoid injury to the ovarian vessels at the hilum. Holding the ovary in the hand, portion of medulla is removed, preserving as much cortex as possible. Ovary, thereafter, is sutured in layers. For the inner layer, purse-string sutures of 4-0, 5-0 nonreactive, absorbable material such as polydioxanone or polyglactin to obliterate the defect should be taken. This can be further strengthened by interrupted "figure of 8" sutures. Using running or baseball sutures of 6-0, 7-0 nonreactive absorbable suture should repair cortex. Care should be taken to avoid leaving any dead space to avoid formation of ovarian hematoma.

Good approximation, precise hemostasis, gentle tissue handling and keeping the tissue moist were the key factors in preventing postoperative adhesion formation. Large amount of intra-abdominal lavage was used, ideally with a physiologic substance, e.g. Ringer lactate solution, following the principles of microsurgery. Postoperative increases in FSH levels and in the emergence of a dominant follicle signified that the surgery was a success.

Wedge resection went out of favor because of the realization that significant postoperative adhesion formation occurred and that initial favorable reports of pregnancy rates were not sustained. It was also noticed that it leaves many women with little ovarian tissue, which results in a poor response to gonadotropins and premature ovarian failure. In different reports following wedge resection it was noted that there was a significant increase in the incidence of ovarian atrophy and almost all patients develop some extensive periovarian and peritubal adhesions.

Laparoscopic Ovarian Drilling—Option Today

For many years, Wedge Resection of the ovaries was the only treatment for patients with PCOS. After Palmer and Cohen made the first attempts in 1972 using Palmer's ovarian biopsy forceps, laparoscopic approach has gained popularity and is now the preferred choice than conventional laparotomy. The procedure can now be done by cautery, diathermy or laser vaporization with a laparoscope and can be performed in conjunction with a diagnostic laparoscopy. The procedure of ovarian drilling using electorcautry via the laparoscope was first described by Gjonnaess, in 1984.

Mechanism of Action

Trauma to the ovary induces a decrease in local androgen production, a fall in E2 and a decrease in positive feedback on LH. This results in spontaneous resumption of the ovarian cycle and hence a higher chance of pregnancy. Trauma to the ovary in any form works and hence may explain why single ovarian drilling also results in

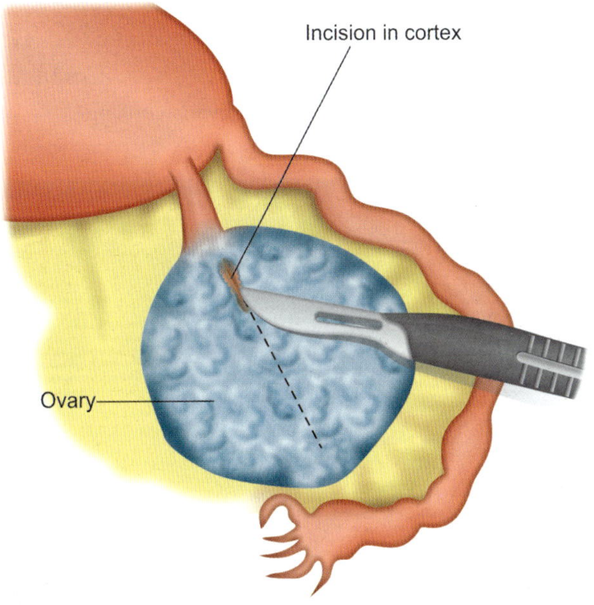

Fig. 2A: Incision on ovarian surface

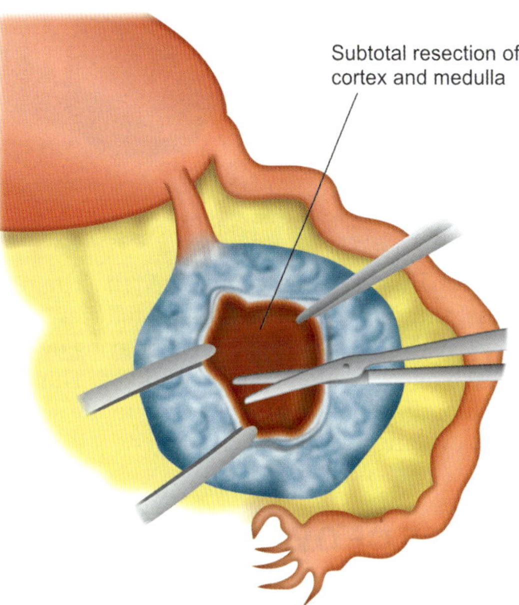

Fig. 2B: Resection of the cortex and medulla

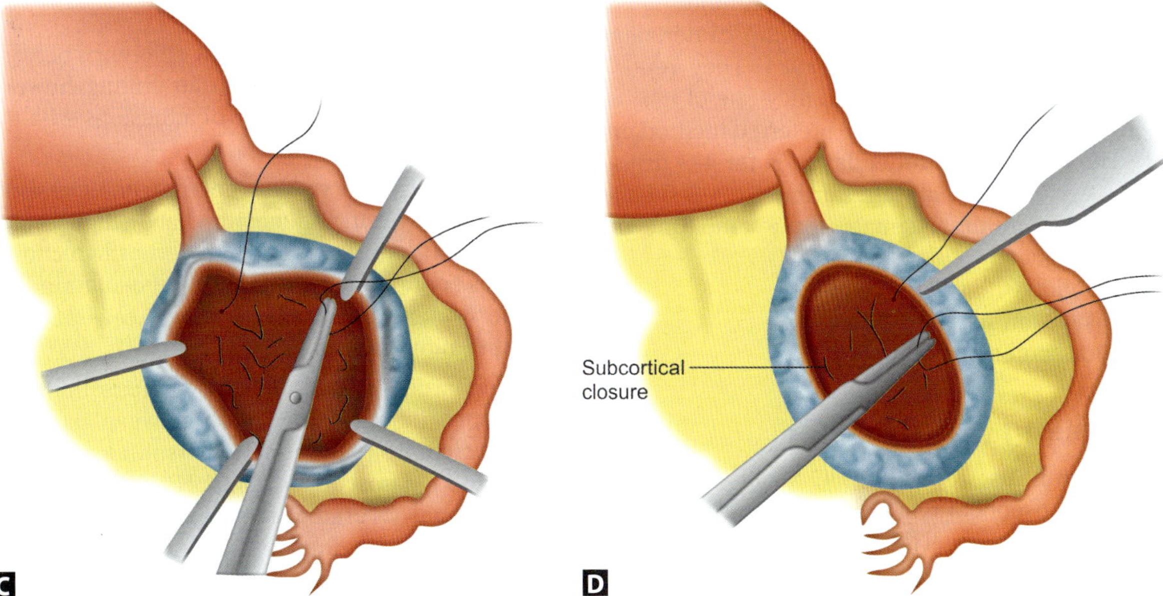

Figs 2C and D: Purse string and figure of 8 sutures to close the defect

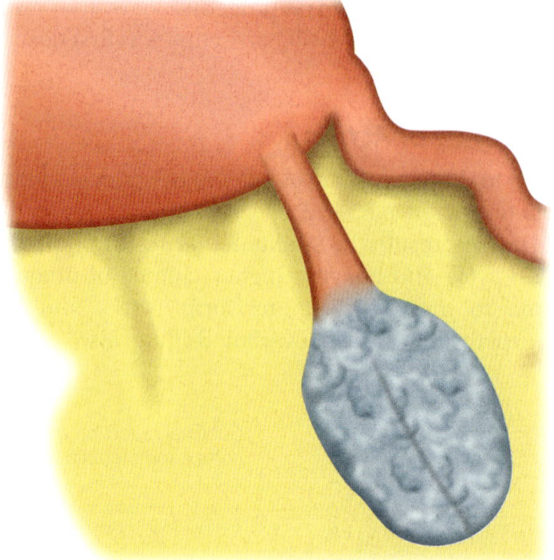

Fig. 2E: Ovarian surface approximated

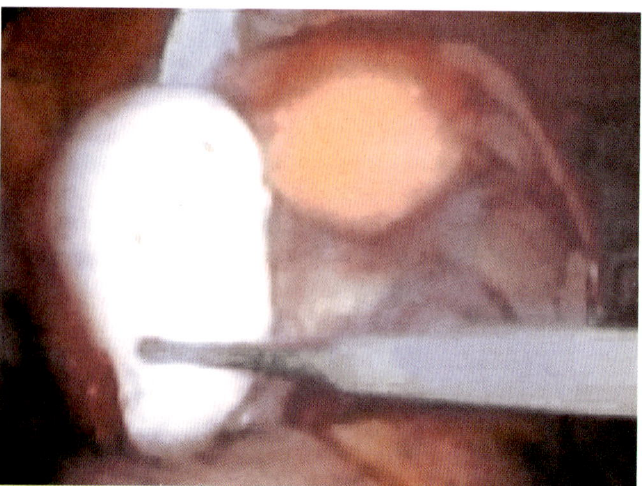

Fig. 3: Electrocautery for ovarian drilling

ovulatory cycles. Brian Cohen hypothesized that drainage of androgens and inhibins from surface follicles could reverse the excessive collagenization of overlaying ovarian cortex and facilitate softening of ovarian tunica. This may help the neighboring follicles to gain access to the surface and normally ovulate.

TECHNIQUES OF OVARIAN DRILLING (FIG. 3)

Electrocautary

a. Using biopsy forceps for ovarian biopsies. This resulted in pregnancy rate of 31.8% within a year time.
b. Multiple punctures using microelectro cauterization, as proposed by Gjonnaess, in 1984. They reported ovulation rate of 92% and pregnancy rate of 69% and abortion rate of 15%. This is the preferred method now.

   The current recommendation is for 4-5 drills in each ovary using 40-50 watts current for 4-5 seconds. This result in minimal damage at the same time gives similar pregnancy rates.
c. Cauterization with small scissors.
d. Slit incisions on surface of ovary.
e. Unilateral cauterization.

Laser Drilling (Fig. 4)

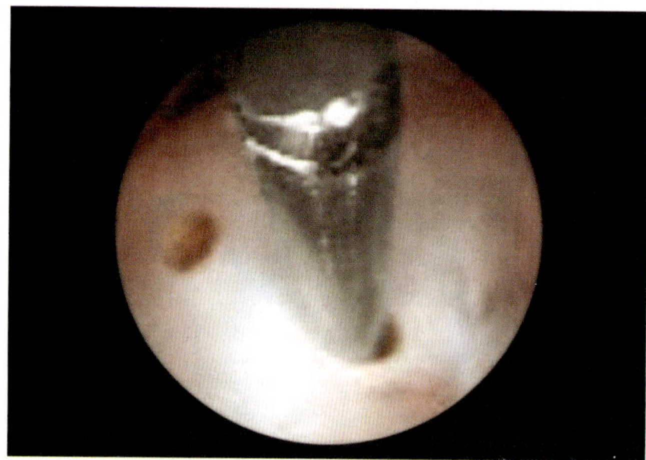

Fig. 4: Laser fiber for ovarian drilling

This has been in use for the last 15 years and different authors have used carbon dioxide (CO_2), argon and yttrium-aluminium-garnet (YAG) lasers. They recommend 5-8 drills, which are 5-10 mm long and 4 mm deep. By and large, there is no significant difference between using electrocautery or laser for ovarian drilling, however-some reports suggest a higher rate of adhesions with the use of lasers.

It is usually reserved for patients with CC resistance and seems to do well in patients who have a high level of serum androstendione. In general, whatever the technique used there is spontaneous resumption of ovulation in 50-70 % of the women and 50% of patients conceive after treatment within 6 months time.

Cocharne Database Review suggests that there is no difference in pregnancy rates between use of medical therapy [controlled ovarian hyperstimulation (COH) with ART] and laparoscopic drilling. However, since the result of meta-analysis of smaller group, larger multicentric trials are required. Also, there is a definite role in patients who has high androgen levels or has shown evidence of ovarian

Box 1 Laparoscopic ovarian drilling

Advantages

1. Eliminates risk of OHSS and multiple pregnancy.
2. Lowers the spontaneous abortion rates.
3. High ovulation and pregnancy rates.
4. Single treatment cycle can result in multiple ovulatory cycles.
5. Decreases the risk of extensive monitoring and high treatment cost using gonadotropins.
6. Lowers the overall cost of treatment.

Disadvntages

1. Need for surgery and anesthesia.
2. Non-permanent ovulatory effect.
3. Higher possibility of postoperative adhesions.
4. Rare cases, excessive use may induce premature ovrian failure.

Abbreviation: OHSS, ovarian hyperstimulation syndrome

hyperstimulation syndrome (OHSS) in previous cycles. Advantages and disadvantages are shown in Box 1.

Transvaginal Hydrolaparoscopy

Fernandez et al suggested use of transvaginal hydrolaparoscopy (THL) for ovarian drilling in clomiphene citrate (CC) resistant PCOS. Operative THL was performed using coaxial bipolar electrode for ovarian drilling in 13 patients. They reported no complications and 6 out of 13 patients started spontaneous ovulation and the remaining seven underwent induction of ovulation. Three spontaneous pregnancy and three after treatment cycles were reported, giving a cumulative pregnancy rate of 33% after THL and no miscarriages were reported. Though early results are promising, larger randomized controlled trial (RCT) are required for its effectiveness to be proven.

Complications of Laparoscopic Drilling

1. Complications of anesthesia
2. Periovarian adhesions
3. Premature ovarian failure due to excessive destruction of ovarian tissue

There are different studies, which quote the risk of adhesions for 0–100%, and this is primarily due to study bias. The average quoted evidence is 19.3%, which can be reduced to 16.5% by use of abdominal lavage.

The incidence of adhesions was higher after use of CO_2 laser as compared to electrocautery.

Ovarian drilling is the current surgical treatment of choice. It can be done laparoscopically by making small holes in the ovarian coating or capsule with a laser or cautery needle. In the first reported series, ovarian diathermy resulted in ovulation in 90% and conception in 70% of the 62 women treated. This shows that procedure yields the same positive effects as wedge resection while preserving much more of the ovarian tissue.

In some women ovulation resumes permanently, while others ovulate intermittently and then return to a state of anovulation. Some women don't respond at all. Hence, it is necessary to appropriately identify the subset of women who will benefit from the procedure.

CONCLUSION

Stein and Leventhal helped us understand the multiorgan dysfunction of the endocrine system, which we call as PCOS. Their management of such women with ovarian wedge biopsy/resection laid the foundation of managing the hyperandrogenemia in women with PCOS. The original procedure is no longer practiced due to the postoperative morbidity involved and is now replaced by minimally invasive method of laparoscopic ovarian drilling. Amongst all the laparoscopic methods suggested, using monopolar electrosurgical current is the most recommended method.

BIBLIOGRAPHY

1. Adashi EY, Rock JA Guzick D, et al. Fertility following bilateral ovarian wedge resection: A critical analysis of 90 consecutive cases of polycystic ovary syndrome. Fertil Steril. 1981;36:320-5.
2. Armar NA, Lachelin GC. Laparoscopic ovarian diathermy: An effective treatment for anti-oestrogen resistant anovulatory infertility on women with polycystic ovaries. BJOG. 1993;100: 161-4.
3. Armar NA, Mcgarrigle HH, Honour JW, et al. Laparoscopic ovarian diathermy in the management of anovulatory infertility in women with polycystic ovaries: Endocrine changes and clinical outcome. Fertil Steril. 1990;53:45-9.
4. Cohen J. Laparoscopic procedures for treatment of infertility related PCOS. Hum Reprod. Update. 1996;2: 337-44.
5. Daya S, et al. Fertil Steril. 1999, Cochrane Database Sys. 2000; 29(2).
6. Farhi J, Soule S, Jacobs H. Effect of laparoscopic ovarian electrocautery on ovarian response and outcome of treatment with gonadotrophins in clomiphenecitrate resistant patients with PCOS. Fertil Steril. 1995;64,930-5.
7. Fernandez H, Alby JD, Gervaise A, et al. Operative transvaginal hydrolaparoscopy for treatment of PCOS: A new minimally invasive surgery. Fertil Steril. 2001;75(3):607-11.

8. Gadir AA, Mowafi RS, Alnaser HM, et al. Ovarian electrocautery verus human menopausal gonadotrophins and pure follicle stimulating hormone therapy in the treatment of patients with polycystic ovarian disease. Clin Endocrinol (Oxf) 1990;33:585-92.
9. Gjonnaess H. Polycystic ovarian syndrome treated by ovarian electrocautery through the laparoscope. Fertil Steril 1984;41(1):20-5.
10. Gjonnaess H. The course and outcome of pregnancy after ovarian elecrocautery with PCOS: The influence of body weight. BJOG. 1989;96:714-9.
11. Goldzieher JW, Axelrod LR. Clinical and biochemical features of polycystic ovarian disease. Fertil Steril. 1963;14:631-53.
12. Halbe HW, da Fonseca AM, Silva P de P, et al. Stein-Leventhal syndrome. Am J Obstet Gynecol. 1972;114:280-1.
13. Heylen SM, Puttemans PJ, Brosens LH. Polycystic ovarian disease treated by laparoscopic argon laser capsule drilling: Comparison of vaporization versus perforation technique. Hum. Reprod. 1994;9:1038-42.
14. Kistner RW, Patton GW. Surgery of ovary. In: Atlas of infertility surgery. Boston, Little, Brown Book Group Ltd; 1975.177.
15. Naether OG, Fischer R, Weise HC, et al. Laparoscopic electrocoagulation of the ovarian surface in infertile patients with polycystic ovarian disease. Fertil Steril. 1993;60:88-94.
16. Naether OG, Fischer R. Adhesion formation after laparoscopic electrocoagulation of the ovarian surface in polycystic ovary patients. Fertil and Steril. 1993;60:95-9.
17. Naether OG. Significant reduction of adnexal adhesions following laparoscopic electrocautery of the ovarian surface by lavage and artificial ascites. Gynaecological Endoscopy 1995;4:17-9.
18. Palmer R, de Brux J. Résultants histologiques, biochemiques et thérapeutiques obtenus chez les femmes don't les ovaires avaient ite diagnostiques Stein-Leventhal a la coelioscopie. Bulletin Federation. Societies Gynaecology Obstetetris Languages Francais. 1967;19:405-12.
19. Predictive value of S. Androstenedione basal levels on the choice of therapy in CC resistant patients with PCOS. J. Gynae. Endocrinol. 2000;14(1):42-9.
20. Stein IF, Duration of fertility following ovarian wedge resection- Stein Leventhal syndrome. West J Surg Obstet Gynecol. 1964;78:124-7.
21. Stein IF, Leventhal ML. Amenorrhea associated with bilateral polycystic ovaries. Am J Obstet Gyne. 1935;29:181-91.
22. Stein IF. Duration of fertility following ovarian wedge resection—Stein-Leventhal syndrome. West JS Obstet Gynecol.1964;72:237-42.
23. Stein IF. Ultimate results of bilateral ovarian wedge resection: Twenty five years followup. Inter of fertility 1956;1:333-44.
24. Weinstein D, Polishuk W. The role of wedge resection of the ovary as a cause of mechanical sterlity. Surgery, Obstetrics and gynecology. 1975;141:417-8.

40.6 OVARIAN CYSTOSTOMY/CYSTECTOMY

Atul Munshi, Sujal Munshi

Ovarian cystectomy in simple terms is defined as removal of cyst without compromising the function of the ovary.

For this, the mass to be enucleated must have a capsule (characteristic of most benign tumor), except endometriotic cysts which needs to be separated from the ovary by sharp dissection.

Benign tumors amenable to these techniques are:

- Benign teratomas (dermoids)
- Serous cystadenomas
- Corpus luteum cysts
- Fibromas.

This modality of treatment is especially useful in following conditions:

a. Young females, where ovarian preservation is to be considered
b. Bilateral ovarian cysts, because if both ovaries removed, it may lead to premature climacterics.

Most ovarian surgeries are for benign disease and can be performed laparoscopically. The major advantages to laparoscopy over laparotomy are reductions in recovery time, hospital stay, cost and adhesion formation, which is particularly important in women in whom fertility is an issue.

A disadvantage of laparoscopic oophorectomy/cystectomy is the potential for spill of cancer cells if the mass is malignant. Unfortunately, neither preoperative clinical and sonographic evaluation nor the laparoscopic appearance of the ovary can reliably predict which masses are malignant. However, it is unlikely that an inadvertent laparoscopic procedure for ovarian cancer will be performed, if patients are carefully selected. Unsuspected ovarian cancer is found in only 0.04% of population.

Situations in which the traditional open method is safer and more appropriate than the laparoscopic approach are when the surgeon and/or assistants are not experienced in the use of an operative laparoscope, when there are dense adnexal adhesions, when the ovary is very large, or when there is a high suspicion of malignancy. Minilaparotomy is an alternative sandwiched approach. Anesthesia, GA/regional anesthesia, is sufficient for these procedures. Local or dissociants anesthesia is associated with difficulties of approach and surgery as ovaries are sensitive to pressure, squeeze and large cutting, tissue destruction.

LAPAROTOMY FOR OVARIAN CYSTECTOMY STEPS OF OPERATION

Abdominal Entry

- Transverse or the longitudinal incision will depend on the size of the ovarian cyst. If malignancy is suspected, vertical incision is preferred.

Exploration of the Abdomen

- Meticulously done, as for staging laparotomy
- Collection of free fluid, if already present or washings [100–200 mL normal saline (NS)] from the peritoneal cavity for cytology.

Extraction of the Enlarged Ovary

- If cyst is large, it is delivered from the wound
- If cyst is small and round ligament, and fallopian tubes are inaccessible easily due to adhesions, procedure is done with in abdomen using a self-retaining retractor to give adequate access.

Cystectomy (Figs 1A and B)

- An elliptical incision is made over the thin ovarian cortex in the axis of the ovary and over its most dependent area.
- After the initial incision, the back of the knife handle or scissors can be used to develop the plane between the cyst wall and the ovarian cortex to shell out the cyst while applying counter traction with an Allis clamp on the cortex. Occasionally, the base of the cyst is very adherent to the ovarian stroma and requires excision with scissors or electrocautery.
- Try to remove the cyst intact; however, if the cyst ruptures, take care to control the spill. This is achieved by packing the surrounding areas with surgical packs. If cyst ruptures the cavity should be copiously irrigated to decrease the risk of both pseudomyxoma peritonei and chemical peritonitis in rare cases.
- After removal of the cyst, the deep tissues of the ovary can be reapproximated or left open (if hemostasis is adequate). The ovarian cortex may appear thin but should not be trimmed because this may remove viable ovarian tissue.

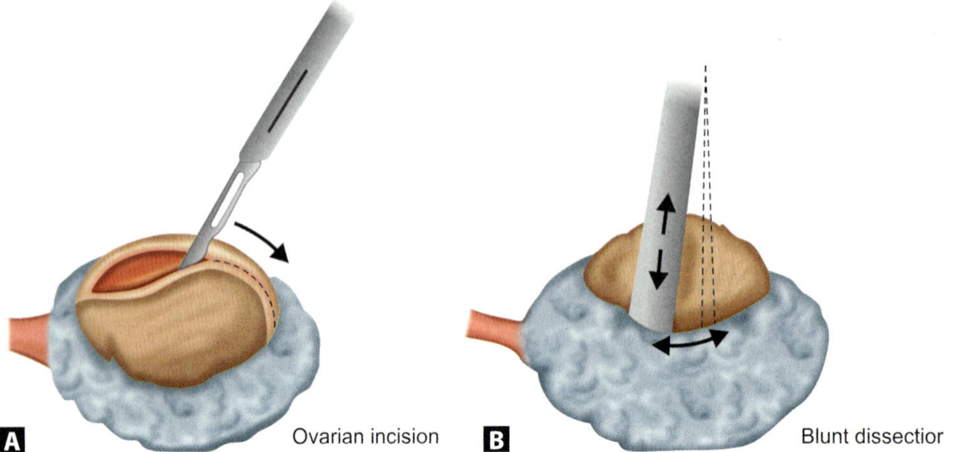

Figs 1A and B: Steps of cystectomy

- Make least number of incisions on the surface of the ovary if multiple cysts are present. An oophorectomy should not be performed even if a major portion of an ovary is removed. Pregnancies have been reported in women with less than 25% of one ovary remaining.

LAPAROSCOPIC OVARIAN CYSTECTOMY (FIGS 2 AND 3)

- A thorough inspection of the abdominal cavity and the ovarian cyst to visually confirm that there is no suspicion of malignancy
- Grasp the utero-ovarian ligament and stabilize the ovary
- The cyst may then be punctured with a 16–18 gauge needle or with cautery, and the cyst contents aspirated to control the contents of the cyst stall in abdominal cavity and to facilitate its removal (Fig. 2)
- The cystotomy is extended to allow introduction of a suction/irrigator and the cyst cavity is irrigated thoroughly. The cystotomy is then extended in the direction of the ovarian axis and the internal walls of the cyst are inspected
- Grasp the cyst wall and dissect it off the ovarian stroma with blunt or sharp dissection
- Incomplete areas of excision can be sharply excised or fulgurated to destroy the lining cells
- Some cysts/neoplasms can be resected and removed intact through a specimen bag or a minilaparotomy incision. The bags can be removed through a secondary trocar or through the infraumbilical trocar insertion site after the trocar has been removed
- If the cyst bed is hemostatic, it can be left to heal by secondary intention. Any suturing that is done should avoid the surface of the ovary. Cautery is also

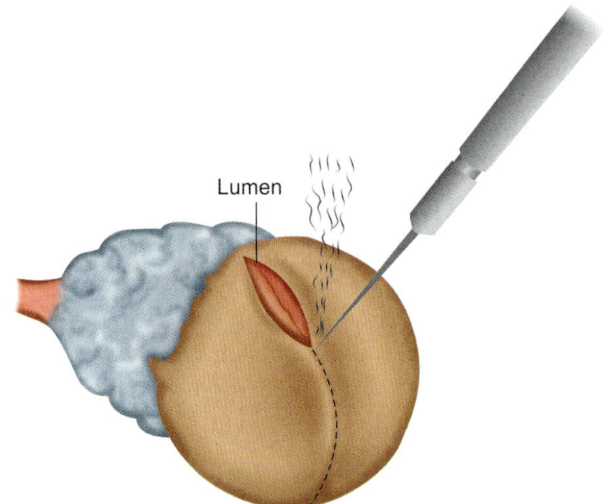

Fig. 2: Extension of cystostomy incision

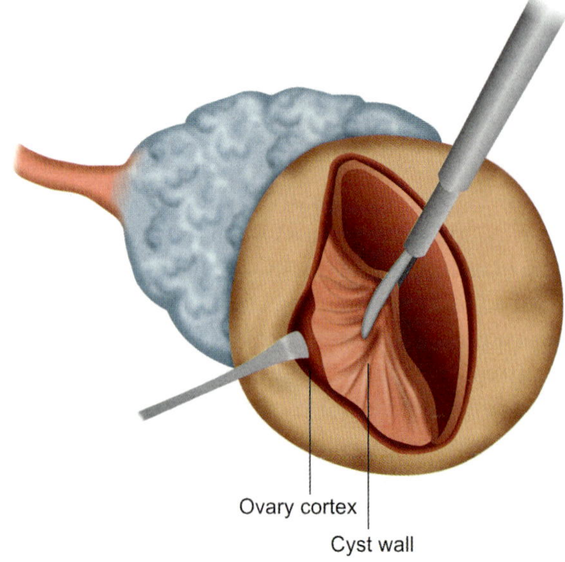

Fig. 3: Dissection of ovarian cyst wall

very effective for hemostasis, but should be kept to a minimum to reduce tissue destruction.

REMOVAL OF A RETROPERITONEAL CYST

- Majority of retroperitoneal cysts and broad ligament cysts are ovarian cysts and have grown retroperitoneally
- Occur after hysterectomy and ovarian conservation, where ovaries become retroperitoneal structures
- In such cases beware of the ureters. Exact position of ureter depends on size of cyst. So identify it in early procedure and follow it for full length of its course across cyst.

Dangers are Injuries to:

- Ureters
- Uterine vessels
- Hemorrhage, because anatomy is distorted.

Concern arises regarding spillage of malignant cells, stem from reports that are cited, cyst rupture as one of the factors that worsened the prognosis in early stage ovarian cancer, although this finding has been questioned by other studies.

BIBLIOGRAPHY

1. Dembo AJ, Davy M, Stenwig AE, et al. Prognostic factors in patients with stage I epithelial ovarian cancer. Obstet Gynecol. 1990;75:263-73.
2. Hulka JF, Parker WH, Surrey MW, et al. Management of ovarian masses. AAGL 1990 survey. J Reprod Med. 1992;37:599-602.
3. Sainz de la CR, Goff BA, Fuller AF, et al. Prognostic importance of intraoperative rupture of malignant ovarian epithelial neoplasms. Obstet Gynecol. 1994;84(1):1-7.
4. Sevelda P, Dittrich C, Salzer H. Prognostic value of the rupture of the capsule in stage I epithelial ovarian carcinoma. Gynecol Oncol. 1989;35:321-2.
5. Sjovall K, Nilsson B, Einhorn N. Different types of rupture of the tumor capsule and the impact on survival in early ovarian carcinoma. Int J Gynecol Cancer. 1994;4:333-6.
6. Webb MJ, Decker DG, Mussey E, et al. Factor influencing survival in stage I ovarian cancer. Am J Obstet Gynecol. 1973;116:222-8.

40.7 TUBAL RECANALIZATION

Parimala Devi

INTRODUCTION

Microsurgical techniques are used for tubal surgery and following are amenable for treatment.

Salpingo ovariolysis, fimbrioplasty, salpingostomy, tubotubal anastomosis, to repair intratubal disease or to reverse tubal sterilization.

As quoted by great surgeon Te Linde's words "microsurgical techniques have to be as simple as possible so that results will be reproducible not only by surgical. Virtuosi but also by all physicians who practice in this field."

Even though laparoscopic route is not much appreciated by many senior surgeons, but not to let this enthusiasm waste or neglect as some procedures by laparoscopy will definitely give better results, e.g. distal tube disease, release of adhesions.

In many cases conventional microsurgery was done without the aid of magnification. Recently, results are improved due to optical aids, discipline of surgery and therapy laser is still in infancy.

PRINCIPLES OF MICROSURGERY

The aim of microsurgery is to produce reconstruction of the anatomical relationships of the tubes and ovaries, with minimal damage to pelvic structures and peritoneum, to achieve healing without postoperative adhesion formation and to leave the patient with functional tube.

FOLLOWING ARE ESSENTIALS FOR SUCCESS OF SURGERY

- *Tissue wetting or irrigation*—tissues dry rapidly and this interferes with healing. To overcome this, constant irrigation is important, Ringers lactate/isotonic solution are commonly used.
- *Careful hemostasis*—intraperitoneal adhesions are usually the result of improper and incomplete hemostasis.
- *Instruments* like operating microscope, bipolar cautery, CO_2 laser play main role in attaining perfect hemostasis.
- *Peritoneal damage*—any small damage in peritoneum also can lead to adhesions, so proper closure is important.
- *Suture material*—tissue reaction from certain absorbable suture can give poor results, adequate care to be practiced in choosing the fine material.

INSTRUMENTS

Operating loupes and microscopes by ZEISS are ideal (Fig. 1).

Operating Microscope

Lower magnification units attached to spectacles can also be used for microsurgery. The magnification is 2-8X, field of view is restricted being 20-100 mm, it keeps changing with head movement, limits the use and many people find them inconvenient to use (Fig. 2).

Features of Operating Microscopes

- Microscopes, single or double headed, are much easier to use for tubal and pelvic microsurgery
- The basic unit with objective lens with focal length of 250-300 mm with a foot operator gives magnification changes of 2-30X, which covers adequately vision and view
- Beam splitter allows a variety of accessories to be attached, i.e. additional eye piece for observer

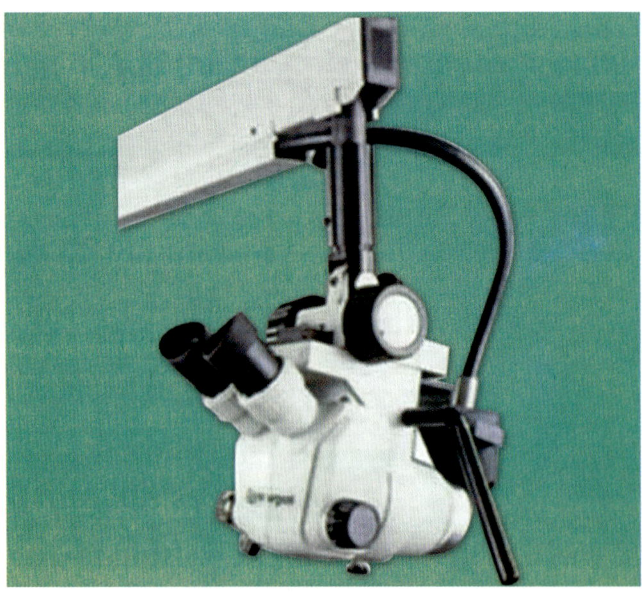

Fig. 1: Operating microscope

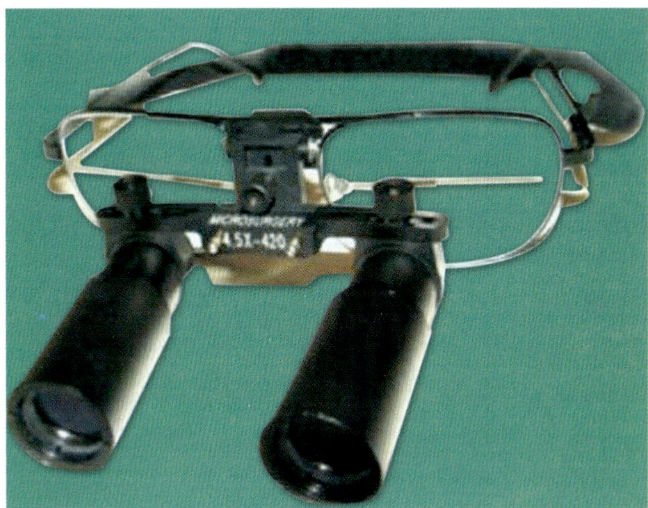

Fig. 2: Magnifying spectacles with 2–10× magnifaction

- Illumination is critical for good microsurgery and most modern microscopes have two cold light source
- The stand is critical part of microscope and modern stand is counterbalanced, easy-to-set and adjust and doesn't come in the way of surgeon.

Tubal Surgery is Traditionally Done by Laparotomy Route

Microsurgical tubal anastomosis has become the standard of care in tubal reapposition and repair in women who have had previous voluntary sterilization.

Laparoscopic or combined laparoscopic hysteroscopic techniques have been used for tubal anastomosis but results have been poor. Minilaparotomy has been an established technique for sterilization operations. It has also a role in ovarian cysts, ectopic pregnancy, hysterectomy and reversal of sterilization. We report the results of our patients in whom tubal surgery was performed by minilaparotomy incision.

METHODS FOR TUBAL PATENCY INVESTIGATIONS

The patency, course and function of the tubes can be, in part, assessed by the following methods:

Hysterosalpingography: A radiopaque substance, such as lipoidal, or a water-soluble medium, such as urograffin, is injected into the uterus through a cervical canula. Imaging of the uterine cavity and tubes is obtained by fluoroscopy and X-ray. The course and patency of the tube and potentially some peritubal adhesions can be assessed; the latter by intraperitoneal pooling of dye. Recently, sonography during intrauterine fluid instillation has been utilized to assess the uterine cavity. This method may also be applicable to assess tubal patency reliably, particularly as contrast agents which allow better visualization of tubal flow become more available.

Laparoscopy: Allows evaluation of the external tubal surface and peritubal pelvic adhesions, and by the addition of chromopertubation (the passage of colored dye), the patency of the tubes can be assessed. Additionally, the presence of a hydrosalpinx or tubal saccluations can be identified.

Salpingoscopy: Allows a panoramic view of the entire tubal mucosa, from the fimbria to the isthmus, and evaluation of intraluminal pathology. It may have a therapeutic role as well in lysing intratubal adhesions and/or treating other tubal pathology. Two types have been utilized in the past: the rigid and flexible salpingoscopes. Currently, narrow fibers are becoming available to allow viewing of the entire tube, thereby allowing examination of the cornual and isthmus segments which were not visible using rigid scopes. Currently, these devices are used in conjunction with laparoscopy or laparotomy to allow manipulation of the tube to facilitate passage of the scopes. If in the future it is possible to view the tubal lumen following transcervical passage without operative intervention, the clinical diagnostic value would increase dramatically.

It is always better to do hysterolaparoscopy to asses the uterine cavity and tubal ostia prior to surgery.

This will adequately give the information to surgeon, such as existing pelvic pathology, tubal status, the method to be followed.

COUNSELING AND CONTRAINDICATIONS

- Women age above 35 years to be made to understand about the lowered fertility and increased risk of fetal abnormality
- Past history of pelvic sepsis leading to frozen pelvis and difficulty in implementing surgery
- Unexpected male infertility and not amenable to treatment
- The low pregnancy rates associated with distal tubal disease may not be acceptable
- Strong motivation, coupled with complete understanding of the chances of success and the risks of tubal surgery, helps to reach the sensible decision by couples.

CONTRAINDICATIONS

1. Serious metabolic disease contraindicating pregnancy, such as advanced renal hepatic, cardiac diseases

2. Pelvic tuberculosis
3. Frozen pelvis
4. Active PID.

Relative Contraindications

Tubal Destruction Following Sterilization

- Less than 5 cm of tubal length is nonfunctional for ovum transport even though corrected by surgery
- Age—35–38 years of patient requires detailed counseling regarding limited outcome
- Previous surgery, i.e. microsurgery
- To save the marriage, many women undergo the surgery, proper and compassionate counseling is important in these cases.

PREOPERATIVE EVALUATION OF COUPLES

- Routine blood hemogram
- X-ray chest to rule out tuberculosis
- Husband's semen analysis, it is utter blunder and unpardanable mistake on the part of the surgeon to do tuboplasty without confirmed good semen report
- Endometrial biopsy for pathalogy for excluding endometrial tuberculosis
- Hysterosalpingogram or laparoscopy with chromotubation to confirm the blocked tubes and to delineate blockade.

STEPS OF OPERATION

- All patients are given GA
- Bladder catheterization performed
- Another number 14 Foley catheter was inserted into the uterine cavity and the bulb inflated
- The catheter slightly withdrawn so that the inflated bulb could get fixed at endocervix thus blocking the cervix completely to avoid any leak
- The end of this catheter was left near the abdominal incision covered in sterile drapper
- The abdomen opened by a 4–6 cm suprapubic transverse incision in the skin and opening the abdomen using Cohen's technique
- The fundus of the uterus is exteriorized using two fingers of right hand and one fallopian tube was exposed, at a time for tubal recanalization
- Atraumatic uterine holding clamp was used to exteriorize the uterus by some surgeons, while performing recanalization or tuboplasty. Whole procedure of recanalization or tuboplasty was virtually performed outside the abdominal cavity (Fig. 3).

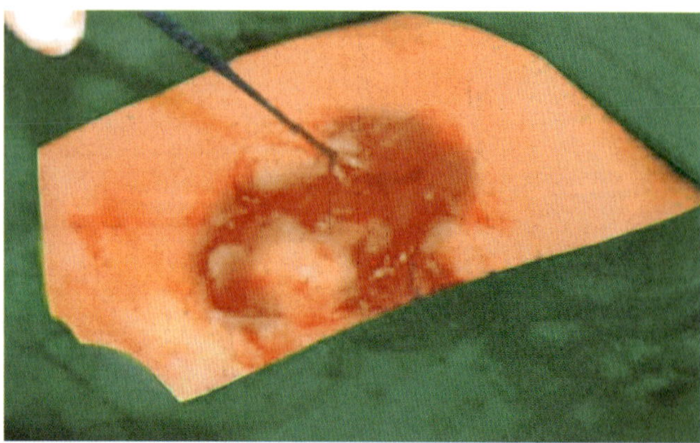

Fig. 3: Recanalization being performed on an exteriorized fallopian tube

No Packs or Retractors Used

- Uterine holding clamp was not used by us at all, in our experience, keeping in view the injury to uterus, exteriorization of uterus was done only with hands of assistant
- The surgical field irrigated intermittently with heparinized Ringer lactate solution/plain normal saline
- The blocked segment of the fallopian tube was excised using scissors
- The dye (methylene blue) injected through intrauterine Foley catheter until it was seen coming out through the medial cut segment of the tube
- Fine epidural catheter inserted through the fimbrial end of the tube and then through the medial segment of the tube into the uterine cavity to facilitate recanalization
- Prolene no 1/0 can also be used as cost-effective material, used as guide to pass through the tube
- The muscularis of the tube stitched together using interrupted 6-0 polyglactin (vicryl) suture with magnification
- The serosa and mesosalpinx stitched with interrupted 5-0 polyglactin (vicryl) suture
- Uterus and fallopian tube were positioned back into the peritoneal cavity
- The epidural catheter is gently pulled out
- The same procedure is repeated on the other fallopian tube after exteriorizing the fallopian tube
- Patency of the tubes was confirmed by injecting dye through the intrauterine Foley catheter which can be seen oozing out through the fimbral end
- The uterus and the tube are then gently pushed back into the pelvis
- Visceral or parietal peritoneum, not stitched
- Rectus sheath was closed using continuous 1-0 polyglycolic (vicryl) suture and the same suture continued as subcuticular skin suture
- Subcutaneous local anesthetic was infiltrated at incision site.

Sedbon et al has devised his own uterine holding clamp to exteriorize the uterus during the procedure. The standard technique of tubal recanalization is by conventional laparotomy as laparoscopic and hysteroscopic techniques for it have not been very successful. Thus, Sedbon et al in their report of 5 cases using fibrin glue had no pregnancies, while Reich in his attempt over 20 anastomosis done by laparoscopic tubal reversal found only two subsequent term pregnancies and three ectopic pregnancies. Dyer and Tregoning performed laparoscopic reconstructive tubal surgery over 177 cases of infertility in a tertiary referral center in South Africa and observed a pregnancy rate of 13.6% with a live birth rate of 9% and ectopic pregnancy rate of 3.4%. They attributed this poor outcome to severity of tubal damage in their population due to mechanical obstruction. Slowely and Coddinton in their comparison of outpatient and inpatient minilaparotomy microsurgical reanastomosis found equal pregnancy rates and outcome in the two groups.

However, Daniell and McTavish performed combined approach of laparoscopy and minilaparotomy and found it to be both safe and cost effective with pregnancy rate of 60%. They could accomplish it as day case procedure. Their complication rate was very low, mostly as a result of good microsurgical techniques, meticulous hemostasis, perioperative antibiotics and early ambulation and discharge from hospital.

With microsurgery, an overall 30–40% pregnancy rate is achieved.

Pregnancy Outcome

- Intrauterine pregnancy (96.66%)
- Ectopic pregnancy (3.33%)
- Term viable pregnancy (96.55%)
- Spontaneous abortion (3.45%).

Incising the Adhesions

- Microsurgery combined with clear visualization and removal of each layer of adhesion is the key to this surgical procedure.
- The adhesions are carefully removed, systematically clearing the pelvis, freeing both fallopian tubes and ovaries, and clearing fimbriae.
- Finally the surface of ovary is cleared with diathermy. Any spots of diathermy are cauterized.
- Laser vaporization of endometrioma and microsuturing of capsule with 6-0 nylon will prevent recurrences of adhesions.
- Common sites of ovarian adhesion are inferior part of ovary to broad ligament.
- Midtubal adhesions will fix the ovary to tube, and on left side adhesions more commonly, will occur to the intestine.
- After removal of adhesions, tubes are tested for chromo tubation and routine postoperative care instituted.
- Pregnancy rates up to 65% are reported.

FIMBRIOPLASTY

This operation is used when there has been distortion of fimbriae by adhesions or partial closure of the fimbriated end of the tube.

Releasing the Fimbriae

- In early stages, 2 or 3 folds of fimbriae are agglutinated and all that is required is dissection down the line of the fused fold using diathermy or laser
- Occasionally, one or two stay sutures are required with 8-0 nylon. Operating microscope is useful in dissection
- Staining the fimbrial folds with 1/1000 methylene blue often helps in identifying normal fimbrial tissues and direction of fimbrial folds.

Salpingostomy/Salpingoneostomy

Salpingostomy/salpingoneostomy means creation of new tubal stroma.

Much has been written about surgery of distal tubal disease and efforts to increase the pregnancy rates.

Technique

Principles of the Procedure

Removal of periampullary and pelvic adhesions—the objective here is to free the tube and restore the mobility to increase the spontaneous ovum pick-up.

FREEING THE TUBE FROM OVARY

Often the distal tube and fimbriae turned down and are adherent to ovary.

Methylene blue via cervical cannula helps in distention of tubes and dissection of rigid, distended tube is more easy.

As much tubal tissue as possible should be conserved.

CREATION OF NEW STOMA

Once you have freed the fimbrial end a small dimple will be seen indicating old ostium. With the tube distended, an opening is made into the hydrosalpinx at the site of the dimple with low power cutting diathermy.

Fimbrial folds of hydrosalpinx are cut linearly and not across.

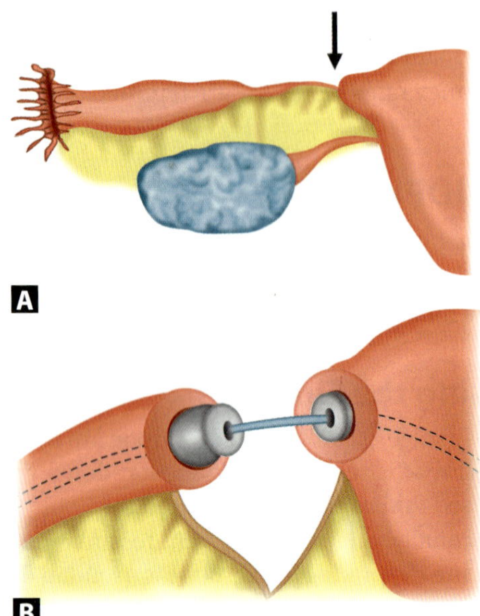

Figs 4A and B: Diagrammatic representation of nylon cannula position at both ends of cut tubal ends

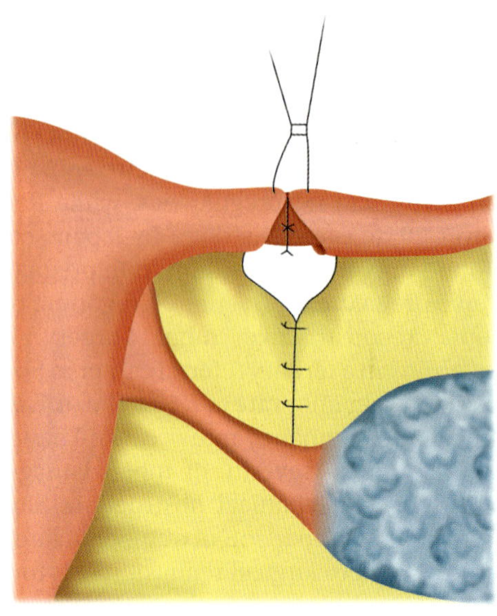

Fig. 5: Diagrammatic representation of suturing of stoma's created

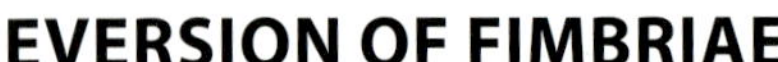

EVERSION OF FIMBRIAE

After control of bleeding either with bipolar or laser the edges of stroma are everted. Traditionally, this is carried out by stay sutures of nylon. One must avoid excessive eversion, as it results in impaired blood supply.

Care to be exercised to restore the relation of ovary to tubes to help ovum pick up.

VARIATION IN TECHNIQUE

Linear Salpingostomy (Figs 4 and 5)

When distal portion of tube has been excised, e.g. after ectopic pregnancy, then diameter of tubal lumen is reduced and there are no fimbriae.

To try and create a "spoon" to collect ovum, the tube is opened laterally for 5-8 mm.

Using the glass rod to protect the tube, incision is made with laser/knife hemostasis is achieved and then few sutures with 8-0 nylon are put to evert the edges of tube to create a spoon end.

Prognosis for this surgery is poor and often need intravenous fluid (IVF) procedure to help achieve pregnancy and secondary closure of linear salpingostomy is a common complication.

PROSTHETIC DEVICES

Studies with tubal splints left in for several weeks postoperatively have been shown to damage the lining of the tube.

Intraoperative splints are recommended but to be removed after 96 hours of surgery.

Table 1: Comparison of various types of surgery and outcome

Type of surgery	Medical terminology	Pregnancy rate	Tubal pregnancy rate
Reconstruct damaged end of tube	Fimbrioplasty	50% over 1–2 years	12% of pregnancies
Cut away scar tissue on tubes or ovary	Salpingolysis ovariolysis	45% over 1–2 years	6% of pregnancies
Make opening in blocked tube	Neosalpingostomy	25% over 1–2 years	25% of pregnancies
Reconnect tubes after tubal ligation	Tubal reanastomosis	50-70% over 1–2 years	4–15% of pregnancies
In vitro fertilization (for comparison)	IVF	50–60% per attempt at our clinic (age < 35, blocked tubes) Our IVF pregnancy rates	1–5% of pregnancies (women with blocked tubes)

Abbreviation: IVF, intravenous fluid

CONCLUSION

The important factors for determining the success of operation were age of the patient, time interval between sterilization and reversal, site of ligation, method used for previous ligation, and the remaining length of the tube after recanalization.

The microsurgical technique should be available at specialized centers to improve the success of reversal surgery. Complications for pregnancy was 41.6% in recanalization group and 20% in tuboplasty group.

The ectopic pregnancy rate was 8.33%. The lower pregnancy rate complications was possibly due to follow-up (some cases were done in last few months only) and non-availability of operating microscope in most hospital. The patients requiring tuboplasty had pathological tubes and high incidence of pelvic infections and tuberculosis, which is responsible for poor pregnancy rate in this group. Low pregnancy rate in tuboplasty were also observed by Dyer and Tregoning due to infection in their population. The pregnancy rate of the present series is almost equal to that after laparotomy in our hospital (mean pregnancy rate 45% in open laparotomy recanalization: unpublished data).

According to published studies, approximate pregnancy rates by 12 months after tubal surgery are shown as in Table 1. These numbers are average figures from a group of women that have had pervious tubal surgery. In real life, each case is unique and should be assessed individually.

The surgeon's approach to adhesions has changed dramatically since the use of microsurgery and operative microscopy.

BIBLIOGRAPHY

1. Bluementhal PD. Laparoscopic sterilization in the supine position using the Ramathibodi uterine manipulator. Fertil Steril. 1995;64:204-7.
2. Daniell JF, McTavish G. Combined laparoscopy and minilaparotomy for outpatient reversal of tubal sterilization. South Med J. 1995;88:914-6.
3. Dyer SJ, Tregoning SK. Laparoscopic reconstructive tubal surgery in a tertiary referral centre. A review of 177 cases. S Afr Med J. 2000;90:1015-9.
4. Flynn M, Niloff JM. Minilaparotomy for the ambulatory management of ovarian cysts. Am J Obstet Gynecol. 1995;173: 1727-30.
5. Hoffman MS, Lynch CM. Minilaparotomy hysterectomy. Am J Obstet Gynecol. 1998;179:316-20.
6. Reich H. Laparoscopic reversal of sterilization (abstract). Second world congress of gynecologic endoscopy. Clermont-Ferrand, France, 1989. pp. 5-8.
7. Ruminjo JK, Lynam PF. A fifteen year review of female sterilization by minilaparotomy under local anesthesia in Kenya. Contraception. 1997;55:249-60.
8. Sedbon E, Delajolinieres JB, Boudouris O, et al. Tubal desterilisation through exclusive laparoscopy. Hum Reprod. 1989;4:158-9.
9. Sharma JB. Minilaparotomy abdominal hysterectomy: A new surgical technique. Obstet Gynecol Commun. 1999;5:28-31.
10. Stovall G, Summitt RL, Bran DF, et al. Outpatient vaginal hysterectomy: A pilot study. Obstet Gynecol. 1992;80:145-9.
11. Tsin D, Mahmood D. Laparoscopic and hysteroscopic approach for tubal anastomosis. J Laparoendosc Surg. 1993;3:63-6.

CHAPTER

41 Uterus

Rajyashri Sharma, Zehra Mohsin, CN Purandare, Madhuri A Patel, Atul Munshi, Sujal Munshi
Harshad Parasnis, SS Sheth, Michael Stark, Sandro Gerli, Gian Carlo Di Renzo, PB PaiDhungat,
GN Allahbadia, Rajalaxmi Walavalkar, Nikhil Purandare, DK Tank, JD Tank , NS Sreedevi

41.1 SURGICAL METHODS OF ABORTION—DILATATION AND CURETTAGE OR EVACUATION

Rajyashri Sharma, Zehra Mohsin

INTRODUCTION

The lack of availability and acceptability of the various contraceptives is resulting in millions of unwanted pregnancies in our country. The spontaneous abortion rate is about 15–20%. The large number of spontaneous and induced abortions make uterine evacuation, the most commonly used procedure. Besides the above indications, it is also used as a diagnostic and therapeutic modality in abnormal uterine bleeding.

The first recorded evidence of abortion is from a Chinese document describing abortions in Royal concubines, where mercury was used to induce abortions about 5,000 years ago. Hippocrates whose famous oath forbid abortions, in his writings describe instruments used to dilate the cervix and curette the uterine cavity. Tertullian, a second century theologian has also described instruments used for procedures similar to dilatation and evacuation. In the middle ages, techniques like abdominal massage were used to induce abortions. Japanese records show methods of induced abortion from as early as the 12th century. Medicine as a discipline since 19th century saw many advances in the field of surgery but physicians in West lobbied for ban on abortion. The Comstock Law (1873) was passed in the USA which prohibited mailing or distribution of information on birth control and abortion, despite women in most parts of the world, dying because of illegal abortions. In 1920, Lenin legalized all abortions in the Soviet Union.

In India, the Medical Termination of Pregnancy (MTP) Act was passed in August 1971 and came into effect from April 1972, which legalized abortions up to 20 week of pregnancy in India. It extends to the whole of India except the state of Jammu and Kashmir. MTP act has laid down guidelines for performing abortions, which are:

- The pregnancy can be terminated by a Registered Medical Practitioner where the length of pregnancy is less than 12 weeks. For pregnancy between 12 weeks and 20 weeks, termination can be done if at least two Registered Medical Practitioners approve of it in good faith
- Pregnancy can be terminated only on the grounds:
  - Medical ground i.e. continuation of pregnancy will endanger the physical or mental health of the mother
  - Eugenic cause i.e. following detection of an abnormal fetus
  - Social cause i.e. if pregnancy is as a result of rape
  - Failure of contraception
- The place for performing the procedure should be:
  - A hospital established or maintained by the government
  - A place approved for this purpose by the government or a district level committee constituted by the government with the chief medical officer as the chairperson.

PREOPERATIVE PREPARATION AND TESTS

Counseling the woman to enable her to make a free and fully informed decision is the most important aspect of the preoperative procedure. The woman needs to be given information regarding issues like the procedure, anesthesia options, pre- and postoperative care and the associated risks. The preoperative workup includes: history of medical disease and drug allergy, e.g. asthma, diabetes.

Simple investigations like hemoglobin (Hb) estimation, urine analysis, blood group and Rhesus (Rh) typing may be done. In elderly patients or in cases where general anesthesia (GA) is to be given, blood sugar, random renal function tests and electrocardiography (ECG) and chest X-ray may be required. The patient should be kept nil orally for at least a period of 6 hours prior to the procedure. A sedative may be given the night before the procedure to alleviate anxiety.

Cervical priming using 400 µg of vaginal or oral misoprostol, 3–4 hours before the procedure is helpful. EI Rafaey et al. have used a higher dose of 600 µg for the same, but a dose of 400 µg appears to be optimal.

Hygroscopic cervical dilators are also used by many for cervical priming. Laminaria tent, a rod made from the seaweed *Laminaria digitata* absorbs fluid from the cervical tissue and swells to mechanically dilate the cervix gradually. It also causes release of prostaglandins which aid in cervical priming. These have to be inserted 4–6 hours before the procedure. The other osmotic dilators are (not available in India):

- Lamicel: This is a cylindrical rod of polyvinyl alcohol sponge impregnated with $MgSO_4$. The advantages of using this are its uniform diameter and hence ease of application and it does not assume the hourglass shape (like Laminaria tent) and so can be easily removed
- Dilapan is a hydrophilic polymer rod which has to be inserted 4 hours before the procedure for effect. The advantage of using these hygroscopic dilators is that they prevent or reduce the risk of cervical trauma. An informed consent signed by the patient or a guardian (in case of a minor or lunatic) is mandatory.

Anesthesia

The options available are:

Paracervical Block

In case, since 1925, many surgeons prefer a paracervical block to avoid complications associated with GA.

Procedure

- 20 mL of 0.5% lignocaine is used (after insuring that there is no known allergy to lignocaine)
- 1 mL of the solution is injected into the anterior lip (12 O'clock position) before using a vulsellum to grasp the cervix
- The area between the smooth cervical epithelium and vaginal tissue is identified and 2 mL of the solution is injected at 3, 5, 7 and 9 O'clock positions. Optional injection sites are 2 and 10 O'clock positions. The needle should go about 3 mm deep into the tissue, and if correctly positioned a swelling and blanching of the tissue can be noted after the injection. Always aspirate before injecting to be sure one is not into a vessel. Wait for 2 minutes before starting the procedure.

Complications

- Injection into a vessel can lead to hematoma formation, anaphylactic shock and even death.

Ketamine Anesthesia

Safe anesthetic, if one is not experienced. This is preferably used in patients of hypovolemia as it increases arterial blood pressure (BP), heart rate and cardiac output. For the same reason, it should be avoided in patients with coronary artery disease (CAD), hypertension, congestive heart failure (CHF), etc. Ketamine is a potent bronchodilator and therefore, a good agent for asthmatics.

- Atropine sulfate/glycopyrrolate, 0.6/0.3 mg intramuscular (IM) is given half an hour before surgery
- Diazepam, 10 mg intravenous (IV) at the time of induction prevents hallucinations
- Monitor vital signs during the procedure and then every 15 minutes till the woman is fully awake
- Ketamine may be given IM, IV or as an infusion. IM dose is 6–10 mg/kg body weight. Anesthesia is reached within 10 minutes and lasts up to 30 minutes
- The IV dose is 1–2 mg/kg given slowly over 2 minutes and the action lasts for 15 minutes.

Complications

- Unpleasant dreams and hallucination may last as long as 24 hours.

Short General Anesthesia

Good for those who are very apprehensive? Anesthesia may be induced with an IV induction agent, with or without a short-acting opioid and maintained via a face mask or laryngeal mask apparatus. Adequate depth of anesthesia is required before cervical dilatation, as vagal stimulation in an inadequately anesthetized patient may lead to bradycardia and laryngospasm.

PROCEDURES

The surgical methods of first trimester abortion are:

Suction and Evacuation

This is still a widely practiced method today. Bladder has to be emptied before the procedure. Shaving the perineum is not required. The vagina is cleaned by either using povidone-iodine or chlorhexidine solution.

After cleaning, a bimanual examination is done to ascertain the size and the position of the uterus.

The anterior cervical lip is held using a vulsellum or tenaculum after the cervix has been exposed using a vaginal speculum (e.g. Sims). Uterine sound is used to delineate direction of uterine cavity (Fig. 1A).

The cervix is then dilated using a metal or plastic dilator. A variety of dilators are available—Hawkin Amber, Hegar, Pratt, or Hanks types of dilators (Fig. 1B). These dilators have to be held in a pen holding fashion and undue force should not be applied. Dilatation is started using the smaller dilators in the set and gradually the larger dilators are used one after the other. The cervix should be dilated approximately 0.5–1 mm more than the size of the suction cannula to be used to allow adequate mobility of the cannula. This is not necessary when an osmotic dilator has been used.

A plastic cannula (Karman's) is then inserted into the uterine cavity (Fig. 1C). The size of the cannula chosen should correspond to the gestational age in weeks, for instance, a 6 mm cannula is chosen for a 6 week pregnancy. The clinician then connects the cannula to a suction machine generating pressure equivalent to 60–70 mm Hg.

The cannula is then rotated at an angle of 360° and moved back 1–2 cm and forth till the entire interior has been evacuated. Evacuation is said to be complete when:

- No more contents are seen coming through the cannula
- The bleeding stops and air bubbles appear in the cannula
- The uterine cavity feels gritty.

Once the procedure is complete, the suction is disconnected and the cannula removed. Many clinicians prefer to use a sharp curette to confirm the completeness of the procedure. Methergin, 0.25 mg, IM may be administered after the procedure.

Examination of the aspirated tissue is mandatory. The clinician must confirm the presence of chorionic villi in the aspirated tissue. Absence of chorionic tissue may indicate an ectopic pregnancy and re-evaluation may be required using other diagnostic modalities, e.g. an ultrasound.

Monitoring the patient is vital and blood loss is an important aspect of postoperative care. Pain relief may be given by using analgesics.

Dilatation and Curettage

The second most common method of first trimester abortion is dilatation and curettage. It is also used for obtaining endometrium for diagnostic evaluation, and is at times therapeutic in cases of dysfunctional uterine bleeding and certain types of spontaneous abortion.

After a bimanual examination at the beginning of the procedure, the cervix is held and dilated by mechanical dilators as previously described. Osmotic dilators may alternatively be used.

After dilatation, a curette is introduced and the cavity is evacuated. Up to 10 weeks, after an initial curettage, the products of conception may be removed using ovum forceps. In later pregnancies, ovum forceps are used first to extract the products followed by a careful curettage evacuation. Blood loss is more with curette as compared to suction evacuation.

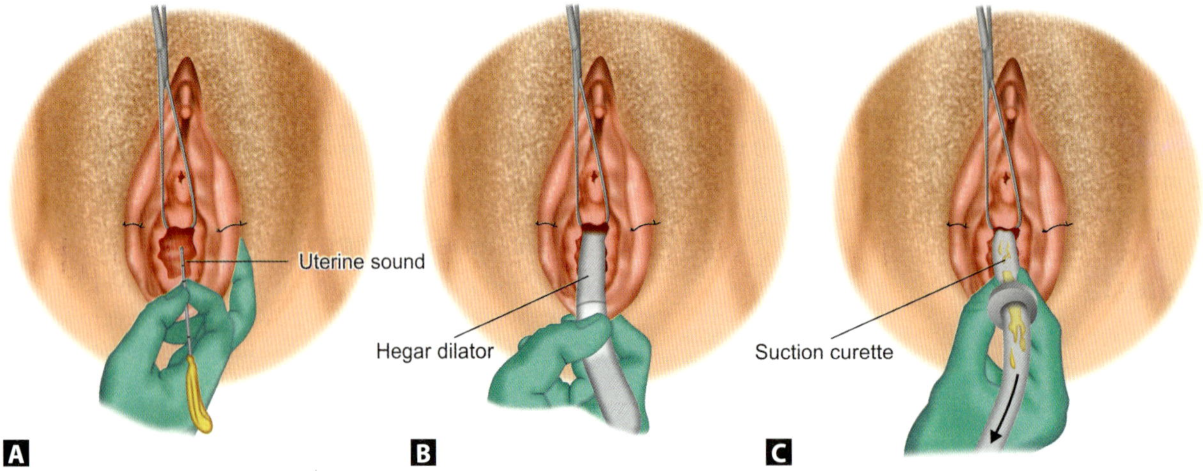

Figs 1A to C: Steps of suction and evacuation: (A) Uterine sound for direction of uterine cavity; (B) Graduated Hegar's dilator used for cervical dilation; (C) Suction of uterine cavity done with Karmen's plastic cannula

Manual Vacuum Aspiration

This is a simple procedure performed by a hand held syringe as a source of suction for removal of the products of conception. World Health Organization (WHO) recommends it as a procedure of choice before 10 weeks. It can be used successfully in 99.5% of cases and carries a minor complication rate of 0.01%. The procedure has the advantages of being short and easy to perform, even in a low resource setting.

Complications

Every woman is advised to report when she has:

- Prolonged cramping
- Prolonged bleeding (> 2 weeks)
- Bleeding more than normal menstruation
- Severe pain
- Fainting
- Fever.

The complications of the procedures have an incidence of 0.5–4.7%. These are:

Perforation

This is suspected when the instrument seems to extend beyond the uterine cavity or there is fat or bowel loop pulled out by the operator.

- If evacuation is complete and there is a small perforation, it heals spontaneously but the patient has to be observed for sometime for signs of hypovolemia. Administer oxytocics (Methergin 0.2–0.5 mg IM) and antibiotics. If intraperitoneal bleeding is suspected, a laparotomy may be required
- If evacuation is not complete, complete the procedure under direct vision either using a laparoscope to visualize the peritoneal cavity during the procedures or a laparotomy
- Administer antibiotics and oxytocics postoperatively
- Bowel injury would require repair or resection and anastomosis depending upon the extent of injury
- In cases of extensive uterine perforation and lacerations hysterectomy may be necessary.

Cervical Lacerations

These are uncommon and should be repaired, if results in excessive vaginal bleeding.

Infection

The risk of infection is around 1.5–4.8%. Treatment may be simple by giving broad spectrum antibiotics along with evacuation of the uterine cavity if the abortion is incomplete.

Serious infections like septic shock have to be managed aggressively by IV antibiotics, fluid management and O_2 at the rate 6–8 liters/minute. Laparotomy is indicated in cases of peritonitis. Suspect gas gangrene if pelvic tissues show gas on X-ray. In such cases, hysterectomy may be necessary.

Incomplete Evacuation

The patient usually presents with prolonged bleeding and the uterine contents will then have to be re-evacuated under antibiotic coverage.

Hypotension

This may be seen due to excessive blood loss, a vasovagal response to pain or following an allergic reaction due to xylocaine sensitivity. Management would be administration of IV fluids and O_2 corticosteroids and whole blood transfusion.

Minor Complications

Postoperative nausea and vomiting has to be managed by antiemetics like metoclopramide or ondansetron. Postoperative pain has to be controlled by available analgesics. Rectal pessary insertion of diclofenac sodium is a good option.

Continuation of Pregnancy

The incidence has been reported around 0.5%. This is usually seen when the procedure is performed very early and fails to suck out the products of conception. It may also result in patients with a uterine anomaly, e.g. uterus didelphys or bicornuate uterus or an ectopic pregnancy. This can be avoided by not doing the procedure very early, the ideal time is between 7 weeks and 10 weeks. Checking the aspirated products will confirm full evacuation.

Delayed Complications

- *Asherman's syndrome* may be managed by hysteroscopic resection of intrauterine adhesions or uterine sounding to break the adhesions followed by insertion of an intrauterine contraceptive device (IUCD) or a number 8 Foley catheter to keep the walls apart. This is followed by combined oral contraceptive (OC) pills given for 2–3 cycles
- *Cervix incompetence* in subsequent pregnancy is managed by cerclage.

The above complications may be avoided by a good history and correct estimation of gestational age following a bimanual examination

- Cervical priming either using prostaglandins or osmotic dilators
- Use of aseptic technique to avoid infections, morbidity.

The mortality due to the procedure is reported to be around 4–6 per 100,000 procedures.

BIBLIOGRAPHY

1. Benson J, Grimes DA, Singh S, et al. Clinical Management of Abortion Complications: A Practical Guide. WHO; 1994.
2. Carbonell JL, Velazco A, Rodriguez Y, et al. Oral versus vaginal misoprostol for cervical priming in first trimester abortion: A randomized trial. Eur J Contracept Rerod Health Care. 2001;6(3):134-40.
3. DA Grimes, IG Ray, CJ Midddleton. Lamicel versus Laminaria for cervical dilation before early second trimester abortion: A randomized clinical trial. Obstet Gynaecol. 1987;69:887-90.
4. El Refaey, Calder T, Wheatley DN, et al. Cervical priming with prostaglandin E1 analogues. Lancet. 1994;343:1207-9.
5. Glenc F. Induced abortion: A historical outline. Pol Tyg Lek. 1974;29(45):1957-8.
6. Government of India. The Medical Termination of Pregnancy Act, 1971 (Act No. 34 of 1971).
7. Grimes DA. Management of Abortion. In: TeLinde's Operative Gynecology. Philadelphia: Lippincot Williams and Wiliams; 1997. p. 8.
8. Holmes P. Tertullian (n.d.): A treatise on the soul. 2006.
9. Li J, Green SM. Anaesthesia and Pain Management. In: van Rooyen M (Ed). Field Medicine: A practical guide for the developing world. New York: McGraw Hill Inc, 2002.
10. Mathai M, Sanghvi H, Guidotti RJ. Paracervical block in MCPC (P1). WHO. 2000.
11. Nonvolatile Anesthetic Agents. In: Morgan GE, Mikhail MS, Murray MJ (Eds). Clinical Anesthesiology, 4th edition. New York, NY: McGraw-Hill; 2006. p. 4.
12. Palaniappan B. Major and minor complications of 1st trimester MTP. In: Manual of MTP. FOGSI, 1988.
13. PD Blumenthal. Prospective comparison of Dilapan and laminaria for pretreatment of cervix in second trimester induction abortion. Obstet Gynaecol. 1988;72:243-6.
14. Unsafe abortion: A worldwide problem in prevention of unsafe abortion, 3rd edition. WHO; 1997.

41.2 MANUAL VACUUM ASPIRATION (MVA)

CN Purandare, Madhuri A Patel

INTRODUCTION

It has been estimated that about 40–50 millions of abortions occur annually in spite of dramatically increased use of contraception over the past three decades. Half of these abortions take place in unsafe circumstances. Ninety-five percent of these occur in developing countries especially in rural area. Globally, about 13% of all maternal deaths occur due to complications of unsafe abortion. In developing countries, the risk of maternal death is several hundred times higher due to complications of unsafe abortion procedures than that of an abortion performed professionally under safe conditions. Complications due to unsafe abortion can also cause serious sequelae for women's health. Almost all the deaths and complications from unsafe abortions are preventable. Therefore, safe abortion services as provided by law, need to be available, with well-trained health personnel. It should also be supported by policies, regulation and a health system infrastructure, including equipment and supplies, so that women can have rapid access to these services.

Dilatation and curettage conventional method of termination of pregnancy in first trimester under GA is more than hundred years old. In spite of increased blood loss and risk of perforation of the uterus due to metal curettage, this method continued under the MTP Act of 1971. Vacuum aspiration of uterine contents has revolutionized technique of MTP and has reduced the risk of complications of D and C. In early seventies, International Projects Assistance Services (IPAS), manufactured and promoted manual vacuum aspiration system (MVA) which was promoted as menstrual regulation (MR) method till 6 weeks of amenorrhea. MR was not much accepted in our country may be because majority of women failed to come before 6 weeks of pregnancy and may be gynecologists too were not comfortable by MR, as there was greater risk of continuation of pregnancy. Now for more than a decade, IPAS has made available a superior version of MR called as MVA and has recently elicited considerable scientific interest as a safe method of voluntary termination of pregnancy up to 12 weeks of gestation. In 1993, Greenslade et al. reported 98% success rate in 5,000 women who underwent early abortion with MVA. Westfall JM et al. reported 99.5% success rate in 1,769 women who underwent early abortion with MVA. Federation of Obstetric and Gynaecological Societies of India (FOGSI)-IPAS multicentric Study in our country reported 98.6% success rate and carried the efficacy and safety of MVA up to 12 weeks of gestation. 94.8% of these procedures were performed under paracervical block with or without sedation.

SURGICAL ANATOMY (FIG. 1)

Manual Vacuum Aspiration (Fig. 2)

It consists of 60 mL syringe with double valve and far superior Karman's cannula ranges from 4 mm to 12 mm sizes. High density polypropylene is used for manufacturing the syringe barrel, the plunger bush and the cannulae causing much better quality and longer durability than the MR system. The syringe can be reused about 65–75 times and the cannulae about 10–12 times. The vacuum generated in the syringe is similar to that produced in electrical suction apparatus i.e. 660 mm of mercury. It has a water displacement capacity of 50 mL in less than a second.

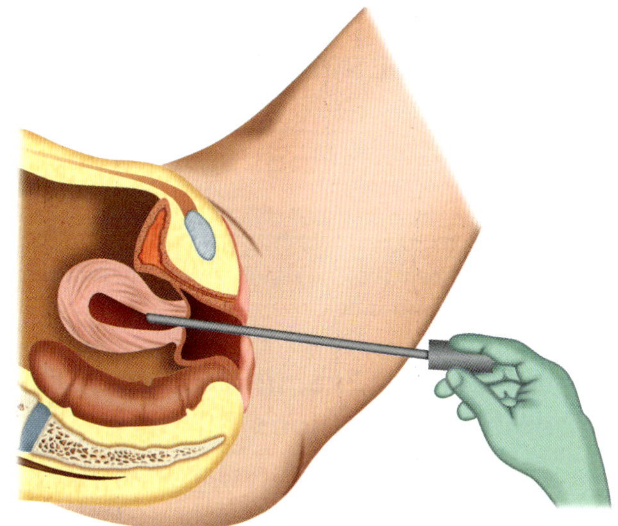

Fig. 1: Surgical anatomy

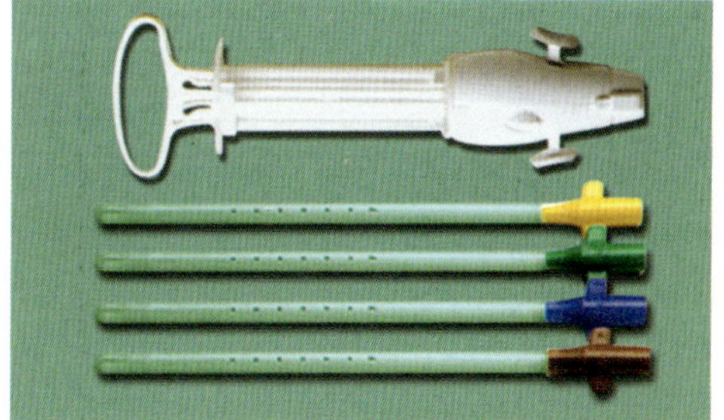

Fig. 2: Manual vacuum aspiration (MVA) instruments

Advantages over Electrical Vacuum Aspiration

- It is as efficient as electrical vacuum aspiration. In 2004, Goldberg AB et al. in the comparative study, a total of 1,726 procedures up to 10 weeks of gestation reported that MVA is as safe as electrical vacuum aspiration for abortion at up to 10 weeks of gestation. In 2003, Dean G et al. reported that physicians and patients found MVA as acceptable as electric vacuum aspiration for elective abortion performed at less than 10 weeks of gestation.
- Very simple
- Portable
- Cheap
- Noiseless
- Sterilized by simple procedure
- Rarely causes perforation: If perforation occurs than vacuum very quickly drops to 10 mm of mercury unlike electrical vacuum aspiration hence, rarely sucking in of the peritoneal contents i.e. bowels, omentum occurs
- Non dependence on electricity source hence, very much advantageous in developing countries, especially in rural areas.

PREOPERATIVE PREPARATION AND TESTS

Careful History Taking

Careful history taking regarding amenorrhea, medical disorders, drug intakes, bleeding disorders, allergies to medication, surgical history, especially previous cesarean section, etc are important.

Careful General Examination and Systemic Examinations

Especially anemia and reproductive tract infection (RTI) should be ruled out.

In 1998, GC Penney et al. reported that the presence of infection in the lower reproductive tract at the time of abortion is a risk factor for post-procedural RTI. Hence, it should be treated before procedure.

Careful Bimanual Examination

For position and size of the uterus.

Laboratory Tests

- Hb estimation, urine analysis
- Blood grouping and Rh typing
- Human immunodeficiency virus (HIV) testing is not mandatory.

Ultrasonography

According to Royal College of Obstetricians and Gynaecologists (RCOG) 2000 ultrasonography (USG) scanning is not necessary in early abortion except when clinically size of uterus is doubtful. Presence of fibroid and ectopic pregnancy, when suspected clinically are other indications for USG scanning.

Information and Counseling

Counseling should be done which will help women to decide, regarding method of MTP and contraception following MTP. Information regarding MVA procedure should be given.

INSTRUMENTS AND SUPPLIES FOR MANUAL VACUUM ASPIRATION

Basic Supplies

- IV infusion set and fluids (Sodium lactate, Glucose, saline)
- Aspiration syringes—10 mL and 20 mL
- Needles (22 gauge spinal for paracervical block, 21 gauge for drug administration)
- Sterile gloves (different sizes as per usage)
- Cotton swabs or gauze pieces
- Water-based antiseptic solution
- Detergent or soap
- Clean water
- Chlorine or glutaraldehyde for disinfection or decontamination of instruments.

Instruments and Equipments

- Sims speculums
- Anterior vaginal wall retractor
- Tenaculum
- Sponge forceps
- Cervical dilators
- Container for antiseptic solution
- Strainer (metal, glass, or gauze)
- Clear glass disk for tissue inspection.

Medication

- Analgesia
- Antianxiety medication
- Anesthetic (lignocaine 0.5–2% or chloroprocaine)
- Oxytocin or ergometrine 0.2 mg.

Manual Vacuum Aspiration Instruments

- 60 mL syringe with double valve
- Karman's cannulae of different sizes range from 4 mm to 12 mm
- Silicone oil for lubricating syringe, if needed.

INDICATIONS

On Medical Ground

Where continuation of the pregnancy might endanger the mother's life or cause grave injury to her physical and mental health in pre-existing maternal disease.

On Eugenic Ground

Where there is substantial risk of the child being born with serious handicaps due to physical and mental abnormalities, especially in cases:

- When previous child or children have been malformed
- When both parents or one parent and previous child or children are mentally defective
- When there is strong family history of disease known to be inherited and child or children are affected
- Isoimmunization to Rh and other blood factors where previous child or children have been affected and husband is proved to be homozygous Rh positive
- Viral disease (especially rubella) during organogenesis period
- Inadvertent exposure of the young fetus to heavy irradiation or to noxious drugs.

On Humanitarian Ground

Where pregnancy is a result of rape.

On Socioeconomic Ground

- Where actual or reasonable foreseeable environments could lead to risk of injury to the health of mother
- Failure of contraceptive device.

PREOPERATIVE ORDERS

- Written informed valid consent
- Inj tetanus toxoid (TT) 0.5 mL intramuscularly
- Cervical preparation: In 1999, BR Pridmore et al. reported that previous gynecological surgery, termination of pregnancy, lower segment cesarean section and the large loop excision of transformation zone of the cervix (LLETZ) procedure, which may result in scarring of the internal cervical os, is a previously unreported risk factor for tearing of the internal os, leading to perforation of the uterus during subsequent surgical abortion procedures. Dilatation of the cervix particularly for these "at risk" procedures should be predominantly passive by the use of oral prostaglandins, such as misoprostol and osmotic dilators
- Sedation IM, half an hour prior to the procedure
- Inj Atropine 0.6 mg IM, half an hour prior to the procedure
- Patient is asked to evacuate bladder
- Prophylactic antibiotics.

Position, Draping

Patient to be put in lithotomy position and aseptically draped.

Anesthesia

Paracervical block with or without sedation: In 1998, P Thonneau et al. reported that use of local anesthesia with vacuum aspiration is safe and effective. In 2005, H Hamoda et al. from USA reported that surgical abortion using MVA under local anesthesia is effective and acceptable to women.

Operative Steps

- Vacuum is created in 60 mL double valve MVA syringe or syringe is charged (Figs 3 to 5)
- Parts cleaned and draped (Fig. 6)
- Bimanual examination is done to confirm size and direction of uterus (Fig. 7)
- Posterior vaginal wall retracted with Sims speculum (Fig. 8)
- Anterior vaginal wall retracted with anterior vaginal wall retractor
- Anterior lip of cervix is caught with tenaculum
- Paracervical block is given at 4 and 8 O' clock positions with lignocaine (Fig. 9)
- Cervix dilated according to size of uterus (Table 1)
- The size of the cannula is selected to snugly fit in the cervical canal
- The cannula is inserted through cervix into the uterine cavity (Fig. 10)
- The charged syringe is attached to the cannula and the pinch valves released allowing the vacuum to get transferred to the uterine cavity
- Contents of the uterus are evacuated by using rotatory and/or back and forth movements of the cannula (Fig. 11)
- Appearance of blood with bubbles (Fig. 12), absence of more products getting aspirated, gritty sensation as the cannula passes over the uterine walls, and feel of uterus contracting around the cannula indicates that uterus is completely evacuated

- The evacuated material is inspected for products of conception (Fig. 13)
- Inj methargine 0.2 mL intramuscularly given
- Inj anti-D, if indicated, is given intramuscularly

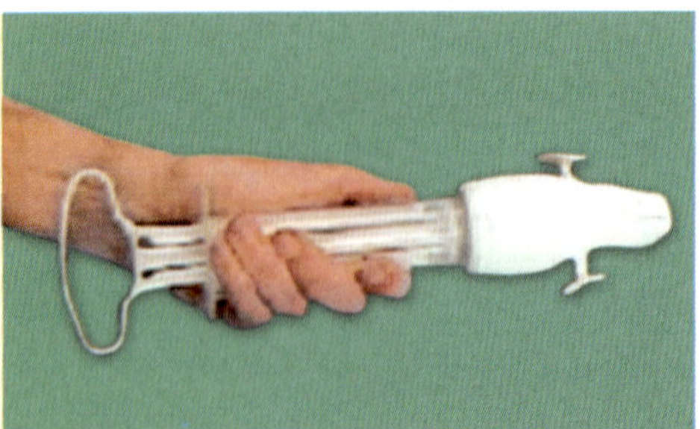

Fig. 3

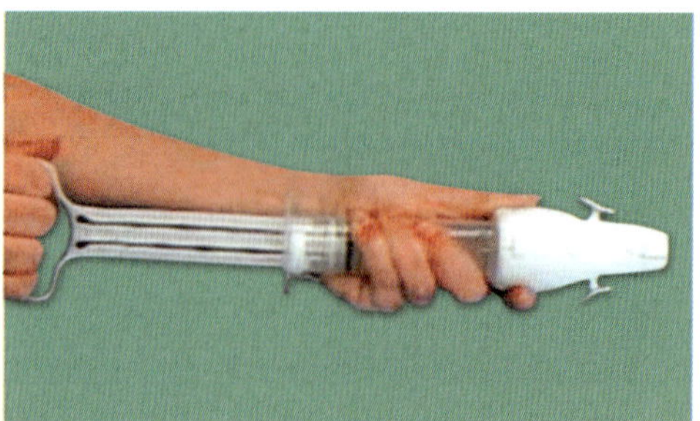

Fig. 4

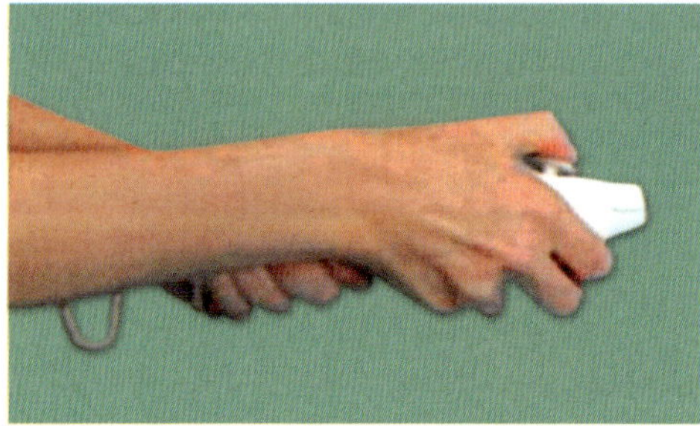

Fig. 5

Figs 3 to 5: Vacuum being created and syringe charged for evacuation

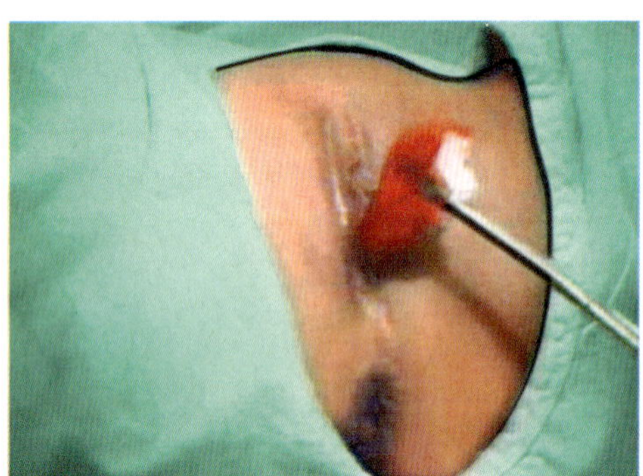

Fig. 6: Cleaned and draped aseptically

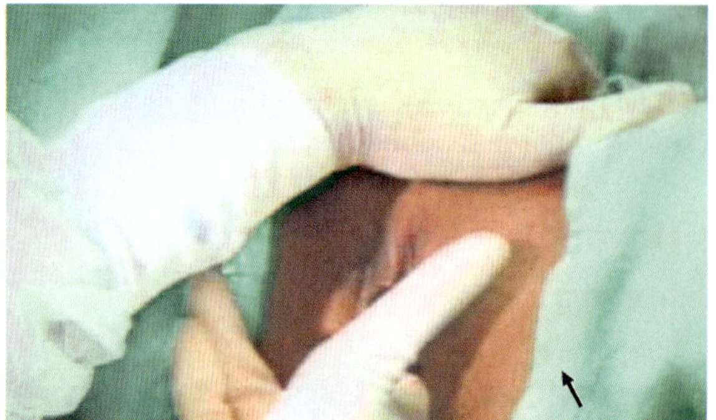

Fig. 7: Bimanual examination

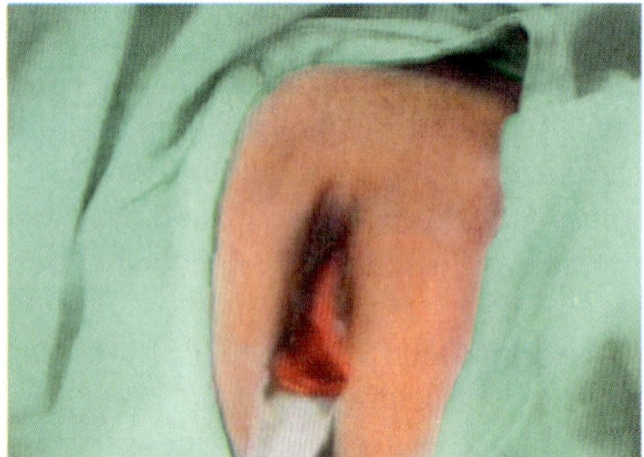

Fig. 8: Retraction of posterior vaginal wall

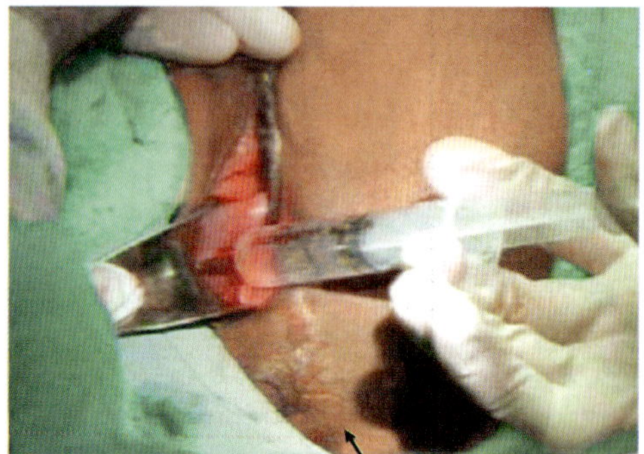

Fig. 9: Paracervical block

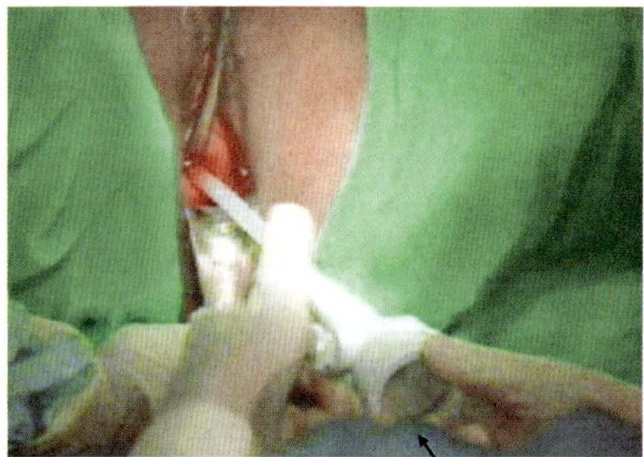

Fig. 10: Cannula in uterine cavity

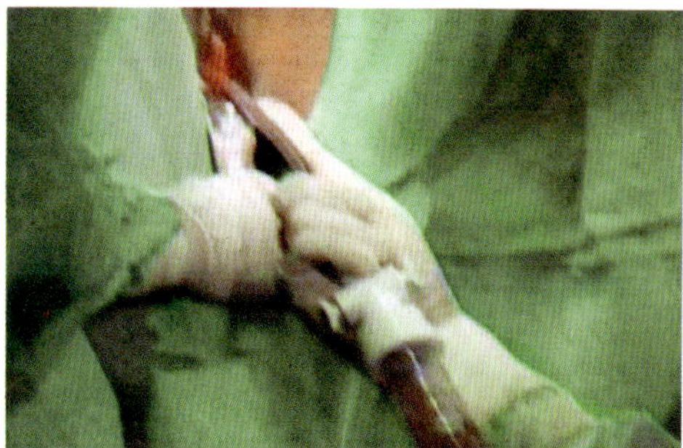

Fig. 11: Products of conception in syringe

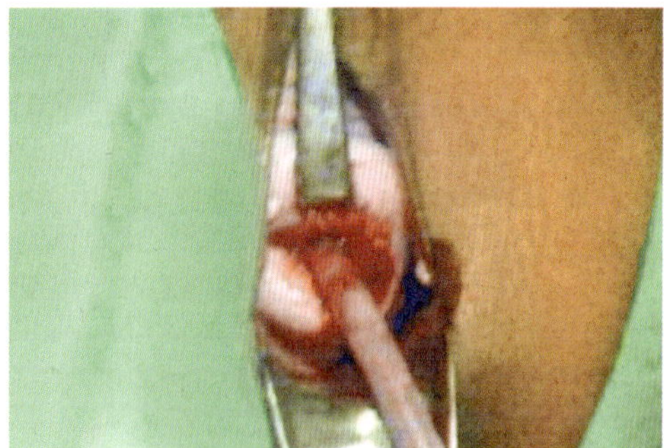

Fig. 12: Blood with bubbles

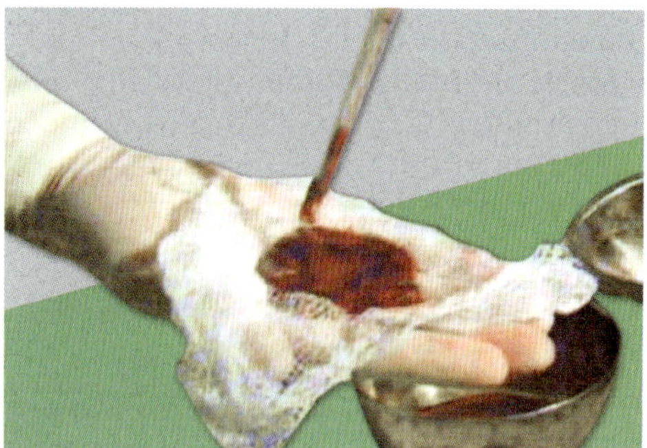

Fig. 13: Inspection of products of conception

Table 1: Usage of corresponding cannula size to uterine size in weeks

Uterine size	Cannula size
4–6 weeks	4–7 mm
7–9 weeks	6–10 mm
9–12 weeks	8–12 mm

POSTOPERATIVE ORDER

- Temperature pulse respiration (TPR) record every half an hour
- BP record every 2 hours
- Watch for bleeding per vaginal (PV)
- Discharge the patient 4 hours after procedure with prescription of oral antibiotics and analgesic
- Patient is called for follow-up after 1 week and after onset of menstruation for contraceptive advice.

COMPLICATIONS

Complication rate increases steeply after 8 weeks of gestation. In 2004, AB Goldberg et al. reported 2.5% complications rate with MVA in the series of 1,002 procedures. In 1998, P Thonneau et al. reported complications after MVA procedure was 2.1%.

Uterine Perforation

Usually, uterine perforation goes undetected and resolves without the need for intervention. In 1989, Kaali et al. reported in their study of more than 700 women undergoing first trimester abortion with laparoscopic sterilization, found that 12 out of 14 uterine perforations were so small that they would not have been recognized if laparoscopy had not been performed.

When uterine perforation is suspected, observation and antibiotics may be all that is required. If the laparoscope is available then under laparoscopy, controlled evacuation of uterus should be completed. If the laparoscopic examination and/or the status of the patient gives rise to any suspicions of damage to bowel, blood vessels or other structures, a laparotomy to repair damaged tissue may be required. In 1999, BR Pridmore et al. reported 0.05% uterine perforation as complications of procedures.

Hemorrhage

Hemorrhage can result from retained products of conception, injury to the cervix or rarely uterine perforation. Treatment will depend upon the cause. In retained products of conception, re-evacuation of the uterus under antibiotic cover is done. Administration of uterotonic drugs to stop the bleeding, IV fluid replacement and in severe cases, blood transfusion, laparoscopy and exploratory laparotomy are necessary.

Incomplete Abortion

It is uncommon with MVA, but does occur. Patient will present with per vaginal bleeding, abdominal pain and signs of infection. Patient requires higher class of antibiotics and re-evacuation of the uterus. In 2005, Sebanti Goswami et al. reported two cases of incomplete abortion in their series of 72 cases, who underwent MVA.

Infection

Infection rarely occurs if performed with proper aseptic precautions. Patient will present with fever, foul smelling vaginal discharge, abdominal or pelvic pain, prolonged vaginal bleeding, uterine tenderness with leukocytosis. Higher class of antibiotics should be started and if there are retained products of conception causing infection then re-evacuation of uterus is done immediately. In 1996, GF Sawaya et al. reported that use of prophylactic antibiotics reduce the risk of postprocedural infection.

Continuation of Pregnancy or Failure of Manual Vacuum Aspiration

Continuation of pregnancy occurs rarely, especially when done before 6 weeks of pregnancy. Careful inspection of the product of conception is necessary after each procedure. If there is failure of procedure then patient will present with continuation of symptoms of pregnancy. On follow-up visit, careful examination is done to rule out continuation of pregnancy. The procedure is repeated or if she comes in second trimester then the second trimester termination procedure is done.

LONG-TERM COMPLICATIONS

- Menstrual disturbances
- Intrauterine adhesions
- Recurrent abortion
- Preterm labor
- Rh isoimmunization
- Infertility
- Chronic pelvic pain
- Ectopic pregnancy
- Endometriosis of vagina and cervix (rare)
- Rupture uterus in next pregnancy, if uterine perforation occurs during present procedure.

If MVA is properly performed then majority of women will not suffer any immediate or long-term effects on their general or reproductive health. In 1997, WHO reported severe complications in very small number of women. In 1999, Houge et al. reported no association between safely induced first trimester abortion and adverse outcome of subsequent pregnancy.

OTHER USES OF MANUAL VACUUM ASPIRATION

- Incomplete abortion and missed abortion: MVA is not widely used for the evacuation of incomplete abortions in Western Europe in spite of its well proven success and safety record. In 2004, R Gazvani et al. reported that MVA is an option in the management of all first trimester pregnancy losses, but in 2006, VK Dalton et al. reported that intrauterine adhesion formation may follow MVA for early pregnancy loss
- As a backup for failure of medical abortion and electrical vacuum aspiration failure
- Endometrial biopsy and endometrial aspiration cytology.

CONCLUSION

Manual vacuum aspiration is the single most promising method which can be widely practiced even in rural areas where the access of medical facilities are limited, high technology equipments are not available and power supply is erratic. It is simple, safe, effective, easily portable, low cost with low maintenance method which can make early abortions safe and easily accessible to women. Therefore, MVA will help to reduce maternal morbidity and mortality remarkably in future.

ACKNOWLEDGMENT

Dr Khyati A Patel

BIBLIOGRAPHY

1. Alan Guttmacher Institute. Sharing responsibilities: Women society and abortion worldwide. New York and Washington DC: The Alan Guttmacher Institute; 1999.
2. Dalton VK, Saunders MA, Harris LH, et al. Intrauterine adhesion after manual vacuum aspiration for early pregnancy failure. Fertil Steril. 2006;85(6):1823.e1-3.
3. Dean G, Carbnas L, Durney P, et al. Acceptability of manual versus electric aspiration for first trimester abortion. A randomized trial. Contraception. 2003;67(3):201-6.
4. Goldberg AB, Dean G, Kang MS, et al. Manual versus electric vacuum aspiration for early first trimester abortion: A controlled study of complication rates. Obstet Gynaecol. 2004;103(1):101-7.

5. Goswami R, Honey E, MacLennan FM, et al. Manual vacuum aspiration (MVA) in the management of first trimester pregnancy loss. Eur J Obstet Gynaecol Reprod Biol. 2004;112(2):197-200.
6. Goswami S, Adhikari S, Sanghamita M. Manual vacuum aspiration. J Obstet Gynaecol India. 2005;55(6):544-5.
7. Greenslade FC, Benson J, Winkler J, et al. Summary of clinical and programmatic experience with manual vacuum aspiration. Adv abortion Com. 1993;3:1-4.
8. Haemoda H, Flett GM, Ashok PW, et al. Surgical abortion using manual vacuum aspiration under local anaesthesia: A pilot study of feasibility and women's acceptability. J Fam Plann Reprod Health Care. 2005;31(3):185-8.
9. Hogue CJ, Boardman LA, Stotland NL, et al. Answering questions about long-term outcome. In: Paul M, Lichtenberg EJ, Borgatta L, Grimes D, Stubblefield PG (Eds). A clinician's guide to medical and surgical abortion. Philadelphia: Churchill Livingstone; 1999; p. 217-28.
10. Kaali SG, Szigetvari IA, Barffai GS. The frequency and management of uterine perforation during first trimester abortion. Am J Obstet Gynaecol. 1989;161:406-8.
11. Parikh MN. Manual vacuum aspiration (MVA). J Obstet Gynecol. 2003;2(5):437-8.
12. Penney GC, Thomson M, Norman J, et al. A randomized comparison of strategies for reducing infective complication of induced abortion. Br J Obstet Gynaecol. 1998;105:599-604.
13. Pridmore BR, Chambers DG. Uterine perforation during surgical abortion: A review of diagnosis management and prevention. Aust NZ J Obstet Gynaecol. 1999;39(3):349-53.
14. RCOG-Royal College of Obstetricians and Gynaecologists. The case of women requesting induced abortion. Evidence based guideline No.7. London: RCOG Press; 2000.
15. Rutgers S. Abortion admission in rural Matebeleland North province. Cent Afr J Med. 2001;47:214-20.
16. Sawaya GF, Grady D, Kerlihowske K, et al. Antibiotics at the time of induced abortion: The case for universal prophylaxis based on a meta-analysis. Obstet Gynaecol. 1996;87:884-90.
17. Thonneau P, Fougeyrollas B, Ducot B, et al. Complications of abortion performed under local anaesthesia. European J Obstet Gynaecol Reprod Biol. 1998;81:59-63.
18. Van Book PF, Cottingham JC. Unsafe abortion: An avoidable tragedy. Best Pract Res Clin Obstet Gynaecol. 2002;16(2): 205-20.
19. Westfall JM, Sophocles A, Burggraf H, et al. Manual vacuum aspiration. Arch Fam Med. 1998;7(6):59-62.
20. World Health Organization. Medical methods for termination of pregnancy. WHO technical report series 871. Geneva; 1997.
21. World Health Organization. Unsafe abortion: Global and regional estimates of incidence of and mortality due to unsafe abortion with a listing of available country data Geneva; 1998.

41.3 ABDOMINAL HYSTERECTOMY

Atul Munshi, Sujal Munshi

INTRODUCTION

Hysterectomy is one of the most commonly performed gynecological surgical procedures worldwide. The national surveillance data from the USA showed that 600,000 hysterectomies were performed yearly, of which approximately 90% were done for a benign condition. In India and other Asian countries with less availability of conservative modalities like balloon therapy, hysteroscopic resection of endometrium to mass population and reluctance for these methods, the number is even higher.

Abdominal hysterectomy (AH) was more common than vaginal route (65% vs. 35%) for many decades. But for past one and a half decade, worldwide vaginal and laparoscopically-assisted hysterectomies are becoming increasingly popular and now secure a larger proportion than ever before amongst all procedures performed.

INDICATIONS FOR HYSTERECTOMY

Benign Diseases

- Abnormal uterine bleeding
- Leiomyoma
- Adenomyosis
- Endometriosis
- Pelvic organ prolapse
- Pelvic inflammatory diseases
- Chronic pelvic pain
- Pregnancy related conditions such as cornual ectopic pregnancy
- Miscellaneous.

Malignant Diseases

- Cervical intraepithelial neoplasm (CIN)
- Invasive cervical cancer
- Atypical endometrial hyperplasia
- Endometrial cancer
- Ovarian cancer
- Fallopian tube cancer
- Gestational trophoblastic tumors.

Traumatic

- Uterine perforation
- Cervical tear, extending to vault
- Rupture uterus.

Obstetrical

- Atonic postpartum hemorrhage (PPH)
- Morbidly adherent placenta
- Contraindications to the vaginal route, including uterine enlargement (uterine weight estimated more than 280 g or uterine size more than 12 weeks); vagina deemed "too narrow" (e.g. vagina narrower than two finger-breadths, especially at the apex); lack of uterine descensus and mobility; presence of adnexal disease; prior pelvic surgery; malignancy; contracted pelvis; and need to explore the upper abdomen. However, these traditional indications for laparotomy have been challenged. When vaginal hysterectomy (VH) is not possible, it is suggested that a laparoscopic approach might avoid the need for abdominal hysterectomy; however, the length of the surgery increases as the scope of the surgery performed laparoscopically increases and these procedures require greater surgical expertize.

The reasons for the hysterectomy, risk and benefits of the procedure, alternatives and outcome should be discussed in detail. Informed consent with thorough exploration of patient preferences and expectations is particularly important. The decision to proceed with hysterectomy is made by woman and her physician based upon functional impairment, childbearing plans, response to medical therapy and discussion of alternatives including:

- Uterine artery embolization and myomectomy may be used to treat symptomatic leiomyoma
- Pain control services may be able to return patients with intractable pelvic pain to a functional status without surgery
- Endometrial ablation may be an effective therapy for excessive uterine bleeding
- Medical therapy with gonadotropin-releasing hormone (GnRH) analogs can help reduce discomfort associated with endometriosis
- Endometrial hyperplasia can sometimes be treated medically with progestins
- Conization (cold knife, loop electrocautery) may be adequate therapy for some women with high grade CIN or cervical carcinoma *in situ* (CIS).

Once the decision for the hysterectomy has been made, physician and the patient must decide whether to proceed abdominally, vaginally or with laparoscopic assistance. The route chosen depends upon the woman's clinical profile and surgeon's personal preference. Risk and benefits of oophorectomy and proposed plan for keeping or removing ovaries should be discussed with patient before surgery.

PREOPERATIVE REQUISITES

- Complete history and physical examination
- Routine blood examination
- Special tests according to patient's medical disease comorbidity
- Chest X-ray in women with cardiorespiratory disease
- Intravenous pyelogram (IVP) or computed tomography (CT) scan of abdomen and pelvis in women with large uterine or extrauterine pelvic mass
- Pap smear to rule out cervical neoplasia
- Recent pregnancy test in reproductive aged women, prior to hysterectomy
- Bowel preparation prior to pelvic surgery to facilitate exposure and reduce trauma to bowel caused by retraction and packing
- Clear liquid diet on the day prior to surgery
- One or two fleet enemas, the evening prior to surgery
- A dulcolax® suppository immediately on arising on the morning of surgery, will evacuate residual feces in sigmoid and prevent contamination of field during surgery (not practiced everywhere)
- IV prophylactic antibiotics given immediately prior to induction of anesthesia, second generation cephalosporins, are commonly used
- If necessary, the pubic and/or vulva hair should be clipped with an electric clipper or even scissors rather than shaved on morning of surgery. Shaving prior to surgery has shown to increase the risk of wound infection and cellulites, due to bacterial colonization of skin
- Informed consent.

TYPES OF HYSTERECTOMY

Depending upon the extent of removal of the uterus and adjacent structures, following types are described (Figs 1A to C).

Total Hysterectomy

Removal of the entire uterus.

Subtotal Hysterectomy (Fig. 1A)

Removal of the body or corpus leaving behind the cervix.

Panhysterectomy (Fig. 1B)

Removal of uterus along with removal of tubes and ovaries of both the sides. The term "hysterectomy with bilateral salpingo-oophorectomy" is preferred.

Extended Hysterectomy (Fig. 1C)

Panhysterectomy plus removal of vaginal cuff.

Radical Hysterectomy

Removal of uterus, tubes and ovaries of both sides, upper one-third of vagina, adjacent parametrium and draining lymph glands of the cervix.

Radical Hysterectomy is further classified depending upon extent of structures removed.

- Type 1: Extrafascial hysterectomy
- Type 2: Modified radical hysterectomy (Wertheim's). Removal of medial half of cardinal and uterosacral ligament and selective removal of enlarged lymph nodes. Less extensive than radical hysterectomy
- Type 3: Radical hysterectomy (Meigs) includes pelvic lymph node dissection along with most of uterosacral and cardinal ligament and upper one-third of vagina is also removed

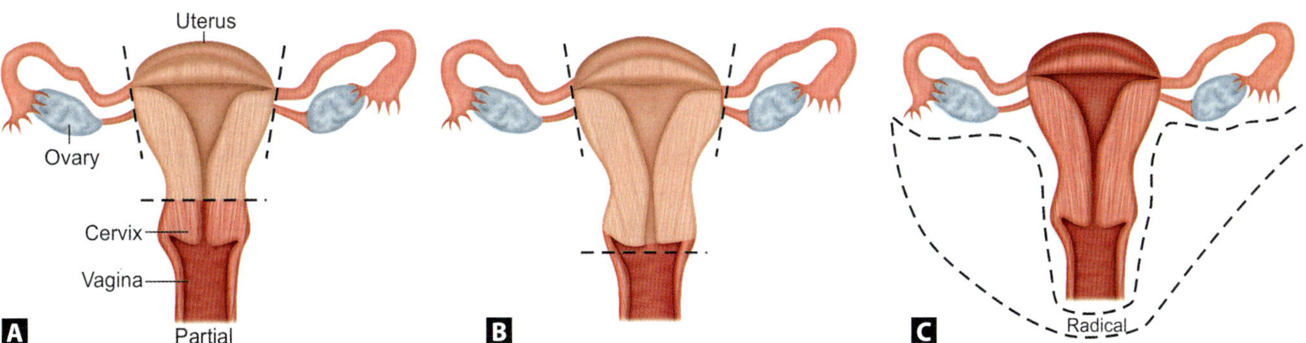

Figs 1A to C: Diagrammatic representation of types of hysterectomy

- Type 4: Extended radical hysterectomy periureteral tissue, superior vesical artery and up to three-fourth of vagina is removed
- Type 5: Portion of distal ureter and bladder are resected
- Mitra's: Pelvic lymph nodes are removed by bilateral extraperitoneal approach.

OPERATIVE TECHNIQUE

Patient is placed in supine position after adequate anesthesia, examination under anesthesia is performed. Foley catheter is recommended in most cases. Vagina cleaned with antiseptic solution. Skin preparations followed by placement of surgical drapes is carried out.

- Skin incision may be transverse or vertical and is determined by variety of factors, such as need for exploration of upper abdomen, size of uterus, presence of prior incision and desired cosmetic results. If prior incision exists, parallel scars are undesirable (Fig. 2)

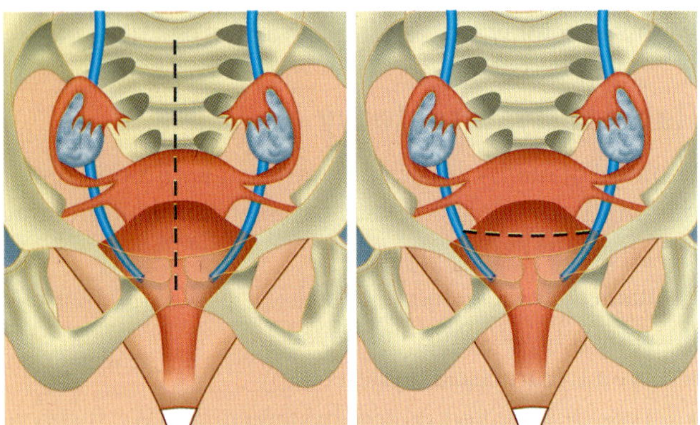

Fig. 2: Vertical and transverse incisions for abdominal hysterectomy

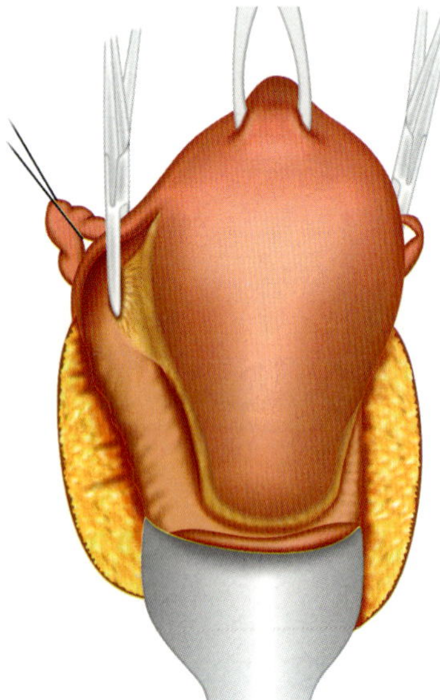

Fig. 3: Holding of uterine cornu to cut round ligament and other supports

- The peritoneal cavity is entered and the upper abdomen and pelvis explored for unexpected pathology and to confirm any suspected pathological findings. Cytological sampling of peritoneal fluid or peritoneal washings, may be collected if indicated because of suspicion of possible spread of malignancy
- The wound edges should be protected with moist laparotomy packs or towels before placing retractor blades
- To begin, the pelvic organs are mobilized by dividing omental, intestinal or abdominal wall adhesions, as indicated
- A large Kelly clamp is placed across each uterine cornu, running down the side of the uterus across the round ligaments. This allows uterine elevation and prevents back bleeding when the round ligaments are divided. The uterus is manually deviated to the patient's left, stretching the right round ligament. The round ligament is suture ligated, clamped and divided (Fig. 3)
- Anterior broad ligament is incised along the vesicouterine fold, separating bladder peritoneum from lower uterine segment (Fig. 4). The retroperitoneum is entered by extending the incision on posterior leaf of broad ligament cephalad, remaining lateral to both the infundibulopelvic ligament and iliac vessels. Blunt or sharp dissection clears the loose connective tissue overlying the external iliac artery
- The ureter is identified crossing the common iliac artery by following the external iliac artery cephalad to bifurcation. Ureter is left attached to the medial or posterior leaf of the broad ligament, so as not to disrupt its blood supply.
- The same procedure is completed on the opposite side. The left ureter is usually more medial than the right. If patient has extensive pelvic disease, the ureter must be dissected down toward bladder as far as necessary.

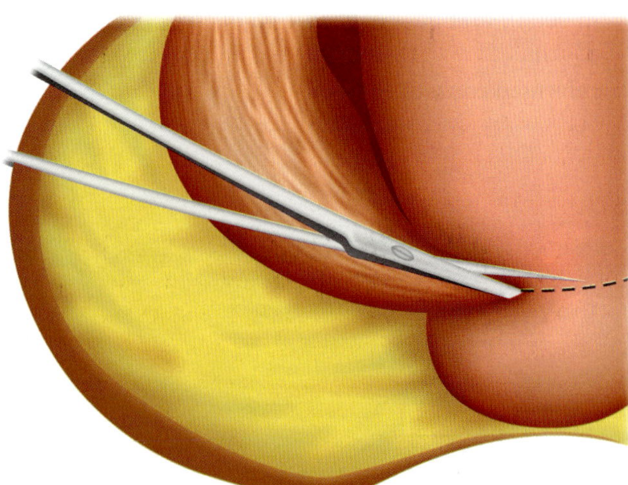

Fig. 4: Opening of vesicouterine fold

The position of the ureter should never be assumed and must always be kept under direct visualization. The perivesical and perirectal spaces may be created to facilitate safe hysterectomy particularly if there is distortion of anatomy by pelvic pathology. Any problems encountered intraoperatively can safely and quickly be addressed when the spaces have been developed

- If ovaries are to be retained, the utero-ovarian ligament on each side is clamped with Heaney's clamp, cut and ligated with both free tie and suture ligature. The medial clamp at uterine cornu will control back bleeding (Figs 5A and B)
- If ovaries are to be removed, infundibulopelvic ligament is cut, ligated with free tie, followed by suture ligature. Tying pedicle before suturing is a good practice as it prevents formation of an expanding hematoma through inadvertent puncture of ovarian vessels
- Bladder is then sharply dissected off the lower uterine segment and cervix. Uterus is then retracted cephalad to one side of pelvis, placing the lower uterine ligaments on stretch. Any loose connective tissue overlying the uterine vessels is sharply removed to skeletonize the vessels and a curved Heaney clamp is placed perpendicular to the uterine artery at the junction of the cervix and body of uterus (Fig. 6). The opposite side is managed in a similar fashion, the uterine arteries cut and suture ligated
- If rectum requires mobilization from posterior cervix, posterior peritoneum between uterosacral ligaments just beneath the cervix and rectum is incised. The cardinal ligament and any remaining broad ligament are divided by placing a straight Heaney's clamp medial to uterine vascular pedicle for a distance of 2–3 cm parallel to the uterus (Fig. 7). Pedicle is cut and ligated with a suture ligature. Procedure is completed on contralateral side. A series of pedicles may be required depending upon the size of the uterus and as well as elongation of cervix
- The pubovesicocervical fascia is then dissected off the lower uterine segment and cervix. A curved Heaney clamp is placed inside the fascia on each side of uterus to incorporate the uterosacral ligaments and upper vagina just below cervix. Care should be taken to avoid foreshortening the vagina. Uterus is resected out using scissors
- Numerous techniques have been described for vaginal cuff closure, one effective method is to place a figure of eight suture of 0 or 2-0 gauge synthetic absorbable suture between the tips of the two clamps. This suture is used for both traction and hemostasis
- Sutures are placed at the tip of each clamp and pedicle is transfixed with suture ligature. This suture incorporates the uterosacral and cardinal ligament at the angle of the vagina. Vaginal cuff can also be left open to heal secondarily (Fig. 8). If this method is used, a running suture is used for hemostasis along the cuff edge. The pelvis is thoroughly irrigated with warm saline or Ringer's lactate solution. Meticulous hemostasis is assured. Urethral and bladder integrity are confirmed. Abdomen closed in layers as per usually done.

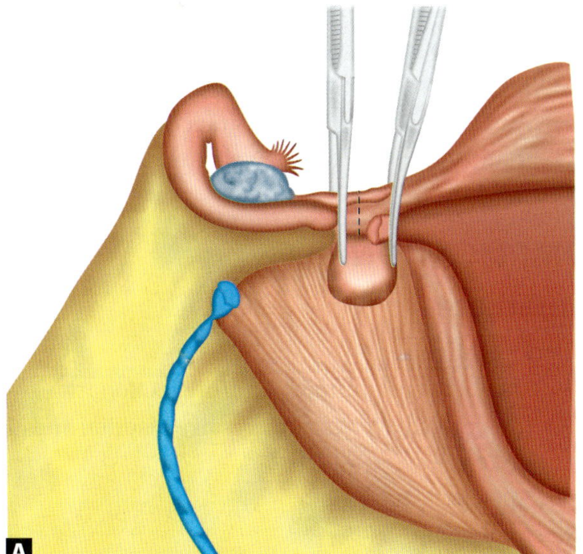

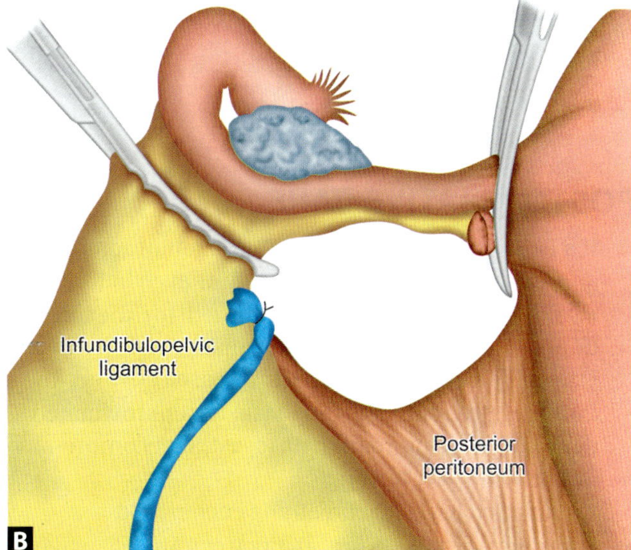

Figs 5A and B: Incision of ligaments at uterine cornu, utero-ovarian ligament and infundibulopelvic ligaments

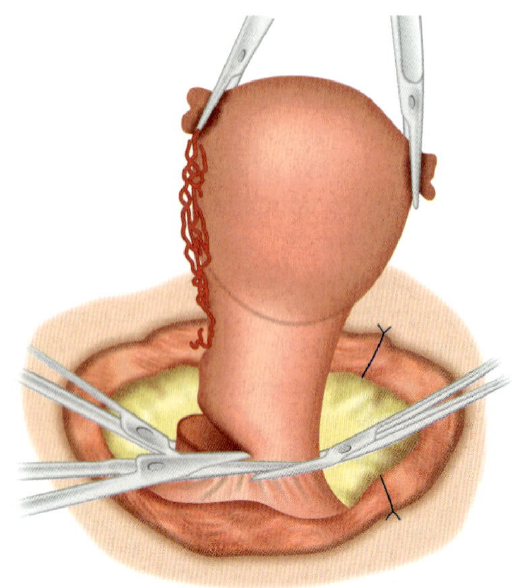

Fig. 6: Dividing uterine artery

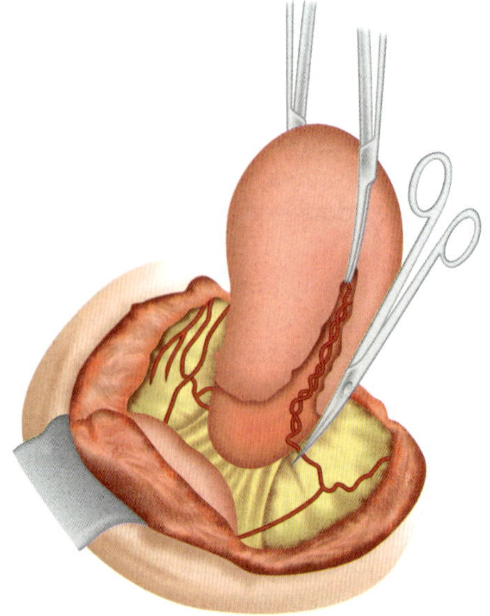

Fig. 7: Colpotomy and dividing the cardinal ligaments

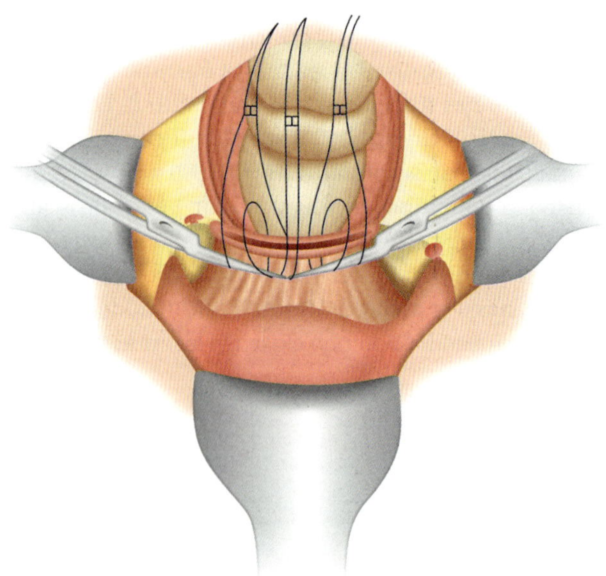

Fig. 8: Suturing of vaginal vault

POSTOPERATIVE CARE

- If a Foley catheter is used, it may be removed any time around morning following surgery or even before that
- IV fluids are generally administered for the first 24 hours to insure that patient remains well hydrated, especially if she experiences any nausea or vomiting
- Postoperative colonic stasis lasts for approximately 3 days but does not require nasogastric decompression or preclude early feeding
- Ambulation and deep breathing encouraged
- For adequate pain control, patient-controlled analgesia can be utilized
- Skin sutures are removed on 7-10th postoperative day.

Instructions on Discharge

- Resume normal daily activity as quickly as possible
- Walking and stair climbing are encouraged
- Tube baths or showers are permissible
- Avoid heavy lifting for 4-6 weeks to minimize stress on healing fascia
- Vaginal intercourse is also discouraged up to 4 weeks to allow the vaginal cuff to heal completely
- Driving should be avoided till full mobility returns and analgesics no longer required
- The patient should inform her surgeon if she experiences:
  - Increase in pain
  - Persistent nausea or vomiting
  - Bleeding heavier than menses
  - Any signs or symptoms of infection i.e. fever more than 101°F, purulent vaginal or wound discharge.

COMPLICATIONS

Immediate

- Perioperative period
  - Hemorrhage—primary and/or reactionary
  - Injury to adjacent structures like bladder, intestine, ureter
  - Anesthetic hazards
- Postoperative
  - Shock—hypovolemic
  - Urinary

- Retention
- Cystitis
- Anuria
- Incontinence
  - Overflow
  - Stress
  - True
- Pyrexia more than 100.8°F
- Hemorrhage, secondary
- Hematoma, cuff or rectus sheath hematous
- Wound dehiscence
- Paralytic ileus and intestinal obstruction
- Phlebitis
- Deep vein thrombosis
- Pulmonary embolism.

Remote

- Vault granulation
- Vault prolapse
- Prolapse of fallopian tube
- Incisional hernia
- Postoperative adhesion formation
- Mortality
- Early surgical menopause, in case of salpingo-oophorectomy done.

SPECIAL CONSIDERATIONS (FOR BENIGN LESIONS)

Age and Parity

An ideal condition is that the patient preferably be in the perimenopausal age group with family completed. However, operation may have to be done under forced circumstances even in comparatively young age group or unmarried or nulliparous women. Contemplating myomectomy is an option.

Total or Subtotal

The preferred surgery is always a total hysterectomy, unless there is a sufficient reason to leave behind cervix. Pap smear must be normal. Indications of subtotal or supracervical hysterectomy are:

- Difficult to remove tubo-ovarian masses
- Pelvic endometriosis involving rectovaginal septum
- Obstetric causes cesarean hysterectomy
- Sudden deterioration of general condition either due to blood loss or anesthetic complications while contemplating to perform total hysterectomy.

ADVANTAGES OF SUBTOTAL OR SUPRACERVICAL HYSTERECTOMY

- Reduced operative and postoperative morbidity
- Reduced vaginal shortening and vault prolapse
- Increased sexual satisfaction.

RISKS

- Cervicitis with abnormal vaginal discharge
- Stump carcinoma (1%).

PRESERVATION OF OVARIES

Amidst controversy, it seems rational to preserve the ovaries in premenopausal women, if they are found healthy. Some, however, continue to remove ovaries beyond 45 years.

ADVANTAGES OF RETAINING OVARIES

- Menopausal symptoms appear less in intensity
- Ovarian function continues till the expected time of spontaneous menopause, so less early incidence of early osteoporosis and atherosclerosis.

DRAWBACKS

- Malignancy or benign neoplasm
- Residual ovarian syndrome
- Chronic pelvic pain and dyspareunia
- Chance of relaparotomy.

EARLY REMOVAL IS REQUIRED

- If the ovaries are diseased in inflammatory process or involved in neoplastic condition with patient around the age of 40 years or earlier
- History of ovarian cancer in first degree relative of patient

Hormone replacement therapy is to be considered when ovaries are removed.

REMOVAL OF FALLOPIAN TUBE

- When the ovaries are removed (salpingo-oophorectomy)
- When the tubes are diseased but ovaries are conserved due to young age (salpingectomy)

BIBLIOGRAPHY

1. Doucette RC, Sharp HT, Alder SC. Challenging generally accepted contraindications to vaginal hysterectomy. Am J Obstet Gynecol. 2001;184:1386-9.
2. Garry R, Fountain J, Mason S, et al. The Evaluate study: Two parallel randomized trials, one comparing laparoscopic with abdominal hysterectomy, the other comparing laparoscopic with vaginal hysterectomy. BMJ. 2004;328:129.
3. Johnson N, Barlow D, Lethaby A, et al. Surgical approach to hysterectomy for benign gynaecological disease. Cochrane Database Syst Rev. 2006;CD003677.
4. Keshavarz H, Hillis SD, Kieke BA, et al. Hysterectomy surveillance—United States, 1994–1999. MMWR Surveill Summar. 2002;51:1-8.
5. Kovac SR. Hysterectomy outcomes in patients with similar indications. Obstet Gynecol. 2000;95:787-93.
6. McPherson K, Metcalfe MA, Herbert A, et al. Severe complications of hysterectomy: The VALUE study. BJOG. 2004;111:688-94.
7. Sizzi O, Paparella P, Bonito C, et al. Laparoscopic assistance after vaginal hysterectomy and unsuccessful access to the ovaries or failed uterine mobilization: Changing trends. JSLS. 2004;8:339-46.

41.4 MODIFIED RADICAL HYSTERECTOMY

Harshad Parasnis

HISTORY

The first radical abdominal hysterectomy (Table 1) for cervical cancer was performed on April 26, 1895 by John G Clark, resident at Johns Hopkins Hospital. In 1898, Ernst Wertheim from Vienna, Austria first developed the radical hysterectomy with removal of the pelvic lymph nodes and the parametrium. In 1912, Wertheim published the outcomes of his first 500 cases, which contributed so much to the development and acceptance of radical hysterectomy that today, his name has become synonymous with the procedure. The operative mortality rate was 18%, and the major morbidity rate was 31%.

In the late 20th century, radiation therapy became the favored approach because of the high mortality and morbidity of the surgical approach. In 1944, Meigs repopularized the surgical approach when he developed a modified Wertheim operation with removal of all pelvic nodes (the Wertheim-Clark plus Taussig's operation).

Table 1: History of radical abdominal hysterectomy

AW Freund (1878)	TAH with removal of enlarged LN
JG Clark (1895)	Radical abdominal surgery
E Wertheim (1898–1905)	Radical abdominal hysterectomy with selective lymphadenectomy
Hidekazu Okabayashi (1921)	Nerve sparing radical hysterectomy
Victor Bonney (1935)	Radical abdominal hysterectomy with routine pelvic lymphadenectomy
Joe E Meigs (1944)	Radical abdominal hysterectomy with BPLND
Richard TeLinde (1950)	Modified radical hysterectomy with BPLND
A Brunschwig (1964)	Pelvic exenteration

Abbreviations: BPLND, Bilateral pelvic lymph node dissection; LN, Lymph node; TAH, Total abdominal hysterectomy

Meigs reported a survival rate of 75% for patients with stage I disease and demonstrated an operative mortality rate of 1% when these procedures were performed by a specially trained gynecologist.

Throughout the 20th century, various modifications have been made for this radical procedure, but the aim remains the same, i.e. "complete removal of central tumor with an adequate margin of tumor-free tissue."

TYPES OF RADICAL HYSTERECTOMY

In order to allay confusion from the various modifications, MS Piver (1974) from Buffalo University classified radical hysterectomy into five classes:

1. Class I: Extrafascial hysterectomy
   This is done for cervical cancer stage IA1.
2. Class II: Modified radical hysterectomy (Telinde)
   This is done for cervical cancer stage IA2.
3. Class III: Radical hysterectomy (Meigs)
   This is done for cervical cancer stage IB to IIA.
4. Class IV: Radical hysterectomy with removal of three-fourth of vagina and complete ureteric dissection.
5. Class V: Class IV procedure with resection of terminal ureter, segment of bladder and rectum. Class IV and V procedures are performed for selected anterior central recurrences.

Though class III hysterectomy has been the standard treatment for stage IB and IIA disease, prospective randomized trial by Landoni et al. have shown that therapeutic efficacy of class II hysterectomy was comparable to that of class III hysterectomy (Table 2) in terms of recurrence free and overall survival. The operative morbidity, especially bladder dysfunction was significantly reduced with class II hysterectomy. However,

Table 2: Hysterectomy of class II and class III

	Piver class II modified radical hysterectomy (Telinde)	Piver class III radical hysterectomy (Meigs)
Uterine artery ligation	At the level of ureter	At the origin from interior iliac artery
Parametria and Paracolpos	Removed at the level of ureter	Removed lateral to ureter
Uterosacral ligaments	Divided midway to rectum	Divided near rectum
Vaginal cuff	1–2 cm removed	≥ 2 cm removed
Preferred in stage	IA1 with LVS, IA2, Stage IB1 Stage IIA	IA2, IB1, IB2, IIA

large multicentric trials are necessary to advocate this as a standard of care.

Lymphadenectomy

The need and extent of lymph node dissection depends upon the stage of the disease.

For stage IA1, the risk of lymph node involvement is low (<1%) hence, pelvic lymphadenectomy is not recommended, unless there is lymphovascular space involvement.

For stage IA2 and IB disease, nodal involvement is 4–10% hence, routine pelvic lymphadenectomy is necessary while performing radical hysterectomy.

ADVANTAGES: RADICAL SURGERY VERSUS RADIATION THERAPY

Radical surgery has the following advantages over radiation therapy:

- Identifies high risk patients who will benefit from adjuvant therapy
- Allows preservation of ovarian function, especially in younger women
- Allows accurate evaluation of the extent of the disease
- Sexual function can be preserved
- Complications of surgery are early as compared to radiation and also easier to treat. Late complications are rare with surgery unlike radiation therapy
- Psychological benefits of removal of tumor
- Ideal radiotherapy unit and expert radiotherapist may not always be available. Incomplete radiation therapy cannot replace good surgical treatment
- Treatment is over in a single sitting with surgery, hence continued patient compliance is obviated.

DISADVANTAGES

- Complications of prolonged surgery and anesthesia are possible
- Surgery does not take care of micrometastases as in radiotherapy
- Sexual dysfunction may result from excessively shortened vagina
- Inoperability in clinically operable cases may further require radiation, hence patient has to undergo unnecessary surgical morbidity
- Postoperative adjuvant radiotherapy may be required, thereby increasing the morbidity
- Risks of thromboembolism, paralytic ileus and RTIs are increased, during surgery.

INDICATIONS OF RADICAL HYSTERECTOMY

- Invasive cervical cancer: Stage IA1 with lymphovascular space involvement, stages IA2 and IB1, selected cases of stage IB2 and IIA
- Invasive vaginal cancer: Stage I and II limited to upper one-third of vagina
- Endometrial cancer: Stage IIB
- Persistent or recurrent cervical cancer after radiation therapy.

CONTRAINDICATIONS

Contraindications to radical hysterectomy include patients who have medical complications and those who refuse surgical treatment. In patients whose religious or personal beliefs prohibit use of blood product transfusion, radiation therapy should be considered as up to 50% cases may require blood transfusion with surgery. The possible requirements for adjuvant radiotherapy (i.e. bulky disease or intraoperative findings of locally advanced disease with overt parametrial involvement or grossly positive pelvic lymph nodes) can be a relative contraindication.

RELEVANT ANATOMY

Knowledge of the relevant anatomy of the pelvis (Fig. 1) is important, especially the pelvic lymph nodes, the course of the ureter (Fig. 2), anatomy of the cardinal and uterosacral ligaments.

The pertinent boundaries for dissection are as follows:

- The paravesical space is bordered:
  - Medially by the obliterated umbilical artery
  - Laterally by the obturator internus muscle
  - Posteriorly by the cardinal ligament
  - Anteriorly by the pubic symphysis
- The pararectal space is bordered:
  - Medially by the rectum
  - Laterally by the hypogastric artery (the internal iliac artery)

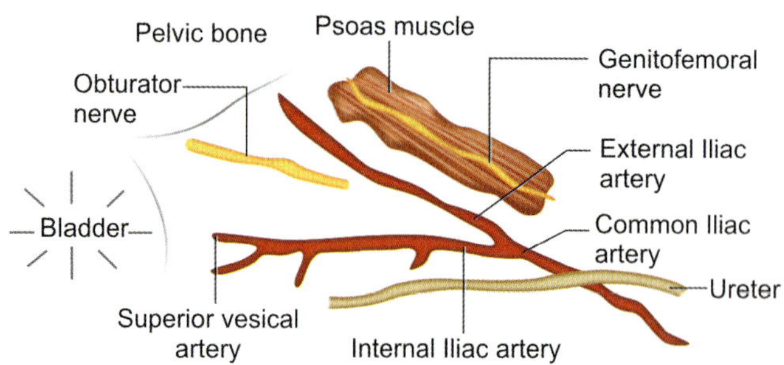

Fig. 1: Anatomy of pelvis—right side

- Posteriorly by the sacrum
- Anteriorly by the cardinal ligament.

- The limits of dissection for pelvic lymphadenectomy are (Fig. 3):
  - Superiorly—2 cm above the bifurcation of common iliac artery
  - Inferiorly—endopelvic fascia
  - Laterally—genitofemoral nerve
  - Medially—bladder and medial side of internal iliac vessel
  - Depth of dissection should be upto the obturator nerve.

The pelvic lymphadenectomy is performed in a systematic fashion.

All fatty tissues are stripped off from the common iliac vessels and the internal and external iliac vessels to the level of the circumflex iliac vein distally, with preservation of the genitofemoral nerve on the psoas muscle. The nodal tissue in the obturator fossa is removed upto the obturator nerve. Care must be taken in the obturator fossa to avoid injury to the obturator nerve or to an accessory obturator vein, which is present in approximately 20% of patients.

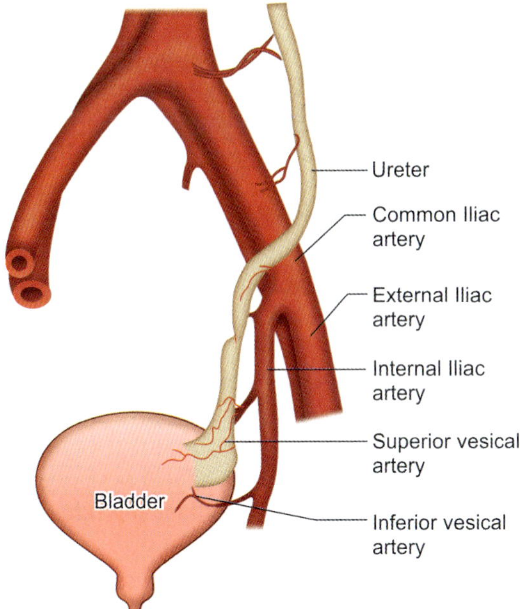

Fig. 2: Course of ureter

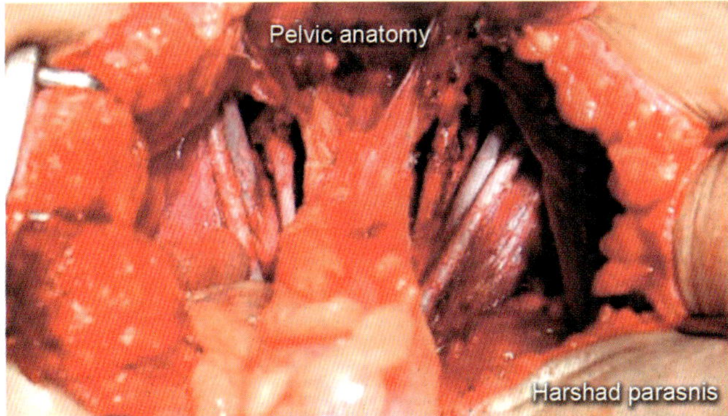

Fig. 3: Pelvic anatomy dissected out at modified radical hysterectomy

Ureteric Dissection

Ischemic necrosis of ureter can be prevented by preserving its profuse collateral blood supply. The ureter should not be denuded of all tissue uptil the adventitia. The lateral aspect of the posterior segment of the vesicouterine ligament needs to be preserved to insure adequate blood supply to the terminal ureter.

PREOPERATIVE EVALUATION

Currently International Federation of Gynecology and Obstetrics (FIGO) evaluation procedures for staging were limited to colposcopy, biopsy, conization of cervix, cystoscopy and proctosigmoidoscopy.

As with any other surgery, careful preoperative risk assessment must be performed. The preoperative workup must include:

- Physical examination for tumor size and extent
- Histopathological confirmation
- Hematological tests: Hemogram, liver function test (LFT), renal function test (RFT), HIV, hepatitis B surface antigen (HbsAg) estimations
- Urine analysis
- X-ray chest to rule out lung metastases
- USG or CT scan for tumor size, extent, enlarged lymph nodes, hydroureter and hydronephrosis
- If clinically indicated, following tests must be performed:
  - IVP
  - Cystoscopy
  - Proctosigmoidoscopy
  - Barium enema
  - Magnetic resonance imaging (MRI) or positron emission tomography (PET)-CT
  - Scalene node biopsy
  - Radioisotope scan.

PREREQUISITES

- Blood compatible with patient's blood ready
- Bowel preparation as for bowel operation
- Gauze packing of the vagina: It converts the vagina into a solid cylinder so that its separation from the bladder and the rectum is facilitated

- Ureteric catheterization is done by some gynecologists, to facilitate ureteric localization and dissection during operation. However, it is not recommended as ureteric epithelium may be crushed while picking the ureter with forceps and may be inadvertently stretched.

TECHNIQUE: STEPS OF OPERATION

- Anesthesia: The operation is done under continuous epidural or spinal anesthesia
- Incision: The abdomen is opened by right paramedian or midline vertical incision which extends from the pubis to above the umbilicus (Fig. 4)
- Assessment of spread and operability: The operability is assessed by exploration of the peritoneal cavity.

The liver surface, under surface of diaphragm, omentum, small and large bowel are examined thoroughly. The kidneys are palpated for enlargement.

- The round and the infundibulopelvic ligaments are divided. The anterior and posterior leaves of the broad ligaments are opened and the paravesical and pararectal spaces are developed by blunt dissection. Parametrial involvement is assessed. Para-aortic lymph nodes are biopsied and sent for histopathological study by frozen section technique
- Pelvic lymph node dissection: After transfixing the round ligaments and the infundibulopelvic ligaments close to the lateral pelvic walls, the pelvic lymphadenectomy is begun. The posterior leaf of the broad ligament is opened up to the pelvic brim with the ureter in the medial portion of the peritoneum. The lymphatic tissue above the common iliac vessels is removed. The external iliac vessels are dissected up to the level of the circumflex iliac vein distally. The obturator space is cleaned of all lymphatic tissue removing all lymph nodes below the bifurcation of the iliac vessels including the hypogastric nodes and the obturator nodes (Fig. 3)
- Bladder and ureteric dissection: The anterior division of the internal iliac artery is traced down and the uterine artery is ligated near its origin. The uterine veins are also ligated. The bladder is dissected off the isthmus, the cervix and the vagina by dividing the uterovesical fold of peritoneum. Lower end of the ureter is identified. The ureteric tunnel is opened by sliding the tips of scissors along the anterior surface of the ureter and gently spreading the blades. The roof of the tunnel is divided between clamps. Anterior and posterior attachments of the broad ligament to the base of the bladder are clamped and divided. Different methods have been adopted for treatment of the denuded pelvic ureter
  - It may be left in its usual retroperitoneal position. In this position, it lies in a pool of serosanguineous fluid and is vulnerable to infection
  - Ureter is suspended from the anterior division of the internal iliac artery, upto the origin of the superior vesical artery, and the exposed segment of the pelvic ureter may be placed intraperitoneally
  - Ureter is placed in a tunnel formed by approximation of the walls of the bladder and the rectum lateral to the ureter.
- Posterior dissection with uterosacral ligation (Fig. 5): The uterus is pulled forward to put the uterosacral ligaments on stretch. The peritoneum of the pouch of Douglas is divided as it gets reflected off the anterior surface of the rectum. The vagina is separated from the

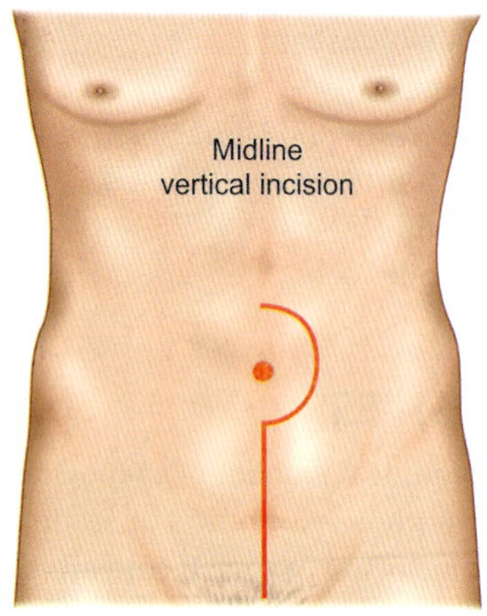

Fig. 4: Abdominal by midline vertical incisions

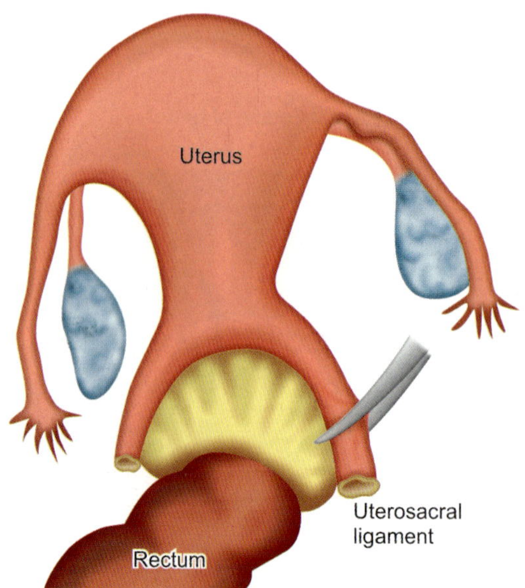

Fig. 5: Removal and division of uterosacral ligaments

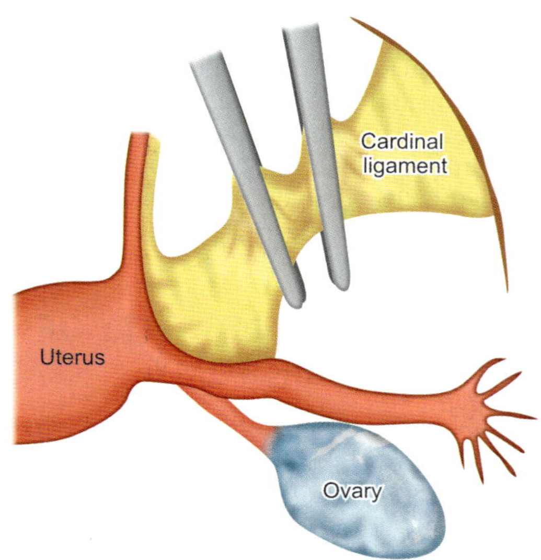

Fig. 6: Dividing cardinal ligament

rectum by blunt dissection and then the vaginal pack is removed. The uterosacral ligaments are divided as far back as possible

- Cardinal ligament ligation: The cardinal ligament is divided on either side at its attachment to the lateral pelvic wall (Fig. 6)
- Paracolpos ligation and opening the vagina: The paravaginal tissue is clamped and divided, so as to free the upper 3–5 cm of the vagina
- Vagina closure: The vault of the vagina is closed by placing a continuous interlocking suture over the cut edges for hemostasis. Drainage from the obturator fossae and the lateral pelvic walls is achieved by continuous low suction drains (constant 10 cm H_2O pressure) brought out by abdominal stab incisions.

POSTOPERATIVE MANAGEMENT

- General care as after an exploratory laparotomy
- Replacement of all the blood lost during operation, if not already replaced intraoperatively
- Continuous bladder drainage for 5–7 days. Prolonged drainage has no therapeutic benefit. After removal of the catheter, residual urine is checked and if it is more than 50 mL, drainage is reinstituted
- The continuous low suction drains are removed when the drainage is less than 50 mL in a 24 hours period which is usually on the 4th or 5th day. Some oncologist prefer not to keep retroperitoneal drains as retrospective as well as prospective studies do not show any advantage with retroperitoneal drains in preventing fistulas or lymphocyst formation.

Follow-Up

Follow-up examinations are done every 3 months for 2 years, and every 6 months thereafter. A speculum examination with Pap test, a bimanual pelvic examination, an abdominal examination and USG are done. Supraclavicular and inguinal lymph nodes are palpated.

COMPLICATIONS

- Hemorrhage—intraoperative and postoperative
- Injury to major blood vessels
- Pelvic infection—urinary tract infection: Cystitis, ascending ureteric infection. Cystitis is due to residual urine, diminished blood supply, and extensive denudation
- Injury to the ureter, bladder and the rectum
- Fistulas—vesicovaginal, ureterovaginal and rectovaginal fistulas due to direct trauma, ischemic necrosis and infection. Urinary fistula occurs in 4.4% cases
- Deep vein thrombosis and thromboembolism
- Edema feet—unilateral or bilateral
- Lymphocyst—it follows extensive excision of lymph nodes and lymphatics and occurs in about 30% cases. It contains clear sterile fluid with high cholesterol levels, and some lymphocytes. It recurs if aspirated and may require a percutaneous drainage or transperitoneal marsupialization
- Urinary stress incontinence—secondary to complete transaction of the cardinal ligaments causing sympathetic denervation
- Operative mortality rate in a good facility is 0.72%.

POSTOPERATIVE EXTERNAL RADIATION

After radical hysterectomy, external radiation is given if the following adverse factors are present:

- Pelvic lymph node metastases
- Presence of lymph vascular space invasion
- Barrel-shaped tumor
- Surgical margin (vaginal) positive for tumor
- Parametrial metastases
- Special histology like adenosquamous or clear cell carcinoma
- Residual pelvic disease after surgery
- Depth of cervical infiltration more than two-third.

MODIFICATIONS

Okabayashi Method

The cardinal principles include performing the posterior procedure prior to anterior procedure, more extensive excision of the parametrium, preservation of the pelvic anatomic nerve bundles and prolonged postoperative bladder drainage. Lymphadenectomy is done after the hysterectomy.

Tokyo Method

The cardinal principles include retrograde pelvic lymphadenectomy to prevent centripetal cellular spread, preservation of the pelvic autonomic nerve bundle under the cardinal ligament and covering the ureter using the walls of the bladder and rectum to prevent adhesion of the ureter to the pelvic wall.

Miami Method

The cardinal principles of this modification of Meig radical hysterectomy include vaginal closure and reconstruction using bladder and rectosigmoid serosa, retroperitoneal drainage through abdominal suction catheters, and suspension of the denuded ureters with ipsilateral obliterated hypogastric artery.

MORBIDITY AND MORTALITY OF RADICAL HYSTERECTOMY

A review of literature of 6,992 radical hysterectomies done throughout the world reveals an overall operative mortality rate of 0.72% and urinary tract fistula rate of 4.4%. In the last few years, the improved techniques have reduced the fistula rate to between 0% and 2%.

BIBLIOGRAPHY

1. Averette HE, Ngoyen HN, Donato DM, et al. Radical hysterectomy for invasive cervical cancer: A 25-year prospective experience with the Miami Technique. Cancer. 1993;71:1422-37.
2. Benedet JL, Anderson MC, Buckley CH, et al. Stage IA carcinoma of the cervix revisited. Obstet Gynecol. 1996;87:1052.
3. Blythe JG, Hodel KA, Wahl TP. A comparison between peritoneal sheathing of the ureters (Ohkawa technique) and retroperitoneal pelvic suction drainage in the prevention of ureteral damage during radical abdominal hysterectomy. Gynecol Oncol. 1988;30:222.
4. Clark JG. A more radical method of performing hysterectomy for the cancer of the uterus. Bull Johns Hopkins Hosp. 1895;6:120.
5. Hopkins MP, Schmidt RW, Roberts JA, et al. The prognosis and treatment of stage adenocarcinoma of the cervix. Obstet Gynecol. 1988;72:915.
6. Jensen PT, Groenvold M, Klee MC, et al. Longitudinal study of sexual function and vaginal changes after radiotherapy for cervical cancer. Int J Radiat Oncol Biol Phys. 2003;56:937.
7. Landoni F, Maneo A, Cormio G, et al. Class II versus class III radical hysterectomy in stage IB-IIA cervical cancer: A prospective randomized study. Gynecol Oncol. 2001;80:3-12.
8. Meigs JV. The Wertheim operation for the carcinoma of the cervix. Am J Obstet Gynecol. 1945;49:542.
9. Okabayashi H. Radical abdominal hysterectomy for cancer of the cervix uteri. Surg Gynecol Obstet. 1921;33:345.
10. Orr JW, Orr PJ, Bolen DD, et al. Radical hysterectomy: Does the type of incision matter? Am J Obstet Gynecol. 1995;173(2):399-405.
11. Piver MS, Rutledge FN, Smith JP. Five classes of extended hysterectomy for women with cervical cancer. Obstet Gynecol. 1974;44:265.
12. Sevin BU, Nadji M, Averette HE, et al. Microinvasive carcinoma of the cervix. Cancer. 1992;70:2121-8.
13. Wertheim E. The extended abdominal operation for carcinoma of the cervix. Am J Obstet Gynecol. 1912;66:169.
14. Whitney CW, Stehman FB. The abandoned radical hysterectomy: A Gynecologic Oncology Group Study. Gynecol Oncol. 2000;79(3):350-6.

41.5 VAGINAL HYSTERECTOMY

SS Sheth

INTRODUCTION

The debate on whether the uterus should be removed vaginally or abdominally was sparked when Langenbeck first performed a vaginal hysterectomy (VH) in 1813. Historically, the reason, gynecological surgery became a specialty in its own right, was its extensive use of the vaginal route. The vaginal approach has always been the hallmark of the gynecological surgeon.

Very often, a hysterectomy that should have been done vaginally is done abdominally only because it is more easily executed and is the favored practice at a particular clinic. It was introduction of laparoscopic surgery, hysterectomy in particular, that has ignited the comparison between routes and techniques. All uteri that can be removed vaginally can be removed by the abdominal route or by laparoscopically-assisted vaginal hysterectomy (LAVH), but the reverse is not true. The famous French surgeon Doyen insisted in 1939 that no one could call himself a gynecologist until he performed vaginal hysterectomy "in private".

Hysterectomy is one of the most common major gynecological operations, with over 100,000 procedures performed annually in England and 600,000 in the United States. All large-scale surveys of hysterectomy practice show that 70–80% of hysterectomies are performed by the abdominal approach, except in uterovaginal prolapse, for which the vaginal route is normally used. A study of more than 37,000 hysterectomies showed that about two-thirds of the operations were abdominal, just over one-quarter were vaginal, and a small proportion, 3.1% were performed laparoscopically.

In Sweden, more than 95% of all hysterectomies that are not performed in conjunction with a uterovaginal prolapse are performed abdominally. Interestingly, Western Australia (WA) has 40% hysterectomies by abdominal route. WA has one of the highest hysterectomy rates in the world but performs proportionately few abdominal hysterectomies compared with most countries.

Generally, the ratio of vaginal hysterectomy to abdominal hysterectomy (AH) varies from 1:3 to 1:4 or less depending on the country, though this ratio is reversed in the hands of experienced vaginal surgeons to 60–90% (e.g. Brown 79%, Bezdek 82%, Hefni 65%, Hewson 80%, Kovac 90%, Magos 57% and Querleu 77%). Decline in AH and LAVH have favorably increased the incidence of VH. In the authors personal series of 7,334 hysterectomies in India, 6,044 (82%) were carried out vaginally, of these 92% were in the absence of uterovaginal prolapse.

The vaginal route is the primary route for hysterectomy provided its superiority is beyond doubt in comparable cases. The scope of selecting one of several options from various types of hysterectomies available, should ideally depend on:

- What is best for the patient, and
- Absence or presence of contraindications. No other factor should interfere in this holistic decision.

ASPECTS THAT COMPEL TO OPT VAGINAL HYSTERECTOMY

Several aspects, cumulatively decide what is the best or choicest to become primary route, are as given below:

Complications

The complication rate for AH is 70% higher than that for VH. More than 20 years later survey in, the UK reached a similar conclusion. Western Australia study of 83,000 hysterectomies shared that the occurrence of a serious complication was 20% lower for vaginal hysterectomies compared with abdominal procedures.

In the Valsartan Antihypertensive Long-term use Evaluation (VALUE) study of 37,298 hysterectomies from the UK, the overall operative complication rate for vaginal hysterectomy was 3.07% while 3.57% of abdominal hysterectomy patients were reported to have a complication of surgery and 6.07% of women treated by LAVH experienced a complication.

One conclusion of the VALUE study is that laparoscopic techniques tend to be associated with higher complication rates than other methods. Major concern is towards urinary tract injuries. Cystotomy and ureteric injury rate is 1.38% and 0.91%, respectively. This rate is far too high when compared with conventional vaginal hysterectomy. In a review of 1,372 articles in the world literature between 1970 and 1996, the incidence of bladder injury was highest with LAVH. Postoperative fever which often matters to patient as well as relatives was significantly higher in the abdominal group (18%) compared with 9% and 8% respectively in the vaginal and LAVH groups. Wound infection, which is unlikely after VH, adds 3.5 days to the hospital stay after AH.

The chances of leaving behind a sponge are remote with VH. However, the collaborative review of sterilization (CREST) study report shows an overall rate for the complication of bleeding of 2.6% with VH and of 1.6% with AH. Blood loss is more when vaginal hysterectomy is associated with repair than without.

According to the data collected by the Centers for Disease Control (CDC) in the USA, excluding pregnancy and cancer-related cases, the mortality rate for a vaginal hysterectomy was 2.7/10,000 procedures, compared with 8.6/10,000 procedures for an abdominal hysterectomy. In an analysis of hysterectomies in the USA, reported least mortality per 10,000 procedure of LAVHs and maximum for abdominal hysterectomy.

Time and Cost

Studies have proved beyond doubt that VH and AH require less operative time and anesthesia time than LAVH or LH. Operation room time is precious and can effect expenses as well as number of admissions to the hospital. The accompanying Table 1 distinctly points that LAVH or LH take longer in performance increasing risk, monetary inputs and efforts. Despite an increase in laparoscopic skills, most gynecologists still find that laparoscopic hysterectomy is technically demanding, takes too long and may need expensive disposable equipment. Thus, when laparoscopic surgery is used more extensively, the costs are higher.

Studies that examined components of total charges indicated that laparoscopic hysterectomy was often more expensive because of the use of disposable instruments, longer operating room and anesthesia times, and intraoperative pharmacy charges. All studies comparing laparoscopic and VH, reported laparoscopic hysterectomy to be more expensive and VH as the least expensive. If 80% or more hysterectomies are performed vaginally, the National Health Service (NHS) hospitals, UK could save as many as 22,000 bed days annually, but the situation is far from the ideal. The cost factor, whether to an individual, his employer or an insurance company, cannot be ignored. In developing countries, cost tilts the balance in favor of not the best.

Table 2 argues in favor of the vaginal route from the study; still only 20–30% of hysterectomies are carried out via the vaginal route in the Western world.

Doucette calculated that a shift of 10% from abdominal to vaginal hysterectomy in the United States would save more than $7.5 million in hospital costs alone. This is an important message, particularly for the developing world. Kovac has contended that if size, access and adnexa are evaluated, 90% of hysterectomies for benign indications could be safely done vaginally, thus saving more than $200 billion each year in the United States—easily more than $1,000 per hysterectomy. Hospital stay did not differ in the laparoscopic and vaginal group but laparoscopic technique proved more expensive than conventional hysterectomy.

Table 1: Summary of meta-analysis distinctly present benefits of technique used

Measure	Statistical significance	Interpretation
Abdominal vs laparoscopic hysterectomy		
Operating time	$p < 0.01$	LH > AH
Anesthesia time	$p < 0.01$	LH > AH
Length of stay	$p < 0.01$	LH > AH
Hospital charges	$p < 0.01$	No difference
Vaginal vs laparoscopic hysterectomy		
Operating time	$p < 0.01$	LH > VH
Anesthesia time	$p < 0.01$	LH > VH
Length of stay	$p < 0.05$	No difference
Hospital charges	$p < 0.05$	LH > VH

Source: Betram DA, Kovac SR, Cruikshank SH. The role of laparoscopy in hysterectomy. J Pelvic Surg. 1997;39:147-58.

Abbreviations: LH, Laparoscopic hysterectomy; AH, Abdominal hysterectomy; VH, Vaginal hysterectomy

Table 2: Complication rates among women aged 15–44 years undergoing hysterectomy by surgical approach

Complication	Complication rate% Vaginal (n=568)	Complication rate% Abdominal (n=1283)
Febrile morbidity	15.3	32.3
Transfusion	8.3	15.4
Atelectasis	1.1	5.9
Ileus	0.2	2.2
Wound dehiscence	0	0.2
Neuropathy	0	0.2
Deep vein thrombosis or Thrombophlebitis	0	0.2

The surgeon needs only standard instruments and sutures, and 80% of the world, i.e. the developing countries, would be better served by gynecologists with knowledge of the techniques of vaginal surgery and expertize in their application. Availability, access, cost and affordability are important aspects of the practice of surgery. The economic benefit and patient friendliness of vaginal surgery are important advantages.

Stay

Hospital stay for VH and LAVH is similar, and both are significantly shorter than for AH. There is no doubt that AH will have hospital stay longer by 24–72 hours and this can matter to patient, relatives, hospital and insurance company. In an interesting study, Summitt et al showed that following simple VH, the total hospital stay could average 9.4 hours with 100% patient satisfaction. This study clearly announced that hospital stay can be considerably reduced, reduced to less than 48 hours.

In short, VH is the procedure associated with the quickest operating time, the shortest hospital stay, and the lowest hospital costs.

Recovery

Vaginal hysterectomy has following favorable facets.

- Hospitalization, pulmonary complications, morbidity, and mortality are reduced
- Discomfort and pain are reduced as a result of minimal or almost no handling of the bowel
- Reduced operative time, better drainage, and simpler anesthesia
- Intestinal: Flatulence, pain, and ileus are less, as are blood loss and shock
- Reduced incidence of thrombophlebitis and emboli
- Hastened recovery as a result of largely extraperitoneal surgery
- No abdominal scar and adhesions.

For any technique route or methodology to become "primary", it has to prove its worth. Worth, value and recognition will come from above benefits.

Blood Transfusion

In a study by Mintz et al, blood transfusions were required in 25%, 12.5%, and 5% of patients undergoing an AH, VH with colporrhaphy, and a VH without repair, respectively. The incidence of blood transfusion is greater with the abdominal rather than the vaginal route; 15.4% with the abdominal and 8.3% with the vaginal route. These rates appear high. Copenhaver also reports increased blood loss with an associated colporrhaphy. Infiltrating the cervix with a vasoconstrictor before VH appears to reduce blood loss. Hewson finds transfusion rate with VH was only 0.38% when compared with 2.1% with AH. In the days tinged with fear of HIV and hepatitis, the gynecologist needs to focus heavily on reducing the incidence of blood transfusion. In the author's personal series, 2.4% women received a blood transfusion because of a low hemoglobin (8–9 g/dL), despite best possible treatment.

Invasion

Trauma associated with surgery needs to be looked at in the proper perspective and just not in the form of punctures and incisions and their size. Even though incisions or cuts are small, it is the handling of tissues for long hours and a woman remaining under anesthesia for disproportionately longer time and bigger cuts on purse and not the greater invasion. Extended operative time and invasion on operation theater occupancy must be considered. These factors play a vital role in many geographical areas and should contribute heavily in the surgeon's choice of hysterectomy.

Morbidity

No surgery can be without complications, or physical price. Operative morbidity, cosmesis and recuperation favor the vaginal approach. It has advantages in recovery, cost, hospital stay, absence of scar and is the least invasive and minimal accessed hysterectomy. Jeffcoate finds advantages in the vaginal route as it is safer, with low mortality, has less postoperative shock and discomfort with early ambulation. There is much less bowel handling, and therefore, ileus and intestinal obstructions are rare.

It is better tolerated by elderly and high-risk patients and with a lesser risk of hernia, adhesions, and wound dehiscence besides providing the opportunity to correct prolapse or laxity. There is definitely less thrombophlebitis, atelectasis and pneumonia, pulmonary embolism and forgotten foreign bodies, though it must be remembered that patients undergoing an AH have more severe disease.

Randomized Studies

A randomized study by Ottosen et al. whose objective was to detect differences in clinical short-term outcome between total abdominal hysterectomy, vaginal hysterectomy and laparoscopic assisted vaginal hysterectomy. Main outcome measures were duration of surgery, anesthesia, time in hospital and recovery time. Mean duration (range) of surgery was significantly longer for LAVH compared with VH and total abdominal hysterectomy (TAH), 102 minutes (50–175), 81 minutes (35–135) and 68 minutes (28–125), respectively. Thus, concluding that traditional VH proved to be feasible and the faster operative technique compared with VH with laparoscopic assistance. The abdominal technique was somewhat faster, but time spent in theater was not significantly shorter. AH required on average a longer hospital stay of 1 day and one additional week of convalescence compared with traditional VH.

A trial in the USA concluded that VH compared with AH and LAVH, scored the most points in terms of patient satisfaction and wellbeing.

There are 20 randomized controlled trials (RCTs) comparing TAH and VH with LH and 16 RCTs comparing LH with TAH. Almost all trials indicate that LH takes more surgical time with lesser stay and shorter recovery period. Conclusion from 27 trials with 3,643 was that where VH is not possible, laparoscopic hysterectomy is preferable to AH, although it brings a higher chance of bladder or ureter injury. Another four studies, though not randomized, clearly suggest that VH should be preferred for hysterectomy, unless specific indications in favor of the abdominal or laparoscopic route are present.

Scar

Just as at laparotomy, laparoscopic hysterectomy or LAVH also leave behind scars though very small. They can stand out if turned into keloid. In contrast, VH has no visible scar. Cuts inflicted to carry out VH are also the same cuts inflicted at AH, LAVH and LH.

Quality of Life and Satisfaction

A more recent prospective study from the technology assessment group at Kaiser Permanente®, which examined quality of life (QOL) measures, found that patients who had VH returned to normal activity much sooner, had more favorable pain, activity, and function outcomes than patients who underwent either LAVH or AH. LH had lower mean increase in quality adjusted life years (QALYs) than VH.

Thus, when all clinical decisions are equal, VH appears to provide the most satisfactory outcomes from the patient's point of view, although QOL outcomes for the laparoscopic procedure were often as favorable and both were superior to AH. Before concluding, results require proof-evidence that convinces and this has accrued out of RCTs and various studies.

All trials point to supremacy of vaginal route for hysterectomy without any scope for offering a flaccid argument with rationale.

When all the parameters tilt the balance heavily in favor of taking the vaginal route for hysterectomy, "decision making" will now necessitate exclusion of contraindications to that route of hysterectomy.

CONTRAINDICATIONS

These are few to take away the option of choosing vaginal route as primary route for hysterectomy. They are:

Common

- Uterus more than 12 weeks size or uterine volume more than 250–300 cm^3
- Restriction of uterine mobility
- Adnexal pathology.

Uncommon

- Cervix flush with the vagina or past Fothergill's operation makes the cervix look most unlike a cervix
- Invasive cancer of the cervix
- Vesicovaginal and/or rectovaginal fistula repair
- Inaccessible cervix: Uncommonly, after repeated uterine surgery, particularly past cesarean section, there are dense adhesions between the uterocervical surface, the bladder and the lower abdominal wall (Fig. 1) an which makes the cervix an inaccessible, approach by the vaginal route. These adhesions can be anticipated by simple speculum examination by the presence of Sheth's cervicofundal sign. With a rise in the cesarean section rate, gynecologists should be aware of such adhesions
- Uterocervical angle of 90° Globular uterus mimicking small melon perched on top of cervical stump typically in angle between the lateral cervical surface and the ascending uterine wall from the cervix. When the angle is reduced from usual 140° or more to 90° or thereabout (Figs 2A and B), chances of failing to perform a VH rise sharply.

Very often vaginal hysterectomy, though recognized as the choicest method, is not performed. Two classic studies give crystal clear picture of operator's weakness.

1. Davies et al reviewed 500 cases of hysterectomies; 76% were by the abdominal route in the absence of an absolute contraindication to vaginal hysterectomy. Reasons given for not taking the vaginal route were absence of prolapse in 76%, presence of fibroid in 45%, and need for oophorectomy in 43%.

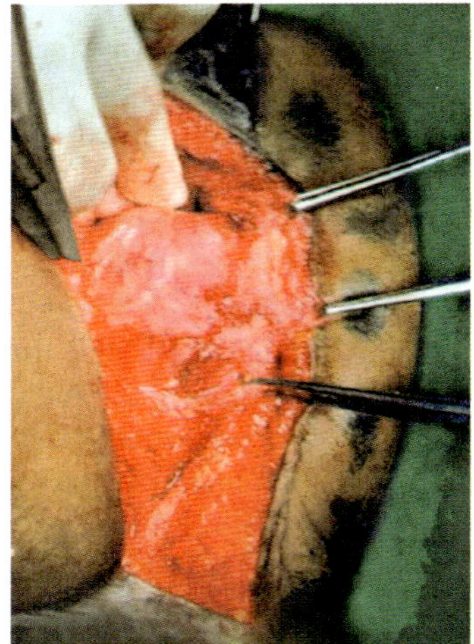

Fig. 1: Classic adhesions seen at laparotomy with cesarean section in the past. Deaver's retractor and Allis forceps on the skin marking at the umbilical level close to the upper end of the right paramedian incision. The uterine fundus of a normal size uterus is well above half way between the symphysis pubis and the umbilicus

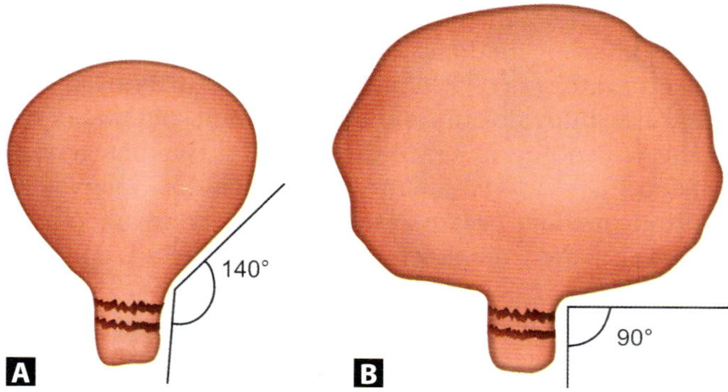

Figs 2A and B: The depicted angle between lateral cervical and uterine borders, greater than 140°, makes access and reach easier. Reduction of the angle toward 90° makes access and reach very difficult or impossible

[***Source:*** Sheth SS. Uterine Fibroids. In: Sheth SS, Studd JWW (Eds). Vaginal Hysterectomy. London: Martin Dunitz Ltd., 2002. pp. 79-94. (permission obtained)]

2. Much can be learned from the experience of Kovac who assessed all his patients scheduled for abdominal hysterectomy by performing a laparoscopy before opening the abdomen. He wanted to determine whether laparoscopy performed immediately before hysterectomy could be used in deciding and finalizing the route of hysterectomy. Assessment of the pelvic findings by laparoscopy changed the decision from the abdominal to the vaginal route in 91% of cases without any complications during surgery. This clearly drives home the fact that careful and thorough assessment is vital in planning this major gynecological procedure. He and his team concluded that preoperative laparoscopy may allow more hysterectomies to be performed by the vaginal route without laparoscopic surgical assistance in lieu of reposing blind faith in the abdominal route as the method of choice.

The gynecologist who opts for LAVH or AH instead a clear indication of VH, often consoles himself with one or other reasons for doing so.

The excuses given for avoiding the vaginal approach and favoring an abdominal or LH or LAVH include:

- There is no uterine prolapse or descent
- The uterus is large. There is a fibroid in the uterus
- The patient is nulliparous
- There is a history of cesarean section or pelvic surgery in the past
- There may be adhesions or endometriosis
- The patient needs an oophorectomy
- Inspection of the abdominal organs, particularly the appendix, is essential.

Let us examine each excuse or reason given for not taking a vaginal route.

EXCUSES

There is no Uterine Prolapse or Descent

Neither absence of prolapse is a contraindication to taking vaginal route for hysterectomy nor presence of prolapse is a prerequisite. Every gynecologist must notice that every freely mobile uterus without pelvic pathology has physiological descent, which permits the start of a VH. Uterine prolapse is pathological descent and non-descent of uterus occurs due to pathological connective tissue, which contraindicates VH. To gain experience in arriving at a decision, the ideal is to seize the opportunity to examine under anesthesia (EUA) every young nulliparous woman undergoing conservative gynecological surgery, as if she is scheduled for hysterectomy.

The Uterus is Large or There is a Fibroid in the Uterus

Uterus may be larger than normal due to several conditions. The most common are uterine fibroids, adenomyosis and dysfunctional uterine bleeding. What matters is that total uterine size is not more than 12 weeks or 250–300 cm^3 volume.

If at examination under anesthesia, particularly on applying traction to the cervix, uterine fundus descends to disappear in the pelvis, and is not palpable per abdomen, the vaginal route should not pose a problem. If one expects a fetus to travel through this very passage, access should not be a problem for a smaller sized uterus.

The Patient is Nulliparous

It is not unusual to find 90% of hysterectomies in the nullipara performed abdominally, as nulliparity creates concern about descent and space. However, after the advent of LAVH, VH percentage has now gone up to 40% from meager 10%.

The author's series of 112 virgins with severe mental handicap who have had VH to eradicate problem of menstrual hygiene, is an example in strong favor of feasibility of VH for nulliparous women. Hysterectomy in a nullipara should not be by laparotomy, unless there is a clear-cut contraindication for VH and unfavorable findings for LAVH. As long as the uterus is less than 12 weeks size, freely mobile and without adnexal pathology, VH should be possible. Nulliparity per se should never contraindicate vaginal hysterectomy.

There is a History of Cesarean Section or Pelvic Surgery in the Past

Previous abdominal or pelvic surgery: Operations performed on the uterus are the most important—cesarean section, hysterectomy and myomectomy demand caution, but in no way contraindicates VH.

It has been observed that when the bladder is adherent following a cesarean in past, it is almost always in central 3/5 and not lateral 1/5. In addition, MRI studies at the level of the cervical isthmus through different planes show a distinct vacant space medial to the line joining the maximally bulging uterus above and the cervix below, with its continuity medially between the uterocervical surface and the bladder until they come extremely close to each other in the midline (Fig. 3). At VH in a patient with history of cesarean, Khung chooses to separate lateral, non-adherent portion of bladder through a surgical window lateral to the midline on the anterior cervix or Sheth's uterocervical broad ligament space (Fig. 4), and the same space is often utilized at the time of AH or LH when separation of bladder in its central portion is difficult or risky. Sizzi and Rossetti note that "a safer approach is from the lateral, the surgical window described by Sheth which allows a safe, sharp dissection, also through laparoscopy, starting from both sides going medially toward the medial portion of the vesicouterine space." The author has routinely used this surgical window for more than 15 years to obtain access to the vesicouterine space during VH in women with a previous history of cesarean section, including many with multiple previous cesarean sections and/or myomectomy in past and rare women with a history of uterine rupture.

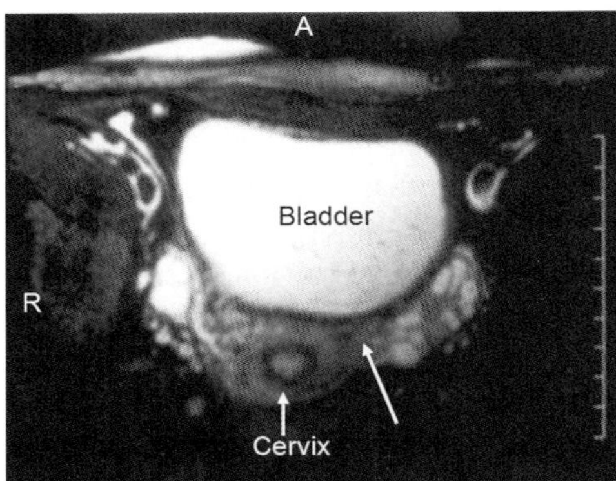

Fig. 3: Transverse section magnetic resonance imaging (MRI) at the isthmic level shows clear space between the bladder in front and the uterocervical surface behind, with continuity laterally between the two leaves of the broad ligament

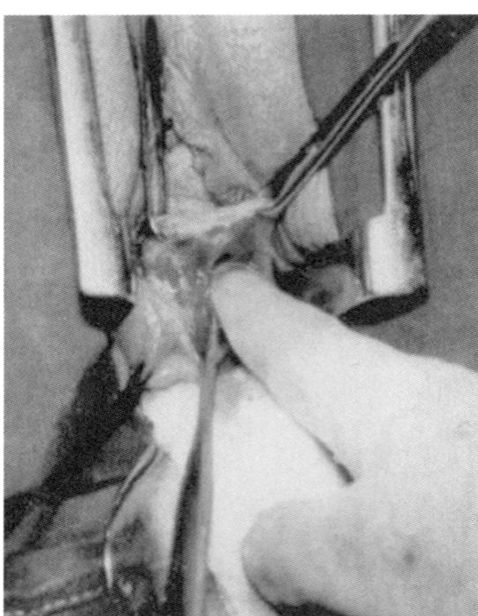

Fig. 4: At vaginal hysterectomy, the finger is on the uterocervical surface, with the bladder anteromedially, as it insinuates further between the two leaves of the broad ligament laterally (surgical window in cases with past cesarean)

There may be Adhesions or Endometriosis

If indicated size uterus is freely mobile with normal adnexa and absence of pelvic pathology, there is no justification to take route or technique other than vaginal route. If doubt and/or anxiety prevails, examination under anesthesia and laparoscopic evaluation will guide the decision making. More often, adhesions are in operator's mind and not in patient's pelvis.

The Patient needs Oophorectomy

Clamping and suturing, pretied ligature placement, automatic stapling devices, bipolar coagulation endoloop sutures and transvaginal endoscopic oophorectomy utilizing endoloop sutures or bipolar electrosurgery have helped surgeons to accomplish oophorectomy vaginally at vaginal hysterectomy without laparoscopic assistance. Objective is to keep invasion at minimum, i.e. do not utilize abdominal access. Author prefers conventional clamping-and-cutting fundibulopelvic ligament and performing salpingo-oophorectomy. This has two prerequisites: (1) To cut round ligament separately, and (2) cut distally, 3–4 cm from the uterus.

Sheth reported 95% success while performing prophylactic oophorectomy at VH in 740 cases. Davies et al. and Hefni and Davies have successfully performed oophorectomy vaginally at VH. Cengiz et al. used laparoscopic evaluation and followed successfully in 64.7% by performing VH using Heaney's technique and salpingo-oophorectomy using Sheth's technique. Kovac and Cruikshank found oophorectomy at VH is possible in great majority and is superior to other approaches.

American College of Obstetrics and Gynecology (ACOG) guidelines clearly define that LAVH is needed only when oophorectomy at VH is difficult. In other words, it can be done at VH and in few cases—in genuinely difficult cases, LAVH rescues.

Inspection of the Abdominal Organs, particularly the Appendix is Essential

This is a very uncommon requirement in a woman undergoing hysterectomy. However, if inspection is the need, diagnostic or evaluatory laparoscopy will answer it the best. After getting clear view of abdominopelvic organs, excluding suspected pathology, gynecologist should then proceed to perform VH.

Having absolved given excuses, let us inspect all the indications and/or associated conditions for which vaginal route can be primary route for hysterectomy.

INDICATIONS OR ASSOCIATED CONDITIONS

For following, in absence of contraindication, vaginal route should be a primary route for hysterectomy and performing alternative is certainly not in the best interest of the patient. These are:

- Uterine prolapse
- Dysfunctional uterine bleeding (DUB)
- Adenomyosis
- Fibroid
- Polyposis
- Carcinoma *in situ* (CIN III) of cervix
- High-risk with early endometrial cancer.

Dysfunctional Uterine Bleeding/Adenomyosis

Dysfunctional uterine bleeding suspected adenomyosis and fibroid can be clubbed together as the ideal set-up for VH when a hysterectomy is indicated and there is no contraindication to this route.

Excepting uterine, absence of pelvic pathology as well as without contraindication for VH, several gynecologists have now taken to perform an LAVH for these conditions, which the author thinks is a gross misuse of high technology. The redeeming feature is, however, that at least the abdomen is not opened like a cupboard!

In a recent paper from England, Hutchon states that he has not done a single AH in the past 6 years in women with a diagnosis of dysfunctional menorrhagia. In his practice of more than 40 years, each and every case of DUB and/or adenomyosis was treated with VH unless genuinely contraindicated. Whether uterus is enlarged due to fibroid or otherwise, what can guide is careful clinical examination, reliable, sonographic uterine volume and examination under anesthesia. Only when the uterine size is unduly large, i.e. greater than 12 weeks size, either debulking at VH or LAVH becomes essential.

Fibroids

In absence of contraindication and irrespective of number of fibroids when the uterus is not larger than 12 weeks or has a total volume not exceeding 250–300 cm^3, the ideal route should be vaginal. The size of a fibroid is not as important as the size to which the uterus is enlarged and how accessible the fibroid is. Edward and Beebe advocate VH for myoma up to 14 weeks size. Navaratil goes on to state: "In general, it can be said that uteri enlarged to the size of a pregnancy of approximately 3–4 months, do not represent a contraindication."

Interestingly, the route for hysterectomy in the presence of uterine fibroids was vaginal in 7.4% of Dicker's series, 81% in Cosson's and 42.6% in Mettler and Semm's series.

In selected cases, debulking is done during VH and/or GnRH is administered (leuprolide acetate 3.75 mg) intramuscularly once a month for two doses to reduce the size of the fibroid; such reduction may be adequate to make the patient fit for VH and take additional benefits.

Data regarding the total uterine volume and exact location of fibroid will be of immense help in decision-making about the route, site for debulking, and uterine delivery. Fundal height can easily mislead the size as because of adenomyosis, uterus may have disproportionately grown in both or other dimensions.

Malignancy

Gyneconcologist will differentiate from others by favoring to take vaginal route for the required hysterectomy for:

- "Select" cases of endometrial cancer early and high risk. Required lymphadenectomy is performed laparoscopically
- Prepare vaginal "cuff" vaginally and turn to abdominal route for required surgery for endometrial cancer. VH is also recommended for very early cancer cervix but is not without rigid limitations, and therefore resorting to alternate route or technique for CIN III is non-gyneconcology.

Associated Obesity

The overall complication rate in the obese was fractionally less and there was no increase in comorbidity. Obesity should per se invite vaginal route and dissuade abdominal approach or assistance. One should go out of his way to spare such abdomen if findings do not contraindicate and permit VH.

Following should never deter gynecologist in taking vaginal route as primary route for hysterectomy:

- Nulliparity
- History of cesarean section
- Oophorectomy
- "High-risk" with early endometrial cancer
- Associated surgery at same sitting (e.g. "Lap" cholecystectomy and VH).

Following can persuade reluctant operator to take vaginal as primary route:

- Ventral scar hernioplasty
- Morbid obesity
- High-risk, e.g. interstitial lung disease which markedly restricts pulmonary function, poor cardiac status, diabetes, and hypertension
- Tuberculous abdomen
- Keloids.

WHAT CAN PROMOTE VAGINAL HYSTERECTOMY AS PRIMARY ROUTE

Examination under Anesthesia (EUA)

This singularly important examination performed just before the start of hysterectomy should form an integral part of the management of a patient needing a hysterectomy. EUA is performed, after placing the patient in the lithotomy position, by careful speculum examination using a vulsellum or tenaculum on the cervix and bimanual examination and not as often performed on a patient lying in supine position. Every VH should be preceded by an EUA and in addition, LAVH or AH should not be considered unless there is a contraindication to VH, which is confirmed under anesthesia. Examination under anesthesia can convert many abdominal and LAVH into simple VH. Bottom line for every gynecologist should be: "Give me reliable findings of examination under anesthesia and I will give you an unambiguous decision on the route for hysterectomy".

Trial Vaginal Hysterectomy

A "trial of forceps" in obstetrics is used when there is a possibility of vaginal delivery, keeping facilities for cesarean section ready. Comparable to this, is the concept of a "trial vaginal hysterectomy" first presented in 1993, with a facility for laparoscopic assistance and/or laparotomy kept available. After careful EUA, there are times when it is felt that VH may be difficult or may fail, despite the absence of well accepted contraindication but an attempt may still be made to proceed with vaginal hysterectomy. Likely to fall in this category are:

- Those with enlarged uterus
- Those who have cesarean section in past
- Nulliparous women
- Operator with doubt and anxiety without reason.

Laparoscopic Evaluation

Laparoscopic evaluation is indicated in patients where there is reason to fear of possible failure to complete VH and/or to gain confidence during the early part of the learning curve. This will pave the way to success.

It is recommended when:

- VH appears to be possible (i.e. not contraindicated), but the surgeon has some doubt or apprehension
- In some cases where a "trial VH" has been planned
- Adnexal pathology: When an experienced vaginal surgeon plans to excise a benign, mobile, adnexal mass at VH, laparoscopy will confirm the earlier findings, exclude malignancy and tuberculosis, and confirm whether removal via the vaginal route is possible.

Preoperative Uterine Volume

When uterus is more than 8 weeks size, it is desirable that the operator religiously utilizes reliably measured uterine volume rather than clinically measured uterine size. Size as measured by gestational fundal height can prove misleading and invite difficulty during VH. Uterine volume will prove to be a better measure of a uterus than fundal height. Even though fundal heights are same, uterine volumes can grossly vary and therefore, so will be surgical demand.

DISCUSSION

The mindset of the practicing gynecologist is vital and pivotal. As an obstetrician, he recommends cesarean section or elective repeat cesarean to keep the perineum, in particular, and pelvic floor, in general, "intact". Interestingly, the same obstetrician in his gynecological practice continues to open the abdomen and perform hysterectomy for a multiparous normal-sized uterus and leaves behind a torn perineum and/or bulging lower third of the posterior vaginal wall rectocele and/or glaring cystocele unattended.

Abdominal hysterectomy is a good choice in cases where the uterus is considered an abdominal organ, where there is associated adnexal pathology, particularly an adherent one or one suspicious of malignancy, and where there is a genuine need to visualize the abdominopelvic organs. In reality, vaginal surgery is the least invasive route because one is using the entrance designed by nature without making any additional cuts—it is kinder to the patient.

Place of LAVH is well crystallized by ACOG guidelines which include:

- Lysis of adhesions
- Treatment of pelvic endometriosis, uterine fibroids that complicate the performance of VH ligation of infundibulopelvic ligaments to facilitate difficult ovary removal and evaluation of the pelvic and abdominal

cavity before hysterectomy. This should inspire operator to take appropriate route.

All the randomized and other studies favor vaginal route and so also are the views of laparoscopic surgeons, whenever VH is possible. It is only when vaginal route cannot be chosen, LAVH or LH and abdominal route need to be considered.

With a personal experience of having performed more than 6,044 vaginal hysterectomies, the author strongly feels that only a genuine contraindication to VH should indicate LAVH or an AH and for every women scheduled for hysterectomy, vaginal route is proved beyond any doubt as primary route. In practice, 80–90% of hysterectomies for nonprolapsed uteri can be carried out via the vaginal route, and only in the remaining 10–20% cases, is LAVH or the abdominal route resorted to.

When a hysterectomy is decided on, every gynecologist should first consider using the vaginal route, which is the least invasive, without any laparoscopic assistance. AH must be reserved for cases in which the vaginal route is contraindicated and LAVH is either risky or difficult. If hysterectomy is possible by all three approaches, in the best interest of the patient the order of preference would be VH, LAVH, and AH. VH differentiates the gynecological surgeon from the general surgeon, who can easily remove the uterus through the abdomen equally competently. If vaginal surgery was marketed to patients as "scarless surgery", perhaps it would become more popular in the consumer-driven society.

Ideal would be to follow words of wisdom "we must continue to train gynecologists to ably perform vaginal surgery and let the public know that fewer laparoscopic techniques and equipment offer no advantage over proven vaginal hysterectomy techniques".

BIBLIOGRAPHY

1. ACOG. Appropriate use of laparoscopically assisted vaginal hysterectomy (Committee Opinion). Compendium of selected publication. Washington DC (USA): The American College of Obstetricians & Gynaecologists Women's Health Care Physicians. 2006;13-4.
2. Boike GM, Elfstrand EP, Delpriore G, et al. Laparoscopically-assisted vaginal hysterectomy in a university hospital: Report of 82 cases and comparison with abdominal and vaginal hysterectomy. Am J Obstet Gynecol. 1993;168:1690-5.
3. Bottle A, Aylin P. Variations in vaginal and abdominal hysterectomy by region and trust in England. Br J Obstet Gynecol. 2005;112:326-8.
4. Cengiz B, Demirel LC, Dokmeci F, et al. Bilateral Salpingo-oophorectomy during vaginal hysterectomy in cases with nonprolapsed uterus: Role of laparoscopy in a residency training program without much vaginal salpingo-oophorectomy experience. J Gynecol Surg. 2002;18:87-93.
5. Davies A, O'Conner H, Magos AL. A prospective study to evaluate oophorectomy at the time of vaginal hysterectomy. Br J Obstet Gynecol. 1996;103:915-20.
6. Hefni AA, Davies AE. Vaginal endoscopic oophorectomy with vaginal hysterectomy: A simple minimal access surgery technique. Br J Obstet Gynecol. 1997;104:621-2.
7. Hospital Episode Statistics. 1994;3(2):415-24.
8. Hutchon DJ. A double-blind randomised trial of leuprorelin acetate prior to hysterectomy for dysfunctional uterine bleeding. Br J Obstet Gynecol. 2000;107:1323-4.
9. Johnson N, Barlow D, Lethaby A, et al. Methods of hysterectomy: Systematic review and meta-analysis of randomised controlled trials. BMJ. 2005;330:1478-85.
10. Jones HW. Hysterectomy rates for benign indications. Obstet Gynecol Survey. 2006;61:577-8.
11. Jones HW. The VALUE national hysterectomy study: Description of the patients and their surgery. Obstet Gynecol Survey. 2002;57:431-2.
12. Khung TTG. Use of Sheth's uterocervical broad ligament space for vaginal hysterectomy in a patient with history of caesarean section. Malaysian J Obstet Gynaecol.1995;4:39-42.
13. Lenihan JP, Kovanda C, Cammarano C. Comparison of laparoscopic-assisted vaginal hysterectomy with traditional hysterectomy for cost effectiveness to employers. Am J Obstet Gynecol. 2004;190:1714-22.
14. Lumsden MA, Twaddle S, Hawthorn R, et al. A randomised comparison and economic evaluation of laparoscopic-assisted hysterectomy and abdominal hysterectomy. Br J Obstet Gynecol. 2000;107:1386-91.
15. Maresh MJ, Metcalfe MA, McPherson K, et al. The VALUE national hysterectomy study: Description of the patients and their surgery. Br J Obstet Gynecol. 2002;109:302-12.
16. Mettler L, Semm K. Vaginale and abdominale hysterektomie an der Universitats-Frauenklinik Kiel. Arch Gynecol Obstet. 1989;245:379-82.
17. Otton GR, Mandapati S, Streatfild KA, Et al. Transfusion rate associated with hysterectomy for benign disease. Aust NZ J Obstet Gynecol. 2001;41:439-42.
18. Quinlan DK. Indications and Contraindications. In: Sheth SS, Studd JWW (Eds). Vaginal Hysterectomy. London: Martin Dunitz Ltd.; 2002. p. 7-14.
19. Rafii A, Samain E, Levardon M, et al. Vaginal hysterectomy for benign disorders in obese women: A prospective study. Br J Obstet Gynecol. 2005;111:223-7.
20. Sheth S, Malpani A. Vaginal hysterectomy for the management of menstruation in mentally retarded women. Int J Gynecol Obstet. 1991;35:319-21.

21. Sheth SS, Paghdiwalla K. Do we need the laparoscopic route? J Obstet Gynaecol India. 2001;51:25-30.
22. Sheth SS, Salvi V. Complications, Morbidity and Mortality of Vaginal Hysterectomy. In: Sheth SS, Studd JWW (Eds). Vaginal hysterectomy. London: Martin Dunitz Ltd.; 2002. p. 341-54.
23. Sheth SS. Concentrate on per via naturales: Spare cesarean section and save the abdomen. Expert Rev Obstet Gynecol. 2006;1:3-5.
24. Sheth SS. Preoperative sonographic estimation of uterine volume: An aid to determine the route of hysterectomy. J Gynecol Surg. 2002;18:13-22.
25. Sheth SS. The place of oophorectomy at vaginal hysterectomy. Obstet Gynecol Survey. 1992;47:332-3.
26. Sheth SS. The scope of vaginal hysterectomy. Eur J Obstet Gynecol Rep Biol. 2004;115:224-31.
27. Sheth SS. Vaginal Hysterectomy. In: Arulkumaran S, Thakar R, Manyonda I (Eds). Best Practice and Research—Clinical Obstetrics and Gynaecology. USA: Elsevier Ltd.; 2005. p. 307-32.
28. Sheth SS. Vaginal hysterectomy. In: Studd J (Ed). Progress in Obstetrics and Gynaecology, 10th edition. London: Churchill Livingstone; 1993. p. 317-40.
29. Sheth SS. Vaginal or Abdominal Hysterectomy. In: Sheth SS, Studd JWW (Eds). Vaginal Hysterectomy. London: Martin Dunitz Ltd; 2002. p. 301-20.
30. Sizzi O, Rossetti A. Overcoming technical limits to laparoscopic hysterectomy. J Gynecol Surg Endosc. 2005.
31. Spilsbury K, Semmens JB, Hammond I, et al. Persistent high rates of hysterectomy in Western Australia: A population-based study of 83,000 procedures over 23 years. Br J Obstet Gynecol. 2006;113:804-9.

41.6 THE TEN STEP VAGINAL HYSTERECTOMY: A METHOD DESCRIPTION

Michael Stark, Sandro Gerli, Gian Carlo Di Renzo

THE TEN STEP VAGINAL HYSTERECTOMY

Any surgical procedure should follow the principle of "nothing lacking, nothing superfluous". All operative steps should have a purpose and be precise. There are many ways to perform an operation. However, the *lex parsimoniae* of William of Ockham (1285–1350) tells that if we face different ways to solve or explain a phenomenon, the simplest way is the right one. Surgery should not be an exception to this rule.

In the last years, abdominal hysterectomies were abandoned in favor of endoscopical operations. At the university hospital of Oslo, for example, the rate of endoscopic hysterectomies increased from 18% to 54% between 2001 and 2005 (including enlarge uteri). Even clinical FIGO stage I endometrial adenocarcinoma have been treated successfully with LAVH in 41% of the patients.

Nevertheless, VH is still a valid alternative to AH even in large uteri. Langenbeck introduced vaginal hysterectomy in 1813. Many modifications and variations of this technique have been reported, based on the authors' interpretation of pelvic anatomy and their own skills and experience. The Porges, Falk, von Theobald, Heaney, Joel-Cohen and Chicago methods, which are common techniques, are carried out with some variations.

To find out whether vaginal hysterectomies can still be optimized and simplified after two centuries of practice and accumulated experience, the six mentioned methods have been evaluated. In the first step, the common steps to all methods have been defined, and in the second step, their necessity has been reassessed. After defining the necessary and optimal steps, their way of performance has been compared to alternatives. As a result, only the re-evaluated, modified and essential steps remained. In the last step, their logical sequence has been defined. The result is the "ten step vaginal hysterectomy". This method was compared in a prospective randomized study with the Heaney-method. It has been shown that the operation time [34,1 minutes (20,5–50) vs. 52,3 (23,3–90) minutes] and the duration of the need for painkillers [29,6 (8–75) vs. 48,7 (19–86) hours] are significantly shorter. This method is logical, easy to learn, perform and teach.

METHOD DESCRIPTION

Each of the ten steps is described with its alternatives and optimal way of performance. In many hospitals, instrument-trays contain many unnecessary instruments that are not used during the operation. The "ten step vaginal hysterectomy" requires only ten instruments. They will be listed for every step.

Vaginal hysterectomies have been recommended for the treatment of endometrial cancer in elderly women, but they are mostly performed for benign conditions. Endometrial malignancy, therefore, should be excluded prior to the operation. This can be done with a preliminary diagnostic curettage or hysteroscopy.

Incision of the Vaginal Wall

The way to perform the incision of the vaginal wall depends on the anatomical findings of the patient.

In a Patient with a Prolapse

Most described methods start with an incision around the cervix, followed by an inverted-T extension toward the orificium urethrae externum and lateral separation of the vaginal wall from the midline. This has been challenged by the Joel-Cohen method which starts the vaginal wall incision under the orificium urethrae externum. This approach was found to be easy and logical compared to the other methods, mainly in multiparae where there are often adhesions around the external os, and when entering to the right cleavage from below might therefore be difficult.

The cervix is grasped with two single-toothed tenaculi. A drop-like incision of the vaginal wall starts under the urethra, continuing laterally and down, encircling the uterine cervix from behind and returning back to the starting point from the contralateral side (Fig. 1). If the depth of the initial incision is correct and the right cleavage found, the vaginal wall will separate easily laterally to the side and backward below the cervix by a gentle traction of surgical forceps (Fig. 2), and this should be nearly bloodless. When the separation of the vaginal wall is completed, the anterior wall colporrhaphy is already prepared.

The tip of the "drop" still covering the bladder is pulled down, peeling the vaginal wall away from the bladder. When performed in the right cleavage, this step should also be nearly bloodless. This step has three main movements rather than six in the other methods.

In a Patient without Prolapse

The cervix is grasped with two single-toothed tenaculi. When there is no or only a small prolapse, a circular incision around the cervix, about 5 mm above the external os is performed, and then, the vaginal wall is separated from the cervix with surgical forceps. An active assistance is needed to help the surgeon to perform this manipulation under good vision.

Instruments: Speculum, two single-toothed tenaculi, scalpel, surgical forceps.

Detaching the Bladder from the Uterus

The border between the anterior wall of the uterus and the bladder must be identified (curved scissors are sometime needed to reach the cleavage). Then, by pushing the bladder up, being always as close as possible to the uterus, it separates and moves up until the anterior peritoneum is exposed. No effort should be made to open the anterior peritoneum. Opening the anterior peritoneum at that stage is not necessary and not recommended because it disturbs the operation dynamics. When the interanatomical relations between the bladder and the peritoneum are not clear due to adhesions, it might also cause damage to the bladder. Bleedings should be carefully controlled. A marked swab can be left under the bladder.

Instruments: Swab, optionally scissors.

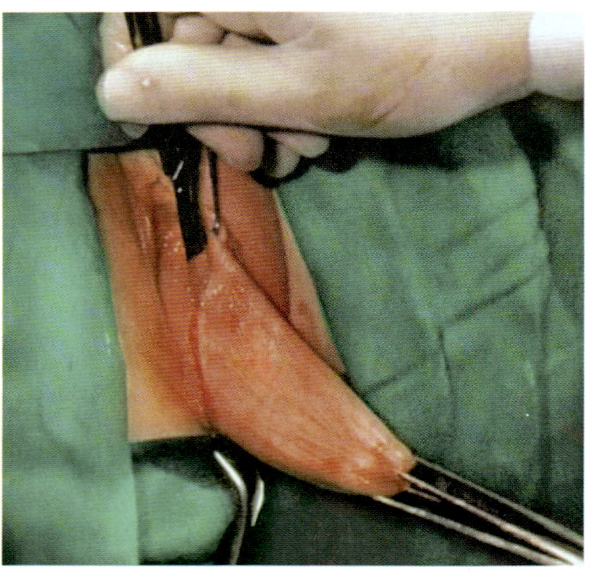

Fig 1: A drop-like incision encircling the uterine cervix

Opening Posterior Peritoneum

To open the posterior peritoneum, the uterus is pulled up. The peritoneum is grasped with surgical forceps and opened with scissors. The scissors are then introduced into the Douglas cavity, and holding each blade with one hand, pulled out while staying open (Fig. 3), so that the backside of the blades expose the insertions of the sacrouterine ligaments.

Instruments: Surgical forceps, scissors.

Dissection of the Lower Part of the Uterus

In opposition to the time honored anatomical approach dealing with each structure separately, the sacrouterine ligaments and the paracervical tissues, which are in different anatomical planes and directions, are clamped together. This is done with the following maneuver: One blade of an open clamp is placed under the insertion of the sacrouterine ligament, the instrument rotates towards the uterus, while the uterus is being contra-rotated. Both anatomical structures are so included between the blades of the closed instrument. Both structures, the relatively bloodless sacrouterine ligament and the paracervical tissues, are cut and ligated leaving the suture material in

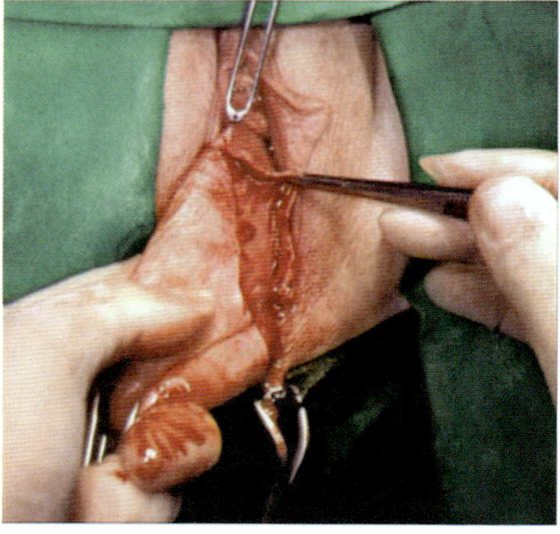

Fig. 2: Using surgical forceps to separate the vaginal wall

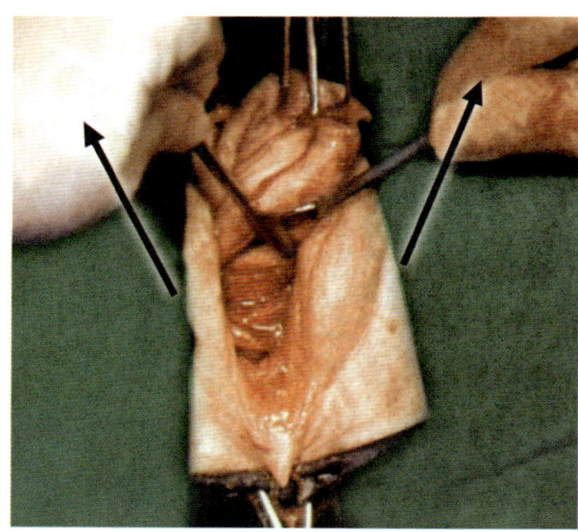

Fig. 3: Opening the posterior peritoneum

its full length. This is repeated on the other side. If properly performed, these steps are safe, bloodless, dynamically correct and time-saving. In most traditional surgical methods for VH, both elements are anyway sutured to each other at the end of the operation (there are exceptions: Some surgeons perform vaginal hysterectomies without ligating the cervical ligaments).

In a patient without a prolapsed uterus, this maneuver will instantly produce a significant prolapse, and with a slight traction, the uterine arteries will get exposed.

Instruments: Wertheim or Heaneys clamp, needle holder, surgical forceps, scissors, two sutures.

Cutting and Ligating the Uterine Arteries

Both uterine arteries are clamped, cut and ligated.

Instruments: Wertheim or Heaney clamp, needle holder, scissors, two sutures.

Opening the Anterior Peritoneum

After both uterine arteries have been cut and ligated, the uterus is pulled down and two fingers are introduced behind the fundus to lift the anterior peritoneum, which can be opened under vision. This will insure the safety of the bladder, as its anatomical relations with the anterior peritoneum are not always clear, in particular after previous cesarean sections.

The access to the fundus in a myomatous uterus is sometimes difficult. In such a case, the surgeon should hold both tenaculi with his left hand while continuously and slowly pulling them down with rotating movements. In most cases, the uterus will descend and be luxated backward until it is possible to insert the right index and middle fingers beyond the fundus and lift the anterior peritoneum. Once in a while, more steps are necessary to separate the parametrium from the uterus. Rising up from the pelvic floor, there is no risk of damaging the ovarian arteries with this rotating and pulling maneuver because the larger the uterus, the longer they are. The decision about the size of a uterus to be removed vaginally, solely depends on the experience of the surgeon and should be taken before starting the operation. The morcellation of the uterus, which is safe and facilitates the removal of enlarged and well-supported uteri, may be performed, where needed. The more experience the surgeon gets with this rotating maneuver, the less often morcellation becomes necessary. In experienced hands, a large uterus should not be a contraindication for VH.

Instruments: Scissors.

Dissection of the Upper Part of the Uterus (and Appendages)

The round and ovarian ligaments and the blood vessels are clamped together and ligated. The ligature should be placed laterally as far as possible from the clamp, leaving the ovarian ligaments as long as possible. The uterus is cut away with scissors medial to the instrument. A ligature is placed beyond the instrument and followed by a transfixion suture between the clamp and the ligature (Fig. 4). This will prevent bleeding, if this transfixion suture comes to slip away or tear by traction. The transfixion suture should never be done before the ligature. The tip of the needle might hit a blood vessel and cause bleeding in the parametrium. The same procedure is done on the contralateral side.

Instruments: Wertheim or Heaney's clamp, scissors, needle holder, surgical forceps, four sutures.

The "non-stage"—Leaving the Peritoneum Open

In 1980s, Harold Ellis showed that closing the peritoneum at the end of abdominal surgery is not necessary. The thin peritoneum does not close end-to-end as skin does. Vascular bridges over peritoneal sutures are focus for ischemia and adhesions. When the peritoneum is left open, the coelum cells will produce a new peritoneum within days. Indeed, leaving peritoneum open in cesarean section proved to cause fewer adhesions than when closing it. It was also shown that the peritoneal closure is not necessary for VH. The British Royal College of Obstetrics and Gynaecology recommended in its guideline number 15 from July 2002 to leave the peritoneum open with evidence level Ib.

The pelvic parietal peritoneum is attached to the pelvic ligaments. The ligation of the ligaments to each other (step 9) will create an additional peritoneal sac between the ligaments and a closed peritoneum, with all its possible consequences.

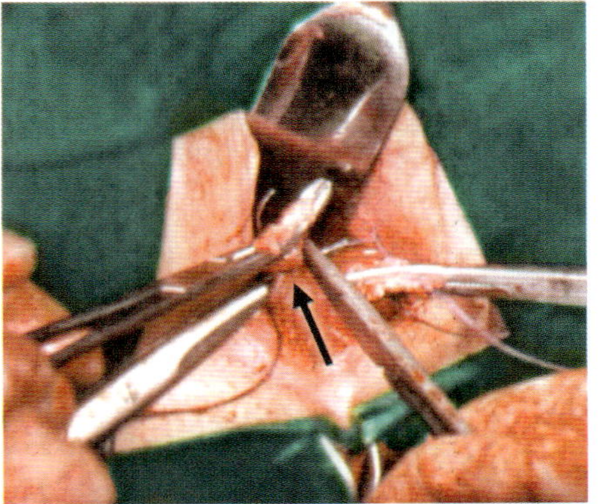

Fig. 4: Transfixion suture between the ligament and the forceps

Another advantage of leaving the peritoneum open is the free drainage into the peritoneal cavity where blood will be absorbed by the peritoneum and the lymph channels.

If an enterocele is to be prevented or repaired, it should be done before continuing the operation.

Reconstruction of the Pelvic Floor

The left and right sacrouterine ligaments with the paracervical tissues as well as the ovarian ligaments are ligated to each other, respectively. An extra suture may be placed to join the sacrouterine ligaments. The decision should be taken according to the particular anatomical relations. The question whether tying the ovarian ligaments to each other causes dyspareunia is still open and should be examined in a prospective study.

Instruments: Scissors, needle holder, surgical forceps, and optionally one suture.

Closing the Vaginal Wall

If a marked swab has been left in step 2, it should be removed before closing the vaginal wall. The vaginal wall is sutured continuously. It is recommended in sexual active women to suture the vagina transversely. This will prevent dyspareunia as the suturing line is on the upper side of the anterior wall.

Instruments: Allis clamp, needle holder, surgical forceps, scissors, one suture.

DISCUSSION

Today, more and more hysterectomies are laparoscopically assisted vaginal hysterectomies, even for big uteri. However, the vaginal route should always be considered when hysterectomy is indicated, because of its quick recovery, the absence of abdominal scar and the short hospital stay.

By acquiring more experience, the number of contraindications for vaginal hysterectomy will decrease. It has been shown that this operation can be performed with nulliparity and with enlarged uterus. Also previous cesarean sections are not considered anymore as contraindication for VH, and there is no justification for LAVH in the presence of significant uterine descent.

In a prospective randomized study, no difference between VH and LAVH has been found concerning estimated blood loss, complications, hospital stay and convalescence. The costs for an LAVH were however, considerably higher.

Many studies compare the outcomes of VH to those of abdominal or LAVH. Campbell et al. compared the three methods in 33,792 operations, with regards to the hospital stay and the involved costs and concluded that "vaginal hysterectomy provides the best patient outcomes, with the shortest hospital stays and lowest complication rates at the lowest cost." The laparoscopically-assisted vaginal hysterectomy is considered an alternative to the abdominal hysterectomy. Shorter hospital stay and less need of analgesia has been reported in the LAVH, but at the same time, there was a higher rate of bladder injuries and a longer operation time when compared to vaginal hysterectomy.

Traditions can prevent new thinking and new surgical developments. No operative step should be a taboo. All surgical procedures should be regularly re-evaluated in the light of new findings in pathology and physiology.

A surgical procedure should be evaluated by examining not only the necessity and way of performance of all its steps, but also their combinations and sequences.

Only few studies explain the outcomes of VH with variations in single operative step. Leaving the parametrium unsutured, resulted in a shorter operation time with no significant differences in other examined parameters. Some advantages were reported where mass closure of the vaginal cuff or morcellation was performed.

The "ten step vaginal hysterectomy" results from the analysis of different methods and is based on up-to-date physiological and anatomical principles. It was shown that this operation is rational and simple. Unnecessary steps are avoided, and the method follows rules of aesthetics and functional minimalism. Only ten instruments and ten sutures are needed and it has been shown that this operation reduced the operation time and the use of painkillers. More randomized prospective studies will be needed to evaluate the late outcome of this method.

BIBLIOGRAPHY

1. American College of Obstetricians and Gynecologists. Appropriate use of laparoscopically-assisted vaginal hysterectomy. Obstet Gynecol. 2005;105(4):929-30.
2. Balfour RP. Laparoscopic-assisted vaginal hysterectomy—190 cases: Complications and training. J Obstet Gynaecol. 1999;19(2): 164-6.
3. Benassi L, Rossi T, Kaihura CT, et al. Abdominal or vaginal hysterectomy for enlarged uteri: A randomized clinical trial. Am J Obstet Gynecol. 2002;187(6):1561-5.
4. Campbell ES, Xiao H, Smith MK. Types of hysterectomy. Comparison of characteristics, hospital costs, utilization and outcomes. J Reprod Med. 2003;48(12):943-9.

5. Claerhout F, Deprest J. Laparoscopic hysterectomy for benign diseases. Best Pract Res Clin Obstet Gynaecol. 2005;19(3):357-75.
6. Cravello L, Bretelle, F, Cohen D, et al. Vaginal hysterectomy: apropos of a series of 1008 interventions. Gynecol Obstet Fertil. 2001;29(4):288-94.
7. Cruikshank SH, Kovac SR. Randomized comparison of three surgical methods used at the time of vaginal hysterectomy to prevent posterior enterocele. Am J Obstet Gynecol. 1999;180(4): 859-65.
8. Dhainaut C, Salomon LJ, Junger M, et al. Hysterectomies in patients with no history of vaginal delivery: A study of 243 cases. Gynecol Obstet Fertil. 2005;33:11-6.
9. Doucette RC, Sharp HT, Alder SC. Challenging generally accepted contraindications to vaginal hysterectomy. Am J Obstet Gynecol. 2001;184 (7):1386-9.
10. Ellis H. Internal overhealing: The problem of intraperitoneal adhesions. World J Surg. 1980;4:303-6.
11. Falk HC, Soichet S. The technique of vaginal hysterectomy. Clin Obstet Gynecol. 1972;15(3):703-54.
12. Gray LA. Introduction. In: Gray LA (Ed). Vaginal Hysterectomy: Indications, Technique and Complications. Springfield, IL: Charles C. Thomas Publisher; 1983.
13. Harmanli OH, Gentzler CK, Byun S, et al. A comparison of abdominal and vaginal hysterectomy for the large uterus. Int J Gynaecol Obstet. 2004;87(1):19-23.
14. Istre O, Langebrekke A, Qvigstad E. Changing hysterectomy technique from open abdominal to laparoscopic: New trend in Oslo, Norway. J Minim Invasive Gynecol. 2007;14(1):74-7.
15. Janschek EC, Hohlagschwandtner M, Nather A, et al. A study of non-closure of the peritoneum at vaginal hysterectomy. Arch Gynecol Obstet. 2003;267(4):213-6.
16. Joel-Cohen SJ. Abdominal and Vaginal Hysterectomy. New Techniques Based on Time and Motion Studies. London: William Heinemann Medical Books; 1972.
17. Kalogiannidis I, Lambrechts S, Amant F, et al. Laparoscopy-assisted vaginal hysterectomy compared with abdominal hysterectomy in clinical stage I endometrial cancer: Safety, recurrence, and long-term outcome. Laparoscopy-assisted vaginal hysterectomy compared with abdominal hysterectomy in clinical stage I endometrial cancer: Safety, recurrence, and long-term outcome. Am J Obstet Gynecol. 2007;196(3):248.e1-8.
18. Kalogirou D, Antoniou G, Zioris C, et al. Vaginal hysterectomy: Technique and results in the last twenty years. J Gynecol Surg. 1995;11(4):201-7.
19. Kudo R, Yamauchi O, Okazaki T, et al. Vaginal hysterectomy without ligation of the ligaments of the cervix uteri. Surg Gynecol Obstet. 1990;170(4):299-305.
20. Leodolter S. The transvaginal surgical school in Austria. Retrospect-present-future. Gynaekol Geburtshilfliche Rundsch. 1995;35(3):142-8.
21. Li Z, Leng J, Lang J, et al. Vaginal hysterectomy for patients with moderately enlarged uterus of benign lesions. Chin Med Sci J. 2004;19(1):60-3.
22. Lipscomb GH, Ling FW, Stovall TG, et al. Peritoneal closure at vaginal hysterectomy: A reassessment. Obstet Gynecol. 1996;87(1):40-3.
23. Meikle SF, Nugent EW, Orleans M. Complications and recovery from laparoscopy-assisted vaginal hysterectomy compared with abdominal and vaginal hysterectomy. Obstet Gynecol, 1997;89(2):304-11.
24. Miskry T, Magos A. Mass closure: A new technique for closure of the vaginal vault at vaginal hysterectomy. BJOG. 2001;108(12):1295-7.
25. Paldi E, Filmar S, Naiger R, et al. Vaginal hysterectomy using the Porges method: Report on 100 cases. J Gynecol Obstet Biol Reprod. 1988;17(2):233-6.
26. Royal College of Obstetrics and Gynaecology. Peritoneal Closure Guideline No. 15; 2002.
27. Schutz K, Possover M, Merker A, et al. Prospective randomized comparison of laparoscopic-assisted vaginal hysterectomy (LAVH) with abdominal hysterectomy (AH) for the treatment of the uterus weighing >200 g. Surg Endosc. 2002;16(1):121-5.
28. Sheth SS. Vaginal or Abdominal Hysterectomy. In: Sheth SS, Studd JWW (Eds). Vaginal Hysterectomy. London: Martin Dunitz Ltd.; 2002.
29. Stark M, Gerli S, Di Renzo GC. The Ten Step Vaginal Hysterectomy. Progress in Obstetrics and Gynaecology. 2006;17,358-68.
30. Stark M. Clinical evidence that suturing the peritoneum after laparotomy is unnecessary for healing. World J Surg. 1993;17(3):419.
31. Summitt RL, Stovall TG, Lipscomb GH, et al. Randomized comparison of laparoscopy-assisted vaginal hysterectomy with standard vaginal hysterectomy in an outpatient setting. Obstet Gynecol. 1992;80(6):895-901.
32. Susini T, Massi G, Amunni G, et al. Vaginal hysterectomy and abdominal hysterectomy for treatment of endometrial cancer in the elderly. Gynecol Oncol. 2005;96(2):362-7.
33. Switala I, Cosson M, Lanvin D, et al. Is vaginal hysterectomy important for large uterus of more than 500 gm? Comparison with laparotomy. J Gynecol Obstet Biol Reprod. 1998;27(6):585-92.
34. Taylor SM, Romero AA, Kammerer-Doak DN, et al. Abdominal hysterectomy for the enlarged myomatous uterus compared with vaginal hysterectomy with morcellation. Am J Obstet Gynecol. 2003;189(6):1579-82.
35. von Theobald P. Simplified vaginal hysterectomy. J Chir. 2001;138(2):93-8.

41.7 VAGINAL HYSTERECTOMY FOR GENITAL PROLAPSE

PB PaiDhungat, GN Allahbadia

INTRODUCTION

Genital prolapse and its management constitute a major part of the practice of gynecology. The literature is very extensive, and moreover shows a continued and progressive development of the methods available for cure of the condition, without the sudden breaks that characterize the history of so many other branches of medicine. For this reason, much of what has been written about prolapse in the past is still valid, and all modern methods are based on the works of many pioneers such as Professor VN Shirodkar and Professor BN Purandare from the Indian subcontinent. At the same time, and in spite of the weight of tradition, the treatment of genital prolapse is essentially a practical discipline—it may legitimately be called a craft—and practice must be based primarily on direct experience. The object of the present chapter is to clarify and systematize a personal experience (of the senior author) gained from some 5,000 vaginal hysterectomies carried out for genital prolapse. One of Descartes rules may be quoted as an apologia.

In the subjects, we propose to study, we must inquire, not what others have taught, nor what we ourselves conjecture, but what we can clearly and evidently see, or what we can infer with certainty: For that is the only way in which knowledge is acquired.

Such a viewpoint demands that constant reference be made to the premises of normal anatomy and physiology, that eponymous operative techniques must not be regarded as anything more than guides, and that, when there is a legitimate choice between various possible procedures, preference is given to the one that will restore the tissues as near as possible to their normal dispositions. The causes of genital prolapse can be divided into two main groups, one being primary and comprising both childbirth and weakness of the walls of the viscera and the supporting tissues, the other being secondary, comprising increased intra-abdominal pressure and postural strains.

INDICATIONS FOR VAGINAL HYSTERECTOMY FOR PROLAPSE

Under certain conditions, a VH combined with an appropriate plastic repair is the operation of choice in the treatment of prolapse. The indications for VH in prolapse fall into two groups: (1) The concomitant indications and (2) the allied indications.

The Concomitant Indications

There are occasions on which the conjunction of some uterine or adnexal lesion and a prolapse renders a VH preferable to the more conservative procedures. A moderately sized fibroid uterus with prolapse or an adenomyotic uterus with prolapse can easily be dealt with via the vaginal route. Lesions of the adnexa would be regarded by most surgeons as contraindications to a VH. As with fibroids, inflammatory appendage disease and ovarian endometriomas are seldom encountered in cases of uterovaginal or total prolapse, for two reasons: (1) By and large prolapse is a disease of parous women in whom adnexal infections are rare and (2) because the pelvic adhesions resulting from these conditions serve to fix the uterus. In addition to the above indications, there are menorrhagias of the perimenopausal age group, with various causes. These are the main concomitant indications in prolapse for VH and, provided that the operation is justified on technical grounds, no other treatment gives such satisfaction, dealing as it does with two distressing conditions using one quite simple procedure.

The Allied Indications

In the selection of cases of prolapse suitable for treatment by a VH, the allied indications and limitations outweigh the concomitant ones. Briefly, if the body of the uterus is substantially involved in the prolapse, and the uterus is not enlarged, the conditions for a VH are satisfied unless there is some overriding indication for preserving the uterus. This means that the operation is best suited to cases of general prolapse and vault prolapse, in which the removal of the uterus is but one step in the exposure necessary to deal with the peritoneal herniation. Such a condition is implied by Palmer's observation that, if the cervix brings the uterosacral ligaments right down to the vulva with it, so that the index finger can be hooked round the ligament, a hysterectomy is indicated.

PROS AND CONS OF THE PROCEDURE

The current technique of VH has evolved from a variety of operations as the major method of surgical treatment for symptomatic uterine prolapse in the presence of cystocele, rectocele, or enterocele. No surgical procedure offers more to the "quality of life" for a woman than a carefully considered and evaluated, but often maligned, hysterectomy. Barnes and Tinkham reported complete satisfaction in most of their patients in whom VH was done.Absence of a scar on the abdomen has an added psychological advantage. Vaginal hysterectomy with adequate and good repair and suspension of the vault gives lasting results, compared with AH or less conservative surgery. The pattern of sexual activity for both the husband and wife is more often than not improved.

There are two major criticisms that are often raised against the operation. One is the high risk of a subsequent vault prolapse and the other that the vagina may be left unduly shortened. Both of these criticisms are legitimate and any technique for a VH must meet them. Vaginal prolapse resulting from a residual enterocele, caused by diastasis of the levator ani muscles and separation of the attachment of the vagina to the levator crura, may be symptomless immediately after hysterectomy, but the degree of prolapse and the severity of symptoms will increase with time. Protrusion of a mass from the vaginal outlet is the symptom that usually causes a woman with a massive recurrent enterocele to seek relief, because walking and sitting are usually difficult. A residual enterocele, which may result in vaginal vault prolapse, occurs far more frequently after vaginal hysterectomy than after an abdominal procedure. Recurrent enterocele usually occurs as a result of a missed enterocele at the time of hysterectomy or if an enterocele is mismanaged during the operation. The incidence of postoperative enterocele is being reduced with better technique and early diagnosis. One of the authors has described a new technique of vault closure to prevent such complications as well as to decrease average operating time by 5–15 minute and hospital stay by 2 days.

THE TECHNIQUE OF VAGINAL HYSTERECTOMY FOR GENITAL PROLAPSE

- The patient who is under anesthesia is given the modified lithotomy position. The parts are painted and draped, and a bimanual examination is done under anesthesia to reassess and grade the genital prolapse. The cervix is now held with a vulsellum and the extent of uterine prolapse is ascertained by firm traction on the vulsellum. Next, the cervix, which was held with the vulsellum, is replaced with two strong sutures of number 2 Barbour linen taken through the entire thickness of the cervix. At this stage, the posterior vaginal wall is depressed with a Sims' speculum
- Once the cervical stitch is complete, the posterior Sims' speculum is replaced with one of the self-retaining specula such as the self-retaining Auvard's speculum; the lateral vaginal walls are retracted using a Jayle's retractor and the anterior vaginal wall by the bladder retractor. All the tissues at this stage are cleaned once again with dilute 5% povidone-iodine solution, including the thread that is kept taut with an artery forceps as a traction suture (Fig. 1)
- The assistant, who is holding the anterior vaginal wall retractor, puts it under tension so that the surgeon can judge the anatomical details—namely, the edge of the bladder, the fold of the vesicouterine ligament, and the vaginal mucosa (Fig. 2)
- The first incision is taken on the anterior vaginal wall just below the level of the vesicouterine ligament. This semilunar incision, made with the scalpel held at an angle of 60° to the horizontal, is deepened by 2–3 mm (Fig. 3)
- The anterior vaginal mucosal flap is held in the midline with the toothed dissecting forceps and lifted up, so that the vesicouterine ligament is visible; this is cut with the sharp, curved, dissecting scissors (Fig. 4) and the bladder is now pushed up with the sponge held on the sponge-holding forceps (Fig. 5)
- The vesicouterine peritoneum is now identified by its shiny, smooth, silky texture, and confirmed by its mobility and transparency; this is held with an artery forceps, cut with sharp scissors, and the incision is extended with the artery forceps inserted in the incision and then opened (Fig. 6). Through this opening into the anterior pouch, an anterior bladder wall retractor is inserted and the assistant holds this against the undersurface of the pubic symphysis (Fig. 7). The important point to remember at this step is that the assistant has to push the bladder retractor against the pubic symphysis, so that along with the bladder, the ureters are moved away and laterally from the area of surgery.

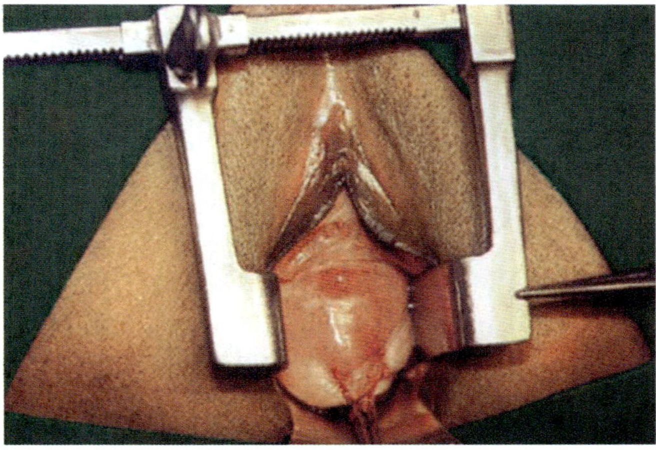

Fig. 1: Tissues are cleaned once again with the dilute 5% povidone-iodine solution, including the thread which is kept taut with an artery forceps as a traction suture

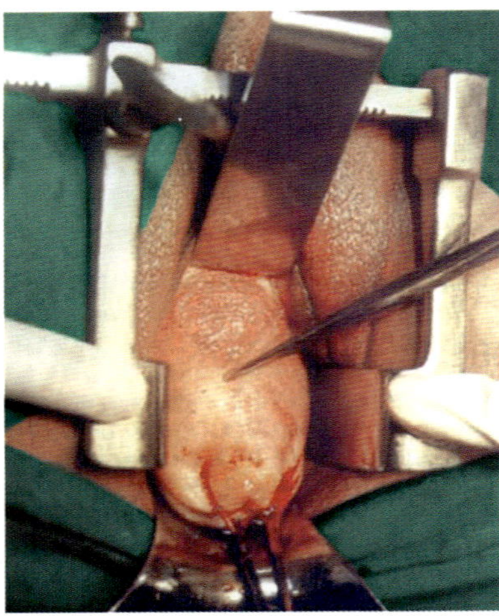

Fig. 2: The anterior vaginal wall retractor is put under tension so that the surgeon can judge the anatomical details: the edge of the bladder, the fold of the vesicouterine ligament, and the vaginal mucosa

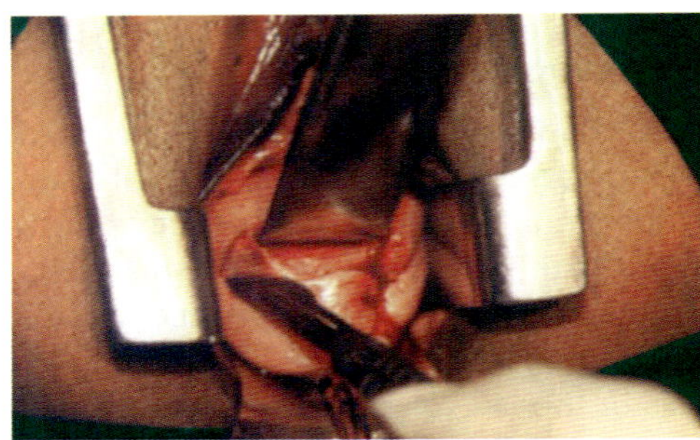

Fig. 3: The first incision is made on the anterior vaginal wall just below the level of the vesicouterine ligament. This semilunar incision, made with the scalpe l held at an angle of 60° to the horizontal, is deepened by 2–3 mm

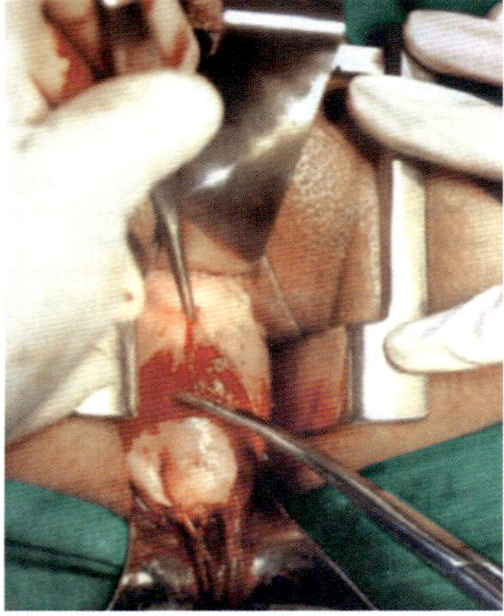

Fig. 4: The vesicouterine ligament is cut with the sharp, curved, dissecting scissors

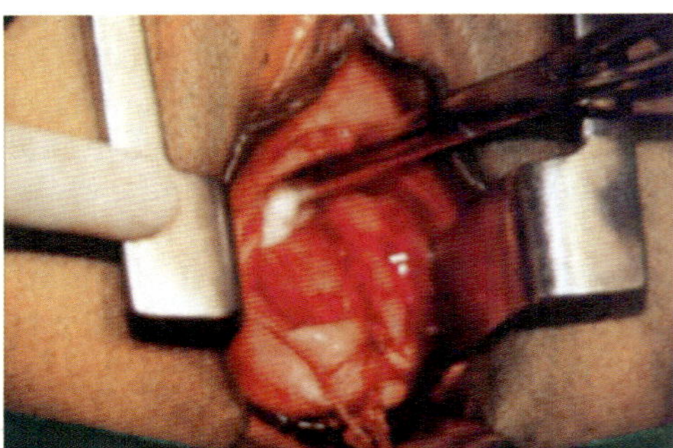

Fig. 5: The bladder is pushed up with the sponge held on the sponge-holding forceps

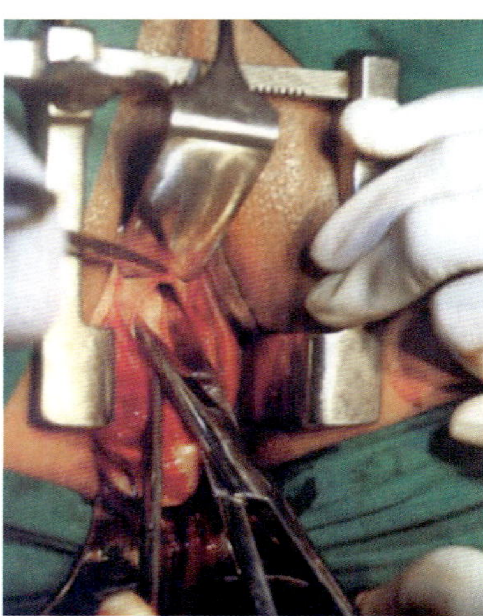

Fig. 6: The vesicouterine peritoneum is held with an artery forceps and cut with sharp scissors; the incision is extended with the artery forceps inserted in the incision and then opened

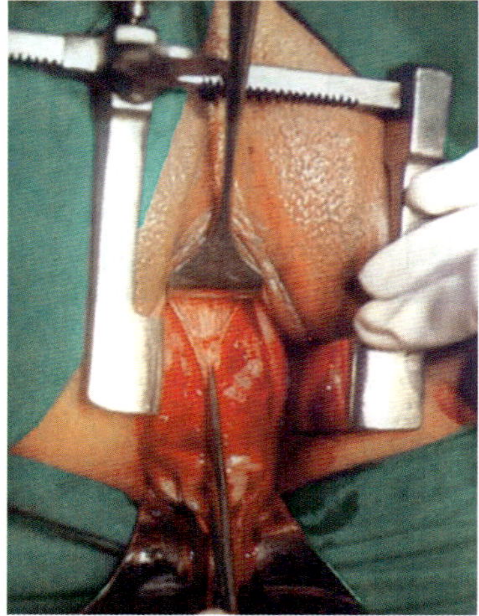

Fig. 7: An anterior bladder wall retractor is inserted into the anterior pouch, and held against the undersurface of the pubis symphysis

- The cervix is now lifted up with the traction sutures and the posterior fornix is inspected. The pouch of Douglas is demarcated by identifying the free fold, which is held with an artery forceps, put under tension, and cut with curved scissors (Fig. 8). The fold is cut such that the mucous membrane and the peritoneum are cut open together. It is important to remember that no dissection is done at this stage
- With a finger in the posterior fornix, the assistant pulls the cervix to the left of the patient and a small portion of the lateral vaginal mucosa is excised (about 2 cm in length and 1 cm in breadth). The right uterosacral ligament is now ligated with number 1 vicryl and cut (Fig. 9). The transverse cervical ligament complex is ligated next and cut. It is important to remember that this ligation is done lateral to the uterosacral ligament pedicle, which is held long, and is included in the subsequent transverse cervical ligament complex ligature, so that the uterosacral ligament gets a double tie (Fig. 10)
- Exactly similar steps are repeated on the left side. Here also the uterosacral pedicle suture is kept long and is held with curved forceps
- The blood supply of the uterus is through the vessels travelling in the broad ligament. Keeping this anatomical fact in mind, the next stitch is taken from the edge of the anterior peritoneum to that of the posterior peritoneum; this is tied lateral to the transverse cervical ligament pedicle (Fig. 11). Then the vessels are cut very close to the uterine body. It is very important to remember that this uterine vessel ligature should be the most lateral stitch in the step of hysterectomy
- A similar procedure is carried out on the right side of the patient, so that the major blood supply of the uterus is ligated
- The assistant pulls the cervix to the right side and one more stitch for the uterine vessel is taken 0.5 cm above the previous one (Fig. 12). This is also cut very close to the uterus. Next, a curved clamp is inserted behind the cornual structures (Fig. 13), threaded with the help of an assistant and the top ligaments are ligated. This pedicle is doubly ligated and then divided. A similar step is repeated on the other side so that the uterus is removed and the pelvic organs such as tubes and ovaries can be visualized clearly (Fig. 14)
- The posterior peritoneum is demarcated by holding the posterior fold of the peritoneum with three tissue-holding forceps, one in the midline and two at the lateral angles. With tension put on these forceps by assistants, the anterior bladder wall retractor is gently eased by the surgeon to pick out the edge of the anterior peritoneum (Fig. 15)
- The peritoneum is now closed with a purse-string suture using a delayed, absorbable 2/0 suture. This suture is taken running from the midline of the anterior peritoneum, via the left lateral angle, corneal structure pedicle, left uterosacral ligaments, left posterior angle, free peritoneal edge in the midline posteriorly, right posterior angle, right uterosacral ligaments, right cornual structures, right anterior angle, and ending at the midline in the anterior leaf of the peritoneum (Fig. 16). This is now tied so that the peritoneal cavity

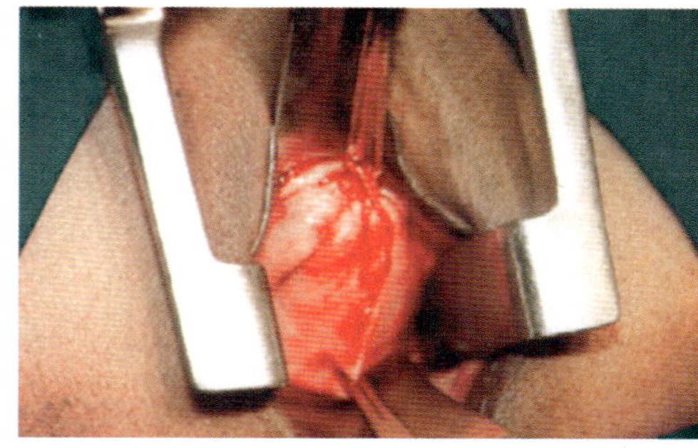

Fig. 8: The pouch of Douglas is demarcated by identifying the free fold, which is held with an artery forceps, put under tension, and cut with curved scissors

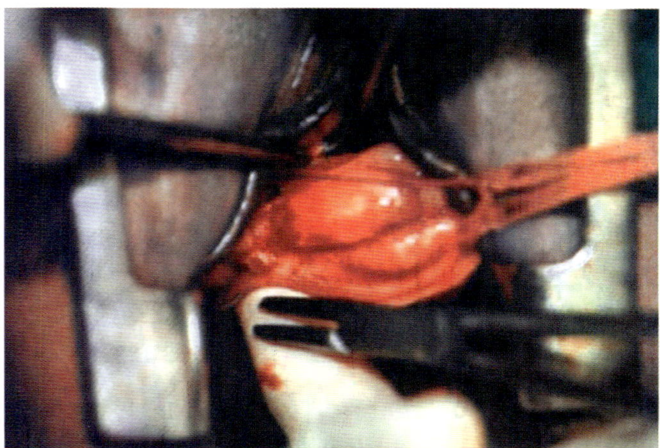

Fig. 9: The right uterosacral ligament is ligated with no. 1 vicryl and cut

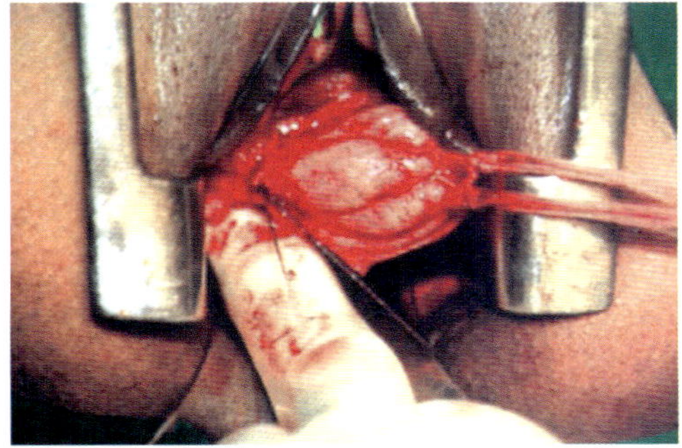

Fig. 10: The uterosacral ligament gets a double tie

is closed. It is important to remember that, when the peritoneum is ligated during the "purse-string", it is distal to the pedicles, so that the pedicles are now outside the peritoneum

- The uterosacral ligaments of either side, which were kept long, are now tied together in the midline and so are the cornual structures. The next step area description of cystocele repair which usually accompanies pelvic relaxation
- The Jayle's lateral vaginal wall retractor is removed. The anterior vaginal wall is held with Allis's forceps at the lower lateral edges and, with a pair of sharp curved scissors, a space is created between the anterior vaginal wall mucosa and the vesicovaginal fascia. The space is created up to the level of the external urethral meatus (Fig. 17). The mucosa under the meatus is held with another Allis's forceps. The mucous membrane is cut in the midline from the lower edge to the external

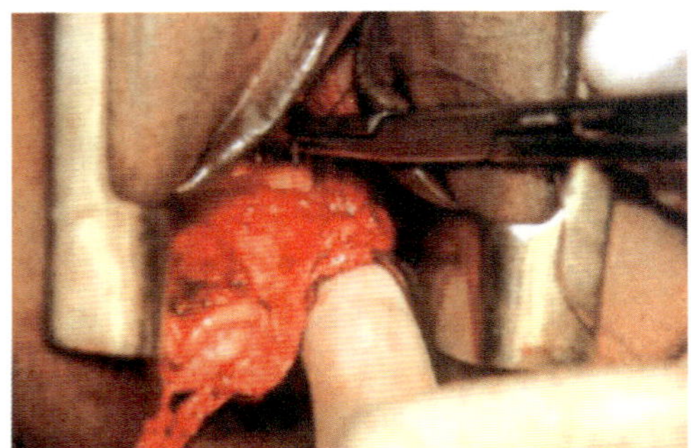

Fig. 11: The next stitch is taken from the edge of the anterior peritoneum to that of the posterior peritoneum, and tied lateral to the transverse cervical ligament pedicle

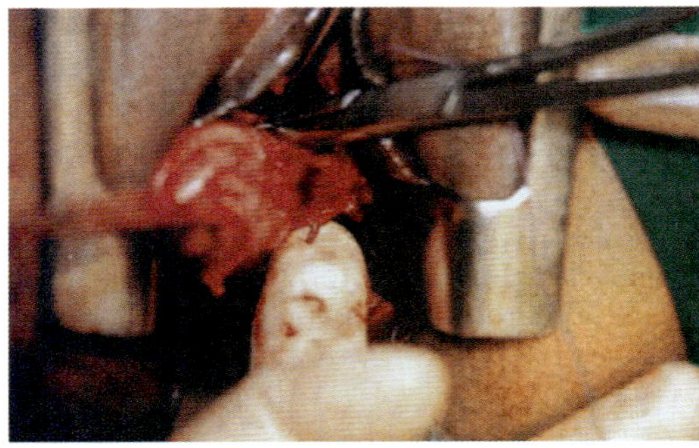

Fig. 12: The cervix is pulled to the right and one more stitch for the uterine vessel is taken 0.5 cm above the previous one

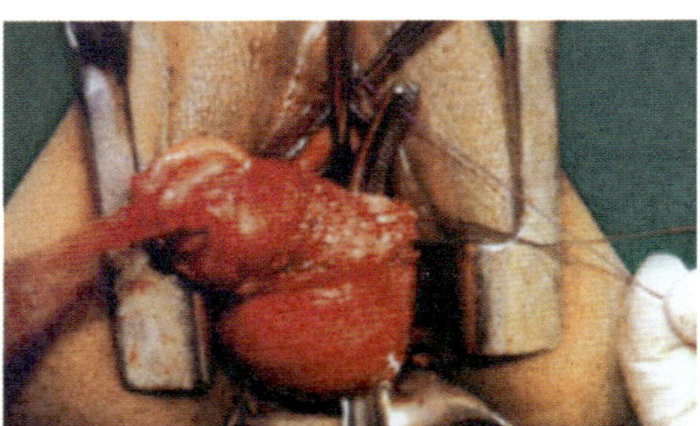

Fig. 13: A curved clamp is inserted behind the cornual structures

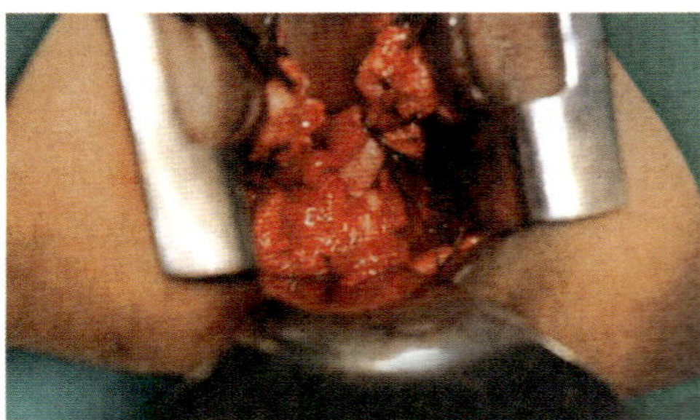

Fig. 14: After the uterus is removed, pelvic organs such as tubes and ovaries can be visualized clearly

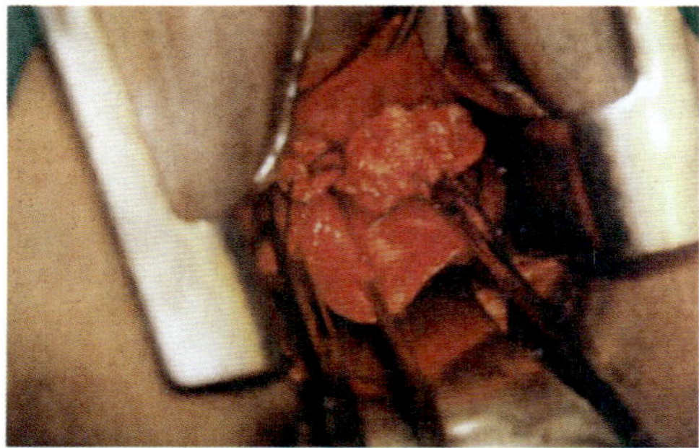

Fig. 15: The anterior bladder wall retractor is gently eased by the surgeon to pick out the edge of the anterior peritoneum

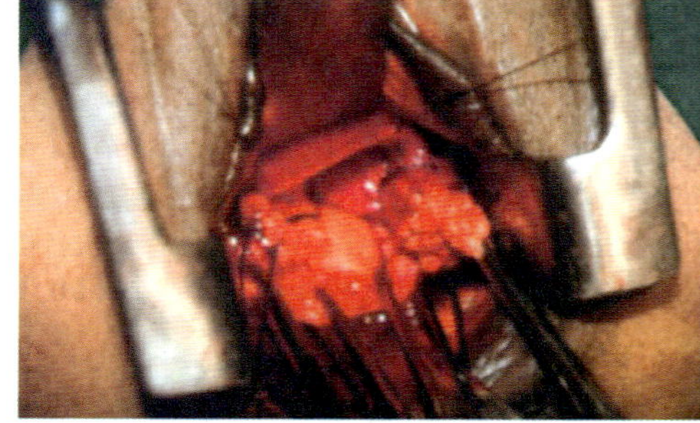

Fig. 16: The peritoneum is closed with a suture running from the midline of the anterior peritoneum, via the left lateral angle, cornual structure pedicle, left uterosacral ligaments, left posterior angle, free peritoneal edge in the midline posteriorly, right posterior angle, right uterosacral ligaments, right cornual structures, and right anterior angle and ending at the midline in the anterior leaf of the peritoneum

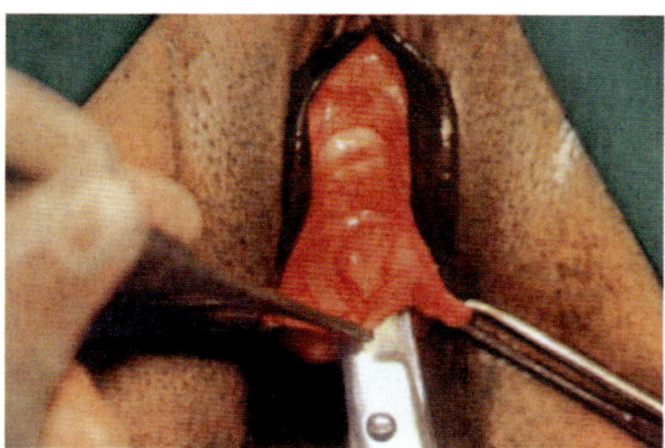

Fig. 17: With a pair of sharp curved scissors, a space is created between the anterior vaginal wall mucosa and the vesicovaginal fascia up to the level of the external urethral meatus

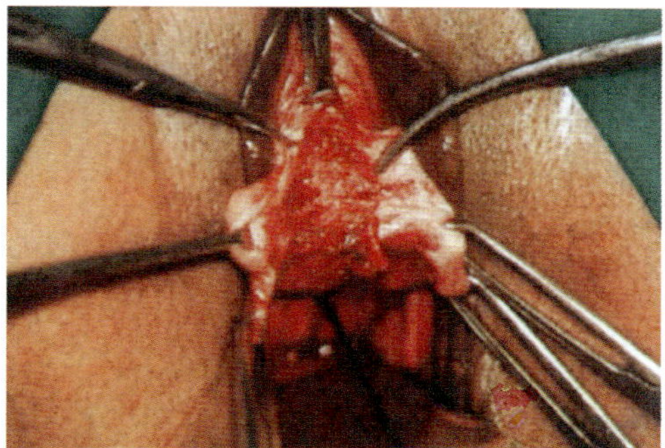

Fig. 18: The edges of the two flaps of the anterior vaginal mucosa are held with one or two additional tissue-holding forceps, depending on the length of the flaps

urethral meatus. This creates two flaps of the anterior vaginal mucosa, the edges of which are held with one or two additional tissue-holding forceps, depending on the length of the flaps (Fig. 18)

- With the edge of the scalpel, a fine incision is taken in the layer between the vaginal mucosa and the vesicovaginal fascia, extending from a little below the urethral meatus to the edge of the flap on either side, thus separating the vaginal mucosa and the prolapsed bladder
- The mucosal edge is held taut with the surgeon's left hand, and using the right thumb covered with a moist swab, the vesicovaginal fascia together with the bladder is pushed away from the vaginal mucosa (Fig. 19). The same procedure is repeated on the opposite side. This blunt dissection is easy up to the level of the vesical pillars where in view of the thickening of the fascia, one has to carry out a sharp dissection by ligating and cutting the pillars. Four hemostatic sutures are taken, two for the paraurethral vessels and two for the paravesical pillars. Then the bladder, paravesical fascia, vesicovaginal fascia, and the edge of the vaginal mucosa can be seen (Fig. 20)
- A purse-string suture is taken from the vesicovaginal fascia, starting from the paraurethral region, the inner surface of the lateral vaginal wall, vesical pillars, the midline which catches the cornual pedicles, the opposite vesical pillar, the opposite lateral vaginal wall, and contralateral paraurethral area. This is tied, making sure that both the assistants release the tension on the edges of the vaginal wall (Fig. 21)
- The vaginal edge is now closed with 1/0 delayed absorbable sutures using a continuous locking stitch or interrupted up to the level of the cornual pedicles
- Then comes the most important step of "vault suspension", which helps in lengthening the anterior vaginal wall and avoiding future vault prolapse. At this stage, the cornual pedicle stitch is taken inside-out bilaterally. The uterosacral stitch is similarly taken inside-out through the vaginal mucosa at the angles. The free ends of the sutures are tied to each other. Thus, suspending the vaginal vault (Fig. 22)
- The surgeon next proceeds to perform the posterior colpoperineorrhaphy. Two Allis's forceps hold the mucocutaneous junction of the posterior vaginal mucosa. A third Allis's forceps holds the posterior vaginal mucosa in the midline up to the level where the repair is to be done. With the toothed dissecting forceps, the perineal skin is held under tension. A horizontal incision is taken with the scalpel, starting from the mucocutaneous junction and extending from one Allis's clamp to the other. Next, a triangular flap is created by incising cranially toward the third Allis's forceps. Now the triangular flap is held taut and, with a pair of curved scissors, the posterior vaginal mucosa is separated from the rectovaginal fascia (Fig. 23). With a moist gauze on the thumb of the left hand, the rectovaginal fascia is separated further from the vaginal mucosa. This is repeated on the opposite side. Excess posterior vaginal mucosa is excised away
- The levator ani and the deep transversus perinei muscles are brought together by two or three sutures of number 1 delayed absorbable suture (Fig. 24). These are interrupted sutures and the muscle bulk is taken vertically rather than horizontally. They are kept long and not tied until the vaginal mucosa has been stitched.
- The posterior vaginal mucosa is stitched with continuous locking suture of 1/0 vicryl. The superficial perineal muscles are approximated with interrupted sutures of 1/0 vicryl to create a neoperineum. Then, the perineal skin is sutured using delayed, absorbable, subcuticular sutures
- A vaginal pack soaked with 5% povidone-iodine and/or antibiotic cream is inserted for 12–24 hours, though this is optional. The bladder is catheterized using a self-retaining Foley catheter for about 48–96 hours postoperatively, depending on the amount of cystocele repair

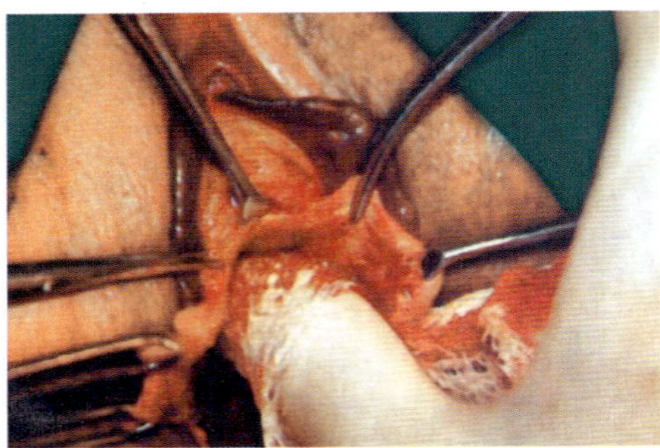

Fig. 19: With the right thumb covered with a moist swab, the vesicovaginal fascia is pushed away from the vaginal mucosa together with the bladder

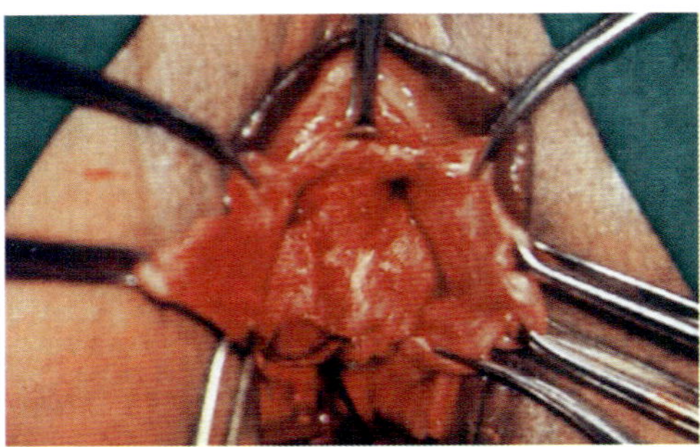

Fig. 20: The bladder, paravesical fascia, vesicovaginal fascia, and edge of the vaginal mucosa can now be seen

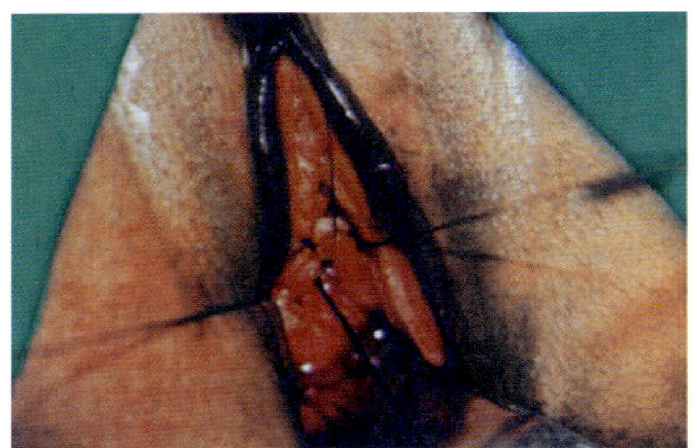

Fig. 21: A purse-string suture is tied, first making sure that the tension on the edges of the vaginal wall is released

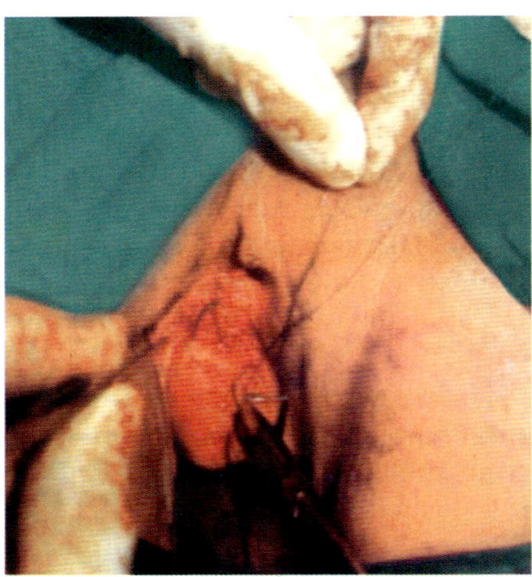

Fig. 22: The free ends of the sutures are tied to each other, suspending the vaginal vault

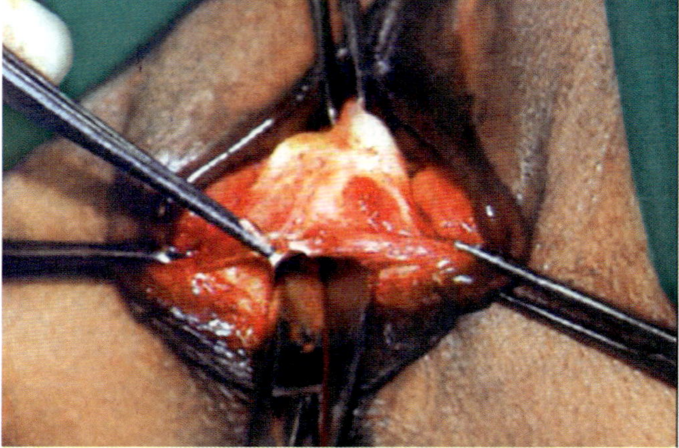

Fig. 23: The triangular flap is held taut and, with a pair of curved scissors, the posterior vaginal mucosa is separated from the rectovaginal fascia

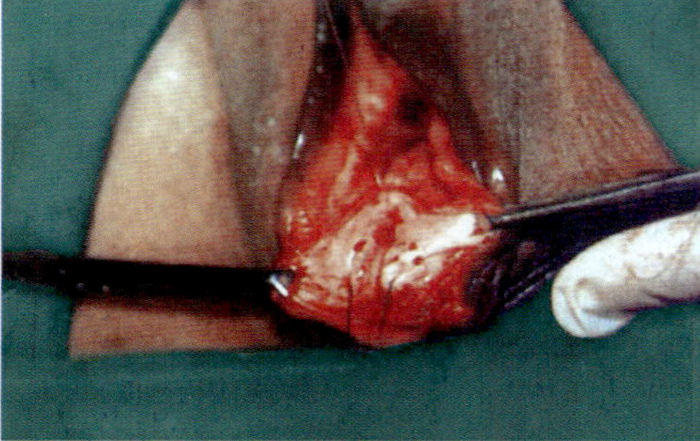

Fig. 24: The levator ani and the deep transversus perinei muscles are brought together by two or three sutures of number 1 delayed absorbable suture

The Intrafascial Technique of Vaginal Hysterectomy

Knowledge about many surgical techniques is essential for proper selection of the type of surgery to be carried out. The intrafascial technique for hysterectomy helps in the preservation of normal anatomical relationships and may diminish significant operative complications. When hysterectomy is carried out for benign disease, preservation of the fascia may improve long-term anatomical and functional results. Intrafascial hysterectomy has evolved with many improvements since its introduction. The surgical technique of vaginal extrafascial hysterectomy, described by Kaser and Ikle, may be followed in certain cases of prolapse with previous abdominopelvic surgery or suspected past adhesive disease. The main principles of vaginal intrafascial hysterectomy as described by Contamin et al. are as follows:

After a circular incision around the cervix and separation of the urinary bladder, the peritoneal cavity is entered anteriorly and posteriorly. Separation of the fascia is started after manual exploration of the pelvis. A transverse incision, 1–2 mm deep is made on the anterior and posterior surface of the cervix at the level of the initial circular incision. The fascia is separated from the cervix by sharp dissection, followed by the perpendicular insertion of closed dissecting scissors between the fascia and cervix up to the level of the internal os. After the fascia is separated laterally, clamps are applied intrafascially. Pedicles are cut and sutured inside the fascial cuff. After the fascial cuff is cut at the 12 and 6 O'clock positions, the cardinal ligaments are cut intrafascially and transfixed. After hysterectomy, the peritoneum is closed to take the pedicles outside the peritoneum. When an enterocele or deep cul-de-sac is present, the posterior vaginal wall is opened in the midline. The peritoneum is mobilized by blunt dissection and the hernia sac resected as high as possible. The right and left cervical fascia and ligaments are sutured together to provide support for the vagina. Additional support may be accomplished by plication of the stretched cardinal and uterosacral ligaments. Palpation of the ureters should be attempted. The vaginal and perirectal fascias are folded in the midline, and the upper portion is attached to the pericervical fascia with the cardinal and uterosacral ligaments.

SPECIAL SITUATIONS

The authors have been successfully carrying out salpingo-oophorectomies or oophorectomies after vaginal hysterectomies for prolapse, using the vaginal route at the same surgical session, whenever indicated. In a recent study, 39 (97.5%) out of the 40 women due to undergo removal of the ovaries were managed successfully via the vaginal route; one woman required laparoscopic removal of one of her ovaries containing an ovarian cyst, which were not diagnosed preoperatively. A variety of techniques was used for vaginal oophorectomy, including salpingo-oophorectomy, oophorectomy without salpingectomy, and transvaginal endoscopic oophorectomy using endoloop sutures or bipolar electrosurgery. Oophorectomy added a mean of 23.4 minute [88.3 vs. 64.9 min, 95% confidence interval (CI) =10.2–36.7 <0.001] to the total operating time, compared with VH alone. No laparotomies were required, and both the complication rate and the postoperative inpatient stay were similar for the two groups. The authors agree with the above study, in that the need to perform oophorectomy should not be considered a contraindication to vaginal hysterectomy.

Vaginal subtotal hysterectomy in combination with sacrospinous colpopexy has recently been described as an option in the management of patients with marked uterine prolapse who desire retention of the cervix. While vaginal subtotal hysterectomy is a simple procedure with low risk of morbidity, controversy remains regarding the value of conservation of the cervix at hysterectomy.

CONCLUSION

Vaginal hysterectomy for genital prolapse is an inherently simple operation if the surgeon follows good surgical principles and has a thorough knowledge of pelvic anatomy. A keen sense of plastic surgery with a good surgical instinct, together with knowledge about dealing with complications, if any arise, is essential for effective cures.

BIBLIOGRAPHY

1. Allahbadia GN, Vaidya PR, Ambrye VR, et al. Sexual function after hysterectomy. Bombay Hosp J. 1993;35:167-72.
2. Allahbadia GN. Vaginal hysterectomy: A new technique of vault closure. J Indian Med Assoc. 1992;90:294-7.
3. Allahbadia GN. Vaginal hysterectomy—a reappraisal. Bombay Hosp J. 1991;33:88-90.
4. Barnes AB, Tinkham CB. Surgical gynaecology. In: Norman MT, Nadelson CC (Eds). The Woman Patient: Medical and Psychological interfaces. New York: Plenum Press; 1978. p. 732-8.
5. Contamin R, Bernard F, Ferrieux J. L'hysterectomie vaginale intrafasciale avec reconstitution de la pario vaginale posteriaire. Gynaecol Pract. 1972;23:17-23.

6. Davies A, O'Connor HM, Magos AL. A prospective study to evaluate oophorectomy at the time of vaginal hysterectomy. Br J Obstet Gynaecol. 1996;103:915-20.
7. Hefni M, El-Toukhy T. Vaginal subtotal hysterectomy and sacrospinous colpopexy: An option in the management of uterine prolapse. Am J Obstet Gynecol. 2000;183(2):494-5.
8. Jaszczak SE, Evans TN. Intrafascial abdominal and vaginal hysterectomy: A reappraisal. Obstet Gynecol. 1982;59:435-44.
9. Kaser O, Me FA. Gynecologic Operations. In: Davis A (Ed). Indications, Technique and Results. New York: Grune & Stratton; 1967. p. 162-7.
10. Malpas P. Genital Prolapse and Allied Conditions. London: Harvey & Blythe Ltd.; 1968.
11. Palmer R. The Anatomy of Genital Prolapse: Dilemmas. New York: Cambridge University Press; 1954. p. 1.

41.8 COMPLICATIONS PECULIAR TO VAGINAL HYSTERECTOMY

CN Purandare, Rajalaxmi Walavalkar, Nikhil Purandare

INTRODUCTION

Vaginal surgery often entails meticulous dissection near the bladder, rectum, ureters, and major blood vessels of the pelvis. Understandably, the more common complications from this surgery relate to injuries to these viscera. Complications occur, either during extensive resections of cancer surgery or when anatomy is distorted due to infection or endometriosis. For the purpose of this chapter, we will be concentrating on complications seen more commonly with vaginal surgeries rather than on complications common with all surgery, e.g. bleeding, infection, etc, also urological or bowel injuries are beyond the remit of this chapter.

VAGINAL VAULT PROLAPSE

Vault prolapse is the downward displacement of the vaginal vault due to loss of apical support. Support to the vault is primarily derived from the integrity of the uterosacral and cardinal ligaments, hence vault prolapse usually follows a hysterectomy for uterine prolapse in which support was not reconstructed or was improperly reconstructed. The incidence of posthysterectomy vaginal prolapse has been shown to be several-fold higher after hysterectomies performed for pelvic relaxation than for those performed for other types of benign disease.

Signs and symptoms include a sensation of pelvic pressure or bearing down, inguinal discomfort, dyspareunia and low-back pain. Symptoms worsen with a gradual increase in size of the prolapse over time. The prolapsed vault may protrude from the vagina, leading to chronic discharge and bleeding from chronic ulceration. Vaginal vault prolapse is frequently accompanied by cystocele, rectocele, enterocele, or a combination of these conditions.

Vault prolapse almost always requires surgical correction because of the symptoms that are disruptive to daily life and sexual function. Pessaries may provide temporary relief of symptoms. Prior to surgery, it is important to rule out any pre-existing symptoms of urinary stress incontinence, as surgical correction of the vault prolapse can exacerbate incontinence hence a patient may need a combined procedure. Coexisting hernias may be due to chronically increased intra-abdominal pressure, which should be dealt with prior to surgery, if possible.

The choice of surgery depends upon the woman's desire to preserve sexual function. In women who are not sexually active and who lead a sedentary lifestyle, colpectomy or colpocleisis may be the options. In women in whom preservation of sexual function is important, the options would be transvaginal sacrospinous vault fixation performed by suturing one or both sides of the vagina to the sacrospinous ligament to support the vaginal apex or transabdominal sacrocolpopexy, i.e. suspension of the vaginal apex from the sacrum using synthetic mesh. The surgeon's expertize also plays a role in determining the surgical approach, as well as the need for other unrelated procedures.

There are only two randomized studies comparing abdominal versus vaginal approach to management of vault prolapse.

In the first trial, 88 women with cervical prolapse or vaginal vault inversion and anterior vaginal wall descent were randomly assigned to vaginal bilateral sacrospinous vault suspension and paravaginal repair or abdominal colposacral suspension and paravaginal repair. There were no significant differences between the groups in morbidity, complications, hemoglobin change, dyspareunia, pain, or hospital stay. However, the vaginal approach was associated with longer catheter use, more urinary tract infections (UTIs), more incontinence, decreased operative time, and lower hospital charges. Surgical effectiveness was more often considered optimal in the abdominal than vaginal group (58% vs. 29%) and unsatisfactory results leading to reoperation occurred twice as often in the vaginal group (33% vs. 16%) after 5 years of follow-up. Reoperation for recurrent incontinence was performed in 12% of the vaginal and 2% of the abdominal groups.

In the other trial, 95 women with vaginal vault prolapse were randomly allocated to abdominal sacral colpopexy or vaginal sacrospinous colpopexy. At a mean follow-up of 2 years, the subjective and objective success rates were similar in both groups (subjective: 94% and 91%, respectively; objective 76% and 69%, respectively). The abdominal approach took longer to perform and recover from, and was more expensive. However, although not a statistically significant difference, vault prolapse to or beyond the introitus occurred in only 2 out of 47 women in the abdominal group versus 8 of 48 women in the vaginal group.

Thus, a common finding for both trials was that the abdominal repair had a better anatomic result, with fewer severe apical recurrences.

VAULT EVISCERATION

Evisceration of the small intestine into the vagina is a rare complication. It may be associated with the Valsalva's maneuver or severe vomiting or coughing. Eviscerations usually occur in the early postoperative period, although in one series of 12 patients, the mean time of occurrence was 27 months (range 5–48 months) after various pelvic surgeries. Symptoms include abdominal-pelvic pain, vaginal bleeding or discharge, pressure in the vagina, and protrusion of bowel, which can become incarcerated.

Acute management involves wrapping the bowel in moist saline soaked towels, administering intravenous (IV) fluids and broad-spectrum antibiotics, and immediate laparotomy with inspection and replacement of the mesentery and small bowel. Any necrotic vaginal mucosa, or bowel, should be resected and the vaginal cuff should be closed.

PROLAPSED FALLOPIAN TUBE

Fallopian tube prolapse is a rare complication of hysterectomy, characterized by vaginal discharge, abdominal pain, pelvic inflammatory disease and vaginal bleeding. Only 80 cases have been described since 1902. The diagnosis is often delayed, and is usually done after a histopathological examination identifies fallopian tube on biopsy. It is often confused with granulation tissue at the vaginal apex. Development of a hematoma or abscess at the vaginal apex is a predisposing factor. If the tissue at the top of the vaginal cuff does not respond to conservative treatment, such as silver nitrate application or cryotherapy, a biopsy of the area is warranted to determine if it is tubal epithelium. Treatment is surgical; the surrounding vaginal mucosa is opened and widely undermined, and the tube is resected. Laparoscopic and vaginal approaches may be used. Fallopian tube prolapse has also been diagnosed in a patient after laparoscopic excision of pelvic endometriosis, without hysterectomy. The prolapsed fallopian tube was preserved by laparoscopic retrieval from the vagina and closure of the vaginoperitoneal fistula. Fallopian tube prolapse may be mimicking aggressive angiomyxoma and thus poses a diagnostic pitfall. An unusual association of fallopian tubal prolapse and herpetic infection has been described in a 37-year-old woman presenting with a small polypoid mass of the vaginal vault, 3 months after abdominal hysterectomy and abdominoplasty. The vaginal mass proved to be the fimbriated end of a fallopian tube, herniated into the vagina. Reintervention 3 months later with resection of a small vaginal "polyp" revealed a residual portion of fallopian tube, with superimposed herpes simplex virus (HSV) infection and marked cytological atypia of surface epithelial cells. HSV-2 immunostaining of viral nuclear inclusions and of atypical cells confirmed the herpetic nature of the infection. In the setting of fallopian tubal prolapse, direct exposure of the herniated fallopian tube to various pathogens in the vagina provides a unique clinical model for salpingitis. In herpetic tubal infections, special attention must be paid to cytological atypia of probable viral cytopathogenic origin, to avoid a misdiagnosis of malignancy.

RECTOVAGINAL FISTULAS

Rectovaginal and anovaginal fistulas frequently result from obstetric trauma. They also occur following an unsuccessful primary repair of a third or fourth degree laceration, from episiotomy infection with formation of a fistulous tract. Rectovaginal fistulas may also result from difficult vaginal hysterectomies, especially those performed for severe endometriosis with involvement or obliteration of the cul-de-sac, and from surgical procedures involving the posterior vaginal wall, perineum, anus, and rectum.

Women suffering from anovaginal or rectovaginal fistulas present with complaints of uncontrollable passage of gas or feces from the vagina. A malodorous vaginal discharge and fecal soiling of the undergarments are also common complaints. Symptoms may be more pronounced when bowel movements are loose. Occasionally, a small fistula may be asymptomatic. It is important to inquire about fecal urgency and fecal incontinence associated with urgency, as this often suggests that the external anal sphincter is also disrupted.

Pinpoint fistulas can be difficult to locate. The use of magnification, such as a colposcope, may be helpful. Lacrimal duct or silver wire probes can also be used to assist in identifying the fistula tract. A few drops of methylene blue dye can be mixed with lubricating gel and massaged into the anterior rectal wall. Alternatively, an enema consisting of warmed saline and a few drops of methylene blue dye can be instilled into the rectum using a genitourinary syringe. Using a peroxide solution will avoid staining the tissues. Proctoscopy may also be useful in visualizing the fistulous tract from the rectal side.

Most rectovaginal and anovaginal fistulas are amenable to early repair. The decision of when to operate should depend upon the status of the involved tissue rather than an arbitrary period of time. Surgical repair should be deferred until there is resolution of any local cellulitis, inflammation, or induration.

There is neither data nor universal agreement regarding the best preoperative regimen for women undergoing rectal surgery. Dietary manipulation should be considered in all women undergoing sphincteroplasty or rectovaginal fistula repair. The ultimate goal is to avoid fecal seeding of the wound during the procedure and to decrease the amount of stool that will pass over the repair in the first few weeks of healing. Institution of a low residue diet should be started 1 week before the scheduled procedure. The stool will become small and hard, thereby eliminating seeding of the fistulous tract with liquid stool just before the intended procedure. A clear liquid diet is usually instituted 48–72 hours before surgery. Mechanical bowel cleansing is routinely recommended. The authors prefer to give oral agents 48–72 hours preoperatively, because giving them closer to the procedure often results in a thin fecal effluent being present at the time of the repair. Either magnesium citrate (32 ounces) or golytely (4–6 liters) can be administered at home. Tap water or phosphate enemas should be given the night before surgery to complete the emptying of the lower colon and rectum. Antibiotic prophylaxis with a single dose of a broad-spectrum antibiotic, such as cefoxitin or cefotetan, 30 minutes before the procedure may be given.

The basic principles essential for successful fistula repair include:

- Wide mobilization of the adjacent tissue planes
- Complete excision of the fistula tract
- Multilayered closure, which reapproximates broad tissue surfaces without tension
- Proper timing of the repair.

Delayed absorbable sutures, such as polyglactin or polyglycolic acid are preferred. The tensile strength is maintained longer and the knot is more secure. Tissue reaction is also less with delayed absorbable suture.

Repair techniques vary significantly by fistula type and etiology. Small rectovaginal fistulas can often be repaired by simple fistulectomy via a transvaginal or transrectal approach. An incision is made around the fistula, which completely excises the fistulous tract and allows mobilization of the vagina, rectum, and rectovaginal septum to create a tension-free closure. Meticulous care must be taken to insure complete hemostasis and closure of all potential dead space.

Trans-sphincteric approach is preferred in anovaginal and low rectovaginal fistulas. Technique involves a midline perineal incision (trans-sphincteric or perineoproctomy) with wide mobilization of the posterior vaginal wall followed by a multilayered closure. Rectovaginal fistulas located above the sphincter complex can also be approached with a transverse transperineal incision. This approach allows the surgeon to preserve the intact internal and external anal sphincter and allows wide mobilization of the rectal and vaginal tissue.

An abdominal approach with sharp dissection of the rectum from the vagina is occasionally needed to repair a rectovaginal fistula located near the vaginal apex. It is imperative that the rectum and vagina be widely mobilized from the fistulous communication. Serosal dissection on the colonic side of the fistula site can be extensive, especially when the defect is large. The fistula should be excised or inverted, followed by multilayered closure of the rectum and vagina.

Colovesical fistulas are rare. They are usually associated with the same conditions and disease processes that cause the high rectovaginal fistulas discussed before. In these instances, a diverting colostomy is almost mandatory to divert the fecal stream and minimize the risks of ascending UTI and renal damage while tissue inflammation subsides.

Postoperatively dietary manipulation should be considered to decrease the amount of stool that will pass over the repair in the first few weeks of healing. A clear liquid diet is prescribed for the first 24–72 postoperative hours. A low residue diet should then be instituted for at least a month. A stool softener should be given for 1 month to lubricate the stool. If the patient complains of constipation, milk of magnesia can be given to encourage a looser stool. Laxatives and enemas should be avoided.

UROGENITAL FISTULAS

Urogenital fistulae in developed countries are typically related to gynecologic surgery, severe pelvic pathology, radiation therapy, or injuries incurred in the healing process. In a series of 126 cases of genitourinary fistulas, 91% followed surgery, primarily abdominal hysterectomy for benign disease. The incidence ranges from less than 0.5% after simple hysterectomy to 10% after radical hysterectomy. Surgical repair is readily accessible and usually successful. In one study of 1,093 women undergoing pelvic operations, ureteral injury occurred in 1.5%. Bladder injuries associated with vaginal surgery are most commonly seen after routine, benign surgery. The incidence of bladder and ureteric injuries are far less than abdominal hysterectomies as can be seen from statistics mentioned above.

This gives a clear message that vaginal hysterectomies should by far be preferred than abdominal route.

The fistulas are usually painless and result in leakage of urine from the vagina. Intermittent leakage, particularly when positional, can be due to ureterovesical fistula, whereas continuous urine loss is more characteristic of vesicovaginal fistulas. Vulvar irritation and recurrent infections are common associated problems. On vaginal examination, the fistula may appear as a small, red area of granulation tissue with no visible opening, or an actual hole may be seen. To find small fistulas, methylene blue may be instilled through a Foley catheter into the bladder, and then have the patient cough or valsalva.

Investigations involving the Moirs test involves placing three cotton swabs in the vagina and then instilling methylene blue through the urethra into the bladder. Cystoscopy with retrograde pyelography is an integral part of assessing lower urogenital tract fistulas. Intravenous pyelography (IVP) is useful for noting any disruption in ureteral integrity. The use of a double balloon urethral catheter under fluoroscopic guidance may be useful for diagnosis of urethral fistula. Ureteral obstruction with upper tract dilation may be seen on IVP, computed tomography (CT), or ultrasound (USG). A dilated ureter or renal pelvis can be present with ureteral fistulas.

Timing of ureteral fistula repair is a controversial issue. Traditional teaching was to delay fistula repair 8–12 weeks after the onset of leakage before attempting any repair. This was to allow recovery from inflammation, infection, and tissue necrosis. Although this might be true for large fistulas resulting from obstructed labor, extensive infection and tissue necrosis are uncommon with small gynecologic fistula. Early excision and repair of the fistulous tract within 1–2 weeks of leakage has become more common. Spontaneous healing of a small (less than 5 mm) lesion in otherwise healthy tissue may occur, if a stent can be placed across the fistula site and left in place for at least 4–8 weeks. Active pelvic infection precludes an immediate surgical approach. Radiology-assisted percutaneous nephrostomy allows temporary urinary drainage until repair can be undertaken.

There are several options for surgical repair. The choice depends upon the surgeon's experience and personal preference, and the specific type of fistula. The patient's specific needs and preferences should also be considered. Most surgeons administer one dose of a broad-spectrum antibiotic prophylactically.

Small post-hysterectomy fistulae can be corrected using the Latzko technique. The use of electrocautery through the cystoscope has been suggested in closing very small (less than 0.5 cm) vesicovaginal fistula tracts.

Various techniques have been described for managing the high vaginal vault fistula. The Mackenrodt technique, the vaginal flaps are raised away from the bladder and preserved for use in the final closure layer. The Martius graft, or labial fibrofatty tissue graft, is most commonly used to reinforce repairs even high in the vaginal vault. Gracilis muscle grafts can also be used on occasion. Abdominal approach involves a transvesical route with separate closure of vagina and bladder. The fistula is resected, the vagina and bladder closed, and omental tissue is interposed between bladder and vagina to separate the suture lines, and act as a neovascular pedicle. The abdominal approach also may be preferred for patients having concomitant abdominal or pelvic procedures.

Fistulas with total urethral loss remain difficult to manage, and repair methods involve mobilization of vulvar and labial tissue to create a neourethra. The repair of ureterovaginal fistulas requires an approach and technique that will both restore normal function of the ureter and close the fistulous defect. A simple ureteral reimplantation or a Boari flap is the most effective repair for most pos-thysterectomy fistulas.

The abdominal approach may a transvesical approach where the dome of the bladder is opened and the fistula tract and ureteral orifices are identified. The bladder serosa is dissected from the vagina and if bowel is also involved then colon through the fistula tract within the bladder mucosa. In cases of bowel involvement even with careful dissection and a multilayered closure, the failure rate is significant. Alternately the posterior bladder can be dissected completely off of the rectum. A multilayered closure of each organ, followed by an omental or muscle interpositional flap, will usually be successful.

Postoperatively, drains and catheters need to be secured to prevent unintentional removal. Antibiotics for prevention of UTIs may be useful. Adequate hydration is important to insure constant fluid flow through the bladder. This prevents any blood clots from blocking the catheter, which leads to bladder distension and disruption of the fistula repair. High volume bladder flow can be achieved by IV fluid administration, intermittent catheter flushing with small amounts of normal saline, or copious oral intake. However, it is unclear how long drains or catheters need to be left in place or if they need to be used at all. Custom has led to drainage for a week or more. A cystogram is ordered to assess repairs of bladder fistulae, while IVPs are used to evaluate ureteral repairs.

SEXUAL DYSFUNCTION

A discussion of sexual function should precede and follow vaginal surgery. If problems are identified with a woman's sex life, then appropriate counseling is warranted as soon as possible, since sexual dysfunction may become worse after surgery or radiation therapy. Vaginal hysterectomy procedures are not associated with long-term subsequent sexual dysfunction. However, one must keep in mind that too much narrowing or shortening of vagina should be avoided in sexually active women.

BIBLIOGRAPHY

1. Benson JT, Lucente V, McClellan E. Vaginal versus abdominal reconstructive surgery for the treatment of pelvic support defects: A prospective randomized study with long-term outcome evaluation. Am J Obstet Gynecol. 1996;175:1418.
2. Carlton CE. Injuries of the ureter. Urol Clin North Am. 1977;4:33.
3. Chaikin DC, Groutz A, Blaivas JG. Predicting the need for anti-incontinence surgery in continent women undergoing repair of severe urogenital prolapse. J Urol. 2000;163:531.
4. Collins CG, Pent D, Jones FB. Results of early repair of vesicovaginal fistula with preliminary cortisone treatment. Am J Obstet Gynecol. 1960;80:1005.
5. Croak AJ, Gebhart JB, Klingele CJ, et al. Characteristics of patients with vaginal rupture and evisceration. Obstet Gynecol. 2004;103:572.
6. Daly JW, Higgins KA. Injury to the ureter during gynecologic surgical procedures. Surg Gynecol Obstet. 1988;167:19.
7. Elkins TE, DeLancey JO, McGuire EJ. The use of modified Martius graft as an adjunctive technique in vesicovaginal and rectovaginal fistula repair. Obstet Gynecol. 1990;75:727.
8. Falk HC, Orkin LA. Nonsurgical closure of vesicovaginal fistulas. Obstet Gynecol. 1957;9:538.
9. Galyer KT, Conaglen HM, Hare A, et al. The effect of gynecological surgery on sexual desire. J Sex Marital Ther. 1999;25:81.
10. Garlock JH. The cure of an intractable vesicovaginal fistula by use of a pedicled muscle graft. Surg Gynecol Obstet. 1928;255:255.
11. Graber EA, O'Rourke JJ, McElrath T. Latrogenic bladder injury during hysterectomy. Obstet Gynecol. 1964;23:267.
12. Hamlin RHJ, Nicholson EC. Reconstruction of the urethra totally destroyed in labor. BMJ. 1969;2:147.
13. Hibbard LT. Surgical management of rectovaginal fistulas and complete perineal tears. Am J Obstet Gynecol. 1978;130:139.
14. Kursh ED. Etiology, evaluation, and endoscopic management of vesicovaginal fistulas. In: Kursh ED, McGuire EJ (Eds). Female Urology. Philadelphia: JB Lippincott; 1994.
15. Kursh ED. Ureteral injuries. In: Kursh ED, McGuire EJ (Eds). Female Urology. Philadelphia: JB Lippincott; 1994.
16. Latzko W. Postoperative vesicovaginal fistulas: Genesis and therapy. Am J Surg. 1992;48:211.
17. Lavy Y, Hamani Y, Lev-Sagie A. Fallopian tube prolapse after hysterectomy. Harefuah. 2002;141(6):530-1.
18. Leenhouts GH, Kylstra WA, Everaerd W, et al. Sexual outcomes following treatment for early-stage gynecological cancer: A prospective and cross-sectional multi-center study. J Psychosom Obstet Gynaecol. 2002;23:123.
19. Lefrancq T, Orain I, Michalak S, et al. Herpetic salpingitis and fallopian tube prolapse. [Article]. Histopathology. 1999;34(6): 19. 548-50.
20. Mackenrodt A. Die operative Heilung grosser Blasenscheiden-fistein. Zentralbl Gynakol. 1894;8:180.
21. Maher CF, Qatawneh AM, Dwyer PL, et al. Abdominal sacral colpopexy or vaginal sacrospinous colpopexy for vaginal vault prolapse: a prospective randomized study. Am J Obstet Gynecol. 2004;190:20.
22. Mann WJ, Arato M, Patsner B, et al. Ureteral injuries in an obstetrics and gynecology training program: Etiology and management. Obstet Gynecol. 1988;72:82.
23. Mant J, Painter R, Vessey M. Epidemiology of genital prolapse: observations from the Oxford Family Planning Association Study. Br J Obstet Gynaecol. 1997;104:579.
24. Moir JC. Personal experiences in the treatment of vesicovaginal fistulas. Am J Obstet Gynecol. 1956;71:476.
25. O'Quinn AG, Degefu S, Batson HK, et al. Early repair of vesicovaginal fistula following preliminary corticosteroid. Presented at the Society of Pelvic Surgeons, New Orleans, November; 1984.
26. Piacenza JM, Salsano F. Posthysterectomy fallopian tube prolapse. Eur J Obstet Gynecol Reprod Biol. 2001;98(2):253-5.
27. Rosenthal DM, Cheung VY. Fallopian tube prolapse after laparoscopic resection of pelvic Endometriosis. [Report]. Obstet Gynecol. 2005;105(4):808-9.
28. Shieh CJ, Gennaro AR. Rectovaginal fistula: A review of 11 years experience. Int Surg. 1984;69:69.
29. Symmonds RE, Hill LM. Loss of the urethra: A report on 50 patients. Am J Obstet Gynecol. 1978;130:130.
30. Tancer ML. Observations on prevention and management of vesicovaginal fistula after total hysterectomy. Surg Gynecol Obstet. 1992;175:501.
31. Thakar R, Ayers S, Clarkson P, et al. Outcomes after total versus subtotal abdominal hysterectomy. N Engl J Med. 2002;347:1318.
32. Varnholt H, Otis CN, Nucci MR, et al. Fallopian tube prolapse mimicking aggressive angiomyxoma. [Report]. Int J Gynecol Pathol. 2005;24(3):292-4.
33. Waaldijk K. The immediate surgical management of fresh obstetric fistulas with catheter and/or early closure. Int J Gynaecol Obstet. 1994;45:11.
34. Waaldijk K. The surgical management of bladder fistula in 775 women in Northern Nigeria. Nymegen: Benda BV; 1989.
35. Wiskind AK, Thompson JD. Transverse transperineal repair of rectovaginal fistulas in the lower vagina. Am J Obstet Gynecol. 1992;167:694.

41.9 TECHNICAL MINUTIAE OF VAGINAL HYSTERECTOMY

DK Tank, JD Tank

INTRODUCTION

Hysterectomy was the most commonly performed major surgery until 1990s and has been second only to cesarean section between then and 2000. A striking feature from many reports is that 70% of these operations and, in a few centers, as many as 85% are done abdominally, whereas only about 30% are done vaginally. The practice style and personal preference of the surgeon, which are dependent on early training, play a significant role in the selection of the hysterectomy type. The absence of clear guidelines for selecting a surgical route, lack of patient knowledge about the options, and inappropriate decision-making all combine to lead to this ratio of 3:1 abdominal versus vaginal operations.

With the inclination to do so, this ratio of 3:1 can be reversed, i.e. 75% of all hysterectomies can be done vaginally. The technical variations suggested in this chapter are the result of the more than 6,900 hysterectomies performed by the senior author. In his practice, he has been successful in performing vaginal hysterectomies in 74% of patients who needed a hysterectomy.

The technique of VH has remained essentially unchanged for almost 100 years. However, minor variations have been suggested by scores of writers to obtain better anatomical and functional results.

Most gynecologists can obtain the degree of surgical dexterity required to perform a vaginal hysterectomy.

However, the major technical barriers to the minds of most surgeons, not only at the initial level of training but even after considerable experience are:

- Reaching and opening of the vesicouterine fold of the peritoneum
- Clamping, cutting, and ligating the uterosacral and Mackenrodt's ligaments when the descent is poor and the space inadequate
- When the uterus is enlarged, or occasionally there is no mobility in spite of securing the cardinal ligaments.

OPENING OF THE ANTERIOR PERITONEUM

The opening of the vesicouterine fold of the peritoneum at VH is a technically demanding step.

In opening the pouch, insight and appreciation of the relationship between the anterior wall of the vagina, urinary bladder, and the cervix are essential. It is also essential to realize that any pathology of the anterior wall of the uterus, such as elongation of the cervix, presence of a myoma, previous surgery such as lower segment cesarean section (LSCS), and post-infection adhesions, changes this relationship (Figs 1A to C).

The level of the incision and its depth are critical to finding the correct plane between the bladder and the cervix or lower uterine body. The standard site for the anterior incision recommended almost universally, is where the vagina blends with the epithelial layer of the cervix. This point can be identified by:

- The loss of rugosity over this area
- The grooved depression felt through the thickness of the vagina
- Moving the cervix anteroposteriorly several times and looking at the point where the mobility of the vagina becomes restricted; the incision is made 2–3 mm above this point.

After the anterior vaginal wall is incised, the cervicovesical fascia is cut. The surgeon usually separates the bladder from the cervix by sharp dissection. Many experts bluntly strip the bladder away from the cervix

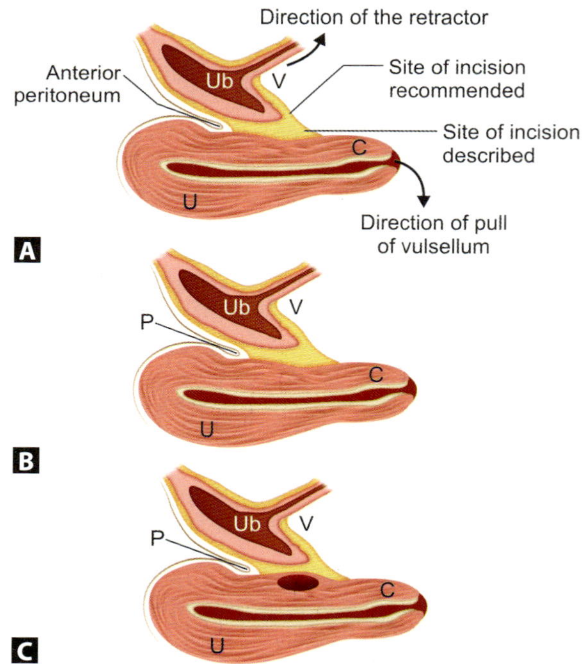

Figs 1A to C: (A) The relationship of the anterior peritoneum in a normal patient; (B) The high position of the anterior peritoneum when the cervix is elongated (thus the site of the incision on the vagina has to be correspondingly higher); (C) The change in relationship of the anterior peritoneum when there is a fibroid on the lower segment (*Abbreviations:* U, uterus; C, cervix; Ub, urinary bladder; V, vagina; P, anterior peritoneum; F, fibroid)

either with a gauze-covered finger or with a sponge. Theoretically, this may result in laceration of the wall of the bladder; however, this problem has rarely been reported.

The authors prefer not to make an arbitrary incision 2–5 mm above the external os, but to select the site of incision after defining the lowermost border of the bladder. When the vaginal wall is a little lax, the lowermost margin of the bladder can be palpated between the index finger and the thumb (Fig. 2).

If the vaginal wall is not lax, it can be felt by pressure of the index finger, and feeling the lower pole of the bladder slipping under the palpating finger (Fig. 3).

A circumferential incision is taken at this level. The direction of traction by the bladder retractor is of paramount importance at this stage. The cervix is pulled downward while the retractor presses the anterior vaginal wall backward. This has two advantages:

1. When the vagina is incised at this level, the vesicocervical ligament is also dissected off with the incision over the vaginal wall
2. As a result of the pressure on the anterior wall, the lower wall of the bladder seems to bulge out and delineates itself in the incision. As a result of the better delineation of the planes, sharp dissection upto the peritoneum becomes easy (Fig. 4).

It is true that in a few cases, sharp dissection may not be possible, especially when the wrong planes have been entered earlier. In these cases, blunt dissection with the finger may help.

Obviously, no attempt is made to open the peritoneum until the bladder is reflected well away. The free peritoneum, which is to be incised to enter the peritoneal cavity, lies a few millimeters above than what appears to be the visceral peritoneum at first sight. The peritoneum is held and pulled downward with an artery forceps, then incised and opened (Fig. 5).

If the bladder wall appears immediately below the incision, it is a simple matter to pick up and dissect the bladder away by sharp dissection to reach the peritoneum.

Occasionally, even the most experienced vaginal surgeon may not be able to enter the correct planes. Difficulty in opening the anterior peritoneum may be overcome in the following ways:

- If the surgeon was unable to open the peritoneum anteriorly, this step is postponed and the posterior cul-de-sac is opened first. Then, the first and second left fingertips are inserted through the posterior peritoneal opening over the fundus of the uterus and the anterior peritoneum is tented over the fingers. It should be highlighted here that this is not possible when there is no descent, unless the cardinal ligaments are clamped and ligated
- If the anterior peritoneum cannot be opened by this method, further clamps are applied, keeping the bladder as far away as possible until the peritoneum is reached

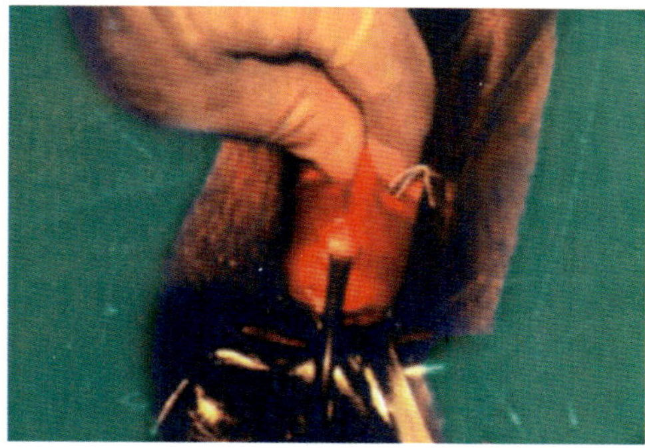

Fig. 2: Surgeon grasping the anterior vaginal wall and defining the edges of the bladder. The lowermost margin of the bladder can be palpated between the index finger and the thumb

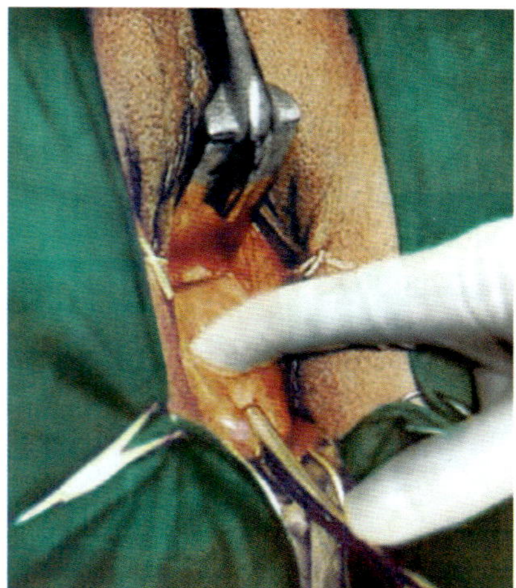

Fig. 3: The palpation of the lower margin of the bladder by pressure against the cervix where the free vaginal wall merges and becomes attached to the cervix. This shows the area upto the lowermost part of which the bladder extends

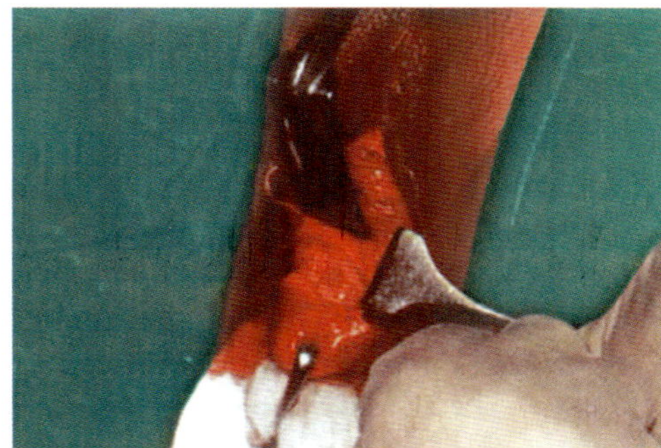

Fig. 4: How the bladder pops out through the incision made in the anterior vagina. Note the direction of the retractor blade, which is downward and backward—giving pressure on the hollow bladder—and the level of the incision

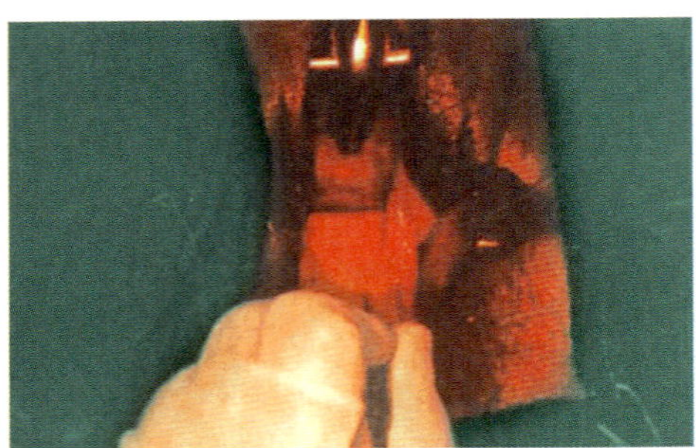

Fig. 5: The delineation of planes at the level of the anterior peritoneum. Just below the retractor, the bladder is seen and below the white line of the bladder the peritoneum can be seen

- In the case of adhesions and fibrosis in this area, particularly when the patient has earlier undergone cesarean section, the cervix is opened by a small longitudinal incision. As a result of the fibrosis, this usually does not bleed. Defining the fibromuscular tissue of the anterior cervical wall, then identifies the exact plane
- If identification is still not possible, a uterine sound is bent in a U-shape and inserted through the posterior peritoneal opening over the top of the fundus; the tip is made to distend the anterior peritoneum as suggested by Hoffman
- The worst scenario, although very rare, would be if one enters the plane between the anterior vaginal wall and the bladder. In this situation, one could dissect between the vaginal wall and the bladder to define the latter.

ELLIPTICAL INCISION

An elliptical incision is made at the cut edge of the vaginal wall and epithelial surface of the cervix, which helps through better exposure of the uterosacral and Mackenrodt's ligaments, improve clamping and ligation (Fig. 6).

When space is limited and the uterosacral ligaments are not well exposed, there is a tendency for these to slip from the clamp. In this situation, a ligature is taken before cutting the pedicle without releasing the clamp. The uterosacral is cut only when one is ready to apply the second ligature. This can be useful in clamp or clampless techniques.

FAILURE OF UTERUS TO DESCEND

Once both the anterior and posterior peritoneum are open and the uterosacral and Mackenrodt's ligament complex is ligated, the surgeon may find that traction applied to the cervix fails to move the uterus further down.

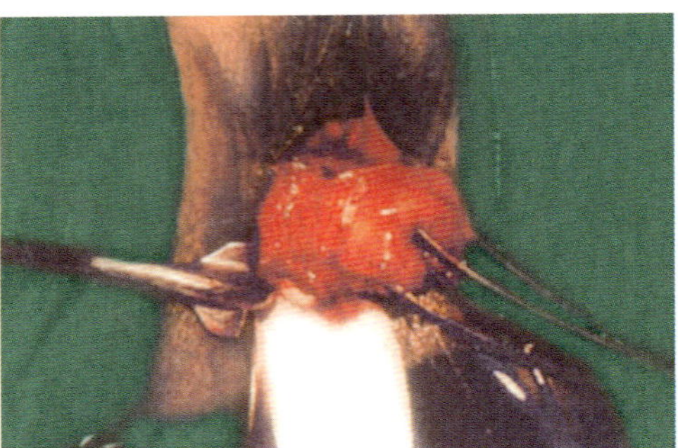

Fig. 6: The elliptical incision used to expose the cardinal—uterosacral ligament complex. The strip of vagina is dissected off with scissors and then the ligaments are clamped

This event requires assessment of the causes, usually a large-sized uterus. The other infrequent causes are:

- Adhesion(s) binding the uterus to intra-abdominal organs or tissues
- Parametrial and broad ligament fibrosis from previous or chronic infections
- Ventrofixation or Gilliam's type uterine suspension
- Pelvic endometriosis.

The choices for the surgeon are:

- To start bisecting the uterus—which mobilizes the uterus to a certain extent or morcellation
- To abandon the vaginal approach to hysterectomy at this point. The operation can be completed either with the help of the laparoscope or by the abdominal route. There is hardly ever the need to convert the vaginal approach to an abdominal one. Most difficulties can be overcome.

Procedures involved in dealing with uteri of large sizes could be:

- Myomectomy
- Bisection or hemisection of the uterus
- Intramural coring
- Morcellation.

When undertaking a VH, the surgeon should be familiar with the technical aspects of these procedures. Morcellation should not be considered as a failure of surgery. It is a part of the technique.

The reported frequency of morcellation performed with VH varies from 0% to 76%. In the authors experience, not many patients require either removal of a myoma or bisection. The senior author had to resort to these techniques in 11% of cases. It is true that, as the indications for VH broaden with the surgeon's experience, these techniques are called upon more often.

Morcellation is usually a bloodless procedure, if it is started after the major vessels supplying the uterus have been ligated. In such circumstances, there is little, if any, additional morbidity. Kammerer-Doak and Mao showed that morcellation significantly increased the duration of the procedure (mean 140 vs. 168 min, p=0.004), but did not increase the duration of hospitalization or rate of perioperative complications [18.6 vs. 17.4%, odds ratio (OR) = 1.09, 95% CI = 0.49–2.35].

In selected patients, transvaginal morcellation is a safe and effective alternative to AH for removal of a moderately enlarged uterus.

In various studies done to show the feasibility of removing large uteri (sizes between 14 weeks and 20 weeks of gestation), a majority of women had macroscopic hematuria. The significance of this happening is not very clear, but it certainly means that the bladder was damaged to a certain extent. Caution should be exercised before attempting such cases vaginally.

SUTURING OF THE VAGINAL VAULT

The handling of the vaginal cuff differs with each surgeon. However, the author believes that there are a few aspects of paramount importance in the suturing of the vault, whatever the technique.

It is mandatory to secure the angles of the vaginal incision separately and in the most secure manner possible. The author also routinely secures the uterosacral pedicle again before suturing the vault. Most often, postoperative bleeding—if it does occur—occurs from these sites. It is often seen that surgeons may be hesitant to suture the anterior vaginal wall with a deep enough bite of the needle. Also, the edges of the incision tend to become inverted and are not always taken well into the suture line. It is important to hold the edges and make sure that the vagina is sutured edge-to-edge. In addition, the posterior bite of the needle has to be deeper than the anterior one. Irrespective of the material used to secure the pedicles, it is of great importance to suture the vagina using polyglycolic acid sutures. This reduces considerably the amount of postoperative discharge that is seen after a hysterectomy.

SURGICAL MICROSCOPY IN VAGINAL HYSTERECTOMY

Would using a magnifying loupe at vaginal hysterectomy help in identifying the bladder from the anterior cervical region when opening the 'A' pouch? An article by Tapia mentioned that magnification may help to perform the following steps: Dividing vesicocervical ligaments, mobilizing the rectum opening, the plica vesicouterine, and opening the pouch of Douglas. The authors, however, have never used this.

INSTRUMENTS AND EQUIPMENT

Since the time that a fiberoptic-fitted Sims' and Auvard's speculum and bladder retractor have been available, they have been used with considerable benefit. The cable coming from the single source has two divisions and an exit light can be used on the speculum and retractor.

A report on the use of a self-retaining vaginal wall retractor during VH claimed that, when the retractor was used, suturing of the cuff and pedicles was easier, because the retractor facilitated good exposure and better visibility.

Electrocautery must be used routinely in vaginal surgery, particularly on the bleeders and the large veins that are seen when there is adenomyosis or vrnyomas. It has a special place in dealing with the bladder pillars and helps in keeping the field clean.

To inject the vaginal wall with either saline or lidocaine (lignocaine), containing epinephrine (adrenaline), from 30 mL to 50 mL, or no epinephrine remains an individual choice. Those who use it believe that a large quantity of solution, up to 50 mL, creates a tourniquet around the area where a circumferential vaginal incision is made, and that adding lidocaine solution reduces postoperative pain. The authors' group feels that it is good to use around 30 mL of saline in dilution 1 in 100,000 to help define the planes better for hemostasis.

SUTURES AND KNOTS

Of the eight varieties of sutures and knots suggested for vaginal surgery, Heaney's transfixion suture for pedicles is most commonly used. However, the authors' group takes simple ligatures and very occasionally horizontal mattress sutures. When clamps are used in a non-descent VH, the authors have noticed that there is a certain retraction of the tissue while taking Heaney's stitch, and some vessels may escape into the bargain.

Another factor is the type of suture material. For a long time, chromic catgut was the material of choice. However, as the new, synthetic, delayed, absorbable, monofilament sutures were developed, they gained widespread acceptance and have now almost replaced chromic catgut. It is worth mentioning here, however, that the knotting property of catgut is superior. Caution is advised when the second knot is placed with polyglycolic acid sutures and care should be taken that the first knot does not loose its grip on the pedicle. As suture technology continues to develop, new and better suture materials will surely emerge. The vagina should preferably be closed with a fine suture material.

CHANGING OVER TO THE ABDOMINAL APPROACH

In the 6,900 cases of the senior author, he had only four occasions to abandon the vaginal route and complete the surgery abdominally. In these cases, the problem was of mobility and not size. This should not be considered a catastrophic event. As a matter of fact, the few ligatures made at the lower end and dissection of the uterovesical and/or pouch of Douglas done vaginally are very useful.

Care has to be exercised to separate the bladder from the upper part of the anterior vaginal wall. Normally, at AH traction on the uterus is available to separate the bladder from the vaginal wall as it is cut; traction exercised normally for pushing up the bladder from the vagina is not available.

A large uterine size (>300 g) was not related to a significant increase in failed VH.

Conversely, failed VH was not size dependent. Furthermore, there was no additional operative morbidity when VH was converted to a total abdominal hysterectomy because of a technical inability to complete the surgery vaginally.

BIBLIOGRAPHY

1. Amy JJ. Vaginal hysterectomy. Natl Med J India. 1997;10:126-7.
2. Dorsey JH, Steinberg EP, Holtz PM. Clinical indications for hysterectomy route: Patient characteristics or physician preference? Am J Obstet Gynecol. 1995;173:1452-60.
3. Hoffman MS, Jaeger M. A new method for gaining entry into the scarred anterior cul-de-sac during transvaginal hysterectomy. Am J Obstet Gynecol. 1990;162:1269-70.
4. Kammerer-Doak D, Mao J. Vaginal hysterectomy with and without morcellation: The University of New Mexico hospital's experience. Obstet Gynecol. 1996;88:560-3.
5. Magos A, Bournas N, Sinha R, et al. Vaginal hysterectomy for the large uterus. Br J Obstet Gynaecol. 1996;103:246-51.
6. Mahmoodian S. Vaginal hysterectomy: The use of a self-retaining retractor. J Okla State Med Assoc. 1994;87:419-23.
7. Mazdisnian F, Kurzel RB, Coe S, et al. Vaginal hysterectomy by uterine morcellation: An efficient, nonmorbid procedure. Obstet Gynecol. 1995;86:60-4.
8. Tapia JE. Surgical microscopy in various stages of vaginal hysterectomy. Zentralbl Gynakol. 1990;112:1331-4.
9. Thompson JD, Warshaw J. Hysterectomy. In: Rock JA, Thompson JD (Eds). TeLinde's Operative Gynecology, 8th edition. Philadelphia: Lippincott-Raven; 1997.

41.10 HEMORRHAGE FOLLOWING HYSTERECTOMY

NS Sreedevi

INTRODUCTION

Hemorrhage is a potential complication in any patient undergoing gynecologic surgery. In patients with normal hemostasis and proper surgical technique, postoperative hemorrhage is a rare occurrence. An experienced surgeon has less trouble from immediate postoperative hemorrhage as his technical ability improves. The division of postoperative hemorrhage into clinical types is valuable in discussing the diagnosis and management.

PRIMARY HEMORRHAGE

This type of hemorrhage is apparent within first 24 hours after operation. This may be the result of lowering of blood pressure (BP) during hypotensive anesthesia. It may also be as a result of failure to control one or more large vessels, often an artery. Another possible cause is the injection of adrenaline to secure a bloodless operative field. When BP rises, hemorrhage may occur from blood vessels which have been cut but never ligated. Primary hemorrhage is most likely to be met with after vaginal surgery, such as repairs.

Hemorrhage immediately after hysterectomy may become apparent in one of the two ways. First, bleeding from vagina may be noted within the first few hours after surgery. Second, less commonly the patient may be noted to have little bleeding from the vagina, but deteriorating vital signs manifested by low BP and rapid pulse, falling hematocrit levels and flank or abdominal pain. The second situation could be due to intraperitoneal or extraperitoneal hemorrhage.

Each situation is approached differently in its evaluation and management. The same general principles to be involved in the diagnosis, stabilization of vital signs, appropriate fluid and blood replacement, and constant surveillance of the patient's overall condition.

Every postoperative patient should be carefully monitored postoperatively for signs of occult bleeding. The intensity and duration of monitoring will depend on the type of surgery and medical condition of the patient.

DIAGNOSIS

The diagnosis is easy when there is evident vaginal bleeding. Occult internal bleeding creates problems in diagnosis, and hence it is a serious postoperative complication after vaginal or abdominal surgery. Occult bleeding does not become evident suddenly in the recovery rooms. The vital signs may remain stable for 12–18 hours after surgery is completed and then severe hypotension may occur.

Symptoms and signs of a considerable blood loss, whether vaginal, intraperitoneal or retroperitoneal are:

- Persistently rising pulse rate unaffected by any drug and unaccountable from any other cause
- Increasing pallor
- Persistent fall in systolic and diastolic BP, although this may be compensated in the initial phases
- Air hunger is a sign of severe hemoglobin deficiency and hence a late sign
- Signs of cerebral vascular anoxemia such as restlessness disorientation, syncope
- Certain symptoms and signs may suggest an intraperitoneal or retroperitoneal bleeding as shoulder pain, abdominal pain, vomiting, shock, and shifting dullness. Furthermore, presence of free fluid in the peritoneal cavity tends to produce a moderate degree of ileus, so that a localized or generalized area of tympanites is present.

In case of small amounts of vaginal bleeding in which vital signs have deteriorated, retroperitoneal hemorrhage should be suspected. Extraperitoneal hemorrhage is manifested by the presence of a palpable fixed tumor, which is tender. The anatomical limits of such an extraperitoneal tumor follow certain definite directions. Clinical examination shows dullness and tenderness in the flanks.

The diagnosis of intraperitoneal bleeding in the postoperative patient is a challenge to the gynecologist. The peritoneal signs are subtle and can be masked by incisional pain and analgesic medications. The peritoneal cavity has enormous capacity for occult blood loss without appreciable abdominal distension. As much as 3,000 mL of blood can be hidden in the peritoneal cavity with only a 1 cm increase in the radius of abdomen.

Ultrasound examination is a rapid, non-invasive, readily available method of confirming the diagnosis of intraperitoneal bleeding. CT scan provides a better visualization of retroperitoneal spaces and can delineate hematomas.

It may be difficult for the surgeon to convince himself or herself that the bleeding is persistent and intervention is urgently needed. Consultation with a senior colleague will be helpful in such a situation.

MANAGEMENT

After vital signs are assessed, the amount of blood loss is determined. The patient should be taken to the operation theater for proper visualization of vagina in case of severe vaginal bleeding. The most likely site of vaginal bleeding is the vaginal angle or cut vaginal edge. The vaginal artery or one of its branches in the lateral fornices is the bleeding vessel. One must realize that the vagina is a distensible organ. If a clot occludes the vaginal introitus, a large amount of blood can distend the vagina and not be evident on a perineal pad. When significant vaginal bleeding is present, the patient should be returned to operating room. Adequate examination should be done under analgesia or anesthesia. The vaginal apex should be inspected. If a bleeding point is seen, it should be ligated from below. Figure of eight sutures are placed to include vaginal mucosa and paravaginal tissue. Care must be taken to avoid the inadvertent placement of a suture into the musculature of the bladder wall, the ureter, or the underlying rectum. If bleeding is not controlled by this technique, it is unwise to continue further suturing. In such cases, bleeding vessels might have retracted well above the vaginal apex and cannot be reached by this approach. Laparotomy may be necessary in such cases. Vaginal pack will not control significant bleeding. A pack may be kept while patient is prepared for laparotomy.

Bleeding from anterior and posterior colpoperineorrhaphy usually is from veins. A fairly tight vaginal pack effectively compresses these vessels and controls the bleeding. It is seldom necessary to re-explore an anterior and posterior colporrhaphy to locate and ligate a specific bleeding vessel.

The question now arises whether the patient should be immediately operated or should be taken for a conservative measure like arterial embolization. If the patient is unstable with a rapid pulse, falling BP, and/or low urine output or if the interval since surgery is short, suggesting fairly larger hemorrhage, re-exploration is the option.

On the other hand, if the patient is stable and bleeding does not appear too brisk, one might consider conservative measures. The decision is based on time from surgery and volume of blood in abdomen or retroperitoneal space by ultrasound estimate. If facilities are available, try to identify the bleeding vessel and embolize the arterial supply by transcatheter interventional radiological technique.

Volume Replacement

Whichever plan is selected, one or more large bore IV lines should be started and fluid replacement instituted. In the immediate management, crystalloids will maintain the cardiac output and renal functions as effectively as colloids. If more than 1,000 mL is required, synthetic colloid replacement such as hemacell are recommended until blood becomes available. The use of 4.5% human albumin solution in such situation is also helpful.

Red cell products are required to correct the loss of oxygen carrying capacity. The oxygen carrying capacity is not compromised until hematocrit falls below 22% (Hb <7 g/L). A Foleys catheter is inserted and urine output has to be measured. Broad-spectrum antibiotics also are started.

Measurement of urine output hourly is a measure of peripheral circulation. The measurement difference between body temperature measured rectally, and peripheral temperature measured on the toe is a very sensitive indication of peripheral perfusion and by inference, blood volume and cardiac output. This can be used widely in intensive care units. Pulse oximetry also helps in assessing the peripheral perfusion. The central venous pressure is a less useful measurement is invasive, requires constant supervision and much more prone to measurement errors.

In patients with pre-existing coagulation defects or in those who have undergone lengthy procedures with a high recorded blood loss, coagulopathies should be considered and a platelet count and coagulation screen performed to aid replacement with appropriate blood products. Fresh frozen plasma (FFP) should be used for replacing the coagulation factors. Cryoprecipitate contains a high concentration of fibrinogen and may be required for massive blood transfusion. After 5–6 units of rapidly transferred red cells, 2 units of FFP should be given without waiting for the coagulation tests. If platelet count is less than 50,000 platelet, transfusion will be required.

Re-exploration

One of the most difficult decisions a gynecologist has to face is to decide when to explore a patient who is bleeding postoperatively. If the patient has a previous abdominal operation, the incision should be reopened. The previous procedure should be reviewed to identify any possible ligatures that were tentative or any troublesome bleeding sites that may have continued to bleed. When the abdomen is opened, the clots should be evacuated and a search instituted to the bleeding sites. Bleeding sites, if any, should be carefully ligated. It is not unusual to find no active bleeding sites after opening. Every attempt should be made to get the pelvis and abdomen completely dry before closing.

During reoperation, patients are at increased risk of ureteral injury. Adequate care should be exercised in clamping and ligating the tissues with distorted anatomy.

At the end ureteral integrity is proved by injecting 5 mL of indigo-carmine dye intravenously and observing efflux of dye from ureteral orifice through cystoscope or by opening the bladder dome.

Bleeding from anterior and posterior colporrhaphy is from veins that have not been secured. A fairly tight pack effectively compresses these vessels and controls the bleeding.

Pelvic Hematoma

Pelvic hematoma developing postoperatively cause serious morbidity, especially if it is large and becomes infected. Hematoma can develop above the vaginal vault, along the pelvic side-wall, in the paravesical space, in the abdominal wall, in the ischiorectal fossa and on the vulva.

A hematoma below the puborectalis muscle attachment will not dissect above into the pelvis but will be limited to the perineum and buttock. A hematoma in the ischiorectal fossa and on the vulva may be obvious on examination when patient complains of pain in the area.

Vault hematoma is a common complication of hysterectomy, particularly by the vaginal route. It has been reported that one-third of patients undergoing hysterectomy will have a hematoma identified by ultrasound and two-thirds of then will develop postoperative pyrexia. These are generally self-limiting and will resolve by a discharge via the vaginal vault in the second week following surgery.

A pelvic hematoma is recognized in a patient whose postoperative discomfort and anemia exceed what is normally expected, whose temperature is progressively increasing and whose postoperative abdominal distension is slow to resolve. If a patient is on anticoagulant therapy, even simple coughing can cause a postoperative pelvic hematoma. Abdominal and pelvic examination reveals a mass. Ultrasound or CT scan can make a definite diagnosis, which is helpful in delineating its exact size and location.

Surgical drainage of hematoma may be required if there is persisting pelvic pain or systemic upset with pyrexia. This can be accomplished by simple drainage through the vaginal vault by probing with a dressing forceps. A small drain can be inserted through the drainage tract and kept in place for 24–48 hours. If drainage cannot be achieved in simple way, drainage under ultrasound or CT guidance or through an abdominal incision may be necessary. Drainage of hematoma will help in expediting the recovery. In some cases, drainage may be difficult or contraindicated. In such cases, infection is not a serious problem, it may be preferable to allow the hematomas to resolve over a few months. This may not be completely resolved and residual fibrosis well persists and continues to cause pain.

Abdominal wall hematomas are also common and tend to be self-limiting. They may cause discomfort on mobilizing, and the spreading bruising that develops in the days following surgery may prove alarming for the patient. Patient should be reassured that this represents old bruising that will resolve with time. Such bruising from the lateral port sites for laparoscopic surgery can also be severe, especially if the port incisions have been widened to remove samples obtained in retrieval bags.

Hypogastric Artery Ligation

One of the methods of controlling severe pelvic hemorrhage is ligation of both hypogastric arteries. It is important to ligate the anterior division of the hypogastric artery distal to the posterior branch because of the major collateral circulation with the aorta and femoral artery—including the lumbar, iliolumbar, middle sacral, lateral sacral, superior and middle hemorrhoidal and gluteal arteries.

In ligating the hypogastric artery, the peritoneum is opened on the lateral side of the common iliac artery near its bifurcation, with the ureter left attached to the medial peritoneal reflection to avoid disturbing its blood supply. The artery is dissected free from the underlying hypogastric vein. Non-absorbable suture is passed around the artery with a right angle clamp and tied. A second suture is placed distal to the initial ligature to avoid recanalization. Discussion of vessel is not essential in this procedure.

Arterial Embolization

Selective angiographic arterial embolization has been used for controlling hemorrhage, after abdominal and vaginal hysterectomy. Selective pelvic artery embolization is a comparatively simple and safe procedure. Success rates of more than 90% are routinely reported when embolization is used for postsurgical hemorrhage. Therefore, embolization rather than surgical ligation is appropriately selected as the primary procedure to control bleeding in patients who are stable or who cannot tolerate another operation.

The disadvantage of embolization is that it requires the expertize of a skilled interventional radiologist. Percutaneous catheterization of the femoral artery under local anesthesia provides direct access in a retrograde manner to hypogastric artery. The site of bleeding can be identified with angiography and fluoroscopy if the rate of bleeding is 2–3 mL/minute or more at the bleeding site. If the bleeding vessel is a vein, venous access for embolization can be obtained through the femoral vein or antecubital vein.

The materials used for embolization are small pieces of gel foams, metal coils, autologous clot, subcutaneous tissue, small silastic spheres, and other hemostatic materials. It is sterile, non-antigenic remains in the vessel for 20–50 days, and forms a fibrin mesh framework on which blood clot can develop. The material is injected under angiographic observation. When it is evident by repeat angiography that the bleeding vessel has been occluded, the catheter is removed and patient is carefully monitored.

OTHER METHODS OF CONTROLLING PELVIC HEMORRHAGE

Antishock Trousers

External counter pressure may be used as a measure to control the bleeding. External counter pressure by means of an inflatable garment wrapped around the legs and abdomen, sometimes called the military antishock trousers (MAST) suit or G suit, or pneumatic antishock garment has been used for the temporary control of acute, profuse intra-abdominal hemorrhage while the patient is being prepared for surgery.

The suit is made of polyvinyl, wraped around the patient and secures with loop and hook fasteners. It contains an abdominal pneumatic bladder that extends from the xiphoid to the pubis, and it has two separate leg bladders. It is inflated to a pressure of 25–40 mm Hg. The disadvantages are: It is contraindicated in patients with pulmonary edema, rupture of diaphragm, and left ventricular dysfunction. Abdominal and/or vaginal examination is impossible unless the garment is removed. If pressures are not carefully monitored, circulation to lower extremities can be impaired sufficiently, to cause progressive muscle necrosis, crush syndrome and death. It is rarely used today.

Logothetopulos Pack

This is an umbrella-type pack used for compressing the retracted bleeding vessels in the pelvis. This is a large pack of loose gauze used in an umbrella manner within the pelvic cavity by tying four corners of the opened gauze together and creating traction as the free end of pack when it is pulled through the vaginal vault. The pack can be kept in place with perineal traction for 24–48 hours until bleeding has ceased. It is removed vaginally by first withdrawing the internal gauze and then the outside bag.

SECONDARY HEMORRHAGE

Secondary hemorrhage is invariably vaginal. The cause of this is sepsis with the resultant erosion of a vessel. This bleeding is difficult to control and after control liable to recur, because the inflammatory reaction tends to hinder the vessel from retraction and it may even erode another vessel. It is futile to attempt to control the bleeding by suturing, as there is intense inflammatory reaction. The needle and suture cut through the friable tissue. This especially applies to vaginal vault bleeding after total abdominal hysterectomy. The most effective treatment is therefore to control bleeding by tight vaginal packing. Application of sponge holding forceps to the bleeding vessels was also advocated in a few cases. The pack on the forceps can be kept for 48 hours.

BIBLIOGRAPHY

1. Abbas FM, Currie JL, Mitchell S, et al. Selective vascular embolization in benign gynecologic conditions. J Reprod Med. 1994;39:492-6.
2. Bergqvist D, Bergqvist A. Vascular injuries during gynecologic surgery. Acta Obstet Gynecol Scand. 1987;66:19-23.
3. Bhatla N. Jeffcoate's Principles of Gynaecology, 6th edition. London: Arnold Publishers; 2001.
4. Bickell WH, Wall MJ, Pepe PE, et al. Immediate versus Delayed Fluid Resuscitation for Hypotensive Patients with Penetrating Torso Injuries. N Engl J Med. 1994;331:1105.
5. Hudson CN, Setchell ME. Shaw's Textbook of Operative Gynaecology, 6th edition. New Delhi: Elsevier; 2001.
6. Monaghan JM, Lopes T, Naik R. Bonney's Gynecological Surgery, 10th edition. London: Blackwell Publishers; 2004.
7. Padubidri VG, Daftary SN (Eds). Shaw's Textbook of Operative Gynaecology, 12th edition. New Delhi: B.I.Churchill Livingstone Pvt Ltd.; 1999.
8. Rock JA, Thompson JD. Te Linde's Operative Gynecology, 9th edition. In: Te-linde (Ed). Philadelphia: Lippincott Williams & Wilkins; 2001.

CHAPTER

42

Laparoscopy

Pranay Shah, Shobhana M, Mala Raj, Malvika Sabharwal, Pranay Shah, Pratap Kumar, Bimal John, Shyam Desai, Nikhil Jani, Nutan Jain, Shilpi Srivastava, Pranay R Shah, Duru Shah, Safala Shroff, Sukhpreet Patel, Mandakini Parihar, Meenakshi Bharath, Pranay R Shah, Pranay R Shah, KK Gopinathan, Fessy Louist, Shlomo B Cohen, Ariella J Setton, Daniel S Seiedman, Jayakrishnan K

42.1A INSTRUMENTATION AND PRINCIPLES OF LAPAROSCOPIC SURGERY

Pranay Shah

INTRODUCTION

During the last 30 years, gynecologic laparoscopy has evolved from a limited surgical procedure used only for diagnosis and tubal ligation to a major surgical tool used to treat a multitude of gynecologic indications. With advances in technology and instrumentation as many as 80% of gynecological operations can now be performed endoscopically.

ADVANTAGES

When compared to conventional open surgery, laparoscopic surgery has the following advantages:

- Rapid postoperative recovery
- Less postoperative pain and reduced need of postoperative analgesia
- Although procedure times are usually slightly longer, hospital stay is less, and often with the same day discharge which equals a faster return to everyday living
- Reduced exposure of internal organs to possible external contaminants thereby reduced risk of acquiring infections and postoperative adhesions
- Less adhesion formation
- Reduced blood loss, which equals less risk of needing a blood transfusion
- Smaller abdominal scars (cosmetic value).

DISADVANTAGES

Fundamentally laparoscopic surgery differs from its laparotomic counterpart only by its particular mode of access. However, it is intrinsically more difficult to perform than laparotomy, due to:

- Indirect palpation of tissues through a finite number of immovable ports
- Restriction of axial freedom
- Replacement of normal stereoscopic three-dimensional visualization by two dimensional video image
- Higher initial expenditure (instrument cost).

Despite these challenges, given proper surgical case selection and the requisite surgical training, it promises to result in at least equivalent results, better cosmesis, less postoperative pain and faster recovery.

For many procedures, such as removal of an ectopic pregnancy, treatment of endometriosis, or ovarian cystectomy, laparoscopy has become the treatment of choice. The advantages of laparoscopy for other procedures, including laparoscopically-assisted hysterectomy and the staging and treatment of gynecologic cancers, continue to be elucidated.

INDICATIONS FOR LAPAROSCOPY

Diagnostic Laparoscopy

Non-acute Conditions

- Evaluation in infertility
- Chronic pelvic pain

- Suspected endometriosis
- Evaluation of Mullerian anomaly
- Prior to tuboplasty.

Acute Conditions

- Acute abdominal pain
- Suspected ectopic pregnancy
- Acute pelvic inflammatory disease
- Torsion of adnexa.

Operative Laparoscopy

In addition to providing diagnostic accuracy, the laparoscope may be used to safely carry out many surgical operations. The indications for these procedures are the same as for laparotomy (Box 1).

Laparoscopies have a more limited place in the primary staging, treatment, and follow-up of patients with gynecological malignancies, but radical hysterectomies, pelvic and para-aortic lymphadenectomies have been performed laparoscopically.

CONTRAINDICATIONS TO LAPAROSCOPY

Absolute

- Mechanical or paralytic ileus
- Large abdominal mass (>24 weeks gestation size)
- Shock
- Medical conditions precluding surgery
  - Severe obstructive airway disease
  - Cardiorespiratory failure
- Irreducible external hernia.

Relative

- Multiple abdominal incisions
- Generalized peritonitis
- Hiatus or diaphragmatic hernia
- Blood dyscrasias and coagulopathy
- Extreme obesity
- Advanced pregnancy.

INSTRUMENTATION

Modern endoscopy exists largely because of technical advances in equipment and instrumentation. The rod lens system, fiberoptic technology and cold light illumination, advanced electronics for gas insufflation and electrosurgical units, video and laser technology and continuous flow, modified urological resectoscope have combined to make advanced endoscopic surgery possible. Although equipment alone seldom ensures success, the lack of it, given the inherent difficulties of the endoscopic approach, makes many procedures unsafe and/or impossible.

The instruments for laparoscopy can be divided into six categories:

Box 1 Operations performed through laparoscopic approach

- Operation on uterus
  - Correction of Mullerian anomalies (rudimentary horn excision)
  - Myomectomy (subserous or intramural)
  - Hysterectomy for benign indications [laparoscopically-assisted vaginal hysterectomy (LAVH), total laparoscopic hysterectomy]
  - Hysterectomy for malignant conditions
- Operations on adnexa (conservative)
  - Ovariolysis or Fimbriolysis or Salpingolysis
  - Puncture of ovarian cysts
  - Polycystic ovary syndrome (PCOS) drilling
  - Ovarian cystectomy
  - Fimbrioplasty
  - Cuff salpingostomy or salpingoneostomy
  - Linear salpingotomy in ectopic pregnancy
  - End-to-end anastomosis (reversal)
  - Removal of paraovarian cysts
- Operations on adnexa (radical)
  - Oophorectomy
  - Salpingectomy (partial or total)
  - Tubal sterilization
  - Adnexectomy
- Laparoscopy in endometriosis
  - Peritoneal deposits coagulation or excision or laser vaporization
  - Endometrioma drainage or fulguration of lining or cystectomy
  - Adhesiolysis (salpingolysis or ovariolysis or omental adhesiolysis)
- Laparoscopy for genital suspension operations
  - Burch colposuspension
  - Sacrofixation of vagina (vault prolapse)
  - Correction of cystocele or rectocele or enterocele
  - McCall culdoplasty
- Other indications
  - Appendectomy
  - Evaluation in ascites
  - Laparoscopy during pregnancy
  - Second-look laparoscopy

1. Optics
2. Light sources
3. Documentation equipment
4. Insufflation equipment
5. Accessory instruments
6. Electrosurgical units or Laser.

Optics

Rod lens system allows a clear undistorted view. Laparoscopes are available in various sizes (2 mm, 5 mm, 10 mm) and viewing angles (0°, 30°) (Fig. 1). The larger the diameter of the optic, better is the panoramic view of the pelvis. Telescope with 30° viewing angle is useful during suturing and complex surgical procedures.

Single puncture telescope has a telescope with a channel which allows passage of 5–8 mm instrument (band applicator for sterilization, scissors, bipolar or monopolar forceps, laser fiber).

Double puncture telescope has optics only. Accessory ports are required to pass instruments to perform surgery.

Light Sources

Enormous technical advances have taken place since the idea of using reflected light in the body cavities was first conceived. At present, there are three types of light sources:

1. Halogen lamp
2. Metal halide
3. Xenon

Illumination suitable for routine diagnostic or operative laparoscopy is well provided by 150/250 watt halogen light (Fig. 2); however, as it produces yellow light, it can cause color distortion. Metal halide lamps emit light at the red end of color spectrum, are cooler than xenon lamps but warm up quickly. Xenon lamp emits light at the blue end of the spectrum, has high intensity that closely resembles daylight, allowing for maximum transmission of true colors.

A fiberoptic cord connects the light source to the telescopes. Although called "cold light", the strong light generates heat to cause a potential burn if the end rests directly on skin or cloth drape.

Documentation Equipment

The advent of video capabilities has contributed greatly to the field of endoscopic surgery. It allows for a panoramic view of the operative site, allowing assistants to actively participate in the surgery. The surgeon can operate in an upright position viewing directly from the monitor, reducing back strain and eye fatigue. It is possible to have a permanent record of the patient's pathology, as well as the surgical techniques used to correct it.

The video monitoring equipment consists of a charged-coupled device (CCD) camera (Fig. 3), a high-resolution color monitor and a video cassette recording (VCR). These modern cameras weigh 2–8 ounces and have more than 375 lines of resolution. They may be single or three chip for three different primary colors. These cameras are thus light in weight, provide accurate color and high resolution and onto the end of the telescopes.

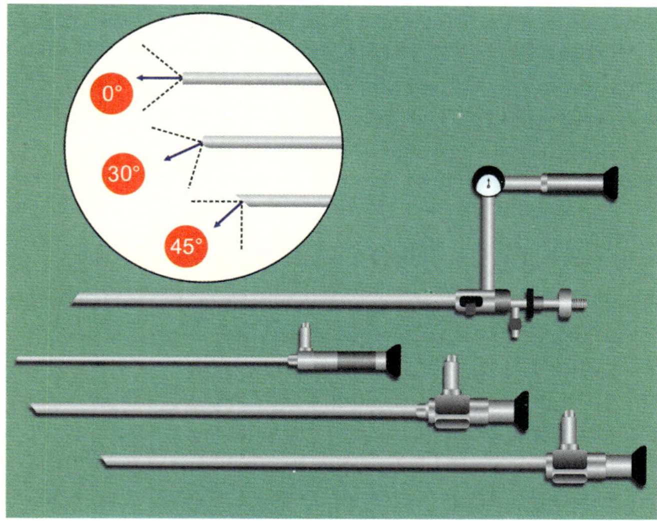

Fig. 1: Various types of telescopes

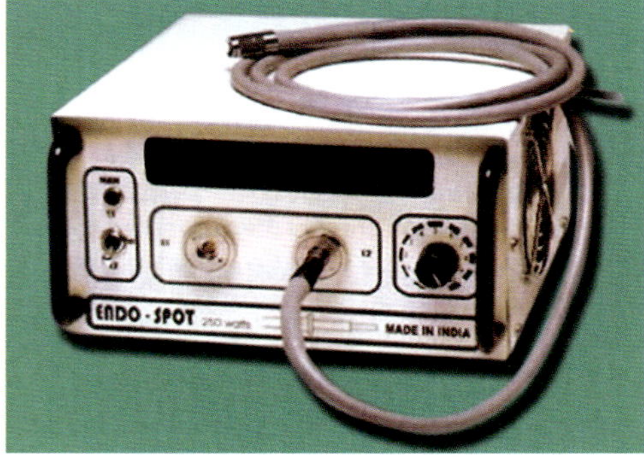

Fig. 2: Halogen light source with cable

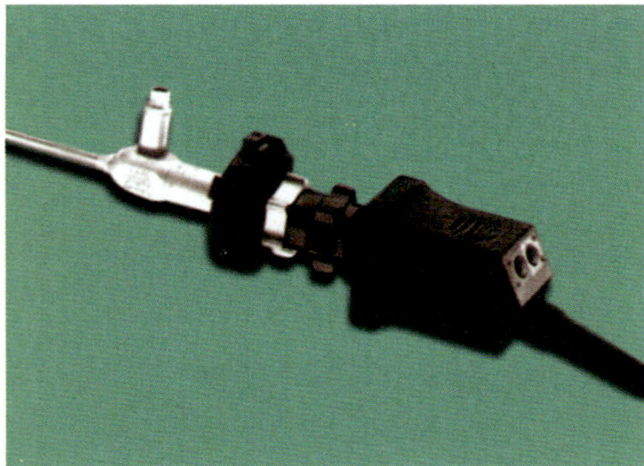

Fig. 3: Charged-coupled device (CCD) camera

Insufflation Equipment

"The key to safety is monitoring intra-abdominal pressure (IAP)". Safe creation of pneumoperitoneum is greatly aided by the development of modern, automatic, high flow (20 L/min), pressure limited insufflators using CO_2 (Fig. 4). High flow insufflators are essential during electrosurgery or laser laparoscopy as the smoke generated has to be rapidly sucked out and replaced with gas to avoid loss in vision. CO_2 gas is cold, which can lead to peritoneal trauma and hypothermia in the patient especially during prolonged surgery.

Thermoflators where preheated gas at body temperature can be delivered to the patient rapidly have been developed.

Accessory Instruments

Trocars

Reusable or disposable trocars in 5 mm and 10 mm sizes are available (Fig. 5). A flap valve is preferable for the primary trocar through which the telescope is inserted. Accessory ports should have flap or trumpet valves; however for suturing silicone valves (Apple Medical Inc.) are preferred. Various devices have been made (endotip, endopath, retractable protective sheaths) to make insertion of the primary trocar safe.

Veress needle: The CO_2 gas is delivered into the abdominal cavity using a spring loaded needle. The inner blunt tip springs out when it enters the peritoneal cavity preventing visceral injury. Disposable needles are also available.

Ancillary Instruments

Blunt probe: It is the simplest instrument used to stabilize or manipulate organs. Probes that are marked in centimeters are useful as the magnification of the laparoscope can make estimation of size difficult.

Graspers: A range of graspers (atraumatic, allis type, spoon forceps, claw forceps) of different sizes and designs is essential in any laparoscopic procedure (Figs 6A to C). Atraumatic forceps hold tube, ovary and bowel delicately. Allis type forceps are essential for performing cystectomy in ovarian cyst or endometriomas. Spoon forceps can be used to extract trophoblastic tissue from salpingostomy site. Claw forceps give a firm grip for tissue extraction through cannula sleeve.

Scissors: Available in various shapes (straight, curved, metzenbaum, hook) (Fig. 7), they are essential for cutting adhesions, dissection and cutting pedicles. Micro-scissors are available for fine dissection and cutting delicate tissues.

Aspirators and irrigators: Needle tipped aspirators are used for aspiration ovarian cysts, cul-de-sac fluid for cytologic or

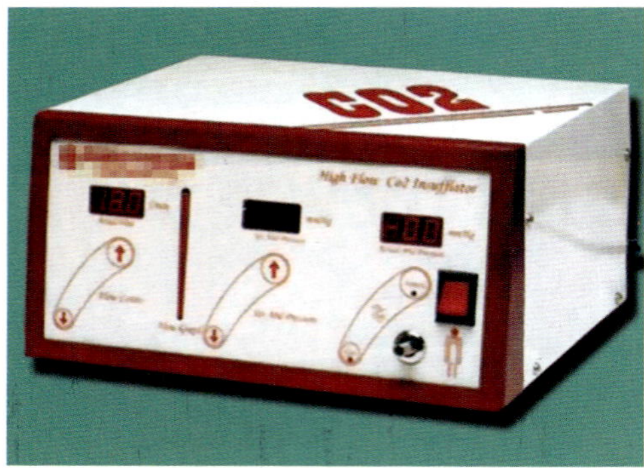

Fig. 4: High-flow electronic insufflator

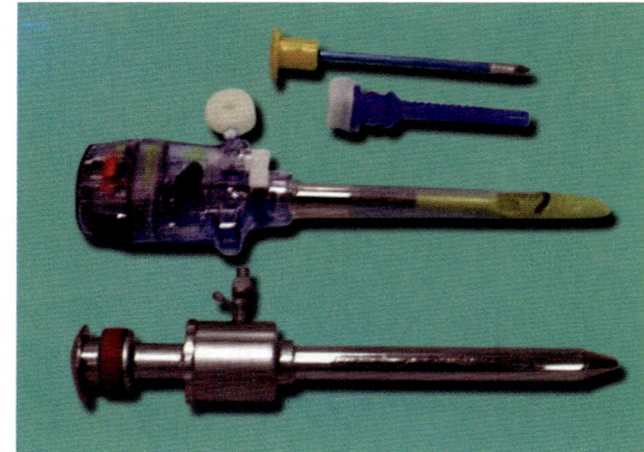

Fig. 5: Trocar and cannula

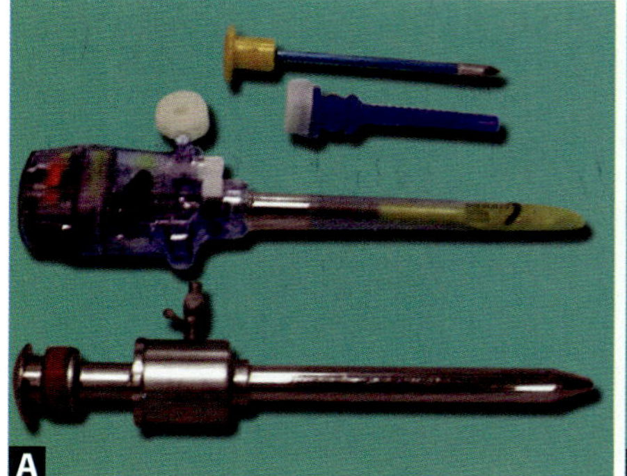

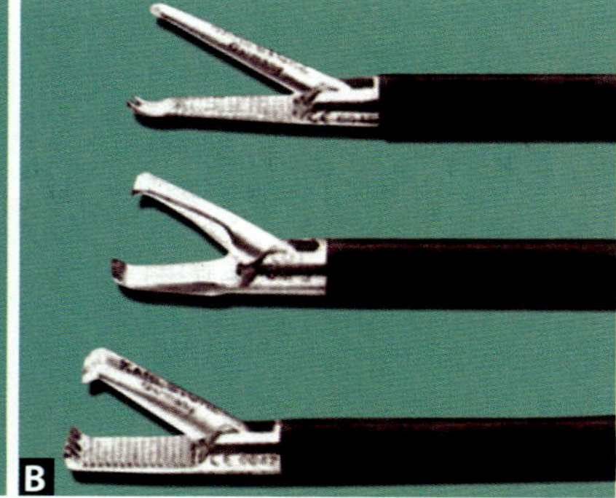

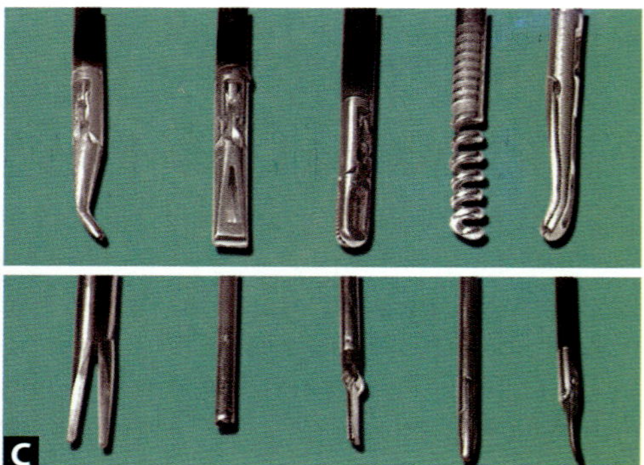

Figs 6A to C: Various types of grasping and holding instruments

microscopic examination. Wide bore suction or irrigation cannulas are used to quickly evacuate hemoperitoneum in an ectopic pregnancy (Fig. 8). Irrigation is essential to maintain a clear view in the pelvis during operative laparoscopy.

Uterine manipulator: It allows the uterus to be placed in desired position (anteverted, retroverted) during laparoscopy (Fig. 9). Some manipulators allow simultaneous chromopertubation which is preferred during tubal testing in infertility patients.

Needle holders with various designs and handle shapes are available for needle handling during suturing. Although suturing is often unnecessary, certain procedures are facilitated by its use (myomectomy, tubal reanastomosis, Burch colposuspension). Any type of suture material or needle can be used laparoscopically. Curved needles make suture placement easier, and are introduced through a strapless trocar sleeve.

Suturing Techniques

Two types of suturing techniques are available:

1. *Extracorporeal suture:* After the suture is passed through the tissue, both ends are brought back out of the peritoneal cavity. A knot pusher is used to push multiple single throws in place much like a surgeon's finger to tighten the knot (Fig. 10).
2. *Intracorporeal suture:* After passing the suture, using classic microsurgical principles and using two needle holders, surgeon's knots are tied to approximate tissues, reconstruct organs or ligate blood vessels (Figs 11A to F).

Clark's Knot Tier

Knot tier or pusher is a simple device that allows safe placement of extracorporeal loop endoscopic sutures in all situations using traditional suturing materials.

Staplers/Endoclips

Instruments that can apply clips singly or in rows are available. Clips are used for hemostasis in small and medium sized vessels. Endo GIA^{TM} staples can cut as well as clip are useful during hysterectomy, but are expensive.

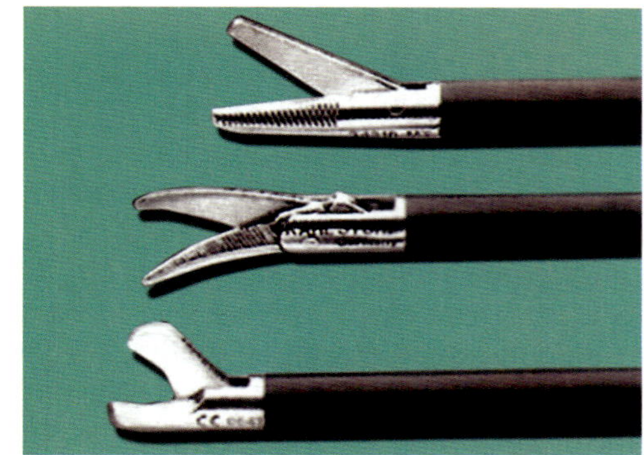

Fig. 7: Straight and curved blade scissors

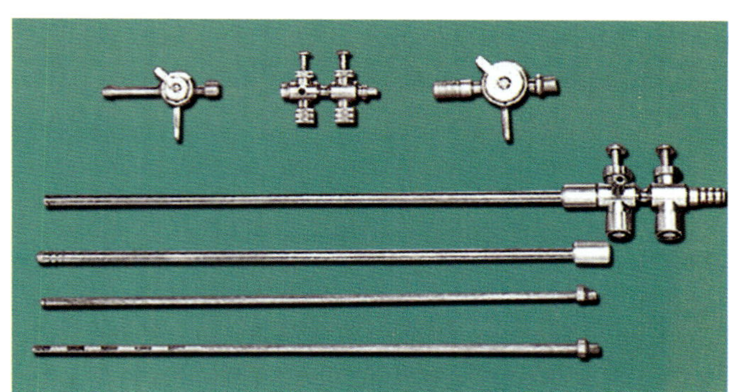

Fig. 8: Suction or irrigation sets

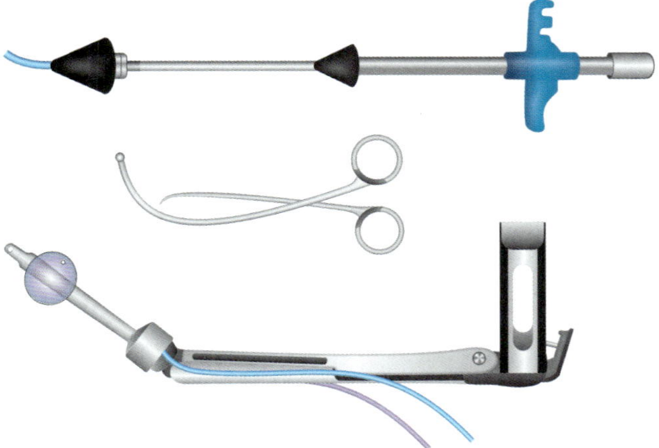

Fig. 9: Uterine manipulators

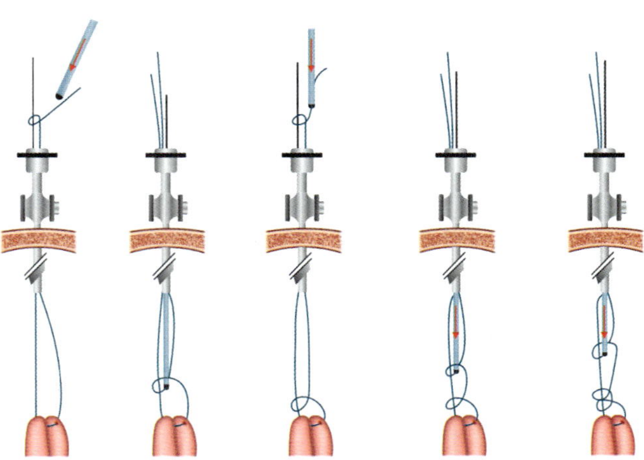

Fig. 10: Extracorporeal suturing

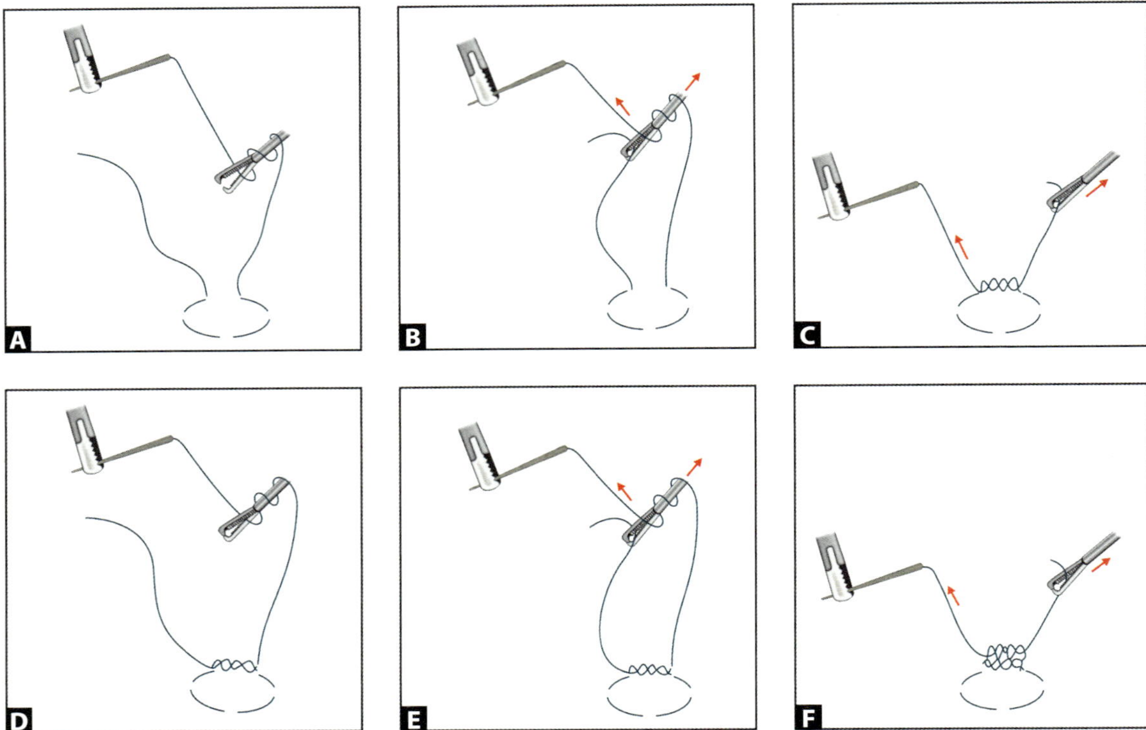

Figs 11A to F: Intracorporeal suturing

CCL Vaginal Extractor

Progress in laparoscopic surgery has been hindered by difficulties encountered during the extraction of tissue masses exceeding the diameter of conventionally used trocars. Transabdominal methods require larger incisions, while transvaginal extractions are associated with CO_2 leakage. These technical difficulties are overcome by the CCL vaginal extractor (Fig. 12A), which enables removal of tissue masses as large as 6–7 cm without loss of gas. The CCL vaginal extractor consists of a trocar fitted with a ball shaped head at one extremity, which adapts well to the posterior vaginal fornix. A groove on the ball guides the surgeon during the intra-abdominal peritoneal incision. After the culdotomy incision, tissue is seized with a grasping forceps introduced through the trocar and removed (Figs 12B to E). Tissue masses may be placed in endobags prior to extraction in order to prevent dissemination and to facilitate passage through incision. The vaginal incision can be closed vaginally. This procedure can be used to extract ovaries, cysts, tubal pregnancies and myomas safely and rapidly.

Electromechanical Morcellator

Endoscopic interventions, which are necessary to remove large sections of tissue, such as myomata or ovaries, still represent a challenge for minimally invasive surgery. Electromechanical morcellator makes it easy to remove even large sections of tissues from the abdomen in only a few minutes through existing incisions (Fig. 13). The morcellator consists of a motor driven cutting tube that can be inserted directly into the abdomen without an additional trocar cannula. Clawed forceps for gripping the tissue to be extracted are inserted into the abdomen through the cutting tube. If the forceps is then pulled back, pressing the tissue against the cutting edge of the rotating morcellator, a cylindrical block of tissue can be cut out and removed through the tube. In excellent cutting effect prevents damage to the architecture, so that reliable histological examinations are also possible.

Electrosurgical Units

"Prophylactic hemostasis takes less time than control of hemorrhage."

Various units are available to provide energy for tissue cutting or coagulation.

- Combined unipolar and bipolar units
- Harmonic scalpel.

There is debate about their relative merits and demerits.

Unipolar Electrocoagulation

In unipolar system, current passes from the instrument to the tissue to a ground plate and then back to the generator (Fig. 14). Depending on the instrument used

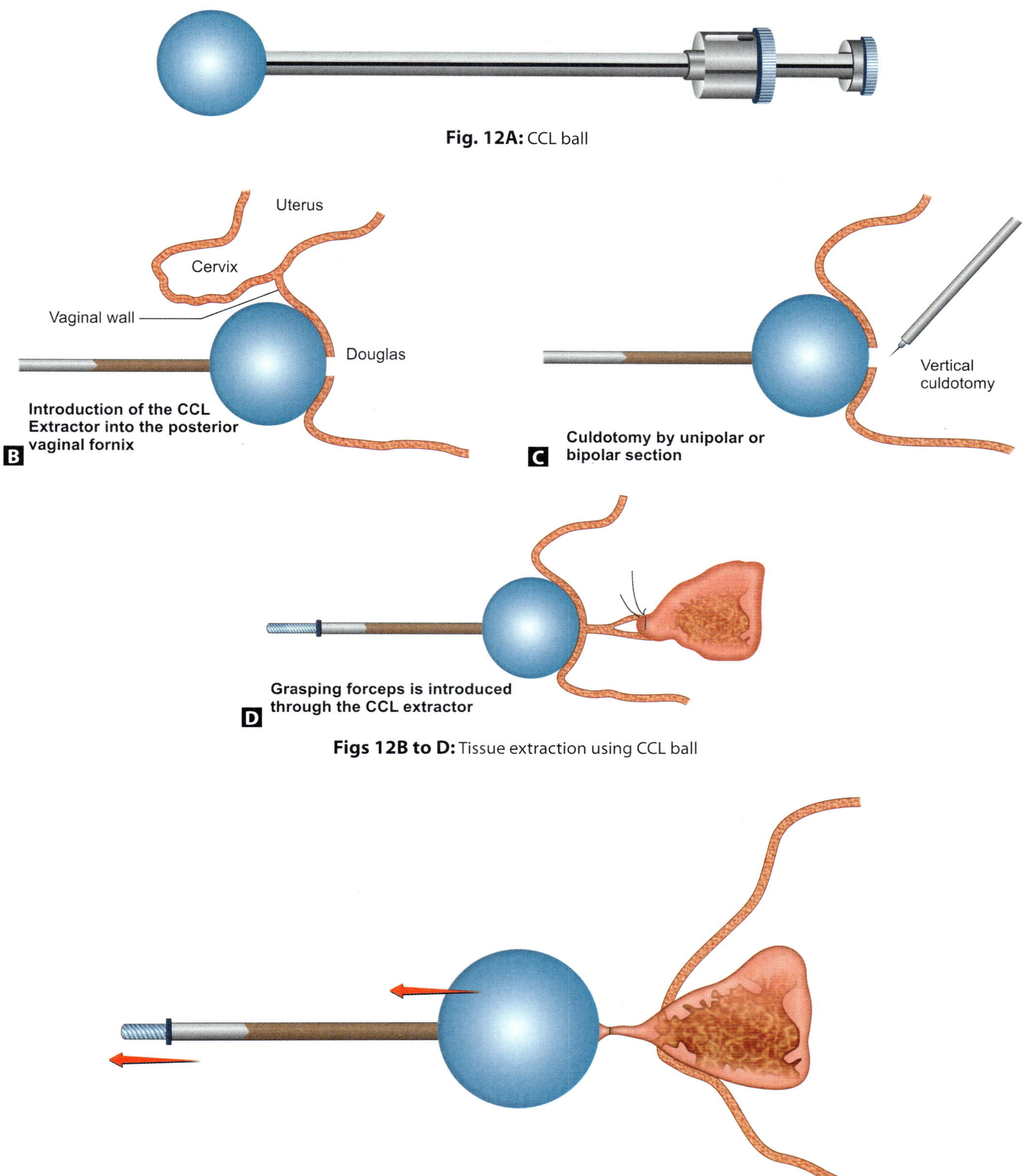

Fig. 12A: CCL ball

Figs 12B to D: Tissue extraction using CCL ball

Fig. 12E: Tissue is extracted together with the CCL ball

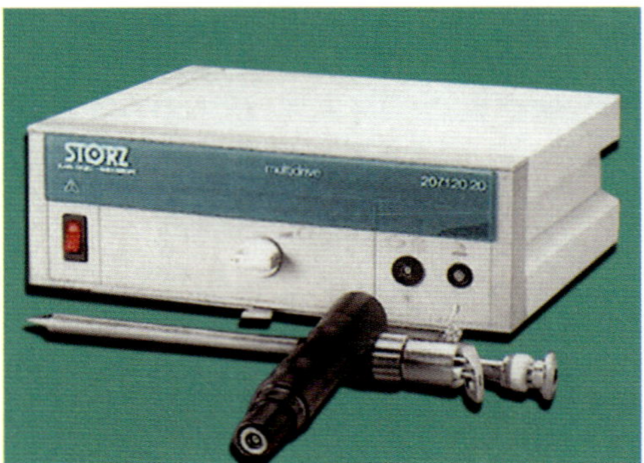

Fig. 13: Electromechanical morcellator

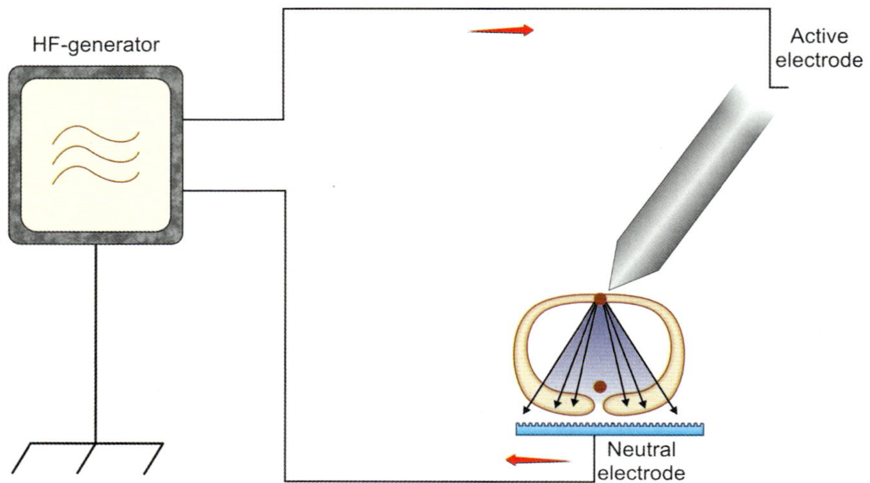

Fig. 14: Monopolar circuit

and current configuration (cutting or coagulation), various different tissue effects can be achieved including cutting, desiccation, coagulation and fulguration.

5 mm instruments are mostly insulated for monopolar use and are safe provided the following precautions are taken:

- Good visual control
- Use lowest wattage necessary
- Short bursts
- Use large properly placed return plate
- Avoid dangerous areas viz. bowel or ureters
- Use all metal or all plastic cannula. Both cutting and coagulation are possible.

Bipolar Electrocoagulation

The bipolar system uses two insulated jaws of instrument to carry the current. The tissue between the jaws completes the circuit, and the tissue is heated (coagulated) by the passage of current (Fig. 15).

This is much safer as the field of coagulation is limited to the contact area of the electrode. Bipolar forceps with 1 mm, 3 mm, and 5 mm jaws are available to provide variable coagulation (Fig. 16A). Kleppinger forceps provide good cooptation and coagulation of large pedicles such as infundibulopelvic or uterine vessels during hysterectomy. Cutting is not possible, however, recently bipolar scissors with ceramic edges has been developed. Other various types of coagulating and cutting instruments available are harmonic scalpel, vessel sealing system ligasure, etc. (Fig. 16B).

Harmonic Scalpel

The instrument operates by means of a blade that vibrates longitudinally at a frequency of 55.5 kHz. The end of the device oscillates at about 50,000 cycles per second, which results in precise cutting, generating neither smoke nor char. The newer devices have a sharp blade that can be rotated at 90° to expose a blunt blade, which will result in a degree of coagulation and will achieve hemostasis without tissue adherence. The device is excellent for laparoscopic myomectomy and is also useful for hysterectomy.

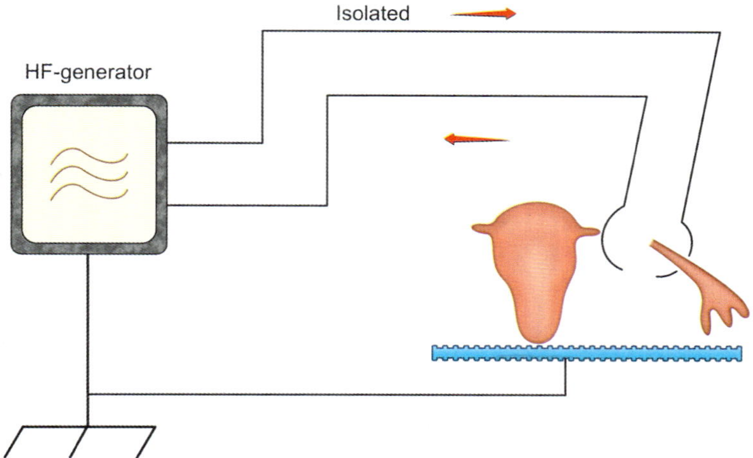

Fig. 15: Bipolar circuit

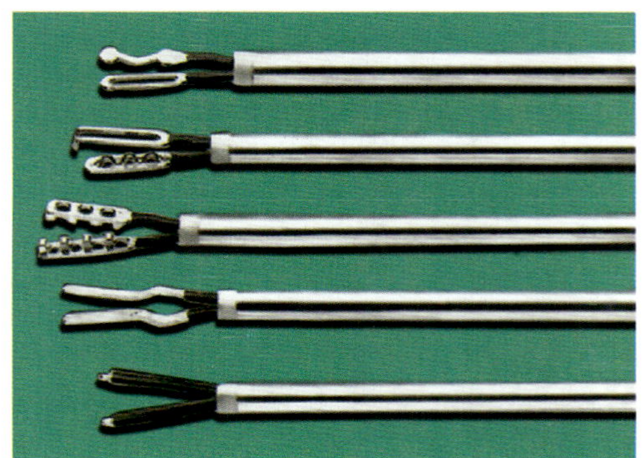

Fig. 16A: Bipolar forceps

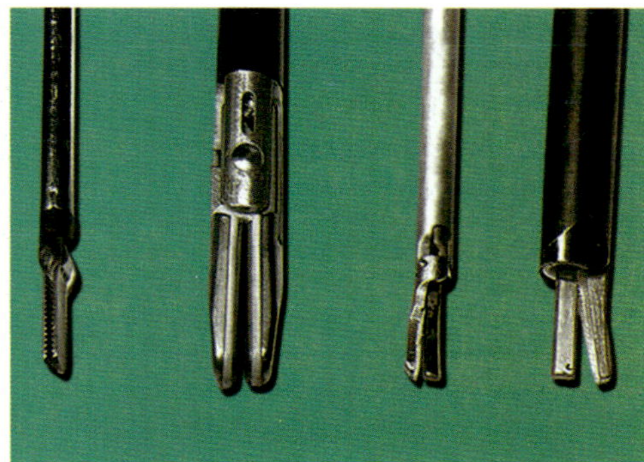

Fig. 16B: Various types of cutting and coagulation instruments

TECHNIQUES OF LAPAROSCOPY

A careful preoperative evaluation is essential before any operative procedure. Indications for the procedure must be reviewed. Contraindications to endoscopic surgery are ruled out. Informed consent should be obtained. The consent form should always contain permission for possible laparotomy.

Laparoscopy should be performed under general anesthesia (GA) with endotracheal intubation. Intraoperative monitoring should include pulse, noninvasive blood pressure amplifier (NIBP), oxygen saturation (SpO_2), electrocardiogram (ECG), and the level of carbon dioxide released at the end of expiration ($EtCO_2$).The OT setup should be designed to optimize efficiency. The OT setup is shown in the diagram (Fig. 17). The OT table should be capable of achieving the steep Trendelenburg position, preferably up to 20°. The instruments are arranged in a mobile cart (Fig. 18).

Patient Position

The patient is placed in a low dorsal lithotomy position with buttocks extended over the end of the table, allowing easier manipulation of the vaginal instruments (Fig. 19). The hips are in extension and abduction and knees slightly flexed with stirrups low, so that the thighs are in line with the abdomen, allowing easy mobility of instruments. The shoulder braces are required to prevent the patient from slipping. The arm on the surgeon's side (preferably both arms) should be tucked by the side to allow greater freedom of movement for manipulation of instruments.

If a prolonged procedure is planned, the legs should be given a compression bandage, to reduce the incidence of thromboembolism.

Primary Trocar Entry

The laparoscopic approach uniquely involves perforating the abdominal wall with a number of conduits to facilitate minimal invasive surgery. Gaining laparoscopic access is therefore associated with some specific risks that would not have occurred if the abdominal or vaginal route had been chosen.

Pneumoperitoneum allows visualization of abdominal and pelvic organs. CO_2 gas is preferred as it is rapidly absorbed and less likely to lead to gas embolism, and

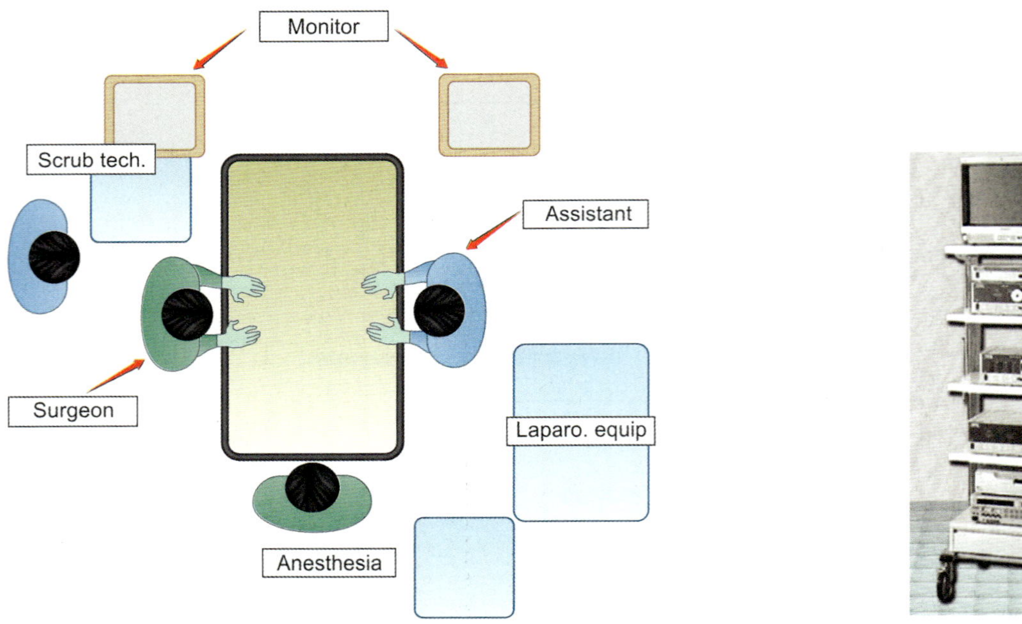

Fig. 17: Operation theater (OT) setup

Fig. 18: Endoscopy cart

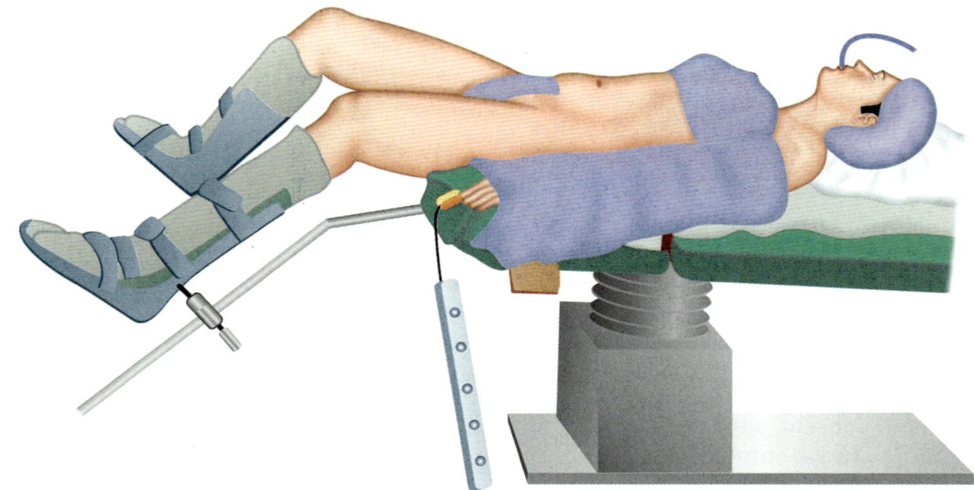

Fig. 19: Patient position

causes less postoperative pain. Insufflation is achieved using a Veress needle only after the patient's stomach and bladder are empty. If any doubt exists, a nasogastric tube to empty the stomach and Foley catheter to empty the bladder are used. It is widely accepted that the most dangerous moment in laparoscopic surgery is during the insertion of Veress needle and sharp primary trocar.

Veress Needle Insertion

A vertical umbilical incision is taken, Veress needle inserted at 45° angle directed in the midline after manually elevating the abdominal wall, and proper placement confirmed.

Palmer's test: A 20 mL glass syringe half-filled with saline is attached to the hub of the Veress needle. The plunger is first drawn back. Failure to aspirate blood or bowel contents confirms that the needle is not in a major splanchnic structure. When this is confirmed the saline is flushed into the cavity. This should be done easily without resistance. The final phase of the test is to withdraw the plunger again. When the needle is correctly situated no fluid will be sucked back into the syringe but when the tip is lying in adhesions or in the abdominal walls the saline will have collected as a pool and can be drawn back.

Pressure test: The CO_2 insufflator is set at low flow (1 L/min) and the abdominal pressure at the beginning of insufflation is recorded. A negative pressure prior to insufflation and low intra-abdominal pressures (<8 mm) during insufflation with good flow suggests correct needle placement.

Loss of liver dullness: After some gas is delivered four quadrant percussion give a tympanic note with the loss of liver dullness.

CO_2 Insufflation

Once the position of the Veress is confirmed, the gas can be insufflated at 3 L/min.

We must understand why the gas is being inserted. The abdominal cavity is distended to raise the abdominal wall away from the underlying structures so that the sharp trocar can be inserted safely into the gas bubble that has been created. What is the safest size bubble we can achieve? Measuring the volume is a less than optimum way to determine how much gas to insufflate. The capacity of the abdominal cavity varies as much as any other human vital statistic and a single arbitrary volume of gas will not produce a similar degree of distention in all shapes and sizes of patient.

Attention should be directed instead to the level of IAP produced by the gas. Three liters of gas produces an IAP of about 10 mm Hg in a woman of average built. It is self-evident that the larger the gas bubble, the larger is the distance between the abdominal wall and the underlying structures, and the safer will be the trocar insertion. Studies in which the distance between the abdominal wall and underlying structures were measured at different abdominal pressures found that the mean distance at 10 mm Hg pressure was 6 cm, while at 25 mm Hg it was 10 cm. More importantly the higher the IAP, the more the abdominal wall is splinted by the contained gas and the less it is deformed by downward pressure. It has been estimated that a trocar insertion requires a force of 4–5 kg. If a standardized force of 4 kg is applied vertically down onto the umbilicus area of a patient with an IAP of 10 mm Hg then the umbilicus will touch the underlying structures making them very vulnerable to damage. When this is repeated at an IAP of 25 mm Hg the force applied indents the abdominal wall in such a way that there is still at least 5 cm gas bubble between the abdominal wall and the underlying bowel.

Primary Trocar Insertion

The Veress needle is removed and the trocar is inserted aiming at the hollow of the sacrum. The laparoscope is inserted, and correct intraperitoneal placement is confirmed. Once the primary trocar is in position, the IAP is reduced to 14 mm Hg.

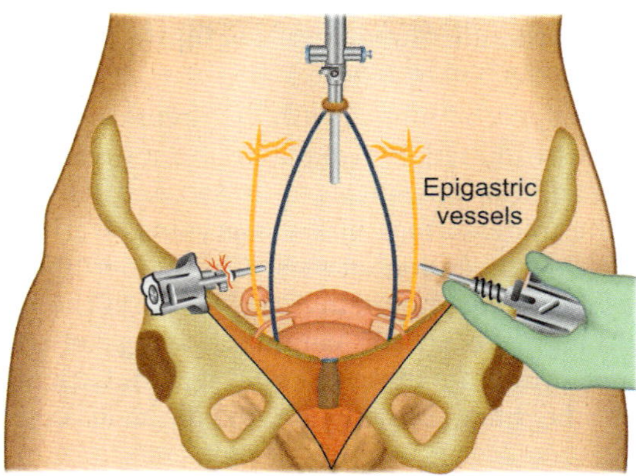

Fig. 20: Additional ports inserted under vision lateral to inferior epigastric vessels

In obese patients, a more vertical angle of the needle is necessary to reach the peritoneum. Patients with previous surgical scars, or organ enlargement may require selection of an alternate site (supraumbilical, left coastal margin) depending on the area at risk.

Secondary trocar insertions: Additional ports are inserted under vision lateral to the inferior epigastric vessels on both sides (Fig. 20). The exact position depends on the surgery undertaken, pathology, patient size, and individual preference.

DIAGNOSTIC LAPAROSCOPY

Diagnostic laparoscopy is now a basic skill which should be learnt by every gynecologist. Direct visualization of the abdominal and pelvic organs allows a definitive diagnosis to be made where clinical evaluation and imaging techniques have failed or are equivocal. One can proceed from diagnostic to operative laparoscopy, and with proper training be able to perform most surgical procedures.

Inspection of the abdominal organs: After insertion of the laparoscope the surgeon should perform a panoramic view of the abdomen to insure that inadvertent damage was not caused by the Veress needle or trocar (Fig. 21).

The inspection is performed in a clockwise direction to visualize the cecum, appendix, ascending colon, liver, stomach, spleen (normal not visualized, unless enlarged), and descending colon. Perihepatic adhesions suggestive of past peritonitis (Fitz Hugh Curtis syndrome) may be noted (Fig. 22). Adhesions may also be present in tuberculous abdomen or previous surgery.

Inspection of the pelvic organs: A 20° Trendelenburg position is given to displace the bowel and omentum in the abdomen and get a clear view of the pelvic organs. A uterine manipulator is inserted in the uterine cavity. It is impossible to perform a complete examination using a single puncture approach. A second puncture with a probe or grasper aids full examination of the fallopian tubes, ovaries and pouch of Douglas.

It is usual to commence with the uterus and proceed in a clockwise direction visualizing the anterior cul-de-sac, right adnexa, posterior cul-de-sac and left adnexa. Inspect the undersurface of the ovary and ovarian fossa for adhesions or endometriosis. Chromopertubation is performed by injecting methylene blue into the uterine cavity through the uterine cannula. Passage of dye can be observed from the fimbrial end (Fig. 23). Lack of tubal filling may be due to obstruction, spasm, or leakage from the cervix.

Peritubal and periovarian adhesions are better visualized by injecting 200 mL of saline in the pelvis for hydroflotation (Fig. 24).

OPERATIVE LAPAROSCOPY

The various operative techniques of laparoscopic procedures are beyond the scope of this chapter. A few common operations are described here.

Tubal sterilization: A 12 mm single puncture laparocator is inserted through the umbilical cannula. Tubal bands are applied on both fallopian tubes about 1 cm from the cornual end (isthmic portion) (Fig. 25).

PCOS drilling: Two accessory ports are used. The ovary is stabilized with an atraumatic grasper. Multiple holes are drilled on the both ovarian surfaces using a high frequency monopolar needle at 40 W pure cut current. Any bleeding can be controlled by inserting the needle in the drilled hole and using coagulation current. The ovaries are cooled using ringer lactate or saline.

Ovarian cystectomy: Laparoscopic treatment is offered for benign ovarian cysts. The cortex is incised using a sharp scissors. Using two graspers traction is given in opposite directions, and the cyst is peeled off from the ovary cortex. Hemostasis is achieved using bipolar forceps. The ovarian cortex usually falls over each other and no suturing is required. The specimen is put in an endobag and retrieved from the abdomen.

Ectopic pregnancy: In an early unruptured tubal ectopic pregnancy (Fig. 26A) linear salpingotomy is performed (Fig. 26B), where preservation of tubal function is desired. The products of conception are flushed out and hemostasis achieved. The incision need not be sutured. Salpingectomy is the treatment of choice for an ectopic pregnancy when preservation of fertility is not desired (Fig. 26C) or when the tube is ruptured or damaged by severe adhesive disease.

Removal of pedunculated myoma: The pedicle is coagulated using bipolar forceps and cut using scissors or monopolar hook. The specimen is removed through the pouch of Douglas or by morcellation.

Myomectomy (subserous or intramural myoma): Dilute pitressin (vasopressin 20 units in 100 cc saline) is injected at multiple sites in the myoma capsule. An incision is

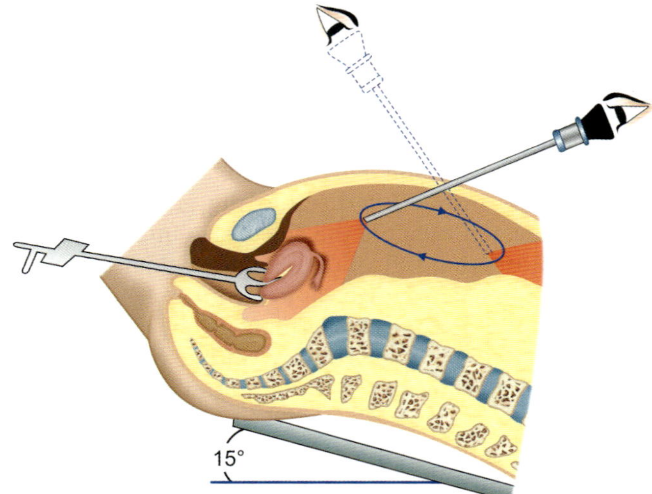

Fig. 21: Panoramic view of the abdomen

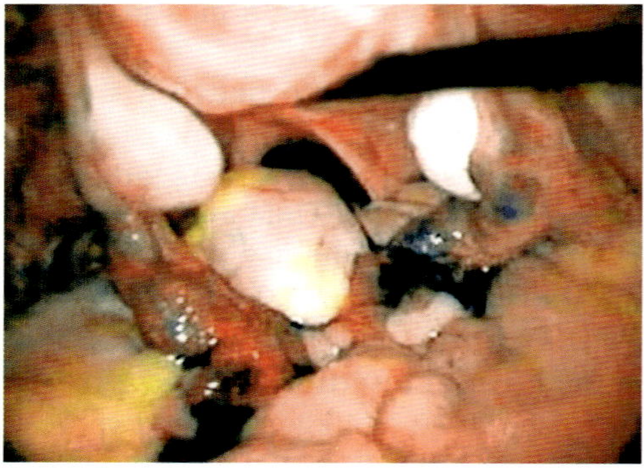

Fig. 22: Fitz Hugh Curtis syndrome

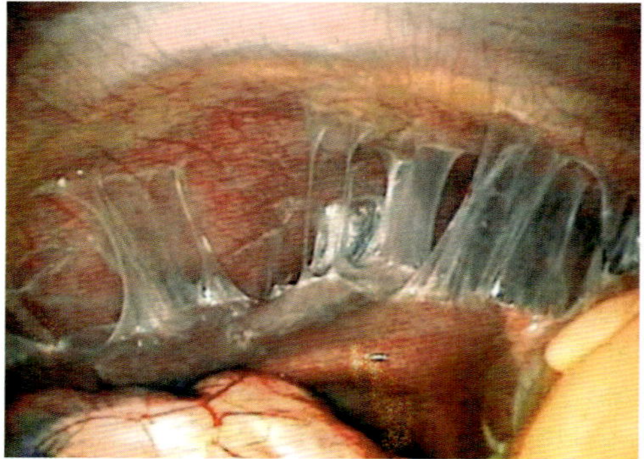

Fig. 23: Chromopertubation test

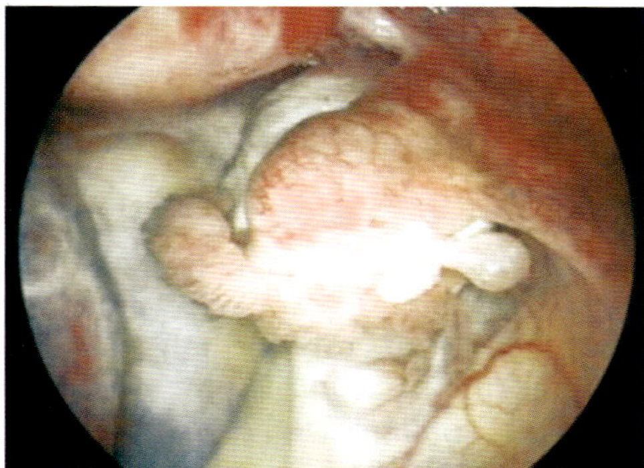

Fig. 24: Hydroflotation

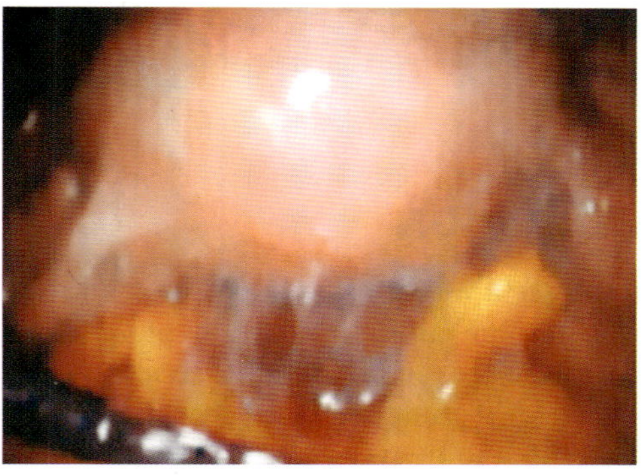

Fig. 25: Laparoscopic tubal ligation (TL) (Yoon bands)

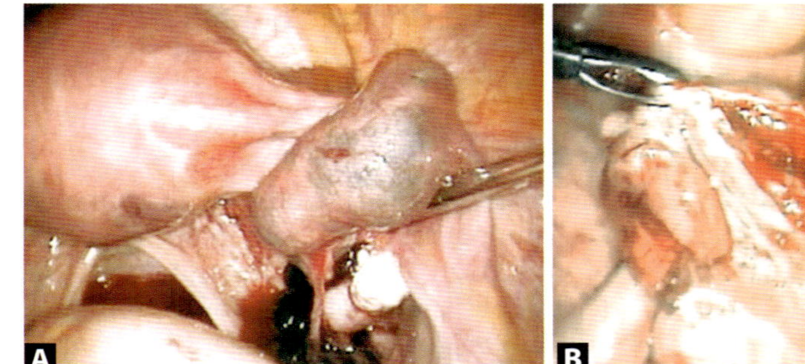

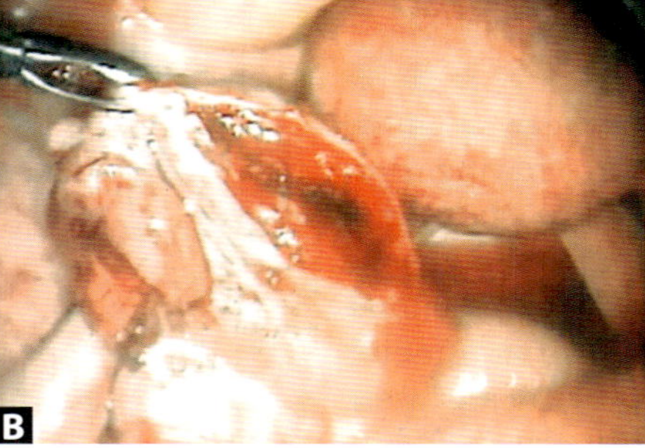

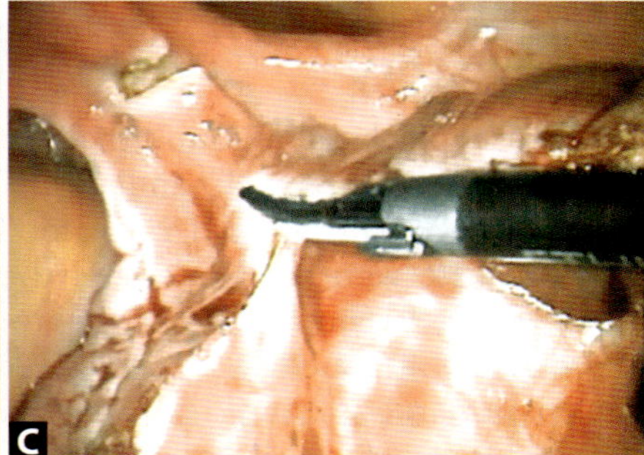

Figs 26A to C: Laparoscopic treatment of ectopic pregnancy: (A) Tubal ectopic pregnancy; (B) Linear salpingotomy; (C) Salpingectomy

made on the serosa overlying the myoma using scissors, monopolar hook, or harmonic scalpel, and extended until it reaches the capsule. The myometrium retracts exposing the myoma. Giving traction on the myoma with a grasper or myoma screw, the myoma is dissected from its capsule and removed. Hemostasis is achieved using bipolar forceps. Myometrium is repaired in two or three layers using extracorporeal or intracorporeal sutures. The specimen is removed through the pouch of Douglas or by morcellation.

Hysterectomy: No consensus exists as to the advantage of laparoscopic hysterectomy over vaginal hysterectomy. In selected cases laparoscopic approach is superior to abdominal hysterectomy. In laparoscopic hysterectomy (LH) all the uterine pedicles are done laparoscopically, whereas in LAVH, the upper pedicles are done laparoscopically and the uterine arteries and uterosacral ligaments are secured through the vaginal route.

ENDOSCOPIC SURGERY TEAM

Endoscopic surgery cannot be performed alone, the quality of the team is critical to the success of the procedure. Not only should the team have a well-trained surgeon, but assistants, scrub nurse, anesthetist who understand the needs and physiology of endoscopy and a trained technician who can keep the equipment in good shape, are vital for success.

42.1B STERILIZATION OF LAPAROSCOPIC INSTRUMENTS

Shobhana M, Mala Raj

INTRODUCTION

Instruments are a major asset and represent a significant share of the total capital spending of a hospital. The practical experience recorded in this chapter together with a description of techniques used in various parts of the globe is intended to help the user to keep the instruments in good working order and preserve their value for many years by ensuring proper care and maintenance.

Case History

A laparoscopic surgeon found that all the cases operated in a particular hospital, ended up with having port site infection. The vaginal instruments, like speculum, vulsellum, etc. were initially kept on the same trolley as the laparoscopic instruments. As a step to prevent infections, the staff was instructed to keep the vaginal instruments on separate trolleys. Swab cultures from the theater were negative for bacteria. In spite of added precautions, the infections continued. Meanwhile, the surgeon had to shift from the hospital. After shifting the hospital, the surgeon stopped getting infected cases. Although in this instance, the cause of recurrent infections remains a mystery, it highlights the fact that adequate sterilization of equipment has a major role to play in any laparoscopic procedure. Since laparoscopy is quite often performed on infertile patients, prevention of infection and its sequelae merit serious consideration.

HOSPITAL PRACTICES IN INDIA

The following protocol outlines the procedure followed at Elite Mission Hospital, Thrissur Kerala (India) for sterilizing laparoscopic equipment.

Storage

Laparoscopic instruments are routinely preserved in an acrylic, multichambered rectangular box. Four formalin (paraformaldehyde) tablets, each 1 gm, are placed in each tray. Instruments are used only when the instruments have been kept in formalin for 24 hours.

After Each Case

After each case, the instruments are washed with tap water. After that they are put in a solution named "cidezyme" for 10–15 minutes. This solution is an enzyme solution. It softens and removes organic encrustations like blood and inspissated secretions. It is a multi-enzyme proprietary preparation, designed to remove proteins, lipids, mucopolysaccharides and carbohydrates. It is used in the hospital in strength of 1:200, i.e. 5 mL in 1 liter of sterile water. For heavier contaminations, 10 mL/liter is used. It is a product owned by 3M, USA and marketed in India by 3M India, 48 to 51 electronic city, Hosur road, Bangalore 561229. After the organic matter is softened, instruments are again washed with tap water and brushes are used to remove dirt from the joints of instruments.

In Between Cases

If there are many cases on the same day, the instruments are kept in 2% Glutaraldehyde (trade names: Cidex, Glutihyde) after thorough cleaning. Instruments have to be kept in glutaraldehyde solution for 20 minutes to achieve sterilization. As an alternative, another solution, orthophthalaldehyde (Cidex OPA®, Johnson and Johnson) has been introduced. Instruments kept in orthophthadehyde have to be immersed only for 5 minutes to achieve sterilization. However, it is costly and will be cost-effective, only if the turnover of patients is high. Glutaraldehyde kills spores, *Pseudomonas*, virus, bacteria, *Mycobacterium tuberculosis*, and fungus. The solution is changed every 14 days or earlier, if there is any color change in the solution. Methylene blue, the dye used for testing the patency of the tubes, is autoclaved once a week.

Before using the instruments for the case, the instruments have to be thoroughly cleaned with sterile water. Personnel using these aldehyde preparations should be careful, as the fumes can be toxic to the eyes and the solution itself can be toxic.

As the instruments tend to stick at their hinges, they are oiled once a month using silicone oil.

REVIEW OF LITERATURE

Transmission of infection from contaminated endoscopic instruments is not very high. However, it is difficult to estimate the actual risk, as the infection may not become apparent until after the patient has been discharged from the hospital. Infection may arise, both from inadequately sterilized instruments, or from solutions used for disinfection. Inappropriate handling of instruments during sterilization could also be one of the factors leading to postoperative infection. Various methods of sterilization are used in different institutions, and practices vary not only from hospital to hospital, but also in various countries. A standard guideline is not available for all instruments. Theoretically, it is deemed necessary to follow the instructions of the manufacturer for sterilizing the particular instrument.

In practice, it may happen that, instruments/scopes are purchased from various manufacturers over the years. There are many indigenous companies which manufacture instruments similar to the ones made by reputed companies. Thus, one may be forced to follow a standard practice for sterilization, for all instruments.

Maintenance of instruments after a surgery essentially involves the three steps:

1. Cleaning,
2. Sterilization, and
3. Storage.

Cleaning

Cleaning essentially means removal of all adherent visible soil from the surface, crevices, joints and lumen of instruments and is normally accomplished using water with detergents or enzymatic products. Cleaning provides better contact with the disinfectant. Heat and some disinfectants like alcohol and aldehydes, are tissue fixatives and may cause lumen or the taps and moving parts of the endoscope to stiffen if the suction channels are not thoroughly cleaned before sterilization or disinfection.

Quality of Water

Water used for cleaning should not be unduly hard. Useful information on the quality of water may be obtained from the local water authority. Water hardness is determined by the amount of calcium and magnesium ions present in the water. Water hardness reduces the rate of killing of certain disinfectants and generally reduces the efficiency of cleaning materials. This occurs because divalent cations (e.g. magnesium and calcium) interact with some disinfectants to form insoluble precipitates. Also, drying of instruments following a post-cleaning rinse with impure water can produce undesirable precipitated residues of the salts dissolved in the water. These residues could cause damage to lens and other components of the scope. Hard water is the locally available water in many centers in India. Most of the centers are using it with apparently no palpable difference in longevity of instruments. However, since many manufacturers advocate the use of demineralized water, it may be prudent to use distilled water, which is available in many parts in huge containers. Cost of maintenance does not hike too much with this precaution. Some cleaning agents are specifically designed for use with hard water. Information about local water quality will aid in selecting an appropriate cleaning agent.

Selection of Cleaning Agents

Cleaning agents remove organic, inorganic and microbial contaminants.

Detergents: A mild alkaline detergent (pH range 8.0–11.5) is more efficient cleaning agent for surgical instruments than neutral pH detergents or surfactant-based detergents.

Enzymatic (proteolytic) cleaners: If exudates or blood have dried or hardened, cleaning with water and detergent will not suffice. For such instruments, soaking in a warm solution of an enzymatic cleaner is required. While using enzymatic products, it must be remembered that using latex gloves does not provide adequate protection and rubber or nitrile gloves are preferable. It's advisable to soak instruments vertically or placed at an angle rather than laying them horizontally in a sink. If an instrument is soaked horizontally, an air bubble is likely to form inside the instrument. On the other hand, soaking an instrument vertically or at an angle establishes a path for the enzymatic cleaner to enter, rise through, and exit the instrument—as long as the solution is deep enough. The solution should be deep enough so that the instrument's entire drive rod is submerged.

Brushes and Accessories for Cleaning

Cleaning accessories should be capable of withstanding regular heat disinfections, or they should be disposable. Adequate supplies of disposable cloths or swabs should be available to allow frequent changing. Cleaning brushes and accessories should be inspected regularly and replaced when worn or kinked.

Preparation during and after Surgery

Already in the operating room, the following preparatory measures should be taken:

- Rinse out hoses and instruments with irrigation channels using sterile rinsing solution when there is heavy soiling
- Remove heavy soiling immediately. If necessary, use a disposable cloth soaked in sterile rinsing solution
- Coagulation instruments should be wiped off with a moist compress on the coagulation surfaces between uses during surgery. Incrustations may be dissolved by briefly immersing in a 3% hydrogen peroxide solution (H_2O_2 solution). Before reusing, rinse off with sterile water and wipe off again
- Instruments should be dismantled directly after surgery and rinsed out with water. If this is not possible, the instruments should be transported assembled to the clean location (dry disposal).

Cleaning must take place within 8 hours to prevent coagulation or contaminants drying out.

Manual Cleaning

Manual cleaning should be done carefully step by step.

- Immediately after use, the laparoscope, fiberoptic light source and cable and plastic tubing with Luer-Lok should be wiped gently with a cloth soaked in 60–90% ethyl or isopropyl alcohol to remove all blood and organic material
- The laparoscopic equipment should be disassembled completely
- Disassembled parts should be placed in a basin of clean water, and mild, nonabrasive soap
- All outer surfaces should be wiped using a soft cotton cloth
- Inner channels should be cleaned with a cleaning brush supplied with the laparoscope kit. Use a circular motion to remove particulate matter. Organic matter hidden in the narrow channels may cause infection later. The brush should not be forcibly pushed against the closed end of the inner tube as this may damage it. A brush that's longer than the shaft of the laparoscopic instrument should be used. The brush should be long enough to enable all the bristles to exit the far end of the shaft. The instrument should be kept submerged under water while performing this task, so that contaminants are not expelled into the room. When finished with cleaning work, the cleaning instruments like brushes should be disinfected. Damaged brushes should not be reused
- All parts should be rinsed thoroughly with clean water (running water or from a basin) three times. A brush should be used to remove soap and particles from the inner channels (soap, if not thoroughly rinsed away, will decrease the effectiveness of the disinfectant)
- There are several ways to flush an instrument's shaft. In centers that have instruments with cleaning ports, most people attach a Luer-Lok syringe filled with enzymatic solution to the cleaning port and flush out the shaft. In this technique, the distal end of the instrument is kept under water level. If the instruments do not have cleaning ports, 3-inch piece of tubing should be affixed over the distal tip. With the tubing securely in place, attach a syringe to the other end of the 3-inch tube and flush. If compressed air is available in the decontamination department, it can be an effective tool for flushing. With a precise nozzle and the ability to control the degree of pressure, air can be forced down the cleaning port using cleaning guns. The air stream can force debris down and out of the shaft. The air used should be sterile to prevent residue on the instruments
- Equipment should be dried with a clean soft cotton cloth or air-dried (Excess water will dilute the disinfectant, decreasing its effectiveness)
- Lenses should be cleaned at least weekly, and more often as needed, but the lenses should not be touched with fingers. A cotton swab soaked in alcohol or acetone should be used to clean the lenses (cotton will not scratch the lens, and alcohol and acetone will not weaken the cement around the lens). The lens should not be touched with fingers (skin oils may damage the lenses). The plastic eyepiece of the laparoscope should be removed prior to cleaning the proximal lens with acetone or 60–90% alcohol (acetone and other organic solvents can severely damage plastic).

Ultrasonic Cleaning

Use of ultrasonic machines for cleaning can help clean instruments much faster and does a more thorough job. These machines use the principle of "cavitation"—which is a by-product of transmitting high frequency sound waves into a liquid medium. Alternating phases of rarefaction and compression during sound wave transmission into a liquid produce and collapse millions of microscopic vacuum cavities each second. The collapse or implosion of these cavities cause high powered microjets of liquid to be propelled throughout the bath removing even the most tenacious particles upon impact. While thorough cleaning of laparoscopic instruments takes 45 minutes on an average, when done manually, an ultrasonic machine can do the job in 15 minutes.

The acoustic cavitation created has the following effects:

- It blasts away the most tenacious soils even when hidden in the smallest crevices
- Accelerates the rate at which soils dissolve by intimately mixing the cleaning solution with the contaminants and attacks the molecular cement by which soils attach themselves to a surface
- The microjet effect from acoustic cavitation prevents the formation of a neutral film on parts, which may have impeded cleaning results
- Acoustic cavitation also raises the temperature of the liquid, which increases the rate of chemical activity of the cleaning solution.

The ultrasonic bath (at 35 KHz) is suited for an especially thorough, mild cleaning of heavily soiled and sensitive parts. The cleaning effect of the ultrasonic also reaches virtually inaccessible instrument channels. The ultrasonic bath can be used manually as well as with a machine. Ultrasonic support of a machine cleaning exists primarily in cyclical washing automats. The duration of manual ultrasonic use should only be as long as dirt is removed, though generally it should not exceed 5 minutes. Prolonged ultrasonic application increases the temperature of the bath and reduces the cleaning effect.

Small parts, such as screws and nuts, which are not tightly fastened, may come loose due to the ultrasonic effect. One should check for completeness. If a cleaning agent is added to ultrasonic baths (use no chlorine-containing agents), especially thorough rinsing is required afterward.

Caution: Ultrasonic cleaning is not permitted for telescopes.

Machine Cleaning

Just like washing machines and dish cleaning machines, many machines are now available for cleaning and disinfection of instruments in the international market. Although many manufacturers claim that manual cleaning is not necessary before keeping instruments in their machines, it may not be entirely true. Machine cleaning always means a greater load on the instrument set than with manual cleaning. The advantage of machine cleaning and disinfection is reduction of risks for the personnel, and, standardization of the cleaning process.

Selection of rinsing programs must be decided with the washer manufacturer.

Due to the partially strong motion of the water in machine cleaning, it is necessary that all parts be fixated in a holder, to prevent damage. For sufficient rinsing out of the instruments, it is necessary that instrument channels be correctly connected. For instruments with a LUER irrigation connection, good rinsing of the jaws is also provided through inside irrigation of the tube. Jointed instruments must be opened in such a way that good rinsing is achieved.

The temperature of the inflowing water should not be above 45°C, since higher temperatures cause coagulation of protein creating problems for cleaning.

Usually, special programs for endoscopic instrument sets (or even for telescopes) are available which are better suited for cleaning and material preservation than general programs. It should be ensured that rigid telescopes are not heated beyond 93°C. Miniature telescopes should not be heated beyond 63°C.

Sterilization and Disinfection

Sterilization and high-level disinfection are two of the commonly used methods used for rendering laparoscopic instruments free of organisms.

Sterilization destroys all microorganisms, including spores.

High-level disinfection (HLD) kills all bacteria, tubercle bacilli and virus, but is ineffective against bacterial spores. HLD could be thermal or chemical.

High-level Disinfection with Chemical Agents

Ideally, one should purchase only instruments that can withstand steam sterilization. However, it is not always feasible and many laparoscopy units have laparoscopes which cannot be autoclaved. The standard method for decontaminating these instruments would be high-level disinfection using chemical agents. Some of the chemicals used for this purpose are:

- 2% glutaraldehyde solution
- Orthophthalaldehyde solution
- Peracetic acid.

Glutaraldehyde

Glutaraldehyde is an aldehyde and is bactericidal, fungicidal and tuberculocidal. Most glutaraldehyde preparations are acidic and become sporicidal only when it has been activated to become alkaline. It takes longer to become sporicidal. It acts at a pH of 7.5–8.5. Some species of mycobacterium and fungi are resistant to glutaraldehyde.

Two percent glutaraldehyde acts as a disinfectant if instruments are soaked in it for 20 minutes at 25°C and as a sterilant with contact for 10 hours. Instruments have to be thoroughly cleaned before soaking in glutaraldehyde solution, as glutaraldehyde sticks to proteinaceous material. Thorough drying is also essential as water can dilute glutaraldehyde. After immersing in glutaraldehyde for 20 minutes, the instruments have to be washed in boiled water. If glutaraldehyde is being used as a sterilant, it has to be washed in sterile water. Immersing the instruments in a basin with water is not adequate. Instruments have to be thoroughly cleaned with water, as glutaraldehyde can be irritating to the tissues. Instruments should be dried before use, as water left on the instruments if exposed to air and handling could lead to infection.

Precautions for personnel: Glutaraldehyde can be toxic to the eyes and there should be facility for washing the eyes immediately just in case it enters the eyes of the staff cleaning it. Wearing goggles while handling the solution would be preferable. Fumes of glutaraldehyde could aggravate asthma. It is toxic to the respiratory tract. Cleaning should therefore take place in a place with good ventilation so that fumes could be let out. Installation of fumehoods to let out the fumes could be useful.

Maintenance: Generally, the solution should be changed every 14 days. However, dilution from water remaining on the device can shorten the reuse time and the solution may have to be changed sooner. When glutaraldehyde is used with automatic disinfecting machines, concentration of glutaraldehyde may reduce every 3 days. It is better to monitor the solution using chemical indicator strips, than to judge the potency of the solution by a change in color as is practised in many places. Testing with chemical strips should be done daily if the solution is used daily, just before use, if the instruments are used every 7 days, and after every 10th case if it is used 30 times per day. Chemical strips should not have undergone expiry date.

Orthophthalaldehyde

Orthophthalaldehyde (OPA), (marketed as Cidex OPA®, Johnson and Johnson in India), a member of the aldehyde family, is a fast acting, high-level disinfectant with tubercidal activity although it has only limited activity against bacterial spores. OPA acts much faster than glutaraldehyde. For example, the mean period of reducing the growth of *Mycobacterium bovis* was 6 minutes with OPA compared to 32 minutes with glutaraldehyde. The high-level disinfectant label claims for OPA at 20°C varies in different countries, as the rules of antimicrobial testing is different in various places. Since it has been introduced only recently, many more studies will be needed for standardization. When used in automatic machines, its minimum effective concentration is reached only after 82 cycles of processing instruments in the machine, as compared to 40 cycles after glutaraldehyde according to the manufacturer. Its advantages over glutaraldehyde are that it is much more stable and is less toxic to personnel.

Peracetic Acid

Peracetic acid or peroxyacetic acid is an oxidizing agent and functions by denaturing protein, disrupting cell wall permeability and oxidizing sulfhydryl and sulfur bonds in proteins, enzymes and other metabolites. It has a rapid, broad-spectrum antimicrobial activity, is not readily inactivated by organic matter and is sporocidal even at low temperatures. This chemical can be corrosive to some metals but additives and pH modifications can reduce this effect. It is considered unstable particularly when diluted.

In Australia, this product is used in an automated processor (Steris System 1®) which is a liquid chemical process capable of sterilization and used to reprocess endoscopes and some accessories. The sterilant, 35% peracetic acid, is diluted to 0.2% and operates at a minimum temperature of 50°C; requiring an exposure time of 12 minutes, with the complete processing cycle taking 25–30 minutes.

Sterilization Procedures

The available procedures are:

- Steam sterilization
- Gas sterilization [formaldehyde, ethylene oxide (EtO)]
- Plasma sterilization
- Chemical sterilization.

Steam Sterilization

Steam sterilization at 134°C is usually the mildest and most inexpensive sterilization method. This also applies to rigid telescopes since the longer required time can have a negative effect on steam sterilization at 121°C. Sterilization is always only possible on clean surfaces.

Steam sterilization is not permissible for the following instrument categories. For these, only methods with a maximum temperature of 65°C, such as gas and plasma sterilization, may be used.

- Non-autoclavable telescopes (the manufacturer would have labeled the telescope "Autoclavable" if it can withstand steam sterilization)
- Telescopes with eyepiece drive mechanism
- Fiberscopes or semiflexible telescopes/Miniature endoscopes
- Fluid light cables
- Video cameras
- Prismatic light deflectors.

Almost all instruments may be sterilized in assembled condition. Screws and connections should be tightened only slightly, so that they may later be easily loosened.

Note: If deactivation of Creutzfeldt-Jakob disease (CJD) is necessary, the sterilization method recommended by World Health Organization (WHO; WHO/CDS/PH/92.104) may be used (18 minutes at 134°C). Extension of the sterilization time up to 1 hour at 134°C is possible in special cases.

Some of the methods used in machine sterilization are:

- Vacuum or prevacuum method
- Gravitation method
- Flash sterilization.

Vacuum or prevacuum method: It consists of four phases:

1. Conditioning phase: The conditioning phase removes air from the chamber by pulling a vacuum and then warms the instruments by injecting steam
2. Sterilization phase: Sterilization takes place at a temperature of 134°C and an operating pressure (Pb) of 2 bar over a period of 5–8 minutes
3. Evacuation phase: The steam is released
4. Drying phase: Drying takes place under renewed application of vacuum over a period of approx. 5 to 20 minutes.

Validated parameters for the prevacuum method:

- Temperature: 270–272°F; 134°C
- Pressure (Pb): 27 psi; 2 bar
- Exposure time: 5 minutes.

Fractioned prevacuum procedure: The fractioned prevacuum procedure also consists of the four previously mentioned phases.

In the conditioning phase, a vacuum is generated up to four times. Steam is then blown in and sterilization takes place at 121°C (250–252°C) or 134°C (270–272°F) in 20 minutes or 5 minutes respectively (minimum times). Before the final drying phase, the steam is removed from the chamber during the evacuation phase. Drying takes place under vacuum.

Validated parameters for the fractioned prevacuum method:

- Temperature: 270–272°F; (134°C)
- Pressure (Pb): 27 psi; 2 bar
- Exposure time: 5 minutes.

Gravitation method: This method is only suitable for smooth and accessible surfaces, not for instruments with channels, gaps or stopcocks. The gravitation method is also made up of four phases:

1. Conditioning phase: Steam is pressed into the chamber and heats the instruments
2. Sterilization phase: Sterilization takes place at a temperature of 121°C and an operating pressure (Pb) of 1 bar over a period of 30–45 minutes
3. Evacuation phase: Steam is released through the outlet
4. Drying phase: Drying takes place under ambient air pressure by heating through the heating jacket of the autoclave.

Validated parameters for the gravitation method:

- Temperature: 270–272°F, 121°C
- Pressure (Pb): 15 psi/1 bar
- Required time: 30–45 minutes.

Disadvantages of Automated Endoscope Reprocessor (AER) Units

The following problems have been reported from the use of AER:

- Incorrect and home-made connection
- Spillage due to incorrect placing of the endoscope in the AER
- Insufficient disinfectant in system
- No water filters used.
- Blocked channels resulting in low or no flow of the disinfectant
- Recontamination of devices from the AER.

Gas Sterilization

Sterilization can be achieved using formaldehyde or ethylene dioxide.

Formaldehyde sterilization: Instruments that have been dried and cleaned are kept in rectangular boxes with at least 8 cm depth. 8% formaldehyde for 24 hours is necessary for sterilizing the instrument.

Sterilization with formalin tablets: In most centers in India, gas sterilization is done by placing formalin tablets in acrylic boxes having one or two compartments with 2–4 tablets of formalin (Paraformaldehyde, a solid isomer of formaldehyde) being placed inside. Time taken for sterilization is 24 hours. If the instruments are to be reused, alternative methods of disinfection, like glutaraldehyde have to be used. We do not have accurate reports of infection rate following the use of this procedure and there are no controlled studies comparing this method with the methods used in the rest of the world. By and large, there is not a very high incidence of postoperative sepsis that could be attributed to infective instruments in centers following this method. Many centers in India continue using it.

This practice is considered inadequate in many parts of the world. There are no correct guidelines for this procedure, as this method is not considered a standard method of sterilization. Some of the reasons given for considering this method insufficient are:

- Formaldehyde is potentially cancer causing and extremely irritating to the skin, eyes, nose, and respiratory tract
- Sterilization with formalin is said to be heavily dependent on relative humidity and temperature, and the use of formalin tablets does not permit any control over these parameters. Formalin does not act well in chambers with low relative humidity
- Concerns are raised about the reach of formalin vapors into lumen of instruments. The possibility of formalin deposited on instruments is also said to be a cause for concern.

Low-temperature steam with formaldehyde (LTSF): This method is used in some countries in Europe and Asia. LTSF sterilizers use formaldehyde at low temperature working at ambient pressure. Glenn, in "surgery in the developing world" describes an indigenous way of using Formalin sterilization. Equipment is left overnight in a refrigerator. Formalin tablets are placed in it at 7 gm/m^3. A light bulb in the refrigerator helps the vaporization process. It is recommended that the area around the refrigerator be well ventilated. After the equipment is removed it has to be washed in sterile water and aerated. All organisms, including human immunodeficiency virus (HIV), are killed in 24 hours. A minimum of at least 12 hours is recommended.

Ethylene oxide sterilization: In EtO sterilization, air is removed by vacuum and ethylene oxide gas is supplied in canisters that are used one per sterilization. Gas sterilization using ethylene oxide involves the use of expensive machinery and is not commonly used.

Method of EtO sterilization: Place the instrument securely on a sterilization sieve. Ethylene oxide gas sterilization has been validated under the following parameters (Table 1):

For gas sterilization with ethylene oxide, the following airing times must be observed for instruments due to gas absorption of the materials (Table 2). When airing in the airing cabinet, the temperature should be maintained between 45°C and 55°C over a period of 12 hours.

Gas Plasma Sterilization

Plasma is the fourth state of matter, distinguished from solid, liquid and gas. Gas plasma is a highly excited body of gas produced by the application of energy to a gas under vacuum, making ions and molecules within the plasma collide to produce free radicals. These are involved in alkylation of the protein in the microbial cell.

The Sterrad® automated sterilization system uses low-temperature H_2O_2 gas plasma to achieve low-temperature, low-moisture sterilization, usually within a 1-hour automated cycle. Special adapters (H_2O_2 boosters) are required for use with devices with lumens to ensure the sterilant gains access to these areas. The system requires the use of nonwoven (noncellulose) polypropylene wraps or packaging.

Instruments with very long narrow lumens, and those closed at one end, are unsuitable for sterilization using hydrogen peroxide gas plasma. Some shorter flexible endoscopes and accessories have been validated for sterilization with this system.

Table 1: Parameters for validation of ethylene oxide gas sterilization

Gas mixture	EtO:HCFC*
Temperature	130°F +
(°F, °C)	54°C + 2°C
Relative air humidity	60 + 20%
Pressure (Pb, psi/bar)	8–10 psi; 0,56–0,7 bar
Exposure time	120 minutes
EtO concentration	600 + 30 mg/L

*Gas mixture consisting of 10% ethylene oxide and 90% chlorotetrafluoroethane (HCFC-124; % by weight)

Table 2: Gas sterilization with ethylene oxide at different temperature

	at 20°C	at 42°C	at 55°C
Telescopes	24 hours	18 hours	12 hours
Rubber items	7 days	4 days	3 days
Plastics/Fiberscopes	5 days	2 days	30 hours

(Minimum time in simple transparent packaging and an application time on the patient of more than 30 minutes).

Chemical Sterilization

Chemical sterilization (STERIS) is a special method, which is particularly suited for thermolabile goods such as fiberscope.

Warning: Parts with a lumen must be prepared together with the STERIS Quick Connect kit. All parts must be thoroughly cleaned before sterilization using the STERIS process, which also applies to the other sterilization methods.

The following product categories have material compatibility and have been validated with the STERIS process.

- Rigid telescopes without working channel, without eyepiece drive
- Semiflexible telescopes without working channel
- Flexible hysteroscopes* and cystoscopes* for adults
- Flexible ureteroscopes*, pediatric cystoscopes* and choledochoscopes*,
- Immersible video cameras
- Illuminated ureteral probes
- Light cable
- Connecting cable.

TESTING FOR STERILIZATION OR DISINFECTION

The sterilization process can be monitored using different ways:

- *Mechanical indicators:* These indicators, which are part of the sterilization equipment, allow the user to observe time, temperature and/or pressure readings during the sterilization cycle.
- *Chemical indicators:* These include:
  - Tape with lines that change color when the intended temperature is reached.
  - Pellets in glass tubes that melt, indicating that the intended temperature and time have been reached.
  - Indicator strips that show that the intended combination of temperature, time and, in an autoclave, steam has been achieved.
  - Indicator strips that show that sterilization chemicals are still effective.
- *Biological indicators:* These indicators use heat-resistant bacterial endospores to demonstrate whether or not sterilization has been achieved. The advantage of this method is that it directly measures the effectiveness of sterilization.

STORAGE

Instruments should always be stored in suitable containers and must be absolutely dry. The place of storage must have normal temperature and air humidity values [30–50% relative humidity (RH); 20°C].

MAINTENANCE

Check for Damages

Even damages, which are barely visible, can impair perfect functioning (e.g. operating property), when it concerns high precision manufacturer's parts.

Insulation Inspection

Laparoscopic instruments quite often have insulations on them. The first 3 inches of the distal tip and the rings are places where cracks appear first. The instrument should be viewed through 360° made to detect these. Pulling back on the insulation should be done to make sure that it has not loosened. Sliding of insulation on the instrument would expose more metal than should be ideally exposed. Exposed metal is dangerous to adjacent organs while performing surgery due to possibility of arcing of current.

After checking over the individual parts, multi part instruments must be assembled. Before the final functional test, the instruments must be cooled down and oiled.

Plastic parts should be checked for discoloration, porosity and flexibility. If the parts show considerable deviations from their new condition, they must be exchanged. This particularly applies to seals. Ensure the patency of channels.

Check jaws and joints especially carefully. The jaws on scissors should allow smooth cutting and forceps should have non-slip edges, aligned properly with one another, and which open and close completely.

Sealing and contact surfaces, e.g. on stopcocks or plungers should be thinly coated with special grease. This thin layer of grease not only serves to lubricate the metal-to-metal surfaces in contact with one another, but also the seal on the stopcocks. Oil is not suitable as sealant. Special silicone or oil-based lubricants should be used, since sterilants cannot penetrate through every silicone or oil.

CONCLUSION

Meticulous disinfection and maintenance of instruments are as important as perfecting the skills of endoscopy. One should be aware of the various equipment that are available locally and internationally, so that the best possible care could be taken to ensure a microbe-free surgery.

BIBLIOGRAPHY

1. Aberline M, Wilson A, Ketts B, et al. Subcommittee members. Infection control task force Glutaraldehyde recommendation No. 11. Victorian advisory committee on infection control; 1998.
2. Cronin W, McIntosh N. High level disinfection: Infection prevention guidelines. Available online from: www.reproline.jhu.edu/english/4morerh/4ip/IP_manual/12_HLD.pdf. [Accessed December, 2013].
3. Keerasuntonpong A, Sitaposa P, Chaiprasert A, et al. Efficiency of the glutaraldehyde test strip for monitoring the concentration of glutaraldehyde in reused solutions for disinfecting endoscopes. J Med Assoc Thai. 2002;85(11):1164-8.
4. Rideout K, Teschke K, Dimich-Ward H, et al. Considering risks to health care workers from glutaraldehyde alternatives in high-level disinfection. J Hosp Infect. 2005;59(1):4-11.
5. Schlutz VK. Using glutaraldehyde safely: outpatient surgery magazine. Connor DO (ED). Available online from: http://www.outpatientsurgery.net/2002/os10/index.shtml. [Accessed December, 2013].
6. Spectrum Surgical Instruments. Tube Scoop: Insider's Guide to Cleaning Lap Instruments. [online]. Available from http://www.spectrumsurgical.com/news/articles/tube_scoop2.htm. [Accessed December, 2013].
7. Verrbrugge GP. Guide to the operation theatre at $25 a patient: Surgery and healing in the developing world. Available from http://www.landesbioscience.com. [Accessed December, 2013].
8. www.cdc.gov/ncidod/hip/dsguide/dsguide.pdfX

42.2 LAPAROSCOPIC DIAGNOSTIC PROCEDURES

Malvika Sabharwal

INTRODUCTION

During the last 3 decades Gynecologic laparoscopy has transcended its boundaries from a limited surgical procedure to a major surgical tool not only for diagnosing but also for carrying out almost all gynecological operative procedures.

Compared with laparotomy, studies have time and again showed laparoscopy to be much safer, patient-friendly, with lesser operative blood loss and shorter hospital stay.

INDICATIONS

- Acute or chronic pain abdomen
- Ectopic pregnancy
- Endometriosis
- Adnexal masses and torsion
- Determination of tubal pathologies
- Any other pelvic pathology
- Oncologic procedures.

PREOPERATIVE PREPARATION AND TESTS

- History and physical examination
- Complete blood count (CBC) with differential and blood group
- Urine analysis
- In patients with known health problems, other tests like liver function test (LFT), electrolytes evaluation may be necessary
- Coagulation profile, if appropriate
- Ultrasonography (USG) of the whole abdomen along with transvaginal ultrasonography (TVS) and Doppler studies and tumor markers in cases of adnexal masses
- ECG and chest X-ray (CXR) in patients with coexisting cardiopulmonary conditions
- Pap's smear, endometrial biopsy, cervical cultures and hysterosalpingogram (HSG) studies, if required in specific cases
- Informed consent.

One Day Bowel Preparation

- Clear liquids a day before surgery
- Laxative and a mild anxiolytic, if required on the night before surgery
- Nil per os (NPO) after midnight
- A shot of intravenous (IV) antibiotic and tetanus toxoid (TT) half an hour before surgery.

Immediate Preoperative Preparation

- IV access
- Bladder catheterization
- Umbilicus preparation cleanses the umbilicus and fix-in a betadine gauze half an hour before surgery.

RISK FACTORS

- Obesity
- Age
- Previous abdominal scars
- Abdominal wall thickness
- Umbilicus—the umbilicus should be examined for signs of umbilical hernia.

Anesthetic Risk Factors

- Time since last oral intake—At least 6 hours, as general anesthesia (GA) and increased IAP during laparoscopy, both may increase the risk of regurgitation and resultant aspiration
- Patients with cardiac and pulmonary ailments.

ANESTHESIA

General anesthesia is routinely preferred as it offers greater comfort to the patient and the surgeon. Especially if extensive diagnostic manipulations are further, required, anesthesia is induced in dorsal position. Minimum monitoring standards should be observed including pulse oxymeter and capnography.

Spinal anesthesia is avoided because:

- Breathing difficulties due to a high block may cause discomfort and breathing difficulties in an awake patient whose diaphragm is already stretched and elevated due to pneumoperitoneum
- Laparoscopic procedures require several changes of patient position during the procedures which may cause cardiovascular instability in a patient whose hemodynamic compensatory mechanisms have been limited by the sympathectomy of regional anesthesia
- Interventional laparoscopy, if needed, requires a higher level of sensory block (T4-T5) which also produces significant sympathetic blockade, causing hypotension.

SURGICAL ANATOMY

For a successful outcome of laparoscopic surgery, a complete knowledge of the laparoscopic anatomy of the pelvic organs is an absolute necessity.

The anterior superior iliac spine and the pubic crest are the superficial landmarks on the abdomen along with the umbilicus, which generally is the site of the primary port.

The umbilicus lies over the bifurcation of the aorta and maybe slightly below it in obese patients. However, in almost all patients, the left common iliac vein lies 4–7 cm below the umbilicus. This is an important landmark for the safe introduction of the Veress needle. Care should be taken as rarely there may be a patent uracus filled with urine.

McBurney's point is the lateral one-third from the anterior superior iliac spinal (ASIS) and the umbilicus. While making the lateral ports, transillumination of the abdominal wall helps in visualizing the superficial vessels but it does not reveal the inferior epigastric vessel. To identify these, we observe the underside of the anterior abdominal wall and follow the round ligament to its exit at the internal inguinal ring. Medial to it the inferior epigastric vessels can be seen. Here, under the peritoneum is the lateral umbilical fold which holds the epigastric vessels. A trocar placed laterally to the McBurney's point can safely avoid injury to these vessels.

On the underside of the anterior abdominal wall one has to visualize the medial umbilical fold which is the peritoneum covering the obliterated umbilical artery. This is a very important landmark for the laparoscopist. Traction given at this obliterated umbilical artery leads on to below the broad ligament to the pelvic side wall to demarcate the superior vesical artery. This leads to the root of the internal iliac artery. Here the superior vesical artery can be seen going on to the internal iliac artery. Medial to this is the uterine artery which goes till the uterus with the ureter clearly seen coursing just beneath it. This knowledge is important for the safe dissection of the pelvic side wall where adhesions are present in cases of inflammation or endometriosis.

On the left pelvic side wall the peristalsis of the ureter can be seen with the pulsation of the internal iliac artery posteriorly.

Position

Trendelenburg position with 30° head low tilt and legs in stirrups at 20–30° to the body is ideal.

Gynecologic laparoscopy procedures are usually performed with the patient in the dorsal lithotomy position to allow vaginal access for uterine manipulation. Most laparoscopists now use boot stirrups specially designed for laparoscopy which avoid pressure on the lateral or posterior aspect of the calf muscles and permit easy positional changes from low lithotomy for laparoscopy to high lithotomy for vaginal procedures, such as hysteroscopy or vaginal hysterectomy. Once the primary trocar is placed, the patient is placed in no more than 20°. Trendelenburg position helps keep the bowel out of the pelvis.

Laparoscopic Access

There is enough evidence to prove that vascular injuries have a seven-fold more chance during the primary or secondary trocar insertion than by the Veress needle.

In a prospective multicentric Dutch study Jansen reviewed 25,764 laparoscopies where five complications were caused by Veress needle and 68 by trocar insertion.

Hence, making the primary port which is the first access site, is a critical step during laparoscopy when most serious unintended injuries occur.

The non-draped abdomen must be inspected for previous scars, and to palpate bony landmarks prior to every primary port placement.

TECHNIQUES OF PRIMARY ACCESS

Five common approaches are:

1. Veress needle insertion followed by a primary trocar insertion
2. Direct trocar insertion
3. Open laparoscopy
4. Expanding access cannulas
5. Endovision.

Direct Trocar Insertion

This refers to inserting the primary trocar without having previously inserted the needle and insufflating the

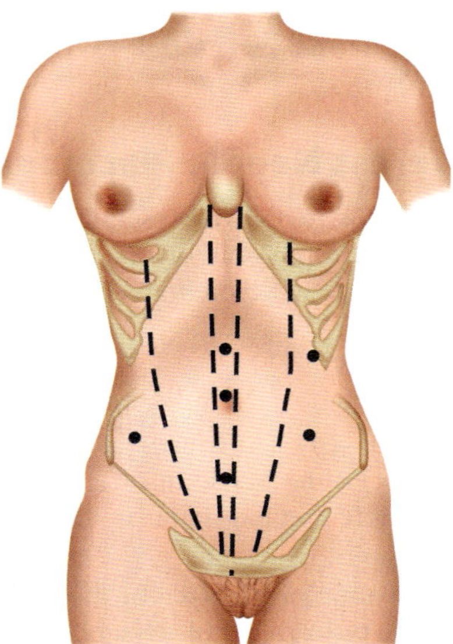

Fig. 1: Sites of introduction of the Veress needle

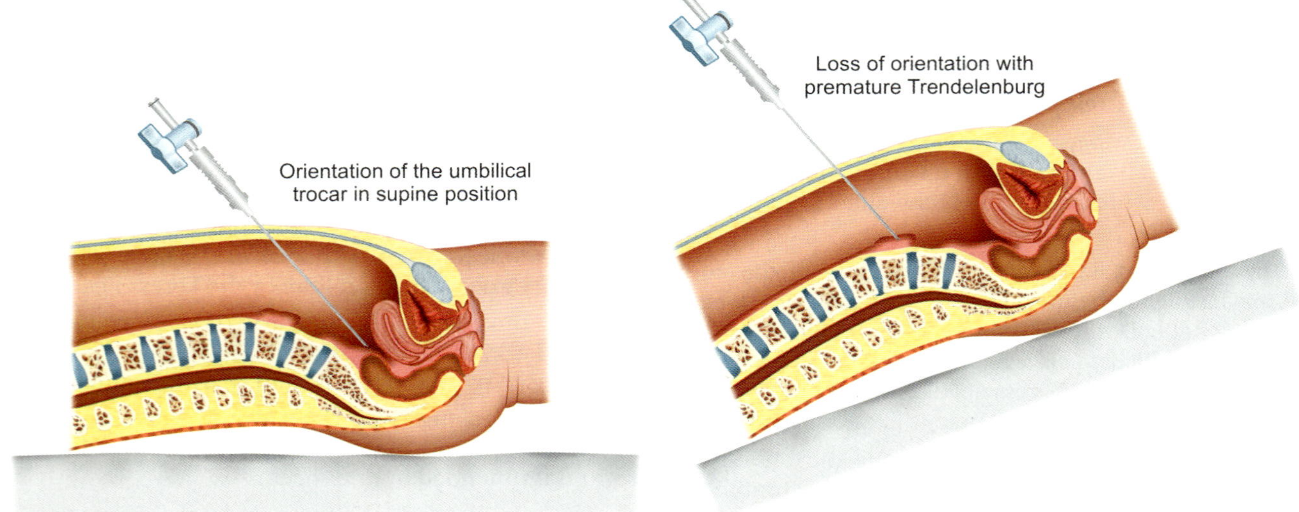

Fig. 2: Insertion of primary trocar is made with patient being supine to avoid vascular injuries

abdomen. The primary trocar is inserted in a manner similar to the veress needle. The advantage is that it avoids extraperitoneal insufflation.

Open Laparoscopy

This involves incising the anterior rectus fascia and bluntly entering the peritoneum with a Kelly or Crile clamp.

Expanding Access Cannulas

It is a relatively new technique for trocar placement and involves the placement of a veress needle for insufflation. After this the needle is removed and reinserted after it is placed into an expandable sleeve and is placed into the peritoneal cavity. The needle is then removed and the cannula is dilated to 5-10 mm to accommodate laparoscopic lens.

Sites of Veress Needle Placement

Usual site of Veress needle placement is intraumbilical, which is the shortest possible distance between the skin and the peritoneal cavity, even in obese patients.

Alternative Sites

- Through umbilicus
- Palmer's point—(the left subcostal margin in the mid-clavicular line) if the pelvic mass is large in size or in cases of multiple previous laparotomies
- McBurney's point
- Transvaginal approach is used by inserting the needle through the posterior cul-de-sac and is effective in patients who have developed preperitoneal emphysema from previous unsuccessful attempts to insert the needle from other sites.

Insertion of Veress Needle

The spring-loaded Veress needle is first tested with the stopcock open so that room air escapes in the abdominal cavity as the peritoneum is penetrated.

The abdominal wall is elevated by manually grasping the skin and subcutaneous tissue to maximize the distance between the umbilicus and the retroperitoneal viscera. The needle is then inserted towards the hollow of the sacrum at an angle of 45°. In patients who are obese, a more vertical approach, approximately 70-800 is required.

Generally two distinct pops are felt when the needle traverses the anterior rectus fascia first, followed by the posterior rectus fascia and the peritoneum. Only a single pop may be felt if the insertion is intraumbilical.

Tests to Confirm the Proper Position of the Veress Needle (Fig. 3)

- Injection and aspiration of the fluid through the veress needle
- Loss of liver dullness in early insufflation
- Hanging drop test
- An unimpeded arc of rotation of the needle to detect anterior abdominal wall adhesions
- Sound of air entering the Veress needle with an elevation of the abdominal wall
- Free flow of gas through the Veress needle
- Observation of the fluctuation of the pressure gauge needle with inspiratory and expiratory diaphragmatic movements.

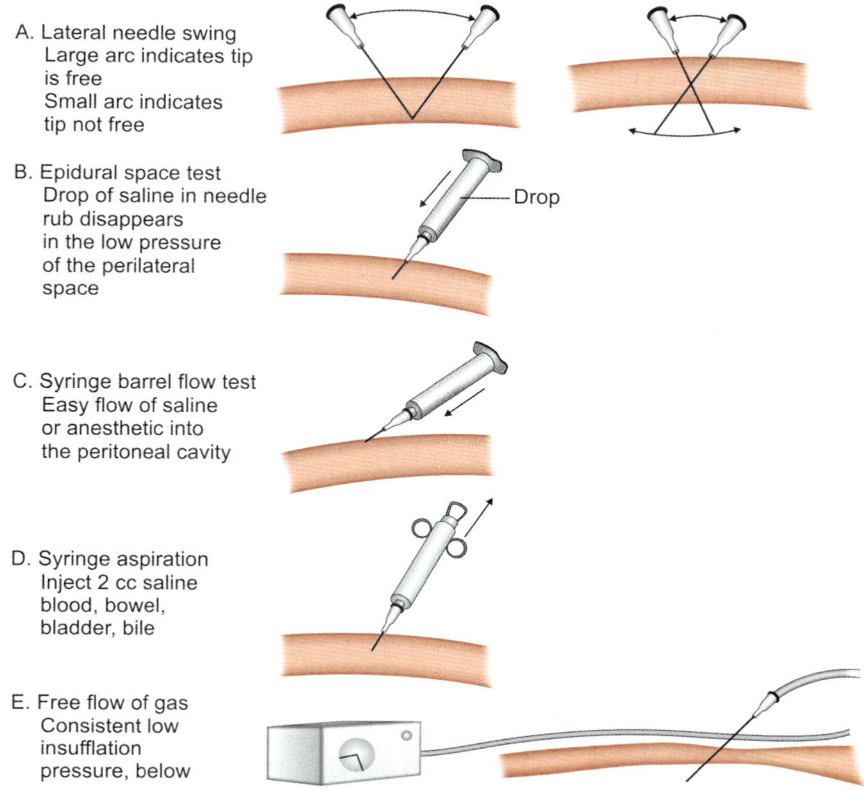

Fig. 3: Various techniques/tests to confirm the proper position of the Veress needle

Improper Veress needle placement and a high flow rate of gas may lead to serious complications. Flow rate should be increased only after confirmation of the correct placement. The intraperitoneal pressure should not exceed 15 mm Hg.

Troubleshooting Tip

If higher pressure is recorded while insufflating, change the needle's position by drawing out or moving the needle sideways slowly to move the tip away from a viscus. One can also lift up the abdominal wall manually. Also saline can be injected to flush out a blocked needle.

Introduction of the Principal Trocar

After creating pneumoperitoneum, the next step is to introduce the principal trocar and cannula to make passage for the telescope. The risks associated with this step are directly related to the force applied.

Successful trocar insertion depends on:

- An adequate incision,
- The trocar's working condition,
- Their proper orientation, and
- Control over the instrument's force and depth of insertion.

Introduction of the Telescope

Telescope should be examined to confirm that the lenses are clear and bright and snugly fitted. Naked eye examination followed by white balance should be done. Once the telescope is inserted, a complete systematic diagnostic panoramis survey of, the whole abdomen should be done.

Introduction of the Ancillary Instruments

In order to avoid trauma to the structures of the abdominal wall, the site of the secondary puncture should be indented with the index finger and observed with the laparoscope in the abdomen. The obliterated umbilical arteries are useful landmarks to avoid major parietal blood vessels. Transillumination of the abdominal wall also helps in identifying the superficial blood vessels. All secondary trocars and cannulae have to be inserted under direct vision of the laparoscope.

Pelvic Exploration

As laparoscopy offers a panoramic view of the whole abdomen, systemic survey of the organs is done. It includes successive observation and assessment of the parietal peritoneum, the visceral surfaces, liver, gall bladder, stomach and diaphragm while the patient is still in the horizontal position. Successively, the transverse, descending and ascending colon and the small bowel are inspected.

The patient is now placed in Trendelenburg position, the cecum and appendix are assessed.

A general panoramic inspection of the pelvis is first performed with the laparoscope kept at some distance from the pelvic contents. The laparoscope is then advanced and the organs are then scrutinized systematically. Manipulation of the uterus in both anteroposterior and side-to-side directions with the use of a probe greatly facilitates a thorough pelvic inspection.

Removal of Instruments and Abdominal Closure

Removal of all laparoscopic instruments and trocars has to be under direct laparoscopic guidance. After a final survey of the abdomen to confirm that there is no unsuspected trauma or bleeding, the laparoscope is removed. With the patient still in Trendelenburg position, the valve of the principal cannula is opened and the gas expelled from the peritoneal cavity. The telescope is gradually and slowly withdrawn keeping in view the proper apposition of the port walls and also to avoid herniation. Keeping the abdominal wall compressed with the nondominant hand, this cannula is removed with the valve in open position.

The published incidence of port herniation is about 0.3–1.3%.

Wound closure is done with the help of glue, sutures or stapler clips.

A smaller telescope, if available, can be used from an ancillary port for visual guidance of the primary trocar removal.

COMPLICATIONS AND MANAGEMENT

Gas embolism: CO_2 embolism is an uncommon but very serious complication. It is usually caused by the inadvertent placement of the Veress needle into a major vessel during attempts to insufflate the abdominal cavity with CO_2.

Prevention: Verify intraperitoneal placement of the Veress needle before insufflation.

Recognition and treatment of a large venous embolization must be immediate. Clinical signs include:

- Decreased $EtCO_2$
- Decreased oxygen saturation
- A loud mill-wheel murmur
- Severe hypotension
- Possible cardiac arrest.

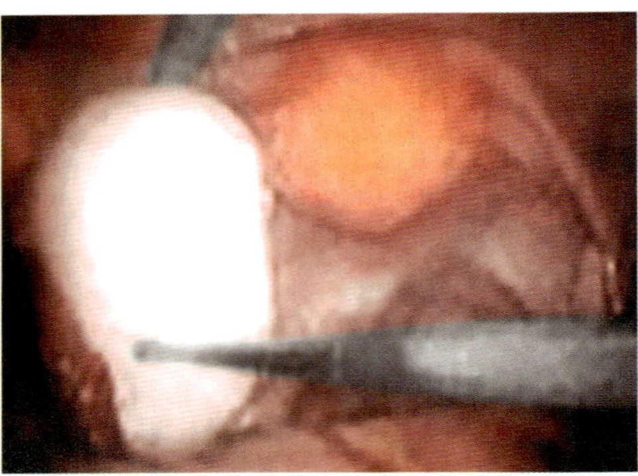

Fig. 4: Bilateral polycystic ovarian syndrome (PCOS) after lap drilling

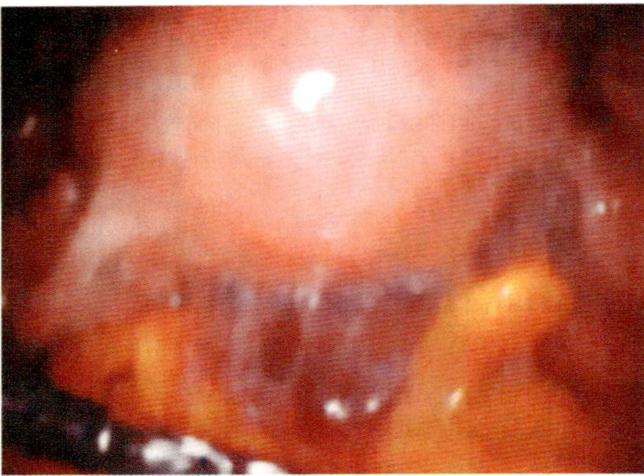

Fig. 5: Adhesions between uterus and pouch of Douglas (POD)

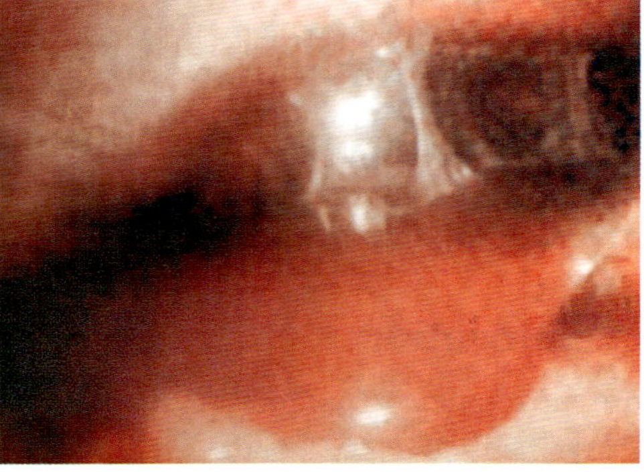

Fig. 6: Flimsy adhesions on undersurface of liver

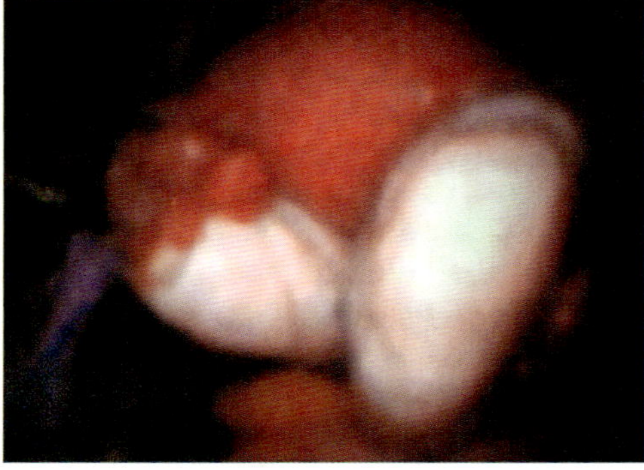

Fig. 7: Polycystic ovaries

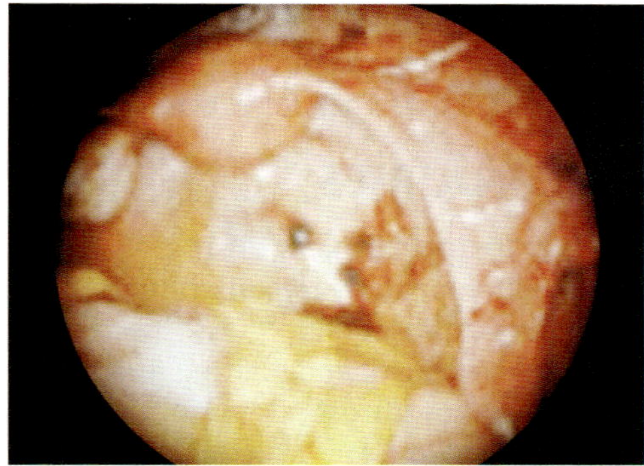

Fig. 8: Endometriosis

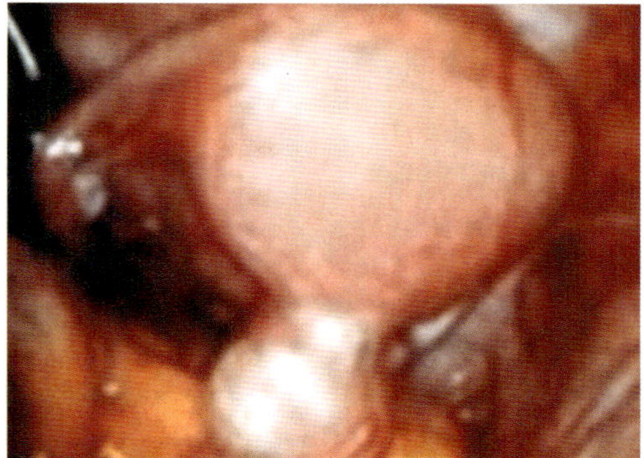

Fig. 9: Subserous myoma

Management

- Immediately stop insufflation
- Remove the needle
- Place the patient in the left lateral decubitus position
- Administer 100% oxygen, and give cardiac support
- The gas embolism may be broken up with external cardiac massage, but definitive treatment is placement of a central line for aspiration of the gas from the right side of the heart and from the pulmonary vasculature.

RETROPERITONEAL MAJOR VESSEL INJURY

Laceration of major abdominal blood vessels is one of the least common but most life-threatening complications in laparoscopy. These occur in approximately 3 cases per 10,000 laparoscopies, may occur during insertion of the Veress or the primary trocar.

When placing the Veress needle, the patient must be in the horizontal position (not Trendelenburg).

Immediate recognition of the injury is paramount.

Signs and Management

- If blood flows from the open Veress needle
- If the patient's vital signs rapidly decompensate after Veress or trocar insertion, prompt action must be taken
- With a retroperitoneal hemorrhage, the peritoneal cavity may not show signs of bleeding. If major vessel injury is a possibility, notify the anesthesiologist in order to place a central line and order blood products, make a midline incision for good exposure, and immediately call a vascular surgeon.

ABDOMINAL WALL VESSEL INJURY

The primary vessels injured are the epigastric vessels (inferior and superficial) and the superficial circumflex iliac vessel.

Prevention

- Know the positions of these vessels and identify the superficial ones by transilluminating the abdominal wall
- The inferior epigastric artery cannot be transilluminated but can be seen intraperitoneally beneath the peritoneum between the insertion of the round ligament at the inguinal canal and the obliterated umbilical artery
- One can improve the chance of successfully avoiding the vessels by placing the trocars lateral to their usual location, which is 5.5 cm from the midline. Therefore, placing the trocars 8 cm lateral to the midline and 8 cm above the pubic symphysis should help to avoid injury to the epigastric vessels
- Additional precautions include using the smallest trocar possible.

Management

Try to coagulate the vessel with electrocautery.

- A Foley catheter can be placed through the trocar and the balloon inflated with saline with upward traction on the catheter, maintained with a clamp on the abdominal side to slow the bleeding until more definitive measures can be performed
- Transabdominal sutures have also been advocated
- Enlarge the incision and selectively ligate the epigastric vessels.

INTESTINAL INJURY

Direct mechanical injury to the gastrointestinal (GI) tract is less common than thermal injuries. Risk of injury is higher with:

- Previous abdominal surgeries or
- A history of abdominal infections, such as pelvic inflammatory disease (PID) or a ruptured appendix.

Prevention

- Displacement of the bowel from the pelvis with a blunt probe
- Blunt dissection of the bowel should be avoided
- Disposable trocars.

Thermal injury to the bowel is not always evident intraoperatively and most intestinal burns less than 5 cm in diameter can be managed expectantly.

If the small bowel injury is not recognized intraoperatively, the patient generally presents on the 3rd or 4th postoperative day with:

- Lower abdominal pain
- Mild fever
- Slight nausea and
- Anorexia.

By the 5th or 6th postoperative day, symptoms include:

- Fever
- Severe pain in the abdomen
- Nausea
- Vomiting
- Constipation
- Raised white cell count and
- Signs of peritonitis.
- Instruments should be checked properly for insulation
- Use of bipolar instruments as much as possible should be done.

BLADDER INJURIES

Intraoperative Signs

- Air in the catheter and urinary bag while insufflation
- Bladder appears pushed by the accessory trocar as it is advanced through the abdominal wall
- Hematuria
- Leak of indigo carmine from the trauma site.

Postoperative Signs

- Decreased urine output
- Hematuria or
- Suprapubic pain.

Treatment

- Empty the bladder before trocar placement
- Small retroperitoneal injuries can be treated with an indwelling Foley catheter for 7–10 days, but larger or intraperitoneal injuries have to be repaired through endosuturing or a laparotomy.

URETERIC INJURIES

These injuries can usually occur during:

- Sharp dissection of an ovary adherent to the sidewall
- Dessication of uterosacrals
- Ligating, transecting or coagulating the uterines
- During removal of fibrosis or endometriotic implants from the ureters
- Performing laparoscopic oophorectomy, presacral neurectomy, lysis of severe bowel or pelvic sidewall adhesions
- Performing hysterectomy
- Vaginal cuff closure.

Symptoms

- Flank pain (secondary to hydronephrosis)
- Urinoma
- Ascites (if the ureter is transected).

Prevention

- Knowledge of proper surgical anatomy of the ureters
- Utmost care in cases of endometriosis and adhesions as the anatomy is distorted in such patients
- In case the ureters are not visualized properly, it should be identified by retroperitoneal dissection.

Management

- Urologist should be immediately consulted
- Retrograde or antegrade stenting should be attempted foremost
- Laparotomy, f/b ureteroureterostomy or ureteroneocystostomy.

CONCLUSION

At its essence, laparoscopy remains an intra-abdominal procedure and so shares all intraoperative and postoperative risks of laparotomy, including infection and injury to the adjacent intra-abdominal structures.

Hence, it is only by meticulous attention to detail, complete familiarity with the instruments, extensive knowledge of the intrapelvic structures as also seen through the laparoscope and thorough experience that laparoscopy can be performed safely, accurately and to the maximum benefit of the patient.

BIBLIOGRAPHY

1. Bouillot JL, Fingerhut A, Paquet JC, et al. Are routine preoperative chest radiographs useful in general surgery? A prospective, multicentre study in 3,959 patients. Association des Chirurgiens de l'Assistance Publique pour les Evaluations medicales. Eur J Surg. 1996;162(8): 597-604.
2. Hirvonen EA, Poikolainen EO, Paakkonen ME, et al. The adverse hemodynamic effects of anesthesia, head-up tilt, and carbon dioxide pneumoperitoneum during laparoscopic cholecystectomy. Surg Endosc. 2000;14(3):272-7.
3. Hurd WW, Wang L, Schemmel MT. A comparison of the relative risk of vessel injury with conical versus pyramidal laparoscopic trocars in a rabbit model. Am J Obstet Gynecol. 1995;173(6): 1731-3.
4. Jansen FW, Kapiteyn K, Trimbos-Kemper T, et al. Complications of laparoscopy: a prospective multicenter observational study. Br J Obstet Gynaecol Scand. 1997;104(5):595-600.
5. Loffer FD. Endoscopy in high risk patients. Am J Obstet gynecol. 1980;55(5):643-8.
6. Loffer FD. Endoscopy in high risk patients. In: Martin DC. Manual of endoscopy. Santa Fe Springs, CA: J Am Assoc gynecol laparosc; 1990. p.43.
7. Mayol J. Garci-Aguilar J, Ortiz-Oshiro E, et al. Risks of minimal access approach for lap surgery. WJ Surg. 1997;21(5):529-33.
8. Nezhat C. Operative gynaecologic laparoscopy-principles and techniques. New York: McGraw-Hill Education; 1995.
9. Rothenberg SS, Georgeson K, Decou JM, et al. Pediatric endosurgery and innovative techniques. 2000;4.
10. Soderstrom RM. Injuries to major vessels during endoscopy. J Am Assoc Gynecol Laparosc. 1997;4(3):395-8.
11. Yim SF, Yuen PM. Randomized double-masked comparison of radially expanding access device and conventional cutting tip trocar in laparoscopy. Obstet Gynecol. 2001;97(3):435-8.
12. Yuzpe AA. Pneumoperitoneum needle and trocar injuries in laparoscopy. A survey on possible contributing factors and prevention. J Reprod Med. 1990;35(5):485-90.

42.3 ADHESIONOLYSIS

Pranay Shah

INTRODUCTION

Peritoneal adhesions can cause bowel obstruction, pelvic pain, and infertility. A major detriment to the success of fertility promoting operations is postoperative adhesion formation. It is important to understand the mechanism of adhesion formation and use optimal techniques for adhesiolysis.

ADHESION FORMATION

Normal fibrinolytic activity usually prevents fibrinous attachments (fibrinous exudates) for 72–96 hours following injury. Mesothelial repair occurs within 5 days of injury. A single cell layer of mesothelium covers the injured raw area replacing fibrinous exudates. However, if the fibrinolytic activity of the peritoneum is suppressed, fibroblasts will migrate, proliferate, and form firm fibrous adhesion with collagen deposition and vascular proliferation. The factors that suppress fibrinolytic activity and promote formation of postoperative adhesions are listed in Box 1.

Postoperative Adhesion Formation

Intraoperatively, the surgeon can minimize adhesion formation through careful tissue handling, complete hemostasis, abundant irrigation, limiting thermal injury, infection prophylaxis, and minimizing foreign body reaction. At laparotomy, even when proper microsurgical techniques are used, adhesion reformation is found at 37–72% of surgical sites and 51% of patients develop new adhesions after reproductive surgery at laparotomy. When performed properly, operative laparoscopy fullfills the major tenets of microsurgery. With few exceptions, operative laparoscopy resulted in fewer reformed and new adhesions.

Box 1 Predisposing factors for adhesion formation

- Ischemia
- Drying of serosal surfaces
- Excessive suturing
- Omental patches
- Traction of peritoneum
- Blood clots retained in peritoneal cavity
- Adnexal trauma
- Infection

LAPAROSCOPIC ADHESIOLYSIS–TECHNIQUE

To perform adhesiolysis, two or three accessory ports are required. Adhesions should be cut close to affected organ at both ends and removed rather than broken. (Fig. 1) Vascular adhesions are coagulated before cutting. Thin, filmsy avascular adhesions are stretched and then cut. Bowel adhesions are severed first followed by periovarian and peritubal adhesions. This approach allows for progressive exposure of pelvic structures. Once the intestines are freed from adjacent structures, they can be pushed cephalad.

Adherent ovaries are freed from the pelvic sidewall, broad ligament, tubes and uterus. Once the ovaries are lifted from the cul-de-sac and mobilized, all peritubal adhesions are removed. Bleeding areas are coagulated using bipolar current at low setting (15–20 W). When there are dense adhesions among different organs (bowel, uterus, ovaries, pelvic sidewall, and anterior abdominal wall), hydrodissection with suction-irrigator probe is useful in creating tissue planes before dissection. Once the pelvic structures are freed and hemostasis achieved, the cul-de-sac is filled with Ringer's lactate and the adnexa allowed to float in clear fluid. Flimsy adhesions that are difficult to identify on the surface of the ovary become visible as they float from the ovarian cortex. These adhesions are grasped and cut.

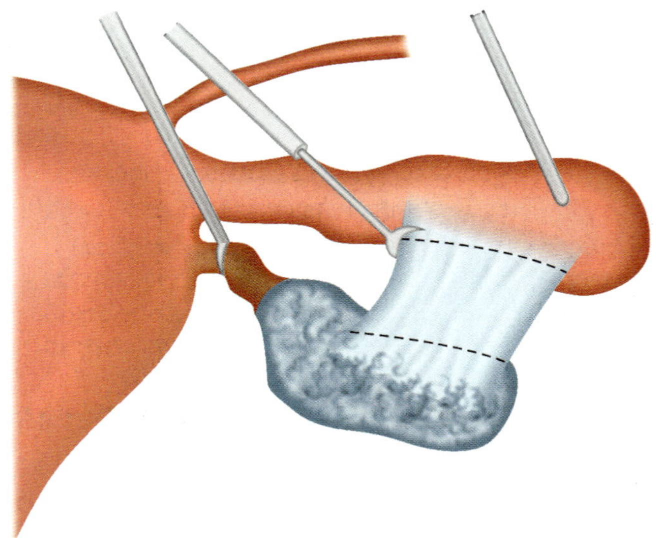

Fig 1: Technique for adhesiolysis

ADHESION PREVENTION—THE VALUE OF ADJUVANTS

A recent Cochrane database systemic review investigated whether pharmacological and liquid agents used as adjuvant during pelvic surgery in infertility patients lead to a reduction in the incidence or severity of postoperative adhesion (re)formation, and/or an improvement in subsequent pregnancy rates. The results of the review are as follows: there is some evidence that intraperitoneal steroid administration decreases the incidence and severity of postoperative adhesion formation; intraperitoneal administration of dextran did not decrease postoperative adhesion formation at second look laparoscopy; there is no evidence that intra-abdominal crystalloid instillation, calcium channel blocking adgents, nonsteroidal anti-inflammatory drugs (NSAIDs) and proteolytics decrease postoperative adhesion formation.

Barrier agents for the prevention of adhesion formation are commercially available. The Cochrane Menstrual Disorders and Subfertility Group investigated the effects of these agents have on postoperative adhesion formation. The 15 randomized controlled trials (RCTs) comprised laparoscopic and laparotomy surgical techniques. Results of the investigation were as follows: oxidized regenerated cellulose Interceed™ (Johnson and Johnson Medical, Somerville, NJ) reduces the incidence of adhesion formation and reformation at laparoscopy and laparotomy in the pelvis; polytetrafluoroethylene Gore-Tex™ (WL GORE and Associates, Flagstaff, AZ) appears to be superior to Interceed™ in preventing adhesion formation in the pelvis but is limited by the need for suturing and later removal; Seprafilm™ (Genzyme, Cambridge, MA) does not appear to be effective in preventing adhesion formation.

If Interceed™ is to be used for prevention of adhesion formation, the intrapelvic fluid should be completely aspirated. A piece of Interceed large enough to cover the at-risk area is placed and moistened with a small volume of irrigant. Complete hemostasis must be achieved prior to placing the material. If hemostasis has not been achieved, the Interceed will turn brown or black and must be replaced as this may actually increase adhesion formation. Animal studies and clinical trials of a gel form of modified hyaluronic acid, a naturally occurring glycosaminoglycan, show evidence for reducing de novo adhesion formation, Intergel™ (Gynecare—Johnson and Johnson Inc. Somerville NJ) is commercially available for open surgery use.

The ideal barrier material should be easy to apply, both in open and laparoscopic surgeries. Additionally, it should be nonreactive, persist during the critical wound re-epithelization period, stay inplace on the target tissue for several days, and eventually be resorbed following peritoneal healing.

Ongoing research suggests that Adept® (icodextrin 4%) may be closest to the ideal profile. A nonviscous liquid, Adept can be used for both open and laparoscopic surgery. Adept is simple to use, being instilled slowly at the end of surgical procedures and used during surgery as an irrigant. A 1.5 liter bag of Adept (enabling 500 mL to be used during procedures with 1,000 mL remaining for instillation at the end of surgery).

A new product, currently undergoing clinical trials, SprayGel™ (Confluent Surgical, Waltham, MA), also meets these criteria. The gel remains intact for the next 5–7 days before breaking down by hydrolysis, and eventual clearance through the kidneys. Preclinical studies of SprayGel™ adhesion barrier demonstrate that it is a remarkably inert, biocompatible material, resulting in no signs of toxicity. In a European myomectomy study, a significant difference was demonstrated in the tenacity of adhesions between the treated and control population, when comparing the initial and second-look laparoscopies. The product is currently under review in a multicenter pivotal clinical trial in US.

The Seprafilm® Adhesion Barrier is a sterile, bioresorbable translucent membrane composed of two anionic polysaccharides, sodium hyaluronate (HA) and carboxymethylcellulose (CMC). It serves as a temporary bioresorbable barrier separating apposing tissue surfaces. When applied within abdominopelvic cavity, it can be expected to reduce adhesions during the early phases of peritoneal wound repair.

SECOND LOOK LAPAROSCOPY

The term "second look laparoscopy" refers to laparoscopy after a primary reconstructive surgery procedure at laparotomy or laparoscopy. The interval between the primary surgery and second look laparoscopy can vary from 3 days to 9 months (usually day 8 postoperative). Fibrosis of unlysed adhesions begins 3 days after serosal trauma and is completed by 21 days. Endoscopic adhesiolysis is performed in an attempt to restore a greater degree of normalacy to the pelvic structures and improve intrauterine pregnancy rates. Studies have suggested that second look laparoscopies effectively reduce peritoneal adhesions, however, its impact on fertility is less certain.

CONCLUSION

Adhesion formation after gynecologic surgery is common. When compared to laparotomy, laparoscopy has been shown to result in less de novo adhesion formation, but adhesion reformation continues to be a problem. Sequelae of intra-abdominal adhesion formation can be fatal, result in infertility and may be a source of chronic pelvic pain.

42.4 ENDOMETRIOSIS

Pratap Kumar, Bimal John

INTRODUCTION

Endometriosis, although first described over 300 years ago in medical literature, continues to vax the gynecologist, and is one of the most common gynecological conditions. Approximately 7–10% of women in the reproductive age-group are diagnosed with endometriosis, with over 38% infertile women and 75–80% women with chronic pelvic pain also being diagnosed with endometriosis. Management of endometriosis focuses on pain relief and restoration of fertility, and includes both medical as well as surgical treatment. The role of laparoscopy in the diagnoses and treatment of endometriosis is constantly evolving, and has become more or less the standard.

LAPAROSCOPY FOR THE DIAGNOSIS OF ENDOMETRIOSIS

Signs and symptoms of endometriosis are nonspecific making the diagnosis of this condition difficult. Laparoscopy is the gold standard test in diagnosing endometriosis in clinical practice. It is a relatively simple and minor procedure when solely used for diagnosis, and done after careful review of medical history and pelvic exam. Referral may be essential for definitive diagnosis of endometriosis by laparoscopy or laparotomy and biopsy, or for surgical ablation. Possible exception to employing laparoscopy for diagnosis is if the disease is visible in the vagina or elsewhere on examination.

Endometriotic implants vary in appearance, and the experience of the surgeon performing laparoscopy is a critical factor in identification. Endometriosis has multiple presentations and histological confirmation of visually identified endometriosis ranges from 9% to 90%. The lesions may appear as black, dark brown or bluish implants or deposits, although even red, serous, and even clear vesicles have been reported. Diagnosing endometriosis solely on visual identification, therefore, can lead to both misdiagnosis as well as over-diagnosis. Howard et al. also described "near-contact" laparoscopy, which results in up to an eightfold magnification of lesions, and can identify atypical implants as small as 400 micrometers (Figs 1 to 4).

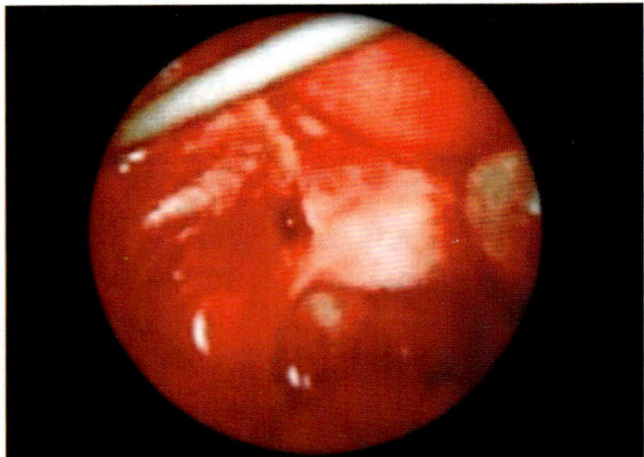

Fig. 1: Red and purple spot of endometriosis on uterosacral

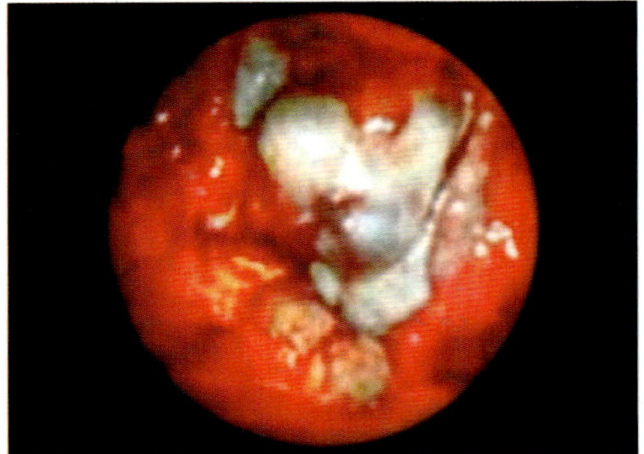

Fig. 3: Chocolate cysts

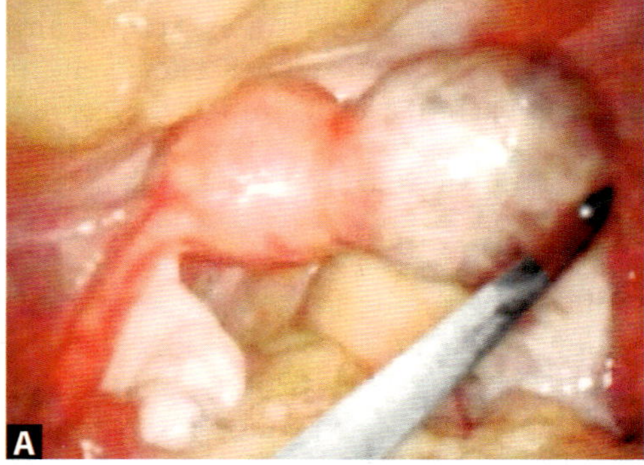

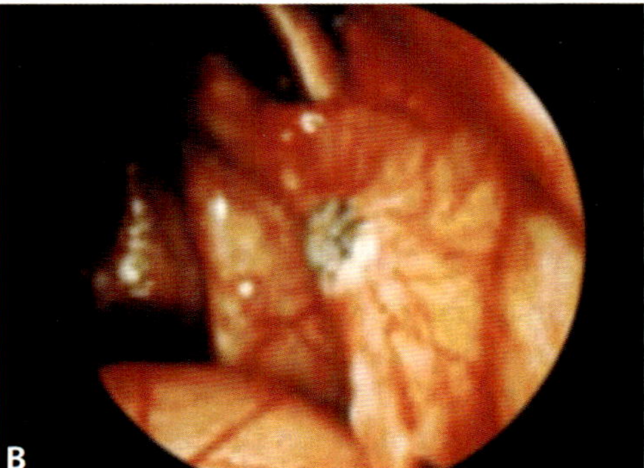

Figs 2A and B: Endometriosis

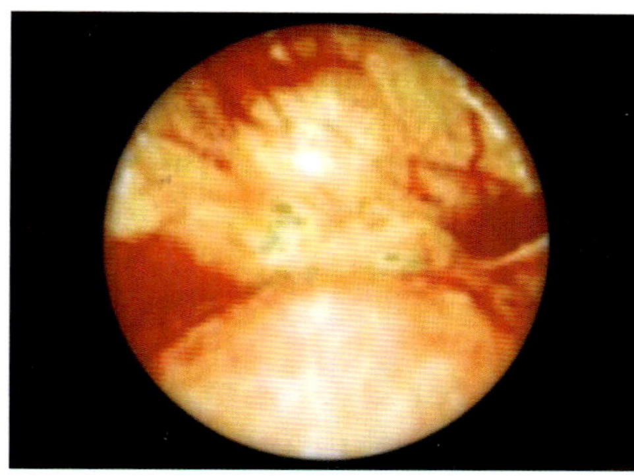

Fig. 4: Dark lesions of endometriosis (Gun powder burns)

DIAGNOSTIC FINDING CONDITIONS ON LAPAROSCOPY

Staging endometriosis can aid in determining the most optimal method of treatment. Depending on the size and depth of the implant, bilaterality and the severity of adhesions, the American Society of Reproductive Medicine (1996) has classified endometriosis as:

- Stage I—Minimal disease
- Stage II—Mild disease
- Stage III—Moderate disease
- Stage IV—Severe disease.

This classification has been reported to have very poor correlation with the severity of symptoms and also lacks reproducibility.

Operative Laparoscopy in Endometriosis

The laparoscopic management of endometriosis usually includes lysis of pelvic adhesions, dissection of ovaries from cul-de-sac or pelvic sidewall, freeing tubal adhesions and chromopertubation to assess patency, fulguration of endometrial implants, resection of endometriomas, and uterosacral nerve ablation or presacral nerve resection for chronic pelvic pain.

A laparoscopy is required if the hormonal treatment used in mild or moderate cases of endometriosis fail, or if endometriosis is severe or debilitating. Patients presenting with symptoms indicative of endometriosis require visual inspection of the pelvis at laparoscopy, and histologic confirmation of at least one lesion. It is recommended that the procedure should be documented in detail, providing the type, location and extent of all lesions in the operative notes, and the findings preferably recorded on video or DVD. Although the evidence is insufficient, laparoscopy is not recommended during or within 3 months of hormonal treatment as it can lead to underdiagnosis.

Parietal and visceral peritoneal adhesions to pelvic organs, bowel and omentum need careful dissection using atraumatic forceps and aquadissection or blunt dissection. Thick or fibrous bands may require cauterization and sharp dissection.

Mild to moderate endometriosis is treated by ablation (cauterizing) of the endometriotic deposits. Diathermy, yttrium-aluminium-garnet (YAG) or carbon dioxide laser and helium thermal coagulator (Helica) are the three electrosurgical devices available. Overall, the recurrence rate is 19% and is similar for all techniques. In Stage III or IV endometriosis, conservative surgery to excise or ablate all endometriotic lesions is recommended.

Genitourinary and GI lesions are best operated by advanced laparoscopic surgeons as involvement of the bladder, ureter, intestine and rectum is common. Careful excision or ablation of all endometriotic spots from the surface of these structures is necessary, and is best done by vaporization, continuous irrigation and hydrodissection.

Surgical Treatment of Pain Associated with Endometriosis

In women with laparoscopically confirmed disease, pain associated with endometriosis is controlled by hormonally suppressing the ovarian function for about 6 months, thereby also reducing the menstrual flow. All hormonal drugs seem to be equally effective in treatment, although their side effects and expense varies and is the criteria for selection for a particular patient. Surgical ablation of endometriotic lesions reduces pain at 6 months compared to diagnostic laparoscopy, but there is no evidence to suggest the need for laparoscopic uterine nerve ablation (LUNA) as well.

Two randomized control trials (RCTs) have addressed pain relief in endometriosis. The first by Sutton et al. RCT compared laser ablation of minimal-moderate endometriosis plus laparoscopic uterine nerve ablation with diagnostic laparoscopy alone for pain relief. At 6 months' follow-up, patients treated surgically reported a significant improvement in symptoms compared to patients who were subjected to only diagnostic laparoscopy (63% vs. 23%).

In the second RCT, Abbott et al. compared laparoscopic removal of endometriotic deposits with diagnostic laparoscopy in women with dysmenorrhea due to endometriosis. They established that laparoscopic excision significantly improved pain symptoms compared with diagnostic laparoscopy at 6 months (80% vs. 32%, $P = 0.002$).

There is sufficient evidence indicating that surgical procedure is effective in relieving pain in majority of the women with endometriosis. Incomplete excision, postoperative disease recurrence or endometriosis not being the real cause for pain, are few reasons why surgical procedures "fail" in some women.

The rather extreme surgical treatment of hysterectomy with bilateral salpingo-oophorectomy, not investigated in RCTs, remains an option, particularly in older women past their childbearing age, or for women who suffer from intractable pelvic pain. In this procedure, care should be taken to ensure that all visible endometriotic tissues are removed. Bilateral salpingo-oophorectomy also results in improved pain relief.

Presacral neurectomy, a procedure during which sympathetic nerves from the uterus are divided, can be effective in women with midline pelvic pain. This procedure involves the interruption of sympathetic innervation of the uterus and central pelvis at the level of the superior hypogastric plexus. This may be performed either by laparoscopy or by laparotomy, but requires more surgical skill than the laparoscopic ablation of uterosacral nerve.

There is insufficient evidence of benefit to justify the use of preoperative or postoperative hormonal treatment as it does not seem to improve pain relief. Similar findings were reported in the Royal College of Obstetricians and Gynaecologists (RCOG) guidelines for the management of endometriosis in 2006 and also in a RCT by Busacca et al. where a postoperative course of the gonadotropin-releasing hormone (GnRH) analog leuprolide acetate depot (3.75 mg) for 3 months did not significantly impact the pain associated with endometriosis. But in a recent clinical review, Farquhar recommended that although preoperative hormonal therapy has no definite benefit, postoperative hormonal therapy helps in reducing endometriotic pain.

Surgical Treatment for Endometriosis Associated Infertility

Two modalities found to be beneficial and supported by evidence-based medicine for the treatment of endometriosis-associated infertility are conservative surgical treatment by laparoscopy and assisted reproductive technology. Surgical treatment increases the chance of conception in women with endometriosis.

In minimal and mild endometriosis, suppression of ovarian function to improve fertility is not effective, but surgical ablation of endometriotic lesions along with adhesiolysis is very effective. Evidence suggests that after laparoscopic treatment, fertility rates improve to around 40–70%, and fertility is inversely proportional to the severity of endometriosis. However, in moderate to severe cases, improvement of fertility rates after surgical treatment of endometriosis has not been established.

A recent Cochrane Database review by Johnson et al. concluded that flushing the fallopian tubes with oil-soluble media improved the pregnancy rates significantly.

Overall, pregnancy rates are highest 6–18 months after surgical treatment of endometriosis.

Preoperative or postoperative hormonal therapy did not improve fertility significantly.

Laparoscopy for Endometriosis in Women of Reproductive Age

Conservative surgical treatment involves removal of the endometriotic implants during laparoscopy or laparotomy, without removing any reproductive organ. It is a good option for women in their reproductive years wanting to become pregnant, and women who are reluctant to use hormonal treatment. Recurrence rates following laparoscopic treatment at two years range from 2% to 47%. The risk increases with the severity of the condition, particularly if endometriosis had affected areas outside the uterus.

Laparoscopic Cystectomy

When compared to procedures like drainage and coagulation of endometriomas, laparoscopic cystectomy for ovarian endometriomas improved fertility rates significantly as well as reduced the chances of recurrence.

Endometriomas less than 2 cm in diameter may be coagulated, laser ablated or excised using scissors or biopsy forceps. All visible lesions and scars must be coagulated or excised from the ovarian surface to prevent recurrence. Cystectomy is recommended for endometriomas of or greater than 2 cm diameter, as simply draining the endometrioma or even partial resection of the cyst wall can cause recurrence due to functional residual tissue in the remaining tissue. The cyst is punctured and the contents aspirated with the suction probe. The cyst wall should be separated and peeled-off entirely from the ovarian stroma to prevent recurrence. Any bleeding vessels from the stroma should be coagulated. The ovarian wall usually does not require closure, but if the defect is greater than 5 cm, suturing, usually a single suture, may be required to approximate the edges. Fibrin sealants may also be used to approximate such large defects without adhesion formation.

Two RCTs also found that laparoscopic cystectomy reduced recurrence of pelvic pain symptoms compared with laparoscopic drainage and electrosurgical ablation of the cyst-wall. Complication rates were similar in both procedures. Even after 26 months postsurgery, no significant differences were seen in cyst recurrence rates (dysmenorrhea: 16% with cystectomy vs.

53% with drainage, P <0.05; deep dyspareunia: 20% with cystectomy vs. 75% with drainage, P <0.05; nonmenstrual pelvic pain: 10% with cystectomy vs. 53% with drainage, P <0.05; cyst: 6% with cystectomy vs. 19% with drainage, P not significant). A second RCT found that laparoscopic cystectomy significantly reduced the recurrence rates of dysmenorrhea compared with laparoscopic coagulation of the endometriotic areas, at the end of 2 years, but found no significant difference in cyst recurrence rate. In this study, 100 women with endometriomas, who either had dysmenorrhea (67 women) or infertility (62 women) were examined. Dysmenorrhea was noted in 15.8% patients with cystectomy compared to 56.7% patients who underwent fenestration and coagulation only (P=0.001). Coagulation or laser vaporization of endometriomas without excision of the pseudo capsule was associated with a significantly higher risk of cyst recurrence. Laparoscopic cystectomy for endometriomas is a better choice than fenestration and coagulation, as cystectomy leads to a lower recurrence of signs and symptom, a lower rate of reoperation, and a higher cumulative pregnancy rate.

Laparoscopic Helium Plasma Coagulation (Helica)

Laparoscopic helium plasma coagulation is a more recent minimally invasive procedure used to vaporize endometrial deposits using an ionized beam of helium gas directed at the endometrial deposits. However, lack of current evidence on the safety and efficacy of this procedure necessitates the use of this procedure only with special arrangements for consent. Until date, there has not been any comparative trial to measure the efficacy of ablation using Helica with that of other electrosurgical devices.

Prognosis of Endometriosis

There is evidence indicating that endometriosis may stabilize or resolve on its own. In a minor study that randomized patients with progestin or placebo, regardless of treatment option followed, follow-up laparoscopy after one year indicated that endometriosis had progressed in 47% of patients, while in 25% the disease resolved, and in another 25% the disease remained unchanged. Natural history of the disease indicates that endometriosis may recur even after surgery, irrespective of whether patients are on hormonal treatment or not. Similarly, there is a tendency for postmenopausal women to develop the condition if they use hormone therapy. It has also been seen that pregnancy rates after conservative surgery in women previously considered infertile due to endometriosis, may be as high as 75% for mild endometriosis, 50–60% for moderate cases, and 30–40% for severe endometriosis.

CONCLUSION

- Laparoscopy is the 'gold standard' for the diagnosis of endometriosis
- Visual identification, although usually adequate, can lead to misdiagnosis, and histologic confirmation of at least one lesion is considered ideal
- Complete ablation of endometriotic lesions reduce disease-related pain, enhance fertility and reduce chances of recurrence
- Laparoscopic uterine nerve ablation does not relieve pain when performed without endometriotic excision.
  - Surgical excision of mild-moderate endometriosis significantly improves fertility, although similar benefit is not established in moderate-severe disease
- Cyst-wall excision of endometrioma = 2 cm is necessary to reduce recurrence and provide better pain relief
- Benefit of pre- and postoperative hormonal therapy is not proven for enhancing fertility, but some RCTs suggest postoperative hormonal therapy reduces endometriotic pain.

BIBLIOGRAPHY

1. Abbott J, Hawe J, Hunter D, et al. Laparoscopic excision of endometriosis: a randomized, placebo-controlled trial. Fertil Steril. 2004;82:878-84.
2. Alborzi S, Momtahan M, Parsanezhad ME, et al. A prospective, randomized study comparing laparoscopic ovarian cystectomy versus fenestration and coagulation in patients with endometriomas. Fertil Steril. 2004;82(6):1633-7.
3. Busacca M, Somigliana S, Bianchi S, et al. Postoperative GnRH analogue treatment after conservative surgery for symptomatic endometriosis Stage III-IV: a randomized controlled trial. Hum Reprod. 2001:16(11):2399-402.
4. Donnez J, Nisolle M. Laparoscopic management of large ovarian endometrial cyst: use of fibrin sealant. Surgery. 1991;7:163-8.
5. Farquhar CM. Extracts from "Clinical Evidence": endometriosis. BMJ. 2000;320;1449-52.
6. Fedele L, Bianchi S, Zanconato G, et al. Long-term follow-up after conservative surgery for rectovaginal endometriosis. Am J Obstet Gynecol. 2004;190:1020-4.

7. Hasson HM: Laparoscopic management of ovarian cysts. J Reprod Med. 1991;56:349-5.
8. Howard FM. The role of laparoscopy as a diagnostic tool in chronic pelvic pain. Bailliere's Best Prac Res Clin Obstet Gynecol. 2000;3:467-94.
9. Johnson NP, Farquhar CM, Crossley S, et al. A double-blind randomised controlled trial of laparoscopic uterine nerve ablation for women with chronic pelvic pain. Br J Obstet Gynaecol. 2004;111:950-9.
10. Johnson NP, Vandekerckhove P, Watson A, et al. Tubal flushing for subfertility. Cochrane Database Syst Rev. 2005;(2):CD003718.
11. Kennedy S, Bergqvist A, Chapron C, et al. ESHRE guideline for the diagnosis and treatment of endometriosis. Hum Reprod. 2005;20(10):2698-704.
12. Laparoscopic helium plasma coagulation for the treatment of endometriosis. National Institute for Health and Clinical Excellence; 2006.
13. Martin DC. Pain and infertility—a rationale for different treatment approaches. Br J Int J Obstet Gynecol. 1995;102 (12):2-3.
14. Mounsey AL, Wilgus A, Slawson DC. Diagnosis and Management of Endometriosis. Am Fam Physician. 2006;74(4):594-600.
15. Olive DL, Pritts EA. Treatment of Endometriosis. N Engl J Med. 2001;345(4):266-75.
16. Osuga Y, Koga K, Tsutsumi O, et al, Role of laparoscopy in the treatment of endometriosis-associated infertility. Gynecol Obstet Invest. 2002;53(1):33-9.
17. Porpora MG, Pultrone DC, Bellavia M, et al. Reproductive outcome after laparoscopic treatment of endometriosis. Clin Exp Obstet Gynecol. 2002;29(4):271-3.
18. Rawson JM. Prevalence of endometriosis in asymptomatic women. J Reprod Med. 1991;36:513-5.
19. Revelli A, Modotti M, Ansaldi C, et al. Recurrent endometriosis: a review of biological and clinical aspects. Obstet Gynecol Surv. 1995;50(10):747-54.
20. Sutton CJ, Ewen SP, Whitelaw N, et al, A randomized, double-blind, controlled trial of laser laparoscopy in the treatment of pelvic pain associated with minimal, mild, and moderate endometriosis. Fertil Steril. 1994;62:696-700.
21. The investigation and management of endometriosis. RCOG, Green-top Guideline No. 24; 2006.
22. Wykes CB, Clark TJ, Khan KS. Accuracy of laparoscopy in the diagnosis of endometriosis: a systematic quantitative review. BJOG. 2004;111:1204-12.
23. Yap C, Furness S, Farquhar C. Pre- and postoperative medical therapy for endometriosis surgery. Cochrane Database Syst Rev. 2004;(3):CD003678.

42.5 ENDOSCOPY IN INFERTILITY

Shyam Desai, Nikhil Jani

INTRODUCTION

A detailed and repeatable visualization of the pelvis has been enabled by way of "Laparoscopy", which has had a great impact on the management of infertility. The advent of endoscopy and improvement in technique and technology with the addition of "Hysteroscopy" to the endoscopic armamentarium has allowed direct visualization of the endometrial cavity, tubal ostia and cervical canal. This has improved our ability to understand, diagnose and treat the various causes of infertility.

We focus on the efficacy and limitations of some of the important fertility promoting endoscopic procedures, restriction of space precludes detailing of technique. Endoscopy can be used for both diagnosis and therapy.

DIAGNOSTIC

As a diagnostic tool, a combined laparoscopic and hysteroscopic examination is the gold standard for the evaluation of infertility (A Golan et al. 1996). Direct visual examination is superior to hysterosalpingography justifying use of the more invasive procedure.

Laparoscopy allows an assessment of tubal patency and also identifies pelvic pathology while hysteroscopy helps in diagnosis of intracavitary lesions. Chromopertubation demonstrating a free spill at the fimbrial end is reassuring, but distension of the tube with blockage at the fimbrial end indicates hydrosalpinx formation, which can be easily detected during chromopertubation.

Development of smaller diameter endoscopies has further simplified the procedure. Microlaparoscopy and minihysteroscopy, performed under local anesthesia or mild sedation have a high degree of diagnostic accuracy despite a smaller visual field, and have been proposed as the first line diagnostic procedures (Campo et al. 1999).

Salpingoscopy and falloposcopy allow evaluation of the tubal lumen. The former is a transfimbrial approach allowing visualization from the ampullary-isthmic junction to the fimbriae. The latter is a transcervical approach allowing assessment of the tubal lumen from the uterotubal ostium to the fimbria. Falloposcopy has the potential to become a standard investigation for infertility since tubes that look normal externally can have lesions of the endosalpinx (M Antony et al. 1996). High cost of equipment has been a major deterrent. Transvaginal hydrolaparoscopy was introduced to assess the tubo-ovarian relationship. Since, it can only view the pouch of Douglas its use is limited.

THERAPEUTIC

The decreased morbidity and shortened hospital stay, an opportunity to diagnose and treat at the same time and a reduction in postoperative adhesion formation has led to the immense popularity of operative endoscopy. Surgeries performed include:

Ovarian Factor

- Polycystic ovary syndrome—Ovarian drilling
- Endometriosis—Ablation
- Ovarian cysts—Excision or cystectomy.

Tubal Factor

- Distal tubal occlusion—Fimbrioplasty, neosalpingostomy
- Proximal tubal obstruction—Transcervical tubal recanalization, reversal of sterilization.

Uterine Factor

- Asherman's syndrome—Adhesiolysis
- Congenital anomalies—Metroplasty, excision of rudimentary horn
- Fibroids—Myomectomy.

Peritoneal Factor

- Adnexal adhesions—Adhesiolysis.

Polycystic Ovary Syndrome

Infertility in polycystic ovary syndrome (PCOS) is related to anovulation. Surgical induction of ovulation was achieved by wedge resection of the ovary. This fell into disrepute because of increased morbidity and postoperative adhesion formation. Endoscopy revived this surgical option in the form of ovarian drilling. Ovulation occurs presumably because of a decrease in stromal mass or disruption of parenchymal blood flow leading to reduction in ovarian androgen production and luteinizing hormone levels (Gjoannaess et al. 1984).

Ovarian drilling can be performed using unipolar needle cautery or laser (Daniell et al. 1989). The ovarian surface is fulgurated at evenly spaced points. Cautery is maintained until the ovarian capsule and cortex is penetrated, 5–6 seconds at each point using a current of 300–400 watts (A Balen et al. 2013). 4–8 punctures are enough with the use of the cautery (Tulandi et al. 1998).

For laser the number of punctures is higher 20–40 (TC Li et al., 1998). Restraint must be used as premature ovarian failure has been reported after too generous a drilling of the ovarian cortex. The peritoneal cavity should be lavaged to reduce risk of adhesions.

Results

To date there is no standardization of the technique. Ovulation rates ranging between 70% and 90% and pregnancy rates of 70% have been reported (Farquhar et al. 2000). The minimum "dose" of diathermy that is required and the modification for each patient needs to be determined.

Prognostic Factors

- Duration of infertility less than 3 years
- Use of diathermy rather than laser
- Pretreatment LH levels more than 10 IU/L
- Age less than 30 years.

Advantages

- As effective as gonadotropin therapy. One time procedure
- Intensive ultrasound monitoring not required
- Reduces risk of multiple pregnancy and ovarian hyperstimulation syndrome (OHSS)
- Increases sensitivity of ovary to stimulation.

Disadvantages

- Adhesion formation
- Possibility of inducing premature ovarian failure.

Recommendation

Cochrane database review states that the value of laparoscopic ovarian drilling as a primary treatment is undetermined. There is insufficient evidence to determine a difference in ovulation or pregnancy rates when compared to gonadotropin therapy in clomiphene resistant women. Multiple pregnancy rates are reduced. None of the modalities of drilling have any obvious advantages (Farquhar et al. 2000).

Endometriosis

Twenty to forty percent of subfertile women have endometriosis. The cause of infertility in endometriosis is debatable. In severe endometriosis distortion of the tubo-ovarian relationship may lead to infertility. In the absence of a mechanical factor, infertility is attributed to ectopic implants inducing a peritoneal inflammatory reaction, an autoimmune response or to related endocrine abnormalities. Surgical treatment involves:

- Ablation or resection of implants
- Correction of abnormal pelvic anatomy
- Management of endometriomas.

Ablation of Implants

Ablation of implants is done by coagulation, vaporization and excision. Coagulation can be achieved by using the unipolar or bipolar electrocautery, the endocoagulator or various surgical lasers. Laser is a more precise delivery system and causes less damage to the adjacent tissues. Results with all the techniques are comparable.

Correction of Tubo-ovarian Relationship

The range of adhesions encountered varies from fine avascular adhesions to extremely dense adhesions that completely obliterate tissue planes. Lysis of adhesions must be meticulous, causing minimal tissue trauma and maintaining complete hemostasis. Adhesions may be lysed by delicate pressure with scissors, aquadissection or blunt and sharp dissection. Vital structures must be clearly identified before dissection.

Management of Endometrioma

Cysts less than 3 cm are usually vaporized or coagulated. Cysts more than 3 cm are dealt with by cystectomy or drainage, stripping of the cyst wall and coagulation of the base and any remnant endometriotic tissue. Simple incision and drainage of the cyst leads to increased rate of recurrence. (H Reich et al. 1986). Extraovarian endometriotic cysts are formed by invagination of the ovarian cortex, therefore, ablation should be limited. Drainage of the cyst with eversion of the cyst wall gives good results (Brosens et al. 1996).

Results and Recommendation

Meta-analysis of literature suggests that in mild and moderate endometriosis laparoscopic ablation is superior to no treatment or medical treatment for infertility management (Adamson et al. 1994). Restoration of the tubo-ovarian relationship improves pregnancy rates with a cumulative pregnancy rate of 70%. Pregnancy outcome with laparoscopy or laparotomy for severe endometriosis does not differ significantly (Adamson et al. 1993) therefore, choice of technique should be based on surgical expertise.

Tubal Occlusion

Occlusion may be fimbrial or cornual.

Fimbrial Block or Hydrosalpinx

Fimbrial agglutination, fimbrial encapsulation and prefimbrial phimosis are sequlae of infection. Collection of fluid within the tubal lumen leads to the formation of hydrosalpinx. Chronic infection like genital tuberculosis is not uncommon in India. The fallopian tubes are the most common sites of involvement. These may form tubo-ovarian masses.

Fimbrioplasty

Distention of the fallopian tube with methylene blue dye facilitates surgery. The tube is stabilized holding the serosa with an atraumatic forceps. A 3 mm alligator forceps is introduced into the tubal ostium. Deglutination of the fimbria is achieved by opening the jaws of the forceps inside the lumen and gently withdrawing it from the tube number of times in different directions (Gomel, 1983).

Correction of prefimbrial phimosis is done by incising the fibrous bands constricting the infundibulum using blended current. Radial incisions are made along avascular points starting at the fimbrial end and going beyond the region of the constriction.

Results: Success rates range from 20% to 50% (Fayez, 1983). Ectopic pregnancy rate is seen in 5%.

Limitations: Forced insertion may lead to mucosal trauma leading to reformation of adhesions.

Neosalpingostomy

After distending the tube with dye the tube is inspected to locate site of scarring. The tube is stabilized and an incision is made extending from the ostium towards the ovary. Two to three radial incisions may be required to expose the fimbria.

Electrocautery, laser or microscissor can be used. Meticulous hemostasis using bipolar cautery and peritoneal lavage are essential to optimize outcome.

Results of reconstructive surgery are optimal when the tubal mucosa shows minimal damage, varying between 58% and 77% (Mage, 1988).

Prognostic factors for surgery are:

- Extent of adhesions
- Nature of adhesions
- Diameter of the hydrosalpinx less than or more than 1 cm
- Macroscopic condition of endosalpinx
- Tubal wall thickness.

Cornual Block

Cornual block occurs in approximately 15% of patients with tubal infertility. The technique of transcervical tubal cannulation was developed by Novy (1988) and it transformed the treatment of cornual occlusion.

A coaxial catheter system is used to access the tubal ostia under direct hysteroscopic vision. The block is removed by moving the catheter with the wire guide in and out of the tubal lumen. Laparoscopic control is maintained to avoid risk of tubal perforation and to facilitate passage of the cannula.

Results: Recanalization is achieved in 80–90% of tubes, and pregnancy rates are in the range of 40%. Compared to tubal microsurgery, the procedure gives better results and is minimally invasive, the ectopic pregnancy rates are also much lower. Pregnancy rates are poor when the wire guide is required to open the block.

Fibroids

Laparoscopy reveals subserous fibroids and bumpy irregularity caused by intramural fibromyomas, whereas hysteroscopy is useful in detecting and treating intracavitary submucous fibromyomatous polyps.

Laparoscopic myomectomy for intramural fibroids in the infertile patient was not encouraged because endoscopic suturing did not give a sound uterine scar. Currently this view is being opposed. Laparoscopic myomectomy for infertility should be attempted by an experienced surgeon.

Hysteroscopic polypectomy and myomectomy enhance fertility and should be the procedures of choice (Varasteh, 1999) for intrauterine lesions.

Adhesiolysis

An inverse relationship exists between the grade of adhesions and the pregnancy rate. Before commencing dissection a careful identification of intra-abdominal structures is essential. Adhesions should be coagulated before division. Thick adhesions should be divided one layer at a time to prevent trauma to underlying structures.

Intrauterine Adhesions

The incidence of infertility due to uterine structural abnormalities and endometrial pathology is approximately 5–10%. Hysteroscopic surgical procedures for intrauterine pathology became popular as they avoided cutting through uterine musculature to enter the cavity.

Hysteroscopic Adhesiolysis

Asherman's syndrome is found in approximately 5% of infertile women. The sine qua non for the development of intrauterine adhesions is endometrial trauma, especially to the basalis layer. The simple movement of the hysteroscope can break mild or minimal adhesions. Thicker lesions require use of scissors or electrocautery.

Laparoscopic control is advocated. Balloon catheter can be used to provide tamponade. The use of intrauterine devices (IUDs) and catheters is not recommended. Conjugated estrogen should be administered after surgery.

Congenital Uterine Anomalies

Incidence is 0.1–1.5%. Müllerian anomalies due to defective lateral fusion may be associated with infertility or repeated pregnancy loss.

Prevalence in women with recurrent pregnancy loss is significantly higher (10–12%). Among congenital anomalies, septate uterus is associated with the highest incidence of reproductive failure.

Metroplasty

The septum can be cut with scissors, electrocautery or a bipolar vaporizer (Versapoint®):

- *Shortening technique (thin septa):* Incision starts from the apex.
- *Thinning technique (wide septa):* Incisions are made along each side of the septum alternately, thinning the septum.

The dissection is complete when the hysteroscope can be moved freely from one cornual recess to the other without intervening obstruction and when both ostia can be visualized simultaneously (Homer, 2000). A small residual septum of less than 1 cm does not impair reproductive outcome (Fedle, 1993). Incision of cervical septum does not lead to cervical incompetence (Nisolle, 1996).

Results of hysteroscopic metroplasty for recurrent pregnancy loss are excellent and superior to those obtained by transabdominal approach. Cumulative pregnancy rate is 80–89% at 36 months and overall miscarriage rate is 15%. Results are not as good when surgery is performed primarily for primary infertility.

Complications: Perforation, uterine rupture in subsequent pregnancy though rare has been reported.

CONCLUSION

The minimal invasiveness, the reduced morbidity and excellent results have assigned endoscopic surgery, the central role in infertility management.

BIBLIOGRAPHY

1. Adamson DG, Pasta DJ. Surgical treatment of endometriosis-associated infertility: meta-analysis compared with survival analysis. Am J Obstet Gynaecol. 1994;171:1488-505.
2. Adamson GD, Hurd SJ, Pasta DJ, et al. Laparoscopic endometriosis treatment: is it better? Fertil Steril. 1993;59:35-44.
3. Antony M, Slangen T, van Herendael BJ. Salpingocopy is an important part of the infertility work-up. J Am Assoc Gynecol Laparosc. 1996;3(3):369-74.
4. Balen A. Polycystic ovary syndrome: mode of treatment. In: Z Shoham, CM Howles, HS Jacobs (Eds). Female Infertility Therapy Current Practice. Switzerland: Informa Healthcare;1998. pp. 45-67.
5. Brosens IA,Van Ballaer P, Puttemans PJ, et al. Reconstruction of the ovary containing large endometriomas by an extra ovarian endosurgical technique. Fertil Steril. 1996;66:517-21.
6. Campo R, Van Belle Y, Brosens I, et al. Office minihysteroscopy. Hum Reprod Update. 1999;5:73-81.
7. Daniell JF, Miller W. Polycystic ovaries treated by laparoscopic laser vaporization. Fertil Steril. 1989;51:232-6.
8. Farquhar C, Vandekerckhove P, Arnot M, et al. Laparoscopic "drilling" by diathermy or laser for ovulation induction in anovulatory polycystic ovary syndrome. Cochrane Database Syst Rev. 2000;(2):CDOOI122.
9. Fayez JA. An assessment of the role of operative laparoscopy in tuboplasty. Fertil Steril. 1983;39:476-9.
10. Fedle L, Arcaini L, Parazzini F, et al. Reproductive prognosis after hysteroscopic metroplasty in 102 women: lifetable analysis. Fertil Steril. 1993;59:768-72.
11. Gjoannaess H. Polycystic ovarian syndrome treated by electrocautery through the laparoscope. Fertil Steril. 1984;41:20-5.
12. Golan A, Eilat E, Ron-El R, et al. Hysteroscopy is superior to hysterosalpingography in infertility investigation. Acta Obstet Gynecol Scand. 1996;75(7):654-56.
13. Gomel V. Salpingo-ovariolysis by laparoscopy in infertility. Fertil Steril. 1983;40:607-11.
14. Homer HA, Li T, Cooke ID. The septate uterus: a review of management and reproductive outcome. Fertil Steril. 2000; 73:1-14.
15. Li TC, Saravelos H, Chow MS, et al. Factors affecting the outcome of laparoscopic ovarian drilling for polycystic ovarian syndrome in women with anovulatory infertility. Br J Obstet Gynaecol. 1998;105(3):338-44.
16. Mage G, PoulyJL, Bouquet de Jolinier J, et al. A. preoperative classification to predict the intrauterine and ectopic pregnancy rates after distal tubal microsurgery. Fertil Steril. 1988;46:807-10.
17. Nisolle M, Donnez J. Endoscopic treatment of uterine malformations. Gynaecol Endosc. 1996;5:155-60.
18. Novy MJ, Thurmond AS, Patton P, et al. Diagnosis of cornual obstruction by transcervical fallopian tube cannulation. Fertil Steril. 1988;50:434-40.
19. Reich H, McGlynn F. Treatment of ovarian endometriomas using laparoscopic surgical techniques. J Reprod Med. 1986;31:577.
20. Tulandi T, al Took S. Surgical management of polycystic ovarian syndrome. Baillieres Clin Obstet Gynaecol. 1998;12(4):541-53.
21. Varasteh NN, Neuwirth RS, Levin B, et al. Pregnancy rates after hysteroscopic polypectomy and myomectomy in infertile women. Obstet Gynaecol. 1999;94:168-71.

42.6 MYOMECTOMY

Nutan Jain, Shilpi Srivastava

INTRODUCTION

Myoma uteri are most common benign uterine tumors encountered in gynecological patients. Computed tomography (CT) and magnetic resonance imaging (MRI) reported an incidence of 20–25% of sexually active and 30–35% of all women irrespective of their age. A genetic and racial predisposition also exists, in women of African origin have 3–9 times greater risk of developing uterine fibroids than Caucasian women who are more likely to have myomas compared to women of Asian origin.

INDICATIONS

The most common indications of myomectomy appear to be as—

- Desire to conserve the uterus
- Severe menorrhagia (large myomas or multiple in number)
- Pressure symptoms leading to abdominal pain
- Rapidly growing myomas
- Myomectomy for infertility in following situations
- Altered tubo-ovarian relationship due to:
  - Intracavitary fibroids
  - Cornual fibroids pressing over the uterotubal junction
  - Significantly large, multiple intramural myomas.

SURGICAL ANATOMY

Uterine leiomyomas are usually diagnosed on physical examination. They may be subserosal, intramural or submucosal in location within the uterus or located in the cervix, broad ligament or on a pedicle (Figs 1A to C).

Grossly, fibroids are discrete nodular tumors that vary in size and number. They may be microscopic or huge. They may cause symmetrical uterine enlargement or they may distort the uterine contour significantly. The consistency of an individual leiomyoma varies from stony hard to soft depending upon the type of degeneration present.

PREOPERATIVE PREPARATION AND SPECIAL PREOPERATIVE TEST

All patients must undergo a complete sonography, which should be a combination of per abdomen, transvaginal and color Doppler sonography (Fig. 2). It is mandatory to know the exact site, size, location and number of myomas. CT and MRI could be indicated in face of multiple myomas to verify their location more precisely. It is extremely important to differentiate an adenomyoma from a myoma to avoid significant surgical difficulty, as adenomyomas do not give a definite surgical plane of cleavage.

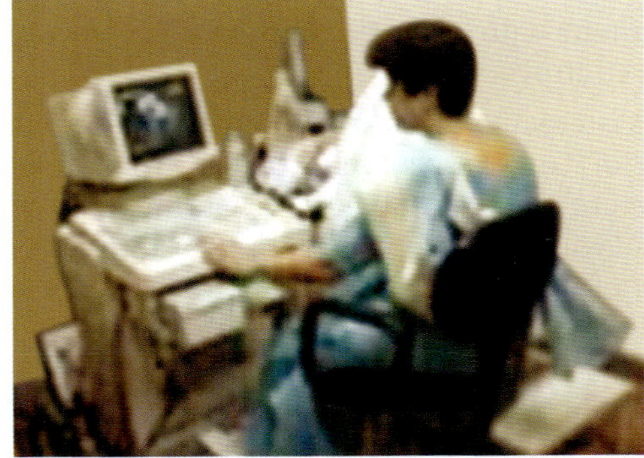

Fig. 2: Transvaginal sonography

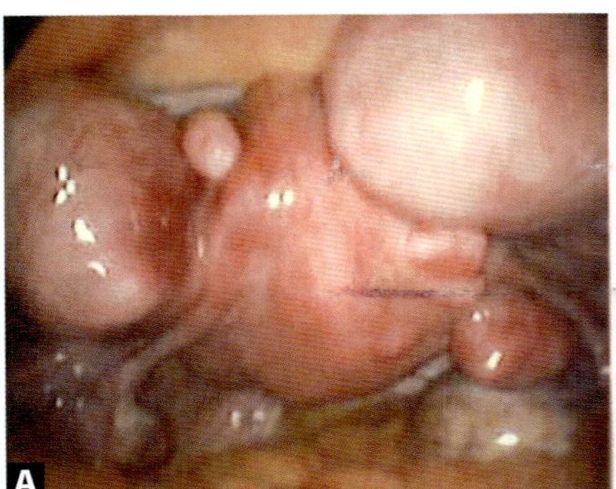

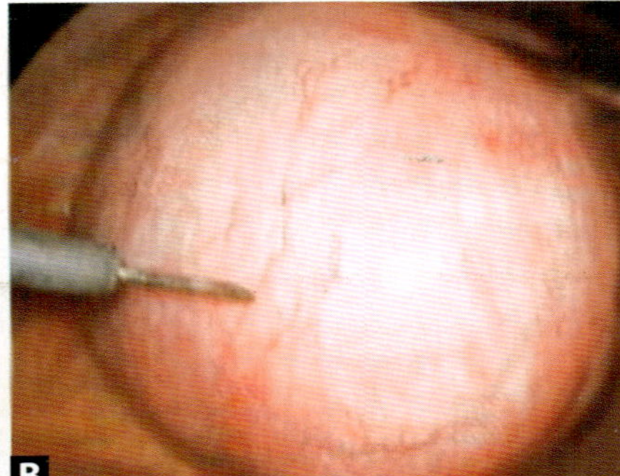

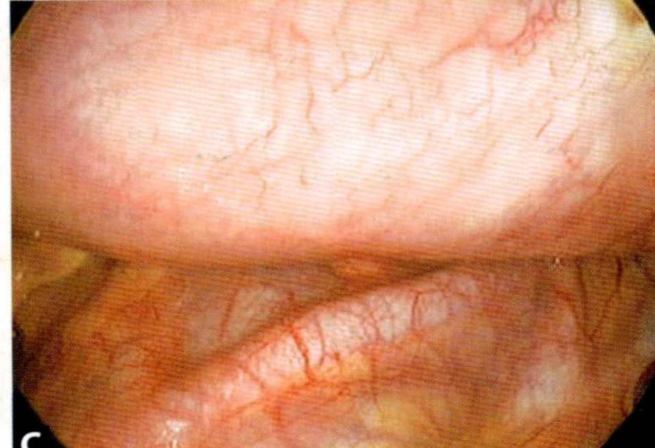

Figs 1A to C: (A) Multiple subserous myoma; (B) Deep intramural myoma; (C) Big myoma over laying the aortic bifurcation

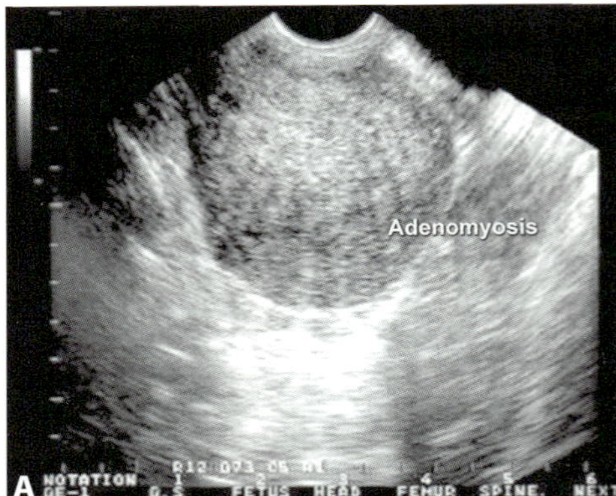

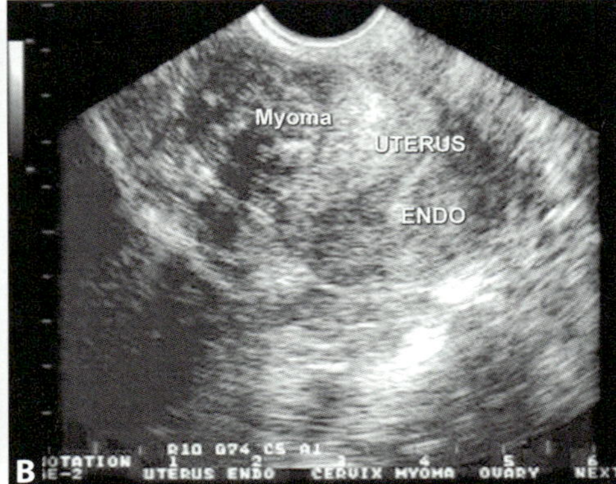

Figs 3A and B: (A) Adenomyosis; (B) Myoma

On ultrasound (USG) an adenomyoma shows a diffuse uterine enlargement with thickened posterior myometrium. There is uniform texture with reduced echogenicity, or irregular cystic spaces 5–7 mm disrupting normal echo pattern (Figs 3A and B). The diagnostic criteria to differentiate the two are with help of CT and MRI. Assessment of uterine cavity and tubal ostia is also important. This is accomplished by hysteroscopy at the time of surgery. Endometrial sampling is also performed if indicated.

MEDICAL PREPARATION

Pretreatment with GnRH agonists before myomectomy remains controversial.

In a systematic review of randomized controlled trials, the use of GnRH analogues before hysterectomy and myomectomy reduces the uterine volume by 40–50% after treatment with GnRH for 3 months. But during surgery the plane of cleavage is lost making enucleation more time consuming so its use largely remains operator dependent. Patients who need laparoscopic myomectomy need rectal and bowel preparation, before operation to deflate the bowel and get more space to work and lessen chances of bowel injury during suturing or morcellation.

POSITION, DRAPING AND INCISION

Once intubated the patient is placed in lithotomy position prepped and draped (Fig. 4) dorsal lithotomy allows the uterus to be easily accessed for hysteroscopy and uterine manipulation.

ANESTHESIA

The safest anesthesia for patient is GA with an endotracheal tube and controlled ventilation (Fig. 5). The expired CO_2 level can be maintained at 35 mm Hg, propofol is commonly used for induction and isoflurane, desflurane or, sevoflurane are used as an inhalation agent for maintenance. Short-acting relaxants are used for relaxation.

N_2O should be avoided as it causes intestinal bloating and compounds the problems of surgical exposure and the risks of bowel injury.

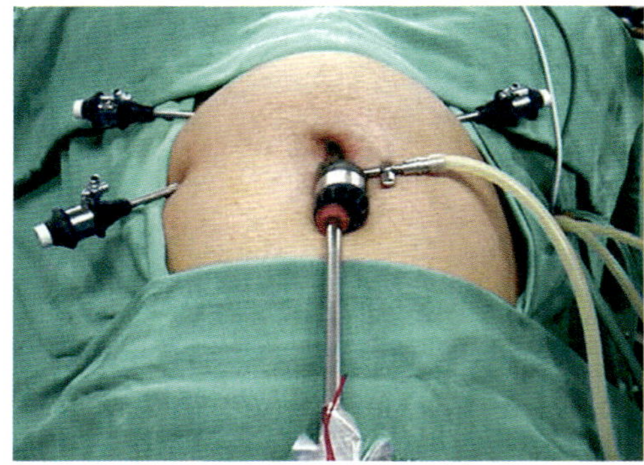

Fig. 4: Port placement

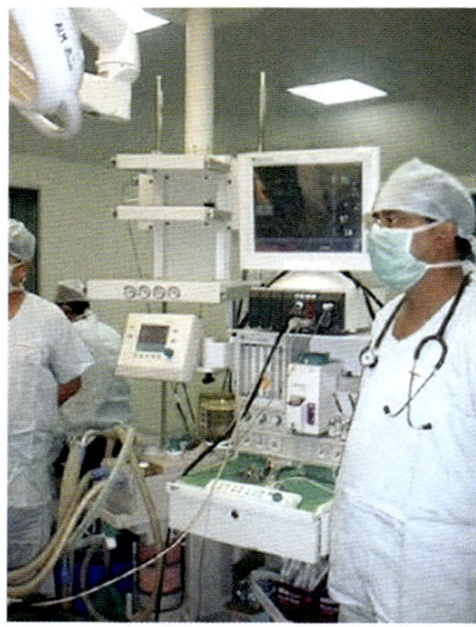

Fig. 5: Equipment for general anesthesia (GA)

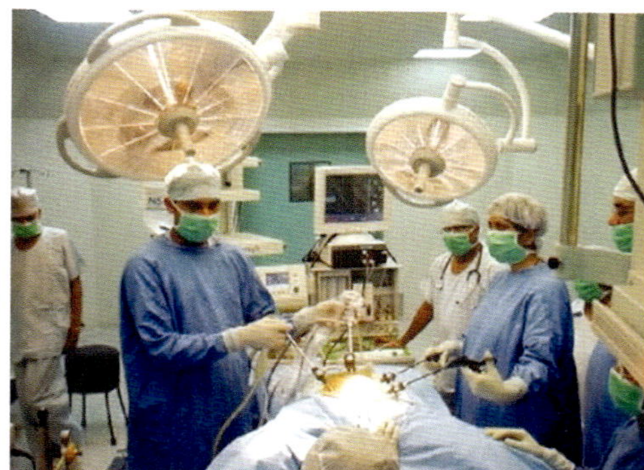

Fig. 6: Port placement theater working

OPERATIVE STEPS

Incision

After intubation 10 mm port is decided to be placed intra-umbilically or supraumbilically depending upon the myoma size, location and number. Accessory ports are also made keeping in mind that the working ports remain above and outside the bigger myomas. Most common port placement is as follows—two port for enucleation and suturing to be placed on the same side (left) as the surgeon stands. One accessory port on right side for the assistant for the purpose of grasping, retraction, suction and irrigation. This is placed any where between the umbilicus and anterior superior iliac spine according to the mandate of the case (Fig. 6).

SURGICAL TECHNIQUES

Following exploration of the pelvic organs and upper abdomen, associated conditions are evaluated, such as endometriosis, adhesions, and ovarian cysts, etc. The laparoscopic procedure is terminated in favor of a laparotomy if the extent of the disease is beyond the scope of the procedure's selection criteria.

The procedure of laparoscopic myomectomy consists of three distinct steps—

1. Disengaging the myoma from its uterine bed
2. Managing the uterine defect
3. Removing the myoma from the abdomen.

DISENGAGING THE LEIOMYOMA

Most of the time a transverse incision is made on the most bulging portion of the myoma with the help of a monopolar needle electrode or harmonic scalpel.

Next, we attempt to develop the cleavage plane between the myoma and its pseudocapsule by applying traction on the myoma and counter traction on the cut edge of the pesudocapsule and cutting or bluntly lysing the connecting bridges. Vascular bridges are coagulated before they are cut. Video magnification is helpful in this regard. A myoma screw is used for manipulation and traction and the prying method of blunt dissection is performed. This involves the placement of a probe or any other instrument that functions as a probe in the cleavage plane to leverage the tumor against the uterine wall and pry it out of its bed firmly, but gently, to avoid rupturing vascular bridges and bleeding. Once the myoma is substantially out of its bed the myoma screw is replaced by the claw forceps and strong traction is applied in various directions to expose remaining bridges and the primary vascular pedicle. When the vascular pedicle is identified, it is coagulated thoroughly with bipolar cautery and cut with sharp scissors to free the myoma (Figs 7A to F).

MANAGING THE OPERATIVE DEFECT

The myoma incision is given transversely over the most bulging part of the myoma. Prior injection of Pitressin reduces the bleeding from incision site. Vicryl 1-0 on a round body, needle is the preferred suture material. A suture about 45 cm in length is loaded on a needle holder and introduced in the peritoneal cavity by the Clarke Reich technique of removing the smaller valveless apple trocars. The angle knot is taken by passing the suture on the upper and lower edges of the myoma bed. Intracorporeal knot is tied making a secure, surgeon's knot. From this point on continuous suturing is done passing the needle from the lower flap to then upper edge without locking. The assistant plays an important role in pulling the slack of the suture and keeping adequate tension on the suture when the surgeon passes the successive sutures. Needle holders in both hands give a much better grip and needle alignment becomes easier. The needle is regrasped as it comes out of the upper flap and is realigned immediately without letting it fall. This adds a lot of speed and convenience to continuous curved needle suturing. It is extremely important to keep aligning the needle as soon as it exits from the upper flap of the myoma bed. Bites in the tissue are taken according to the thickness of the myometrial bed and keeping in mind that it gives good anatomical closure without being too bulky or too thin, both of which will result in either inadequate or bad tortuous suture line. Sutures should be placed evenly, bringing the tissue together without excessive tension or malalignment of layers. First layer is thus completed by passing running non-locking suture from one end of the myoma bed to other where it is anchored by a square knot. If the myometrial defect is small and adequate suture length still remains, the same suture is used to stitch the superficial myometrium and serosa up to the starting point of the first layer at the angle. While suturing the superficial layer it is extremely important to pass the sutures at an even distance and take almost same amount of tissue in each bite of two give a neat look to finished suture line a good anchoring square knot is used and can be tied to tail end of first knot given at start of the suturing. So, in this way, there is only one knot in the entire myoma bed (Figs 8A to F). The amount of adhesions formed per suture line is directly proportional to the number of knots. Lesser the number of bulky knots, lesser the adhesions formation. Copious irrigation and lavage is done and complete hemostasis achieved. No adhesion barrier is used. About 2 liters of Ringer's lactate (RL) is left for hydrofloatation.

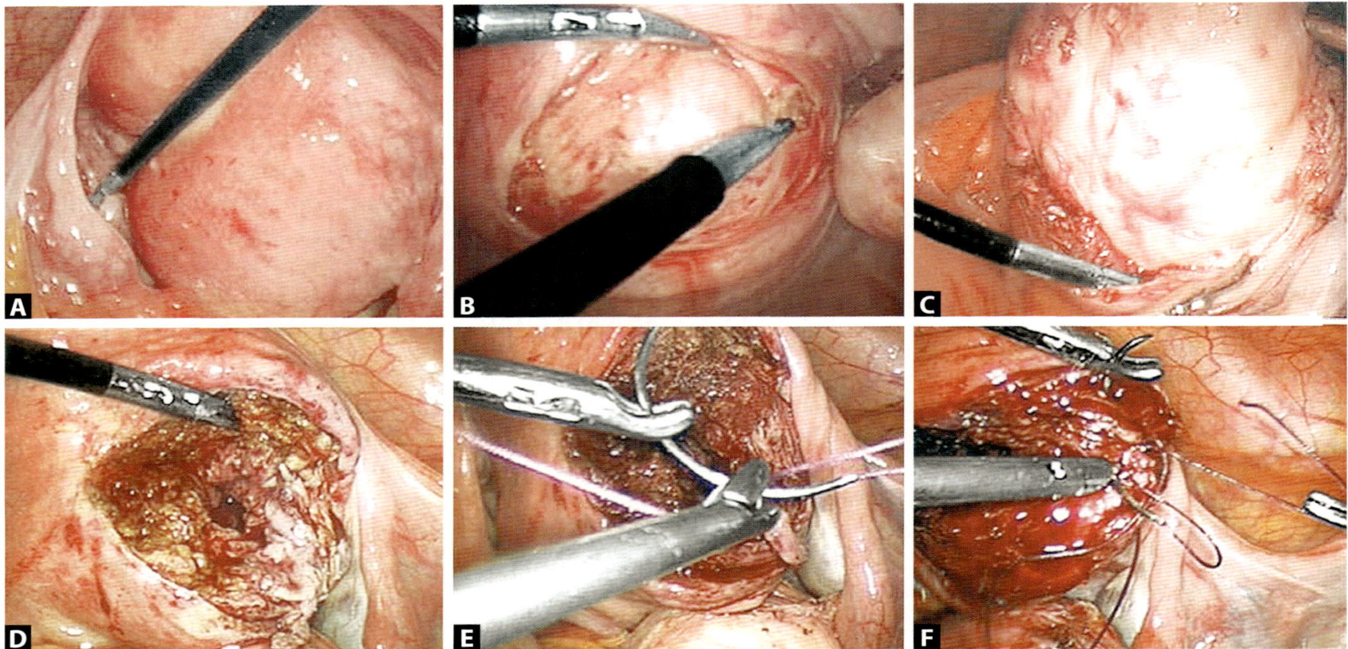

Figs 7A to F: (A) Initial appearance of myoma; (B) Transverse Incision given over the myoma by monopolor hook; (C) Enucleation of the myoma; (D) Cavity after removal of myoma; (E) Position of the needle; (F) Passing the needle

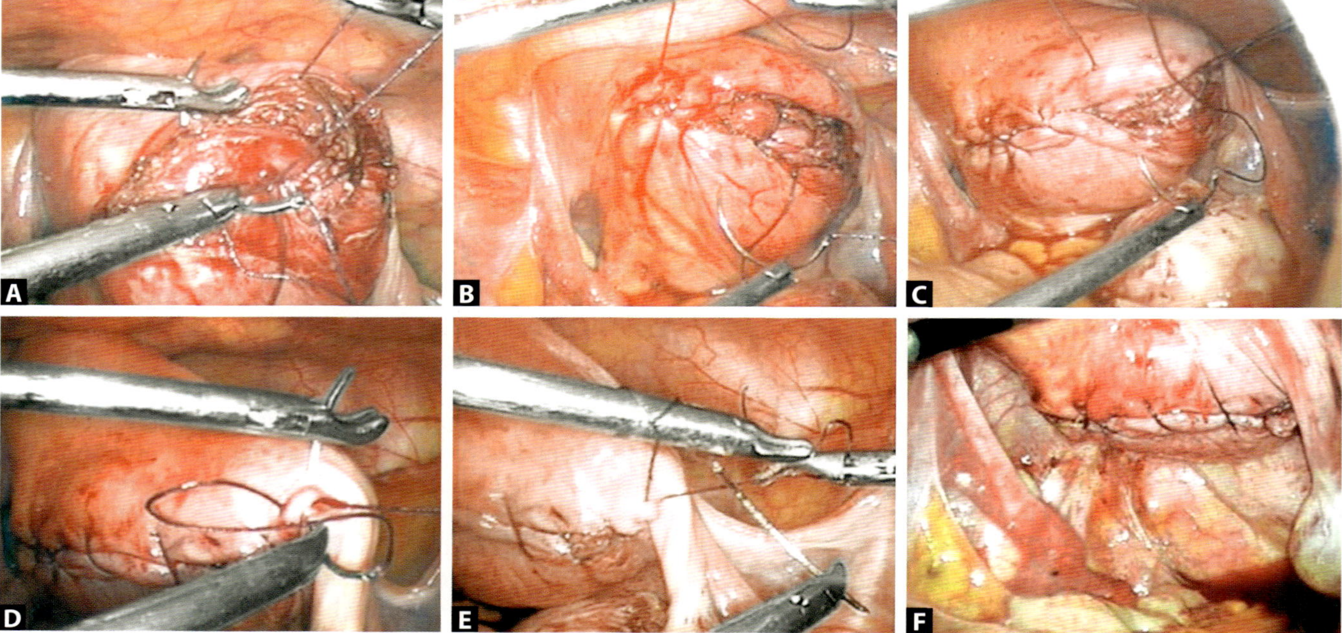

Figs 8A to F: (A) First layer in progress; (B) First layer is completed; (C) Second layer in progress; (D) Second layer almost completed; (E) Tying the knot;, (F) Final picture of myomectomy

REMOVING THE MYOMA

Following myomectomy, individual myomas are stored in cul-de-sac in preparation for removal from abdomen. There are three distinct modalities of removal.

1. *Motorized morcellator:* The electromechanical morcellator consists of motor cutting device inserted in the abdomen with the help of trocar and cannula. Sawhle morcellator is usually of 12 mm sleeve. There are also 15 mm and 20 mm sleeves for bigger tissue masses. Electromechanical morcellation quickly removes tissue from the abdomen and makes the tissue retrieval much easier.
2. *By posterior colpotomy:* We can make a colpotomy incision over CCL vaginal extractor placed in the vagina and then remove myoma by grasping with a 10 mm claw forceps inserted in colpotomy wound. Now push the myoma deep in the pouch of Douglas laparoscopically and making a colpotomy incision per-vaginum straight away on the vaginal mucosa bulging over the myoma. It is very simple and the myoma is easily pushed out within a minute or so. Posterior colpotomy wound is sutured by 2-0 vicryl vaginally.
3. *By minilap incision, laparoscopic-assisted minilap myomectomy:* Laparoscopic-assisted myomectomy appears to be safer and relatively simpler procedure in the hands of experienced laparoscopists as well as novices since the much dreaded steps of myomectomy, i.e. suturing and morcellation can be completed by minilap route.

Technique

Initially laparoscopy is performed, Pitressin injected over the myoma. Transverse incision given by monopolar hook or ultrasonic shears and myoma partially enucleated by traction of myoma screw. 3–4 cm Pfannenstiel minilap incision is given. Through this minilap incision enucleation morcellation and suturing of beds carried out of all multiple and big myomas (Figs 9A to D). After achieving complete hemostasis the minilap incision is sutured back laparoscope reinserted and thorough suction irrigation and lavage done.

It should be planned preoperatively and there is no sudden conversion on table from laparoscopic myomectomy to laparoscopic assisted minilap myomectomy.

It appears to be a patient friendly procedure giving all the benefits of laparoscopy with the help of small 3–4 cm incision, which heals, in postoperative phase.

COMPLICATIONS

Laparoscopic myomectomy has been noted to have immediate as well as late complications. They are as follows:

- Hemorrhage
- Lost, needles and small myomas
- Conversions to laparotomy

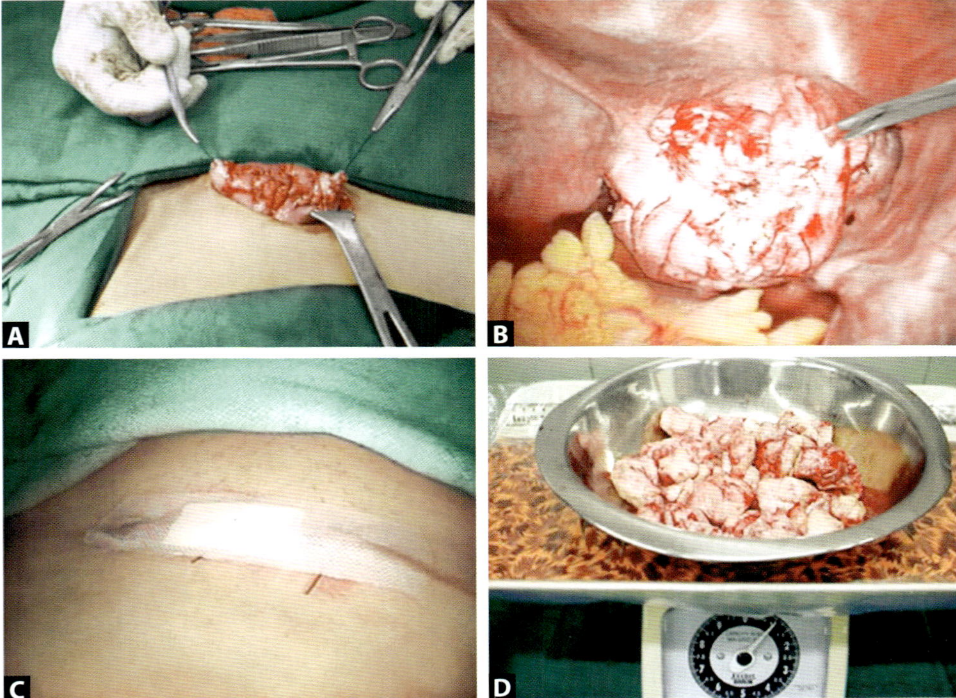

Figs 9A to D: (A) Completed suturing of myoma bed; (B) Uterus after completed myomectomy; (C) Final appearance of minilap incision; (D) Weight of the myoma

- Hysterectomy (rare)
- Morcellator injury
- Scar dehiscence during pregnancy.

CONCLUSION

Laparoscopic myomectomy has become a common laparoscopic procedure the order of the day. It offers several advantages over laparotomy including less operative trauma and blood loss, reduced postoperative morbidity, shorter hospital stay and recovery time, earlier return to normal activity, fewer postoperative adhesions, better cosmetic scars, improved patient compliance and better pregnancy outcome. Furthermore, the magnification of that video laparoscopy provides allows for careful microsurgical dissection of tissues, the development of avascular planes, and the occlusion of blood vessel before they are transected. Moreover, pregnancy rates are consistent with myomectomy via laparotomy.

BIBLIOGRAPHY

1. Alexander GD, Noe FE, Brown EM. Anesthesia for pelvic Laparoscopy. Anesth Analg. 1969;48:14-8.
2. Fedele L, Bianchi S, Dorta M, et al. Transvaginal sonography in the diagnosis of diffuse adenomyosis. Fertil Steril. 1992;58:94-7.
3. Miller CE, Davies S, Johnston M. Presented at the 27th Annual Meeting of the American Association of Gynecologic Laparoscopists, Atlanta, GA. November 10–15, 1998. Miller CE. Laparoscopic Myomectomy with uterine reconstruction is a safe surgical procedure.
4. Nezhat C, Nezhat F, Bess O. Laparoscopically assisted myomectomy: a report of a new technique in 57 cases. Int J Fertil. 1994;39:39-44.
5. Nezhat C, Nezhat F, Silfen S. Laparoscopic Myomectomy. Int J Fertil. 1991;36:275-80.
6. Nezhat C. Laparoscopic myomectomy complications (Letter). Int J Fertil. 1992;37:64.

42.7 TOTAL LAPAROSCOPIC HYSTERECTOMY

Pranay R Shah

INTRODUCTION

Hysterectomy is the one of the most frequently performed major gynecological procedure. The uterus traditionally has been removed by either the vaginal or abdominal route. The first planned vaginal hysterectomy was performed by "Conrad Langenbeck" in 1813 and the first abdominal hysterectomy by "Clay and Koeberle" in 1863. The techniques were progressively refined over the remainder of the 19th century and by the early years of the 20th century had become established as the "classic" techniques and have been passed down essentially unaltered to successive generations of gynecological surgeons. In spite of the obvious advantages of the vaginal technique, about 75% of the hysterectomies are accomplished abdominally. In the UK Vaginal Abdominal Laparoscopic Uterine Excision (VALUE) study, Hall et al. reported that in 1995 some 74% of 15,379 hysterectomies performed for dysfunctional uterine bleeding (DUB) were by the abdominal route. A national survey of hysterectomies performed in Finland indicated that 93% of 9,095 hysterectomies were abdominal. The route of hysterectomy is usually determined by the skill, experience, and preferences of the operating gynecologist. Most consider vaginal hysterectomy should be considered for specific indications and that abdominal hysterectomy can be used for every indication and can be considered to be "default operation".

Vaginal hysterectomy is sometimes contraindicated due to severe endometriosis, adnexal pathology, suspected malignancy, pelvic adhesions, prior abdominal surgery, previous cesarean section or fibroids. Many gynecologists find that vaginal hysterectomy is technically more difficult (and more dangerous) in younger women with a well supported uterus and some will only perform a vaginal hysterectomy when there is significant uterine prolapse.

The optimum approach to hysterectomy would be to retain the advantages of the abdominal route, which include clear visualization and the ease of manipulation of the adnexal structures, and to combine these features with the principal advantage of vaginal hysterectomy, namely avoidance of a large abdominal incision (Table 1). The use of laparoscopic techniques now permits this combined approach. The extent of laparoscopic and vaginal dissection should be based on the surgeon's preference and the experience with laparoscopic surgery.

Harry Reich's paper on laparoscopic hysterectomy in 1989 stimulated a great interest in proper scientific evaluation of all forms of hysterectomy. Since then various techniques for hysterectomy using laparoscopy have been developed (Box 1). We regard the division of the uterine artery and the cardinal ligament as the most difficult and critical step of the operation. The procedure is termed laparoscopic-assisted vaginal hysterectomy (LAVH) if the uterine vessels are secured by the vaginal route (Fig. 1) and laparoscopic hysterectomy (LH) if the uterine vessels are secured laparoscopically (Fig. 2). In addition, if the uterosacral and cardinal ligaments are also secured laparoscopically and the cervix completely freed from the vagina using laparoscopic techniques, the procedure is called total laparoscopic hysterectomy (TLH) (Fig. 3).

A hysterectomy, regardless of the approach, is performed in seven consecutive steps.

The steps are as follows:

1. Bilateral desiccation or ligation and cut of the round ligaments and dissection of the broad ligament
2. Bilateral desiccation or ligation and transection of the tube and utero-ovarian ligament if the adnexa are to be preserved, or bilateral desiccation and transection of the infundibulopelvic ligaments if adnexa are to be removed

Table 1: Advantage and disadvantages of abdominal, vaginal and laparoscopic-assisted vaginal hysterectomy (LAVH)

	Abdominal	Vaginal	LAVH
Exposure	Excellent	Limited	Excellent
Assoc Pelvic Disease	Easily treated	Reduced access	Easily treated
Incision	Large abdominal	Vaginal	Key hole abdominal
Hospitalization (days)	3–4	2–3	1–2
Cost	Average	Least	More expensive
Morbidity (%)	30	10	10
Surgical expertise	Average gynecologist	Average gynecologist	Expert endoscopist
Oophorectomy	Easy	Possible, difficult	Easy

Box 1 Classification: Stages of laparoscopic hysterectomy (Johns and Diamond)

Stage 0: Diagnostic laparoscopy performed, but no laparoscopic surgery required before a vaginal hysterectomy (VH).

Stage 1: Laparoscopic adhesiolysis or excision of endometriosis before VH.

Stage 2: Either one or both adnexa, including the infundibulopelvic ligaments, freed laparoscopically prior to VH.

Stage 3: Bladder dissected from the uterus laparoscopically prior to VH.

Stage 4: All the above + uterine arteries transected laparoscopically prior to VH.

Stage 5: Anterior and posterior colpotomy and freeing of the whole uterus performed laparoscopically.

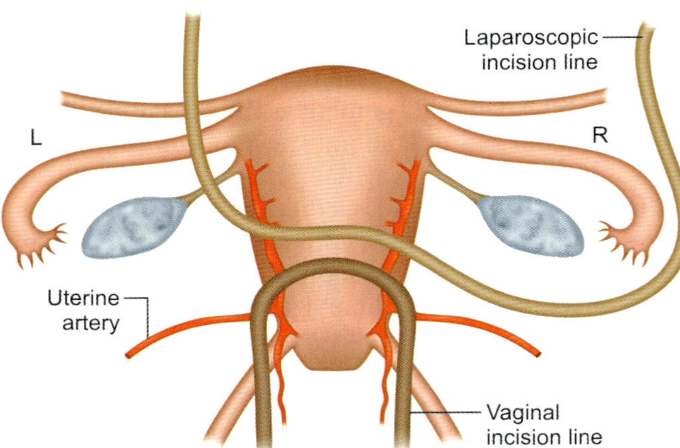

Fig .1: Stage 3—Laparoscopic-assisted vaginal hysterectomy (LAVH) with laparoscopic mobilization of adnexa and vaginal securing of uterine arteries and uterosacral and cardinal ligaments

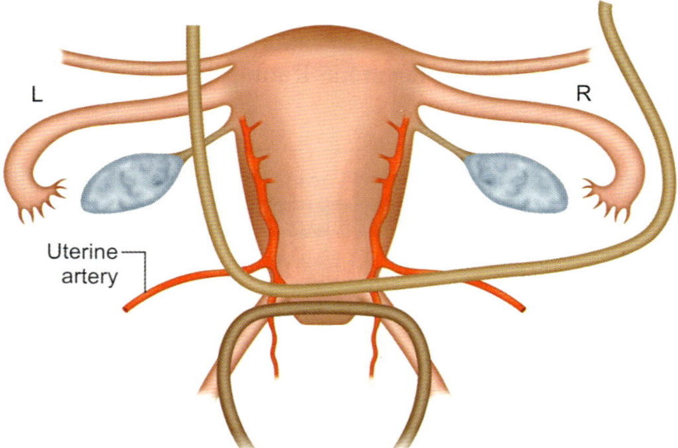

Fig. 2: Stage 4—Laparoscopic hysterectomy (LH). This stage includes laparoscopic division of uterine arteries but vaginal division of uterosacral ligaments

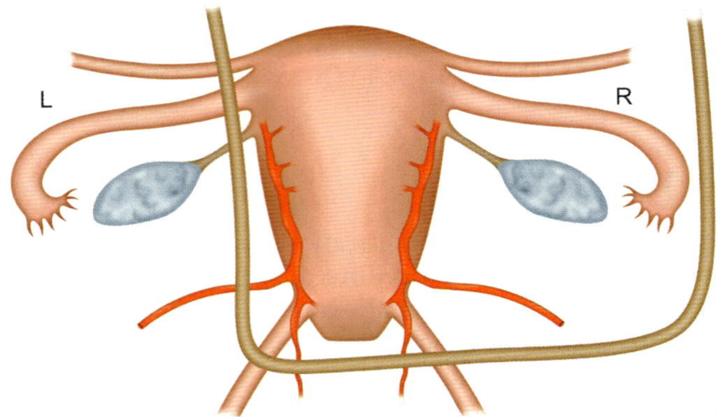

Fig. 3: Stage 5—Total laparoscopic hysterectomy (TLH). This stage involves the complete mobilization of the uterus laparoscopically including uterosacral and cardinal ligaments combined with laparoscopic opening of anterior and posterior cul-de-sac. Vaginal closed laparoscopically or vaginally

3. Bilateral desiccation or suture ligation, and transection of the uterine vessels
4. Preparation of the bladder flap and severing the bladder pillars
5. Bilateral desiccation or ligation, and transection of the cardinal-uterosacral ligament complex
6. Anterior and/or posterior culdotomy and separating the cervix from the vagina
7. Closure of the vaginal vault.

INDICATIONS

The indications for LAVH and LH are yet not defined and each team involved with these procedures is currently evaluating its own experience. The need for laparoscopic hysterectomy may vary according to the individual gynecologist's practice. Those who routinely perform the majority of their hysterectomies by the vaginal route may perhaps find fewer indications than those who usually employ the abdominal technique. Replacing abdominal hysterectomy (AH), however, appears to be the most persuasive reason for attempting this less invasive approach.

LAVH is especially useful in the following circumstances:

- *To remove the ovaries:* In clinical practice few oophorectomies are carried out via the vaginal route since it is generally considered more difficult than via the abdominal route. Oophorectomy cannot be guaranteed at the time of VH even by those who promote the technique. Laparoscopic approach can be employed where oophorectomy is not possible by vaginal approach alone.
- *To evaluate an adnexal mass:* A preliminary laparoscopy helps to determine the etiology of the mass. It can facilitate the removal of ovary, tube or adnexa if indicated, and allows the surgeon to complete the procedure vaginally.

- To evaluate the pelvis in patients with history of pelvic inflammatory disease (PID), endometriosis or pelvic adhesions, malignancy: Pathologies are confirmed at laparoscopy in only 50%. If pelvis is normal, a VH can be safely accomplished, avoiding an unnecessary laparotomy. If pathology is confirmed, it can be corrected laparoscopically and then one can proceed for a VH.

Total Laparoscopic Hysterectomy

With our initial experience with laparoscopic-assisted vaginal hysterectomies, we learned that LAVH had a reduced chance of success in the following situations:

- Narrow pubic angle
- Narrow vagina
- High and immobile uterus. TLH is the method of choice in such situations. However, TLH has few advocates because separating the cervix from the vagina is difficult. The use of a vaginal tube (delineator) simplifies this step and makes the TLH procedure more feasible, safe and a reproducible technique.

Vaginal Tube—A Novel Idea

A blue polypropelene tube of 35 mm in diameter is introduced in the vagina to expose the cervicovaginal junction after the vesicouterine fold of peritoneum is dissected (Fig. 4). The stretched vagina falls away from the cervix as monopolar diathermy cuts over the tube rim. The tube guides the incision, and the plastic protects adjacent structures. As upward traction is obtained on the vault, the ureters tend to fall away from the uterine artery, thus protecting them while the uterine vessels are coagulated or sutured. The uterosacral ligaments are cut close to its insertion to the cervix. As the ligament complex is not disturbed, there is no need to perform a culdoplasty following the hysterectomy. The distal end of the tube has a valve that maintains pneumoperitoneum and allows 5 mm/10 mm instruments to be introduced.

Preoperative Evaluation or Preparation

Preoperative evaluation is done as for any major surgery. Informed consent with a possibility of laparotomy is obtained. Bowel preparation included a liquid diet for two days preoperatively with bowel cleansing using Peglac on the night prior to surgery. Milk and fizzy drinks are avoided. Bowel enema is avoided.

OPERATION TECHNIQUE

Patient Position

After suitable GA is administered, the patient is put in a low dorsolithotomy position (extension at hips and flexion at knees, so that the thighs are almost in line with the trunk) with 1–20° Trendelenburg.

For the vaginal portion, the patient's legs are readjusted in candy-cane stirrups for better access. This will require redraping.

Insertion of Ports

A vertical 10 mm intraumbilical incision is made and trocar inserted by direct technique or after pneumoperitoneum is created and 10 mm 0° telescope introduced. For LAVH two trocars are inserted lateral to the obliterated umbilical ligament and 2–3 cm above and medial to the anterior superior iliac spine as recommended by Harry Reich (Fig. 5). Higher placement can be obtained if the uterus is bulky. An additional trocar is introduced parallel to the umbilical port in the midclavicular line to assist in uterine mobilization later on during the procedure as recommended by Garry especially in cases requiring TLH (Fig. 6). Uterus is manipulated using a modified Valtchev manipulator (Fig. 7).

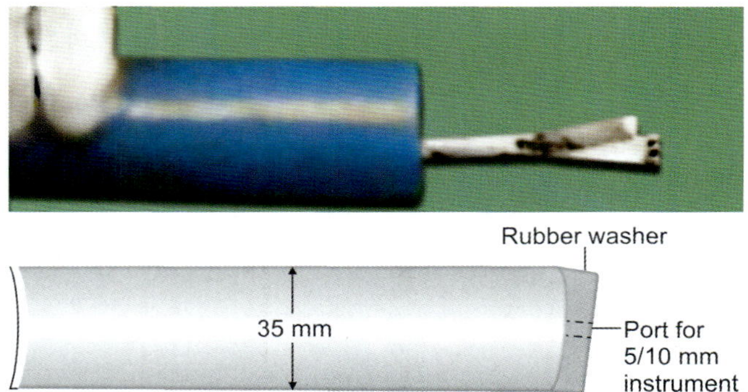

Fig. 4: Polypropelene tube 35 mm in diameter for colpotomy

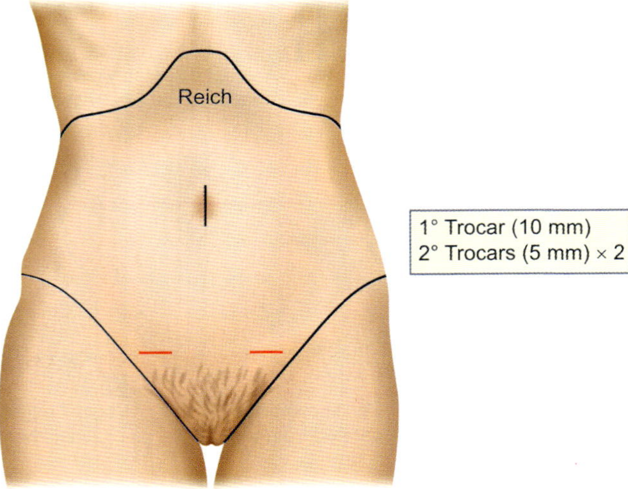

Fig. 5: Reich's recommended portal of entry

Garry
1° Trocar (10 mm)
2° Trocars (5 mm) × 3

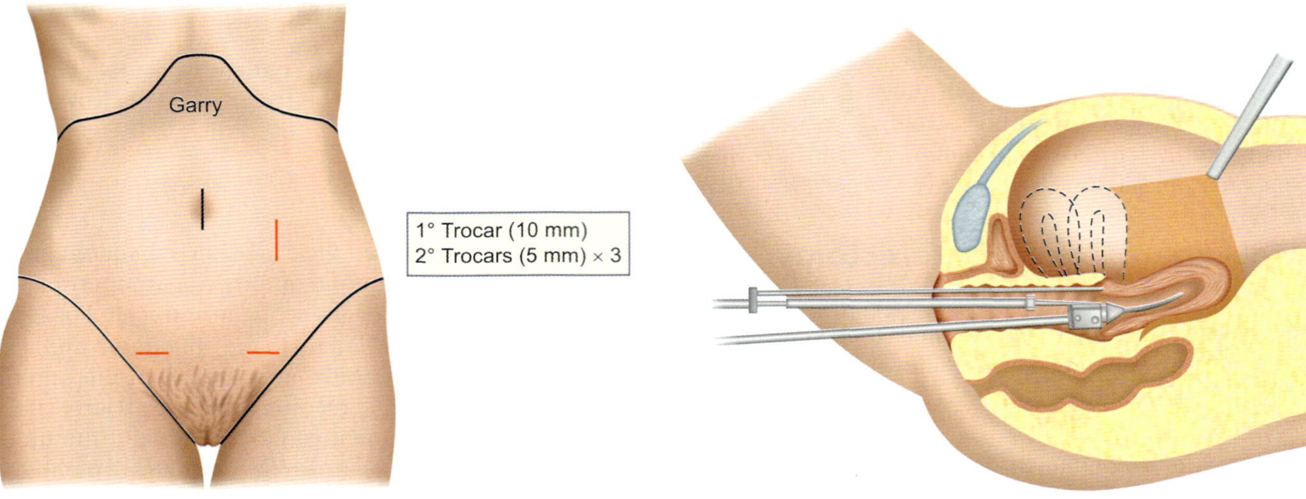

Fig. 6: Garry's modifications to the recommended points of entry for total laparoscopic hysterectomy (TLH)

Fig. 7 : Valtchev manipulator in situ

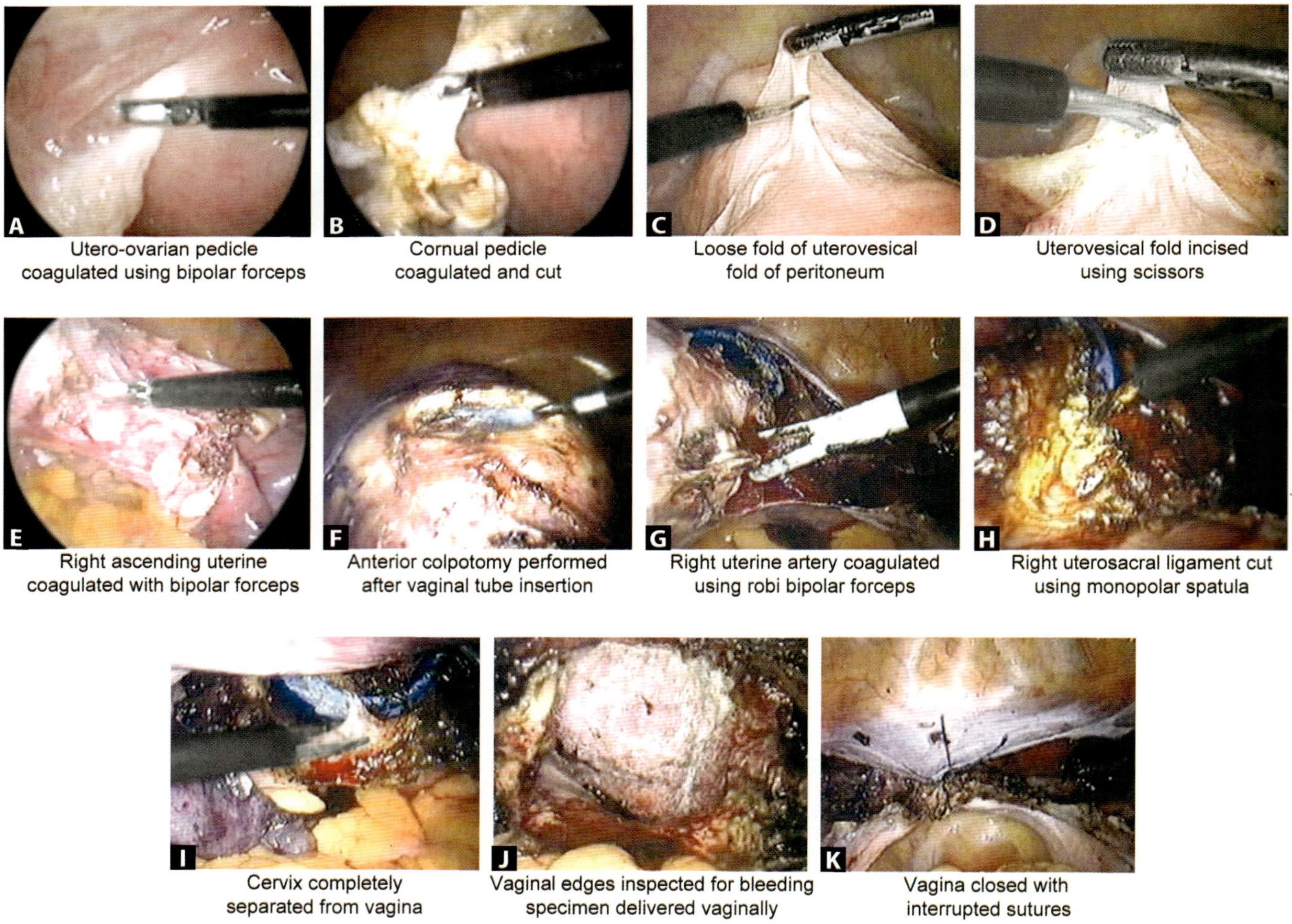

A
Utero-ovarian pedicle coagulated using bipolar forceps
B
Cornual pedicle coagulated and cut
C
Loose fold of uterovesical fold of peritoneum
D
Uterovesical fold incised using scissors
E
Right ascending uterine coagulated with bipolar forceps
F
Anterior colpotomy performed after vaginal tube insertion
G
Right uterine artery coagulated using robi bipolar forceps
H
Right uterosacral ligament cut using monopolar spatula
I
Cervix completely separated from vagina
J
Vaginal edges inspected for bleeding specimen delivered vaginally
K
Vagina closed with interrupted sutures

Figs 8A to K: Steps of laparoscopic hysterectomy

Instruments

Five millimeter graspers, straight and curved scissors, 5 mm bipolar forceps, monopolar hook/spatula, 5 mm suction irrigation cannula, myoma screw, uterine manipulator.

Needle holders, knot pusher (if suturing is required), vaginal tube.

Operative Steps

Laparoscopically-assisted Vaginal Hysterectomy (Figs 8A to K)

After preliminary visual examination, any adhesions if present are divided. Adnexal pathology like endometrioma, TO mass, hydrosalpinx, ovarian cyst is dealt with. Tubo-ovarian pedicle and round ligament are desiccated using bipolar forceps and cut. Alternatively, a window can be made between the round ligament and infundibulopelvic ligament and vicryl suture, passed through it for an extracorporeal ligature. When ovarian conservation is required, the utero-ovarian ligament, fallopian tubes and round ligament are cauterized and cut. Uterovesical fold is opened using sharp dissection and bladder is mobilized. Broad ligament is dissected open and ascending uterine vessels are coagulated and cut. If the procedure is planned in an LAVH, anterior and posterior colpotomy is performed using a sponge-stick. A monopolar needle or hook is used to incise the vagina till the sponge is visible. Packing the vagina around the uterine manipulator can prevent gas leakage. Rest of the hysterectomy can be completed vaginally.

Total Laparoscopic Hysterectomy

If it is thought that the vaginal route is not feasible, you could proceed to perform a TLH. The uterine manipulator is now removed and a stay suture is placed on the cervix using strong linen or black silk. The vaginal tube is now introduced to encircle the cervix. When pushed cranially, the laparoscopic surgeon will notice the vault delineated and made prominent. Bladder mobilization is completed using blunt and sharp dissection. This step is especially useful in patients with previous cesarean section.

Uterus can now be manipulated using a myoma screw inserted through the port parallel to the umbilicus. At 3 O'clock and 9 O'clock uterine vessels entering into the uterus are coagulated with bipolar centry and cut. As the vessels are tackled very medially, the chance of thermal injury to the ureters is greatly reduced. A monopolar hook/needle/spatula is used to incise the vagina over the tube starting at 12 O'clock and working around 360° to circumcise the vagina separating the cervix from the vaginal attachments. The uterosacral ligaments are incised flush with the cervix. The uterus is now delivered vaginally using the traction suture. In cases of uterine enlargements, the uterus can be morcellated or bisected and delivered. A pack is introduced in the vagina, pneumoperitoneum reinstated and hemostasis achieved from vaginal margins using bipolar coagulation. Vagina can be closed laparoscopically using continuous sutures or vaginally in the standard fashion using no. 1-0 vicryl.

At any stage when the surgeon feels comfortable, the vaginal part of the surgery can be performed to complete the rest of the hysterectomy. There is no advantage in continuing to perform the procedure laparoscopically, if it can be safely accomplished vaginally.

The laparoscope is reinserted, thorough lavage given using Ringer's solution, clots removed and hemostasis reconfirmed after reducing intra-abdominal pressure. The trocars are removed under vision and absence of bleeding from the ports confirmed. An indwelling bladder catheter was introduced and left in place for a day.

POSTOPERATIVE CARE

Three doses of perioperative broad spectrum antibiotics (Omnatax/Metrogyl, Augmentin) are administered intravenously. Most patients can be started oral liquids after 12 hours, and are discharged after 48 hours. They are advised follow-up after 1 week and can resume routine duties after 15 days.

RESULTS

Laparoscopic hysterectomy accounts for only 4–8% of hysterectomies even in developed countries like USA, UK, and Australia (Table 2). There have now been at least six randomized controlled studies comparing laparoscopic and abdominal hysterectomy. These all show quicker recovery, less complications, and less patient discomfort with the laparoscopic approach. At the same time, there have been two small RCTs comparing vaginal hysterectomy to LH. Both show similar pain with reduced costs from vaginal hysterectomy. This would clearly be expected, since there is minimal equipment required for vaginal hysterectomy when compared to that required for LH.

Clearly, as more gynecologists have become comfortable doing laparoscopic hysterectomies, it has increased the numbers of vaginal hysterectomies, which they perform without laparoscopy. This has reduced the overall numbers of abdominal hysterectomies being performed. As a gynecologist begins to do LH, he gains more confidence and skill at vaginal surgery. It is northwhile having a laparoscope in the abdomen looking from above while trying to do difficult vaginal surgery. This enhances visibility, improves safety, and encourages the surgeon to be more aggressive.

Table 2: Comparison of type of hysterectomy in different countries

Country	Total Hysterectomies	LAVH/TLH	Vaginal	Abdominal
		(%)	(%)	(%)
USA, 1991	731,000	4	24	72
UK, 1995	34,700	5	21	74
Australia, 1995	19,702	8	35	57

Abbreviations: LAVH, Laparoscopically-assisted vaginal hysterectomy; TLH, Total laparoscopic hysterectomy

One reason frequently quoted against laparoscopic hysterectomies is the higher rate of complications associated with the procedure. Harkki-Siren et al. reviewed all laparoscopic hysterectomies performed in Finland over a 2-year period. Major complication rate was 3.5%. The rate of ureteric injury appeared to be high (13.9 per 1,000 for LH, 0.4 per 1,000 after AH and only 0.2 per 1,000 after VH). This represents an astonishing 35-fold higher rate of ureteric injury after laparoscopic than AH. Other reports of ureteric injury include those by Saidi et al. (2 per 1,000 in 489 LAVH), Deprest et al. (4.2 per 1,000 in 4,502 LAVH cases reviewed) and Scottish Audit (8 per 1,000 from 458 cases). Most of the studies reviewed here were performed during the "World Learning Curve for Laparoscopic Hysterectomy". Certainly in none of the cases was the surgeon as experienced in the new technique as he/she was in the conventional technique that was being compared. The VALUE study clearly indicated the importance of experience in influencing outcome. In our study the complication rate was low, comparable to other techniques and could be safely performed in all the selected cases. The combination of increasing experience, better equipment, and much greater attention to the technical details of the procedure, have allowed a transformation in results from unacceptable to levels significantly better than accepted standards.

CONCLUSION

Surgeons with appropriate skills can replace more than 90% of abdominal hysterectomies by vaginal or laparoscopic hysterectomy. Introduction of the simplified technique (vaginal tube) to perform total laparoscopic hysterectomy would improve its acceptability in indicated cases to complete the surgery safely and effectively.

BIBLIOGRAPHY

1. Deprest JA, Munro MG, Konincke PR. Review on laparoscopic hysterectomy. Zentralblatt Gynakol. 1995;117:641-51.
2. Hall V, Overton J, Hargreares J, et al. The VALUE national hysterectomy study: description of the patients and their surgery. Br J Obstet Gynecol. 2002;109:302-12.
3. Harkki-Siren P, Sjoberg J, Makinen J, et al. Finnish national register of laparoscopic hysterectomies: a review and complications of 1,165 operations. Am J Obstet Gynecol. 1997;176;118-22.
4. Lengebrekke A, Eraker R, Nesheim BJ, et al. Abdominal hysterectomy should not be considered as a primary method for uterine removal: a prospective randomised study of 100 patients referred to hysterectomy. Acta Obstet Gynae Scand. 1996;75:404-7.
5. Lumsden MA, Hawthern R, Davis J. BJ of Obs and Gynaec 1998;105(517);60.
6. Marana R, Busacca M, Garcia N. J of Am Asso of Gynec Laparoscopists. 1997;4(55).
7. Nezhat F, Nezhat C, Gordon S, et al. Laparoscopic versus abdominal hysterectomy. J Reprod Med. 1992;37:247-50.
8. Olsson JH, Ellstrom M, Hahlin M. A randomised prospective trial comparing laparoscopic and abdominal hysterectomy. Br J Obstet Gynaecol. 1996;103:345-50.
9. Phillips JH, John M, Nayak S. Comparison of laparoscopically assisted vaginal hysterectomy and bilateral salpingo-oophorectomy with conventional abdominal hysterectomy and bilateral salpingo-oophorectomy. Br J Obstet Gynecol. 1993;100:698-700.
10. Raju KS, Auld BJ. A randomised prospective study of laparoscopic vaginal hysterectomy versus abdominal hysterectomy each with bilateral salpingo-oophorectomy. Br J Obstet Gynecol. 1994;101:1068-71.
11. Reich H, Decaprio J, Mc-Glynn F. Laparoscopic hysterectomy. J Gynecol Surg. 1989;5:213-6.
12. Richardson RE, Bournos N, Magos AL. Is laparoscopic hysterectomy a waste of time? Lancet. 1995;345:36-41.
13. Saidi MH, Sadler RK, Vancaillie TG, et al. Diagnosis and management of serious urinary complications after major operative laparoscopy. Obstet Gynecol. 1997;87:272-6.
14. Sheth SS. The place of oophorectomy at vaginal hysterectomy. Br J Obstet Gynecol. 1991;98:662-6.
15. Summit RL, Stovall TG, Gary LH, et al. Randomized comparison of laparoscopy-assisted vaginal hysterectomy with standard vaginal hysterectomy in an outpatient setting. Obstetrics and Gynecology 1992;80:895-901.
16. Sutton C. Hysterectomy: a historical perspective. Balleres Clin Obstet Gynecol. 1997;11(1):1-22.
17. Wilcox LS, Koonin LM, Pokras R, et al. Hysterectomy in the United States, 1988–1990. Br J Obstet Gynecol. 1994;99:402.

42.8 PCOS SURGICAL MANAGEMENT

Duru Shah, Safala Shroff, Sukhpreet Patel

INTRODUCTION

The symptoms attributable to chronic anovulation are the main reasons that women with polycystic ovary syndrome (PCOS) present themselves to the clinicians. Not surprisingly, a major complaint is the infertility that accompanies PCOS. Historically, PCOS has been described by Stein and Leventhal in 1935, which identified the association of polycystic ovaries with hirsutism, amenorrhea and obesity. Prior to the availability of ovulation inducing agents, laparotomy with bilateral ovarian wedge resection (OWR) rapidly gained popularity. Surgical ovarian wedge resection was the first established treatment for anovulatory PCOS patients but was largely abandoned because of the risk of postsurgical adhesion formation. Ovulation rates obtained with OWR were excellent. But several investigators noted postoperative adhesions that gave suboptimal pregnancy rates. Hence, today OWR is all but obsolete having been replaced by other modalities of treatment.

It was replaced by medical ovulation induction with clomiphene and gonadotropins. However, patients with PCOS treated with gonadotropins often have a poly-follicular response and are exposed to the risks of OHSS and multiple pregnancies. Although effective, it is an expensive, stressful and time-consuming form of treatment requiring intensive monitoring. Hence, the new surgical therapy, laparoscopic ovarian "drilling" gained popularity since it avoids or reduces the use of gonadotrophins for inducing ovulation. The procedure can be done on an outpatient basis with less trauma and fewer postoperative adhesions. It has been claimed in many uncontrolled observational studies that it is followed, at least temporarily, by a high rate of spontaneous postoperative ovulation and conception, or that subsequent medical ovulation induction becomes easier.

A PRACTICAL APPROACH TO OVULATION INDUCTION

The "antiestrogenic compounds" (primarily clomiphene citrate) are the most commonly used agents for ovulation induction, as the "first line" of treatment for women with PCOS-related anovulatory infertility. The ovulation rate with clomiphene is more than 80%. However, 15–20% women remain anovulatory despite treatment with incremental doses of clomiphene. Furthermore, in spite of a high ovulation rate, the pregnancy rate is only between 40% and 50% and the abortion rate is as high as 30–40%.

In the patients resistant to clomiphene citrate, gonadotrophin therapy has traditionally been the next step. "Gonadotropins" have the same disadvantages as clomiphene citrate, which includes increased rates of multiple gestation and spontaneous abortions. The risk of ovarian hyperstimulation syndrome, a well known complication with use of human menopausal gonadotropin (hMG), also necessitates careful monitoring during its administration.

The prevalent complications of ovarian hyperstimulation syndrome and multiple pregnancies can largely be avoided by administering follicle-stimulating hormone (FSH) in a low dose and individualized regimen. Hyperinsulinemia can be corrected by weight loss or insulin-sensitizing agents, such as metformin, which alone or in combination with other agents are capable of restoring ovulation. Advice about weight loss is critical in modern management of PCOS and infertility.

According to current data, metformin has gained popularity as first-line management in clomiphene citrate-resistant women with PCOS. If ovulation does not occur within several months after treatment with metformin, after the evaluation of all pros and cons related to each treatment, laparoscopic ovarian drilling or gonadotropins may be considered as an effective option according to patient choice.

An alternative to medical approach is surgical treatment. The most popular treatment is laparoscopic ovarian drilling. Operative laparoscopy has renewed the interest in the surgical approach to ovulation induction in patients resistant to clomiphene or hMG therapy. The results are promising with a high ovulation rate ranging between 70% and 90% and a pregnancy rate of 70%. Advocates of laparoscopy claim a lower risk of postoperative adhesions compared to laparotomy. Other arguments in favor of the laparoscopic approach include the minimal morbidity associated with the procedure and virtually no cyclic monitoring of ovulation induction. In addition there is no increased risk of multiple gestation and ovarian hyperstimulation. Some studies have noted a lowered rate of miscarriage after LEOS than medical therapy. It has also shown to produce significant endocrine changes with better results in obese patients with higher preoperative luteinizing hormone (LH) values and LH-FSH ratio.

Several "methods of laparoscopic treatment" have been studied, including ovarian electrocauterization, laser drilling, and multiple biopsy. Each of these methods share a common goal of creating focal areas of damage to the ovarian cortex and/or stroma, with the most extensively studied method being laparoscopic electrocoagulation of the ovaries (LEOS). However, there is no standard technique among different reproductive surgeons. The aim of newer studies is to compare different laparoscopic techniques and study the hormonal profile, ovulation rate and pregnancy rate after surgery. Takeuchi et al. performed a prospective, randomized study of infertile women with PCOS and compared a group who underwent laparoscopic ovarian drilling using a harmonic scalpel laser to a group who underwent laparoscopic ovarian drilling using a neodymium-yttrium-aluminum-garnet (Nd:YAG) laser. Change in the hormonal profile after surgery, ovulation rate and pregnancy rate were compared between both groups. LH and testosterone serum levels and the LH-FSH ratio showed a statistically significant reduction after surgery, and the spontaneous ovulation rate was 94% in both groups. The cumulative pregnancy rates within 2 years of follow-up were 77% in those who underwent laparoscopic ovarian drilling using a harmonic scalpel laser and 60% in those who underwent laparoscopic ovarian drilling using a Nd:YAG laser. This study shows that the technique of laparoscopic ovarian drilling using a harmonic scalpel resulted in ovulation and conception without major complications.

Malkawi et al. studied how many punctures per ovary are needed to improve the reproductive outcome? To evaluate the biochemical, clinical and reproductive results after laparoscopic ovarian drilling they carried out a different number of punctures in the ovaries. They concluded that five, instead of more than or equal to 10, punctures per ovary are sufficient to ameliorate the hyperandrogenic status in these women, improving their clinical and reproductive outcome.

Currently, the choice of the "number of punctures" to be applied at laparoscopic ovarian drilling (LOD) is empirical. Historically, the amount of ovarian tissue removed during bilateral ovarian wedge resection varied between one-third and three-quarters depending on the size of the ovary. Some gynecologists apply the same principle to LOD by empirically making different numbers of punctures in each ovary depending on its size. Between 3 punctures and 25 punctures have been reported with power settings between 30 watts and 400 watts. As a general principle, increasing the amount of thermal energy delivered to the ovarian stroma may increase the efficacy of the procedure but at the expense of increasing the risk of ovarian atrophy.

Gjonnaess reported that ovulation occurred more frequently if five or more holes were applied compared with three holes per ovary. However, others found that four diathermy holes per ovary were sufficient to achieve good results and that no improvement was achieved when applying more holes. There are a number of difficulties in comparing the experience of various authors due to variation in the techniques used in LOD, including:

- Using different instruments (needles, scissors, biopsy forceps, etc.) to deliver the energy to the ovary
- Applying different amount of energy to the ovary (measured in joules, equivalent to power in watts multiplied by the duration of electricity applied in seconds per puncture)
- Distribution of the thermal energy, either localized to a few holes or more widely spread over many holes with varying depths of penetration.

Calculation of Thermal Energy

Gjonnaess in 1984 correlated the ovulation rates after LOD to different numbers of points cauterized. He reported that the best results [ovulation rate = 96.7% (n = 30)] were obtained when the number of points were more than five per ovary (>10 points per patient). However, this referred to the use of biopsy or sterilization forceps applied against the ovarian surface and activating the electricity at 200–300 watts for 3 ± 1 sec. Hence, the amount of thermal energy delivered to each ovary, on an average, was 250 watts × 3 s × more than 5 = more than 3750 joules. Armar in 1990s found that four diathermy holes per ovary were sufficient to achieve good results and that no improvement was achieved when applying more holes. This referred to the use of a specially designed needle to penetrate the ovary with activation of the electricity (40 watts) for 4 seconds at each point. The amount of thermal energy delivered to each ovary was 40 watts × 4 secs × 4 = 640 joules, which is significantly lower than that used by Gjonnaess. Another study compared the amounts of thermal energy used where 2, 3, 4, 5, 6, 7 punctures were applied. The calculation of thermal energy was watts applied × no. of seconds × no. of punctures. It is important that the comparison between different studies should take into consideration the total amount of thermal energy delivered to each ovary, not just the number of holes made in the ovary.

Threshold Dose

The application of two holes per ovary, equivalent to the delivery of 300 joules, was found to produce significantly poorer results than the other groups, measured in terms of restoration of menstrual regularity, ovulation rate and conception rate. The threshold dose may therefore be higher than two punctures per ovary.

Plateau Dose

The plateau dose refers to the lowest dose at which all subjects who will respond are observed to respond.

There does not appear to be significant differences in the outcomes (menstrual pattern, ovulation and conception) of groups where 2–6 punctures are applied. It seems that three punctures (450 joules) per ovary produce results as good as higher numbers of punctures. A prospective dose-finding study is required to estimate more accurately the optimal amount of energy required for LOD.

Excessive Thermal Energy

Ovarian atrophy and failure is a rare complication of LOD. A case of severe ovarian atrophy following LOD has been reported in which eight punctures were created at 400 watts for 5 sec per each puncture, equivalent to 16,000 joules. It is, therefore, possible that application of excessive amounts of thermal energy to the ovary during LOD will produce irreversible damage to the ovary, leading to ovarian failure.

FSH is considered to be a reasonable marker of ovarian reserve and function. It seems possible that the application of seven or more punctures per ovary represents an excessive amount of thermal energy used for LOD and should therefore be discouraged.

Depth of Penetration of Energy

Where a significantly greater amount of thermal energy (>3,750 joules per ovary) was applied, it was done so using a pair of biopsy or sterilization forceps, which applied the thermal energy to the ovarian surface and the depth of penetration was therefore between 2 mm and 4 mm, i.e. superficial. In contrast, the depth of penetration using the specially designed ovarian diathermy needle (Rocket of London) is up to 8 mm. Similar instruments used by others, found that the amount of thermal energy used to produce a good result was approximately 640 joules per ovary. It is, therefore, possible to conclude that with deeper penetration during LOD, the amount of thermal energy can be reduced without compromising the outcome. Furthermore, achieving good results with deep penetration using low energy supports the hypothesis that LOD works by destroying androgen-producing ovarian stroma.

Preoperatively the routine tests for any laparoscopic surgery are performed along with the special hormonal investigations such as day 3 FSH, LH, prolactin, total testosterone and dehydroepiandrosterone (DHEAS).

Postoperative Monitoring

Following ovarian diathermy, women are asked to keep a record of their menstrual cycle. If the patient started a menstrual period within 6 weeks of the surgery, a blood sample is taken on day 2 of that cycle for measurement of serum concentrations of LH, FSH, testosterone, androstenedione and sex hormone-binding globulin (SHBG). Another blood sample is taken on day 21 of the same cycle for measurement of serum concentration of progesterone. Ovulation is diagnosed when the progesterone level is more than 30 nmol/L. Two more mid-luteal phase blood samples are taken in the subsequent cycles to measure serum progesterone levels. If spontaneous menstruation does not occur during the 6 weeks following surgery, a random blood sample is taken to measure all the above hormones.

In order to comprehend the mechanism of action of LEOS, it is necessary to understand the pathophysiology of polycystic ovarian disease (PCOD).

PATHOPHYSIOLOGY OF POLYCYSTIC OVARIAN DISEASE

Elevated LH levels may stimulate androgen production in stromal and hyperplastic thecal cells in the ovarian follicle. Although abundant substrate for estrogen synthesis is available, the low levels of FSH in the follicle prevent induction of aromatase activity and result in a lack of ovarian estrogen production. As granulosa cell mitosis and follicular growth require an estrogenic follicular microenvironment, follicular maturation is arrested. High intra-ovarian androgen levels may also contribute to follicular atresia. Peripheral availability of ovarian testosterone that is converted by 5-α reductase in the skin to dihydrotestosterone, accounts for acne and hirsutism in these women. Increased androstenedione secretion leads to increased acyclic production of estrogens, principally estrone by aromatization in peripheral tissues. This chronic high estrogen feedback at the level of the hypothalamo pituitary axis is positive for LH-FSH ratio of 2.5 or more. Thus the inappropriate gonadotrophin secretion is secondary to abnormal steroid feedback rather than a primary abnormality at the level of the pituitary (This has been amply supported by studies that demonstrate normal negative and positive feedback responses to estrogen administration).

MECHANISM OF ACTION OF "LEOS" IN OVARIAN OVULATION INDUCTION

The mechanisms responsible for the ovulation inducing properties of "LEOS" have as yet to be satisfactorily elucidated. Various hypotheses have been suggested, based on the hormonal changes observed after LEOS:

- Marked decrease in circulating levels of androgens, i.e. androstenedione and testosterone

- Decrease in levels of DHEAS
- Decrease in circulating levels of estradiol
- Reduction in the concentration of immunoreactive LH as well as in LH bioactivity
- Decrease in LH-FSH ratio
- Central opioid and dopaminergic control over gonadotropin secretion appears to remain unaffected by LEOS
- Temporary decrease in inhibin levels which reach baseline values in one week
- Significant reduction in serum concentration of homocysteine.

Possible Mechanisms

- *Destruction of ovarian stromal elements* and release of androgen rich follicular fluid from the puncture of subcapsular cysts causes a fall in local and circulating levels of androgens. Decrease in substrate for follicular aromatase and damage to the follicle walls itself, produces a fall in circulating estradiol levels, release of the pituitary from negative feedback of estradiol on FSH, producing positive feedback effects on LH secretion and normalization of LH-FSH ratio leading to follicular development followed by ovulation.
  The observations which support the above hypotheses are:
  - Pituitary LH secretion in response to infusions of GnRH is reduced postoperatively, compared to the preoperative response
  - Ovulation rates and continuation of ovulatory cycles are best in patients in whom LH levels are high preoperatively, proving that the decrease in LH levels is directly proportional to the success of LEOS
  - Pregnancies occur more often when the follicular fluid is rich in androgen content at the time of surgery
- Transvaginal ultrasound guided follicular aspiration of subcapsular cysts without causing significant stromal damage has yielded a 50–85% ovulation rate and 50% pregnancy rate. This may suggest that removal of the androgen rich follicular fluid eventually helps to restore LH-FSH ratio
- *Hyperemia* associated with the postoperative healing process may play a role by increasing the delivery of gonadotropins to the ovary
- The side on which ovulation occurs after "LEOS" is randomly distributed even when only one ovary is treated. Thus, it means that whatever the effects are at the ovarian level, the mechanism responsible for ovulation seems to exert itself through systemic routes.

OUTCOME ANALYSIS OF LEOS

The results are promising with a high ovulation rate ranging between 70% and 90% and a pregnancy rate of around 70%. Majority of patients have spontaneous ovulation after surgery.

The crude pregnancy rates after ovarian drilling in one study varied between 52% and 80% with electrocoagulation and 0–56% with laser. Using life table analysis, Heylen et al. reported pregnancy rates of 68% and 73% respectively at 12, 18 and 24 months after laparoscopic treatment with argon laser. Li et al. reported a cumulative pregnancy rate of 54%, 62–68% respectively at 12, 18 and 24 months using argon laser. Felemban et al. reported in a recent study a pregnancy rate of 54%, 68% and 82% respectively at 12, 18 and 24 months using insulated needle cautery for ovarian drilling. In our personal series the ovulation rate achieved was 82% and a 58% pregnancy rate.

Table 1 shows the summary of conceptions following LEOS.

Three-dimensional (3D) sonographic characterization of polycystic ovaries has been performed recently, including the study of the effect of laparoscopic ovarian drilling on ovarian volume. Ovarian volume decreased, and an increase in intraovarian flow intensity after laparoscopic electrocautery has been observed. Besides, hormonal levels correlated well with changes of 3D sonographic features. Therefore, 3D USG may be a useful adjunct and noninvasive method for correlating clinical parameters with the blood flow alterations in polycystic ovary syndrome patients.

In our experience of 296 prospectively studied cases of LOD till 2005, the ovulation rate was 82% and pregnancy rate of 58%.

The routine protocol for management of infertile PCOS patients is to begin with insulin sensitizing agents along with ovulation stimulating drugs for 6 months (33% pregnancy rate). In case the patients do not respond, they are subjected to LOD (58% pregnancy rate).

PREDICTIVE FACTORS OF LEOS

Although LOD has been widely used to induce ovulation in women with PCOS, predicting the clinical response to this treatment remains to be elucidated further. Amer et al. carried out a study to identify factors that may help to predict the outcome of LOD. The results showed that women with body mass index (BMI) more than or equal to 35 kg/m^2, serum testosterone concentration more than or equal to 4.5 nmol/L, free androgen index (FAI) more than or equal to 15 and/or with duration of infertility more than 3 years seem to be poor responders to LOD.

Table 1: Summary of conceptions following laparoscopic ovulation induction

Author	Year	N	Method	Ovulation (%)	Pregnancy (%)
Aakvaag and Gjonnaess	1985	58	LEOS	91	42
Greenblatt and Casper	1987	6	LEOS	83	67
Vander Weiden and Alberda	1987	11	LEOS	82	45
Sumioki et al	1988	7	Biopsy	86	57
Daniell and Miller	1989	85	CO_2/KTP	71	56
Yanagibori et al	1989	6	Nd/YAG	—	50
Abdel Gadir et al	1990	29	LEOS	87	48
Keckstein et al	1990	27	Nd:YAG	70	37
Tasaka et al	1990	11	LEOS	91	36
Utsunomiya et al	1990	16	Biopsy	94	50
Kovacs et al	1991	10	LEOS	90	40
Rossmanith et al	1991	11	Nd:YAG	72	36
Gurgen et al	1992	40	Nd:YAG	70	50
Ostrzenski	1992	12	CO_2	100	75
Armar and Lachelin	1993	50	LEOS	92	62
Campo et al	1993	23	Biopsy	61	56
Verhelst et al	1993	17	CO	82	65
Tiitinen et al	1993	10	LEOS	70	20
Greenblatt and Capser	1993	8	LEOS	100	88
Szilagyi et al	1993	4	Nd:YAG	75	25
Balen and Jacobs	1994	10	LEOS	100	40
Gjonnaess	1994	219	LEOS	92	69
Naether et al	1994	206	LEOS	77	70
Heylen et al	1994	44	Vaporization	—	73
Shah DS	1997	125	LEOS	82	58
Al Took et al	1997	—	Drilling	—	52–80
Li TC et al	1998	31	Argon	—	68
Li TC et al	1998	80	LEOS	—	68
Felemban	2000	112	LEOS	73	54–82
Takeuchi S et al	2003	17	Harmonic	94	77
Scalpel					
Al-Fadhli R	2004	—	LEOS	80	50–60
Cleemann L	2004	—	LEOS	61	
Api M	2005	45	Drilling	93	64
Yildirim M	2004	134	Minilaparotomy and ovarian wedge resection		78–90

Abbreviations: LEOS, Laparoscopic electrocoagulation of the ovaries; Nd:YAG, Neodymium-yttrium-aluminum-garnet laser; KTP, Potassium-titanyl-phosphate

In LOD responders, serum LH levels more than 10 IU/L appeared to be associated with higher pregnancy rates. Marked obesity, marked hyperandrogenism and/or long duration of infertility in women with PCOS seem to predict resistance to LOD. High LH levels in LOD responders appear to predict higher probability of pregnancy.

FACTORS INFLUENCING POSTOPERATIVE OVULATION INDUCTION AFTER TREATMENT WITH LEOS

- Presence of any additional factors responsible for infertility
- Patients with elevated LH levels (≥ 10 mIU/mL) seem more likely to conceive postoperatively, while those with absence of postoperative fall of LH levels are unlikely to ovulate
- Early resumption of anovulatory state postoperatively is associated with return to the pretreatment hormonal milieu and indicates the need for other therapeutic modalities
- Overweight patients experience a lower rate of ovulation than patients with normal body weight
- Smoking adversely affects the pregnancy rates is these patients
- Metformin improves insulin resistance, reduces androgen levels and significantly increases the ovulation and pregnancy rates in infertile women, following LOD.

ADVANTAGES OF LEOS

- LEOS yields a better ovulation rate and pregnancy rate than other modalities of laparoscopic surgery for ovulation induction in patients with PCOS
- It has been suggested that patients who had previously developed OHSS during gonadotropin therapy, either ovulate spontaneously or with clomiphene citrate (CC) after LEOS and even the incidence of OHSS reduces in subsequent gonadotropin cycles.

COMPLICATIONS

Adhesion Formation

Adhesion formation was a significant complication of Osler–Weber–Rendu syndrome (OWR) which was due to tissue handling and serosal trauma at laparotomy. Adhesions resulted in non-availability of ovarian surface for ovulation and peritoneal ovum transport was hindered. LEOS has gained importance as it is expected to minimize adhesion formation postoperatively (Table 2).

The definite etiology of pelvic adhesion formation is not clearly well known, but the following risk factors have been incriminated in this process:

- Intra-abdominal infection
- Tissue hypoxia or ischemia
- Tissue drying
- Rough manipulations of tissues during surgery
- Presence of reactive foreign body
- Presence of intraperitoneal blood
- Dissection of prior adhesions.

Adjuvants for Adhesion Reduction

Adhesion formation and reformation are still an unavoidable event in reproductive pelvic surgery in spite of the variable skills in microsurgery, endoscopic or laser surgery. This fact necessitates the search for an adjuvant(s) that can be used in the perioperative period. The field of these adjuvants becomes large enough to require a classification (Box 1).

Fibrinolytic Agents

Fibrinolytic agents act directly by reducing the fibrinous mass and indirectly by stimulating plasminogen activator activity.

Table 2: Adhesion formation rates with laparoscopic electrocoagulation of the ovaries (LEOS) as noted by various workers at second-look laparoscopy

Author	Year	No. of points	Method	No. of points with adhesion/No. of points undergoing second-look scopy
Naether et al.	1993	199	LEOS	19.3%
Gurgen	1991	7	LEOS	85.3%
Shah Duru	2003	207	LEOS	12%
Yildirim M	2004	44	Minilaparotomy and ovarian wedge resection	11.4%

Box 1 Classes of adhesion-reduction adjuvants and their proposed mehanism of action

I. Fibrinolytic agents (fibrinolysis, stimulation of plasminogen activators)
   - Fibrinolysin
   - Streptokinase
   - Urokinase
   - Hyaluronidase
   - Chymotrypsin
   - Trypsin
   - Pepsin
   - Plasminogen activators

II. Anticoagulants (prevention of clot and fibrin formation)
   - Heparin
   - Citrates
   - Oxalates

III. Anti-inflammatory agents (reduce vascular permeability, reduce histamine release and, stabilize lysozomes)
   - Corticosteroids
   - Nonsteroidal anti-inflammatory agents
   - Anti-histamines
   - Progesterone
   - Calcium channel blockers
   - Colchicine

IV. Antibiotics (prevent infection)
   - Tetracyclines
   - Cephalosporins

V. Mechanical separation (surface separation, hydroflotation)
   - Intra-abdominal Instillates:
     - Dextran
     - Mineral oil
     - Silicone
     - Vaseline
     - Crystalloid solutions
     - Carboxymethylcellulose
     - Hyaluronic acid
     - Chelated hyaluronic acid
     - Poloxamer
   - Barriers:
     - Endogenous tissues:
       - Omental grafts
       - Peritoneal grafts
       - Bladder strips
       - Fetal membranes
     - Exogenous materials:
       - Fibrin glue
       - Polytetrafluoroethylene
       - Oxidized cellulose
       - Oxidized regenerated cellulose
       - Gelatin
       - Rubber sheets
       - Metal foils
       - Plastic hoods

Anticoagulants

Heparin is the most widely investigated anticoagulant used for prevention of adhesions. Its mechanism of action is probably through one of the following: first, heparin may interact in the clotting cascade by a combination with antithrombin III. Second, heparin directly stimulates the activity of plasminogen activators, thereby promoting breakdown of fibrin clots once they form. Lastly, heparin may act by binding to fibroblast growth factor (FGF) leading to considerable improvement in healing of cutaneous wounds. Heparin has been added to peritoneal irrigants with concentrations of around 5 U/mL. In a study, a significant reduction in adhesion formation was only observed with the combination of Interceed (TC7) and heparin where Interceed was utilized as a carrier to deliver heparin to traumatized surfaces.

Anti-inflammatory Agents

This group of agents were used to reduce the initial inflammatory response to tissue injury and hence, subsequent adhesion formation. This goal is probably achieved through the capability of these agents to reduce vascular permeability, inhibit synthesis and release of histamines and/or stabilize lysosomes. Anti-inflammatory agents that have been investigated included corticosteroids, nonsteroidal agents, progesterone and progestogens, antihistaminics and calcium channel blockers.

Nonsteroidal anti-inflammatory drugs (NSAIDs) act through several postulated mechanisms. NSAIDs have an antiprostaglandin effect, thereby blocking the adhesiogenic action of prostaglandins instilled intraperitonealy. They have also been shown to inhibit platelets' aggregation, leukocyte migration and phagocytosis, and lysosome release. Tolmetin, a NSAID was presumed to enhance macrophage function, and hence, allow rapid phagocytosis of tissue debris or fibrin. Tolmetin and ibuprofen have also been shown to increase fibrinolysis through decreasing the secretion of plasminogen inhibitors resulting in enhanced plasmin production. Results support the view that there is a common mechanism through which NSAIDs act to prevent adhesions.

Antibiotics

The rationale behind the use of antibiotics is prophylaxis against infection, and hence the inflammatory response, that leads to adhesion development. Systemic broad-spectrum antibiotics, particularly cephalosporins, were widely used in the past. Nowadays, tetracyclines are commonly used to protect from *Chlamydia*, a potentially infectious organism in the female genital tract.

Unfortunately, there is no sufficient published data supporting this practice.

Mechanical Separation

Mechanical separation of peritoneal surfaces of the pelvic organs during the early days of the healing process postoperatively was a practical way to prevent postoperative adhesions. This separation may be accomplished by intra-abdominal instillates and barriers whether endogenous tissue or exogenous material.

Crystalloid Solutions

Crystalloid solutions were the most commonly used instillates put into the abdominal cavity after completion of the surgical procedure. In addition to its mechanical action in separation of the raw peritoneal surfaces, crystalloid solutions dilute fibrin and fibrinous exudate released from the traumatized surfaces.

Unfortunately, crystalloid solutions are absorbed from the peritoneal cavity at an estimated rate of 35 mL/hr. Thus a volume of 500 mL will be absorbed within about 14 hours and 5 liters of crystalloid solution are needed to cover the first 6 days postoperatively. The process of peritoneal repair, fibrin deposition, and adhesion formation extends quite beyond the time during which a reasonable volume of crystalloid persists. The other drawback is the possible increased risk of infection with instillation of such a large volume of fluid into the peritoneal cavity.

In an attempt to prolong the period of instillate persistence inside the peritoneal cavity, more viscous solutions have been tried in both experimental and clinical studies. A "32% dextran-70 solution" (Hyskon) was among the most commonly used viscous solutions. Usually 200 mL of it is instilled into the posterior cul-de-sac at completion of the surgery. Hyskon acts as a siliconizing agent, coating raw surfaces. As an osmotic agent, it results in hyrdroflotation of the pelvic viscera, and additionally it stimulates plasminogen activators. Complications reported from its use include anaphylaxis, pleural effusion, vulvar edema, transient liver function abnormalities, wound separation, disseminated intravascular coagulation, and abdominal bloating after its instillation.

Carboxymethylcellulose

Carboxymethylcellulose is a high molecular weight polysaccharide that acts as an adjuvant for prevention of adhesion by coating the intraperitoneal surfaces and creating hydroflotation of intra-abdominal structures. A novel CMC sponge has been developed for prevention of surgical wound adhesions. Hyaluronic acid is a glycosaminoglycan that under aqueous conditions forms a viscous solution.

Exogenous Barriers

Exogenous barriers such as metal foils, plastic hoods, silk and rubber sheets were used in the past to reduce postoperative adhesions. However, these substances have been abandoned because of lack of success and the need for its removal by a second surgical procedure.

Fibrin Glue

Fibrin glue is a combination of highly concentrated fibrinogen, thrombin, calcium, and factor VIII. It is postulated that fibrin glue acts by separating the raw surfaces through its rapid sealant effect.

Surgicel®

Surgicel® is an oxidized regenerated cellulose (ORC) that was initially designed as a hemostatic agent. It was investigated as an adjuvant for prevention of adhesions because it is easy to apply and becomes a gel within hours after application. Initial studies showed that Surgicel® is effective in preventing adhesions in rat cecal trauma model. However, other studies failed to realize any reduction in adhesion formation.

Interceed

Interceed is an "altered relative" to Surgicel®, also composed of oxidized regenerated cellulose but differs in several characters including its degree of oxidation, weave, and smaller pore size. Interceed becomes a gel about eight hours after its intra-abdominal application. The material usually cannot be identified in the field within 3–4 days, and usually is degraded by the body without evidence of a foreign body reaction at the site of application. Interceed is metabolized into glucose and glucoronic acid within a few days.

To evaluate the efficacy of Interceed in prevention of postsurgical ovarian adhesions many studies were carried out. One such study was by Franklin and The Ovarian Adhesion Study Group. It was a multicenter randomized study including 55 patients with bilateral ovarian disease. One ovary was randomly wrapped with Interceed at the completion of laparotomy and the other was left uncovered. At the time of second-look laparoscopy, they found that treatment of ovaries with Interceed significantly reduced the occurrence and severity of postsurgical ovarian adhesions. As regards laparoscopic ovarian surgery, Interceed was found to be safe and effective also in reducing the incidence of postoperative adhesion formation in patients undergoing laparoscopic ovarian cystectomy. These results are consistent with most studies.

A modified version of Interceed is neutralized Interceed (nTC), that is blood insensitive, has also proved efficacious in reducing adhesion formation and reformation in animal studies. The results using the nTC7 Interceed are comparable to those obtained with Interceed in combination with heparin.

Following LEOS, translucent adhesions judged of limited consequence to the normal tubo-ovarian relationship were noted.

Animal research on pigs (Naether et al., unpublished data) suggested that one major effect of LEOS is an increase in ovarian blood supply and adhesion formation which are classified as mild to minimal.

In women failing to conceive postoperatively a follow-up laparoscopy was performed. A high incidence of mild adhesion formation was documented. However, their extent and severity was not influenced by the number of ovarian punctures; however, the left ovary appeared more prone to develop severe adhesions than the contralateral one.

LOD with laser appears to produce more adhesion formation than electrocoagulation. Table 2 shows the rate of adhesion formation in various studies during second-look laparoscopy.

Filmy adhesions confined to the ovarian surface do not seem to affect the success rate of the surgery. However, because of consequences of intra-abdominal adhesions such as abdominal pain and small bowel obstruction, adhesion prevention is necessary. Felemban et al. suggest that the best method for decreasing adhesion formation is with the use of an insulated needle electrode, which minimizes injury to the ovarian surface. As the insulated part of the needle is inside the ovarian stroma, thermal injury to the surface of the ovary is limited.

Thus, although a high rate of adhesion formation is undeniable, adhesiolysis may not improve subsequent pregnancy rates (or perhaps that the adhesions are not of sufficient severity to prevent conception).

Interceed, a widely used therapeutic agent to prevent adhesions formation after conservative operative procedures on the reproductive organs, was not of benefit in preventing adhesion formation after electrocauterization.

One recent study suggests "microlaparoscopy" as a cost-effective alternative with the advantage of significantly less adhesion formation than with the conventional operative laparoscopy (24% vs. 48%, $p < 0.05$). This may be due to reduced exposure and amount of CO_2, which has minimal effect on peritoneal microcirculation and cell protective systems, which are proposed mechanisms for adhesion formation and closely related to peritoneal injury.

Some questions still need more investigations to be answered: Why some patients are more susceptible for adhesion formation and others are not? Can those patients be identified preoperatively? Which stage of adhesion formation is more suitable to interfere with by an agent to reduce it? Further studies are needed, but the results thus far appear quite promising.

OTHER COMPLICATIONS

Ovarian Atrophy

In addition to adhesion formation, a case of unilateral ovarian atrophy has been reported following the procedure and even questions regarding the potential for including epithelial ovarian cancers have been raised.

Abortion Rates

Rate of spontaneous abortions in women with PCOS is elevated as compared to women without PCOS and is approximately 30%. This could be due to elevated levels of LH in many of the women. The rates of abortion did not change in patients with PCOS having normal LH values. The excess LH may allow premature resumption of meiosis resulting in a prematurely aged oocyte. Such postmature oocytes are associated with lower rates of fertilization, cleavage and implantation (as has been observed in vitro fertilization). Further, adverse effects of elevated LH levels on the oocyte might be mediated via changes in the antral steroidogenic environment, such as premature progesterone production. No differences have been noted in ovulation or pregnancy rates in patients treated with LEOS as compared to medical therapy. However, it is noted that the group treated with LEOS had fewer cycles with multiple dominant follicles, consistently lower luteal phase testosterone levels and lower rates of early pregnancy loss. Gjonnaess reported early pregnancy loss in 14.3% of 89 patients who conceived following laparoscopic electrocautery. While Abdel Gadir et al. reported an early pregnancy loss in 3 out of 14 (21.4%) patients treated with LEOS and 55.4 and in the hMG group. Felemban had a miscarriage rate of 7.7% in his study of LEOS.

On the other hand, Gjonnaess has proposed LEOS as the first line of treatment for all patients of PCOS, undergoing laparoscopy for any reason even if pregnancy is not desired at that time. He has noted that majority of the patients continue to have ovulatory cycles for up to 10 years following electrocautery and a pregnancy rate of 89% in anovulatory cases of PCOS. In Gjonnaess series, those patients who underwent the procedure had no difficulty of conceiving after a period of 2 years of contraception after LEOS.

Cleemann et al. used LOD as a first line of treatment, as a second line of treatment after patients were proved resistant to clomiphene or as a third line of treatment after failed ovulation induction with gonadotropins. This strategy with diagnostic laparoscopy and LOD as the first line of treatment of infertility in women with PCOS shortened the time to pregnancy for many women, reduced the need for medical ovulation induction and enabled diagnosis of those women with anatomic infertility, who could achieve pregnancy only by in vitro fertilization treatment.

While the considerable experience of Gjonnaess should not be discounted, more controlled studies have to be performed to judge the efficacy of the procedure. These studies do provide compelling preliminary evidence that LEOS is comparable (or even superior) to available methods of ovulation induction for that small group of PCOS patients who are resistant to clomiphene citrate therapy. Little is known about the long-term effect of LEOS on the age of menopause and risk of ovarian cancer.

Hyperprolactinemia

Hyperprolactinemia after ovarian cauterization may be considered as a possible cause of anovulation in women with polycystic ovaries and improved gonadotropin and androgen levels. The cause of hyperprolactinemia is unknown. Hormonal assay particularly prolactin (PRL) in anovulatory patients after ovarian cauterization is recommended.

In view of the above facts, LEOS should be reserved for patients unresponsive to clomiphene citrate therapy, who cannot or do not wish to undergo gonadotropin therapy. Nevertheless, the high pregnancy rate, and economic aspect of the procedure offer an attractive management for patients with PCOS.

CONCLUSION

Notwithstanding the shortcomings of the available data, there seem to be some real benefits of LEOS for carefully selected patients who fail to respond to clomiphene citrate therapy.

LEOS has to be performed in patients when all other available options have been exhausted, taking into consideration the possibility of adhesion formation as well as the cost and risk associated with any operative procedure. Thus, it would be in the interest of the patient, to perform LEOS after a complete infertility evaluation and a determined attempt with clomiphene citrate therapy. LEOS can have a place in the therapeutic armamentarium of the clinician, only when it has been shown to do no harm to the patients' fertility potential and long-term health and all noninvasive options have been explored.

BIBLIOGRAPHY

1. Aakvaag A, Gjonnaess H. Hormonal response to electrocautery of the ovary in patients with polycystic ovarian disease. Br J Obstet Gynaecol. 1985;92:1258-64.
2. Abdel Gadir A, Alnaser HM, Mowafi RS, et al. The response to patients with polycystic ovarian disease to human menopausal gonadotropin therapy after ovarian electrocautery or a luteinizing hormone-releasing hormone agonist. Fertil Steril. 1992;57:309-13.
3. Abdel Gadir A, Khatim MS, Alnaser HM, et al. Ovarian electrocautery: responders versus non responders. Gynecol Endocrinol. 1993;7:43-8.
4. Abdel Gadir A, Khatim MS, Mowafi RS, et al. Hormonal changes in patients with polycystic ovarian disease after ovarian electrocautery or pituitary desensitization. Clin Endocrinol. 1990;33:585-92.
5. Abdel Gadir A, Mowafi RS, Alnaser HM, et al. Ovarian electrocautery versus human menopausal gonadotropins and pure follicle stimulating hormone therapy in the treatment of patients with polycystic ovarian disease. Clin Endocrinol. 1990;33:585-92.
6. Al Took S, Tulandi T. Surgical management of PCOS. J Soc Obstet Gynaecol Can. 1997;19:721-9.
7. Al-Fadhli R, Tulandi T. Laparoscopic treatment of polycystic ovaries: is its place diminishing? Curr Opin Obstet Gynecol. 2004;16(4):295-8.
8. Al-Ojaimi EH. Endocrine changes after laparoscopic ovarian drilling in clomiphene citrate-resistant women with polycystic ovarian syndrome. Saudi Med J. 2004;25(12):2063.
9. Al-Took S, Platt R, Tulandi T. Adhesion related small bowel obstruction after gynecologic operations. Am J Obstet Gynaecol. 1999;180:313-5.
10. Amer SA, Li TC, Ledger WL. Ovulation induction using laparoscopic ovarian drilling in women with polycystic ovarian syndrome: predictors of success. Hum Reprod. 2004;19(8):1719-24.
11. Api M, Gorgen H, Cetin A. Laparoscopic ovarian drilling in polycystic ovary syndrome. Eur J Obstet Gynecol Reprod Biol. 2005;119(1):76-81.
12. Armar NA, Lachelin GC. Laporoscopic ovarian diathermy: an effective treatment for antioestrogen resistant anovulatory infertility in women with the polycystic ovary syndrome. Br J Obstet Gynecol. 1993;100:161-4.
13. Armar NA, McGarrigle HH, Homour J, et al. Laparoscopic ovarian diathermy in the management of anovulatory infertility in women with polycystic ovaries, endocrine changes and clinical outcome. Fertil Steril. 1990;53:45-9.
14. Balen AH, Jacobs HS. A prospective study comparing unilateral and bilateral laparoscopic ovarian diathermy in women with the polycystic ovary syndrome. Fertil Steril. 1994;62:921-5.
15. Campo S, Feli A, Lamanna MA, et al. Endocrine changes and clinical outcome after laparoscopic ovarian resection in women with polycystic ovaries. Hum Reprod. 1993;8: 359-63.
16. Campo S, Felli A, Lamanna MA, et al. Endocrine changes and clinical outcome after laparoscopic ovarian resection in women with polycystic ovaries. Hum Reprod. 1993;8:359-63.
17. Cleemann L, Lauszus FF, Trolle B. Laparoscopic ovarian drilling as first line of treatment in infertile women with polycystic ovary syndrome. Gynecol Endocrinol. 2004;18(3):138-43.
18. Dabirashrafi H. Complication of laparoscopic ovarian cauterization. Fertil Steril. 1989;52:878-9.
19. Daniell JF, Miller W. Polycystic ovaries treated by laparoscopic laser vaporization. Fertil Steril. 1989;51:232-6.
20. Daniell JF, Miller W. Polycystic ovaries treated by laparoscopic ovarian laser vaporization. Fertil Steril. 1989;51:232-6.
21. Donesky BW, Adashi EY. Surgically induced ovulation in PCOS: wedge revisited in the age of laparoscopy. Fertil Steril. 1995;63:439-63.
22. Felemban A, Tan SL, Tulandi T. Laparoscopic treatment of polycystic ovaries with insulated needle cautery: a reappraisal. Fertil Steril. 2000;73(2):266-9.
23. Frank S, Adams J, Mason H. Ovulatory disorders in women with polycystic ovarian syndrome. Clin Obstet Gynecol. 1985;12: 605-32.
24. Garcia J, Jones GS, Wentz AC. The use of clomiphene citrate. Fertil Steril. 1977;28:707-17.
25. Gjonnaess H. Ovarian electrocautery in the treatment of women with polycystic ovary syndrome (PCOS): factors affecting the result. Acta Obstet Gyn Scand. 1994;73:407-12.
26. Gjonnaess H. PCOS treated by ovarian electrocautery through the laparoscope. Fertil Steril. 1984;41:20-5.
27. Gomel V, Yarali H. Surgical treatment of polycystic ovary syndrome associated with infertility. Reprod Biomed Online. 2004;9(1):35-42.
28. Greenbaltt E, Casper RF. Endocrine changes after laparoscopic ovarian cautery for polycystic ovarian syndrome. Am J Obstet Gynecol. 1993;156:276-85.
29. Greenblatt EM, Casper RF. Adhesion formation after laparoscopic ovarian cautery for polycystic ovarian syndrome: lack of correlation with pregnancy rate. Fertil Steril. 1993;60:766-70.
30. Greenblatt EM, Casper RF. Adhesion formation after laparoscopic treatment of PCOS: lack of correlation with pregnancy rate. Fertil Steril. 1993;60:766-70.
31. Gurgan T, Kisnisci H, Yarali H, et al. Evaluation of adhesion formation after laparoscopic treatment of PCOD. Fertil Steril. 1991;56:1176-8.
32. Gurgen T, Urman B, Aksu T, et al. The effect of short-interval laparoscopic lysis of adhesions on pregnancy rates following Nd:YAG laser photocoagulation of polycystic ovaries. Obstet Gynecol. 1992;80:45-7.
33. Heylen SM, Puttemans PJ, Brossens IA. PCOD treated by laparoscopic argon alser capsule drilling. Comparison of vaporization versus perforation technique. Hum Reprod. 1994;9:1038-42.

34. Homburg R. Management of infertility and prevention of ovarian hyperstimulation in women with polycystic ovary syndrome. Best Pract Res Clin Obstet Gynaecol. 2004;18(5):773-88.
35. Keckstein G, Rossmanith W, Spatzier K, et al. The effect of laparoscopic treatment of polycystic ovarian disease by CO2–Laser or ND:YAG laser. Surg Endosc. 1990;4:103-7.
36. Keckstein J, Rossmanith W, Spatzier K, et al. The effect of laparoscopic treatment of PCOD by CO2 laser or Nd-Yag laser. Surg Endosc. 1990;4:103.
37. Kocak I, Usa A. Effects of metformin on insulin resistance, androgen concentration, ovulation and pregnancy rates in women with polycystic ovary syndrome following laparoscopic ovarian drilling. J Obstet Gynecol Res. 2006;32(3):292-8.
38. Kovacs G, Bucklar H, Bangah M, et al. Treatment of anovulation due to polycystic ovarian syndrome by laparoscopic ovarian electrocautery . Br J Obstet Gynecol. 1991;98:30-5.
39. Kovaks G, Buckler H, Gangah M, et al. Treatment of anovulation due to PCOS, laparoscopic ovarian cautery. Br J Obstet Gynecol. 1991;98:30-5.
40. Kucuk M, Kilic-Okman T. Hormone profiles and clinical outcome after laparoscopic ovarian drilling in women with polycystic ovary syndrome. Med Sci Monit. 2004;11(1):CR29-34.
41. Li TC, Saravelos H, Chow MS, et al. Factors affecting outcome of laparoscopic ovarian drilling for PCOS in women with anovulatory infertility. Br Obstet Gynaecol. 1998;195:338-44.
42. Lobo RA, Paul L, Granger L. Clomiphene and dexamethasone in women unresponsive to clomiphene alone. Obstet Gynecol. 1982;60:497-501.
43. Luciano AA, Maier DB, Koch EL, et al. A comparative study of postoperative adhesions following laser surgery by laparoscopy versus laparotomy in the rabbit model. Obstet Gynecol. 1989;74:220-4.
44. Luciano AA. Laparotomy versus laparoscopy. Prog Clin Biol Res. 1990;358:35-44.
45. Malkawi HY, Qublan HS. Laparoscopic ovarian drilling in the treatment of polycystic ovary syndrome: how many punctures per ovary are needed to improve the reproductive outcome? J Obstet Gynaecol Res. 2005;31(2):115-9.
46. Merchant RN. Treatment of PCOD with laparoscopic low watt bipolar electrocoagulation of the ovaries. J Am Assoc Gynecol Laparos. 1996;3:503-8.
47. Mercorio F, Merrcorio A, Di Spiezio Sardo A, et al. Evaluation of ovarian adhesion formation after laparoscopic ovarian drilling by second-look. Fertil Steril. 2008;89(5):1229-33.
48. Mio Y, TodaT, Tanikawa M, et al. Transvaginal ultrasound-guided follicular aspiration in the management of anovulatory infertility associated with polycystic ovaries. Fertil Steril. 1991;56:1060-5.
49. Naether O, Baukloh V, Fisher R, et al. Long-term follow-up in 206 infertility patients with polycystic ovarian syndrome after laparoscopic electrocautery of the ovarian surface. Hum Reprod. 1994;9:2341-9.
50. Naether OG, Fisher R, Weise HC, et al. Laparoscopic electrocoagulation of the ovarian surface in infertile patients with PCOD. Fertil Steril. 1993;60:88-94.
51. Ostrzenski A. Endoscopic carbon dioxide laser ovarian wedge resection in resistant polycystic ovarian disease. Intl J Fertil. 1992;37:295-9.
52. Persanezhad ME, Alborzi S, Zolghadri J, et al. Hyperprolactinaemia after laparoscopic ovarian drilling: an unknown phenomenon. Reprod Biol Endocrinol. 2005;3:31.
53. Portuondo JA, Melchor JC, Neyro JL Periovarian adhesions following ovarian wedge resection or laparoscopic biopsy. Endoscopy. 1984;16:143-5.
54. Rossmanith WG, Keckstein J, Spatzier K, et al. The impact of ovarian laser surgery on the gonadotropin secretion in women with polycystic ovarian disease. Clin Endocrinol. 1991;34:223-30.
55. Rossmanith WG, Keckstein J, Spatzier K, et al. The use of ovarian laser surgery on GnRH secretion in women with PCOD. Clin Endocrinol (Oxf). 1991;34:223-30.
56. Sagle M, Bishop K, Ridly N, et al. Recurrent early miscarriages and ovaries. Br Med J. 1988;297:1027-8.
57. Shah DS. Laparoscopic electrocauterisation of ovarian surface: does is it really help? Personal communication (unpublished) 1997.
58. Sumioki H, Utsunomyiya T, Matsuoka K, et al. The effect of laparoscopic multiple punch resection of the ovary on hypothalamopituitary axis in polycystic ovary syndrome. Fertil Steril. 1988;50:567-72.
59. Szilagyi A, Hole R, Keckstein J, et al. Effects of ovarian surgery on the dopaminergic and opioidergic control of gonadotropin and prolactin secretion in women with polycystic ovarian disease. Gynecol Endocrinol. 1993;7:159-66.
60. Takeuchi S, Futamura N, Takubo S, et al. Polycystic ovary syndrome treated with laparoscopic ovarian drilling with a harmonic scalpel. A prospective, randomized study. J Reprod Med. 2003;48(4):307.
61. Tan SL, Farhi J, Homburg R, et al. Induction of ovulation in clomiphene resistant PCOS with pulsatile GnRH. Obstet Gynecol. 1996;88:221-6.
62. Tasaka K, Sakata M, Kurachi H, et al. Electrocautery in polycystic ovary syndrome. Horm Res. 1990;33(2):40-2.
63. Taskin O, Sadik KS, Onoglu A, et al. Adhesion formation after microlaparoscopic and laparoscopic ovarian electrocoagulation for PCOD. J Am Assoc Gynecol Laparosc. 1999;6(2):159-63.
64. Tiitinen A, Tenhunen A, Seppala M. Ovarian electrocauterisation causes LH-regulated but noninsulin-regulated endocrine changes. Clin Endocrinol. 1993;39:181-4.
65. Toyoda N, Limieusx S, Lewis GF, et al. Correction of hyperandrogenemia by laparoscopic ovarian cautery in women with PCOS is not accompanied by improved insulin sensitivity or lipid-lipoprotein levels. J Clin Endocrinol Metab. 1999;84(11):4278-82.
66. Tulandi T, Took S. Surgical management of PCOS. Clin Obstet Gynaecol. 1998;12(4):541-53.
67. Tulandi T, Watkin K, Tan SL. Reproductive performance and three dimensional ultrasound volume determination of polycystic ovaries following ovarian drilling. Int J Infertil. 1997;42:436-40.

68. Unlu C, Atabekoglu CS. Surgical treatment in polycystic ovary syndrome. Curr Opin Obstet Gynecol. 2006;18(3):286-92.

69. Utsunomiya T, Sumioki H, Taniguchi L. Hormonal and clinical effects of multifollicular puncture and resection on the ovaries of polycystic ovary syndrome. Horm Res. 1990;33(2):35-9.

70. Van der Weiden RM, Alberda AT. Laparoscopic ovarian electrocautery in patients with polycystic ovarian disease resistant to clomiphene citrate. Surg Endosc. 1987;1:217-9.

71. Verhelst J, Joostens M, Ven Der Meer S, et al. Clinical and endocrine effects of laser vaporization in patients with polycystic ovarian disease. Gynecol Endocrinol. 1993;7:49-55.

72. Vizer M, Kiesel L, Szabo I, et al. Assessment of three-dimensional sonographic features of polycystic ovaries after laparoscopic ovarian cauterization. Fertil Steril. 2007;88(4):894-9.

73. Weerakiet S, Srisombut C, Choktanasiri W. Eficacy of laparoscopic ovulation induction in PCOS. J Med Assoc Thai. 1999;82(8):760-4.

74. Yanagibori A, Kojima E, Ohtaka, et al. Nd:YAG laser therapy for infertility with a contact type probe. J Reprod Med. 1989;34: 456-60.

75. Yildirim M, Noyan V, Bulent Tiras M, et al. Ovarian wedge resection by minilaparatomy in infertile patients with polycystic ovarian syndrome: a new technique. Eur J Obstet Gynecol Reprod Biol. 2003;107(1):85-7.

42.9 LAPAROSCOPIC STERILIZATION (COAGULATION RINGS AND CLIPS)

Mandakini Parihar, Meenakshi Bharath

"Family planning could bring more benefits to more people at less cost than any other single technology now available to the human race."—UNICEF Report

INTRODUCTION

For both men and women, surgical sterilization is a popular and well-established method of contraception. It offers highly effective protection against pregnancy; it carries a very low risk of complications when done according to accepted medical standards; and as a once only procedure, it eliminates the need for long-term contraceptive supplies. Males and female sterilizations can be carried out as outpatient procedures because the modern techniques are safe and simple. Since this form of contraception if intended to be permanent, informed choice and adequate counseling are crucial.

Female sterilization is a surgical procedure used to end women's ability to become pregnant. The procedure involves ligation with or without resection or blocking of both the Fallopian tubes, so that egg and sperm cannot meet. For many couples female sterilization is the most widely used contraceptive method in the world. Of 202 million married couples that have been sterilized for contraception worldwide, 163 million are women and out of this, 161 million are in developing countries (WHO 1994). In spite of the fact that vasectomy is safer and easier method of permanent contraception, female sterilization is being performed 4 times more commonly throughout the world. Thus female sterilization, as a most popular method of contraception effects the world's demography status in a big way. It is more significant in Indian context, as Indian National Family Planning Program has focused primarily on female sterilization especially till 1996. As a contraceptive method and surgical procedure involves a large population, all clinicians need to have adequate knowledge of all aspects of female sterilization.

HISTORY OF THE PROCEDURE

Dr J Bhundell of London first performed tubal ligation in 1823. At first, it was used to be practiced only for therapeutic reasons and was not widely used for voluntary sterilization of women until the 1930s. Voluntary sterilization was still infrequently asked for till the 1950s. It was only in 1960s that tubal ligation was promoted for sterilization and now this contraceptive method of permanent contraception has grown rapidly.

Currently, laparoscopy (using Fallope ring, bipolar laparoscopy, Filshie clip) is the most popular method of female sterilization in nonpregnant women. Periumbilical minilaparotomy (Pomeroy, Parkland) is the most common in the immediate postpartum period. Historical progression of sterilization procedures is given as in Appendix on page 613.

EVOLUTION OF FAMILY PLANNING PROGRAM IN INDIA

India was the first country in the world to adopt a National Family Planning Program as far back as 1951.

"But we have failed in its proper implementation." With a population of more than 1,050 million people, India is the second most populous country in the world, next only to China, whereas it is seventh in land area. Indian population has been steadily increasing since 1921 and is currently increasing at the rate of 16 million each year and is projected to reach 1.53 billion by year 2050s. The rampant population growth has been viewed as the greatest obstacle to the economic and social advancement of the majority of people in our under developed world.

The Indian Family Program has evolved throughout the years from 1952 to 2000 yet we have not succeeded in slowing Indian rapid population growth to a population replacement. One of the major reasons for failure is supposed to be the emphasis of family planning program on sterilization as method of contraception in initial phase and compromised quality of sterilization in Government hospital and camp setup at the same time (Mariya Kagan, 2000).

In the National Family Health Survey found that of the 36.2% of eligible couples using any modern method, 30.7% had been sterilized and only 5.5% were using temporary methods. Thus sterilization is six times more common than all other methods combined. During 2000-2002, 4.73 million couples accepted female sterilization as their family planning method in India.

TIMING OF THE FEMALE STERILIZATION PROCEDURE

- "Interval sterilization should be the method of preference for all tubal sterilizations done." It should preferably be performed within 7 days after the menstrual period is over (in the follicular phase of

the menstrual cycle). However, if the sterilization is done in premenstrual phase, counseling regarding the possibility of existing conception should be ensured and follow-up with the next menstrual period is mandatory
- "Postpartum sterilization" should preferably be done within 48 hours to 7 days of delivery. However, the procedure may be performed at any other time provided there is no infection or contraindication
- "Sterilization with medical termination of pregnancy (MTP)" can be performed concurrently. However, post-MTP tubectomy should not be done in camp conditions
- "Sterilization following spontaneous abortion" can be performed, with antibiotic coverage, in the absence of anemia and infection.

Laparoscopic tubal ligation should not be done concurrently with second trimester abortion and in postpartum period.

TECHNIQUES OF STERILIZATION

Widespread demand for simple, effective and inexpensive female sterilization procedure, which can be performed on an outpatient basis, has encouraged both medical practitioners and researchers to evaluate variety of methods of tubal occlusion and to develop new one. At present, following approaches and techniques are available:
- Abdominal approach
  - Conventional laparotomy
  - Minilaparotomy
  - Laparoscopy
- Transvaginal
  - Colpotomy
  - Culdoscopy
- Transcervical approach
  - Hysteroscopy
  - Quinacrine instillation (no longer recommended).

In this chapter, we will be restricting discussion to laparoscopic sterilization using clips, bands and cautery.

LAPAROSCOPIC STERILIZATION

Female sterilization with use of an operating laparoscope is getting more and more popular, because it has been found to be a safe, simple and effective procedure, which can be performed through one or two very small incisions on the abdomen, can be performed under GA, or under sedation and local anesthesia on an outpatient basis. "However, this procedure needs special instrument and special training."

Laparoscopic tubal occlusion procedures—guiding principles:
- The surgeon and staff must be well-trained, skilled and competent in the techniques they are using
- Appropriate and safe anesthesia
- Proper use of uterine elevator
- Clinic and operation theater (OT) should be well equipped with drugs and equipment to handle life-threatening situations and other emergencies
- An exploratory laparotomy set should always be ready along with necessary IV fluids at all times
- All instruments and equipment must be in optimum working order before starting any procedure
- Strict asepsis must be maintained
- No infected person should be allowed to enter sterile area. No one should enter without change of clothes, footwear, cap, and mask
- Patients should be carefully screened and selected
- Tubal occlusion should be carried out in the isthmic region of the Fallopian tube, 2.5 cm away from the cornual region, which will give better recanalization results, if needed
- Postoperatively patient should be monitored in the recovery area or ward for minimum of 6 hours.

Follow-up

The first follow-up is after 3–7 days. She should be encouraged to attend the clinic for first follow-up. If not, then she should be advised to go to the nearest health facility for a check-up of:
- Examination of surgical site
- Suture removal (if nonabsorbable sutures are used)
- Ensure comfort and privacy of patient
- Adequate records should be maintained at service center
- Discharge card should be given to each patient with detailed notes and operative findings and follow-up treatment and follow-up date mentioned
- Also give instructions to report to the clinic or a nearby dispensary in case of any missed period and to rule out possibility of pregnancy.

Instruments Used for Laparoscopic Sterilization

- A gynecological minor surgery set
- *Laparoscope*—using a 5 mm or 10 mm diameter with in-built lens and prism as well as fiberoptics light bundle system to transmit cold light source from an external source so that the direct visualization of the uterus and other pelvic structures. The single puncture laparoscopes are of two main types:

- Straight type with in-built operating system used for applying bands on the Fallopian tubes
- Angled type in which view finder is set off from the main part and has a special sheath for introducing operating instrument
- If double puncture technique is used then, the band applicator is pushed through second trocar placed about 6 cm above pubic symphysis. Most medical institutions in our country now have switched to the double puncture technique. This avoids the blind spot effect seen with single puncture telescopes

- Fiberoptics external light source with cable
- Gas insufflation apparatus to produce controlled pneumoperitoneum. Ideally only carbon dioxide should be used for creating a pneumoperitoneum. However, in many areas in our country CO_2 is not easily available and hence, the GOI guidelines permit the use of air for pneumoperitoneum during laparoscopic tubal ligation, without use of cautery
- Verres needle to introduce gas or air for pneumoperitoneum safely
- Trocar and cannula through which laparoscope is introduced. Additional trocar for the second puncture to introduce the applicator/bipolar forceps
- Uterine manipulator
- Applicator for applying the band or clips
- If using cautery, then a suitable bipolar forceps for cauterizing the Fallopian tubes.

Anesthesia

The woman usually receives light sedation to relax her. Then either local anesthesia 1% lignocaine is used in the local area along with paracervical block or a suitable short GA depending on the facilities available.

Preoperative Instructions

- The patient must bathe and wear clean and loose clothing to the OT
- The patient must not ingest anything by mouth 4–6 hours prior to surgery
- On the morning of surgery, she must empty her bowels, and before entering the OT, empty her bladder
- The client must remove nail polish, jewelry or hairpins before entering the OT
- She must also remove her glasses, contact lenses and dentures
- A responsible adult must be available to accompany the patient home after the surgery.

Procedure

- After voiding the urine, the patient is placed in the modified lithotomy position with the thigh at 45° angle to the body. Abdomen and vagina are cleaned with antiseptic solution and draped
- A bimanual P/V examination is performed and paracervical block given. The cervix is held with vulsellum and uterine elevator or Hulka's tenaculum, which combines a tenaculum and uterine elevator, is introduced. These devices enable the assistant to manipulate the uterus for better access and visibility of Fallopian tubes during the procedure
- The table is titled to a 30° Trendelenburg position, the operator if right handed stand on the left side of the patient. After giving anesthesia a small nick is made with a fine scalpel into the umbilicus. This is ideal as there is deficient rectus sheath at this point and hence, entry of primary trocar becomes very easy
- The surgeon elevates the abdominal wall with his left hand and Veress needle is introduced through small incision, which is directed towards the mid pelvis at an angle of about 60° to the body (care must be taken to see that it is not pushed perpendicularly so that injury to the aorta is avoided)
- For determining that the needle is in peritoneal cavity, first aspirate air by attaching 5 mL of syringe then 5 mL of saline is injected and the negative pressure should draw the drop of saline from the edge of the needle into the abdominal cavity
- About 2–3 liters of CO_2 or N_2O gas or air is introduced slowly from a cylinder at a pressure of about 10 mm of mercury. In tube ligation camp set up, it is air which is usually used
- After gas insufflation, Veress needle is removed and skin incision enlarged transversely/horizontally to the size of the telescope being used. After elevating the abdominal wall manually with the left hand, the trocar is boldly inserted through incision with right hand into the pneumoperitoneum with a controlled thrust directed towards the mid pelvis at an angle of 60° to the body surface. The obturator is removed from the trocar and the laparoscope with the light cable is introduced (Figs 1A and B)
- The pelvic structure now visualized, tubal grasping forceps is inserted through special channel. The tube is grasped at the isthmic portion away from the utrotubal junction and then it can be occluded by any of the following methods:
  - Tubal ring: Tubal ring (Sialistic band—the Fallope ring) is most widely used mechanical occlusion device. It is made of silicon rubber with 5% barium sulphate. Outer diameter is 3.6 mm, inner diameter is 1.0 mm and thickness 2.2 mm. Fallope ring was

developed to eliminate hazard of electrocautery during laparoscopy and at the same time providing a simple tubal occlusion method surpassing the effectiveness of clips.

If double puncture technique is used then, the band applicator is pushed through second trocar placed about 6 cm above pubic symphysis.

Most medical institutions in our country now have switched to the double puncture technique. This avoids the blind spot effect seen with single puncture telescopes.

Specially designed band ligator can be loaded with two-Fallope rings. After identifying Fallopian tube, tong of band applicator is extended and tube grasped in the isthmic area. The Fallopian tube is now drawn into applicator and band is pushed over knuckle of tube by moving the applicator. The tongs are than released and tube is dropped (Figs 1C and D).

While applying the bands, the following steps should be adhered to:

- Band applicator with mounted bands should be seen through the laparoscope
- Prongs should be released under vision only. Posterior prong should go behind the tube and lift the posterior lip of the broad ligament
- Draw the tube up slowly and smoothly into the sleeve of the laparoscope after proper identification. The site of occlusion should be 2–2.5 cm away from the cornual region
- Press the trigger to push the bands from the outer prongs on to the Fallopian tube
- Simultaneously advance the band applicator, which will prevent tearing of the tube
- Disengage the prongs from the Fallopian tube and withdraw the prongs in the inner barrel under vision
- Band the other tube in a similar way
- Fallope siliastic band placed on the tube (Fig. 2)

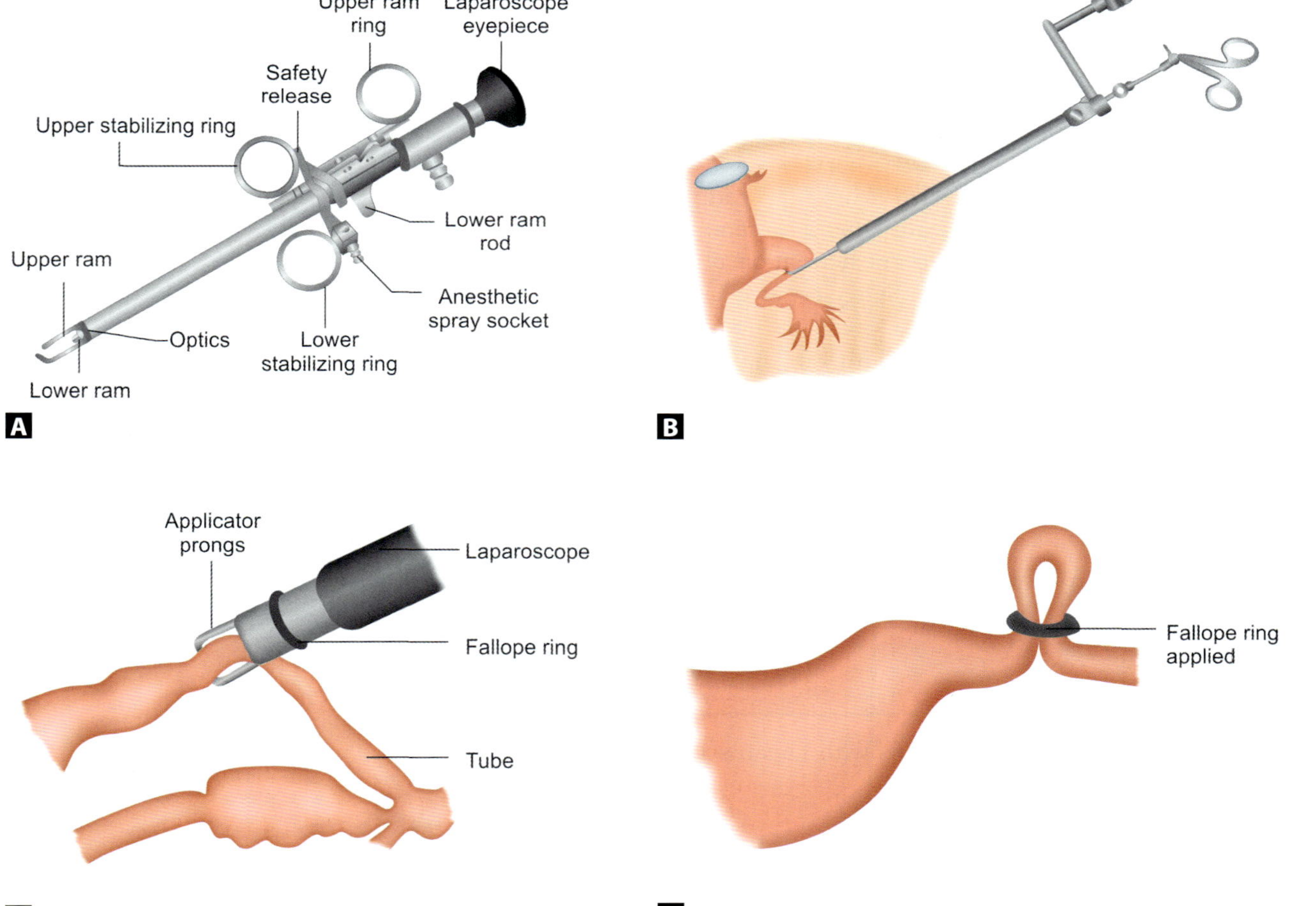

Figs 1A to D: (A) Single puncture operating laparoscope; (B) Laparoscopic sterilization by single-puncture technique; (C) The tube is picked up by operating laparoscope, to be drawn in so as to push the silastic band in the loop of tube; (D) Silastic band is placed on the tube

Clips

Clips are not available in India and hence not used routinely.

However, in expert hands it is a simple procedure. They are of two types— (1) Filshie's clip and (2) Hulka's clips.

The clip is applied at the isthmic area and acts as a mechanical barrier. Since the area of destruction is minimal, it has the best results if recanalization is needed.

- Spring loaded Hulka's clips—It is made of two plastic jaws with interlocking tooth. It is placed in isthmus of tube (Figs 3 and 4A)
- Filshie clip—Silicon tentanium clip (Fig. 4B)
- Electrocoagulation—It involves use of high frequency electric current to coagulate and block the tube. Unipolar electrocoagulation damages 20-50% of each Fallopian tube. Bipolar coagulation destroys less tubal tissues.

Usually in camp setups, electrocoagulation is not recommended because of risk of thermal burn.

- Both the tubes should be visualized to assess the adequacy of the loops and site of the bands and the presence of any hemorrhage and injury to the adjacent structures (if tubes are thick or fixed, the operator may switch to minilap)
- The laparoscope is withdrawn from the cannula under vision and then the trocar should be removed along with the cannula to prevent herniation of the omentum, after the gas is completely removed from the peritoneal cavity
- Entry site should be closed with a suture or clip.

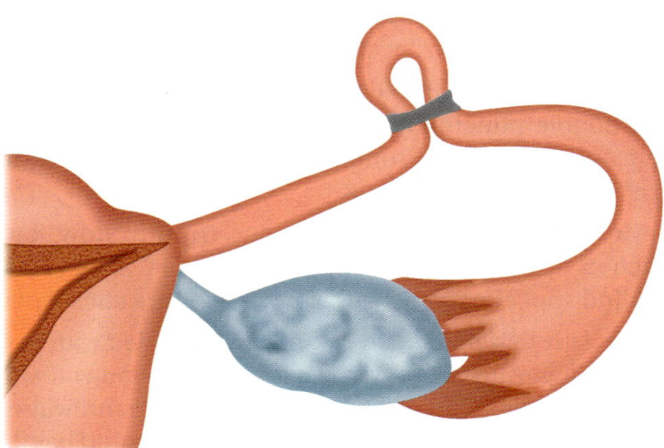

Fig. 2: Graphic representation of Fallope ring in situ

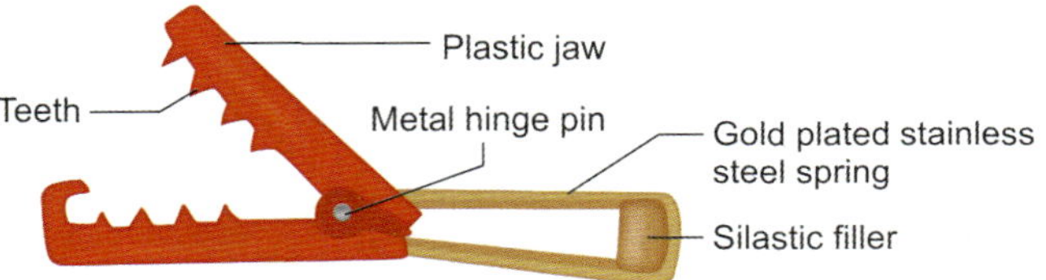

Fig. 3: Hulka clip

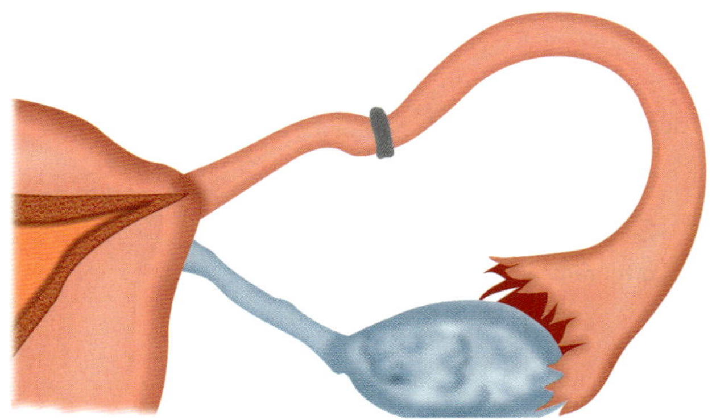

Fig. 4A: Hulka clip graphic representation

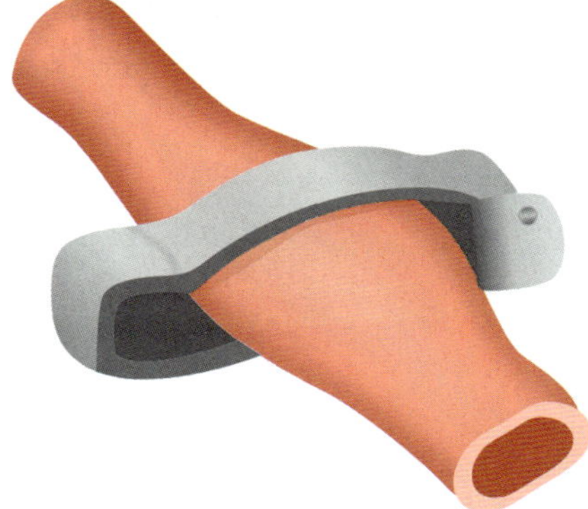

Fig. 4B: Filshie clip graphic representation

Complications (Box 1 and Table 1)

Box 1 Factors directly related to frequency of complications

- Surgical expertise
- Facility of operating room
- Aseptic care
- Proper choice of case
- Care taken by surgical team

WHO 1994 manual complications with Laparoscopic TL are rare in expert hands.

Minor complications are:

- Wound sepsis
- Abdominal wall hematoma
- Surgical emphysema
- Uterine perforation and
- Postoperative pain.

Table 1: Advantage and disadvantage of laparoscopy

Advantages		Disadvantages	
1.	Very low complication rate in trained hands	1.	Complications, if do arise, may be serious
2.	Quicker, takes 5–15 min	2.	Insufflation of abdomen with gas can cause chest and shoulder pain, rarely gas embolism and cardiopulmonary distress technique
3.	Very small scar	3.	Specially learning needed
4.	Less pain full	4.	Specialized equipment needed
5.	Postoperative recovery faster	5.	Equipment is expensive and difficult to maintain and repair
6.	Good for camp setup	6.	Not recommended in the immediate postpartum period or after a IInd trimester medical termination of pregnancy (MTP)
7.	Incidental diagnosis of other diseases	7.	Very obese patient, patient with pelvic adhesion and previous operative scar need special caution

Major complications are:

- Anesthetic hazard causing cardiorespiratory embarrassment and even death
- Unintended laparotomy: Unintended laparotomy occurs with 1–2% of laparoscopic procedures; most of these conversions are attributable to technical inability to complete the laparoscopic procedure rather than to complications of the procedure
- Bowel injury: Bowel injury can occur during insertion of the insufflation needle or trocar or during electrocoagulation. All bowel injuries must be managed actively and immediately
- Vascular injury: Vascular injury can occur during insufflation needle or trocar insertion. Injury to a large vessel is a life-threatening emergency. Perform an immediate laparotomy with direct pressure over the injury to control bleeding until repair (usually by a vascular surgeon) can be performed
- Visceral (bowel, bladder and uterus) injuries: Organ injuries can occur from sharp trauma (e.g. insufflation needle, trocar, scalpel), blunt trauma (e.g. from adhesiolysis), or electrical-thermal trauma. Injuries can also occur during inadvertent application of the occlusion device to the incorrect structure. If recognized at the time of occurrence, injuries to the bowel and bladder (which are more common in the presence of adhesions) are relatively easy to manage and will not result in long-term adverse sequelae. Injuries to the uterus, most often caused by uterine manipulators, do not usually lead to adverse sequelae unless bowel or bladder has been perforated simultaneously
- Patient regret: Poststerilization regret is a complex condition often caused by unpredictable life events.

Risk factors for regret need to be identified and addressed during the presterilization counseling.

- Mortality: The risk of death from tubal sterilization is 1–2 cases per 100,000 procedures; most of these are complications of GA. The most common cause of death during laparoscopic tube ligation appears to be hypoventilation related to anesthesia. Cardiopulmonary arrest and hypoventilation are reported as the leading cause of death in most cases. Sepsis as a cause of death from laparoscopic sterilization is directly related to bowel perforations or electrical bowel burns
- Failure rate: The typical failure rate following female sterilization by tubal ligation (Fig. 5) and laparoscopy in USA is 0.4% in the first year (WHO 1994). In India, large studies reported a failure rate of 0.2–1.13% following laparoscopic sterilization (Bhiwandiwala et al. 1982, Chi et al. 1980). The failure rate are much higher in inexperienced hands and in camp setup more so if the client are not properly selected or if the operations are performed too hurriedly. Although sterilization is highly effective and considered the definitive form of pregnancy prevention, it has a failure rate during the first year of 0.1–0.8%. At least one-third of these are ectopic pregnancies. The risk of pregnancy varies by patient age at sterilization and by method, with the highest risk among young women sterilized with bipolar coagulation. Overall, women sterilized at

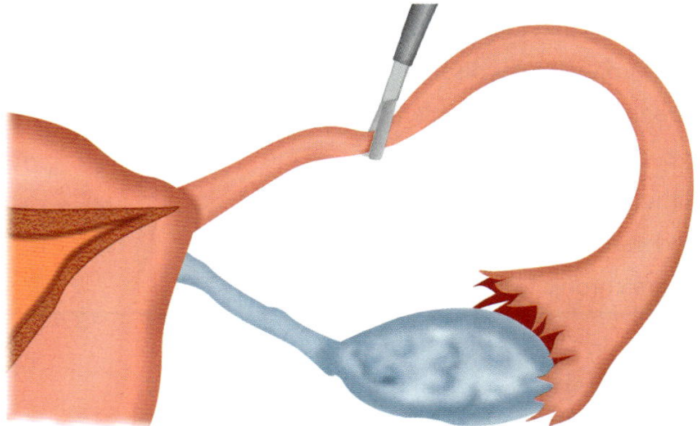

Fig. 5: Bipolar forceps grasping the isthmus for tubal ligation—graphic representation

age 34–44 years were half as likely to become pregnant after sterilization compared to women sterilized at age 28–33 years and were approximately one third as likely to become pregnant as women sterilized at age 18–27 years. Several studies suggest that the risk is highest after bipolar coagulation, with more than 50% of pregnancies being ectopic.

Selection of Cases—Government of India Guidelines for Sterilization (Table 2)

Eligibility Criteria for Sterilization

- The client must have been married
- Male clients should ideally be below the age of 60 years
- Female clients should be below the age of 45 years and above 22 years
- Although the number of children the couple has, is not a necessary criterion, they should have at least one child, whose age is above one year
- Clients or their spouses must not have undergone sterilization in the past (not applicable in cases of failure of previous sterilization)
- Clients must be in a perfectly normal state of mind so as to understand the full implications of sterilization
- Mentally ill clients must be certified by psychiatrist and consent should be given by the legal guardian or spouse.

However, "WHO guidelines" differs here and says that special counseling needs to be done in the following circumstances and special precautions taken.

Table 2: World Health Organization (WHO) medical eligibility criteria for female sterilization

Contraindication–No permanent contraindication	
*Delay the procedures**	
Known or suspected pregnancy	Following pregnancy condition
Active pelvic infection	Puerperal sepsis
Acute systemic infection	Prolonged rupture of membranes
Active liver disease	Pregnancy with persistent hypertension
Skin infection at operative area	Antepartum or postpartum hemorrhage
STD infection	Severe trauma to genital tract
Severe anemia	Postpartum psychosis
Acute respiratory disease	Unhealthy newborn/stillbirth
Current cerebrovascular or coronary artery disease	Recent septic abortion
Complicated valvular heart disease	Severe postabortal hemorrhage (delay should be for at least six weeks after delivery or abortion)
Malignant trophoblastic disease	
Any other temporary operative risk	
Any psychiatric condition that may impair decision making	
*Special precaution/Refer client***	
Conditions that increase anesthetic risk	*Conditions that increase surgical difficulties and risk*
Past cardiovascular disease	Endometriosis
Chronic respiratory problem BP >160/100 mm Hg	Past pelvic infection
Hyperthyroidism	Past complicated abdominal or pelvic surgery
Diabetes with vascular disease	Marked obesity
Moderate anemia (Hb <7 gm/dL)	Umbilical hernia
Severe chronic liver disease	Coagulation disorder

Source: IPPF Medical Bulletin. 1999;33(4).

* Condition must be treated and resolved before operation

** Refer to center with facilities for general anesthesia and experienced surgeon and staff

Abbreviations: STD, Sexually transmitted diseases; BP, Blood presseure

- Client is young
- Few or no children
- Have not talked with spouse
- Spouse opposes sterilization
- Not married
- Having marital problems.

Assure Voluntarism

A woman's decision to use voluntary sterilization should be well-informed and freely made so she should be counseled for:

- The specific surgical procedure emphasizing, what the women will experience during and after surgery
- Permanent nature
- Very small risk of pregnancy after sterilization
- A woman's right to change her mind anytime before the procedure
- The fact that no penalties will be imposed or any other benefits withheld, if, woman decides against sterilization.

Medical Eligibility Checklist

Cases for contraception are selected nowadays on the basis of WHO medical eligibility criteria (WHO, 1996).

Delay—means delay female sterilization. The condition must be treated or resolved before female sterilization. Till than temporary contraceptive methods should be provided.

Refer—means refer client to a center. Where an experienced surgeon and staff can perform the procedure in a setting equipped for GA.

Caution—means the procedure can be performed in a routine setting but with extra preparation and precaution depending upon the condition.

If no condition requires delay or referral, female sterilization can be postponed in routine setting by minilaparotomy or laparoscopy.

CONCLUSION

Voluntary surgical contraception is the "permanent method" of contraception. It is a highly effective and safe method, which offers long-term coverage. Female surgical contraception is more prevalent in India than male surgical contraception. It should be used judiciously, with proper counseling and explaining the permanent nature of the procedure along with the small risk of failure. Laparoscopic sterilization should be restricted to interval voluntary sterilization or along with first trimester MTP, or in camp settings. Proper selection of the case with proper counseling is the key to success.

APPENDIX

Historical Progression of Sterilization Surgery

- In 1823, Blundell first suggested tubal ligation for sterilization before the Medical Society of London
- In 1880s in Toledo, OH, Lungren was first to ligate a woman's tubes
- In 1876, Porro performed a cesarean hysterectomy with the secondary intention of sterilization
- In 1885, Thomas suggested tubal ligation as opposed to Porro's operation for sterilization
- In 1895, Dührssen used a double ligature and was the first to perform tubal ligation via colpotomy
- In 1897, Kehrer and Buettner divided the tubes between the sutures
- In 1898, Ruhl cut the tube 5 cm from the uterus and sutured the ends to a vaginal incision
- In 1898, Rose removed the tubes at the cornua
- In 1919, Madlener crushed and ligated the tubes with nonabsorbable suture
- In 1924, Irving published his method in which the proximal portion of the severed tube is buried in a small myometrial tunnel on the anterior uterine surface
- In 1930s, colleagues posthumously published the Pomeroy technique in the New York State Journal of Medicine
- In 1940s, Hajime Uchida developed his technique, which can be performed as an interval or puerperal procedure. He subsequently reported on his personal experience with more than 20,000 tubal sterilizations over 28 years without a known failure
- In 1936 in Switzerland, Bosch performed the first laparoscopic tubal occlusion as a method for sterilization
- In the 1960s, the era of laparoscopy began, which led to unipolar electrocoagulation tubal sterilization, the Hulka spring clip, the Yoon's plastic, Fallope ring, and bipolar cautery.

BIBLIOGRAPHY

1. Bhatt R. Camp laparoscopic sterilization death in Gujrat State, India 1978–1980. Asia Oceanica J Obstet Gynaecol. 1991;17(4):297-301.
2. Bhiwandiwala PP, Mumford SD, Feldbbum PL. Laparoscopic tubal ligation. Am. J Obstet Gynaecol. 1983;145:684.
3. Chi IC, Laufe LE, Gardner SD, et al. Tubal sterilization. Am J Obstet Gynecol. 1980;736:68.
4. Dawn CS. Scope of Culdoscopic tubal clipping. J Obstet Gynaecol India. 1972;22:437-9.
5. Govt of India. Annual Report 2003–2004, Ministry of Health and Family Welfare, New Delhi; 2004..
6. Govt of India. Year Book Family Programme in India 1996–1997, Ministry of Heath and Family Welfare, New Delhi; 2003.
7. Gupta. Contraception-Past Present Future. In: Parihar M, Gandhi AB (Eds). New Delhi: Jaypee Brothers Medical Publishers; 2006.
8. Hatcher RA, Rinechart W, Blackburn R, et al. The Essentials of Contraceptive Technology, Baltimore: John Hopkins School of Public Health; 1997.
9. Hatcher RA, Trussel J, Stewart F, et al. Contraceptive Programs. Baltimore, USA: The John Hopkins School of Public Health; 1999.
10. Hubert D. IIPF Med Bulletin. 1998;32(4):3.
11. Huezo CM, Carignam CS. Medical and Service guidelines for Family Planning, 2nd edition. International Planned Parenthood Federation (IPPF) and World Health Organization (WHO); 1997.
12. ICMR. In: Collaborative study on sequels of tubal sterilization in India. New Delhi: Council of Medical Research; 1982. pp. 88.
13. IIPF. IIPF Med Bulletin. 1996;30(5):1
14. IIPF. IIPF Med Bulletin. 1999;33(4):3.
15. Kagan M. Contraception in India: the need for improved quality and diversity of contraceptive option, Science and Technology in the Global Arena. 2000;303-5.
16. Liskin L, Blackburn R, Rutledge AH, et al. Minilaparotonomy and Laparoscopy: safe, effective and widely used. Population Reports, Series C, No. 9. Baltimore; John Hopkins University, Population Information Program; 1985.
17. Malvalankar D, Sharma B. The quality of care in sterilization camps: evidence from Gujrat. In: Koenig MA, Khan ME (Eds). Improving Quality of Care in Indian Family Welfare Programme. New Delhi: Population Council; 1999. pp. 293-313.
18. Mattingly RF, Thompson JD (Eds). Te Linde's Operative Gynaecology, 6th edition. Philadelphia: Lippincott; 1985. pp. 421.
19. Mroueh A. Out patient tubal sterilization by operative culdoscope. J Med Leban. 1972;25(3):233-6.
20. Peterson HB, Xia Z, Hughes JM, et al. The risk of ectopic pregnancy after tubal sterilization. US Collaborative Review of Sterilization working group. N Engl J Med. 1997;336(11):762-7.
21. Population Reports-Voluntary female sterilization series 10. Baltimore: Jhon Hopkins University; 1990.
22. Purandare BN. Development and Implementation of Sterilization programme, paper presented at the second International conference on voluntary sterilization, Geneva, Switzerland. 1973;28:16.
23. Rahman MM, Mamun AA. Direct trocar insertion: alternative abdominal entry technique for laparoscopic surgery. M Med J. 2003;12(1):45-7.
24. Rao KB, Mallik PE, Swami R. Proceedings of 6th Asian Congress of Obstetrics and Gynaecology Kualalumpur; 1974.
25. Townsend JW, Khan ME, Gupta RB. The Quality of Care in Sterilization Camp of U.P. In: Koenig MA, Khan ME (Eds). Improving Quality of Care in India's Family Welfare Program. The Challenges Ahead. New Delhi: Population Council; 1999. pp. 314-30.
26. Wheeless CR, Katayam KP. Te Linde's Operative Gynecology, 6th edition. In: Mattingly RF, Thompson JD (Eds). Philadelphia: Lippincott; 1985.
27. WHO. Contraceptive Method Mix, Geneva; 1994.
28. WHO. Female sterilization, Geneva. 1994;94.2(Rev 1).
29. WHO. Medical eligibility criteria for contraceptive use, Geneva; 1996.
30. WHO. Progress in human reproduction and researches, Geneva. 1994;31.
31. Yoon IB, King TM. The Laparoscopic Fallope Ring Technique. Advances in Planned Parenthood. 1975;(10)3:154-9.

42.10 LAPAROSCOPIC BURCH COLPOSUSPENSION

Pranay R Shah

INTRODUCTION

Three types of urinary incontinence exist: (1) stress incontinence, (2) detrusor instability, and (3) overflow.

Stress urinary incontinence (SUI) is defined as urinary loss which occurs with sudden elevations of intra-abdominal pressure without detrusor contractions. Stress urinary incontinence may improve with surgery, but the other two do not. Therefore, an accurate diagnosis is imperative.

Three types of SUI are:

1. One associated with hypermobility of the urethrovesical junction (bladder neck), often called genuine stress urinary incontinence
2. Intrinsic sphincter deficiency
3. Fixed urethra with failure of the intrinsic sphincter. Hypermobility accounts for 80–90% of all cases of SUI.

The urethra lies on pubocervical fascia, which stretches between the pelvic sidewalls at the level of the arcus tendineus fascia pelvis. The intact fascia creates a hammock, which allows the urethra to be compressed with increased intra-abdominal pressure. If the fascia is detached, torn or stretched, it no longer provides support, leading to inferior rotation of urethra.

METHODS OF EVALUATION OF URETHRAL SUPPORT

Clinical Examination

It involves inspection of the urethra and bladder neck while the patient is at rest and then during maximum straining. Rotational descent of the bladder neck can be easily demonstrated. Leakage of the urine with increased intra-abdominal pressure can also be demonstrated, provided the patient has a full bladder. It is important to note that urinary leak in some patients can be demonstrated only when the patient is standing. The character and timing of leakage should be noted.

Q Tip Test

It is a test to evaluate urethral axial mobility. A sterile lubricated cotton-tipped swab is placed in the urethra up to the bladder neck. The resting angle of the urethral axis is first measured. The patient is then asked to strain maximally and the angle of excursion of the swab is measured. If the maximum straining angle is more than 30°, it signifies urethral hypermobility. It is indicative of hypermobility and not diagnostic of SUI.

Bonney's Test

The test aims at seeing if the uplift of the uretherovesical junction will stop the urinary leak. With the patient in dorsal position, light pressure is applied at the sides of the urethra.

Lateral Urethrocystography (Micturating Cystourethrogram)

Urinary bladder is filled with radiopaque contrast medium through a urethral catheter and then taking lateral radiographs at rest, while straining and during micturition. In a normal person, the posterior urethrovesical angle is lost during voiding so that the urethra and the trigone come into line opening up the bladder neck. In patients with incontinence, the posterior urethrovesical angle is lost. This may be apperent when the woman is standing or sitting quietly in severe cases; in mild cases, it is apparent only with straining.

Cystourethroscopy

Endoscopic examination can be used in identification of poorly functioning urethras, e.g. scarred urethras in which the lumen remains throughout the examination making visualization of the bladder interior possible from the distal urethra.

Urethral Pressure Profile

It involves measurement of the pressure along the entire urethral length using a special catheter with 3 microtip pressure transducers placed 6 cm apart pulling it out from the bladder to the outside through the urethra at a fixed rate. All along the transducers keep measuring the intravesical pressure till it enters the urethra when the pressure rises and peaks at the point of maximum urethral pressure. The difference between the maximum urethral pressure and intravesical pressure gives the maximum urethral pressure.

Maximum urethral closure pressure = Maximum urethral pressure – intravesical pressure.

Leak Point Pressure

It is the total intravesical pressure required to produce SUI in a patient. Patients with leak point pressure (LPP) less than 60 cm of water have severe incontinence due to intrinsic sphincteric deficiency.

MANAGEMENT OF SUI

- Kegel's exercises aim to strengthen the striated urogenital sphincter and support to proximal urethra
- Electric nerve stimulation involves passage of electric current either transvaginally or transrectally in a continuous or intermittent manner to the pelvic floor muscles causing their contraction and reflex inhibition of detrusor activity.
- Pharmacological agents:

α adrenergic agonists	Ephedrine (25–50 mg qds), pseudoephedrine HCL (30-60 mg qds) Imipramine (10–25 mg tds)
Anticholinergic agents	Propantheline bromide (15–30 mg qds) Hyocyamine sulphate (375–750 mg bd)

  Calcium channel blockers Terodiline HCl 12.5–25.0 mg bd)
- Estrogen replacement: Therapy in postmenopausal patients
- Treatment of moderate to severe SUI is almost always surgical. More than 200 different surgeries have been described so far for correction of SUI. This itself suggests that an ideal surgery applicable to all patients has not been devised yet (Box 1).

Box 1 Classification of operations for stress urinary incontinence (SUI)

- Anterior colporrhaphy with Kelly's plication
- Abdominal bladder neck suspension procedures designed to correct urethral hypermobility.
  - Retropubic bladder neck suspension
    - Marshall Marchetti Krantz
    - Burch colposuspension
  - Paravaginal bladder neck suspension
    - Paravaginal defect repair
    - Vaginal obturator shelf procedure
  - Needle suspension procedures
    - Pereyra procedure
    - Pereyra modifications, e.g. Raz, Stamey, etc.
- Operations to correct Intrinsic Sphincteric Deficiency
  - Sling operations
  - Organic materials: Autologus (rectus sheath, fascia lata) Heterologous (porcine, ox dura)
  - Synthetic (polypropylene)
  - Suburethral sling operations [transvaginal tape (TVT), T-SUIT)
  - Artificial urinary sphincter
  - Periurethral injections (Teflon, Autologous fat, Urethrin)

Until recently there was a consensus, especially among gynecologists, that retropubic colposuspension (Burch's procedure) is the surgical treatment of choice for patients with genuine stress urinary incontinence who have intact uretheral sphincters but whose urethrovesical junction is displaced. For those patients who have a poor urethral sphincteric mechanism, suburethral sling procedures will be more appropriate.

The goal of incontinence surgery is a reduction of the hypermobility and restoration of normal anatomy at the urethrovesical junction and proximal urethra. Surgery for urethral hypermobility has evolved. The retropubic procedures are the most popular, based on the belief that these procedures have excellent immediate results and better long-term durability than other approaches do here. The Tanagho modification of the Burch colposuspension is probably the most commonly used technique. In this procedure, no dissection is carried out within 2 cm of the urethra or bladder neck. The fatty tissue along the lateral aspect of the vaginal fornix is removed. This allows fibrosis to occur. Sutures are tied loosely to avoid necrosis of the fascia and to avoid compression or kinking of the urethra.

THE SURGICAL TECHNIQUE OF THE BURCH PROCEDURE (TANAGHO MODIFICATION)

- A urethral catheter should be placed. Because the balloon helps to identify the urethrovesical junction, a 30 mL balloon, which is easier to palpate than a 5 cc balloon, is used
- Four trocars are placed. The primary trocar usually is placed in an intraumbilical location. Three 5 mm punctures are made in the abdomen. The lower pair of punctures is made lateral to the deep inferior epigastric vessels, and the upper is placed lateral to the abdominal rectus muscle at about the level of the umbilicus
- After the cul-de-sac is obliterated, the parietal peritoneum between the lateral umbilical ligaments are incised approximately 3 cm superior to the pubic symphysis (Fig. 1). It is dissected away from the anterior abdominal wall toward the pubic bone, and the retropubic space is entered
- The following anatomic landmarks are identified: the pubic symphysis, Cooper's ligaments, the obturator neurovascular bundle (aberrant obturator vessels are seen), the obturator foramina, the arcus tendineus fasciae pelvis, and the arcus tendineus fascia levator ani
- The bladder is mobilized medially to reveal the paravesical fat, which is dissected away from the pearly white pubocervical fascia (Figs 2A and B), where sutures are placed. Caution is exercised to avoid dissection within 2 cm of the urethra

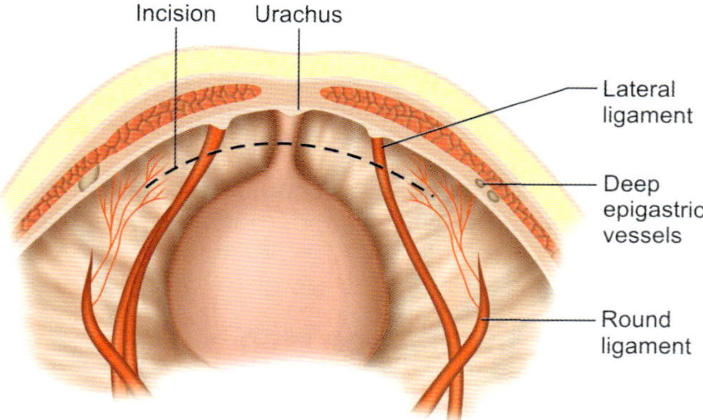

Fig. 1: Peritoneal incision to enter space of Retzius

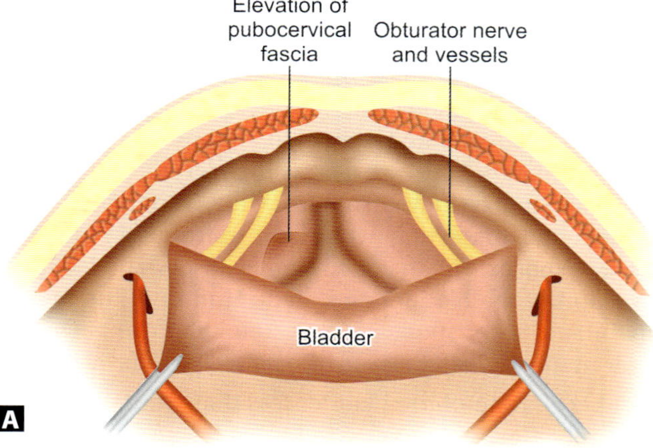

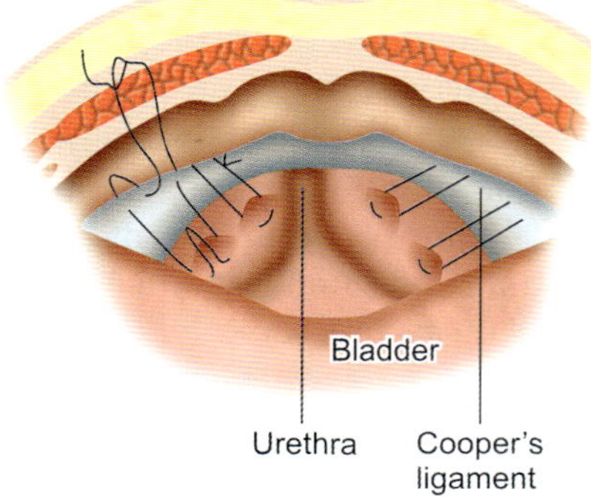

Figs 2A and B: Dissection in paraurethral space and placement of sutures

- The optimal locus for suture placement is at the level of the midurethra and urethrovesical junction (Fig. 3). The urethra may be identified by palpating the catheter, and the urethrovesical junction can be identified by palpating the catheter balloon. The surgeon can identify these sites by placing the index and middle fingers of the nondominant hand in the vagina. Both fingers are initially placed on the same side of the urethra, and then the fingers are pushed superiorly

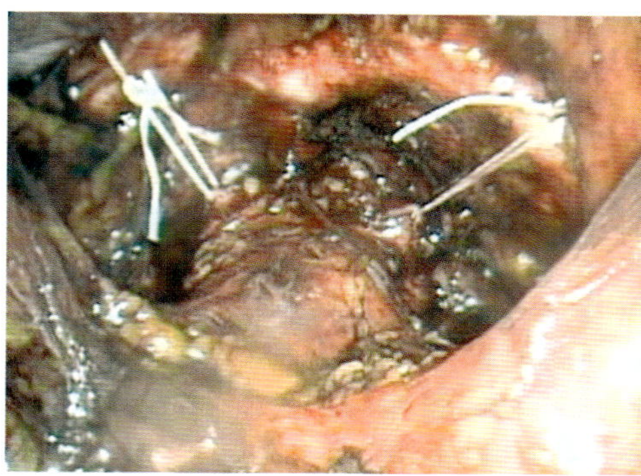

Fig. 3: Laparoscopically placed sutures at midurethral level

- A suture is passed through Cooper's ligament immediately superior to the location where it will pass through the anterior vaginal wall fascia. A double loop of suture is passed through on the fascia approximately 2 cm lateral to the midurethra. Tenting the fascia helps to identify the proper loci for placing the sutures and to better view the bladder. Placing the pubocervical fascia on tension helps to drive the suture needle through the fascia. A similar technique is used to place a suture at the level of the urethrovesical junction but lateral to the first midurethral suture. This step is carried out bilaterally. Permanent suture material, such as No. 2 Goretex is most commonly used. The suture knots are tied extracorporeally and tightened with a knot pusher. We have used a single stitch at the level of urethrovesical junction bilaterally with good results
- The parietal peritoneum incision is closed using continuous suture
- The bladder may be inspected with cystoscopy to ensure that no sutures have been passed through the detrusor muscle. Efflux of indigo carmine dye documents ureteral patency
- Lastly, the bladder is drained with an indwelling urethral or suprapubic catheter because normal micturition is disrupted temporarily

Success of the Burch retropubic urethropexy is dependent on stabilizing the pubocervical fascia, which supports the urethra. Determining the correct degree of tension in these sutures and the urethrovesical angle is subjective and continues to be the part of the procedure. If the urethrovesical junction is pulled too high, the urethra may be kinked, which interferes with normal urine flow. Some quantitative measures may help with this determination. When tied properly, the supporting sutures form loops and do not approximate Cooper's ligament and fascia. When a cotton-tipped swab is placed into the urethra, it should be horizontal to the floor or point slightly upward and should have some mobility.

In 1995, Liu reported long-term results of laparoscopic procedures. Sixty-five percent of patients stated that they were markedly improved. Twenty-four percent stated that they continued to have leak but were better than before surgery. Ten percent reported that they were not improved. These data are comparable with those reported for open Burch colposuspension.

COMPLICATIONS OF BURCH COLPOSUSPENSION

Burch Colposuspension (Table 1)

Table 1: Major complications of laparoscopic Burch colposuspension

	% Ou et al. n=165	% CY Liu n=196	% Ross n=148	% Lyon n=179
Bladder injury	1.8	2.1	1.4	.22
Hemorrhage	1.2	0.5	1.4	0.0
Urinary retention	1.2	2.1	N/A	1.1
Detrusor instability	2.4	2.1	2.0	24.8
Ureteral obstruction	0.0	0.5	0	1.1

Source: 24th World Congress American Association of Gynecologic Laparoscopists (AAGL), Orlando, FL (November 1995).

INTRAOPERATIVE COMPLICATIONS

Extraperitoneal Method

Surgeons experienced with the extraperitoneal approach cite as its advantages faster dissection, decreased chance of bladder injuries, and the option of regional anesthesia. Potential disadvantages are bleeding, tearing into the peritoneum resulting in a pneumoperitoneum that may restrict the surgeon's view, subcutaneous emphysema, and the inability to explore the pelvis and perform other intra-abdominal procedures. Keeping the insufflation pressure to less than 8–10 mm Hg can minimize subcutaneous emphysema, a potential complication by this approach.

Trocar placement for the Laparoscopic Burch procedure is usually more cephalad and lateral, which allows angulation for suturing, or adequate distance in which to use a stapling device. Direct visualization of the inferior epigastric vessels is essential while placing accessory trocars, to minimize transection and bothersome bleeding from the insertion of accessory trocars.

Although trocar site herniation may occur at any site, it is most common with trocars greater than 10 mm. Trocar movement, removal and replacement may cause fascial tears as large as 2 or 3 cm. Partial and complete small bowel obstruction secondary to herniation through these fascial defects has been reported. Numerous fascial closure devices are available to simplify closing these trocar sites. We recommend suture closure of fascia for any trocar site exceeding 5 mm.

Urinary tract infections secondary to catheterization can be minimized with administration of prophylactic antibiotics.

Intraperitoneal Approach

Access to the space of Retzius from the abdominal cavity requires exiting anterior to the bladder and medial to the umbilical ligaments.

Bladder Injury

Bladder injury is one of the most common complications noted during the early learning curve for the Laparoscopic approach. The bladder may be filled with 250–400 cc of methylene blue-stained saline to outline the bladder's superior margin and avert any inadvertent cystotomy. A bladder injury may result from the initial peritoneal incision and dissection within the retropubic space or during exposure of the paravaginal fascia. To facilitate retraction of the bladder and identification of the proper site for sutures or staples, the operator can use his or her finger in the vagina to elevate the paravaginal fascia.

A perforation of the bladder less than 5 mm in length should heal spontaneously with continuous drainage for seven to ten days. In contrast, larger defects require closure. Repair of the defect can be accomplished by using either intraperitoneal or extraperitoneal suturing techniques with Vicryl. Using a pretied loop suture may close perforations on the dome of the bladder.

After repairing the bladder, continuous drainage is recommended for seven to ten days. The bladder heals rapidly, and this complication should not require abandonment of the laparoscopic approach.

Bleeding

Dissection in the space of Retzius is almost bloodless if carried out in the proper plane. In most cases, excessive bleeding indicates that the dissection is too close to the bladder. The correct dissection should lie within the loose areolar tissue anterior to the bladder. Hemorrhage may occur from injury to the obturator or inferior epigastric vessels. For example, injury to the venous plexus located along the attachment of the lateral vaginal fornices may lead to troublesome bleeding. Bipolar coagulation will control most bleeding. Laparoscopic clips or hemostatic agents can be used if the bleeding persists or appears close to vital structures.

Urethral Vasculature

Suture or mesh attachment to the paravaginal fascia should be made 1.5–2.0 cm lateral to the urethrovesical junction to avoid the neurovascular supply to the urethra. Prior bipolar desiccation before suture placement or staple fixation over paravaginal tissue prevents troublesome bleeding. Urethral injuries may occur from injudicious dissection. In addition, inaccurate suturing or stapling can cause injury. A large Foley catheter with a 25 cc bulb may be placed before beginning the procedure to aid in identifying the urethra and the bladder neck.

EARLY POSTOPERATIVE COMPLICATIONS

Return of normal voiding function varies considerably. Transient voiding difficulties have a reported incidence as high as 25%. Urinary retention may be related to partial outflow obstruction, postoperative edema, or narcotic use. Patients who have a history of such problems are at higher risk. If a posterior colporrhaphy has been performed in combination with the Burch, spontaneous voiding is often delayed secondary to irritation of the levator muscles and inability to completely relax the pelvic floor. This problem will usually resolve itself in time. Patient reassurance along with either continuous or intermittent self-catheterization is recommended. A small percentage of patients will have a more prolonged delay of spontaneous voiding. This effect may be the result of overelevation of the bladder neck that produces kinking or compression of the urethra. It is important to understand that no absolute position of the urethra is associated with continence. The amount of urethral mobility affects development of this condition. Therefore, adequate support of the urethra, not excessive elevation, is the surgical goal. It is not necessary to tightly approximate paravaginal fascia to Cooper's ligament. At the end of the procedure, a 1 cm space should remain between the urethra and the symphysis.

Detrusor instability is a recognized complication of the Burch procedure. Patients should be aware that they might have postoperative incontinence secondary to detrusor instability even though the stress component has been corrected.

Preoperative urodynamic studies have shown a 15–30% concurrence of instability with genuine urinary stress incontinence. A postoperative incidence of 2–28% is associated with the laparoscopic Burch. The exact pathophysiology is unknown, but some cases may relate to overcorrection and partial outflow obstruction. Patients may be treated with drug therapy, bladder training, and behavior modification.

Ureteral injury is rare, but a few cases have been reported. Obstruction may occur due to kinking of the ureter from the acute elevation of the anterior vaginal wall. Suture ligation injury arises only rarely because of the inferior insertion of the ureters into the bladder trigone. The common symptoms associated with Ureteral injury include flank pain, fever, and anuria, which usually appear in the first 48–72 hours. An intravenous pyelogram may show hydronephrosis and site of obstruction. Therapeutic options include cystoscopic antegrade stent placement, percutaneous nephrostomy with or without retrograde stent placement, and reoperation to alleviate the obstruction.

If sutures or staples are placed into Cooper's ligament, groin pain may occur. Expectant management and analgesics are traditional means of treatment. If symptoms persist, reoperation to remove the offending suture or staple should be delayed if possible. This waiting period allows adequate time for scarring and fixation, so that the outcome of the surgery is not jeopardized.

LATE POSTOPERATIVE COMPLICATION

The most challenging late postoperative complication is the development of genital prolapse. Incidence of uterine descent and the formation of an enterocele and/or rectocele were reported to range from 5 percent to 20 percent in a large series of open Burch procedure cases. Wiskind reported that 26% (35 out of 131 patients) required another procedure for associated prolapse. The same intrinsic weakness of the pelvic floor that leads to urinary stress incontinence predisposes these women to develop problems related to vaginal prolapse, later in life. In addition, pulling the vagina anteriorly, thereby exposing the vaginal apex and posterior vaginal wall to the direct vector of intra-abdominal pressure may alter the vaginal axis.

It is imperative to identify all sites of prolapse preoperatively and correct these defects during the initial operation. Concurrent laparoscopic culdoplasty, i.e. uterosacral ligament fixation and Moschcowitz stitches can effectively close a deep cul-de-sac and reduce the incidence of this complication. When performing a culdoplasty, the ureters must be identified, or culdoplasty should be done after mobilizing ureters. If necessary, a relaxing incision can be made in the peritoneum to ensure that the ureters are not pulled in and obstructed. Bladder calculi may occur from either permanent stitch or staple placement into the bladder. Careful dissection and proper stitch and staple placement should prevent this complication. In addition, cystoscopic evaluation of the bladder prior to completion of the case may identify errant sutures or staples. Simple removal and replacement are all that is necessary at the time of surgery. Late identification of a suture or staple in the bladder may be managed cystoscopically.

The use of synthetic mesh and staples is not new to surgery. Mesh has been used for the repair of hernia defects for many years. Different materials have been used, with the most popular and widely used being polypropylene mesh (Prolene and Marlex). This monofilament plastic, which offers minimal elasticity or stretch capacity, is nonallergenic, nononcogenic, resistant to infection, and resistant to rejection. Most importantly the mesh is a weave in which interstices between the fibers allow immediate fibroblastic in growth. As a consequence, it provides a framework promoting the formation of scar tissue. The mesh itself will support up to 250 lb/in, and the tissue growing on it will further enhance the support.

In his original paper, Burch used absorbable suture material to perform his surgery. Many surgeons today continue to use absorbable suture material. Obviously, the suture does not maintain the support: rather, the scarring associated with healing provides the foundation for long-term success. Many authors have commented on ways to increase the scarring by removing fat from the space of Retzius, using reactive suture material or other agents, and even encouraging bleeding. It seems logical that the use of mesh would provide a reasonable alternative.

CONCLUSION

The surgical treatment of urinary stress incontinence is a challenging and frustrating, but rewarding pursuit. Patients are eternally grateful when an uncomplicated long-term cure is achieved. Complications and failures occasionally do occur, however, and are an inseparable part of surgery. It is the surgeon's responsibility to be aware of and recognize these potential complications and pitfalls. He or she must know how to avoid complications if possible and manage them when required. For their part, patients must understand that success cannot be guaranteed and that new problems or worsening of their condition may occur. One must be careful to prevent general complications related to any laparoscopic surgery like complications from trocar entry and injury, vascular injury, bleeding, infection, injury to various organs, etc.

BIBLIOGRAPHY

1. Abrams P, Blaivas JG, Stanton SL, et al. Standardization of terminology of lower urinary tract function. Br J Obstet Gynaecol. 1990;97(6):1-6.
2. Beck RP, McCormick S, Nordstrom L, et al. The fascia lata sling procedure for treating recurrent genuine stress incontinence. Obstet Gynecol. 1988;72:699-703.
3. Bergman A, Ballard CA, Koonings PP, et al. Primary stress urinary incontinence and pelvic relaxation: Prospective randomized comparison of three different operations. Am J Obstet Gynecol. 1989;161:97-101.
4. Bergman A, Elia G. Three surgical procedures for genuine urinary stress incontinence: five-year follow-up of a prospective randomized study. Am J Obstet Gynecol. 1995;175:66-71.
5. Burch JC. Cooper's ligament urethrovesical suspension for stress incontinence. Am J Obstet Gynecol. 1968;100:764-74.
6. Capozzi JA, Beckenfild JA, Cherry JK, et al. Repair of inguinal hernia in the adult with prolene mesh. Surg Gynaeco obstet. 1988;167:124-8.
7. Clarke AL, Gregory T, Smith VJ, et al. Epidemiologic evaluation of reoperation for surgically treated pelvic organ prolapse and urinary incontinence. 2003;189(5):1261-7.
8. DeLancey JO. Structural support of the urethra as it relates to stress incontinence: The hammock hypothesis. Am J Obstet Gynecol. 1994;170:1713-23.
9. Drutz HP, Baker K, Lemieux MC, et al. Retropubic colpourethropexy with transabdominal anterior and/or posterior repair for the treatment of genuine stress incontinence and genital prolapse. Int Uro Gynecol J. 1991;2:201-7.
10. Ericksien BC, Hagen B, Eik-Nes SH, et al. Long-term effectiveness of the Burch colposuspension in female urinary stress incontinence. Acta Obstat Gynecol Scand. 1990;69:45-50.
11. Ferriani RA, Silva de Sa MF, Dias de Moura M, et al. Ureteral blockage as a complication of Burch colposuspension. Report of six cases. Gynecol Obstet Invest. 1990:29:239-40.
12. Galloway NTM, Davies N, Stephenson TP, et al. The complication of colposuspension. Br J Urol. 1987;60:122-4.
13. Gittes RF, Loughlin KR. No-incision pubovaginal suspension for stress incontinence. J Urol. 1987;138:568-70.
14. Horbach NS, Blanco JS, Ostergard DR, et al. A suburethral sling procedure with polytetrafluoroethylene for the treatment of genuine stress incontinence in patient with low urethral closure pressure. Obstet Gynecol. 1988;71:648-57.
15. Horowitz IR. Whats new in gynaecology and Obstetrics. J Am Coll Surg. 2003;197(4):612-9.
16. Hurt WG. Retropubic urethropexy or colposuspension. In: Hurt WG (Ed). Urogynaecologic Surgery. Gaithersburg: Aspen; 1992. pp. 81-95.
17. Kadar N, Reich H, Liu CY, et al. Incisional hernias after major laparoscopic gynecologic procedures. Am J Obstet Gynecol. 1993;168:1493-5.
18. Kelly HA, Dumm WM. Urinary incontinence in women without manifest injury to the bladder, 1914. Int Urogynecol J Pelvic Floor Dysfunct. 1998;9(3):158-64.
19. Kieswetter H, Fischer M, Wöber L, et al. Endoscopic implantation of collagen (GAX) for the treatment of urinary incontinence. Br J Urol. 1992;69:22-5.

20. Kohorn EI. The surgery of stress urinary incontinence. Obstet Clin North Am. 1989;16:841-52.

21. Korda A, Ferry J, Hunter P. Colposuspension for the treatment of female urinary incontinence. Aust NZ J Obstet Gynecol. 1989;29:146-9.

22. Kung RC. Laparoscopic treatment of urinary incontinence. Obstet Gynecol Clin North Am. 2004;31(3):539-49.

23. Marshall VF, Marchetti AA, Krantz KE. The correction of stress incontinence by simple vesicourethral suspension. Surg Gynecol Obstet. 1949;88:509-18.

24. Maulik TG. Kinked ureter with unilateral obstructive uropathy complicating Burch colposuspension. J Urol. 1983;130:135-6.

25. Ou CS, Beadle EM, Presthus JB. Laparoscopic bladder neck suspension using hernia mesh and surgical staples. J Laparoscopic Surg. 1993;36:563-6.

26. Pereyra AJ, Lebherz TB, Growdon WA, et al. Pubourethral support in perspective modified Pereyra procedure for urinary incontinence. Obstet Gynecol. 1981;59:643-8.

27. Raz S, Klutke CG, Golomb J. Four-corner bladder and urethra suspension for moderate cystocele. J Urol. 1989;142:712-5.

28. Richardson AC, Lyon JB, Williams NL. Treatment of stress urinary incontinence due to paravaginal fascial defect. Obstet Gynecol. 1981;57:357-62.

29. Stamey TA. Endoscopic suspension of the vesical neck for urinary incontinence in females. Ann Surg. 1980;192:465-71.

30. Tanagho EA. Colpocystourethropexy: the way we do it. J Urol. 1976;116:751-3.

31. Vancaillie TG, Schuesslern W. Laparoscopic bladder neck suspension. J Laparoscopic Surg. 1991;1:169-73.

32. Vierhout ME, Mulder AF. De novo detrusor instability after Burch colposuspension. Acta Obstet Gynecol Scand. 1992; 71:414-6.

33. Webster GD, Perez LM, Khoury JM, et al. Management of type III stress urinary incontinence using artificial urinary sphincter. Urology. 1992;39:499-503.

34. White GR. An anatomic operation for the cure of cystocele. Am J Obstet Dis Wom Child. 1912;56:289-90.

35. Wiskind AK, Creighton SM, Stanton SL. The incidence of genital prolapse after the Burch colposuspension. Am J Obstet Gynecol. 1992;167:399-404.

36. Wiskind AK, Stanton SL. The Burch colposuspension for genuine stress incontinence. In: Thompson JD (Ed). TeLinde Operative Gynecology. Philadelphia: Lippincott; 1993. pp. 1-13.

42.11 LAPAROSCOPIC PARAVAGINAL REPAIR

Pranay R Shah

INTRODUCTION

The paravaginal defect is a result of detachment of the pubocervical fascia from its lateral attachment to the fascia of the obturator internus muscle at the level of the arcus tendineus fascia of the pelvis (white line) (Figs 1 and 2). It can be unilateral or bilateral. Eighty percent of the urethrocystoceles are due to paravaginal defects.

Ninety five percent of patients with paravaginal defects also have stress urinary incontinence (SUI). The paravaginal repair operation re-establishes the lateral pelvic sidewall attachments of the pubovesicocervical fascia and restores stability of the hammock by correcting the anatomic defect. However, the paravaginal repair is not an operation to correct SUI, but rather a procedure designed to correct cystocele or cystourethrocele.

OPERATION TECHNIQUE

Under GA with endotracheal intubation, the patient is placed in a low dorsolithotomy position. A 16 Fr Foley catheter with 30 mL balloon tip is then inserted into the bladder. A 10 mm laparoscope is inserted through a vertical intraumbilical incision. Three 5 mm punctures are made in the abdomen. The lower pair of punctures are made lateral to the deep inferior epigastric vessels, and the upper is placed lateral to the abdominal rectus muscle at about the level of the umbilicus. After a careful inspection, the patient is placed in a 15–20° Trendelenburg's position. All visible pathologies, such as endometriosis or adhesions, are excised, and a hysterectomy and/or salpingo-oophorectomy is performed, if indicated. Prior to the initiation of the paravaginal repair, the entire pelvic floor is carefully surveyed both by viewing the pelvis through the laparoscope and by performing digital vaginal examinations simultaneously. Posterior and middle compartment defects, such as enterocele, and vaginal vault prolapse are first repaired laparoscopically and a low rectocele and perineorrhaphy are performed vaginally.

A transverse incision is then made on the parietal peritoneum approximately 3 cm above the symphysis pubis in between the two umbilical ligaments with laparoscopic scissors or monopolar hook. The parietal peritoneum is dissected away from the abdominal wall toward the pubic bone, and the retropubic space is entered. Anatomic landmarks, such as symphysis pubis, the obturator foramen, and the obturator neurovascular bundle are identified. The paravaginal defect can be seen detached from the arcus tendineus fascia of the pelvis. As much paravaginal fat as possible is removed to promote fibrosis and scar formation in the paravaginal area. The prominent paraurethral vascular plexus usually can be seen after the fat has been excised.

The bladder is then mobilized medially and the pubocervical fascia exposed. The ischial spine can be located digitally by placing the operator's finger inside the vagina while viewing through the laparoscope. During the mobilization of the bladder, the assistant places his or her fingers in the vagina and lifts the lateral vaginal sulcus to facilitate the dissection.

The separation of the lateral vaginal sulcus from the pelvic sidewall can be easily appreciated laparoscopically (Fig. 2). Permanent 2-0 prolene sutures are used to suture the lateral vaginal sulcus to the arcus tendineus fascia of the pelvis (white line), placing a full thickness stitch through the vagina (Fig. 3). The sutures are tied extracorporeally and tightened with a knot pusher. An assistant pushes

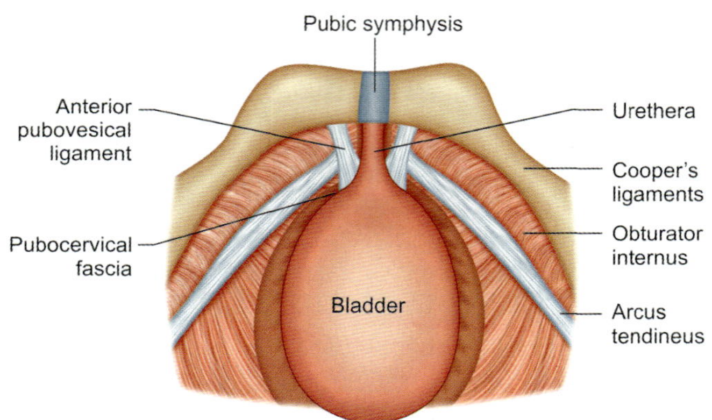

Fig. 1: Normal anatomy of space of Retzius

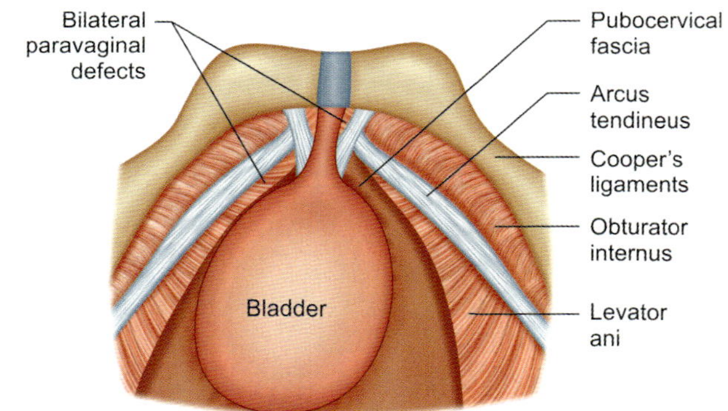

Fig. 2: Lateral vaginal wall defects result in cystourethrocele as seen from the space of Retzius

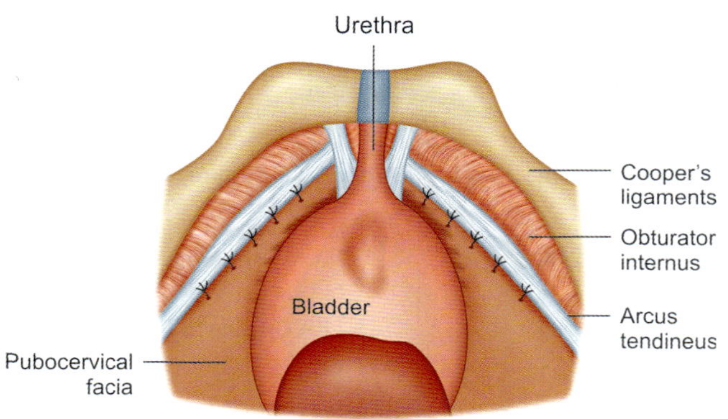

Fig. 3: The reapproximation of the pubocervical fascia to the obturator internus at the arcus tendineus fascia pelvis

the vaginal sulcus to the sidewall, so that the knot can be tied with less tension. The fascia and arcus are closely approximated as opposed to the loose approximation during the retropubic urethropexy.

Troublesome bleeding can occur when the needle penetrates the paraurethral vascular plexus, which runs longitudinally along the axis of the vagina. This bleeding invariably will stop when the sutures are tied. To avoid contamination of the operative field by the blood, the first paravaginal suspension stitch should be placed as close to the ischial spine as possible. Figure-of-eight sutures are used to obtain a better hemostasis and suspension. Further 3–4 stitches are placed through the vaginal sulcus and the arcus tendineus fascia ventrally toward the symphysis pubis. The last stitch should be as close as possible to the pubic ramus. Injury to the pudendal nerve and vessels can be avoided by placing the first stitch through the white line 1.5 cm ventral to the ischial spine.

If the urethrovesical junction is not well supported and the patient has an SUI, additional Burch stitches should be placed to elevate the ureterovesical (UV) junction. The entire retropubic space is then thoroughly irrigated and hemostasis achieved by electrosurgery. No drains or suprapubic drainage are necessary. The peritoneal defect is closed with 2-0 vicryl. Cystoscopic examination is performed to ensure that no suture is inside the bladder, and to ascertain the integrity of both ureters.

The laparoscopic approach to paravaginal defect is not a solitary procedure; rather, it is part of a larger operation in which the whole pelvic floor is reconstructed. Laparoscopy provides better visualization of pelvic floor defects, as well as greater precision in placing strategically important stitches in the repair of paravaginal defects. Richardson et al. reported that 95% of patients had a satisfactory result following paravaginal repair for cystocele and urethrocele. They noted that this technique provided an anatomic correction of cystocele and urethrocele, relief of stress urinary incontinence, preservation of normal voiding, and no persistent voiding dysfunction. They also demonstrated that the incidence of de novo detrusor instability was less than with other procedures. Subsequently, in 1989, Baden and Shull found a 95% restoration of anatomy with paravaginal suspension. They emphasized that all defects must be corrected. Liu described repairing paravaginal defects and other pelvic floor defects concomitantly. He recommended a combined paravaginal and Burch procedure.

42.12 COMPLICATIONS OF LAPAROSCOPIC SURGERIES: VERESS NEEDLE INJURIES, TROCAR INJURIES AND VASCULAR INJURIES

KK Gopinathan, Fessy Louist, Shlomo B Cohen, Ariella J Setton, Daniel S Seiedman, Jayakrishnan K

Veress Needle Injuries

KK Gopinathan, Fessy Louist

INTRODUCTION

The method employed to gain access to the abdominal cavity during laparoscopy still remains as one of the most debated topics among laparoscopic surgeons. Since the injury rates are low, the size of clinical trials required to demonstrate that one technique is safer than another is large. In a study by Mintz of nearly 100,000 cases, a bowel injury rate of 0.3/1,000 and vascular injury rate of 0.5/1,000 was reported. Another study of above 100,000 cases by Harkki-Siren et al. reported a bowel injury rate of 0.3/1,000 and vascular injury rate of 0.1/1,000. Even though the injuries during laparoscopic entry are rare, when they do occur, can have serious sequelae needing laparotomy, bowel resection, vascular grafts and even death.

Janos Veress, a respiratory physician, invented Veress needle in 1930s to create pneumothorax in pulmonary tuberculosis. It is the most common instrument used to create pneumoperitoneum in laparoscopy. The important points to be noted in Veress usage will be discussed here.

APPROPRIATE CASE SELECTION

Proper selection of cases for laparoscopy reduces any sort of complications during laparoscopy.

PATIENT PREPARATION

It is important to note the history and scars of previous surgeries to avoid complications prior to surgery. Bladder catheterization is advised to avoid injury to distended bladder. Just to avoid Veress injury there is no need for routine bowel preparation. However bowel preparation is advisable in patients undergoing advanced laparoscopic procedures.

Anesthesia

At the time of induction of anesthesia, insufflation of air or oxygen by mask should not be carried out as distention of the stomach may take place. A distended viscous is more prone to trauma as the Veress needle is inserted. Some even advocate routine usage of Ryle's tube deflation of stomach before Veress insertion.

The Conventional Approach

- Check the Veress needle for patency and check the CO_2 insufflator before insertion. Palpate the abdominal wall of the patient for any mass. Always make sure the patient is in horizontal position during Veress needle insertion
- Make a skin incision at the base of the umbilicus. The incision is made on the skin alone as the abdominal wall is thinnest here and the parietal peritoneum is most firmly attached here
- The Veress needle is grasped like a dart, with the tap open. This will facilitate air to enter the negatively pressured abdominal cavity when the Veress is inserted
- Abdomen is lifted anteriorly and in a caudal direction.
- The Veress is inserted at an angle between perpendicular and 45° towards the pelvis, aiming towards the sacral hollow in the midline. Usually it is inserted for a short distance and we can feel the Veress incising the rectus sheath and peritoneum as two distant resistances.

Confirmation of Proper Veress Insertion

Even though several techniques have been described for these, none of them are fool proof.

- *Saline insufflation test:* About 5 cc saline is taken in a syringe and attached to Veress needle and aspirated. If no blood or fecal matter is seen, the saline is injected and attempt is made to aspirate it. Dissemination of the saline in the peritoneal cavity prevents its aspiration. The aspiration of blood or bowel contents occurs if a major splanchnic organ is entered. The ease of the initial infiltration suggests that the needle is free in the cavity, rather than against adhesion
- *Hanging drop test:* A small amount of saline is placed on the top of the Veress needle tip, the abdominal wall is elevated, if Veress tip is intraperitoneal, the negative pressure thus created will cause the saline to be sucked in.

CO_2 Insufflation

Initially low flow is used for CO_2 insufflation. Usually a flow rate of 1 L/min is used. The intra-abdominal pressure is preset to 14–15 mm Hg. The venous return and blood pressure is usually not affected at this pressure.

Minimizing Vascular Injuries

Surface Anatomy

The umbilicus is not a fixed anatomical landmark. The top of the iliac crests corresponds to L_4 vertebrae. In 80% of cases the aortic bifurcation lies within 1.25 cm of L_4 vertebrae. Iliac crests, which are easily palpable, must be used as the surface marker for the aortic bifurcation.

Body Mass Index

The importance of body mass index (BMI) is that in patients with low BMI, the great vessels lie as little as 2.5 cm below the umbilicus. So in these patients abdominal wall should be elevated to increase the distance from umbilicus to aorta. Some even advocate to hold the Veress on the shaft rather than on barrel, which will reduce the length of needle to be inserted.

In patients with high BMI, since there is increased thickness of the abdominal wall, there is an increased risk of preperitoneal insertion of the Veress needle. This is more especially in patients with BMI more than 30. Hurd et al. found out that in these patients the average distance from the base of the umbilicus to the aorta is 13 cm. So in these patients it is advisable to introduce the Veress needle more perpendicularly.

Patient Position

The aortic bifurcation is more caudal in Trendelenburg position as compared with supine position. Also the angle of introduction of Veress to the horizontal plain varies in Trendelenburg position, increasing the chances of damage to major vessels.

Abdominal Wall Lifting

Routine lifting of the abdominal wall is done by many surgeons. But some surgeons advocate mechanical elevation of the abdominal wall during Veress insertion. Even though it increases the distance to the great vessels, it may increase the risk of preperitoneal insufflation of gas, which may complicate the entry procedure.

Minimizing Bowel Injuries

Injuries to the bowel during laparoscopic entry is classified into two groups:

1. Type I—Damage to normally located bowel
2. Type II—Damage to bowel adherent to the abdominal wall.

De novo occurrence of periumbilical adhesions is very less, 0.5% compared to 31% in cases with previous midline laparotomy. Also in cases of previous Pfannenstiel incision 6.9% and in cases of previous laparoscopy 0.8% of periumbilical adhesions are reported.

Management of Bowel Injuries

In a study conducted by Bishoff et al. 69% of bowel injuries are not recognized at the time of surgery. Usually they become apparent 12–36 hours after surgery, but by that time patient would have been discharged already. Nonthermal injuries usually present earlier than thermal injuries. Also trauma to small bowel present earlier than large bowel trauma.

If there is no tearing, with just insertion of Veress needle into bowel, conservative management with antibiotics and observation is advised.

Bowel injuries by Veress needle may not present with classic features of fecal peritonitis. They may present with pain around the trocar site, diarrhea or abdominal distention. Also they may present with abdominal pain, ileus, nausea and vomiting. Leukocytosis may not be there and there can be even leukopenia. Even after discharge, if the patient develops worsening of pain or postoperative pyrexia, great suspicion of bowel injury must be there and patient must be advised to return to hospital.

ALTERNATE TECHNIQUES FOR ESTABLISHING PNEUMOPERITONEUM

Direct Insertion

This technique first proposed by Dingfelder in the late seventies. The primary trocar is inserted directly with gas tap open and making use of the negative pressure in the abdomen. The advantage of this technique is that the laparoscope can be inserted to view the cavity when entered. Once safe entry is confirmed, rapid insufflation of gas can be done. This decreases the incidence and complications of preperitoneal insufflation. In a population with low risk for type II bowel injury, this may be a better technique, but may be associated with a higher risk of type II bowel injury.

Open Technique

This technique was first described by Hasson in early 70s. Here an intraumbilical minilaparotomy incision is made initially before introducing the main trocar. Even though a survey of members of American Association of Gynecologic Laparoscopists (AAGL) showed that this technique has reduced the risk of major blood vessel injury but the incidence of bowel injury is not reduced. In some studies it showed even a higher incidence of bowel injury. This may be due to the high-risk cases in which this technique is employed.

Gasless Laparoscopy

In this technique the initial step is the same as open laparoscopy. After entering the peritoneum, with a variety of devices the abdominal wall is elevated. The only major advantage described is the possibility of decrease in tumor metastasis in malignancy compared to pneumoperitoneum.

Optical Veress

This allows visualization of the abdominal wall layers during introduction into the peritoneal cavity. There is no evidence that they reduce type II bowel injuries.

Rapidly Expanding Sleeves

First a blunt trocar of 1.5 mm diameter containing the expandable sleeve is inserted as in the conventional technique, through a 3 mm skin incision to enter the abdominal cavity. A tapered dilator is then inserted that expands the sleeve up to 12 mm if necessary. Larger study results are needed to establish its safety.

Alternative Entry Sites

The most accepted alternate entry sites are Palmer's points, which are:

- 3 cm inferior to the left costal margin in the midclavicular line, and
- The ninth left intercostal margin in the anterior axillary line.

The advantages of these sites are that in the upper abdomen, especially over left hypochondrium, the parietal peritoneum is sufficiently adherent and is usually devoid of adhesions. But care must be taken to ensure there is no splenomegaly and in intercostal space Veress is inserted on the superior border of tenth rib to avoid injury to the neurovascular bundle on the inferior undersurface of the ninth rib.

Other less used alternate sites for Veress insertion are subumbilical, suprapubic, pouch of Douglas, transuterine and midway between umbilicus and symphysis pubis.

CONCLUSION

Even though different abdominal wall entry techniques are there, the most accepted is the Veress needle. But all have their own pitfalls and advantages. So the entry technique must be tailored to the individual patient. The international group of laparoscopic gynecologists and surgeons compiled a consensus document on laparoscopy entry techniques. These are summarized below.

Consensus Document on Laparoscopy Entry Techniques

- Identify risks of bowel adhesion
- If at high-risk of bowel adhesion, exclude splenomegaly and introduce a microlaparoscope at Palmer's point
- Ensure the bladder is empty
- Check the abdomen for masses and the position of the aorta
- Many feel the patient should be horizontal during all entry procedures
- Primary incision should be made through skin only, at the base of the umbilicus
- Check the Veress is sharp, has a good spring action and allows gas to flow
- The umbilicus should be elevated during insertion of the Veress
- Insertion of the Veress should stop as soon as the peritoneal cavity is entered
- Tests (saline aspiration, gas flow pressure readings) should be performed to establish the Veress in the peritoneal cavity
- The Veress needle should not be swung under the peritoneum
- CO_2 should be insufflated to 25 mm Hg until all trocars are inserted
- The primary trocar should be introduced through the base of the umbilicus
- Once the laparoscope is inserted, a 360° survey should be performed to exclude bowel or vascular trauma.

BIBLIOGRAPHY

1. Anon. A consensus document concerning laparoscopic entry techniques: Middlesborough. Gynecol Endosc. 1999;8:403-6.
2. Audebert AJ, Gomel V. Role of microlaparoscopy in the diagnosis of peritoneal and visceral adhesions and prevention of bowel injury associated with blind trocar insertion. Fertil Steril. 2000;73:631-5.
3. Batemon B, Kolp L, Heoger K. Complications of laparoscopy—operative or diagnostic. Fertil Steril. 1996;66:30-5.
4. Bhoyrol S, Mori T, Way LW. Radially expanding dilatation. A superior method of laparoscopic trocar access. Surg. Endosc. 1996;10(7):775-8.

5. Bishott J, Allat M, Kirkels W, et al. Laparoscopic bowel injury Incidence and clinical presentation. J Urol. 1999;161:887-90.
6. Briel J, Plaiser P, Meijer WS, et al. Is it necessary to lift the abdominal wall when preparing a pneumoperitoneum? A randomized study. Surg Endosc. 2000;14:862-4.
7. Byron JW, Fujiyoshi CA, Miyozawa K. Evaluation of the direct trocar insertion techniques at laparoscopy. Obstet Gynecol. 1989;74:423-5.
8. Desai SV, Kurian JA. Gynecological Endoscopic Surgery: Current concepts. New Delhi: Jaypee Medical Publishers (P) Ltd.; 2002. 65-8.
9. Dingtelder J. Direct trocar insertion without prior pneumoperitoneum. J Repro Med. 1978;21:45-7.
10. Garry R. Towards evidence-based laparoscopic entry techniques. Clinical problems and dilemmas. Gynecol Endosc. 1999;8: 315-26.
11. Garry R. Towards evidence-based laparoscopic entry techniques. Gynaecol Endosc. 1999;8:403-6.
12. Gray H. Anatomy of Human Body. Philadelphia: Lea & Febiger Publishers; 1985.
13. Harkki-Sirem P, Syoberg J, Korki T. Major complications of laparoscopy. A follow-up Finnish study. Obstet and Gynecol. 1999;94:94-8.
14. Hill DJ, Maher PJ. Direct cannula entry for laparoscopy. J Am Assoc Gynecol Laparosc. 1996;4:77-9.
15. Hulka J, Petersontt HB, Phillips J, et al. Operative laparoscopy AAGL 1993 membership survey. J Am Assoc Gynecol Laparosc. 1995;2:133-6.
16. Hulka J. Major vessel injury during laparoscopy. Am J Obstet Gynecol. 1980;138:590.
17. Mintz M. Risks and prophylaxis in laparoscopy survey of 100,000 cases. J Reprod Med. 1997;18:269-72.
18. O'Donovan PJ, Downes GRE, McGurgan P (Eds). Advances in Gynecological Surgery. London: Greenwich Medical Media; 2001. p. 169-85.
19. Palmer R. Safety in laparoscopy. J Repro Med. 1974;3:1-5.
20. Reich H, Levie M, Mc Glynm F, et al. Establishment of pneumoperitoneum through the left ninth intercostal space. Gynecol Endosc. 1995;4:141-3.
21. Watson D, Mathew G, Ellis T, et al. Gasless laparoscopy may reduce the risk of Port site metastases following laparoscopic tumor surgery. Arch Surg. 1997;132(2):166-8.

Trocar Injuries

Shlomo B Cohen, Ariella J Setton, Daniel S Seiedman

INTRODUCTION

Laparoscopic surgery even in the hands of the most skilled and cautious surgeons is associated with a low degree of risk 11.1% in various surveys. The complication rate depends on the difficulty of the procedure.

The most critical point of laparoscopy, concerning the complications, is the abdominal cavity entry with the Veress needle or trocars. In a series of 2,324 laparoscopies, more than half of the complications were from the insertion of Veress needle or the trocars, rather than from the actual procedure. Other studies suggest that from one-third to half of the complications, are of this origin.

PREVENTION OF COMPLICATIONS

Patient Selection

The first step for prevention of complications is the right choice of appropriate candidates for the operation. Relative contraindications for laparoscopy are numerous, although they can be reduced with improvement in the skills and experience of the surgeon.

Those conditions can include morbid obesity, severe adhesions, previous abdominal operations, cancer, abdominal hernia, pregnancy (over 16 weeks), hypovolemic shock and bowel perforation with generalized peritonitis.

Nevertheless, there are some situations where laparoscopy can be undertaken in spite of commonly accepted contraindications. For example, hypovolemic shock due to ruptured ectopic pregnancy, or bleeding hemorrhagic corpus luteum, where the pneumoperitoneum helps controlling the bleeding source. Another example will be peritonitis due to appendicular or gastroduodenal perforation, where laparoscopy is considered a safe procedure.

Assessment of Risk for Adhesions

There are a few groups of patients who are at high-risk for adhesions: Patients with previous abdominal operations, patients with pelvic inflammatory device (PID), endometriosis, and patients with inflammatory bowel disease. Abdominal adhesions can present a risk factor for trocar insertion injury during laparoscopy. Abdominal adhesions are more common after midline incision than after Pfannenstiel incision. Bowel adhesions after midline incision are most common above the umbilicus. The surgeon must consider the possibility of the presence of adhesions in these high-risk patients.

Gastric and Bladder Emptying

The stomach may be distended after prolonged manual ventilation, or when endotracheal intubation is difficult. The distended stomach might be punctured itself; especially when the Veress needle is inserted in the upper abdomen, but also when it is inserted through the umbilicus. The stomach can also displace the transverse colon downward, which increases the risk of an intestinal puncture.

An over distended bladder is also at risk for injury. Placing a nasogastric tube and a Foley catheter, before the procedure, may eliminate the risk for those injuries.

Positioning of the Patient

Proper positioning of the patient is important for the safety of the patient. Correct positioning will give the surgeon the comfort and good visualization, and minimize the risk of injury.

The patient is placed in the low lithotomy position, the legs supported in stirrups, and the buttocks protruding slightly from the edge of the table, the knees in slight flexion and leaning on pads, so protected from neural injuries, the arms are placed near the patient's side in adduction.

The Veress needle and the trocar insertion should be inserted when the patient is in a horizontal position, so the great vessels will be positioned more cephalic and posterior, and thereby will be less vulnerable to injury. A prospective study found that the aortic bifurcation is more likely located caudal to the umbilicus in the Trendelenburg than in the horizontal position.

The rest of the operation is usually performed in the Trendelenburg position, allowing optimal visualization of the pelvic organs.

Insertion of the Insufflation Needle

The insufflation needles are modifications of the hollow needle designed by Veress.

The preferred site for the insertion of the needle is in, or close to the umbilicus, where the abdominal wall is the thinnest.

A 3 mm incision is made by a scalpel, and the abdominal wall is elevated by the surgeons. The needle is placed in the midline so it can directed between the iliac vessels, therefore in average weight women, it will be directed at a 45° angle to the spine, and in obese patients, the angle will be closer to 90°.

The needle should be held with the tips of the fingers, and steadily guided so the needle enters the fascia and the peritoneal cavity.

In cases of suspected intra-abdominal adhesions around the umbilicus, it is preferable to choose a different site for the insertion of the needle. Optional sites are—palmer point [left upper quadrant (LUQ), left costal margin after decompression of the stomach)], Douglas pouch, or fundus of uterus.

Examining the right position of the Veress needle is essential before insufflation. First, listening to two "clicks", when the needle passes through the rectus fascia and the peritoneum. Then using a syringe with saline, attached to the Veress needle, the surgeon will try to aspirate, and then inject some saline. If blood or intestine contents are aspirated, then the needle will be misplaced in a blood vessel or intestine, respectively. If there is resistance to injection of saline, the needle may be misplaced in the omentum, for instance. If the needle is placed appropriately, no contents will be aspirated and the saline will be easily injected.

Another way of demonstrating the position of the needle is by creating a negative intra-abdominal pressure, there by elevating the abdominal wall, after putting a drop of saline over the open end of the needle. The drop will be aspirated when elevating the abdominal wall.

Other signs for reassuring the right placement of the needle may be checked after starting the insufflation with CO_2. The pressure measured should be less than 10 mm Hg usually when starting insufflation. The earliest reassuring sign is the loss of liver dullness (unless there are adhesions in the area). Then, the abdomen should be distended symmetrically. Compression of the xiphoid lightly will increase the pressure measured by the insufflator.

By umbilical insertion of the Veress needle, the organs that are at increased risk are the bowel and omentum, especially if previous adhesions exist. The bladder and the stomach, if not emptied are at risk, too. When the needle is placed in the upper abdomen, it can puncture the pleural cavity, stomach, liver, or spleen.

Veress needle injuries are normally not apparent until gas insufflation, when abnormal high pressure appears.

After introducing the laparoscope, an examination of the middle and upper abdomen, around the insertion site, should be performed, looking for signs of needle induced trauma—punctures, hematomas and collections of gas.

Insertion of Primary Trocar

The introduction of cannulas is necessary for the insertion of laparoscopic instruments into the peritoneal cavity.

The cannula is a hollow tube with a valve mechanism, to prevent loss of intraperitoneal pressure. The trocar is a long instrument, passed through the cannula, allowing penetration of the abdominal wall.

The trocar should be pyramidal-tipped shape, and sharp, and the skin incision should be large enough, so no excessive force will be needed to introduce the trocar through the abdominal wall. One study shows less bleeding in trocar site, and less incisional hernia, using a cone-tipped non-cutting reusable trocar rather than sharp cutting disposable one. Another study shows an increased risk for vessel injury with pyramidal versus conical-tipped trocar.

New blunt-tipped devices exist now, that may limit the risk of injury.

Some surgeons prefer insufflating the gas up to 20 mm Hg, creating an adequate pneumoperitoneum for a safer trocar introduction, with less risk of injuring intra-abdominal organs. After introducing the cannulas and moving the trocars out, they reduce back the pressure to around 12 mm Hg, minimizing the hypercarbia effect by that.

There are some reports of using an abdominal wall retractor and optical trocar to minimize the injuries.

There are a few ways for introducing the cannulas into the abdominal cavity:

- Open laparoscopy (minilaparotomy or Hasson's technique)
- Secondary puncture—after creation of pneumoperitoneum by Veress gas insufflation
- Primary puncture—direct insertion of trocar without previously insertion of intraperitoneal gas.

Open laparoscopy allows the surgeon to observe adhesions in the entry site, and either perform adhesiolysis or choose a different entry site, though, open laparoscopy cannot prevent all insertion injuries, as the intestine can be adherent in the insertion site too. Open laparoscopy reduces the serious vascular or visceral injuries in patients with previous abdominal surgeries. It prolongs the surgery in between 5 minutes and 25 minutes. Even in patients with no previous operations, open laparoscopy reduces the rate of major vascular injuries.

Direct insertion of trocar, without previous creating of pneumoperitoneum, is complicated with less minor complications than introducing the Veress needle first, (6% vs. 22%), but there is no difference concerning major complications. Another study, recording 937 laparoscopic procedures performed using the direct trocar insertion technique showed no major complications, and minor complication decreasing from 5.3% to 1.3%, as department experience increased. Other studies, including one with 6,173 records of laparoscopies, showed no difference between the different methods concerning the complications. The direct insertion has the advantages of rapid creation of pneumoperitoneum, less cost, reduced risk of gas embolism, and it allows immediate recognition of major blood vessel injuries.

The position of the patient, as mentioned before, should be supine rather than Trendelenburg position during the insertion of the first trocar.

Insertion of Accessory Trocars

In most laparoscopies, there is need for introduction of accessory cannulas. The insertion site is chosen according to the disease, the kind of operation, the body build of patient, previous operation sites, and of course, the preference of the operator. The most common site is in the midline of the lower abdomen, 2–4 cm above the symphysis pubis (not too close to the symphysis, so the mobility of the instruments won't be limited). Other useful sites are lower quadrants, after locating the inferior epigastric vessels.

The insertion of the accessory trocar should be always done under direct vision, in order to avoid injury of bowel and blood vessels.

The most common complication made by insertion of accessory trocars in the lower quadrants, is injury of inferior epigastric vessels (superficial and deep) that run lateral to the rectus muscle.

Three methods to avoid injuring these vessels are:

1. Transillumination of the abdominal wall, so that the superficial vessels can be seen. In women with normal weight, a single vessel can be seen 5 cm from the midline in more than 90%, and a second vessel can be seen about 8 cm from the midline in 51% of patients. The technique is less useful in obese patients.
2. Visualization of the deep inferior epigastric vessels is important to avoid their injury. They are located deep to the rectus sheath, in between the umbilical ligaments (obliterated umbilical arteries) medially, and exit point of the round ligament into the inguinal canal, laterally. The trocar should be directed so avoiding the vessels if they are seen, and if not, the cannula should be placed 3–4 cm lateral to the medial umbilical ligament, or lateral to the lateral margin of the rectus abdominis muscle directing the trocar under vision, so avoiding the inferior epigastric vessels, seen by the laparoscope
3. Placing a 22 gauge spinal needle through the skin, observing the entry with laparoscope, before insertion of the trocar, will reassure the safe location of entry.

There are reports of using Doppler intraoperatively to avoid abdominal wall vessels injury.

The trocar should be directed toward the sacral hollow. If it is directed medially, the abdominal wall vessels can be injured. It can go down the pelvic side-wall or to the posterior peritoneum.

The smallest cannula needed should be used to decrease risk of injury.

Controlled force should be used, in order to avoid laceration of the bladder, uterus or bowel.

Complications of Trocar Insertion

Gastrointestinal Complications

The stomach, small bowel and colon are vulnerable to Veress and trocar insertion injuries, more often in pre-existing adhesions due to previous operations or inflammation, causing adhesions between intestine and the abdominal wall in or next to the insertion site. Distended stomach can be injured itself, or can displace the colon caudally, and increasing its risk for injury.

Insufflation Needle Injuries

Needle injuries are normally not apparent until gas insufflation when abnormal high pressure appears, or after insertion of laparoscope. Probably, many of them are unnoticed, and have no further complications.

The injury can be identified by increased filling pressure, asymmetrical distention of the abdominal cavity, feculent odor, or aspiration of intestinal contents.

If the injury is recognized, the needle should not be removed, and another insertion site should be found in order to enter a laparoscope and identify and repair the intestinal injury. The technique chosen for repair depends on the organ involved and the operator's skills. Some can be repaired laparoscopically and some require laparotomy.

Establishing a Pneumoperitoneum

Complications are made by insufflating CO_2 into the stomach or intestine, instead of the peritoneal cavity. Stomach or bowel insufflation is recognized by asymmetric distention, belching or passage of flatus. If these happen, gas is allowed to escape, and after inserting the laparoscope, the suspected perforated area is examined.

Pneumo-omentum is a common benign occurrence unless a vessel is lacerated. It is recognized by high filling pressure. Elevating the abdominal wall or withdrawal of the needle will usually release the omentum. After introducing the scope, an initial examination of the omentum and the omental vessels is performed to find lacerations.

Trocar Injuries

Puncture of the intestine with the trocar is potentially serious because of the large diameter of the trocar. Stomach distention can be created by difficult or prolonged intubation, and can be prevented by preoperative gastric suction when difficult intubation or when upper quadrant insertion site is used.

Puncture of the bowel is recognized by feculent odor or by seeing the mucosa when inserting the laparoscope. When the trocar passes through the lumen, as in cases of an adherent loop of bowel, however, recognizing the injury may be delayed until peritonitis, enterocutaneous fistula, abscess or death occurs. Therefore, direct visualization of the removal of the first cannula is crucial.

Once the injury is recognized, the cannula should be left in place so avoiding spillage of intestinal content, and for easier location of the laceration.

Bowel injuries by the trocar should be repaired as soon as recognized, either by suture made in a laparoscopic way, or if the injury is more extensive, conversion to laparotomy and performing resection of the bowel and reanastomosis, is needed.

Preoperative bowel preparation in high-risk patients is important and can minimize the need for colostomies.

Hemorrhagic Complications

Great Vessel Injury

The most dangerous hemorrhagic complications are injuries to the great vessels, including: The aorta, vena cava, common iliac arteries and veins, and the internal and external iliac arteries and veins. A prospective study that examined the location of aortic bifurcation in relation to the umbilicus, found that in Trendelenburg position, the bifurcation will be caudal to the umbilicus in 33% of cases, while only in 11% in supine position.

Vascular injuries are the main cause of mortality from laparoscopy, and for emergency laparotomies.

Most of these injuries occur by the insertion of the insufflation needle, although rarely, they can be secondary to primary or accessory trocar insertion.

The diagnosis will be made by blood coming from the insufflation needle, and patient developing instability, and profound hypotension. Sometimes, the diagnosis is delayed as bleeding is contained in the retroperitoneum.

If bleeding is suspected, the needle should be left in place, while immediate preparations for blood transfusions and for laparotomy are made. Once performing laparotomy, immediate compression on the aorta and vena cava should be made below the renal vessels for temporary control. Then, the management will be according to the vessel that was injured, and the extent of injury.

Abdominal Wall Vessel Injury

The most common injured vessels are the superficial inferior epigastric, in their course in the lower quadrants, usually injured by the accessory trocars. The bleeding can be recognized immediately, seeing blood running down the cannula, or formation of abdominal wall hematoma. Diagnosis can be delayed by tamponade of the bleeding by the trocar, until its removal.

The bleeding usually stops spontaneously, and expectant management is reasonable. Otherwise, sutures or electrocoagulation usually solve the problem.

The more serious bleeding is that of the deep inferior epigastric vessels, that branch from the external iliac arteries and veins. The bleeding here is more extensive, especially if retroperitoneal bleeding occurs and not immediately diagnosed. Diagnosis can be made intraoperatively by recognition of blood coming out of the cannula, or formation of hematoma, or postoperatively by recognition of hematoma in incision site, or hemodynamic instability, or in rare cases, pararectal or vulvar mass.

Delayed recognition of bleeding can be prevented by removal of trocars under vision.

Deep epigastric bleeding can be controlled by sutures, in the figure of eight, or with a straight needle, with the trocar in place. The suture needs to be removed after 24 hours in order to avoid cutaneous necrosis.

Another option is introducing a bipolar forceps through the opposite trocar, and coagulation of the vessels.

If recognized postoperatively, local pressure should be used, and only if hematoma grows or instability develops, then exploration is needed.

More laterally than the deep epigastric, the deep circumflex iliac vessels are located. Not often they are encountered in the laparoscopic surgery.

Intraperitoneal Vessel Injury

Other intraperitoneal vessels can be damaged by the entry into peritoneal cavity or during the operation. Sometimes, there is delay in recognition because of the limited visual field, spasm of the vessels or tamponade by the gas. Therefore, before ending the operation, all the areas of the operation should be examined for bleeding, and careful hemostasis should be made.

Gas Embolism

If a large vessel entry is not recognized on insertion of the insufflation needle, and insufflation is started, a gas embolism and even death can occur.

The presentation is of sudden bilateral mydriasis, cardiorespiratory distress with cardiac bradycardia or arrhythmia, and a specific murmur. The patient should be placed in left lateral decubitus for a possible cardiac puncture to release the gas.

Bladder Complications

Injury of the bladder can occur from a trocar perforation. Preoperative drainage of bladder, usually prevents that kind of injuries.

Small injuries, if made, in size of 1–2 mm, may be treated by immediate repair, or with bladder catheterization for 5–7 days. If a larger injury is made, it can be repaired laparoscopically or in an open procedure, if the area of the trigone is involved with catheterization for 10–14 days. Cystography should be performed before removal of catheter.

Abdominal Wall Complications

Incisional Hernia and Wound Dehiscence

There are reports of incisional hernia after laparoscopy. The incidence reported is around 1%, and the risk factors are the trocar diameter, mainly more than 10 mm, the trocar design, and pre-existing fascial defects.

The incisional hernia can be classified into several types—the early onset type, that occurs immediately after the operation, and can be either asymptomatic or cause bowel obstruction, the late onset type, that occurred several months after the operation, mostly with local bulging and no bowel obstruction, and a third type with protrusion of intestine or omentum.

Richter's hernias contain only a portion of the intestine in the defect, so the diagnosis is usually delayed.

The symptoms of incisional hernia are variable, including asymptomatic situations, pain caused by incomplete obstruction, and diffuse peritonitis if incarceration occurs. Rare complication is necrotizing fasciitis.

The diagnosis will be made by the clinical situation, and may be confirmed by ultrasound or computed tomography (CT).

The management of hernia with evisceration always requires surgery, either by laparoscopy if diagnosed immediately and the bowel has no evidence of necrosis, or by laparotomy, if perforation is suspected, including repair or resection of intestine.

Prevention of the hernia can be achieved by closure of port site defects of or more than 10 mm, especially in lateral location.

Emphysema

The most common extraperitoneal site insufflated by mistake is the preperitoneal space. If this is recognized early, the gas supply is disconnected, and the gas is allowed to escape. The needle is removed and re-inserted. If it is not recognized early enough, gas will be filled in the preperitoneum and cause subcutaneous emphysema.

It will be recognized after the insertion of the laparoscope—a spider-web appearance of the tissue.

The emphysema can extend to the mediastinum, and cause cardiac function problems, that will require stopping of the procedure, and letting the CO_2 escape.

SUMMARY

This section reviews the complications associated with abdominal entry during laparoscopy.

This section also reviews techniques for prevention of these complications. Attention to risk factors, habitus of the patient, and to the procedure itself, may reduce markedly the incidence of the complications.

BIBLIOGRAPHY

1. Amara DP, Nezhat C, Teng NN, et al. Operative laparoscopy in the management of ovarian cancer. Surg Laparosc Endosc. 1996;6:38-45.
2. Angelini L, Lirici MM, Papaspyropoulos V, et al. Combination of subcutaneous abdominal wall retraction and optical trocar to minimize pneumoperitoneum related effects and needle and trocar injuries in laparoscopic surgery. Surg Endosc. 1997;11:1006-9.
3. Baadsgarrd SE, Bille S, Egeblad K. Major Vascular injury during gynecologic laparoscopy. Acta Obstst Gynecol Scand. 1989;68: 283-5.
4. Bateman BG, Kolp LA, Hoeger K. Complications of laparoscopy—operative and diagnostic. Fertil Steril. 1996;66:30-5.
5. Berek JS. Gynecologic Endoscopy. In: Munro MG, Brill AI (Eds). Novak's Gynecology, 13th edition. Philadelphia: Lippincott Williams and Wilkins; 2002. p. 711.
6. Bloom DA, Ehrlich RM. Omental evisceration through small laparoscopy port sites. J Endourol. 1993;7:31-2.
7. Brill AI, Nezhat F, Nezhat CH, et al. The incidence of adhesions after prior laparotomy: A laparoscopic appraisal. Obstet Gynecol. 1995;85:269-72.
8. Byron JW, Fujiyoshi Ca, Miyazawa K. Evaluation of the direct trocar insertion technique at laparoscopy. Obstet Gynecol. 1989;74:423-5.

9. Chapron CM, Dubuisson JB, Ansquer Y. Is total laparoscopic hysterectomy a safe surgical procedure? Hum Reprod. 1996;11:2422-4.
10. Chapron CM, Pierre F, Lacroix S, et al. Major vascular injuries during gynecologic laparoscopy. J Am Coll Surg. 1997;185:461-5.
11. Chi I, Feldblum PJ, Baloh SA. Previous abdominal surgery as a risk factor in interval laparoscopic sterilization. Am J Obstet Gynecol. 1983;145:841-6.
12. Clough KB, Ladonne JM, Nos C, et al. Second look for ovarian cancer: Laparoscopy or laparotomy? A Prospective comparative Study. Gynecol Oncol. 1999;72:411-7.
13. Crawford DL, Phillips EH. Laparoscopic repair and groin hernia surgery. Surg Clin North Am. 1998;78:1047-62.
14. Cueto J, Diaz O, Garteiz D, et al. The efficacy of laparoscopic surgery in the diagnosis and treatment of peritonitis: Experience with 107 cases in Mexico city. Surg Endosc. 1997;11:366-70.
15. Dixon M, Carrillo EH. Iliac vascular injuries during elective laparoscopic surgery. Surg Endosc. 1999;13:1230-3.
16. Fahlenkamp D, Rassweiler J, Fornara P, et al. Complications of laparoscopic procedures in urology: Experience with 2,407 procedures at 4 German Centers. J Urol. 1999;162:765-70.
17. Franks AL, Kendrick JS, Peterson HB. Unintended laparotomy associated with laparoscopic tubal sterilization. Am J Obstet Gynecol. 1987;157:1102-5.
18. Fried M, Peskova M, Kasalicky M. The role of laparoscopy in the treatment of morbid obesity. Obes Surg. 1998;8:520-3.
19. Harkki-Siren P, Kurki T. A nationwide analysis of laparoscopic complications. Obstet Gynecol. 1997;89:108.
20. Holzinger F, Kleiber C. Trocar site hernias: A rare but potentially dangerous complication of laparoscopic surgery. Chirurg. 2002;73:899-904.
21. Hulka JF, Levy BS, Parker WH, Philips JM. Laparoscopic assisted vaginal hysterectomy: American Association of Gynecologic Laparoscopists 1995 membership survey. J Am Assoc Gynecol Laparosc. 1997;4:167.
22. Hurd WW, Wang L, Schemmel MT. A comparison of the relative risk of vessel injury with conical versus pyramidal laparoscopic trocars in a rabbit model. Am J Obstet Gynecol. 1995;173:1731-3.
23. Jansen FW, Kapiteyn K, Trimbos-Kemper T, et al. Complications of laparoscopy: A prospective multicentre observational study. Br J Obstet Gynecol. 1997;104:595.
24. Jirecek S, Drager M, Leitich H, et al. Direct Visual or blind insertion of the primary trocar. Surg Endosc. 2002;16:626-9.
25. Lee PI, Chi YS, Chang YK, et al. Mini laparoscopy to reduce complications from cannula insertion in patients with previous pelvic or abdominal surgery. J Am Assoc Gynecol Laparosc. 1999;6:91-5.
26. Leibl BJ, Schmedt CG, Schwartz J, et al. Laparoscopic Surgery complications associated with trocar tip design: Review of literature and own results. J Laparoendosc Adv Surg Tech. 1999;9:135-40.
27. Leng J, Lang J, Huang R, et al. Complications in laparoscopic gyneco ogic surgery. Chin Med Sci J. 2000;15:222-6.
28. Losanoff JE, Richman BW, Jones JW. Trocar site hernia, complicated by necrotizing fasciitis — case report and review of the literature. Hernia. 2003;7:220.
29. Lowry PS, Moon TD, D'Alessandro A, et al. Symptomatic port site hernia associated with a nonbladed trocar after laparoscopic live-donor nephrectomy. J Endourol. 2003;17:493-4.
30. Mac Cordick C, Lecuru F, Rizk E, et al. Morbidity in laparoscopic gynecological surgery: Results of a prospective single centre study. Surg Endosc. 1999;13:57.
31. McKernan JB, Champion JK. Access techniques: Veress needle-initial blind trocar insertion versus open laparoscopy with a Hasson Trocar. Endosc Surg Allied Technol. 1995; 3:35.
32. Morrison CP, Wemyss-Holden SA, Iswariah H, et al. Lateral Laparoscopic port sites should all be closed: The incisional "spigelian" hernia. Surg Endosc. 2002;16:1364.
33. Munro MG. Laparoscopic access: Complications, technologies and techniques. Curr Opin Obstet Gynecol. 2002;14:365-74.
34. Nezhat C, Siegler A, Nezhat F, et al. Operative Gynecologic Laparoscopy—principles and techniques. In: Complications, 2nd edition. New York: McGraw-Hill Professional; 2000. p. 365.
35. Nezhat F, Brill AI, Nezhat CH, et al. Laparoscopic appraisal of the anatomic relationship of the umbilicus to the aortic bifurcation. J Am Assoc Gynecol Laparosc. 1998;5:135-40.
36. Nezhat FR, Silfen SL, Evans D, et al. Comparison of direct insertion of disposable and standard reusable laparoscopic trocars and previous pneumoperitoneum with Veress needle. Obstet Gynecol. 1991;78:148-50.
37. Nezhat FR, Tazuke S, Nezhat CH, et al. Laparoscopy during pregnancy: A literature review. J Soc Laparoendosc Surg. 1997;1:17-27.
38. O'Sullivan GC, Murphy D, O'Brein MG, et al. Laparoscopic management of generalized peritonitis due to perforated colonic diverticula. Am J Surg. 1996;171:432-4.
39. Plaus WJ. Laparoscopic trocar site hernias. J Laparoendosc Surg. 1993;3:567-70.
40. Quint EH, Wang FL, Hurd WW. Laparoscopic transillumination for the location of anterior abdominal wall blood vessels. J Laparoendosc Surg. 1996;6:167-9.
41. Rosen DM, Lam AM, Chapman M, et al. Methods of creating pneumoperitoneum: A review of techniques and complications. Obstet Gynecol Surv. 1998;53:167-74.
42. Saville LE, Woods MS. Laparoscopy and major retroperitoneal vascular injuries. Surg Endosc. 1995;9:1096.
43. Servais D, Aslthoff H. Fatal carbon dioxide embolism as a complication of endoscopic interventions. Chirurg. 1998; 69:773-6.
44. Soriano D, Yefet Y, Oelsner G, et al. Operative laparoscopy for management of ectopic pregnancy in patients with hypovolemic shock. J Am Assoc Gynecol Laparosc. 1997; 4:363-7.
45. Tonouchi H, Ohmori Y, et al. Trocar site hernia. Arch Surg, 2004;139:1248.

46. Usal H, Sayad P, Hayek N, et al. Major vascular injuries during laparoscopic cholecystectomy: An institutional review of experience with 2,589 procedures and literature review. Surg Endosc. 1998;12:960-2.
47. Whiteley MS, Laws SA, Wise MH. Use of a hand-held Doppler to avoid abdominal wall vessels in laparoscopic surgery. Ann R Coll Surg Engl. 1994;76:348.
48. Wolfe BM, Gardiner BN, Leary BF, et al. Endoscopic cholecystectomy: an analysis of complications. Arch Surg. 1991;126:1192-6.
49. Woolcott R. The safety of laparoscopy performed by direct trocar insertion and carbon dioxide insufflation under vision. Aust NZ J Obstet Gynecol. 1997;37:216-9.
50. Yerdel MA, Karayalcin K, Koyuncu A, et al. Direct trocar insertion versus Veress needle insertion in laparoscopic cholecystectomy. Am J Surg. 1999;177:247-9.

Vascular Injuries

Jayakrishnan K

INTRODUCTION

Although uncommon with experienced laparoscopists, vascular injury leading to hemorrhage is a possibility. Injury to the aorta, vena cava and iliac vessels can result in rapid blood loss. It is important to have an intravenous (IV) access of reasonable size even though the procedure may be considered to have a low potential for blood loss. It should be remembered that a retroperitoneal hematoma may result in major blood loss without a great deal of blood being visible in the peritoneal cavity. Particular attention should be paid in the case of an inexperienced surgeon or in the case of a patient in whom difficulty in placement of needle or trocar is anticipated.

The development of the laparoscope marshaled in a new era in terms of both diagnostics and therapeutics, often eliminate the need for open abdominal surgery. However, as with all developing techniques, as usage increases, so does the number of reported associated complications. Although relatively few, minor complications are reported in as many as 5.1% of laparoscopic procedures and major complications in more than 2.3% (Kane and Krejis, 1984). Complications related to laparoscopic procedures include ureteric injury (Cheng, 1976, Hunter and McCartney, 1993, Grainger et al, 1990) as well as damage to other internal organs including the bowels, bladder and uterus (Yuzpe, 1990). Vascular trauma has also been associated with the placement of trocars where the incidence of injury to the vessels of the anterior abdominal wall (Hurd et al., 1993) occurs with greater frequency than injury to deep vessels such as the aorta and iliac vessels (Baadsgaard et al, 1989). Despite the use of relatively standardized techniques and increasing surgeon experience, complications related to the insertion of trocars still occur.

BLOOD VESSEL INJURY

The Veress needle may penetrate omental or mesenteric vessels or any of the major abdominal or pelvic arteries or veins. Minor vascular injuries involving the omental or mesenteric vessels are difficult to prevent as it is impossible to insure that the omentum is not close to the abdominal wall during blind insertion of the insufflating needle.

Injury may be suspected if blood returns up the open needle or if free blood is seen in the peritoneal cavity after insertion of the laparoscope. If blood returns up the needle and the patient's condition is stable, the site of injury may be investigated laparoscopically. The needle should be left in place and a 5 mm laparoscope introduced through a suprapubic cannula. Minimal bleeding may usually be controlled by bipolar coagulation or a laparoscopic suture. Laparotomy is not usually necessary except in the case of injury to the superior mesenteric artery. Such injury requires repair by a vascular surgeon (Bassil et al, 1993).

Injury to the major vessels may be prevented by lifting the abdominal wall, angling the needle toward the pelvis, once the initial thrust through the fascia has been made and by inserting only as much of the needle as necessary. Thin patients and children are at particular risk of this injury.

Withdrawal of blood on aspiration following insertion of the needle should allow early detection of blood vessel injury. If injury to a vessel such as the aorta, inferior vena cava or common iliac vessel is suspected, the needle should be left in place to mark the site of the injury and laparotomy performed through a midline incision. There is usually a large hematoma which obscures the site of the injury. The aorta should be compressed with a clamp or hand until a vascular surgeon arrives to perform definitive surgery.

Dramatic collapse may result from penetration of a major vessel but the bleeding may not be immediately evident, if it is retroperitoneal. The loose areolar tissue anterior to the aorta can allow accumulation of a considerable amount of blood before frank intra-abdominal bleeding is seen. A thorough search must be made to determine the extent of vessel damage. This includes retraction of bowel to expose the aorta above the pelvic brim which is the most common site of perforation. Failure to do so may result in continued bleeding and formation of a large hematoma leading to a second episode of shock, some hours later.

REPAIR OF MAJOR VESSEL INJURY

The first priority is to perform a laparotomy and compress the aorta. This goal is achieved with an assistants's hand, an aortic compressor or a vascular clamp. The field is cleared of blood in quick motion. The vessel is found and a finger is placed over it for hemostasis till repair materials are gathered.

The smaller vessels that produce significant bleeding e.g. middle sacral or inferior epigastric are ligated. Larger vessels are repaired with 4/0 Prolene® over a Dacron® reinforcing bolster. Larger defects need interposition graft. This work is done by a trained cardiovascular surgeon.

If a large artery is clamped for over 10–15 minutes, systemic anticoagulation with heparin should be considered.

Once the patient reaches the recovery room, careful neurovascular assessment is done of the lower limbs in addition to the usual intensive care support. After 4–6 weeks after an arterial injury, Doppler flow studies would be helpful in characterizing the flow through the repaired vessel.

CONCLUSION

The avoidance of vascular injury during placement of lateral trocars is of paramount importance.

The following recommendations are made:

- In accordance with Hurd et al, 1994, in the absence of laparoscopic anatomical landmarks to guide placement, lateral trocars should be inserted at least 5 cm above the pubic symphysis and 8 cm from the linea alba
- The placement of the patient in Trendelenburg position should only be carried out after trocar insertion
- The use of insufflation to achieve a pneumoperitoneum with a pressure of 25 mm Hg, allows for a safer and easier entry technique
- Safe trocar entry in the absence of pneumoperitoneum can only be achieved in thin patients with lax abdomens where direct manual abdominal lift can be insured
- The trocar found to offer the safest use is the short disposable palm trocar as it requires only half the force for insertion
- Finally, an in-depth knowledge of the anatomy of the vasculature of the anterior abdominal wall is one of the cornerstones for safe trocar placement.

MEDICAL ANALYSIS

Injuries that occur at the initiation of laparoscopy can be best categorized into two types: (1) Damage to vessels; and (2) damage to visceral organs, i.e. bowel or bladder. Vascular injuries have been reported to occur at a rate of 0.11–0.25% in an analysis of 77,604 cases. Injuries occur more frequently as a result of the placement of the insufflating needle than from primary trocar placement. A review of the literature in 1995 by one researcher identified 20 reported major vascular injuries, 12 out of which were caused by the insufflation needle. Another article reported a total of 7 vascular injuries in 5 patients. Three of the injuries were from the insufflation needle insertion. In a Canadian questionnaire, responders noted 109 injuries from the insufflation needle, 104 primary trocar injuries, and 61 secondary trocar injuries. In a 1996 report of 103,852 laparoscopies, 83% of vascular injuries, 75% of bowel injuries, and 50% of local hemorrhages were caused by the primary trocar insertion.

SUMMARY

A major vascular injury at laparoscopy is a dangerous surgical complication. A thorough anatomic knowledge and understanding will reduce the risk of the procedure. Should an injury occur prompt diagnosis and treatment will help to limit the morbidity and mortality that could result from the rare major vessel injury at laparoscopy.

BIBLIOGRAPHY

1. Baadsgaard SE, Bille S, Egeblad K. Major vascular injury during gynecologic laparoscopy. Acta Obstet Gynecol Scand. 1989;68:283-5.
2. Bilgic S, Sahin B. Rare arterial variation: A common trunk from the external iliac artery for the obturator, inferior epigastric and profunda femoris arteries. Surg Rad Anat. 1997;19:45-7.
3. Cheng YS. Ureteral injury resulting from laparoscopic fulguration of endometriotic implant. Am J Obstet Gynecol. 1976;15:1045-6.
4. Grainger DA, Soderstrom RM, Schiff SF, et al. Ureteral injuries at laparoscopy: Insights into diagnosis, management, and prevention. Obstet Gynecol. 1990;75:839-43.
5. Hunter RW, Mccartney AJ. Ureteric injuries at laparoscopic hysterectomy. AM J Obstet Gynecol. 1993;169:752.
6. Hurd WW, Bude RO, DeLancey JO, et al. Abdominal wall characterization with magnetic resonance imaging and computed tomography: The effect of obesity on the laparoscopic approach. J Reprod Med. 1991;36:473-6.
7. Hurd WW, Bude RO, DeLancey JO, et al. The relationship of the umbilicus to the aortic bifurcation: Implications for laparoscopic technique. Obstet Gynecol. 1993;80:48-51.
8. Hurd WW, Bude RO, DeLancey JO, et al. The location of abdominal wall blood vessels in relationship to abdominal landmarks apparent at laparoscopy. Am J Obstet Gynecol. 1994;171:642-6.
9. Hurd WW, Hurtcau JA. Practical Manual of Laparoscopy and Hysteroscopy. Berlin: Springer; 1997.
10. Hurd WW, Pearl Ml, DeLancey JO, et al. Laparoscopic injury of abdominal wall blood vessels: A report of three cases. Obstet Gynecol. 1993;82:673-6.
11. Jakubowicz M, Czarniawska-Grzesinska M. Variability in origin and topography of the inferior epigastric and obturator arteries. Folia Morph. 1996;55:121-6.
12. Kane MG, Krejis GJ. Complications of diagnostic laparoscopy in Dallas: A 7-year-prospective study. Gastro Endosc. 1984;30:237-40.

13. Loffer FD, Pent D. An alternative technique in penetrating the abdomen for laparoscopy. J Reprod Med. 1974;13:37-40.
14. Levy BS, Soderstrom RM, Dail DH. Bowel injuries during laparoscopy. Gross anatomy and histology. J Reprod Med. 1985;30:168-72.
15. Nordestgaard AG, Bodily KC, Osborne RW, et al. Major vascular injuries during laparoscopic procedures. Am J Surg. 1995;169:543-5.
16. Soderstrom RM, Levinson C, Levy B. Complications of operative laparoscopy. In: Soderstrom RM (Ed). Operative Laparoscopy: The Master's Technique. New York, NY: Raven Press; 1993. p. 187-98.
17. Usal H, Sayad P, Hayek N, et al. Major vascular injuries during laparoscopic cholecystectomy. Surg Endosc. 1998;12:960-2.
18. Yuzpe AA. Pneumoperitoneum needle and trocar injuries in laparoscopy: A survey on possible contributing factors and prevention. J Reprod Med. 1990;35:485-90.

CHAPTER

43

Hysteroscopy

Pranay Shah, Nandita Palshetkar, Rishma Pai, Abha Majumdar, Tejshree Singh, PG Paul, Tony Thomas

43.1 FUNDAMENTALS OF HYSTEROSCOPY: INSTRUMENTATION, PRINCIPLES AND TECHNIQUE

Pranay Shah

INTRODUCTION

Hysteroscopy is the inspection of the uterine cavity by endoscopy. It allows for the diagnosis of intrauterine pathology and serves as a method for surgical intervention (operative hysteroscopy). Hysteroscopic procedures were first described by Pantaleoni in 1869. Although it was one of the first endoscopic procedures to be performed, it took over 100 years for refinements in instruments, distension media, electronic hysteroflators before hysteroscopy was accepted as a modality of treatment for intrauterine pathology.

ADVANTAGES

Operative hysteroscopy has in many ways superceded laparoscopy in meeting the minimal invasive criteria. It uses the endocervical canal, the body's natural passage, to gain entry into uterine cavity. Nonhysteroscopic techniques to treat intrauterine septa and adhesions are obsolete. Submucous myoma removal no longer requires a hysterotomy. Cornual and interstitial tubal obstruction is also managed hysteroscopically. Endometrial ablation or resection is considered as an acceptable alternative to hysterectomy for treatment of abnormal uterine bleeding.

Since the 1990s, hysteroscopy has finally found its proper niche and every practicing gynecologist must learn the skills of hysteroscopy.

DISADVANTAGES

If used properly, there are no disadvantages of this procedure.

INDICATIONS

Diagnostic hysteroscopy is indicated in evaluation of the uterine cavity in patients with:

- Infertility (to evaluate abnormal hysterosalpingograms— filling defects, adhesions)
- Abnormal uterine bleeding (menorrhagia, irregular bleeding, postmenopausal bleeding)
- Mullerian abnormalities (in patients with recurrent pregnancy loss—septate uterus, "T" shaped uterus)
- Lost or misplaced intrauterine devices (IUDs).

INDICATIONS OF OPERATIVE HYSTEROSCOPY

- Targeted endometrial biopsy (suspected tuberculosis, endometrial carcinoma)
- Removal of polyps, submucous myoma
- Adhesiolysis
- Metroplasty (incision of uterine septum)
- Removal of misplaced IUD or foreign body
- Tubal cannulation in cornual or interstitial block

- Treatment of dysfunctional uterine bleeding (DUB) [endometrial ablation, transcervical resection of the endometrium (TCRE)]
- Sterilization (electrocoagulation or tubal plugs to block the tubes cornual ends).

CONTRAINDICATIONS

- Recent or active pelvic inflammatory disease (PID)
- Acute cervicovaginal infection
- Active uterine bleeding (causing poor visibility)
- Current intrauterine pregnancy.

EQUIPMENT FOR HYSTEROSCOPY

Telescope and Sheath

The hysteroscope system is comprised of a rigid telescope that is used together with an outer sheath for instillation of the distension media. Telescopes of different diameters (2–4 mm) and variety of viewing capability (0°, 12°, 30°, 70°) are available.

The most popular hysteroscope is a 4 mm 30° telescope with a 5.5 mm outer sheath for diagnostic hysteroscopy (Fig. 1). A 6.5 mm double channel continuous flow sheath is available and is useful when the uterine cavity is bleeding. The same telescope can be used with operative hysteroscopy sheath and resectoscope.

Operative Hysteroscope

The internal lumen of the sheath must be of adequate size to allow passage of the telescope and an operative instrument, e.g. scissors, biopsy forceps, catheters and coagulation electrode (Figs 2A and B). The external sheath diameter ranges between 3.5 mm and 7 mm to allow for passage of telescope, operative instruments and liquid distention media.

Resectoscope has been used by urologists for many years. Since 1990, it has been used in a modified form by gynecologists to perform operative procedures such as excision of submucous myomas, polypectomy, division of uterine septa and endometrial ablation or resection.

The Resectoscope

The resectoscope (Figs 3A and B) has five parts:

1. The 4 mm telescope, preferably with a 12° lens (30° can also be used).
2. A continuous flow outer sheath that has an inflow and an outflow stopcock. The outflow holes are located at the distal end of the sheath.
3. An inner sheath, which is inside and connected to the outer sheath. It has an insulated ceramic tip.
4. The working element is called an Iglesias-type element, allowing one handed operation. The working element is held with the fingers on the handgrip and the first digit of the thumb in the thumb ring. Pushing on the ring moves the electrode forward approximately 2 cm and the spring brings it back.
5. Electrodes: There are a variety of electrodes (cutting loop, ball, barrel, knife, vaportrode) that utilize unipolar electrosurgical systems. A cable connects the electrode to the electrosurgical generator.

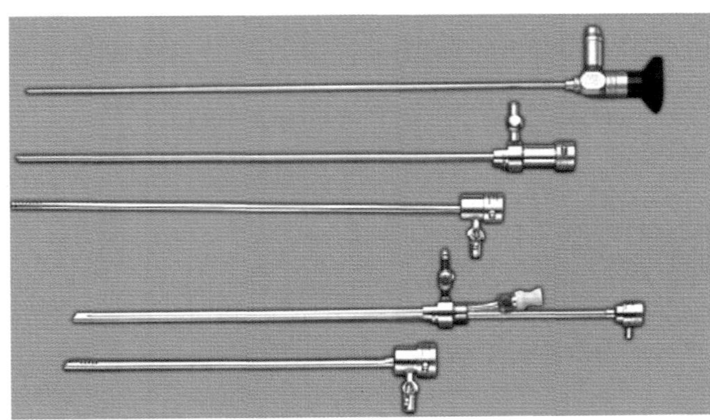

Fig. 1: Hysteroscope with diagnostic sheath

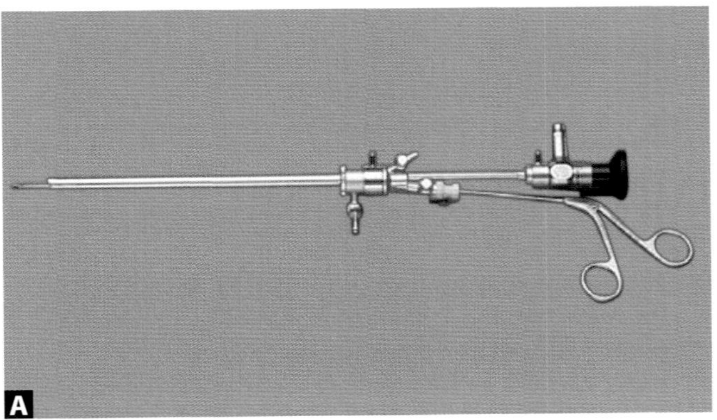

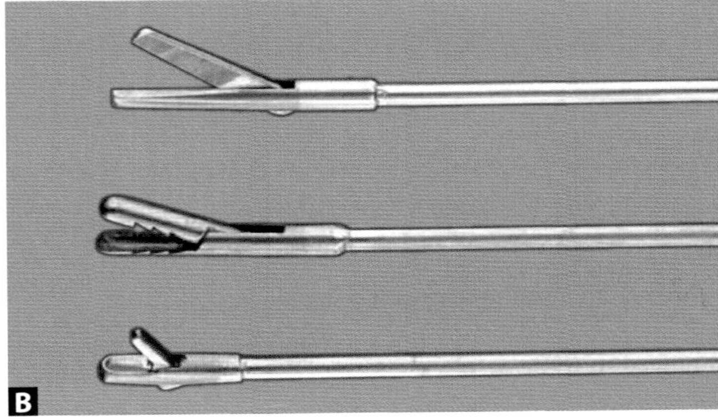

Figs 2A and B: (A) Operative hysteroscope with instrument through the operative channel; (B) Operative hysteroscopic instruments

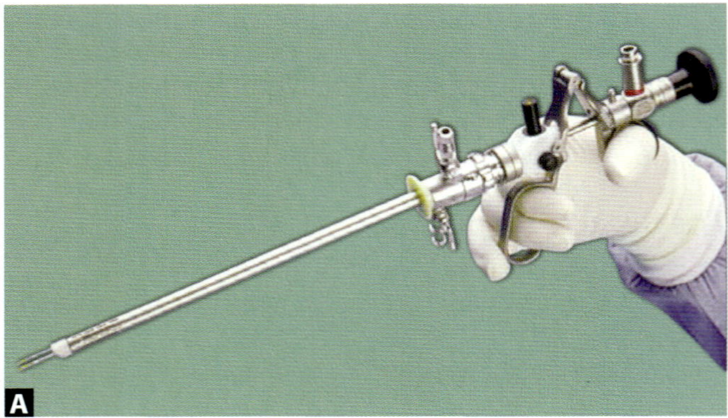

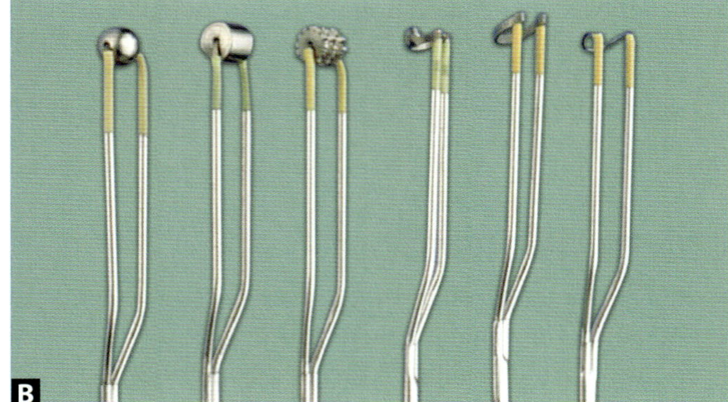

Figs 3A and B: (A) Resectoscope; (B) Accessories with resectoscope

The cutting loops come in different diameters ranging from 0.010" to 0.015" wire. The thinner the wire, the higher the power density and the faster the cut with less coagulation. However, the thin wires will bend and break easily. Cutting loops are primarily used to shave or remove polyps, submucous myomas.

The loop should not be used to cut mechanically. Never use the loop without activating the current.

Monopolar desiccation electrodes with ball or barrel configurations have a substantially larger surface area and are typically used to perform focal hemostasis or endometrial ablation. The roller ball, because of its smaller size, provides 1 mm of surface contact as opposed to 3 mm of contact area for the barrel. The smaller size produces a higher power density and therefore a deeper burn over a smaller area.

Ancillary Equipment

The light source, computer-controlled display (CCD) camera, recording device and electrosurgical unit are same as used in laparoscopy.

Distension Media

Hysteroscopy provided little information until safe, effective distention was developed. Uterine cavity is a potential space. Distention media enables to separate the uterine walls and obtain a panoramic view. Liquid distention media when used in continuous flow, flush out the blood, blood clots and debris formed during operative hysteroscopy and resectoscopy.

The Media

Gaseous: The media are of two types:

1. Gaseous media
2. Liquid media.

Gaseous: Carbon dioxide (CO_2) is used for diagnostic hysteroscopy. It is inexpensive, non-messy, readily available and has refractive index same as air, giving a clear view. In presence of blood or mucus, it can cause a distorted view. It needs an expensive electronic hysteroscopic insufflator for safe delivery of gas at correct flow rate (30–60 mL/min) and pressure range (100–120 mm Hg).

Liquid:

- *Saline and Ringer's lactate* are physiologic, iso-osmolar and isotonic. Until very recently, they were used only during diagnostic hysteroscopy or operative hysteroscopy without the use of electrosurgical systems, as the presence of electrolytes precluded the use of these solutions during monopolar electrosurgical operations.
  The recent development of bipolar intrauterine surgery, explicitly designed to avoid use of electrolyte free solutions, has encouraged the use of normal saline solution for hysteroscopic surgery
- *Glycine* is a simple amino acid that is mixed with water as a 1.5% solution. It is readily available, cheap, and provides fairly good visibility. Like all nonviscous distention media, it is miscible with blood and requires continuous-flow irrigation. It is a non-electrolyte solution and can be used during monopolar electrosurgery. As it is hypo-osmolar and hypotonic, if it intravasates into the vascular tree in significant amounts; it can produce profound hyponatremia and hypervolemia, with pulmonary edema, cerebral edema, heart failure and death.

FLUID DELIVERY SYSTEMS

The systems used to control flow and pressure during hysteroscopy are as follows:

- *Pressure cuff:* These devices, similar to a sphygmomanometer, are inflated around the bag, exerting pressure on it (Fig. 4)
- *Electronic suction and irrigation pump:* Hamou® Endomat® is a automatically controlled suction and

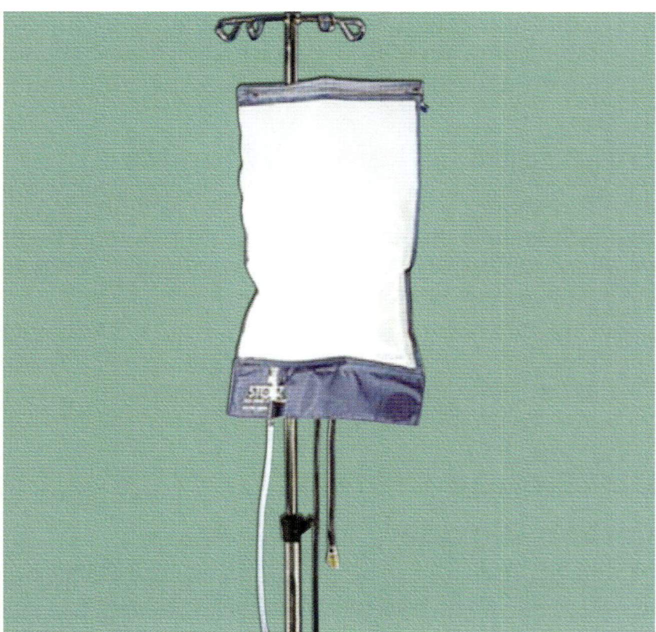

Fig. 4: Pressure cuff

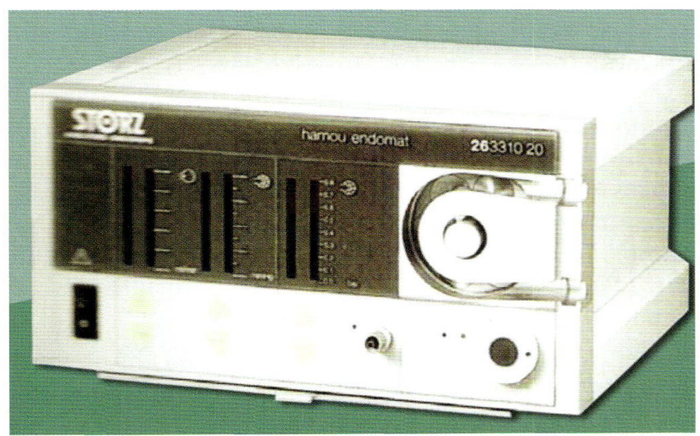

Fig. 5: Hamou® Endomat®

irrigation pump which can maintain a clear field of view and constant uterine distention during hysteroscopic surgery (Fig. 5).

TECHNIQUE OF HYSTEROSCOPY

Patients can be scheduled for diagnostic hysteroscopy after obtaining a detailed patient history, performing a physical examination, discussing choice of anesthesia, and obtaining informed consent. Hysteroscopy should be done in the postmenstrual period as the endometrium is thin, which facilitates intracavity viewing, bleeding is minimal and pregnancy is ruled out.

Although, hysteroscopy in the office setup can be done without anesthesia or paracervical block, in most cases we prefer to do under general anesthesia (GA).

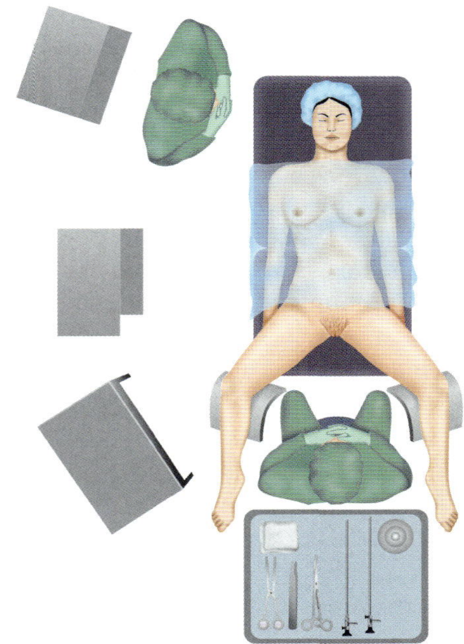

Fig. 6: Hysteroscopy setup

If combined with laparoscopy, a GA with tracheal intubation is preferred.

Position: Patient is placed in standard lithotomy position with legs apart to obtain vaginal access (Fig. 6).

COMPONENTS OF HYSTEROSCOPY

The Hysteroscope

There is a range of hysteroscopes starting from 1.2 mm flexible hysteroscope with a 2.5 mm diagnostic sheath, to the standard 4 mm scope with a 5 mm diagnostic sheath. The 1.2 mm scope is a flexible scope, which can be easily passed into the uterine cavity without dilatation. However, it is very fragile and generates a small image. Neither does it allow any degree of operative work to be performed. On the other hand, a standard 4 mm Hopkins scope is rigid and gives a very good image. In case of doing operative procedures, it needs to be combined with an operative sheath with a diameter of 7.0–8.5 mm, necessitating anesthesia and cervical dilatation procedures. In order to overcome the above shortcomings, there have evolved two systems that can be effectively utilized for diagnostic and operative office hysteroscopy. With these systems it is possible to perform operative procedures such a polypectomy, adhesiolysis, tubal cannulations and myomectomies (< 2 cm):

The Bettochi Hysteroscope (Karl Storz)

- The standard Bettochi hysteroscope with Hopkins based rods lens system is a miniature version of the famous Hamou® 2 hysteroscope. The scope has an external diameter of 2.9 mm. It can be used as a panoramic hysteroscope (1x) as well as as a micro-contact hysteroscope (80x). For diagnostic purpose, it can be used with a single flow outer sheath of 3.6 mm or a continuous flow outer sheath of 4.4 mm. In case of operative office hysterescopy, it can be combined with a continuous flow operative sheath of 3.9 mm × 5.9 mm (average diameter 5 mm). This sheath has an operative channel to accommodate five French instruments to pass through.

- The modified Bettochi: This is a new version with a 1.9 mm diameter optic along with corresponding smallar diameters for diagnostic and operative sheath.

The Versascope System (Johnson and Johnson)

The versascope is a flexible telescope made up of a set of 50,000 fused optical fibers, providing a 0° field of vision with an outer panoramic angle view of 75°. The scope has an external diameter of 1.8 mm and length of 28 cm. The density and optical quality of the image system produces an image, which is similar to the conventional rod lens panoramic hysteroscope. The scope is used with a continuous flow diagnostic cum operative sheath, which has an outer diameter of 3.5 mm and a distal curvature of 10°. A proximal collar is rotatable. This allows manipulation of the scope for full peripheral viewing, without disturbing the instrument position. The operative channel has an expandable instrument channel which can easily accommodate instruments till 7 French in diameter. This operative channel also simultaneously functions as an independent outflow port for continuous flow during the procedures.

Unlike Storz, the Versascope has got a disposable sheath. However, in practice the sheath can be reused, after resterilization in cidex, at least 10–20 times, making the instrument much more cost effective. Both the scopes come with fiberoptic cables.

Light Source

There are various light sources, one can use for illumination:

- Halogen: This is 150–250 W cold light source and is sufficient for vision. However, it tends to give off a reddish tinge to the image
- Xenon: A 175 W xenon light source provides an outstanding illumination and enables a good depth of field. Although the light is extremely hot at its source, most of the heat gets dissipated along the length of the fiberoptic cable. Despite this, a significant amount of heat can be generated at the distal tip. This can cause thermal injury to the patient or burn paper drapes or clothing with prolonged contact. Hence, one should keep the intensity of the light as less as possible.

Endoscopic Camera and Monitor

In office hysteroscopy, the image size is quite small. Hence, it is preferable to use cameras with zoom system to select the appropriate size of the picture. A single chip endoscopic camera is sufficient for diagnostic and minor operative work. A three-chip camera will not be of additional help, unless it has additional filters to eliminate the pixelization and digitalization of the image.

DISTENTION SYSTEMS

Carbon Dioxide

Carbon dioxide gas has been routinely used to distend the cavity in an office setting. The gas insufflators use low gas flow rate and are easy to maintain. It gives excellent visualization. The gas is rapidly absorbed and cleared by the lungs. With proper criteria for pressure and flow rate, there is a very low incidence of CO_2 intoxication or embolism. However, the gas has major disadvantages. The CO_2 often leaks around the hysteroscope, making diagnosis difficult. A mild contamination of the lens by blood or mucus can form troublesome bubbles, during the use of CO_2. This can greatly obscure the picture clarity. Besides this, CO_2 use necessitates the use of a dedicated gas hysteroflator. One cannot use laparoscopic insufflators, which have high flow rate. Inadvertent use of these laparoscopic insufflators can lead to CO_2 embolism and even death.

In case one wants to use CO_2 for distention, the pressure should be kept in the 100–120 mm Hg range with a flow rate of 30–60 mL/min, corresponding to a final working intrauterine pressure of 40–80 mm Hg.

Ionic media: In case one comes across intrauterine pathology and wants to perform intrauterine procedures, one cannot do it.

Hence with office hysteroscopy, it is best to use fluid distention systems rather than CO_2 gas distention for visualization of the uterine cavity.

Fluid Distention Media

These can be used for both diagnostic and operative purposes. These consists of the high viscosity high molecular weight liquid media (hyskon) or the low viscosity low molecular weight media (saline or glycine).

- *High viscosity media:* High molecular weight dextran has been used in the past. However, it is viscous and messy in consistency and if not cleaned from the instrument, can immobilize moving parts of the hysteroscope. If the amount exceeds 500 mL there is a risk of pulmonary edema, disseminated intravascular coagulation (DIC) or anaphylaxis. This medium is rarely used in present day practice

- *Low viscosity media:* They can be of two types: non-ionic media and ionic media.
  - *Non-ionic media:* These are mediums such as glycine, mannitol, or sorbitol. Glycine is easily available and frequently used. One can use monopolar as well as bipolar current with these solutions. However, the biggest problem with these solutions is water intoxication and fluid overload, especially if the net fluid intravasation into the patient exceeds 800–1,000 mL. Therefore, it is critical to measure accurately the input-output of the distention media. As soon as the intravasation exceeds 1,000 mL, the procedure should be stopped. In an office setting, this is a rare, as in operative hysteroscopy.
  - *Ionic media:* These mainly consist of saline or Ringer's lactate. These are safe media and can be easily used with operative procedures such as mechanical surgeries with scissors or forceps, versapoint bipolar coagulation or the standard bipolar coagulation. These media, coupled with continuous flow sheaths with inflow and outflow channels, are preferred for both diagnostic as well as therapeutic (barring monoplar cautery probes and monopolar resection) visualization of the uterine cavity.

Distention Machines

There are various distention systems that can be used. These are:

- Gravity
- Pressure cuff
- Hysteromat
- Endomat®
- Total input output system.

Of these, the Endomat® is the ideal system, especially for office hysteroscopy purposes, as it correctly maintains intrauterine pressure to around 70 mm Hg, thus preventing peritoneal reflux and resultant discomfort. However, a simple pressure cuff can also do the trick.

ENERGY SOURCES

Mechanical Energy

These are in the form of 2 mm semi-rigid, sharp as well as blunt scissors, biopsy forceps and the myoma screw. These instruments can be passed through the operating channel to obtain biopsy specimens, transecting base of small polyps, excising uterine septa and synechiae.

Unipolar

This has been the traditional energy used for operative hysteroscopy. However, one cannot use this energy in the office hysteroscopy as the fully conscious patient will not tolerate it and will complain of pain.

Bipolar Versapoint

This bipolar cautery, marketed by Johnson and Johnsons has many advantages:

- It can be used with saline thus eliminating the side effects of using glycine
- The electrodes can easily pass through the operative channel of office hysteroscopy
- Instant vaporization and desiccation can eliminate resection chips
- Decrease in the amount of blood loss
- The pain is minimal if you restrict the surgery to the endometrial layer.

DIAGNOSTIC HYSTEROSCOPY

Procedure: Cervix is held with vulsellum and dilated using Hegar's dilator. The hysteroscope is inserted in the cervical canal and advanced under vision till it enters the uterine cavity. A systematic evaluation of the cavity is done observing the fundus, tubal ostia, anterior and posterior wall, and cervix canal. Any irregularity in the cavity (Fig. 7), adhesions (Fig. 8), polyps (Fig. 9) or myomas (Fig. 10) and uterine septum (Fig. 11) are noted.

Inadequate visualization is usually due to over-dilatation of cervix causing leakage of distention media and inadequate distension, excessive bleeding, and uterine perforation.

Operative Hysteroscopy

Hysteroscopic biopsy forceps can be used for targeted biopsy in patients with suspected tuberculosis or endometrial carcinoma. Hysteroscopic scissors is used to cut adhesions and uterine septum. A 6F catheter can be passed through the operative channel of the operative sheath and tubal ostia cannulated (Fig. 12).

Resectoscope loop can be used to shave submucous myomas and perform endometrial resection. Roller ball is used to perform endometrial ablation and knife can be used to cut dense adhesions and thick uterine septae.

COMPLICATIONS OF HYSTEROSCOPY

Complications of hysteroscopy occur when contra-indications are ignored or when the procedure has been incorrectly performed on well chosen patients.

Fortunately they are not common and many large series report no serious complications. When complications do occur, most arise during operative rather than diagnostic hysteroscopy.

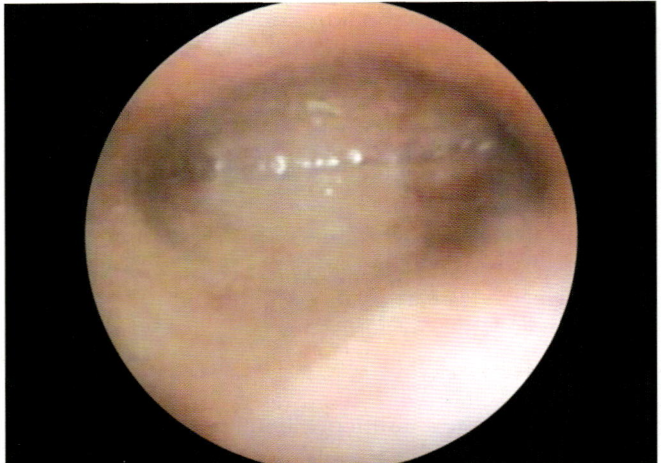

Fig. 7: Hysteroscopy—normal cavity

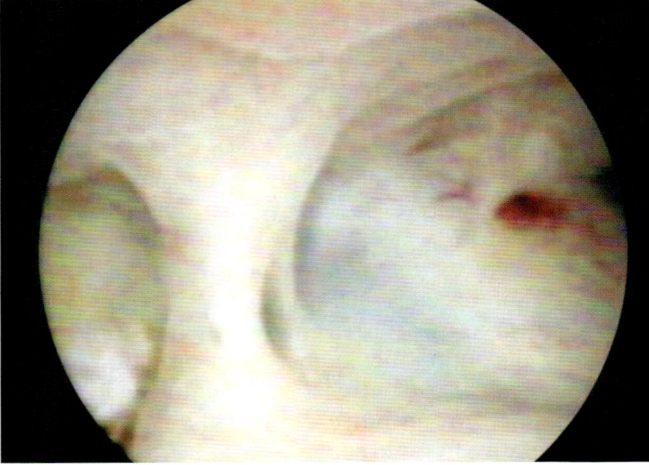

Fig. 8: Hysteroscopy—adhesions

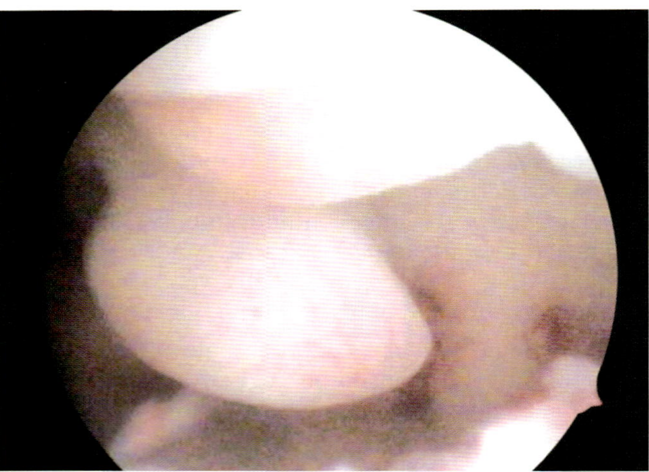

Fig. 9: Hysteroscopy—polyp

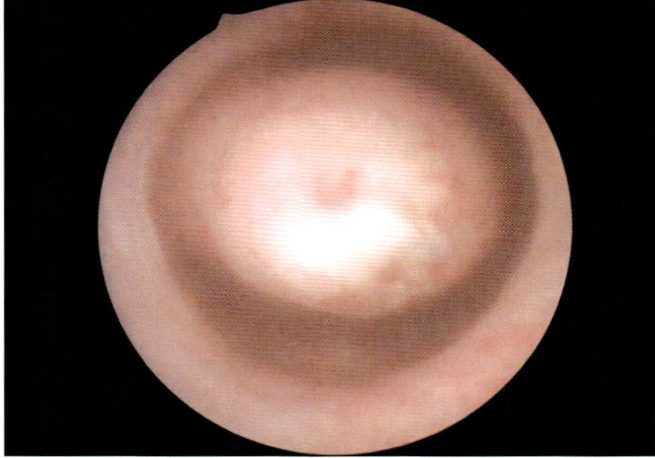

Fig. 10: Hysteroscopy—fibroid

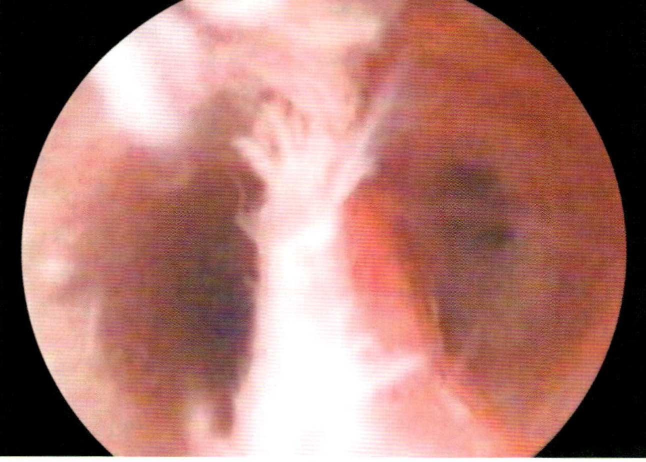

Fig. 11: Hysteroscopy—septum

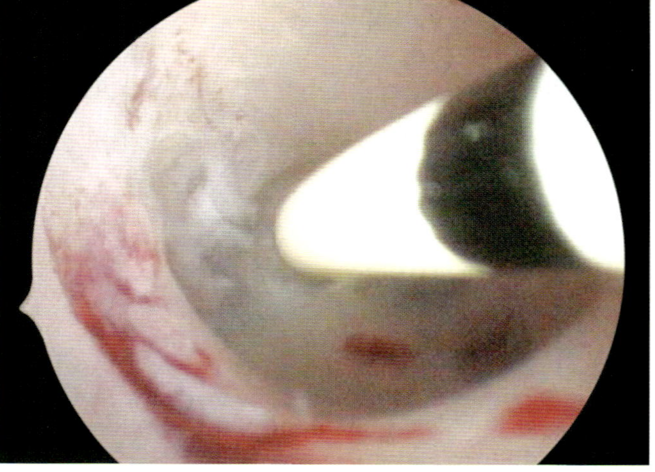

Fig. 12: Tubal cannulation

Anesthetic complications: The risks to the patient from the anesthetic are similar to those from any other operation.

Patient position: Incorrect positioning of the patient may result in:

- *Nerve injuries:* Brachial plexus injury may result from incorrectly placed shoulder restraints or from leaving the patient's arm abducted on an arm board. Pressure on the peroneal nerve by lithotomy stirrups may result in paresthesia and foot drop.
- *Damage to soft tissue:* The surgeon should ensure that no part of the patient is in contact with metal parts of the table because these can act as return plates for electrical energy and burns can occur at the point of contact.
- *Deep venous thrombosis:* Deep vein thrombosis (DVT) can result from prolonged compression of the calves by the leg supports. The surgeon should ensure that the type of support is appropriate and well padded. If DVT is suspected, the advice of a physician should be sought and appropriate anticoagulant therapy instituted.

Distention Media

Complications produced by the distension media are specific to hysteroscopic surgery. It is essential that all the operating room staff is cognizant of the side effects of the distention media and that responsibility for accountancy of fluid media is placed on a designated member of staff.

Carbon dioxide: Cardiac arrhythmia, and rarely gas embolism, may occur with diagnostic hysteroscopy.

Liquids

Saline may be used in diagnostic hysteroscopy but only nonelectrolyte fluids should be used with electrosurgery because of the risk of producing burns to other organs. All low-molecular-weight fluids may produce fluid overload. Accountancy of fluid input and output is mandatory in any hysteroscopic procedure. The severity and management of fluid overload depends on the nature of the medium in use.

Saline overload produces a simple hypervolemic state which may be treated by insertion of a central venous line, administration of a diuretic, oxygen and, if necessary, cardiac stimulants.

Glycine overload may produce nausea and vertigo, hyponatremia, transient hypertension followed by hypotension associated with confusion and disorientation. Excessive overload may produce elevated blood ammonium levels leading to encephalopathy, and rarely death. Hyponatremia should be treated with administration of diuretics and hypertonic saline solution combined with monitoring of serum electrolyte levels until normality has been restored. Encephalopathy requires hemodialysis to be performed.

Surgical

Complications of surgery may arise during the operation or be delayed. Intraoperative complications include uterine perforation and hemorrhage.

Traumatic Injuries of the Uterine Cervix and Corpus

Injuries related to hysteroscopy are more common during operative than diagnostic procedures because more dilatation is necessary for inserting the larger-diameter operative hysteroscopes.

Cervical tearing by the tenaculum during dilatation is a common event without significant sequel. Treatment is suturing if the bleeding is brisk. Laceration of the lateral margins of cervical canal and lower uterine segment may also occur during dilatation. They become a source of fluid intravasation. Lacerations may be avoided by inserting laminaria tents or giving tablet misiprostol 400 μg orally or 200 μg vaginally, the night before surgery.

The cervix or uterus may be perforated during dilatation or insertion of the hysteroscope. This is a potential problem, especially in an acutely anteflexed or retroflexed uterus and in women with a stenotic cervix. It will limit the ability to complete the procedure as adequate distention cannot be achieved. It can be prevented by maintaining appropriate techniques of dilatation and inserting the scope under vision.

Simple perforation may be made with a cervical dilator with the hysteroscope or non-electrical instruments. Simple perforation rarely causes any further damage and may be treated conservatively by observation and appropriate broad spectrum antibiotics. Laparoscopy may be considered to exclude bleeding.

Complex perforation occurs with electrosurgical instruments and are associated with thermal injury to adjacent structures including bowel or large vessels. If the perforation has been caused by an electrosurgical instrument, laparoscopic examination or laparotomy to exclude bowel or vascular injury is mandatory.

Delayed complications include infection, discharge and adhesion formation.

INCIDENCE OF COMPLICATIONS

The complication rate in diagnostic hysteroscopy is low and was estimated by Lindemann to be 0.012%. Complications from operative hysteroscopy are more common and potentially more serious.

43.2 HYSTEROSCOPY IN INFERTILITY

Nandita Palshetkar, Rishma Pai

INTRODUCTION

Hysteroscopy is a very simple and well established procedure which allows direct visualization of the endometrial cavity and tubal ostia. Moreover, it can also be used to treat the intrauterine lesions in the same sitting. Till recently, hysteroscopy has been a hospital or outpatient surgery center procedure, usually necessitating GA or regional block. With newer advances in optics, hysteroscopes with smaller diameter are now available, thus reducing the need for major anesthesia and making office-based hysteroscopy a reality. Office hysteroscopy is a safe, efficient and routinely practiced procedure worldwide.

Diagnostic Indications

- The hysteroscopy can be routinely combined with a concomitant laparoscopy, while investigating a case of infertility
- It can also be used as a routine procedure prior to undergoing assisted reproductive technology (ART)
- It can be used in patients who have an abnormal hysterosalpingography (HSG) or sonohysterography
- It can be used in infertile patients associated with Asherman's syndrome (Koch's, PID, etc.)
- Women presenting with secondary infertility because of recurrent abortions.

Therapeutic Indications

- Hysteroscopy can be used effectively to remove submucous fibroids, endometrial polyps and polypoidal endometrium
- It can be used in connection with the laparoscope to try and perform tubal cannulation [Fallopian tube recanalization (FTR)] and reversal of the tubal block
- It can diagnose mullerian anomalies such as septate, subseptate or bicornuate uterus. It can also be used to effectively treat some of these conditions
- Hysteroscopic adhesiolysis for Asherman's syndrome.

HYSTEROSCOPY IN AN OFFICE SETTING

In this technique, hysteroscopes with outer sheath diameters varying from 1.2–5 mm are used in an office based setting without or with minimal local anesthesia to perform diagnostic and limited operative hysteroscopic work.

The patient should be examined in the counseling room and informed about the hysteroscopy. It is necessary to perform this procedure in a room which has got access to oxygen and emergency resuscitation trolley. This is in anticipation of an occasional vasovagal shock or anaphylaxis secondary to the usage of local anesthetic.

Recovery room: Following this procedure, a recovery room with reclining chairs is necessary for the patient to recuperate for 30 minutes to 1 hour prior to getting discharged. It should be ideally performed in the early or mid-proliferative phase of the cycle. The bleeding has stopped and the endometrium has not grown enough to obscure the vision of the hysteroscope. One can do it any time, provided patient is not pregnant.

Contraindications

There are no real contraindications except pregnancy, acute PID and cervical cancer.

Premedications

Most of the time the procedure can be performed without giving any medication. Occasionally, one can give nonsteroidal anti-inflammatory drugs (NSAIDs), either orally or rectally, 1 hour before the procedure. Occasionally, a mild sedative may be administered intramuscularly.

Patient position: Normally, the patient is in dorsal lithotomy position. An adjustable electronic table is ideal for giving comfortable position. As has been mentioned, very few need some degree of anesthesia, if at all one can give a paracervical or intracervical block.

Cervical Preparation

One can do vaginal preparation with povidone-iodine. Some units are not preparing the vagina with any antiseptic. However, this is a risky move and can lead to PID. One can expose the cervix with a bivalve speculum, which can be removed after hysteroscope enters the uterine cavity. This gives flexibility of moving the hysteroscope much more easily. Instead of using the speculum, one can insert the hysteroscope into the vagina without using the speculum. Once the vagina distends with media, one can locate the cervix and gently pass the hysteroscope into the uterine cavity.

The hysteroscope is gently inserted through the external os and the endocervical canal is inspected, distention of cavity is obtained using gas or fluid media, the distention allows visualization of the cavity which appears as a darkspot. The hysteroscope is directed towards the dark spot (spot at 6 o'clock) until the cavity is entered. Systemic inspection of the cavity is performed keeping the pressure between 60 mm Hg and 100 mm Hg. Examination of fundus, anterior, posterior and lateral walls, both ostia and endocervical canal is done.

Precautions: There should be no air bubbles when using liquid as distention media, pressures should be below 100 mm Hg to prevent pain; air bubbles to be sucked out when using versapoint.

Complications

There are hardly any complications with diagnostic hysteroscopy. These are:

- Inadequate visualization: Mainly due to lack of flow of the distention media, as well as non-use of continuous flow sheath
- Perforation: This is hardly the case with office hysteroscopy as one enters the uterine cavity under vision
- Infection is rare: An adequate prophylactic antibiotic cover will prevent infection
- Bleeding: This is rare with office hysteroscopy.

HYSTEROSCOPY IN AN OPERATION THEATER SETTING

These procedures are carried out in the operation theater. The size of the hysteroscope optics is 4 mm with a 30° oblique view. The diagnostic scope along with its sheath has a diameter of 5 mm, while the operative hysteroscope with a 2 mm operating channel is about 7 mm in diameter. The versapoint bipolar resectoscopes or the standard monopolar resectoscopes are 9–10 mm in diameter. Due to its larger sizes, besides giving GA, one needs to dilate the cervix. Barring this and the configuration of the resectoscope, the remaining instrumentation is similar to that which has been described in the section of office hysteroscopy instrumentation. A detailed description of the resectoscopes is given below:

Operative Resectoscopy

The size of the whole assembly is 26 French. It consists of:

- The external outflow sheath for efflux of the distention medium
- The internal inflow sheath for influx of the distention medium
- The standard 4 mm diameter Hopkins hysteroscope
- The working element with either monopolar or bipolar electrodes:
  - The monopolar electrodes are either in the shape of loops, ball, cylinders or knife. Normally a good high frequency generator with a blended cutting
  - Coagulating current of 80–120 W or a pure cutting current of 100–120 W is used
  - The bipolar versapoint electrodes are in the form of loop or cylinder. The current is automatically controlled by the bipolar generator
  - The distention media is in the form of 1.5% glycine for the monopolar resectoscopes. In case of bipolar resectoscopes, one can use normal saline. Please note that the normal saline should never be used with monopolar resectoscopes. The uterine distention should be maintained between 90 mm Hg and 150 mm Hg. It is important to use a safe distention system, such as the Endomat®, which controls the flow, pressure and calculates the fluid intravasation into the patient's circulation, while performing septum resection or myoma resection. Although many operators use gravity or pressure cuff sytems, these can be dangerous and can cause mortality. Many European nations have made it compulsory for doctors to use an Endomat® during resectoscopy. In any case, a strict maintenance of input minus output of distention fluid is desired. One should become cautious when the deficit crosses 750 mL and stop the procedure at 1,000–1,100 mL. These safeguards can prevent pulmonary edema, cerebral edema and the dreaded transuretheral resection of the prostate (TURP) syndrome, which can occasionally lead to mortality.

In the bipolar resectoscopes, saline is used as a distention medium. If proper precautions are not taken, this can also lead to pulmonary edema. However, unlike glycine complications, this can be rapidly reversed with intravenous (IV) frusemide.

DISCUSSION

In the early days, hysteroscopy was performed for purely diagnostic reasons, especially if there were symptoms or findings on clinical or radiological examination [abnormal ultrasound, HSG or computerized axial tomography (CAT) scan/magnetic resonance imaging (MRI)] suggestive of an intrauterine pathology. However, there have been recent studies that have shown an abnormal hysteroscopic finding in patients with previous normal ultrasonography (USG)/HSG findings. This has prompted many clinicians to routinely perform hysteroscopy in association with a diagnostic laparoscopy. Although, this may not be universally acceptable, there is a definitive consensus of routinely performing a hysteroscopy prior to an ART procedure. It is also indicated in patients with recurrent implantation failures following ART.

Operative hysteroscopic procedures related to infertility may be done in the following circumstances:

- Asherman's syndrome
- Severely stenosed cervix
- Intrauterine adenomatous polyps
- Submucous myomas
- Fallopian tube recanalization
- Genital malformation: Septate or subseptate uterus
- Foreign body in the uterine cavity
- Hysteroscopic embryo transfer (ET).

Asherman's Syndrome

Asherman's syndrome, first described around 1920, is characterized by the development of intrauterine adhesions (IUAs) following infection or uterine curettage for postpartum hemorrhage or incomplete or missed abortion, with subsequent damage to the basalis endometrium. In India, these adhesions are commonly seen in patients with genital tuberculosis. These adhesions can cause infertility, recurrent pregnancy loss, hypomenorrhea, amenorrhea, ectopic pregnancy, preterm labor, abnormal placentation and fetal demise, if pregnancy is achieved.

It is demonstrated on HSG as single or multiple lacuna-shaped filling defects of variable size in uterine cavity. These filling defects are characterized by their irregularity, angulated form, very sharp contours, homogeneous opacity and persistent appearance on several exposures taken at various intervals. Hysteroscopy is used to confirm the HSG findings and permits surgical correction as well. These adhesions are classified, based on the hysteroscopic findings according to the IUA classification of the European Society for Gynecological Endoscopy (ESGE) as given below.

Grade/Extent of Intrauterine Adhesions

I. *Thin or filmy adhesions:*
   - Easily ruptured by hysteroscope sheath alone
   - Cornual areas normal.

II. *Singular dense adhesion:*
   - Connecting separate areas of the uterine cavity
   - Visualization of both ostia normal
   - Cannot be broken by hysteroscope sheath.

IIa. *Occluding adhesions only in the region of the internal os:* Upper uterine cavity normal.

III. *Multiple dense adhesions:*
   - Connecting separate areas of the uterine cavity
   - Unilateral obliteration of ostial areas of the tubes.

IV. *Extensive dense adhesion with (partial) occlusion of the uterine cavity:*
   - Both tubal ostial areas (partially) occluded.

V. *Extensive endometrial scarring and fibrosis:*
   - In combination with grade I or grade II adhesions
   - With amenorrhea or pronounced hypomenorrhea.

Va. *Extensive endometrial scarring and fibrosis*:
   - In combination with grade III or grade IV
   - Adhesions
   - With amenorrhea.

Treatment of IUAs by blind intrauterine procedures such as dilatation and curettage (D&C) can deteriorate the possibilities for hysteroscopic treatment by creating a false passage or perforation and reducing the amount of residual endometrium, required for adequate regeneration after adhesiolysis. Thin or flimsy adhesions can be lysed under direct vision by pushing in the hysteroscope sheath. More substantial adhesions will require division by sharp instrumentation. The hysteroscopic semi-rigid scissors are the instrument of choice as they do not employ a current, thereby reducing the risk of damage to the surrounding endometrium.

Areas of healthy endometrium are often scant in Asherman's syndrome, and it is essential to maintain their integrity so that re-growth of the endometrium is possible postoperatively. Adhesions are divided at their midpoint allowing the cut edges to retract.

Thick vascular and dense adhesions are incised using resectoscopes utilizing the thin electrosurgery (Collin's) knife. Monopolar current using 90–100 W cutting or 30 W coagulating current is used. Alternatively bipolar versapoint cautery can also be used.

In situations, where the adhesions completely obliterate the uterine cavity, selective dissection should begin at the internal os creating a neocavity, and then proceeding towards the fundus and tubal ostia. The uterine contour must be followed closely during the dissection. Concomitant laparoscopy should be used in order to avoid uterine perforation.

Postoperative balloon catheter or plastic intrauterine contraceptive devices (IUCDs) can be used in cases of severe adhesions to avoid apposition of the uterine walls. Estrogen is usually prescribed postoperatively for 1–3 months to hyperstimulate the endometrial lining. An HSG is obtained at the completion of hormonal therapy to assess the uterine cavity and decide upon the course of care. The results of hysteroscopic treatment of IUAs depend upon the type and the extent of adhesions. The more extensive and severe the adhesions, the more difficult they are to treat and therefore, the more difficult it is to achieve a viable pregnancy. The worst prognosis is in those who have suffered from genital tuberculosis. Of those women who become pregnant, about 40–80% will have a normal pregnancy.

Fallopian Tube Cannulation and Recanalization

Tubal pathology is one of the common causes of infertility. Proximal tubal occlusion constitutes 25–30% cases of tubal pathology.

Proximal tubal occlusion can be classified as:

- Nodular: Salpingitis isthmica nodosa (SIN) or endometriosis
- Non-nodular:
  - True fibrotic
  - Pseudo-occlusion: Polyps (15–19%), hypoplastic tubes, synechiae, mucosal alteration (10–15%).

In about 50% of the infertile patients with proximal tubal block, there are tubal plugs due to amorphous material responsible for occlusion. Remaining 50% of the patients have true pathological block. Until the recent past, laparotomy with microsurgical reconstruction was the only choice to overcome proximal tubal occlusion.

Though microsurgical reconstruction and tubocornual anastomosis is associated with good pregnancy rates (57%) it is a prolonged surgery, associated with significant postoperative morbidity, and prolonged hospital stay. After the introduction of operative hysteroscopy, hysteroscopic cannulation for proximal tubal occlusion has attracted a great deal of interest.

Unfortunately, the conventional methods used to study tubal patency, such as HSG or the direct observation by laparoscopy and selective chromopertubation, frequently do not allow differentiation between an insufficient filling of the tubes, tubal spasm or a true mechanical obstruction. The selective tubal cannulation technique, with hysteroscopic guidance is highly useful in the diagnosis of tubal patency or in the confirmation of partial or total proximal tubal disease. This procedure permits precisely reaching the diagnosis of the tubal obstruction due to the presence of a true pathology or simply functional, or secondary to a tubal spasm; besides it also works as a therapeutic procedure since in the first case, it permits the lysis of lax adhesions and the removal of the amorphous material that obstructs the tube and permits the catheterization. Distal tubal disease with rigid tubes as a result of infection, especially tuberculosis and presence of hydrosalpinx on ultrasound are the relative contraindications of this procedure.

As proximal tubal cannulation requires simultaneous laparoscopy to confirm the status of the distal Fallopian tubes, as well as negotiation of the block, GA is preferred. Diagnostic survey of the uterine cavity is carried out to note the anatomy and to rule out intrauterine pathologies like adhesions, especially near the ostium, polyp, submucous fibroid, etc. Mesh-like adhesions can be seen in some patients, which cannot be detected on HSG. Laparoscopic inspection of pelvis is then carried out, especially to note the distal tubes to ascertain the cause and type of obstruction. Laparoscopy also allows evaluation of rest of the pelvis. If the distal tubes appear normal, only hysteroscopic cannulation should be performed. Diseased distal tubes are associated with poor outcome of the hysteroscopic cannulation.

Procedure

After dilating the cervix to no. 8 mm Hegars, the operating channel with the 4 mm hysteroscope is introduced into the uterine cavity with continuous flow of saline to distend the uterine cavity. Simple cannula with the guidewire inside is then introduced through the operating channel. One-sided tubal ostium is then identified and the tip of the hysteroscope is brought in near proximity to the ostium. The tip of the cannula is then advanced near the ostium under constant hysteroscopic visualization. Guidewire is then advanced into the ostium for about 1–1.5 cm to negotiate the cornual block. Guidewire should not be pushed further as it may result in perforation due to sinusoidal shape of the intramural portion of the Fallopian tube. The Terumo guidewire is relatively stiff and should not be used to cannulate the distal Fallopian tube. After introduction of the guidewire into the intramural portion, the cannula is railroaded over the guidewire to fix the tip of the cannula into the proximal part of the intramural portion. Guidewire is then removed and dye is injected through the proximal portion of the cannula. Simultaneous visualization by laparoscopy can identify the exit of the dye through the fimbrial end of the tube. Cannula is then removed and the same procedure is repeated on the other side.

Advantages

- Works as therapeutic procedure, which permits the lysis of lax adhesions and removal of amorphous material, and permits catheterization
- Differentiation between the spasm of the tube, true pathological block and the functional block
- Low rate of complications
- Low cost
- Valuable information about the proximal and distal tubes.

When compared to microsurgical anastomosis in patients with normal distal tubes, intrauterine pregnancy rates are similar and ectopic pregnancy rates are lower in the cannulation group. One year patency rates in non-pregnant patients are higher in the anastomosis group (80% vs 33%). Recurrence of the tubal obstruction is seen in 50% of the patients in 6 months of time after the cannulation.

UTERINE SEPTUM RESECTION

Uterine septa cause reproductive failure in about 25% of patients with this condition. Septate uterus is apparently linked to a high rate of fetal loss generally occurring in the first half of pregnancy. It has been proposed that miscarriages may be due to vascularization problems at the implantation site, especially if located in the septum itself.

Uterine septum resection in a patient presenting with infertility is as yet controversial. Most of us, including the author, would resect such septae.

To differentiate between bicornuate and septate uterus, HSG and hysteroscopy, apart from a clinical examination are useful imaging techniques. Three-dimensional (3D)/four-dimensional (4D) ultrasound, and especially MRI, is also now advocated for diagnosing and correctly classifying Müllerian abnormalities and malformations. Laparoscopy, however, continues to be the method of choice as it affords a definite differential diagnosis and distinguishes between bicornuate and septate uterus.

Several different procedures have been adopted and yield more or less the same results. The basic concept involves hysteroscopic transcervical observation of the uterine septum followed by resection.

Scissors are the most commonly used method for septum resection. Division is performed systematically from side to side until the uterotubal openings can be seen and bleeding is observed at the myometrical junction. Once septal division is complete, the intrauterine pressure of the distending fluid can be decreased; if arterial bleeding occurs, selective coagulation can be performed with a 7F ball-tipped electrode. If bleeding has occurred, the resectoscope can be used to coagulate selectively each bleeding arteriole.

The final goal is to produce a satisfactory uterine cavity. The most delicate part of the procedure is probably the decision when to stop the resection in order to prevent damage to the myometrium and immediate complications, such as perforation, or more delayed difficulties, e.g. the postoperative formation of synechiae. Simultaneous laparoscopic control is also extremely suitable for this purpose. Recently, it has been proposed to use ultrasound for precise preoperative measurement of the septum, which can easily be distinguished from the myometrium, and subsequent continual monitoring of the operation, so that an extremely precise decision can be made about when to stop resecting so that the myometrium is not affected. Preoperative treatment with danazol or leutinizing hormone-releasing hormone (LHRH) antagonists decreases the bleeding at the time of resection. The author uses scissors to cut the septum and bipolar versapoint cautery to cauterize the bleeders.

Follow-up examination should be performed 1–2 months after the operation depending on the type of postoperative management used. A second look hysteroscopy can be performed at this time. The full-term pregnancy rate obtained by various authors ranges from 70% to 80%, which is very similar to the results of traditional laparotomic metroplasty with the techniques proposed by Tomkins, Te Linde and Jones.

Advantages of Hysteroscopy

- The operation may be performed as an office procedure without hospitalization of the patient
- No scar tissue remains on the abdominal and uterine walls
- There is a lower rate of intra- and postoperative morbidity compared to traditional surgery
- There is no reduction in the volume of the uterine cavity.

Submucous Myoma

Protrusion of a myoma inside the uterine cavity with anatomical distortion of the cavity, with the symptoms like menorrhagia or associated infertility, is the most common indication for a hysteroscopic myomectomy.

Intrauterine myoma can be classified as per the ESGE:

Grade 0: Pedunculated Myoma or myoma limited within the cavity or has small base.

Grade 1: Myoma with parial intramural development, with more than 50% of intracavitary component. Angle of protrusion between the myoma and the uterine wall less than 90°.

Grade 2: Predominantly, intramural myoma with cavitary component less than 50%. Angle of protrusion between the myoma and the uterine wall is greater than 90°.

Preoperative Diagnostic Assessment

An accurate transvaginal ultrasound examination is most of the times sufficient to diagnose an intracavitary fibroid. However, the gold standard is of course a diagnostic hysteroscopy performed under gas distention viz. CO_2 rather than a liquid distention. Use of CO_2 as distention media also helps to distinguish between polyps and myomas. An ultrasound may give a clue to the intramural extent of the myoma. It is also important to assess the amount of myometrial tissue between the outer border of the myoma and the serosal surface of the uterus. A tissue of at least 1 cm thickness indicates a much easier and safer removal during surgery. However, newer studies have shown that a thickness as less as 0.6 cm is also good enough. It has been demonstrated that increase in the thickness as the resection progresses.

The techniques used are either the standard monopolar resectoscope-glycine method or the new bipolar versapoint vaporization-resectoscope-saline method.

In the latter method, saline can be used instead of glycine to decrease the complications of bowel burns and fluid overload.

Resection of Submucous Fibroids

The loop is placed behind the myoma to be resected and then withdrawn with application of the current. Sometimes a backward and forward movement can be used in conjunction and tandem to facilitate the fast removal of the myoma under vision. The extent of completion is identified by the presence of the adjacent endometrial surface.

Various methods are being suggested for the removal of intramural extension of the myoma, as this may present more technical difficulties during removal. However, depending upon the size, the commonly used method remains the same as the use of cutting angled loop. The slicing technique helps, but one may have to gauge the extent of resection intermittently so as to avoid over-resection. If one can see the myometrium, the procedure can be considered complete in that area. Coagulation of the base of myoma is usually recommended by a roller ball or cylinder to prevent hemorrhage, especially in case of larger myomas with large intramural component. Myometrial contraction, however, is sufficient to arrest the hemorrhage in most cases.

The administration of gonadotropin-releasing hormone (GnRH) analogues preoperatively helps reducing the size and vascularity of the fibroid. In case of a large intramyometrial component, one can stop the procedure, give a postoperative GnRH agonist and perform a repeat resection few weeks or few months after the primary procedure.

A second look hysteroscopy may be performed after 2–3 months of a primary procedure to evaluate the cavity in cases for infertility or before intravenous fluid (IVF).

ADENOMATOUS POLYPS

These may vary from very small 1–2 mm polyps to large 2–3 cm polyps. The small polyps may be located in the region of the ostia. They may be blocking the ostial opening, thus causing a pseudocornual block during chromopertubation of methylene blue at laparoscopy or during HSG. The small polyps may also cause foreign body reaction in the endometrium, which is bad enough to result in infertility, especially in those patients selected for ART.

As these polyps are soft, they can be easily removed by using a combination of scissors and grasping forceps. Alternately, they can be desiccated—vaporized using versapoint bipolar cautery. Very rarely, one has to use the resectoscopes for removal of large polyps.

Stenosed Cervical Canal

This condition often presents itself in nulliparous patients with smaller than normal size uterus, in patients with polycystic ovary syndrome (PCOS), in postmenopausal women wanting children who have restarted their menstruation following hormonal replacement therapy and in women who have had a history of difficult previous ET or intrauterine insemination. In these patients it is wise to make use of smaller sized mini hysteroscopes. Sometimes one needs to do a vaginoscopy, visualize the cervix, increase the cervical diameter by using sharp scissors and then negotiate the hysteroscope under vision into the uterine cavity. One can also make use of prostaglandin (PGE_2, misoprostol) tablets and insert them in the vagina, 1 day prior to the surgery. The prostaglandin tends to soften the cervix, thus making it easier to perform a hysteroscopy.

Intravenous Fluid and Embryo Transfer

Hysteroscopy, as a routine examination, should be performed before the first in vitro fertilization-embryo transfer (IVF-ET) cycle in all patients. A statistically significant difference in pregnancy rate was found between women who underwent hysteroscopy before IVF-ET cycle and in women who did not undergo the procedure. Hysteroscopic revision of the cervical canal results in easier ET and improves pregnancy rates in patients with cervical stenosis and histories of difficult ET. Many groups have performed ET under hysteroscopic control, with excellent results.

CONCLUSION

Assessing the endometrial cavity is an integral part of the infertility evaluation. It appears that hysteroscopy is the most sensitive method amongst the tools to evaluate the cavity, recognizing the benefits of hysteroscopy from both a diagnostic and therapeutic viewpoint, the clinician must decide in which setting to perform the procedure.

Thus to conclude, "the hysteroscope which was literally looking for an indication a decade ago has become an indispensable tool today".

- Alan Decherney, 85.

BIBLIOGRAPHY

1. Doldi N, Persico P, Di Sebastiano F, et al. Pathologic findings in hysteroscopy before in vitro fertilization-embryo transfer (IVF-ET). Gynecol Endocrinol. 2005;21(4):235-7.
2. Hallez JP. Single-stage total hysteroscopic myomectomies: indications, techniques, and results. Fertil Steril. 1995;63(4): 703-8.
3. Pabuccu R, Ceyhan ST, Onalan G, et al. Successful treatment of cervical stenosis with hysteroscopic canalization before embryo transfer in patients undergoing IVF. a case series. J Minim Invasive Gynecol. 2005;12(5):436-8.
4. Porcu G, Cravello L, D'Ercole C, et al. Hysteroscopic metroplasty for septate uterus and repetitive abortions: reproductive outcome. Eur J Obstet Gynecol Reprod Biol. 2000;88(1):81-4.
5. Römer T. Surgical interventions. In: Operative Hysteroscopy: A Practical Guide (Pocket Guides for Gynaecologists), 2nd edition. Berlin, Germany: Walter de Gruyter; 2011. pp. 24-108.
6. Shamma FN, Lee G, Gutmann JN, et al. The role of office hysteroscopy in vitro fertilization. Fertil Steril. 1992;58(6):1237-9.
7. Tantini C, Tiso E, Napolitano AC, et al. GnRH analogues for preparation of hysteroscopic metroplasty. Gynaecol Endoscopy. 1996;5:161-3.
8. Vilos GA. Intrauterine surgery using a new coaxial bipolar electrode in normal saline solution (Versapoint): a pilot study. Fertil Steril. 1999;72(4):740-3.
9. Valle RF. Office hysteroscopy. Clin Obstet Gynecol. 1999;42(2): 276-89.

43.3 HYSTEROSCOPIC-GUIDED BIOPSY POLYPECTOMY AND MYOMECTOMY

Abha Majumdar, Tejshree Singh

INTRODUCTION

Hysteroscopy is a minimally invasive intervention that can be used to diagnose and treat many intrauterine and endocervical problems. Hysteroscopic polypectomy, myomectomy and directed endometrial biopsy are just a few of the commonly performed procedures. Given their safety and efficacy, diagnostic and operative hysteroscopy have become standards in gynecologic practice.

SURGICAL ANATOMY

Endometrial Polyps

- Endometrial polyps are localized overgrowths of the endometrium that project into the uterine cavity. They develop because of excessive multiplication of the endometrial cells, may be hormonally dependent and increase in size depending upon estrogen levels
- Polyps may be sessile or pedunculated and rarely include areas of neoplastic growth. Specifically, adenomatous hyperplasia and endometrial adenocarcinomas have been reported in only 0.6% of cases of endometrial polyps
- They can usually be detected on an ultrasound scan on second or third postmenstrual day or in mid-cycle, when estrogen levels are maximal and the endometrium is echogenic
- The prevalence of polyps is estimated to be 10–24% in hysterectomy samples. Endometrial polyps are rare among women younger than 20 years of age
- The incidence of these polyps rises steadily with increasing age, peaks in the fifth decade and then declines after menopause.

Fibroids

- These are well-circumscribed, noncancerous tumors arising from the myometrium of the uterus. In addition to smooth muscle, leiomyomas are also composed of extracellular matrix, i.e. collagen, proteoglycan, fibronectin
- Fibroids are the most common solid pelvic tumors in women, causing symptoms in approximately 25% of reproductive-aged women. The overall prevalence increases to over 70%, inclusive of asymptomatic fibroids. These are usually detected in women in their 30s and 40s and may shrink after menopause in the absence of postmenopausal estrogen replacement therapy.
- These are classified by their location in the uterus:
  A. Subserosal ones are located just under the uterine serosa and may be pedunculated or sessile
  B. Intramural fibroids are found predominantly within the myometrium but may distort the uterine cavity or cause an irregular external uterine contour
  C. Submucous fibroids are located just under the uterine mucosa and may be either pedunculated or sessile
- Tumors in subserosal and intramural locations comprise the majority (95%) of all leiomyomas; submucous leiomyomas make up the remaining 5%
- Although this classification scheme is widely used by clinicians, it suffers from the limitation that few leiomyomas are actually a single "pure" type. Most leiomyomas span more than one anatomic location and, therefore, are hybrids, e.g. a predominantly intramural leiomyomas with a submucous component
- Transformation of uterine leiomyomas to uterine leiomyosarcomas is extremely rare, and in fact, many researchers and clinicians believe this type of transformation never occurs. Uterine leiomyosarcomas are found in approximately 0.1% of women with leiomyomas and are reported to be more frequently associated with large or rapidly growing fibroids.

Thickness of the Uterine Wall

This knowledge allows the surgeon to manipulate the surgery on the basis of the area of the uterus where surgeon is operating. The uterus is longer and thicker in reproductive-aged women than in postmenopausal women.

PREOPERATIVE PREPARATION

Appropriate surgical management always begins with accurate history taking, physical examination, and careful work-up of the suspected problem. In preparation for hysteroscopic procedures the following considerations may be useful (Table 1).

Laboratory Studies

Apart from general health tests, the following tests are required:

- *Blood typing and screening:* With the risk of hemorrhage approaching 7–8% in some surgical hysteroscopic procedures, a sample in the blood bank increases the

Table 1: Considerations for hysteroscopic procedure

Location	Mean (mm)	Range (mm)
Anterior wall	22.5	17–25
Posterior wall	21	15–25
Fundus	19.5	15–22
Isthmus	10	8–12

efficiency of access to replacement of blood products, if needed

- *Electrolyte determinations:* In patients with medical disorders that predispose them to metabolic abnormalities, e.g. diuretic use, electrolytes should be tested preoperatively. Some surgeons routinely obtain baseline levels in case a significant deficit of distention medium occurs, especially with a hyposmolar solution, whereas most obtain electrolyte levels intraoperatively or postoperatively only if a clinically significant fluid deficit occurs. The ultimate decision should be based on the type of case, the surgeon's skill, the suspected fluid absorption, and the ability to accurately ascertain fluid deficits in the operating room
- Determination of *human chorionic gonadotropin (hCG) levels* is mandatory in any woman of reproductive age to exclude pregnancy
- *Cervical cultures:* May be taken depending on the prevalence of *Chlamydia* and gonorrhea in the population and a wet smear for bacterial vaginosis and trichomoniasis are recommended
- *Papanicolaou test:* A normal or abnormal Pap smear that has been appropriately evaluated is required because trauma to the cervix may alter the appearance of any existing abnormalities.

Imaging Studies

- Ultrasound of the lower abdomen is done postmenstrually to evaluate the size and shape of the uterus, endometrial thickness, fibroids [location (Figs 1 and 2), whether distorting the uterine cavity (Figs 3A and B) as well as endometrial polyps (Fig. 4)]
- Hysterosalpingogram or sonohysterosalpingogram is used for evaluating the uterine cavity and patency of Fallopian tubes. However, to selectively look at the uterine cavity, sonohysterography or saline-infused sonography and 3D ultrasound appear to have a better predictive value than that of hysterography for determining the location and size of fibroids and endometrial polyps (Figs 5A and B)
- Computed tomography (CT) scan or MRI: These are not usually needed unless the findings on ultrasound are inconclusive.

Antibiotic Prophylaxis

Prophylactic antibiotics are not indicated unless the patient has clinically significant cardiac disease or a history of tubal occlusion due to PID.

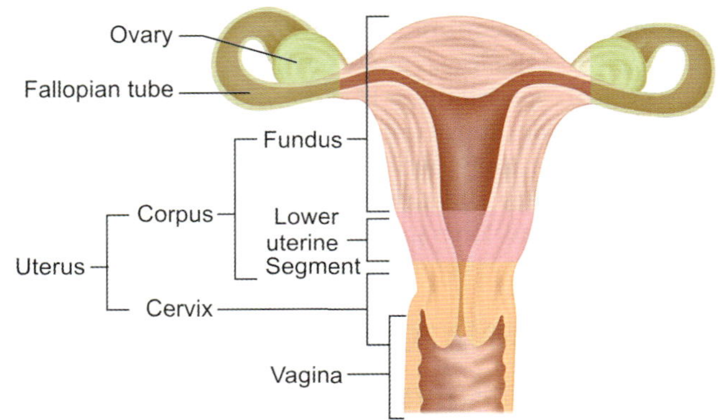

Fig. 1: Anatomical division of reproductive canal

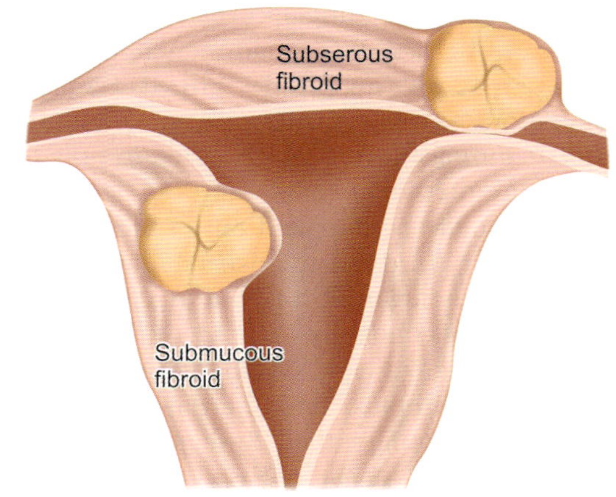

Fig. 2: Submucous and subserous fibroids

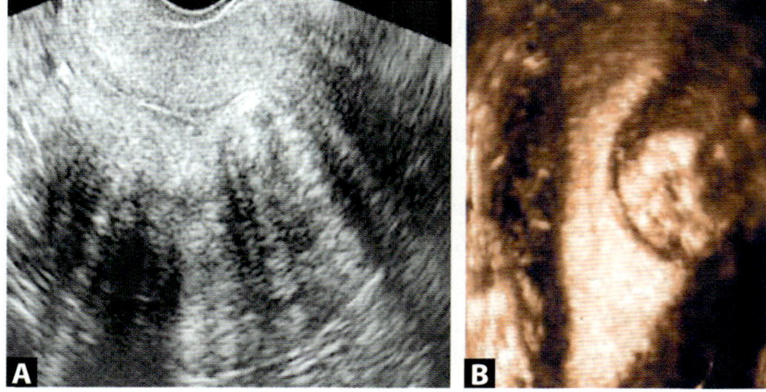

Figs 3A and B: Ultrasound image of submucous fibroid

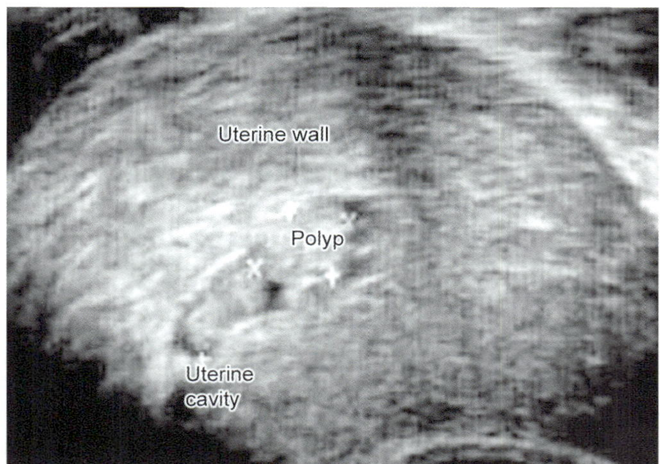

Fig. 4: Uterine polyp as seen during an ultrasound scan

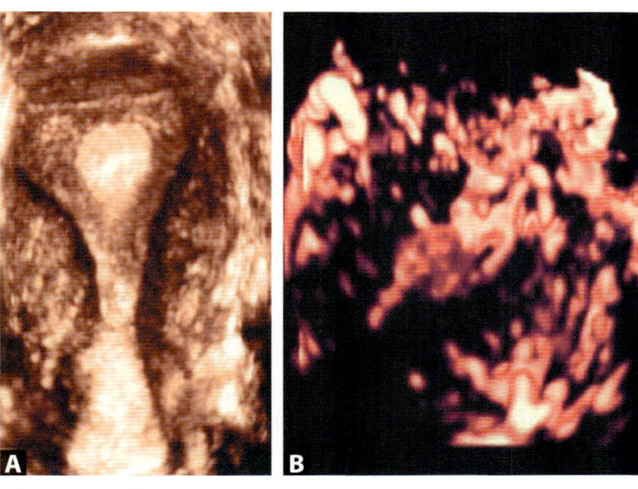

Figs 5A and B: Three-dimensional (3D) depiction of (A) a polyp and (B) Doppler flows

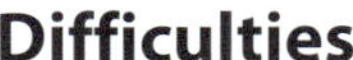

Difficulties

Cervical Stenosis

In patients with known cervical stenosis or tortuous cervical canals, preoperative vaginal or oral misoprostol, or intraoperative vasopressin 1% administered paracervically, may be used to assist in cervical dilation.

Large Uterus

A uterus longer than 10 cm makes the case difficult, because the length of the hysteroscope is typically 35 cm, and it must traverse the length of the uterus, cervix and vagina while maintaining a position outside the introitus with enough distance to attach the camera and manipulate the fluid inflow-outflow valves and the surgical instruments. Also, maintaining intrauterine pressures in large cavities is more difficult than with small cavities.

Preoperative Medications to Reduce the Size of Fibroids

- *Gonadotropin-releasing hormone agonists:* For large submucosal fibroids, the use of an GnRH agonist decreases uterine volume by approximately 30%. It may decrease blood loss and allow for an easier and more complete resection, though some data suggest that the change in tissue quality may make the procedure technically more difficult than before, negating other benefits
- *Gonadotropin-releasing hormone antagonists:* The primary advantage over GnRH agonists is that antagonists have a faster onset of action
- *Other medical therapies:* This group includes androgenic agents like danazol, progestins, oral contraceptive progestin pills and antifibrotic drugs (pirfenidone). However, these medications do not consistently decrease uterine or fibroid volume.

CONTRAINDICATIONS

In general, hysteroscopy is avoided in patients with the following findings:

- Active cervical or uterine infection
- Severe medical conditions precluding surgery
- Pregnancy.

CONCERNS FOR HYSTEROSCOPY IN SPECIFIC SITUATIONS

- Myomectomy of transmural lesions
- Use of glycine in patients with liver disease
- Use of sorbitol in patients with severe diabetes
- For lesions larger than 3 cm, patients must be counseled about possibility of a staged procedure.

INTRAOPERATIVE DETAILS

Anesthesia

- The type of anesthesia used depends on the procedure, the patient's level of anxiety, and the anesthesiologist's expertise
- Simple diagnostic procedures can be completed without anesthesia, with a paracervical block alone, or with mild sedation
- For extensive procedures or for patients with a low pain tolerance, general or regional anesthesia is indicated. If electrosurgery is to be performed, sufficient anesthesia must be given to ensure that the patient does not move

with uterine stimulation because of the risk of uterine perforation and intraperitoneal injury.

Positioning

- The patient is placed in the dorsal lithotomy position and prepared and draped in a sterile manner
- Unless a laparoscopy is also planned, the patient's thighs should be positioned at a 90° angle to the pelvis to create enough space for the surgeon to manipulate the hysteroscope. The patient's perineum should be just past the edge of the table, with the coccyx and sacrum well supported on the flat surface of the table. The patient's legs should be secured in the leg stirrups to avoid any abrupt movements, which can cause nerve or muscle injury to the patient or potential injury to the surgeon
- The surgeon should be seated with the operative field and hysteroscope at the level of his or her abdomen. If it is positioned higher, the surgeon's shoulders become fatigued, and if it is positioned lower, the instrument is hard to maneuver and is likely to become contaminated.

Hemostasis

- Use of cold distention media at 5°C causes vasoconstriction and reduces blood loss. However, the patient's core body temperature substantially decreases and may interfere with the anesthesia process
- Vasopressin in dilute solution (i.e. 1%) can be injected paracervically to help constrict the cervical and lower uterine branches of the uterine artery and its collaterals, reducing blood loss and fluid deficits.

Bladder Catheterization

At the discretion of the surgeon, the bladder may need to be emptied with a rubber or metal catheter by using sterile technique.

Examination Under Anesthesia

Bimanual examination should always be performed before the endocervix and uterus are dilated and entered. This examination aids the surgeon in assessing angles and preventing perforation.

Cervical Dilation

- The cervix is manually dilated with metal dilators to the same diameter as the outer diameter of the outer sheath of the hysteroscope. A tenaculum/volsellum is placed on the anterior lip of the cervix while dilating to help straighten the uterocervical angle
- In cases of acutely anteverted uterus, it may be necessary to remove the vaginal speculum to ease dilatation
- Avoid creating a false cervical passage that could make it difficult to continue with the surgery. If the surgeon is unsure of the path of the cervical canal, lacrimal duct probes or flexible uterine sounds or urethral boogies should be used to determine the correct angle. Ultrasonographic guidance for dilation may be helpful in severe cases.

Visualization of the Uterine Cavity

After the cervix is dilated, the hysteroscope is inserted into the endocervical canal and advanced into the uterine cavity with the distention medium flowing under direct vision to limit the risk of perforation. The tenaculum on the cervix is left in place to help in manipulating the uterus and the vaginal speculum is removed to increase maneuverability of the hysteroscope. If the cervix is dilated too much and fluid is leaking extensively, a purse-string suture can be placed around the cervix using 0 vicryl to limit this leakage. The suture should be removed at the end of the procedure.

TECHNIQUES

Hysteroscopic-directed Biopsy

- Routinely, a 5–10 mm hysteroscope is used with isotonic sodium chloride distention medium. A 30° scope is preferable to clearly visualize the tubal ostial region. The ability to introduce small surgical instruments through an operating channel is optimal
- Office procedures can be performed with a 2.5–3 mm flexible or rigid hysteroscope attached to isotonic sodium chloride solution in a bag or 20–50 mL syringe. Some new models have a small operating channel through which a thin-wired biopsy forceps can be placed. This channel is enough to sample suspected areas
- Dilatation and curettage has traditionally been considered as standard for the investigation of abnormal uterine bleeding. The two main disadvantages of D&C are most cases require GA and it is a blind procedure, which can miss focal lesions. It has been observed that 60% of patients have less than half the uterine cavity curetted and 16% have less than a quarter during routine D&C. Therefore, hysteroscopy with guided endometrial biopsy should replace D&C for cases of abnormal uterine bleeding
- Hysteroscopy is also becoming an integral part of the infertility work-up
- Hysteroscopic surgery is safe and effective for postmenopausal women with benign intrauterine lesions

- There is a controversy regarding the possibility that reflux of endometrial cells during fluid-based hysteroscopy, might cause retrograde dissemination of malignant cells into the peritoneal cavity. Data support a correlation between fluid-based hysteroscopy and the presence of cancer cells in the peritoneal cavity. However, it cannot be determined whether peritoneal washings "turned positive" as a result of hysteroscopy or whether they were present prior to this procedure, as the rate of positive peritoneal cytology is similar in both instances.

Hysteroscopic Polypectomy (Figs 6 to 10)

- It has been shown that curettage alone is not sufficient for detection and extraction of endometrial polyps. Curettage alone detected endometrial polyps in only 43% out of all cases of polyps diagnosed by hysteroscopy
- The ease of surgery depends upon the situation of the polyp as well as the presence of a broad or thin pedicle. Polyps on the uterine fundus are more difficult to handle, as it is difficult to see the pedicle, especially with large polyps
- A hysteroscopic scissor is adequate for most of the polyps; however, if the pedicle is vascular, electrocautery can be used for removal or for achieving homeostasis.

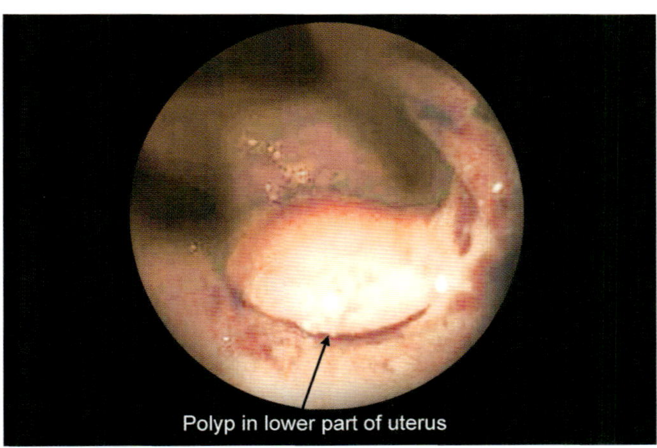

Fig. 6: Uterine polyp as seen during hysteroscopy

Hysteroscopic Myomectomy

Instrumentation: Several instruments may be used for hysteroscopic myomectomy. They include the resectoscope (Fig. 11), which is by far the most common, scissors and the laser.

Monopolar Cautery

- The resectoscope is a specialized instrument with a monopolar, double-armed electrode and a trigger device for use in hypotonic, nonconductive media, such as glycine. It cuts and coagulates tissue by means of contact desiccation with resistive heating. The depth of thermal damage is based on several factors: endometrial thickness; speed, pressure, and duration of contact during motion; and power setting.

A thin electrode can cut tissue, whereas one with a large surface area, such as a ball or barrel, is best suited for coagulation for hemostasis.

Bipolar Cautery

- The Versapoint system uses bipolar circuitry for electrosurgery which can be performed in isotonic conductive media. This system includes a spring tip for hemostatic vaporization of large areas, a ball tip for precise vaporization and a twizzle tip for hemostatic resection and morcellation of tissue. There is also a cutting loop similar to traditional resectoscope.

Laser

- Several fiber optic lasers are available for gynecologic use, including potassium-titanium-phosphate (KTP), argon, and neodymium-doped yttrium-aluminum-garnet (Nd:YAG) lasers. They all have different wavelengths, though the KTP and argon lasers have similar properties.

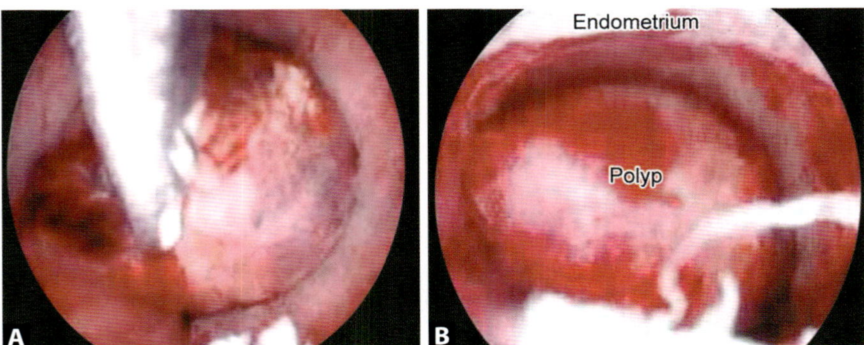

Figs 7A and B: Hysteroscopic polypectomy

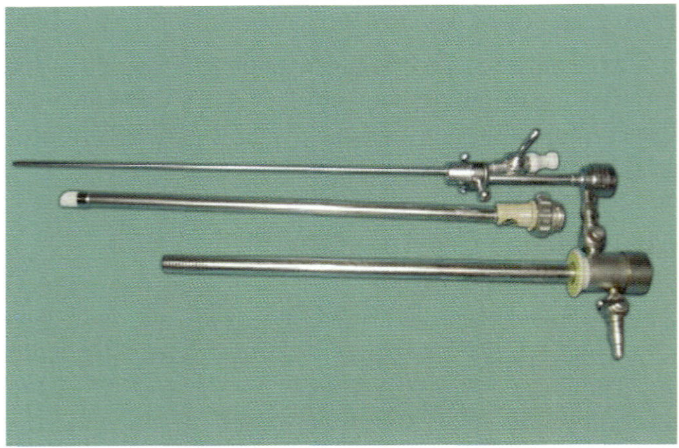

Fig. 8: Diagnostic hysteroscopy unit

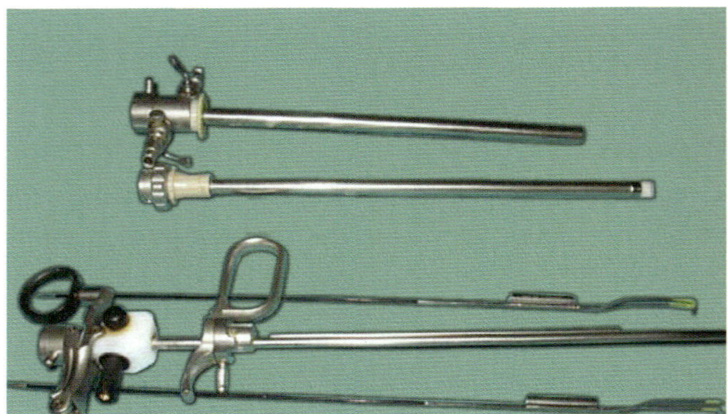

Fig. 9: Operative hysteroscopy unit

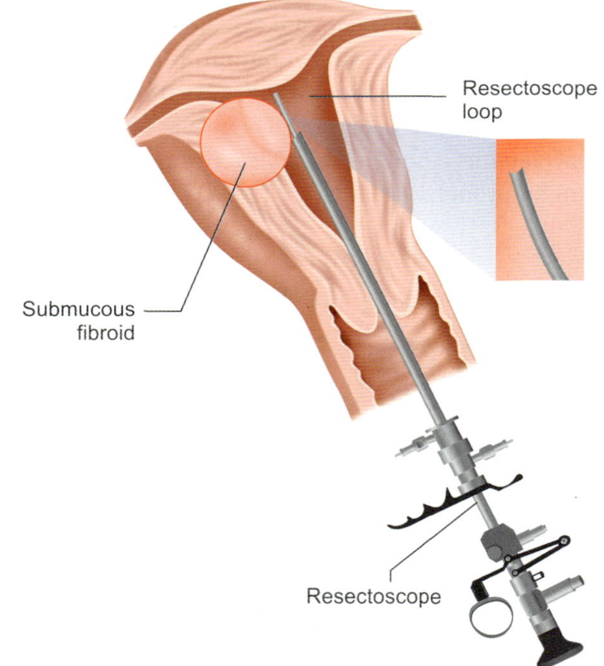

Fig. 11: Resectoscope

Distention Media

The advantage of fluid over gas is the symmetric distention of the uterus with fluid and its effective ability to flush blood, mucus, bubbles and small tissue fragments out of the visual field. Both low-viscosity and high-viscosity medium can be used for distention. A pressure of 75–100 mm Hg is usually adequate for the distention of the uterus.

Pressures higher than this can increase the risk of intravasation of medium.

Technique (Figs 12 and 13)

- It is essential to take care while resecting a fibroid with a resectoscope, to limit the resection to only the fibroid without resecting the adjoining endometrial

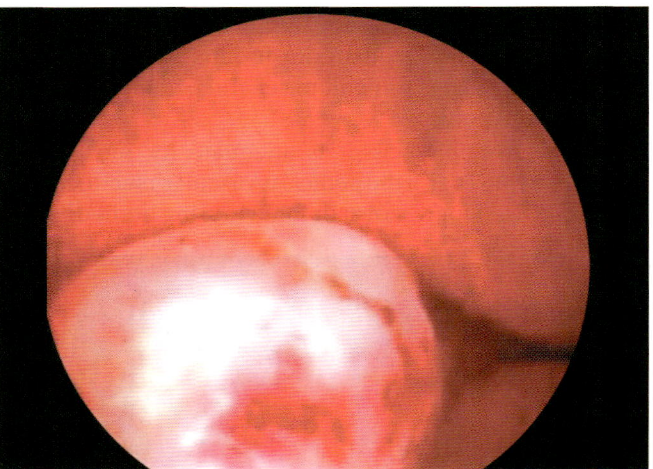

Fig. 10: Distending uterine cavity revealing a polyp

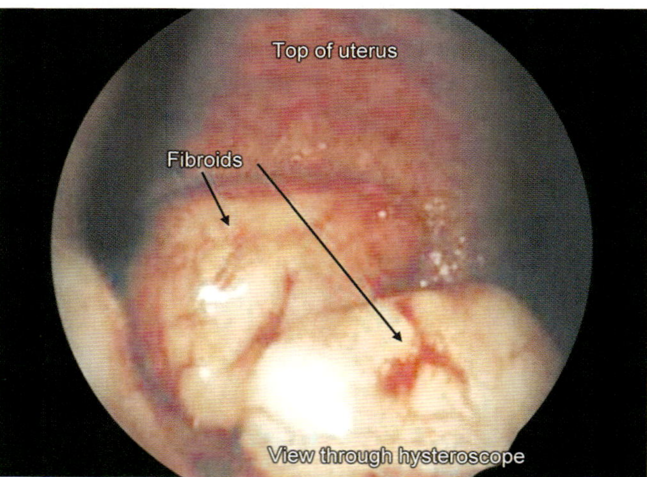

Fig. 12: Hysteroscopic view of two submucous fibroids

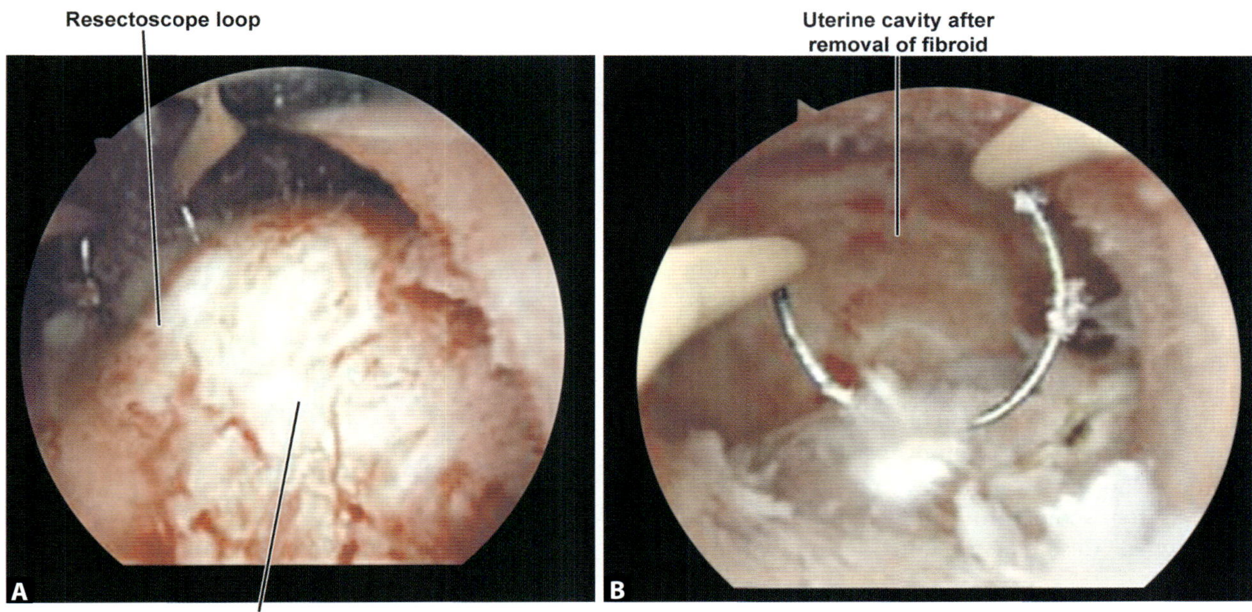

Figs 13A and B: Hysteroscopic resection of a fibroid with a resectoscope

tissue, especially in women desiring to conceive. After the superficial portion of the fibroid is resected, its intramural portion may begin to evert inside the endometrial cavity. Surgeons should apply their skill and experience to estimate how many passes they will continue to resect to avoid uterine perforation. The loop can often be used to separate the fibroid from the pseudocapsule, facilitating its removal and helping to identify normal myometrium and endometrium to avoid coagulation

- For resection of a submucosal fibroid, high cutting power is required. Using the cutting mode at 80–100 W provides clean cuts through the fibroid and facilitates a rapid technique. Power settings lower than this do not allow for easy resection and only delay completion of the procedure, with resulting fluid deficits
- Resection of a predominantly intramural fibroid poses the risk of intravasation of media due to prolonged procedure time.

NEWER DEVELOPMENTS

Improvements in hysteroscope design have improved the effectiveness of inflow-outflow tracts, for example the Resection Master resectoscope incorporates a suction channel and a pump to aid in removing chips of tissue during resection. This feature improves visibility and may decrease operating time otherwise spent emptying the pieces from the endometrial cavity. Other instruments on the forefront include a hysteroscopic morcellator which may reduce myomectomy time by morcellating and removing tissue in one movement under direct visualization.

POSTOPERATIVE DETAILS

General Care

- *Diet:* Patients can be allowed clear liquids as early as 3 hours after surgery. Once the patient tolerates liquids, she can be allowed normal diet
- *Pain:* Patients typically report cramping after the procedure. A single dose of NSAIDs reduces postoperative discomfort. Opioid derivatives can be added, if needed, for severe pain. Peritoneal discomfort may occur if a substantial amount of the distention media enters the abdominal cavity by way of the Fallopian tubes. This discomfort generally subsides within 24 hours
- Broad-spectrum antibiotic for 3–5 days
- *Discharge:* Most patients can go home within few hours, once they have passed urine. Patients may have some light-to-heavy spotting for a few days to a couple of weeks, depending on the procedure performed.

Special Care

- Following hysteroscopic myomectomy, the patient may pass small pieces of tissue which may cause cramping
- Removal of extensive adhesions or fibroids raises the possibility of adhesion formation in the uterine cavity.

Use of high-dose estrogen is advocated to encourage endometrial growth over any denuded areas. Ethinyl estradiol 0.05–0.1 mg or conjugated estrogen 2.5–5 mg daily for 25 days, followed by progesterone supplementation for last 6–12 days is typically sufficient

- To prevent the juxtaposition of the inner uterine walls during the initial phase of the healing process, placement of an intrauterine catheter (Malecots or Foleys) is recommended. A pediatric Foley catheter with the balloon filled with 15–20 mL of sterile water may be used because it has the added benefit of providing tamponade to any areas that may be bleeding. The exterior end of the catheter is capped, placed along the thigh and the patient is given doxycycline 100 mg twice daily until the catheter is removed 3–7 days later
- Patients who have large myometrial wall defects after a hysteroscopic procedure should be counseled for elective Cesarean section during subsequent pregnancy.

COMPLICATIONS

An accepted rate for all complications during surgical hysteroscopy is 3.8% with myomectomy having the highest incidence of complications.

Mechanical Complications

A. *Cervical lacerations:* Tearing of the tenaculum/volsellum from the cervix during difficult dilatation.
   - Relatively atraumatic instruments, such as ringed forceps, can be used to prevent this complication
   - Preoperative medications may help to decrease resistance during dilation
   - In addition, ultrasonographic guidance may help to direct dilating maneuvers
   - Use small-diameter and flexible hysteroscopes can ultimately limit the need for excessive dilation.

B. *Uterine perforations:* This is the most common complication of hysteroscopic myomectomy with incidence rates of approximately 0.7–0.8%.
   - Risk factors for perforation include cervical stenosis, acute uterine anteflexion or retroflexion, infection, myomas of lower uterine segments and synechiae
   - A small midline or fundal injury with a blunt instrument does not have clinically significant sequelae if bleeding is minimal, but large rents or those caused by sharp or electrosurgical instruments may result in a need for diagnostic laparoscopy to completely evaluate the patient for bleeding or visceral injury
   - Lateral perforations involve risk of injury to vessels and should be further inspected with diagnostic laparoscopy or interventional radiology and/or angiography.

C. *Electrical or laser injury* to the bowel or bladder if suspected, laparoscopy or laparotomy is required for complete evaluation.
   - The risk of peritonitis, sepsis and death are most often associated with unrecognized and untreated thermal injuries to the surrounding viscera
   - Some of these thermal visceral injuries occur without apparent perforation of the uterus
   - For procedures in which electrical or laser energy is used, the surgical tip should be kept in direct view to avoid thermal injury.

Media-related Complications

A. *Gas embolism:* The risk of gas embolism is the primary complication associated with the use of CO_2 as the distention medium with devastating results and circulatory collapse.

B. *Intravasation of media:* The risk of absorption of media is minimal under normal operative conditions. Risk factors for clinically significant intravasation of fluid include:
   - Prolonged operative procedures
   - Use of large volumes of low-viscosity media
   - Resection of fibroids or myometrial trauma that results in open uterine venous channels or unidentified perforations
   - Intrauterine pressure greater than the patient's mean arterial pressure.

C. *Fluid overload:*
   - *Electrolyte containing media* rarely cause overload, except when excessive intravasation occurs. This is relatively easy to treat. These fluids, however, are uncommonly used in operative procedures
   - *Nonelectrolyte, hypotonic media,* which are nonconductive are most often used for prolonged, complicated electrosurgical procedures. These media have relatively serious adverse effect profiles. When large volumes of these solutions are absorbed, subsequent hyponatremia, hypervolemia, pulmonary edema, cerebral edema, and cardiovascular collapse can occur. Absorption of nonelectrolyte solutions must be closely monitored throughout operative hysteroscopy. For every liter of hypotonic media absorbed, the patient's serum sodium decreases by 10 mEq/L. If the patient's sodium level is less than 120 mEq/L, she is at increased risk for having serious complications and the procedure should be terminated immediately. Forced diuresis with furosemide 40 mg IV, fluid restriction, and

administration of 3% sodium chloride at a rate to correct hyponatremia by 1.5–2.0 mOsm/L/hour is required. Frequent assessments of the patient's sodium levels every 30 minutes may be appropriate to follow-up this titration
- *High-viscosity media* cause clinically significant overload in long surgical procedures. The maximal absorption should not exceed 500 mL. This overload does not respond to diuretic treatment because kidneys poorly excrete the medium. Plasmapheresis may be required. Pulmonary edema and DIC can occur as a result of fluid overload, toxic effects on the pulmonary capillaries, and/or probable anticoagulant effects.

D. *Destruction of instruments:* Occurs mainly with high-viscosity media.

E. *Allergic reactions:* Anaphylaxis is a rare complication reported mostly with dextran 70 (1 in 1,500–300,000 patients). Treatment includes diphenhydramine, epinephrine, steroids, and possible fluid and ventilatory support.

Bleeding

Bleeding during or after surgery is the second most common complication of hysteroscopy (0.25% of all cases).

- Distention media by itself may yield enough pressure to cause hemostasis during a procedure
- The coagulating effects of surgical instruments can aid in controlling bleeding during surgery
- If bleeding persists after surgery, a 30 mL Foley catheter balloon filled with 15–30 mL of fluid can be inserted into the cavity. This balloon can easily be removed 24 hours later. Antibiotic prophylaxis should be given if a foreign body is placed in the uterus
- Vasopressin and misoprostol are alternate medications that can help with vasoconstriction and uterine contractions
- As a last resort, embolization of the uterine artery or hysterectomy is an option for definitive management.

Infection

Infection is an uncommon complication of hysteroscopy even with solutions like dextran 70, which is a polymerized sucrose.

- If a patient has a preexisting infection or a significant history of PID, treatment before surgery is recommended
- If indicated, antibiotics should be used to prevent subacute bacterial endocarditis
- Cystitis and endometritis are rarely associated with hysteroscopic procedures, and should be treated with standard protocols.

CONCLUSION

Operative hysteroscopy has revolutionized the management of benign intrauterine pathologies. It has not only reduced operative morbidity but also made subsequent obstetrical outcome favorable in women desiring future reproduction. However, good equipment with proper distention of the uterine cavity and surgical expertise is the key to successful hysteroscopy and it is wise to know ones limitations before undertaking complex and prolonged hysteroscopic procedures.

BIBLIOGRAPHY

1. Borten M, Seibert CP, Taymor ML. Recurrent anaphylactic reaction to intraperitoneal dextran 75 used for prevention of postsurgical adhesions. Obstet Gynecol. 1983;61(6):755-7.
2. Brill AI. Energy systems for operative hysteroscopy. Obstet Gynecol Clin North Am. 2000;27(2):317-26.
3. Cooper JM, Brady RM. Intraoperative and early postoperative complications of operative hysteroscopy. Obstet Gynecol Clin North Am. 2000;27(2):347-66.
4. Cooper JM, Brady RM. Late complications of operative hysteroscopy. Obstet Gynaecol Clin North Am. 2000;27(2): 367-74.
5. Gebauer G, Hafner A, Siebzehnrübl E, et al. Role of hysteroscopy in detection and extraction of endometrial polyps: results of a prospective study. Am J Obstet Gynecol. 2001;184(2):59-63.
6. Gimpelson RJ. Hysteroscopic treatment of the patient with intracavitary pathology (myomectomy/polypectomy). Obstet Gynecol Clin North Am. 2000;27(2):327-37.
7. Hacker NF. Uterine cancer. In: Berek JS, Hacker NF (Eds). Practical Gynecologic Oncology, 2nd edition. Philadelphia, USA: Lippincott Williams & Wilkins; 1994. pp. 285-326.
8. Indman PD. Instrumentation and distention media for the hysteroscopic treatment of abnormal uterine bleeding. Obstet Gynecol Clin North Am. 2000;27(2):305-15.
9. Jansen FW, Vredevoogd CB, van Ulzen K, et al. Complications of hysteroscopy: a prospective, multicenter study. Obstet Gynecol. 2000;96(2):266-70.
10. Jedeikin R, Olsfanger D, Kessler I. Disseminated intravascular coagulopathy and adult respiratory distress syndrome: life-threatening complications of hysteroscopy. Am J Obstet Gynecol. 1990;162(1):44-5.
11. Leather AT, Savvas M, Studd JW. Endometrial histology and bleeding patterns after 8 years of continuous combined estrogen and progesterone therapy in postmenopausal women. Obstet Gynecol.1991;78(6):1008-10.

12. Loffer FD. Contraindications and complications of hysteroscopy. Obstet Gynecol Clin North Am. 1995;22(3):445-55.
13. Luciano AA. Power sources. Obstet Gynecol Clin North Am. 1995;22(3):423-43.
14. Marlow JL. Media and delivery systems. Obstet Gynecol Clin North Am. 1995;22(3):409-22.
15. Morrison DM. Management of hysteroscopic surgery complications. AORN J. 1999;69(1):194-7.
16. Obermair A, Geramou M, Gucer F, et al. Does hysteroscopy facilitate tumor cell dissemination? Incidence of peritoneal cytology from patients with early stage endometrial carcinoma following dilatation and curettage (D&C) versus hysteroscopy and D&C. Cancer. 2000;88(1):139-43.
17. Petrozza JC,. Attaman JA. (2013). Hysteroscopy. [online] Available from emedicine.medscape.com/article/267021-overview. [Accessed January, 2014].
18. Shushan A, Protopapas A, Hart R, et al. Diagnostic and therapeutic advantages of hysteroscopic surgery in management of intrauterine lesions in postmenopausal women. J Am Assoc Gynecol Laparosc. 2001;8(1):87-91.
19. Shushan A, Rojansky N. Should hysteroscopy be a part of the basic infertility workup? Hum Reprod. 1999;14(8):1923-4.
20. Tulandi T, al-Took S. Endoscopic myomectomy. Laparoscopy and hysteroscopy. Obstet Gynecol Clin North Am. 1999;26(1):135-48.
21. Vercellini P, Zaina B, Yaylayan L, et al. Hysteroscopic myomectomy: long-term effects on menstrual pattern and fertility. Obstet Gynecol. 1999;94(3):341-7.
22. Zerbe MJ, Zhang J, Bristow RE, et al. Retrograde seeding of malignant cells during hysteroscopy in presumed early endometrial cancer. Gynecol Oncol. 2000;79(1):55-8.

43.4 HYSTEROSCOPIC PROXIMAL TUBAL CANNULATION

PG Paul, Tony Thomas

INTRODUCTION

Tubal disease accounts for 25–35% of infertility in women. Proximal tubal obstruction and occlusion account for 10–25% of tubal factor. The traditional treatment for this condition is uterotubal implantation or tubocornual anastomosis. The term pregnancy rate reported for uterotubal implantation is 11–15%, which is very poor. In 1980s, there was a transition from macrosurgical techniques to microsurgical anastomosis. Microsurgical tubocornual anastomosis is technically difficult, but in experienced hands it gives a pregnancy rate of 57% and 11% ectopic pregnancy rate. But both surgical procedures involve laparotomy resulting in significant patient discomfort and convalescent period. IVF is another alternative for tubal factor infertility, but it is inconvenient to the patient, is time consuming and results in 30–35% pregnancy per attempt. Additional procedures are required for subsequent pregnancies.

Development of a minimally invasive technique for correction of proximal tubal block began with interest in transcervical tubal sterilization. Since then, a variety of instrument and techniques have been developed for cannulation of Fallopian tube. Fallopian tubal cannulation can be done by hysteroscopic, fluoroscopic or sonographic techniques.

PATHOPHYSIOLOGY OF PROXIMAL TUBAL OCCLUSION

The Fallopian tubes are 7–14 cm long and the intramural segment ranges from 1.5 cm to 2.5 cm with an average diameter of 100 μm. The intramural portion of the tube is divided into two segments: A proximal segment, approximately 1 cm in length which follows a straight path, and a 1.5 cm distal segment, which is sinuous. The course of the intramural tube is tortuous in 69% of the hysterectomy specimen in one study. The thick muscular wall and convoluted intramural course make the uterotubal junction a likely site for blockage by uterine debris.

Tubal obstruction can be due to chronic salpingitis, SIN, intratubal endometriosis, amorphous material (mucus plugs), or spasm. Most of the proximal tubal obstructions are thought to be caused by inflammatory process or endometriosis which leads to local fibrosis. But only in seven out of 18 cases, where surgically resected segment of the occluded tube showed an organic pathology. The rest of cases the tubes appeared normal or patent with moderate fibrosis or inflammation, but were patent. So a surgical correction is not warranted in majority of proximal tubal blocks since there is no true block. This is the basis for tubal cannulation.

DIAGNOSIS OF PROXIMAL TUBAL OCCLUSION

Proximal tubal blockage, suggested by failure of contrast medium to enter the intramural or isthmic portion of either tube, is diagnosed in 10–20% of HSGs performed for infertility. There are no pathognomonic radiographic findings to confirm the presence of tubal obstruction or occlusion. Characteristic findings are seen only in SIN, where a stippled or honeycombed appearance on HSG indicates retained contrast medium in small diverticular projections. Some investigators suggest that selective salpingography may serve as a diagnostic test. If tubal patency is established, then obstruction likely was due to spasm or mucous debris. In support of this, Letterie and Sakas evaluated histologic findings in 15 patients (27 tubal segments) at laparotomy after failed tubal cannulation. They found that 93% of these patients had severe disease, suggesting that tubal cannulation might distinguish functional obstructions from true occlusion.

So confirmation of proximal tubal blockage requires a second HSG, selective salpingography or chromopertubation by laparoscopy.

TUBAL CANNULATION

Now it is proposed that the functional proximal tubal obstructions are due to some sort of "tubal plugs". This is the basis for the newer technique of tubal cannulation by hysteroscopy, sonography or fluoroscopy.

Selective salpingography consists of passing a catheter through the cervix into the proximal tubal ostium, then injecting contrast medium directed to ostia. Increased pressure generated by direct injection may overcome obstructions associated with plugging. Selective salpingography usually is performed under fluoroscopic guidance.

There are several reports of tubal cannulation using abdominal and transvaginal ultrasound guidance. The image is inferior to that obtained with fluoroscopy but air bubbles flowing into the cul-de-sac are an unequivocal sign of tubal patency.

Tubal cannulation by hysteroscopic control offers a number of advantages over other techniques. First is the guidance of tubal catheter into tubal ostia is simple because it is done under direct vision. Second, since it is done along with a laparoscopy the presence of distal tubal disease can be diagnosed and treated simultaneously. So it offers a one-step evaluation and treatment in infertile patient with proximal obstruction.

HYSTEROSCOPIC CANNULATION

Hysteroscopic cannulation is a relatively simple technique. Different custom made catheter systems are available. Essentially, it consists of a flexible guidewire to negotiate the intramural portion of the tube and a cannula to direct it towards the tubal ostia. A flexible or rigid hysteroscope can be used. Hysteroscopic cannulation is done under GA if a simultaneous laparoscopy is performed.

Technique

A diagnostic laparoscopy is performed first to look for any other pelvic pathology. Severe pelvic adhesions and hydrosalpinx are contraindications for hysteroscopic cannulation. Any pelvic pathology is corrected first and then hysteroscopy is performed. We use 5 mm Bettochi hysteroscope with a 5 Fr operating channel. Hysteroscopy is performed and the tubal ostia identified (Fig. 1). Cannulation is usually done with a Novy's cannulation set and it is introduced through the operating channel. The introducer is removed and replaced with the inner catheter. The hysteroscope and outer catheter are positioned in such a way that, if the inner catheter is pushed, it should enter the ostia (Fig. 2). The flexibility of guidewire is altered by varying the length of the guidewire protruding from the outer catheter. The guidewire is now pushed into the ostia for 2–3 cm, always keeping the outer catheter almost in a straight line for easy sliding (Figs 3 and 4). Camera is shifted

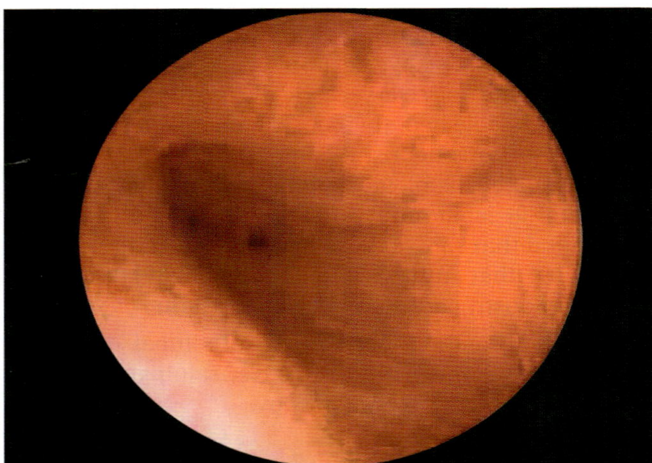

Fig. 1: Visualization of tubal ostia

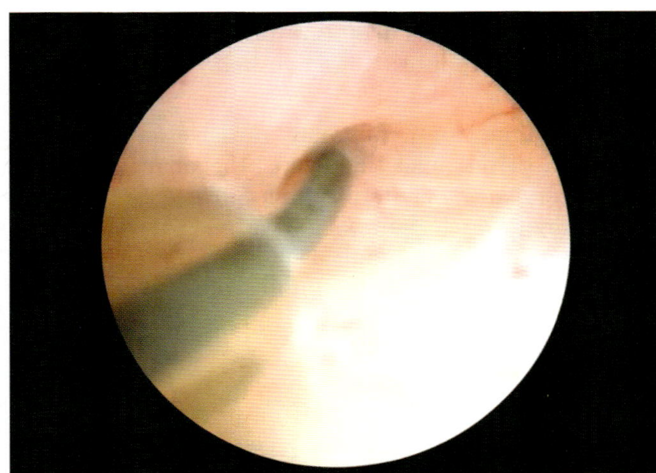

Fig. 2: Inner guidewire pointing towards the tubal ostia

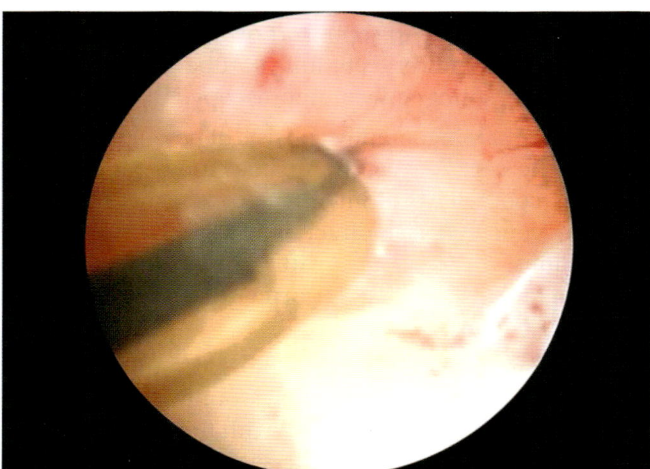

Fig. 3: Outer catheter stabilizes the guidewire

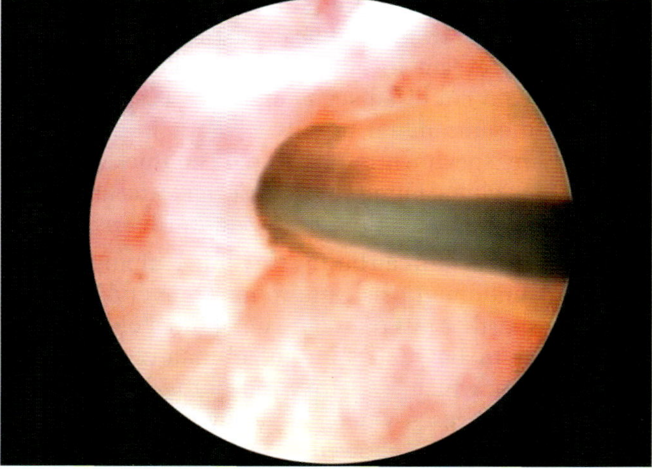

Fig. 4: Outer catheter is hitched against the ostia and guidewire

to laparoscope and further pushing of the inner catheter can be done under laparoscopic control (Fig. 5). If difficulty is encountered, the isthmic portion of the Fallopian tube can be straightened with a grasper. It is not necessary to cannulate the ampullary portion of tube because it can damage the delicate mucosa. The procedure is repeated on the other side. Hysteroscope is withdrawn and chromopertubation done and observed through laparoscope to confirm the result of cannulation.

Novy's cannulation set is designed for single use and its inner catheter is spoiled after single use. A urological catheter like Terumo guidewire (Radifocus guidewire M diameter 0.89 mm) can be used as inner catheter with the Novy's outer catheter and author finds it a better alternative.

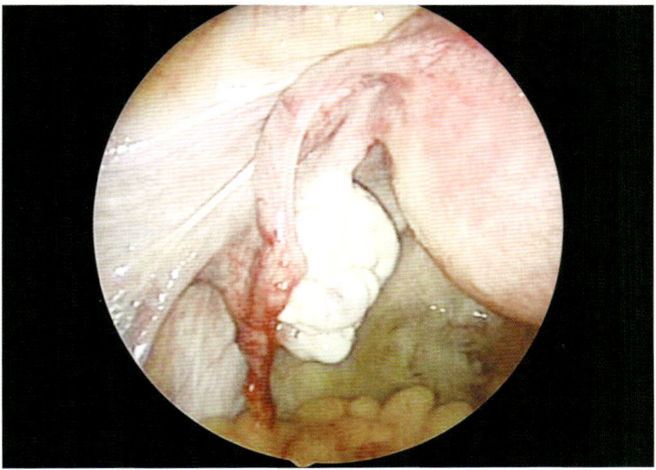

Fig. 5: Guidewire is seen in the proximal part of the tube and wire is pushed further

COMPLICATIONS AND CONTRAINDICATIONS

Perforation is reported in up to 10% of attempted procedures. Use of appropriate flexible catheter may decrease the risk of perforation. When perforation occurs, it is left to heal spontaneously. Infection is rare.

Transcervical tubal cannulation should not be performed in presence of known pelvic infection. A marked distorted uterine cavity may make the procedure technically difficult. The procedure should not be attempted in patients with known distal tubal disease as it can increase the chance of developing an ectopic pregnancy.

We had reported our initial experience of hysteroscopic cannulation in 31 cases (58 tubes) of proximal tubal obstruction. At least one tube could be cannulated in 26 cases (83.9%). Associated distal tubal disease was present in three cases patients conceived after hysteroscopic cannulation. Five of these patients had associated pathologies. There were no ectopic pregnancies. We had performed hysteroscopic cannulation in 164 cases subsequently with similar results.

CONCLUSION

Proximal tubal block is common infertility problem and needs confirmation by a repeat HSG or laparoscopy. Considering the simplicity of the procedure, hysteroscopic cannulation should be tried as the first procedure for proximal tubal block. If the procedure is not successful or a pregnancy is not achieved, IVF is recommended. Laparotomy and microsurgical anastomosis is indicated in few situations where other simpler methods fail and technical expertise is available.

BIBLIOGRAPHY

1. Dubuisson JB, Chapron C, Ansquer Y, et al. Proximal tubal occlusion: is there an alternative to microsurgery? Hum Reprod. 1997;12(4):692-8.
2. Letterie GS, Sakas EL. Histology of proximal tubal obstruction in cases of unsuccessful tubal canalization. Fertil Steril. 1991;56(5):831-5.
3. Musich J, Behrman SJ. Surgical management of tubal obstruction at the uterotubal junction. Fertil Steril. 1983;40(4):423-41.
4. Paul PG, Jeevanraj Rani JS. Hysteroscopic cannulation for proximal tubal obstruction. JOGI. 1998;48:65-7.
5. Platia MP, Krudy AG. Transvaginal fluoroscopic recanalization of a proximally occluded oviduct. Fertil Steril. 1985;44(5):704-6.
6. Rock JA, Katayama KP, Martin EJ, et al. Pregnancy outcome following uterotubal implantation: a comparison of reamer and sharp cornual wedge excision techniques. Fertil Steril. 1979;31(6):634-40.
7. Sulak PJ, Letterie GS, Coddington CC, et al. Histology of proximal tubal occlusion. Fertil Steril. 1987;48(3):437-40.
8. Sweeney W. The interstitial portion of the uterine tube—its gross anatomy, course, and length. Obstet Gynecol. 1962;9:3-8.
9. Thurmond AS. Selective salpingography and fallopian tube recanalization. AJR Am J Roentgenol. 1991;156(1):33-8.
10. Winfield AC, Pittaway D, Maxson W, et al. Apparent cornual occlusion in hysterosalpingography: reversal by glucagon. Am J Roentgenol. 1982;139(3):525-7.

CHAPTER

44

Bladder, Urethra and Incontinent Surgery

Rooma Sinha, Sanjay Sinha

INTRODUCTION

A large number of operations have been devised for stress urinary incontinence (SUI) but over the last few years most of the attention has been focused on two operations—(1) the Burch Colposuspension and (2) the Pubovaginal Sling. Several other operations which were commonly performed earlier are no longer in vogue owing to poor long-term outcome. The advent of synthetic tapes has revolutionized surgery for stress incontinence and the seminal work of Ulmsten and colleagues in devising the tension-free vaginal tape will be recorded as a significant landmark in the evolution of stress incontinence surgery. Currently, there is a large multicentric trial sponsored by the National Institutes of Health (NIH) in the USA which is recruiting patients for randomized comparison of the Burch and Rectus Fascia Sling operations. This is a proof of concept trial and aims to establish whether a sling-like procedure should be the treatment of choice for uncomplicated stress incontinence. Conceptually, the sling has the potential to treat intrinsic sphincter deficiency (ISD) in addition to hypermobility and since some element of ISD seems to be mandatory for a leak, we have always favored the sling over the Burch operation. Most long-term recurrences are related to ISD and not surprisingly, slings give the best long-term outcome. The tension-free tape procedure is based on the pubovaginal sling and is now the most commonly performed operation worldwide for stress incontinence. Several newer modifications are available now, such as the transobturator tapes and crossover tapes. For these reasons, we have chosen the rectus fascia sling as the procedure to be discussed in detail in this chapter. Key points regarding other procedures follow later.

THE PUBOVAGINAL SLING OPERATION FOR STRESS INCONTINENCE

Surgical Anatomy

Normal urinary continence is a function of the bladder, urethra, external sphincter and the surrounding muscle and fascial supports. When an individual is at rest (not voiding), the bladder is normally completely relaxed and the outlet is active thus preventing leak of urine. When one goes to the toilet to void urine, there is a signal from the brain indicating that this is the socially appropriate time to pass urine. This signal travels via the pontine micturition center through the spinal cord to the lower urinary tract. This leads to two simultaneous events. There is relaxation of the outlet mechanism followed a fraction of a second later, by a coordinated bladder contraction. This leads to a unimpeded emptying of the bladder at safe pressures. Any additional stress to the outlet such as during a cough, is accompanied by a series of events which prevent leakage of urine. This include a passive transmission of pressure to the proximal urethra and bladder neck, a contraction of the pelvic floor, a rise in tone of the striated sphincter and a compression and kinking of the urethra against the board-like fascial support. All the mechanisms which prevent excessive mobility of the urethra and ensure adequate pressure transmission prevent what is termed as the "hypermobility" of the urethra, while all the urethral functions which provide a good "water seal" mechanism prevent what is termed as "intrinsic sphincter deficiency". It has been suggested that a normal urethra would not permit leak of urine even in the face of significant hypermobility and hence, some element of ISD may be necessary for any leak to occur. This concept is important both in terms of explaining long-term recurrences (which urodynamics have proven to be due to ISD) as well as in decision regarding which surgery is most appropriate.

The intrinsic sphincter mechanisms consist of the urethral mucosa, submucosa, muscle and the rich venous plexuses in the wall. These lead to good coaptation of the urethra and as well as a compressive force to prevent leakage. The normal pliability of the mucosa and submucosa with their rich vascular plexus is important. Estrogens play an important role in the health of these tissues. There is probably no "internal sphincter" in women that is equivalent to that found in men. It is possible that an arrangement of smooth muscle fibers at the bladder neck may help in continence in women.

The striated sphincter mechanism consists of circumferentially arranged rhabdosphincter fibers which are thinner posteriorly. These fibers are thickest at the level of the mid-urethra and fan out distally to cover about 80% of the length of the urethra. The posterior fibers are deficient in the proximal and distal third of the urethral length. The rhabdosphincter consists of slow twitch fibers that can provide a tonic occlusion of the urethra. In contrast, the distal urethral sphincter comprised has fast twitch fibers that occlude the urethra in the face of rapid rises in intra-abdominal pressure.

The anatomic support of the urethra and bladder are crucial in preventing urinary incontinence. The key supporting structure is the levator fascia which forms condensations around the neurovascular bundles that go to the pelvic viscera. The pubourethral ligament attaches the midurethra to the posterior aspect of the pubic bone and prevents its backward and downward rotation. The urethropelvic ligament has two leaves—(1) the endopelvic fascia on the abdominal side and (2) the periurethral fascia on the vaginal side. These form the main support for the urethra. Similarly, the vesicopelvic fascia has an endopelvic fascial layer on the abdominal side and a perivesical fascia on the vaginal side. This provides posterior support to the bladder and bladder neck. The pubocervical ligament is another name given to this tissue which supports the bladder and uterine cervix to the pelvic sidewall. The upper zone of this fascia supports the bladder, the midzone supports the trigonal level and the lower zone supports the bladder neck. The pelvic diaphragm supports the pelvic viscera and prevents descent. A complete discussion on the pelvic support is out of the scope of this chapter. Urethral closure during intra-abdominal "stress" is dependent on appropriate transmission of pressure rises to the proximal urethra and bladder neck with a compression against the unyielding urethropelvic ligament. This is the essence of DeLancey's hammock hypothesis. In women with stress incontinence, there is a shearing force due to abdominal pressure rise that causes the bladder neck and posterior urethra to open up. In normal women, the urethropelvic ligament support prevents a shearing force that could potentially open up the urethra by allowing a separation of the anterior and posterior walls of the urethra. In women with successful incontinence surgery, the most striking feature observed is a restoration of the mid-urethral pressure hump. Mid-urethral support by a tape prevents opening up of the urethra during rises in intra-abdominal pressure and kinks the urethra to prevent leak.

Preoperative Evaluation

Preoperative evaluation must focus on the following:

- The type of incontinence: Stress, urge or mixed
- Voiding diary
- Assessment of pelvic anatomy including pelvic floor strength.

Hence, the following answers must be available:

- Is it stress incontinence?
- Is there associated voiding dysfunction? This might have an impact on the treatment, prognosis or complications that one might encounter. For instance, presence of a major intrinsic sphincter deficiency component would dictate a suburethral sling placement (synthetic or autologous) rather than a retropubic procedure. It may also impact the prognosis of the patient since patients with ISD do not have as good a long-term outcome with any procedure as those with predominant hypermobility. An underactive detrusor may suggest the possibility of voiding difficulty following surgical treatment of incontinence.
- Is there associated pelvic floor dysfunction such as cystocele, enterocele, rectocele, anal sphincter incompetence or vault prolapse? Lack of identification of these problems with a narrow focus on the stress incontinence alone, can lead to a very unsatisfied patient following surgery.

For these reasons a complete evaluation of the patient with history, physical examination, and stress test should be performed. Ultrasonogram (USG) should be performed and the residual urine checked. Urodynamics gives important diagnostic and prognostic information and is routinely recommended prior to any invasive therapy (Fig. 1).

Indications

Slings can be used to treat all forms of stress incontinence. Traditionally, they have been used primarily in patients with ISD. However, of late there is a trend toward slings as a treatment option for primary presentation of stress incontinence in women with hypermobility. The rationale for this shift in management approach is the recognition that long-term recurrences are primarily related to ISD. Slings are also indicated in women with concomitant pelvic organ prolapse. Patients with failed procedures such as needle suspension or Burch operation should also be offered slings. In all these situations the sling carries a success rate in excess of 85%. In women with a urethral diverticulectomy or urethral loss such as after a urethra-vaginal fistula repair, an autologous sling is the treatment of choice. Synthetic slings may carry a much higher incidence of erosion in these circumstances. "In girls with myelodysplasia or incompetent bladder outlets secondary to anatomical malformations, the autologous sling is the treatment of choice." In such situations, the safety of the bladder as a reservoir must be documented by urodynamics prior to surgery.

Position

Lithotomy.

Anesthesia

Spinal or general.

Technique

A 3-inch transverse incision is made just above the pubis below the pubic hairline down to the surface of the rectus fascia, which is dissected free of subcutaneous tissue. Two parallel horizontal incisions are made 2 cm apart in the midline of the rectus fascia about 2 cm above the pubis and extended superolaterally toward the iliac crest in the direction of the fascial fibers. The wound edges are retracted to obtain a sling of about 12–16 cm. The undersurface of the fascia is freed from muscle. A suture of prolene no. 1-0 is tied to each end using a running horizontal mattress placed at right angles to the direction of the fascial fibers (Fig. 2). The ends are not divided until the entire dissection

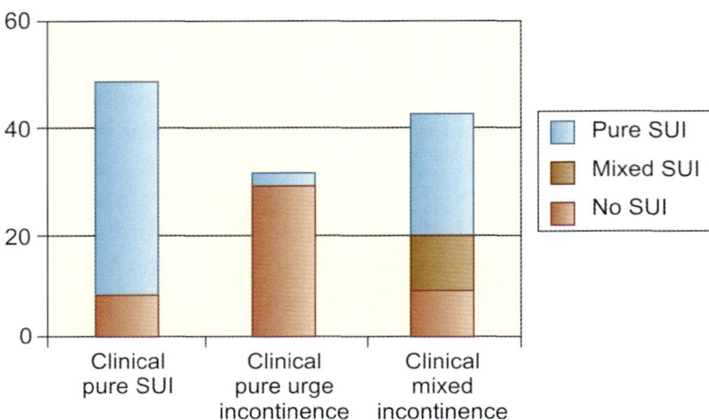

Abbreviation: SUI, Stress urinary incontinence

Fig. 1: Urodynamics data for 121 adult women with urinary incontinence presenting between November 2004 and October 2006 at Medwin Hospital. A clinical diagnosis of stress urinary incontinence (SUI) led to misdiagnosis in a significant number of patients (8/48 in the pure SUI patients and 9/42 in mixed incontinence group and missed 2 patients presenting as pure urge)

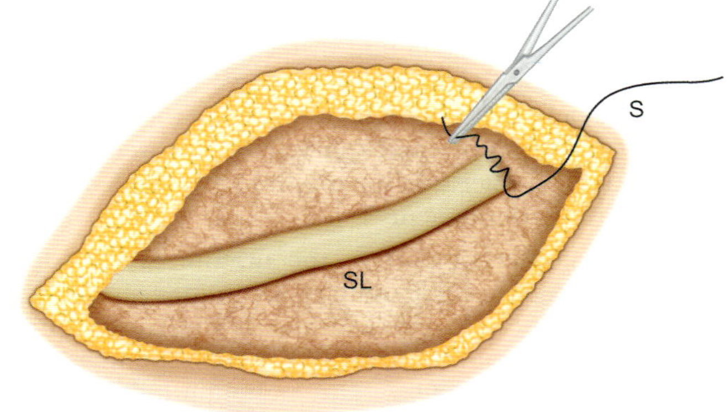

Fig. 2: Harvesting a strip of rectus fascia. This is usually possible even in patients who have previously undergone lower abdominal surgery. Prolene no. 1 mattress suture (S) should be placed at each end of the sling (SL)

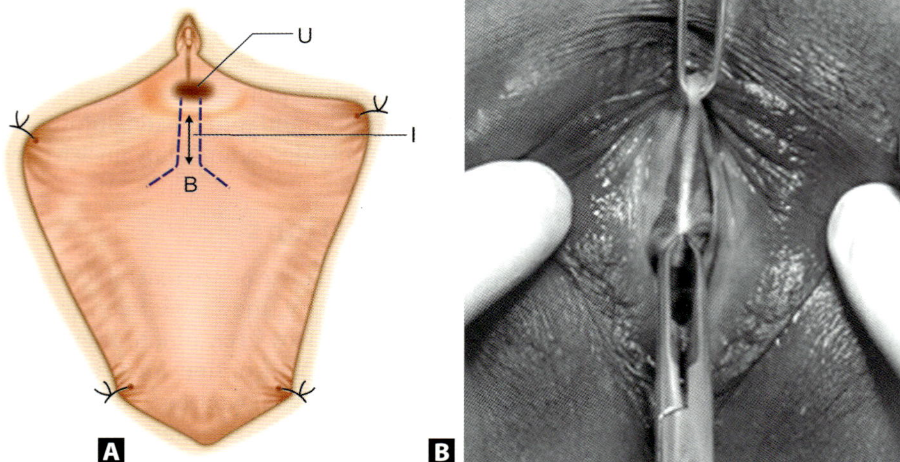

Figs 3A and B: A short vertical incision (I) is made over the mid-urethra. The Foley catheter and its balloon help to identify the precise location of the urethra and bladder neck (B)

is done. Thereafter, the fascial strip is excised and placed in a basin of saline. The wound is packed temporarily and the vaginal surgery is commenced. Alternatively, a second team can simultaneously start the vaginal dissection.

A Foley catheter is inserted into the bladder. The bladder neck can be identified by placing gentle traction on the Foley catheter and palpating the balloon. Either a vertical short incision (author's preference) or a gently curved horizontal incision is made in the anterior vaginal wall (Figs 3A and B). This incision should be made superficial to the pubocervical fascia. Placing Allis clamps on either end of the proposed incisions helps. The proper plane is identified by noting the characteristic shiny white appearance of the undersurface of the anterior vaginal wall (Fig. 4). The Metzenbaum scissors are pointed in the direction of the patient's ipsilateral shoulder until one can feel the pubic bone (Figs 5A and B). During this part of the dissection, it is important to stay as far lateral as possible to insure that the urethra, bladder, and ureters are not injured. One can point the concavity of the scissors laterally and exert constant lateral pressure with the tips of the scissors against the undersurface of the vaginal epithelium. Blunt dissection can be performed to create a space up to the pubic bone. The authors perform this part of the surgery in a manner similar to that done for synthetic tapes.

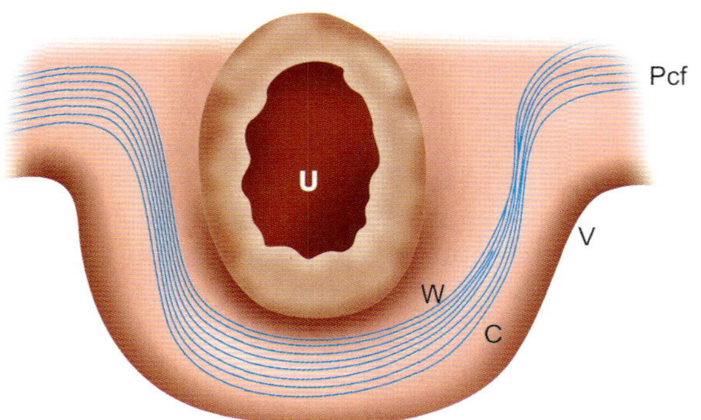

Fig. 4: The correct plane (C) of dissection is a shiny layer superficial to the pubocervical fascia (Pcf). The layer deeper to the fascia is also shiny but dissection in this wrong (W) plane endangers the urethra (U)

An Allis forceps is applied to the inferior edge of the rectus fascia in the midline and traction is given. The right index finger dissects under the fascia, lateral to the rectus and under the pubic bone. The left index finger is placed in the vagina simultaneously to bluntly retract the bladder neck medially. The two fingers can come close to each other with some intervening tissue. At this point a curved long artery forceps is placed from the abdominal side to perforate the endopelvic fascia and enter the vagina. This is done while protecting the bladder continuously using the left index finger. The clamp is used to pull up the suture attached to one end of the harvested rectus strip. The procedure is repeated on the other side. Two small stab wounds are made in the rectus fascia just above the pubis and the sling is brought through them on either side.

Cystoscopy is performed to ensure that the urinary tract is safe and then the vagina is closed using 2:0 chromic catgut. The vagina should be closed before the sling is tied since adequate access may become difficult once the sling is tied and the bladder neck moves up to a higher and less accessible location. The sling sutures are tied to each other over the inferior leaf of the rectus fascia. The sling is tied without any tension and it should be possible to comfortably insert an instrument between the sling and the rectus. It is usually possible to place two fingers comfortably between the sutures and the rectus fascia.

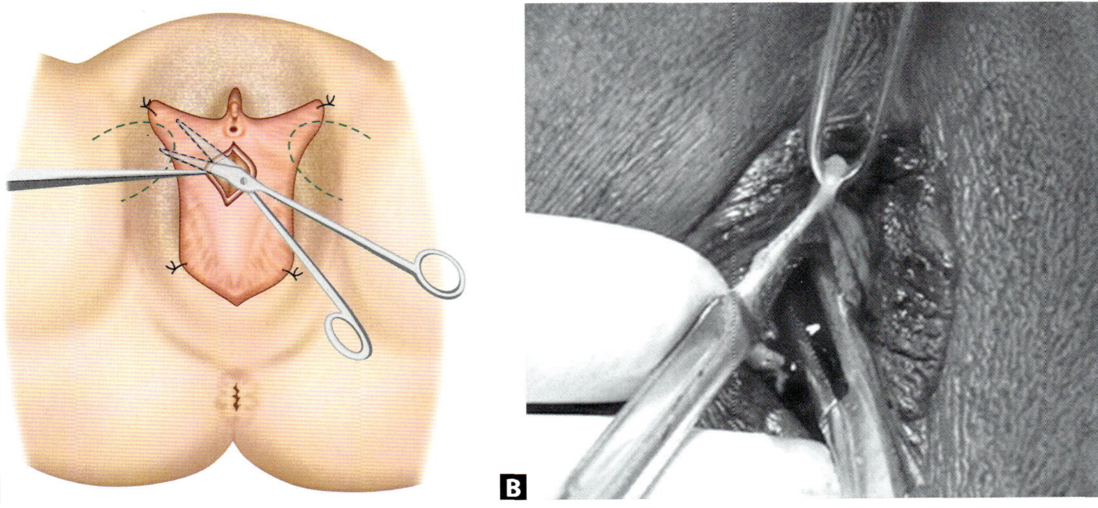

Figs 5A and B: Dissection proceeds in a direction toward the ipsilateral shoulder. A combination of sharp and blunt dissection is performed until the finger can palpate the ischiopubic ramus

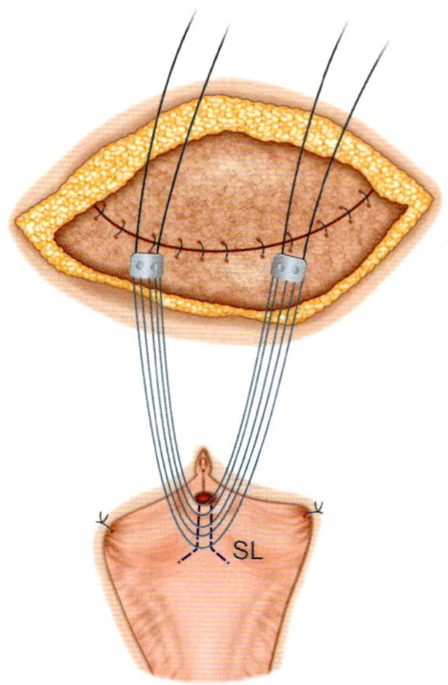

Fig. 6: The sling (SL) is tied over the inferior leaf of the rectus using nonabsorbable prolene suture which had initially been placed into each end of the sling, in a tension-free manner similar to a synthetic tape

The sling is placed in a tension-free manner, just like the tension free tape (Fig. 6). One can place a heavy pair of scissors between the sling and the urethra [similar to the tension-free vaginal tape (TVT)] to ensure that the sling is not under tension and close the vagina after the sling is tied. In special situations where there is severe ISD, one may elect to keep the sling snug and encourage the patient to perform clean intermittent self-catheterization (CISC). In such patients, CISC should be taught to the patient prior to surgery. In the usual stress incontinence, the authors feel that this is unnecessary. A vaginal pack is usually not left. Voiding trials are begun as soon as the patient is comfortable, usually on the 1st or 2nd (author's preference) postoperative day.

Complications and their Management

Sling Erosion

Sling erosion may be vaginal bladder or urethral (rare). Erosion is much less common with autologous material as compared to synthetic material. The American Urological Association (AUA) Stress Incontinence Panel reported 12 erosions out of 1,715 patients with autologous material (0.7%) versus 41 out of 1,515 patients who underwent synthetic slings (2.7%). Erosions may occur due to incorrect placement of the sling, either through the lumen of, or too close to the mucosal lining of the urinary tract. It may be due to excessive tension on the sling, poor quality of vaginal tissue or inadequate cover during closure. Erosion presents as dysuria, urinary frequency, urgency, vaginal discharge, bleeding or discomfort or with perineal pain. There may be dyspareunia. In most situations, erosion can be dealt with by trimming the exposed tape either vaginally or cystoscopically with closure if there is a vaginal erosion. Rarely, more extensive removal may be necessary unless there is intractable infection or discharge.

Retention

Urinary retention is uncommon after sling surgery provided the sling is kept without any tension. The reported incidence is about 2–12% with most studies now reporting figures closer to the lower value. In the event of prolonged retention, one may resort to dilatation of the urethra in an effort to loosen the sling or division of the sling (recommended). Some of these women may develop recurrent stress incontinence. Some women may develop retention even if the sling is not too tight. These women are having an underactive detrusor. Hence, all women with urinary retention should undergo urodynamics evaluation. In women with underactive detrusor, the treatment is CISC. A clue to this disturbing complication may be evidence of slow flow with a low detrusor pressure during the preoperative urodynamics evaluation. All such women must be counseled regarding the possible need for postoperative intermittent catheterization.

Detrusor Overactivity

Postoperative storage symptoms are not uncommon. These may be de novo in women who did not have any such symptoms or may represent persistence or aggravation of pre-existent symptoms. The initial urodynamics may again give a clue to this problem. This problem is perhaps related to the periurethral dissection that is part of all these procedures. Treatment consists of anticholinergic medication and fluid management. A voiding diary can be very helpful in understanding the problem. Urge incontinence may be an important cause for "failure" of stress incontinence surgery and should always be kept in mind.

Others

Recurrent urinary infection, incisional hernia, vaginal discharge, hematoma formation, thromboembolism are some of the rare complications that may follow.

Other Forms of Slings: Synthetic Vaginal Tapes

Over the last few years, this group of variants of the pubovaginal sling has become the most widely performed procedure for stress incontinence. These were pioneered by Ulmsten and coworkers in the late 90s. The most widely used tapes are macroporous polypropylene tapes which are placed under the mid-urethra in a tension-free manner using especially designed needles. The tapes are covered in a plastic sleeve to allow free introduction. The sleeve is removed after placement. The American Medical Systems' (AMS) tapes come with an absorbable tensioning suture with carrier knots that allows easier adjustment after sleeve removal, and this should be necessary.

The procedure can be carried out under general, spinal or local anesthesia. The patient is positioned in the lithotomy position and an incision is made in the vagina over the mid-urethra. Thus the incision is about 1.5 cm long and is located 1 cm proximal to the meatus. Dissection is carried out on either side in the plane as previously described until the pubic ramus is reached. The bladder is emptied with a catheter.

Tension-Free Vaginal Tape (TVT®, Johnson and Johnson)

The bladder is retracted away using a bladder retractor that is provided with the kit. This retractor is threaded into a Foley catheter and placed into the bladder through the urethra. The retractor is angled such that it is lying along the thigh on the side on which the needle is about to be inserted. The trocar is attached to the tape and is passed through the urogenital diaphragm in a posterior direction. One can feel the characteristic "give" of the diaphragm as the needle traverses it. At this point, the needle is rotated to go behind the pubic symphysis. The needle must hug the back surface of the bone as it moves up, to minimize injury to the bladder or other pelvic structures (Fig. 7). Cystoscopy should be performed to ensure integrity of the bladder after each trocar passage. Following the cystoscopy, the trocar is pulled through along with the tape and the tape is grasped by a hemostat and cut. The same maneuver is performed on the other side. A heavy pair of scissors is placed between the tape and the urethra at the time of sleeve removal so as to prevent inadvertent tightening of the tape (Fig. 8). There should be visible space between the tape and the urethra and must scrupulously avoid the temptation to make the tape tight. Excessive tightness of the tape can cause troublesome voiding symptoms, retention and urethral erosion.

Suprapubic Arc Tape (SPARC, AMS®)

In SPARC, the needles are disposable, thinner and passed suprapubically to the vagina. There is no need for hydrodissection or a catheter guide and the suprapubic incision is small stab wound rather than an incision. The cystoscopy can be done once after passing both needles rather than after each needle pass. There is no limitation regarding patient position in contrast to TVT where a 15-degree limitation of leg elevation is recommended. The sling need not be connected until the positions are confirmed. There is an absorbable tensioning suture that permits adjustment of sling tension.

The suprapubic stab wounds are marked close to the midline at the level of the symphysis pubis. One may infiltrate the retropubic space and anterior vaginal wall with local anesthetic or saline but the author does not do this routinely. A clear understanding of retropubic

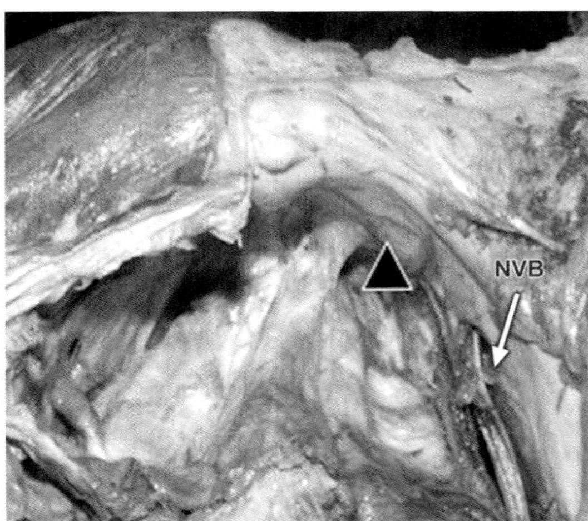

Fig. 7: Cadaveric dissection view from India's first cadaver dissection workshop on female pelvic floor reconstruction held in March 2006 at Hyderabad. Needle entry point (arrow head) is well away from the obturator neurovascular bundle (NVB)

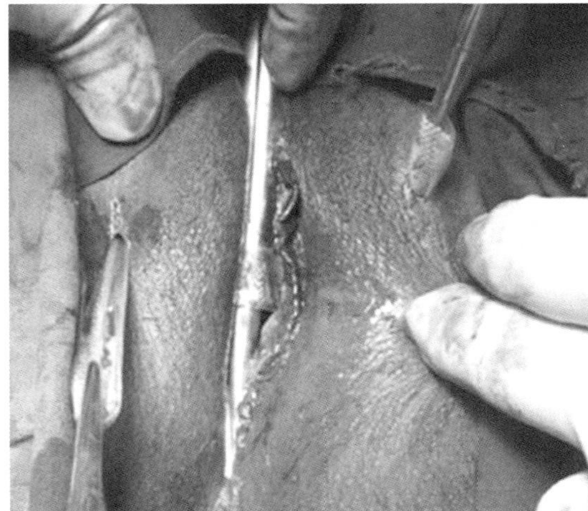

Fig. 8: A heavy pair of scissors is placed between the urethra and the tape to prevent excessive tightening at the time of removal of the sleeve covering the tape. Ideally, a visible space should be left between the tape and the urethra

anatomy is important in avoiding injury to vascular structures. The obturator vessels and inferior epigastric vessels are generally at a safe distance in a lateral location. The SPARC tape is placed from the retropubic space down to the vagina (Fig. 9). One may place a clamp over the midline to mark out the midpoint of the tape but in contrast to the TVT, this is usually not necessary for the SPARC as there are clear markings along the outer aspect of the tape.

The authors do not believe in a cough test for "tensioning". The tape should be placed tension-free with visible space between the urethra and the tape. The tape should lie flat along the mid-urethra. A heavy pair of scissors or similar instrument is placed between the tape and the urethra when the plastic sheaths are removed from either side of the tape. After the plastic sheaths are removed, the tape is cut at the surface of the abdominal skin, and the abdominal and vaginal wounds are closed. A Foley catheter is placed, and a voiding trial is done once the patient can ambulate comfortably to the bathroom. Alternatively, one may not place a Foley catheter at all.

Monarc® Transobturator Tape (American Medical Systems®)

The Monarc is a subfascial hammock placed across both the obturator foramina in a manner that supports the urethra. It is placed in an outside-in manner. The tape is similar to the SPARC. The Monarc comes with disposable helical needles, one for each side. The patient is placed in the lithotomy position and the vaginal dissection is carried out exactly in the same manner as for a TVT or SPARC. Next the medial border of the obturator foramen is palpated at the level of the clitoris, just below the pubic attachment of the tendon of the adductor longus. One may feel the pubic ramus and the medial border of the obturator foramen between two fingers kept within and outside the vagina. A small stab incision is made in the skin at this level and the helical needles are passed, one by one. The author prefers to perform a cystoscopy at each needle passage although the company product insert mentions this as optional. To pass the needle of the second side one must complete the tape passage of the other side and remove the needle. The tape is placed below the urethra in much the same manner as the SPARC (Fig. 10). However, since the tape is far away from the retropubic space and other major vascular structures, it is much less likely to damage the urinary tract or blood vessels. Hence, such complications appear to be fewer with the Monarc as compared to the TVT. The tape is placed tension free with a heavy pair of scissors preventing the tape from becoming too taut when the sleeves are removed. The tape is cut flush at the medial aspect of the thigh and closure proceeds as usual. The patient can void on the same or next day.

Outcome of Slings

Pubovaginal rectus fascia slings have excellent long-term results with upwards of 80% remaining continent beyond 5 years. In a comparison of vaginal wall slings with rectus fascia sling, the long-term outcome showed a trend toward better outcome with rectus slings (73% vs. 61%) despite a much shorter follow-up of the vaginal wall sling patients (70 months vs. 45 months).

Results of cadaveric fascia have been unsatisfactory with 32% recurrence at 14.8 months. Even with small intestinal submucosa (SIS), the short-term results are

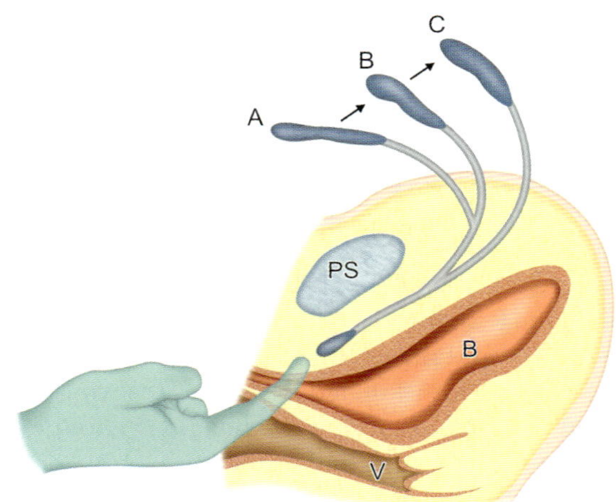

Fig. 9: The suprapubic arc tape (SPARC) needle is initially inserted with the hub pointing toward the surgeon (A). As the needle is guided down the back of the symphysis, the needle hub moves cranially (B) till it is pointing in the direction of the roof (C). The needle is guided on to the nondominant hand which is placed in the vagina (V). Staying close to the pubic symphysis (PS) avoids damage to the urinary tract

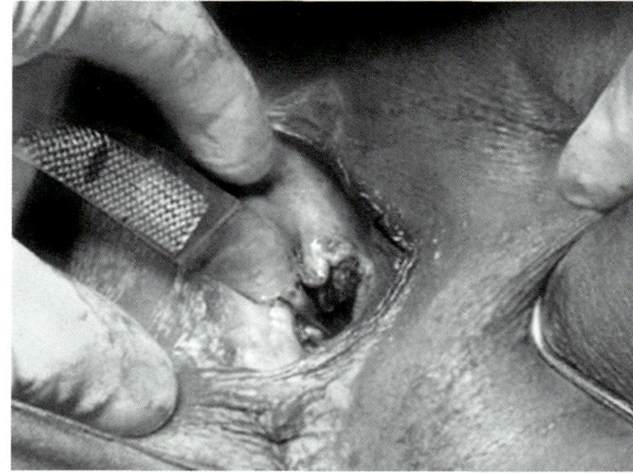

Fig. 10: Monarc® tape attached to the helical needle in preparation for withdrawal back through the obturator foramen. The wrist movement for withdrawal is reverse of that for needle placement

unsatisfactory with 3 out of 15 patients needing reoperation by 1 year. In both these series, at re-exploration, none or little of the initial sling material was found on histological examination. There was little tissue reaction seen.

Synthetic suburethral slings are now the most commonly performed procedure for SUI and have been studied in detail (Table 1). In a comparison of TVT with the Burch colposuspension, where 344 women were randomized across 14 centers in UK, there was no difference in pad test and questionnaire outcomes at 2 years.

In a comparison of TVT and transobturator tape (TOT), there was no difference in short-term outcome at 1 year with respect to cure (84% vs. 90%), bladder outlet obstruction (14% vs. 11%). There were no bladder injuries in the TOT group compared to 3 in the TVT group (not statistically significant).

Long-term data of TVT is now available and at an average follow-up of 91 months, 81% had objective cure. Sixty four of the original 90 women were available for analysis. There was de novo urgency in 6%.

Urethral erosions are very rare and no case was reported in a recent series of 316 patients. Vaginal erosions are commonest and occurred in 5% of the same series of patients. Postoperative urgency can occur in up to 15% of women in the long-term and the risk factors are parity, age and history of cesarean section. This symptom can be as bothersome as the preoperative SUI with which the patient presented in the first place.

TVT results in the elderly more than 75 years are significantly poorer compared to younger cohorts in long-term follow-up (mean 5.7 years). It was also poorer in women with severe obesity [body mass index (BMI) >35] compared the less and nonobese group. In these two groups, the success rates were 56% and 52% respectively as compared to the about 80% success rate in the comparative groups.

Table 1: Medwin Hospital data on synthetic vaginal tapes. 33 out of the 34 patients had a satisfactory correction of incontinence over a maximum follow-up of 6-and-a-half years. Three (9%) patients had postoperative de novo urgency needing anticholinergic therapy

Total synthetic tapes	34 (Retropubic 11, Transobturator 23)
Outcome	
Failure	1 (no need for pads but incontinence which is bothersome)
Bleeding	1 (wrong plane; corrected immediately, no transfusion)
Nonhealing sinus	1 (bilateral, retropubic tape)
Vaginal erosion	1 (spontaneous healing)
Tape breached vagina	1 (covered by local flap)

BLADDER BUTTRESS OPERATIONS

This includes a range of procedures all of which use some form of midline plication of tissues on the anterior vaginal wall. The procedure was described by Kelly in 1912. In addition to the Kelly plication, other names of similar procedures include anterior colporrhaphy and anterior repair. The continence rates for these procedures are clearly lower than more established procedures and as such this operation can no longer be recommended for the treatment of stress incontinence. It is, however, often performed in conjunction with other procedures for completing a comprehensive pelvic floor reconstruction, chiefly for the correction of a central defect cystocele.

The patient is positioned in the lithotomy position under spinal or general anesthesia. A midline vaginal incision is made down from a point about 1 cm proximal to the urethral meatus till the level of the cardinal ligaments. The vesicopelvic fascia is dissected and reapproximated in the midline using absorbable sutures. The excess anterior vaginal wall is excised and the vagina may be packed.

Although, the procedure appears to give a good "lift" to the bladder neck and proximal mid-urethra, the vagina is a very distensible structure and tends to drop off with time. The backboard support provided by this repair to the urethrovesical unit is insufficient. Also, the degree of lift is much lesser. Hence, this procedure leads to a much higher incidence of failure. These procedures show a progressive and sharp decline in success rates with time. The risk of recurrent incontinence was 2.5 times higher than Burch suspension in a study of 932 patients across 9 trials. In this pooled analysis, women offered anterior colporrhaphy had a 41% failure rate as compared to 17% for those offered Burch colposuspension. Hence, anterior colporrhaphy should not be offered to women for SUI.

RETROPUBIC OPERATIONS

This includes the Marshall Marchetti Krantz (MMK) operation, the Burch colposuspension and the paravaginal fascial repair. In all these operations, the paraurethral vaginal wall is suspended to a structure in the retropubic area—the symphysis pubis in MMK, the Cooper's ligament in Burch colposuspension and the arcus tendineus fascia pelvis in paravaginal repair. The Burch procedure can also be performed laparoscopically. The Burch is the most common operation in this group and is the reference standard against which most other operations for stress incontinence are compared. Hence, this operation is described.

The patient is placed in an exaggerated lithotomy to permit access to the abdomen and vagina simultaneously by the surgeon and the patient is draped accordingly. A Pfannenstiel incision is given and the retropubic space of Retzius is developed. The bladder is gently displaced medially by a sponge on a stick and the urethrovesical junction is identified by palpating a Foley catheter balloon. The surgeon inserts the fingers of the nondominant hand in the vagina to elevate the bladder neck area about 2 cm lateral to the urethrovesical junction. The overlying fibrofatty tissue is dissected away and (usually) three prolene sutures are placed between the vaginal wall minus the mucosa and the Cooper's ligament (Fig. 11). These sutures may not completely approximate the vaginal wall to the ligament. The fingers in the vagina can feel the lift given to the anterior vaginal wall by the sutures and the vaginal finger elevation should be continued until all sutures have been placed.

Burch procedure is clearly superior to anterior repair and needle suspension at 5 year follow-up. Between 85% and 90% are continent at 1 year with at least 70% continent at 5 years. There are very few studies comparing Burch with MMK operation and Burch procedure had a better long-term outcome. The Burch procedure is equally effective as the sling operations.

Laparoscopic Burch has been offered with the objective of offering a less invasive procedure than the open Burch with lesser morbidity. However, the procedure is yet to prove itself. There is no standardization in terms of the technique used and most studies comparing it to the standard Burch find it inferior in the short and medium term. This disparity is likely to widen with long-term data since there is a continued divergence in the medium term data. The technique of laparoscopic Burch makes a difference. A single suture technique was associated with a higher failure rate than two sutures (65% vs. 89%). However, even at 1 year, the results show inferior continence rates compared to the open Burch. For a procedure for which results are now being seen in terms of 10–15 year outcome, this would most likely, translate into unacceptable continent rates in the long-term.

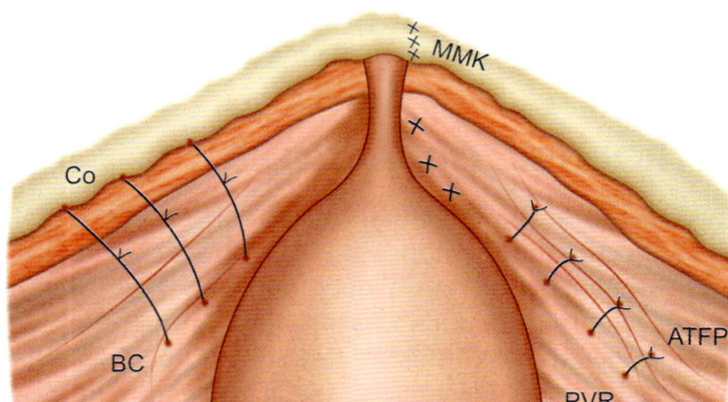

Fig. 11: In the Marshall Marchetti Krantz (MMK) operation, three sutures are given to suspend the paraurethral vaginal wall to the pubic symphysis. The Burch procedure (BC) uses fixation to the Cooper's ligament (Co) while in the paravaginal repair (PVR), fixation is performed to the arcus tendineus fascia pelvis (ATFP).

A recent multicentric study from Australia showed similar outcome between laparoscopic and open Burch suspension groups at 2 years and beyond. The procedure was done in the same manner as an open procedure. The blood loss was lesser and the time for surgery significantly longer in the laparoscopic group. A recent Cochrane analysis of 21 studies suggested that the operation might be as good as the open surgery at 2 years and that a two-suture technique was better than one. However, with the advent of synthetic tapes that give perhaps a better outcome with even lesser morbidity, the future of this operation is uncertain. There is a distinct reduction in the number of reports published with this operation in recent times and this probably reflects the smaller number of patients that are now being offered this procedure.

BLADDER NECK SUSPENSION

These are a group of procedures in which a suture is passed on either side of the bladder neck by means of specially devised long needles and is tied up at the abdominal wall usually at the rectus fascia level. It includes the Stamey procedure and its variants the Pereyra and Gittes bladder neck suspension. These procedures should no longer be offered since they have a significant medium term recurrence risk and there are much more durable, low morbidity procedures available. Briefly, a small midline vaginal incision is given and the periurethral area dissected on either side of the proximal urethra and bladder neck. The endopelvic fascia is pierced to enter the retropubic space and number 1 prolene sutures are passed through the lateral free edge of the periurethral fascia and endopelvic fasica. These sutures are brought up to the rectus level by means of an especially designed long needle such as the Stamey needle. These sutures are tied over the rectus in the midline. Cystoscopy is performed to ensure safety of the urinary tract and to confirm the precise location of the needle. Electively, a Q-tip test may be used to judge the degree of lift during suture tightening.

These procedures also have a high failure rate of 29% at 1 year compared to 16% for Burch colposuspension. The relative risk of failure was 2.1 times in this pooled analysis of 784 women from nine trials. Our own data at Medwin with needle suspensions was equally dismal with 4 recurrences out of 23 patients at an average follow-up of 2.9 years. The 23 patients who underwent bladder neck suspension included Gittes' in 19 patients, Stamey's in 3, and a

Microvasive bone anchor in one. One recurrence occurred in 6 months and required repeat surgery. There were no intraoperative complications and the mean hospital stay was 2.7 days. Bone anchor vaginal procedures have shown dismal results with postoperative complications in terms of pubic pain, osteitis pubis, osteomyelitis as well as poor long-term outcome.

PERIURETHRAL INJECTIONS

These procedures entail the injection of a periurethral bulking agent to achieve a physical coaptation. These procedures are less effective but have low morbidity and are indicated in women who are unfit or unwilling for a more invasive procedure. They are particularly suitable for women with ISD. The injection causes an increase in the bladder outlet resistance with increase in closure pressure and leak point pressures. Various agents have been used such as collagen, fat, durasphere, teflon and silicone. Fat is easily available and compatible but is quickly phagocytosed leading to low success rates. Collagen can easily be administered but is also biodegradable and needs repeated injection. Allergy testing is also required. Durasphere is non-degradable but difficult to inject. Teflon has had several reports of migration and particles have been documented in the regional lymph nodes and even the lung.

The injection can be made by either the transurethral route or the paraurethral route under endoscopic control using an appropriate needle and injection system under local anesthesia (Fig. 12). Injections are made on either side of the bladder neck until coaptation is achieved.

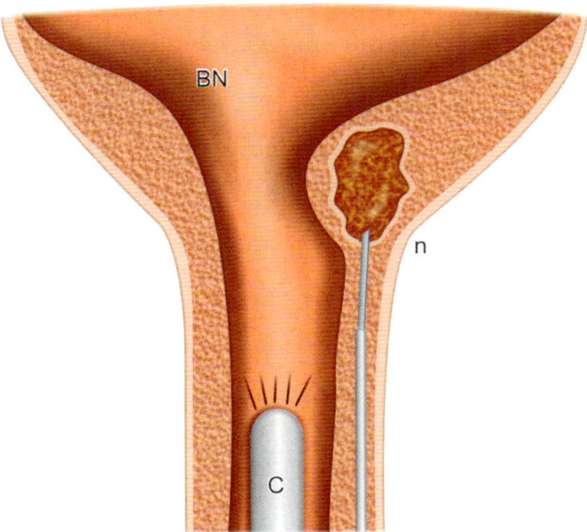

Fig. 12: Paraurethral injection under endoscopic control using a specially designed needle (n) achieves visible coaptation of the urethral wall at the level of the bladder neck (BN)

Several periurethral bulking agents have been tried but the one used most often has been collagen, which is US Food and Drug Administration (FDA) approved. Results are unpredictable and several injections might be necessary. Continence rates in the short-term vary from 7% to 83%. Other agents used are autologous fat, teflon and silicone. 3 year follow-up data shows continence rates of 21% for durasphere and 9% for collagen, too poor to recommend. There are no comparisons available to standard therapy but case series would suggest that this procedure should not be offered for primary stress incontinence.

ARTIFICIAL URINARY SPHINCTER

This is indicated only as a "last resort" in women with multiple failed procedures. The AMS® 800 is the most common sphincter used. It has a three-piece design with a pump, reservoir and cuff. A complete description of the procedure is outside the scope of this chapter. There are very few reports of the use of this device in SUI. By and large, in women with simple incontinence this is an overtreatment, while in women with multiple failed recurrences, this is often fraught with device erosion and the need for revision.

FACTORS INFLUENCING THERAPY

Surgeon must be experienced with the type of surgery being planned. The following factors may influence the choice of the surgeon:

- Intrinsic sphincter deficiency versus hypermobility. If hypermobility predominates, both pubovaginal sling and Burch colposuspension are equally effective. However, if ISD predominates, a pubovaginal sling is more effective. In patients with a very low abdominal leak point pressure, a little extra "snugness" of the sling may be indicated.
- Urodynamics findings of underactive detrusor may make one extra cautious to avoid obstructing the urethra during the procedure. It might also dictate a counseling for possible postoperative clean intermittent catheterization.
- Need for concomitant surgery such as an abdominal hysterectomy, may influence the choice. However, it is "not" an automatic choice to perform a Burch colposuspension merely because the abdomen was being opened. The most appropriate operation must be performed in each situation.
- Lifestyle of the patient is important. A young and very active patient may be better suited to a sling.
- Age, life-expectancy and overall medical condition may dicate the use of minimal therapy, such as a collagen injection.

OCCULT URINARY INCONTINENCE

Stress incontinence may be masked by pelvic organ prolapse. The distortion of the lower urinary tract and pressure effect of pelvic organ prolapse (POP) within the vagina may prevent a woman from leaking despite having stress incontinence. It is also possible that some of the women with stress incontinence following POP surgery, the incontinence is de novo. Overall, about 11% women show demonstrable SUI after POP surgery. Viewed from the opposite perspective, about 40% of women coming for stress incontinence surgery have POP.

Urodynamic testing prior to POP surgery may unmask stress incontinence. These studies are done after reducing the prolapse and may be done with a pessary in place. Such evaluation may save the woman from repeat surgery and the surgeons from unnecessary embarrassment.

MIXED URINARY INCONTINENCE

Thirty to fifty percent of all patients with incontinence present with a mixed picture and this group has historically had a poorer outcome. Mixed urinary incontinence is defined as a stress related urine leak along with the symptoms or urgency with or without urge incontinence. One must, of course, remember that stress incontinence may present as urgency due to a urethral trickle of urine during periods of stress. As a rough guide, one-third of patients present with pure stress incontinence, urge incontinence and mixed incontinence each. Anticholinergics help in two-third of patients and helps in all but the most severe incontinence group. Schrepferman showed that the outcome following pubovaginal sling surgery could be stratified based on the initial urodynamics findings in women with mixed incontinence. In those with low pressure detrusor overactivity (defined as detrusor overactivity of less than 15 cm H_2O), 90% of women had resolution of urgency; in those with urgency alone ["sensory" urgency, a term which is no longer recommended by the International Continence Society (ICS)] about 60% have a resolution. In those with high pressure detrusor overactivity, only 30% have resolution.

RECURRENT STRESS URINARY INCONTINENCE

Recurrent stress urinary incontinence may occur due to suture breakage, continued pelvic floor weakness and most important, development of significant ISD. The proportion of women with ISD varies from 13% at initial presentation to 25% in women who have failed one surgery and 75% in those who have failed two or more surgeries for stress incontinence. The outcome of Burch procedure reflects this data. While the success rate of primary Burch is around 80%, the success of a second Burch procedure is about 25% and that of a third procedure close to 0%. Hence, Burch operation should not be offered to women with recurrent SUI unless it can clearly be demonstrated that recurrence has occurred in a setting of hypermobility without ISD. This is likely to occur chiefly in women who were offered needle suspension or anterior repair earlier.

STRESS INCONTINENCE SURGERY COMBINED WITH OTHER PELVIC SURGERY

Synthetic tape procedures can be combined with other pelvic procedures with safety. In a large series of 687 patients across 41 hospitals, 59 had concomitant surgery with similar outcomes in terms of efficacy and complications in both the groups at 2 years follow-up. In a series of 15 patients who underwent transvaginal sacrocolpopexy along with tension-free tape, the outcome was similar to historical cohorts undergoing tape alone except for a high rate of initial retention. One-third patients had retention and this could last for up to 6 months. In a recent series of the Monarc transobturator tape, patients with concomitant surgeries did as well as those who underwent tape alone with excellent satisfaction on validated questionnaires. There was a lower complete cure rate with concomitant surgery perhaps reflecting the severity of the pelvic floor dysfunction (74% vs. 57%).

BIBLIOGRAPHY

1. Abdel-Fattah M, Sivanesan K, Ramsay I, et al. How common are tape erosions? A comparison of two versions of the transobturator tension-free vaginal tape procedure. BJU Int. 2006;98:594-8.
2. Amaye-Obu FA, Drutz HP. Surgical management of recurrent stress urinary incontinence: a 12-year experience. Am J Obstet Gynecol. 1999;181:1296-307.
3. Carey MP, Goh JT, Rosamilia A, et al. Laparoscopic versus open Burch colposuspension: a randomised controlled trial. BJOG. 2006;113:999-1006.
4. Chrouser KL, Fick F, Goel A, et al. Carbon coated zirconium beads in beta-glucan gel and bovine glutaraldehyde cross-linked collagen injections for intrinsic sphincter deficiency: continence and satisfaction after extended followup. J Urol. 2004;171:1152-5.

5. Dean NM, Ellis G, Wilson PD, et al. Laparoscopic colposuspension for urinary incontinence in women. Cochrane Database Syst Rev. 2006;3:CD002239.
6. deTayrac R, Deffieux X, Droupy S, et al. A prospective randomized trial comparing tension-free vaginal tape and transobturator suburethral tape for surgical treatment of stress urinary incontinence. Am J Obstet Gynecol. 2004;190:602-8.
7. Glazener CM, Cooper K. Anterior vaginal repair for urinary incontinence in women. Cochrane Database Syst Rev. 2001;(1):CD001755.
8. Glazener CM, Cooper K. Bladder neck needle suspension for urinary incontinence in women. Cochrane Database Syst Rev. 2004;2:CD003636.
9. Hellberg D, Holmgren C, Lanner L, et al. The very obese woman and the very old woman: tension-free vaginal tape for the treatment of stress urinary incontinence. Int Urogynecol J Pelvic Floor Dysfunct. 2007;18:423-9.
10. Holmgren C, Nilsson S, Lanner L, et al. Frequency of de novo urgency in 463 women who had undergone the tension-free vaginal tape (TVT) procedure for genuine stress urinary incontinence—a long-term follow-up. Eur J Obstet Gynecol Reprod Biol. 2007;132(1):121-5.
11. Lapitan MC, Cody DJ, Grant AM. Open retropubic colposuspension for urinary incontinence in women. Cochrane Database Syst Rev. 2005;20(3):CD002912.
12. Mellier G, Mistrangelo E, Gery L, et al. Tension-free obturator tape (Monarc Subfascial Hammock) in patients with or without associated procedures. Int Urogynecol J Pelvic Floor Dysfunct. 2007;18:165-72.
13. Nilsson CG, Falconer C, Rezapour M. Seven-year follow-up of the tension-free vaginal tape procedure for treatment of urinary incontinence. Obstet Gynecol. 2004;104:1259-62.
14. Owens DC, Winters JC. Pubovaginal sling using Duraderm graft: intermediate follow-up and patient satisfaction. Neurourol Urodyn. 2004;23:115-8.
15. Persson J, Wolner-Hanssen P. Laparoscopic Burch colposuspension for stress urinary incontinence: a randomized comparison of one or two sutures on each side of the urethra. Obstet Gynecol. 2000;95:151-5.
16. Richter HE, Varner RE, Sanders E, et al. Effects of pubovaginal sling procedure on patients with urethral hypermobility and intrinsic sphincteric deficiency: Would they do it again? Am J Obstet Gynecol. 2001;184:14-9.
17. Rodrigues P, Hering F, Meler A, et al. Pubofascial versus vaginal sling operation for the treatment of stress urinary incontinence: a prospective study. Neurourol Urodyn. 2004;23:627-31.
18. Schraffordt Koops SE, Bisseling TM, van Brummen HJ, et al. Result of the tension-free vaginal tape in patients with concomitant prolapse surgery: a 2-year follow-up study. An analysis from the Netherlands TVT database. Int Urogynecol J Pelvic Floor Dysfunct. 2007;18:437-42.
19. Schrepferman CG, Griebling TL, Nygaard IE, et al. Resolution of urge symptoms following sling cystourethropexy. J Urol. 2000;164:1628-31.
20. Shaker DA, De Boer F. Performance of the tension free vaginal tape procedure when combined with sacrospinous fixation for apical prolapse. J Obstet Gynaecol. 2006;26:663-6.
21. Tennstedt S. Urinary Incontinence Treatment Network. Design of the Stress Incontinence Surgical Treatment Efficacy Trial (SISTEr). Urology. 2005;66:1213-7.
22. Ward KL, Hilton P. UK and Ireland TVT Trial Group. A prospective multicenter randomized trial of tension-free vaginal tape and colposuspension for primary urodynamic stress incontinence: Two-year follow-up. Am J Obstet Gynecol. 2004;190:324-31.
23. Wiedemann A, Otto M. Small intestinal submucosa for pubourethral sling suspension for the treatment of stress incontinence: first histopathological results in humans. J Urol. 2004;172:215-8.

CHAPTER

45 Small Bowel, Colon and Appendix in Gynecological Surgery

Lakhvinder Singh

INTRODUCTION

In the medical field rapid super-specializing and subspecializing, the interdisciplinary issues are becoming more and more problematic. A working knowledge of adjacent field is required. A gynecologist may be required to face complex gastrointestinal (GI) or colorectal problems as a missed diagnosis or as a part of the gynecologic condition. Though this is a teamwork but desired help might not be available. This chapter mentions few scenarios where the boundaries of specialties become blurred.

GASTROINTESTINAL CONDITIONS SIMULATING GYNECOLOGIC CONDITIONS

Various GI conditions pose a differential diagnosis in women of reproductive age group. If not diagnosed early, may be encountered on the operating table. Though the list is long, the major culprits are mentioned here.

DIVERTICULITIS

Colonic diverticulitis may be confused with pelvic inflammatory disease (PID). These two processes generally do not occur in the same age group; however, rarely diverticulitis may occur in women younger than 40 years of age. Patients with acute diverticulitis present with pain, altered bowel function, fever, and leukocytosis. Tenderness and guarding are usually localized to the left lower quadrant. One in five patients with acute diverticulitis also has signs and symptoms of colonic obstruction. Treatment for unruptured diverticulitis and PID are similar, and include intravenous (IV) fluid resuscitation, bowel rest, and broad-spectrum antibiotic coverage for anaerobes, gram-negative rods, and enterococci. Diagnostic computed tomography (CT) scan clarifies whether a pericolonic abscess is present, and CT-directed drainage of an abscess expedites recovery and avoids surgical exploration in most cases. Nasogastric decompression is necessary in the setting of obstruction. If obstructive symptoms persist, or if bowel perforation has occurred, surgical exploration is warranted. If bowel perforation results in generalized peritonitis, consideration is given to diverting colostomy, with extensive irrigation and drainage of the peritoneal cavity.

APPENDICITIS

This poses the frequently encountered diagnostic dilemmas as both are common between second decade and third decade of life. Whereas cervical motion tenderness is helpful in the diagnosis of PID and right-sided pain on rectal examination is helpful in the diagnosis of appendicitis, but it is not pathognomonic. Peritoneal irritation from any source can be elicited by manipulation of the pelvic organs, so that manual manipulation of the cervix elicits an intensely painful response (cervical motion tenderness) in women with either PID or appendicitis. Similarly, rectal examination may illicit pain in a woman who has PID. Acute appendicitis will be overlooked by clinicians who assume the ailment is PID after finding cervical motion tenderness. Historical suggestive of lateralization of pain from umbilicus to McBurney's point with progressive anorexia raises suspicion for appendicitis. A history of prior PID, multiple sexual partners, recent acquisition of a new sexual partner, recent menses, and physical findings of a purulent cervical discharge suggest PID. Radiographic studies may be needed to clarify the diagnosis because acute appendicitis is a surgical emergency; PID, however, may be initially treated with broad-spectrum antibiotics and supportive care. Spiral CT scan has gained acceptance as an accurate determinant of the appendiceal anatomy. Contrast CT imaging is also invaluable in the diagnosis of pelvic abscess. Bilateral pelvic abscesses are more characteristics of PID than an appendiceal process.

Appendectomy as a surgical procedures is explained in Figures 1 to 5.

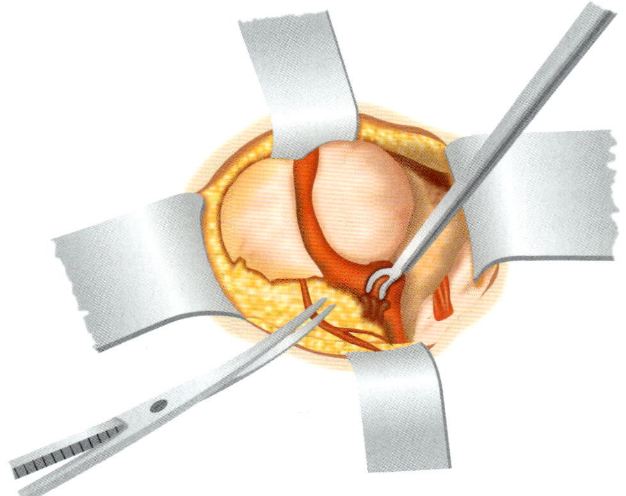

Fig. 1: After opening the abdomen and exposing the right lower abdominal region, the appendix is identified and when necessary adhesions are dissected sharply to provide complete appendix mobility

Helpful hint: When the appendix is adhesed or retrocede, scissor or cautery dissection should be used to mobilize it and separate it from the adherent or overlying colon.

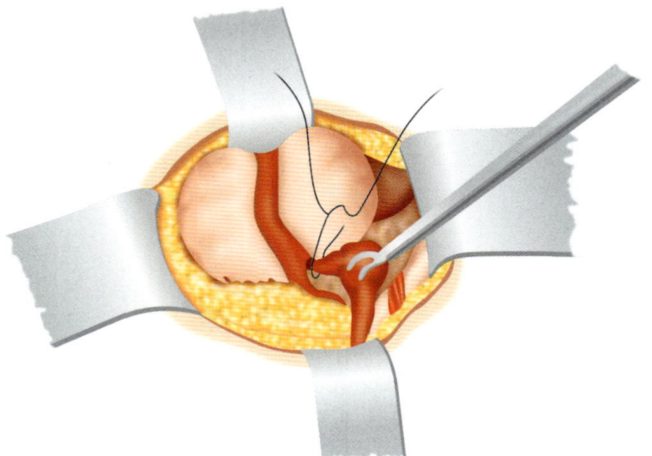

Fig. 2: The base of the appendix is crushed and then doubly ligated with chromic ligatures

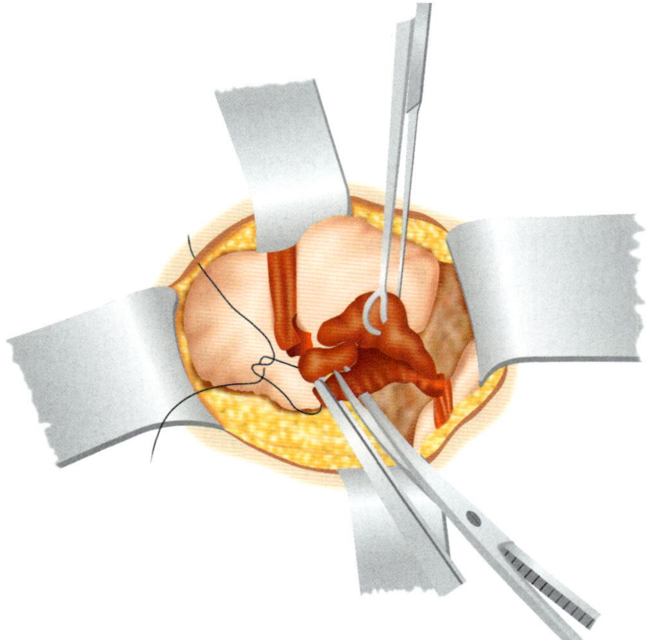

Fig. 3: If the mesoappendix is thin, it can be singly clamped and ligated; however, if it is broad, two or more clamps might be needed to ligate the appendiceal blood supply

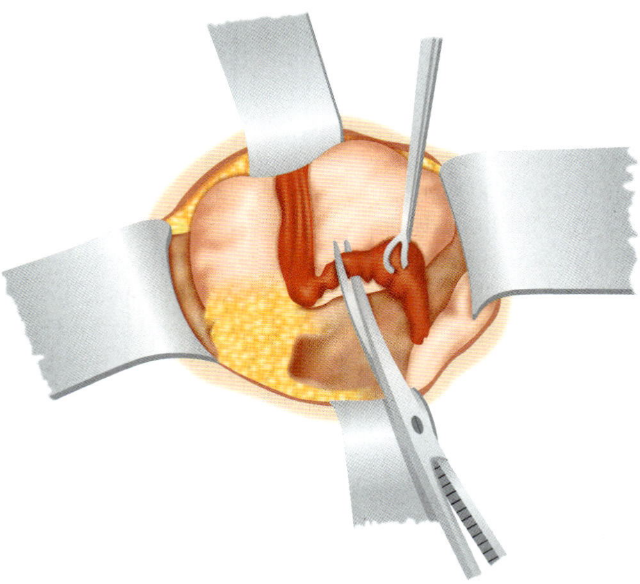

Fig. 4: The appendix is incised several millimeters distal to the chromic ties placed at its base and removed from the operative field

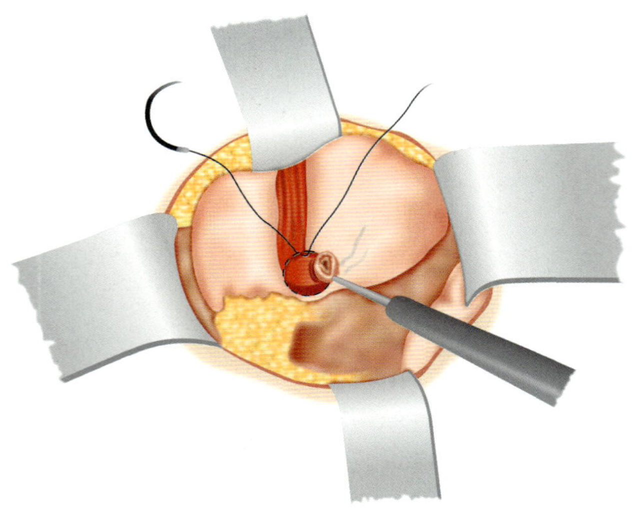

Fig. 5: The author favors both electrocautery of the base of the appendix and a 3-0 silk purse-string suture to bury the appendiceal stump followed by copious irrigation with saline or water

MECKEL'S DIVERTICULUM

Meckel's diverticulum represents a residual portion of the vitelline (yolk) duct and is present in 1% of women. Diverticula average 5 cm in length and are located along the antimesenteric border of the ileum within 2 feets of the ileocecal valve. They are lined by ileal type mucosa, but at least one in five cases have ectopic pancreatic or gastric tissue. Acute symptoms result from inflammation, hemorrhage, or obstruction in approximately 5% of Meckel's diverticula. Inflammation and hemorrhage result from gastric acid secretion, and obstruction follows intussusception or torsion. Presenting signs and symptoms may mimic acute appendicitis or PID. Most complications from Meckel's diverticula are during early childhood, and the likelihood of problems significantly decreases with advancing age. Accordingly, most surgeons believe resection of an asymptomatic Meckel's diverticulum in adulthood is unnecessary. Some recommend prophylactic removal if encountered during surgery, because morbidity associated with resection is low. It is generally agreed, however, that resection should be undertaken if the individual has previously been symptomatic, if the diverticulum is unusually long or has a narrow neck, or if thickening at the tip suggests ectopic gastric mucosa. Resection is accomplished by excising the base of the diverticulum with transverse closure of the enterotomy. Care is taken to avoid unnecessary resection of bowel wall to prevent luminal narrowing.

VOLVULUS

Sigmoid volvulus is an acute malrotation that presents with sudden onset of intense pain, similar to that of ovarian torsion. Volvulus is generally accompanied by constipation, abdominal pain, and distention. Nausea and vomiting may occur. Volvulus is most commonly seen after the age of 60 years; however, cases in young individuals have been reported. Flat plate abdominal radiographic features are that of a markedly dilated, gas filled sigmoid colon. Barium enema shows a tapered obstruction at the rectosigmoid junction with a typical bird's beak deformity. Sigmoid volvulus can usually be corrected nonoperatively with sigmoidoscopy or cautious barium enema. If volvulus is discovered at the time of surgery, initial management consists of untwisting the loop of bowel and observing for viability. Resection is infrequently necessary and should be reserved for devitalized bowel. Cecal volvulus is rare and tends to occur in the elderly population. This too is best managed by derotation, and resection is reserved for nonviability.

Pelvic Malignancies

Colorectal carcinomas may be difficult to distinguish from other pelvic malignancies. Advanced colorectal carcinoma may invade the vagina and/or bladder producing symptoms suggestive of a gynecologic or urologic problem. Advanced ovarian, cervical, and endometrial cancers may also invade surrounding organs leading to rectal bleeding. Resultant inflammation, tissue necrosis, and abscess formation contribute to the diagnostic dilemma. Historical information, thorough physical examination, colonoscopy or barium enema, cystoscopy, CT scan, and tissue biopsy can clarify the origin of pelvic malignancies in most cases.

Inflammatory Bowel Disease

Inflammatory bowel disease includes Crohn's disease (regional enteritis) and ulcerative colitis. Crohn's disease is an inflammatory process of uncertain etiology that usually involves the small bowel. It most frequently occurs in young adults with symptomatic onset during the late teens, but may occur at any age. Those affected have intermittent diarrhea, intestinal cramping, and weight loss. The extent of intestinal symptoms generally enables the clinician to distinguish inflammatory bowel disease from PID. Clinical findings, such as a functional ovarian cyst, may lead to overdiagnosis of a gynecologic disorder and result in unnecessary surgery. Gynecologic surgery is best avoided if possible in Crohn's patients because of the high risk of intestinal complications, even if the bowel is uninjured. Medical management is the mainstay of treatment because there is a high recurrence rate that follows surgical resection.

Therapy consists of bowel rest, nutritional support with total parenteral nutrition (TPN), and anti-inflammatories such as sulfasalazine and corticosteroids. Surgery is reserved for patients whose disease is complicated by obstruction, perforation, fistula, or hemorrhage. Affected areas of the small intestine may be interspersed by normal segments of bowel. The appearance of Crohn's intestine is thickened walls with dull, purple-red discoloration, inflammatory exudate, and adherent mesenteric fat. If surgical resection is necessary, only the involved segments of bowel are removed. Because of the high rate of anastomotic dehiscence following resections for Crohn's disease, some surgeons advocate stricturoplasty as an alternative to resection. Stricturoplasty is accomplished by opening the bowel longitudinally and closing transversely, creating a wider lumen. The appendix is eventually affected by Crohn's disease and ulcerative colitis in 25% and 50% of cases, respectively. Prophylactic appendectomy may be considered if the terminal ileum and cecum are not involved by active disease at the time of exploration. Fistulae (i.e. enterocutaneous, enterovaginal, enterovesical) are frequently associated with inflammatory bowel disease and its surgical management. Surgical correction is reserved for problematic fistulae that fail to respond to extended medical management. The intestinal defect, as the source of fistulous drainage, must be corrected for any chance of successful resolution.

GYNECOLOGIC CONDITIONS THAT AFFECT THE GASTROINTESTINAL TRACT

Extensive endometriosis may involve the small or large intestine. Inflammation from small bowel endometriosis may result in adhesions, with painful peristalsis and intermittent or complete obstruction. Rectal implants and invasive endometriosis can manifest clinically as cyclic pain, intermittent diarrhea, bleeding, and pain associated with bowel movements. Rectovaginal endometriosis can cause perineal discomfort and a tender palpable mass on rectovaginal examination, which could mimic a perirectal abscess.

Pregnancy, either ectopic or intrauterine, must be considered in any symptomatic woman of reproductive age. Serum beta human chorionic gonadotropin (β-hCG) can be obtained rapidly in most hospital settings to rule out pregnancy. Tubo-ovarian abscess and adnexal torsion are often difficult to distinguish from inflammatory GI conditions such as appendicitis or diverticulitis. All of these conditions may cause fever, nausea, anorexia, diarrhea, pain, and leukocytosis. Gynecologic infections may also adversely affect the intestinal tract, causing inflammation, adhesions, and obstruction. The fundamental history and physical examination help clarify the situation and separate gynecologic from GI disorders in most cases.

Preoperative Bowel Preparation

The surgical morbidity of GI procedures is probably reduced in patients who undergo mechanical and antibiotic bowel preparation prior to surgery. The objectives of preoperative bowel preparation are to reduce enteric volume and bacterial load. Potential benefits include better operative handling and exposure, reduced infectious complications, and enhanced anastomotic healing. A good mechanical bowel preparation does eliminate stool and gas from the colon, thus improving exposure and making it easier to pack the bowel out of the operative field. Mechanical cleansing also allows for better visibility during intraoperative colonoscopy, if needed. The literature, however, is inconclusive as to whether or not bowel preparation consistently reduces operative morbidity. Various bowel preparations have been proposed and used, including mechanical cleansing alone versus mechanical preparation plus oral antibiotics, with or without parenteral antibiotics. In the past, such agents as castor oil, senna, bisacodyl, and magnesium citrate were used, but frequently resulted in inadequate bowel cleansing. Large volumes of isotonic solution and osmotic agents such as mannitol were more effective in bowel preparation; however, the prohibitive side effects included electrolyte and fluid abnormalities, nausea, vomiting, and abdominal distention. Newer mechanical preparations usually consist of either polyethylene glycol or sodium phosphate. Polyethylene glycol is an effective, osmotically balanced solution that causes fewer electrolyte and fluid abnormalities. The major disadvantage is that 4 L must be consumed. Many patients are unable to complete this preparation because of the large volume and the resultant GI symptoms. Sodium phosphate has the advantage of being an effective cathartic while only requiring 90 cc of oral liquid. In randomized clinical trials (RCTs) comparing polyethylene glycol to sodium phosphate, patients who took sodium phosphate had significantly less trouble drinking the solution and reported less abdominal discomfort. Sodium phosphate provided a significantly better preparation for colonoscopy. This trend was also observed in surgical patients, although not statistically significant. Polyethylene glycol and sodium phosphate should be used cautiously in debilitated patients and those with cirrhosis, renal impairment, electrolyte abnormalities, or ascites. They should not be used in patients with renal failure, congenital megacolon, bowel obstruction, or congestive heart failure.

Nonabsorbable or minimally absorbed oral antibiotics have traditionally been used in bowel preparation to reduce the intraluminal colonic flora. It is presumed that reduction in the bacterial load causes less peritoneal contamination and complications if the bowel is opened during surgery. Following colorectal surgery, cultures from wound infections and intraperitoneal abscesses most commonly reveal aerobic bacteria and other coliforms, such as *Escherichia coli, Streptococcus faecalis, Pseudomonas, Klebsiella,* and *Proteus,* and anaerobes, such as *Bacteroides* and *Clostridia*. In some randomized trials of oral preoperative neomycin and erythromycin compared with no oral antibiotics, the infection rate was significantly decreased. The patients studied had also been given a mechanical preparation plus IV antibiotics. Other clinical studies have not shown an additional benefit to oral antibiotics when IV antibiotics are used. Similarly, oral antibiotics alone have not been proven to be superior to IV antibiotics alone for infection prophylaxis. Oral ciprofloxacin compared with no oral antibiotic has been noted to reduce postoperative infections. Metronidazole with either erythromycin or neomycin has also been effectively used. There is no data to support that one regimen is superior to another. In selected patients, the bowel preparation regimen that we prefer is summarized in Table 1.

There are few randomized trials comparing mechanical bowel preparation with no preparation. The utility of bowel preparation is called into question with collective retrospective data from trauma surgeries involving colonic injury and from emergent colorectal surgery for bowel obstruction. A recent review of 2,964 unprepared patients who underwent primary repair of colon injury reported an anastomotic leak rate of only 2.3%. Despite lack of consistent evidence supporting reduced morbidity, there is a general consensus regarding the potential benefit, such that the majority of gynecologic oncologists, surgical oncologists, and colorectal surgeons continue to recommend a preoperative bowel preparation.

Positioning the Patient

Examination under anesthesia facilitates evaluation of anatomy and may clarify the likelihood of intestinal involvement by disease. Low dorsal lithotomy position is used if there is an expectation of possible rectosigmoid resection and anastomosis.

Proper positioning reduces the risk of injury. The anesthetized patient is placed with her hips at the end of the table and buttocks extending several centimeters beyond the table end. Padding is secured below the coccyx to avoid pressure point injury. Careful positioning ensures the thighs are slightly flexed and the weight of the legs is distributed evenly, with no pressure points from the stirrups. Lithotomy position also allows access for intraoperative pelvic examination and provides easy

Table 1: Bowel preparation for surgery

Your surgery is planned for:
Day____________ Date____________ Time____________
Follow these instructions on the day before surgery:
Day____________ Date____________

6:00 am	Only clear liquid foods today. Clear liquid foods would include beef or chicken broth, plain Jell-O, hot tea, popsicles, 7-Up, or clear fruit juices. Do not eat or drink any milk products. Do not eat or drink anything you cannot see through. Do not drink any alcoholic beverages.
10:00 am	Take one Reglan 10 mg pill. This will help keep your stomach from being upset by the other medicines. You may repeat this every 4 hours, if needed for nausea.
11:00 am	(1) Drink half of the 3-ounce bottle of Fleet Phospho-soda. This is a strong laxative and will cause you to have diarrhea. (2) Take one of each of the antibiotic pills, Neomycin and E-mycin.
2:00 pm	Take one Reglan 10 mg pill.
3:00 pm	(1) Drink the second half of the bottle of Fleet Phospho-soda. (2) Take the second dose of each of the antibiotic pills, Neomycin and E-mycin.
6:00 pm	Take one Reglan 10 mg pill.
7:00 pm	Take the third dose of each of the antibiotic pills, Neomycin and E-mycin.
12:00 Midnight	No eating, drinking, or smoking between now and surgery.

We understand this bowel preparation may be difficult for you. However, we strongly encourage you to follow all of these steps as outlined. A proper bowel preparation may help maximize your effective healing and minimize your chance of problems after surgery. If you have any questions about these instructions, please call our office.

exposure to assess bladder or rectal integrity after pelvic dissection. Additionally, an assistant or surgeon can be positioned between the stirrups to elevate the vaginal apex or assist with a rectal anastomosis, or to enable dissection in the para-aortic and upper abdominal areas.

INTRAOPERATIVE CONSIDERATIONS

Lysis of Adhesions

Adhesions may be associated with prior surgical procedures, trauma, irradiation, infection, bleeding, or chemical irritants. Prior gynecologic surgery is the most frequently noted predisposing factor. After surgery, desiccated tissue surfaces in direct opposition are those at greatest risk for adhesion formation. History alone is not predictive, in that certain individuals have adhesions without identifiable predisposing factors. Others have a predilection for an exaggerated healing response and excessive adhesion formation.

Adhesiolysis may be necessary to mobilize the bowel, expose the surgical field, and circumvent obstruction. Constricting adhesive bands require transection. It is best to start with translucent adhesions that can be sharply lysed without difficulty. As adhesions become more dense, efforts are made to isolate a window such that an index finger and thumb can be placed behind and in front of the adhesion, respectively. Gentle blunt tissue dissection by rubbing the index finger and thumb back and forth helps to identify translucent adhesive bands that can be sharply lysed. There is often a recognizable white line between adhesions and their peritoneal attachment, which identifies a safe tissue plane for dissection. Another plane ideal for sharp dissection is one followed in close parallel proximity to a recognizable structure, such as along a loop of small bowel. Inadvertent tissue injury is less likely with adhesiolysis close to the bowel wall than with cutting through the center of dense adhesions. Controlled traction and countertraction facilitates isolation and dissection, but excessive force is avoided. With dense adhesive bands, excessive force may literally tear a hole in the bowel wall, which may go unrecognized during surgery.

Intestinal Injury in Open Gynecologic Surgery

Most intestinal injuries in gynecologic surgery occur during abdominal procedures. One comprehensive clinical review estimated that 37% of injuries occurred during entrance into the peritoneal cavity, and 35% during lysis of adhesions. Ten percent of injuries occurred during laparoscopic procedures, 9% during vaginal surgeries, and an additional 9% during dilatation and curettage as a consequence of uterine perforation. Enterotomy refers to a full-thickness opening in the bowel wall such that the lumen is entered. Enterotomy may be an incidental occurrence during dissection or an intentional orchestrated maneuver during GI surgery. Unintentional enterotomies are best avoided by cautious entry into the peritoneal cavity and meticulous dissection of adhesions. Adequate visualization and access are necessary for safe adhesiolysis. Ongoing visual and manual bowel inspection is advisable to ensure there is no compromise to wall integrity. If an inadvertent enterotomy occurs, the affected bowel must be mobilized from surrounding tissues to allow adequate exposure and a tension free repair. Although it is generally best to repair an enterotomy immediately, if the dissection is particularly difficult, it is advisable to finish the dissection so the extent of injuries can be assessed. The initial impression of a single enterotomy can be incorrect. Mobilization of tissues from the surrounding area may demonstrate multiple enterotomies within a single bowel segment or involvement of more than one loop of bowel.

If an enterotomy is not immediately repaired, it should be marked with a suture of 3-0 silk tied loosely with the tails left long for easy identification. Eventual suture repair should be accomplished in a transverse direction to avoid excess narrowing of the lumen. This is most important in the small bowel. Staple repair is also acceptable if luminal diameter is not compromised. If multiple enterotomies occur within a localized segment of small bowel, the best plan may be to resect the damaged segment rather than individually repair three or four injuries. Resection of an affected bowel segment may also be necessary if the blood supply is compromised, if greater than 50% of the circumference is injured, if irregular edges preclude reapproximation, or if repair would result in excessive luminal narrowing (Figs 6A to C).

In general, small bowel injury with intraperitoneal contamination by enteric content is associated with less morbidity than similar occurrence in the large bowel. Historically, large bowel injury (colostomy) with gross intraperitoneal contamination has been managed by diverting colostomy, with delayed surgical repair and colostomy closure after several months. Collective clinical experience from scheduled procedures and trauma surgeries have demonstrated that immediate repair without colostomy is associated with acceptably low morbidity. Suture and staple closure techniques, as well as segmental resection with anastomosis, have been successfully used. Furthermore, some studies suggest that immediate recognition and repair of intestinal injury is associated with less morbidity than the diversion techniques previously thought to be mandatory.

Aggressive peritoneal irrigation and administration of IV broad-spectrum antibiotics reduce bacterial count.

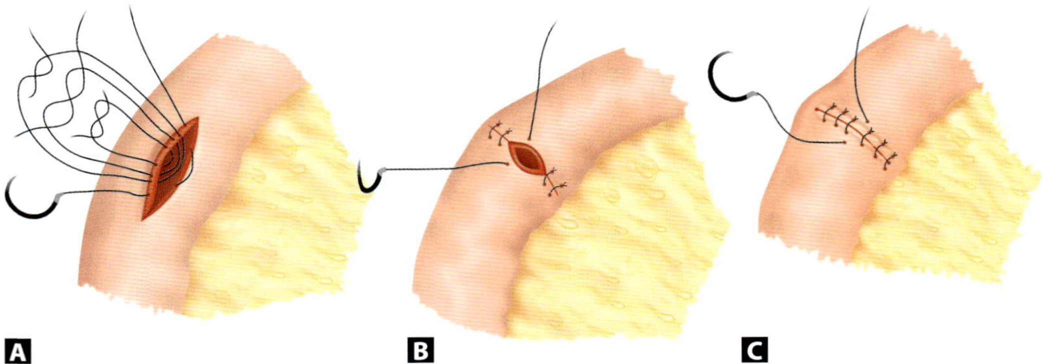

Figs 6A to C: Steps: (A) When suturing an intestinal injury through the full thickness of bowel wall, it is advisable to do so in a fashion that increases rather than decreases the intestinal caliber. The demonstrated full-thickness bowel laceration along the long axis of the intestine is repaired so as to avoid narrowing the lumen. When the bowel mucosa is intact but the muscularis is disrupted, a one-layer of interrupted 3-0 silk suture should be performed by reapproximating the serosal edges without changing the orientation of the injury; (B) A two-layer interrupted closure with 3-0 silk sutures is recommended for a through-and-through injury of the bowel wall. The final sutured layer encompasses all layers of bowel; (C) The second seromuscular layer imbricates and completely cover the first layer of sutures

Helpful hint: With thermal injuries the damaged tissue should be imbricated approximately 5 mm beyond the visible injury. However, with more severe injury, resection and repair of injured tissue is required. Alternatively, the laceration can be repaired with a TA-55 stapling device. Again, care must be taken to insure that the bowel is not compromised. This approach is best used for colonic laceration in which satisfactory lumen caliber can be maintained more than for small bowel lacerations.

Peritoneal drains should not be placed in the immediate vicinity of an anastomosis, because this can actually impede healing.

However, there may be therapeutic benefit from suction drains in dependent regions, such as the pelvis and pericolic gutters, which prevent accumulation of fluid. A diverting colostomy is indicated when a full-thickness colonic injury occurs in those who have undergone irradiation, who are profoundly malnourished, or whose condition is unstable from shock or sepsis.

Intestinal Injury during Endoscopic Procedures

Gastrointestinal injury during laparoscopy can occur with introduction of the insufflating needle or trocar, and during cautery or sharp dissection. Good clinical judgment is necessary to determine which patients are appropriate candidates for laparoscopy. Previous surgeries, inflammatory conditions, and prior irradiation increase the risk of injury from enteric adhesions, which fix intestine to the abdominal wall. Oxygenating the patient via bag-mask in preparation for intubation can distend the stomach below the level of the umbilicus, placing it at risk for injury. Nasogastric decompression before introduction of a Veress needle or trocar reduces this risk. In the presence of enteric adhesions, the laparoscopic trocar can be inadvertently placed into the stomach, transverse colon, or small intestine. Perforation is recognized by nonidentification of intraperitoneal structures, visual characteristics of intraluminal tissue, and reflux of enteric content. If perforation occurs, it is prudent to leave the trocar in position and convert to an open laparotomy. It is much easier to recognize injuries using the trocar to guide identification of the affected anatomy (Fig. 3).

Cautery or sharp dissection can result in enterotomy, which commonly occurs during adhesiolysis. The skill and comfort level of the laparoscopic surgeon determines whether the defect can be successfully repaired laparoscopically or whether laparotomy is required. The most serious laparoscopic intestinal injuries are those that go unrecognized at the time of surgery. Thermal injury from electrocautery or laser can have a potentially disastrous outcome. With electrosurgical injury, a progressive zone of tissue destruction extends well beyond the area of thermal contact, resulting in tissue necrosis and perforation 72–96 hours after surgery. Perforation may be signaled by high fever, leukocytosis, nausea, vomiting, and a generalized ill appearance. Signs of peritonitis are present on examination. Flat plate X-ray studies may be of limited benefit in the early postoperative period, because intraperitoneal air can persist for 7 days following surgery. CT scan using water-soluble contrast is better suited for this evaluation and should demonstrate extravasation of contrast material into the peritoneal cavity with possible abscess formation. If perforation is suspected or confirmed, urgent re-exploration is warranted. Hypovolemia, electrolyte abnormalities, and anemia should be aggressively corrected. Broad-spectrum antibiotics are administered and nasogastric decompression is performed as the patient is prepared for surgery. At surgery, aggressive irrigation is necessary to enhance visibility. Copious enteric exudate causes a profound inflammatory response and generalized matting together of intraperitoneal content. Inspection of the small bowel is begun at the ileocecal junction and is done proximally in a hand over hand fashion. Careful examination of the bowel and mesentery is continued to the ligament of Treitz, followed by thorough inspection of the large intestine. The stomach and proximal small bowel are also inspected. In contrast to sharp enterotomy, which can be repaired primarily, significant thermal injury is best corrected by resection of affected bowel. At the very least, a wide margin of bowel wall is removed beyond any visible thermal injury. Because of enteric contamination, other necrotic tissues such as fulgurated endometriotic implants are at high risk for abscess formation and should be excised.

Intestinal Injury during Uterine Curettage

It is estimated that most uterine perforations go unrecognized; therefore, injury to pelvic viscera may also go unrecognized. If fundal perforation occurs during sharp or suction curettage, intestine and mesentery can be drawn into the uterine cavity by the curette. Evisceration as a consequence most commonly occurs during dilatation and curettage of the gravid uterus. Tactile feedback may suggest products of conception, when in fact what is felt is prolapsed abdominal viscera.

Recognition of this injury warrants immediate surgical exploration. With the abdomen open, the bowel is retrieved by gentle traction from above. The surgical objectives are to control hemorrhage from the uterine injury, thoroughly inspect the bowel, repair injuries, and complete the uterine evacuation. In women of reproductive age, hysterectomy is avoided unless uterine preservation poses a significant threat to her health.

RADIATION INJURY

Radiation therapy for gynecologic cancers can cause intestinal injuries that require surgical correction. Also, damage from prior irradiation contributes to complications during other surgical procedures. The intestinal tract is adversely affected by radiation during treatment and soon thereafter (acute injury) or remote from treatment (late injury). The acute phase is associated with small bowel irritability, cramping, and diarrhea, with onset generally 2–3 weeks after initiation of therapy. Injury to the large bowel manifests acutely as proctosigmoiditis, with resultant pain, tenesmus, frequent bow movements, and bleeding. Low residue diet, antispasmodics, and anti-inflammatories are helpful in uncomplicated cases. In more severe cases, debilitating symptoms can adversely affect lifestyle. Intestinal adhesions, fibrosis, obstruction, perforation, abscess, and fistulae are potential late complications.

Surgery in previously irradiated patients warrants special attention and is best performed by those experienced in this regard. Whenever possible, the surgical incision is made in a location beyond the radiation field. Extensive lysis of adhesions is best avoided, and dissection should be confined to the minimum area necessary to complete the surgical objectives. If obstruction occurs, consideration is given to intestinal bypass as opposed to extensive mobilization. Resection is avoided unless the anastomosis can be completed with nonirradiated bowel segments. This objective is often theoretical, because damaged bowel may appear normal and yet have significant microscopic endarteritis and vasculature obliteration. The characteristic pale, thickened bowel wall, telangiectatic vessels, and strictured lumen need not be present to indicate significant radiation injury. If resection is unavoidable, the suture line can be reinforced by wrapping the anastomosis with omentum, which elicits support of exogenous blood supply.

A vesicovaginal or rectovaginal fistula may develop if there is extensive damage to the intervening tissue. The time course of fistula occurrence is usually between 6 months and 24 months after therapy, but it may present years after irradiation. The mechanism of late radiation injuries is believed to be obliterative vascular injury with compromised blood flow and tissue necrosis. Post-irradiation rectovaginal fistulae are complex problems that rarely heal with simple excision, mobilization, and closure, such that they are probably best corrected using a three-staged approach. First, a diverting ileostomy or colostomy is performed to redirect the colonic content, reduce bacterial infiltration, and allow resolution of inflammation. Several months later, the objectives of the second surgery are complete resection of the fistulous tract and surrounding damaged tissue plus neovascularization via an omental flap or myocutaneous graft. The goal of the eventual third surgery is reversal of the diverting ostomy to re-establish normal intestinal continuity.

POSTOPERATIVE CONSIDERATIONS

Some surgeons use routine postoperative nasogastric decompression to reduce nausea, vomiting, and abdominal distention and to enable healing of bowel anastomoses. These prophylactic objectives differ from the therapeutic goals of nasogastric decompression used to alleviate symptoms and expedite recovery from an existing ileus or small bowel obstruction. The literature, however, does not support routine postoperative use. Nasogastric tubes increase patient discomfort and increase the risk of occurrence of sinus infections and epistaxis. A meta-analysis of selective versus routine nasogastric decompression after elective laparotomy included 26 trials and 3,964 patients. Routine postoperative decompression was associated with an increased incidence of pneumonia, atelectasis, and fever. Abdominal distention and vomiting were increased in selectively treated patients who did not have nasogastric tubes, and eventual tube insertion was required in 5–7% of patients in this group. Nasogastric tube reinsertion was required in 2% of routinely decompressed patients. There was no significant difference in the occurrence of wound infections, wound dehiscence, or anastomotic leaks. The authors of this analysis concluded that, through the selective use of nasogastric decompression, only 1 in 20 patients require a nasogastric tube.

Early Postoperative Oral Feeding

There is a wide spectrum of practice patterns among surgeons regarding postoperative diet. For many decades, the conventional approach has been to wait for auscultation of bowel sounds before providing clear liquids and to wait for the occurrence of flatus before giving solid food. Inpatient managed care pressures and successful outpatient recovery following laparoscopic procedures have challenged clinicians to re-evaluate traditional postoperative feeding regimens. Current trends are toward much more aggressive early postoperative feeding, even in the setting of bowel resection and anastomosis. Some RCTs have shown early feeding to be associated with increased frequency of nausea and vomiting, whereas others have shown no difference. The overall rates of ileus, anastomotic complications, and times required for return of bowel function are generally comparable. Early postoperative feeding, however, has not consistently resulted in shorter average length of hospital stay.

Supplemental Nutrition

Perioperative nutritional support is indicated in patients who have been without nutrition for more than 7 days, in patients who are malnourished (weight loss exceeds 15% of usual weight), and when expected duration of recovery is longer than 10 days. TPN has extended the lives of numerous surgical patients and enabled the resumption of normal lifestyle in many.

Long-term parenteral nutrition, however, has morbidity that is not insignificant. The need for indwelling central venous access puts patients at risk for catheter sepsis and other catheter-related complications. Metabolic derangements and pancreatic or hepatic dysfunction are common. Intestinal mucosal atrophy results from nonuse in patients who are reliant solely upon parenteral nutrition.

Use of the gut for nutrition is advisable whenever possible. The advantages of enteral tube feeding over TPN include no requirement for venous access, enhanced intestinal lymphatic function, reversal of mucosal atrophy, decreased risk of bacterial translocation, and stimulation of intestinal adaptation. Adaptation is the process whereby the villous height and crypt depth increase, with gradual bowel dilation and lengthening, resulting in increased absorptive surface area. Enteral feeding is not indicated in patients with a nonfunctional intestinal tract or intestinal obstruction, or in those at high risk for aspiration.

Acute Gastric Distention

Acute gastric distention results from inhibition of gastric peristalsis. Postoperative gastric distention more commonly occurs after surgical manipulation in the vicinity of the stomach. Patients at increased risk are those who are diabetic, elderly, or medically debilitated. Short-term postoperative nasogastric decompression can prevent and manage this problem in those who are at high risk. Stimulatory agents such as metoclopramide may expedite gastric emptying in the nonobstructed patient.

Ileus

Postoperative ileus is a mechanical dysfunction in which the normal anterograde GI peristalsis is disrupted. Ileus may involve any segment of the digestive tract, including the stomach, small bowel, or colon. In fact, ileus is most frequently a large bowel dysfunction, in that the colon is generally the last segment in the GI tract to regain function after pelvic surgery. Postoperatively, the stomach and small intestine usually resume activity within 8 hours. At times, active small bowel peristalsis is noted at the conclusion of even complex abdominal procedures. In contrast, the colon may take 48–72 hours to regain function. Colonic dysfunction generally resolves from proximal to distal, such that rectosigmoid activity is the last to return.

Factors that predispose to ileus or worsen the severity of ileus include dehydration, electrolyte abnormalities, diabetes, long-term laxative use, bowel manipulation during surgery, extensive retroperitoneal dissection, general anesthetic agents, narcotic analgesics, immobility, urinary or GI leak, peritonitis, abscess, and hematoma. Some degree of adynamic ileus results from all intra-abdominal procedures. With return of bowel function, peristaltic pains are often severe, such that many patients describe them as being worse than surgical pain. Normal recovery of bowel function is evident by gradual increase in appetite, tolerance of oral nutrition, and flatus.

Significant delay in bowel function associated with worsening gas pains, nausea, and vomiting is suggestive of clinically significant ileus. Physical examination confirms abdominal distention with diffuse discomfort, hypoactive bowel sounds, and tympanic percussion. Correction of contributing factors and supportive care

are the cornerstones of management. Therapeutic interventions include bowel rest, IV hydration, correction of electrolytes (i.e. potassium, sodium, and magnesium), physical activity, and judicious use of narcotic analgesia. If good bowel sounds for 24 hours or more suggest that colonic dysfunction is a predominant underlying factor, transrectal colonic stimulation (e.g. docusate sodium or stimulating enema) may be helpful. Patients with vomiting, those not responding to supportive measures, and those with evidence of gastric or small bowel dilatations on X-ray study benefit from nasogastric decompression. Decompression is generally continued until flatus ensues and abdominal distention resolves.

Adynamic ileus must be distinguished from a mechanical small bowel obstruction. If the patient has not passed flatus within 4–5 days or does not respond to conservative measures, then the possibility of a mechanical small bowel obstruction should be considered. Early in the disease process, radiographs may provide little assistance in clarifying the diagnosis because the changes of postoperative ileus and early obstruction are similar. However, after 3–5 days, plain abdominal radiographs with supine, upright, and/or lateral recumbent views will help distinguish ileus from mechanical small bowel obstruction. The typical radiographic pattern of an ileus is that of intermittent air found throughout the GI tract, including the colon and rectum. Upright views may show air-fluid levels within the small bowel and stomach, and, occassionally, the transverse colon. In contrast, radiographic characteristics of mechanical small bowel obstruction include proximal distended loops with a paucity or absence of gas in the colon. The dilated small bowel loops with air-fluid levels may follow a stair-step pattern from the right lower quadrant to the left upper quadrant in parallel with the anatomic base of the small bowel mesentery.

With intermittent or partial small bowel obstruction, some gas is seen in the colon. Conversely, if the obstruction is in the proximal small bowel, there may be no distended loops at all. Radiographic studies can at times clarify the type of obstruction (mechanical vs. nonmechanical), the extent of obstruction (partial vs. complete), and the location of obstruction (stomach vs. small bowel vs. colon). If the diagnosis remains unclear, a water-soluble contrasted GI study with small bowel follow-through can clarify the situation and localize the point of obstruction if present. Contrast material may also stimulate peristalsis and has been reportedly therapeutic in some cases of paralytic ileus.

Small Bowel Obstruction

Intraperitoneal adhesions is the most common etiology of intestinal obstruction. Malignancies and hernias are also frequent extrinsic causes. An estimated 85% of all small bowel obstructions are secondary to one of these three conditions.

Intraluminal causes include tumors, polyps, gallstones, and bezoars. Obstructive intramural strictures can complicate irradiation or inflammatory bowel disease.

Early postoperative obstruction deserves a trial of nonsurgical management. Nasogastric decompression, supportive care, and correction of underlying contributing factors are as described for adynamic ileus. Supine position with legs flexed helps relax rectus abdominus muscles to facilitate examination. Early in the course of obstruction, there may be minimal to absent distention. Proximal obstruction may also manifest with minimal abdominal distention. High-pitched bowel sounds with metallic tones and rushes are suggestive of an obstructive process. Hypoactive or absent bowel sounds are more suggestive of paralytic ileus. Hypoactive bowel sounds may also occur with intestinal fatigue from long-standing obstruction, closed loop obstruction, or pseudo-obstruction. Fewer than half of obstructed patients manifest the classic triad of rebound tenderness, guarding, and rigidity. Also, the physical findings of focal tenderness and guarding are neither sensitive nor specific in confirming underlying obstruction or ischemia.

The duration of asymptomatic intervals between peristaltic pains may suggest the level of obstruction. Peristaltic waves tend to be 3–5 minutes apart in high obstruction, whereas in distal obstruction, 10–15 minutes may lapse between episodes.

Radiographically, small bowel distended by gas outlines the valvulae conniventes (plicae circulares), which traverse the entire diameter of the dilated bowel lumen. Valvulae conniventes are closely spaced and may appear to interdigitate. In contrast, distended colon highlights the haustra, which partially traverse the bowel lumen and are spaced more widely apart.

The central abdomen is occupied by distended small bowel loops, whereas the abdominal periphery houses the colon. In the decompressed patient, character of gastric aspirate suggests the potential anatomic site of obstruction. Gastric outlet obstruction produces clear gastric secretions. Bilious output is suggestive of obstruction in the proximal to mid small bowel, or a colonic obstruction with a competent ileocecal valve. Feculent drainage is characteristic of a distal small bowel obstruction, or colonic obstruction with an incompetent ileocecal valve. Intestinal obstruction leads to an accumulation of intraluminal fluid and gas with distention proximal to the occlusion. It is estimated that more than 70% of air in the GI tract is from swallowing. Accordingly, distention is significantly worsened by swallowed air. With progressing distention comes tension and venous compression. Arterial inflow continues, resulting in blood accumulation within the bowel wall and lumen. Protein-rich fluid exudes from the capillaries, adding to tissue edema. Malabsorption combined with intestinal secretion further exacerbates intraluminal fluid collection.

In the setting of complete obstruction, up to 7–8 L of fluid can accumulate, including 50% of plasma volume and 30% of circulating blood volume. Mucosal integrity is disrupted and enteric bacteria traverse the defective bowel wall, seeding the peritoneum. If the process goes uncorrected, intestinal viability is irreversibly damaged as tissue necrosis ensues.

If a decision is made for operative intervention, preparation concentrates on correction of hypovolemia, anemia, and electrolyte imbalances. Broad-spectrum antibiotics may suppress bacterial translocation and delay intestinal ischemia. Upon exploration, the point of obstruction is identified and corrected. All necrotic bowel must be resected. It is not always possible, however, to discern the viability of bowel in the setting of obstruction. Visible characteristics such as tissue color, extent of edema, and peristalsis are not consistently reliable. Active bleeding from the cut bowel edge is a more accurate indicator. Intraoperative Doppler testing of the antimesenteric border should provide characteristic arterial pulsations. Absent Doppler sounds do not necessarily indicate inadequate arterial blood flow. In this setting, viability can be confirmed by IV 10% fluorescein (15 mg/kg), followed in 10 minutes by Wood's lamp illumination. Observation of bowel wall fluorescence suggests adequate blood flow to support anastomotic healing. Bowel segments that are less than 2 cm in diameter with no fluorescence can be preserved, but should not be included in the anastomosis. Larger areas of non-fluorescence suggest ischemia and likely require resection.

Large Bowel Obstruction

The vast majority of large bowel obstructions are due to malignancy or inflammatory conditions. This is in contrast to small bowel obstructions for which adhesions are the principal etiology. The gynecologic surgeon may encounter large bowel obstruction from a primary colon or a gynecologic malignancy, ulcerative colitis, diverticular disease, pelvis abscess, or radiation injury. The onset of most colonic obstructions is insidious because of gradual luminal narrowing, which manifests clinically as decreased caliber stools, constipation, and bleeding. Progressive obstruction leads to obstipation, abdominal distention, colicky pain, nausea, and vomiting. Radiographic studies reveal a dilated colon proximal to the point of obstruction. If the ileocecal valve is incompetent, the distention extends proximally into the small bowel as evident by dilated bowel loops with air-fluid levels. A more serious closed loop obstruction occurs when the ileocecal valve is competent. The cecum is commonly involved, and, as cecal dilation exceeds 10–12 cm, the risk of perforation increases significantly. Preoperative endoscopy or water-soluble contrast study can clarify the etiology and location of obstruction.

Barium enema should not be performed in the setting of acute obstruction or suspected perforation to avoid barium peritonitis. If necessary, any viable segment of large bowel proximal to the point of obstruction can be exteriorized as a colostomy.

Ogilvie's syndrome (acute colonic pseudo-obstruction) is a dysfunction of colonic peristalsis. Clinical presentation may be indistinguishable from a large bowel obstruction. The mechanism of colonic pseudo-obstruction is theorized to be an imbalance between the proximal and distal colonic innervation. Parasympathetic innervation from the vagus nerve supplies the colon proximal to the splenic flexure. In contrast, the left colon receives parasympathetic innervation from the sacral plexus (S2 to S4). Most commonly, only the right colon is dilated. Ogilvie's syndrome is seen more commonly in elderly and debilitated patients and in those who are on narcotics and phenothiazine or tricyclic antidepressants. Supportive care includes hydration, correction of electrolyte abnormalities, and GI decompression (nasogastric tube, rectal tube). Sequential radiographs are used to monitor cecal dilation to assess the risk of perforation. Endoscopic decompression or tube cecostomy are preferred alternatives to exploration, because surgical morbidity is significant. If necessary, intraoperative colonic decompression can be accomplished using an 18-gauge needle passed obliquely through the *Taenia coli* and attached to suction. Decompression facilitates exteriorization of the bowel for diverting colostomy.

Fistulae

Postoperative intestinal fistulae are an especially challenging problem for patients and clinicians. An enterocutaneous or enterovaginal fistula may be difficult to confirm, even when clinical findings are strongly suggestive of a fistulous communication. The high-pressure bowel defect may be small with only intermittent drainage, thus obscuring localization. Oral administration of charcoal or of brilliant blue or carmine red dye confirms the diagnosis if characteristic color change is observed in the effluent. Clarification of the fistulous tract can be aided by a fistulogram. Contrast material is injected transcutaneously, and the pattern of flow is evaluated radiographically. Excessive force during injection is avoided to prevent dislodgment of the bowel from its adherence to the abdominal or vaginal wall. Initial nonoperative management of fistulae in selected cases has gained wide acceptance. The fundamentals of conservative management include correction of underlying inflammatory processes and electrolyte abnormalities, nutritional support, and maintenance of adequate hydration. The more proximal the fistula, the greater the potential for physiologic derangements, and they are less likely to close spontaneously with conservative management. Gastric, duodenal, and proximal jejunal fistulae can cause potentially fatal physiologic disturbances and thus require prompt intervention. Distal ileal or colonic fistulae are generally well tolerated and tend to close spontaneously if predisposing factors are circumvented. There must be no abscess, peritonitis, distal bowel obstruction, or foreign body within the fistulous tract. Prior irradiation is likely to preclude spontaneous healing.

Approximately two-thirds of distal fistulae are expected to heal within 6 weeks if no complicating factors persist. A fistula that persists beyond 6 weeks is unlikely to heal without operative intervention. Depending on the clinical situation, it may be reasonable to wait an additional 1-2 months to optimize nutritional status and allow for resolution of inflammation.

The appropriate time for surgical intervention must be individualized. The surgical objectives are to completely excise the fistulous tract and resect the affected bowel segment whenever possible. In certain circumstances, such as irradiated bowel or extensive adhesions, the fistula could be more aptly addressed by bypassing the diseased area.

Dehiscence and Evisceration

Surgical steps are shown in Figures 7 to 10.

Dehiscence implies postoperative wound separation and most commonly involves only the skin and subcutaneous tissue (superficial or incomplete dehiscence). Complete (deep) wound dehiscence refers to separation of the fascia and usually manifests with skin and subcutaneous disruption as well. Fascial disruption generally occurs between the 5th and 10th postoperative day, and is estimated to occur in approximately 1 in 200 high-risk patients. Complete dehiscence is most frequently associated with suture tearing through the tissue and is suspected in the setting of copious serous or serosanguineous drainage from the abdominal wound. The incision is explored with a sterile swab or gloved finger to assess for fascial defects. A small defect (1-2 cm) in an otherwise intact fascia with no associated bowel extrusion may be reapproximated with an interrupted fascial suture. Larger fascial defects and all defects with bowel herniation (evisceration) require immediate surgical attention.

Evisceration is an acute full-thickness wound disruption through which abdominal contents extrude and most commonly includes loops of distal small bowel and omentum. Evisceration is rare following laparoscopic procedures but should be suspected with a palpable or visible hernial defect and serosanguineous fluid drainage. Concomitant problems may include abnormal bowel function, nausea, vomiting, or evidence of bowel incarceration. CT and ultrasound (USG) imaging are useful if the diagnosis is uncertain. In preparing the eviscerated patient for surgery, she is kept in supine position and the

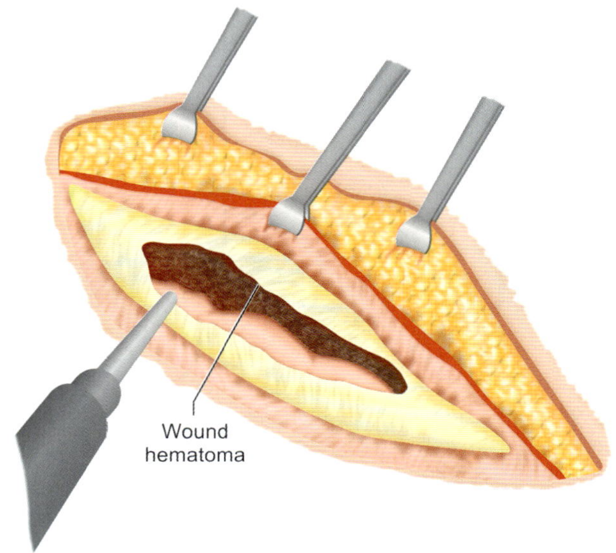

Fig. 7: The preparation and sterile draping of the abdomen, staples and sutures are removed, thereby permitting easy separation of previous incision and access to the peritoneal cavity inspection should help identify the etiology of the dehiscence and residual suture material should be removed. A hematoma should be evacuated and the wound carefully irrigated with several of saline followed by an antibiotic solution. If the peritoneal cavity is open, it should also be irrigated copiously with antibiotics

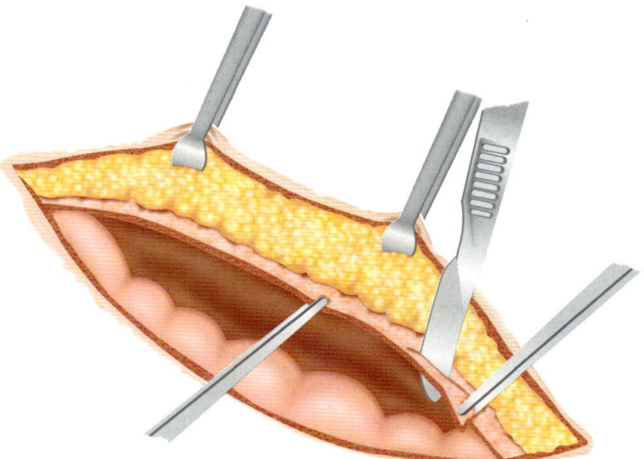

Fig. 8: The fascial edges should be freshened with a knife or scissors along the full length of the dehiscence

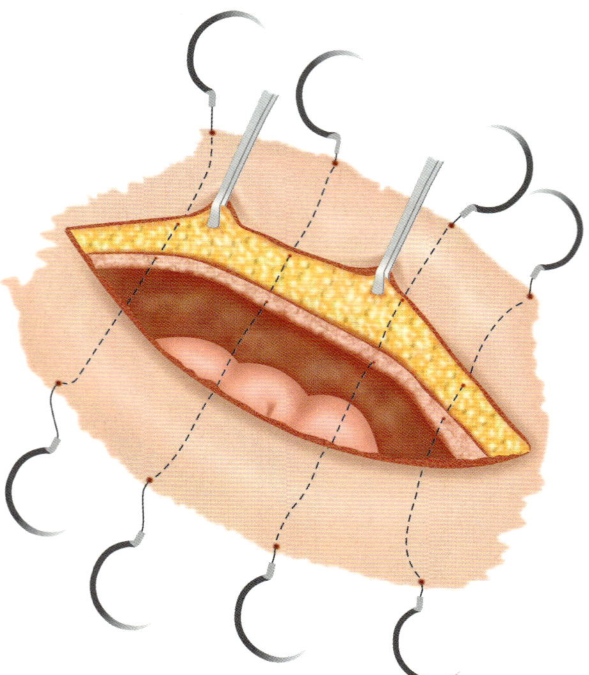

Fig. 9: Number 2 nylon or prolene retention sutures should be placed approximately 2-inch intervals 3–4 cm from the wound edge and through-and-through all abdominal wall layers

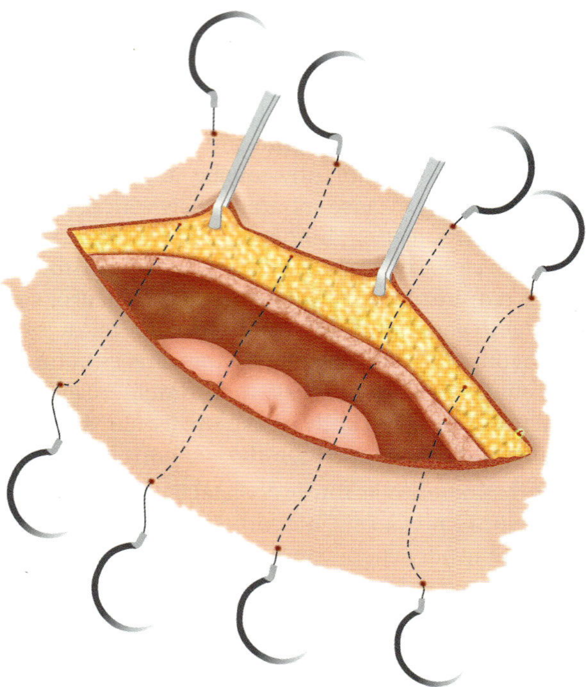

Fig. 10: The fascia then should be approximated with interrupted 0 nylon or prolene sutures placed a full centimeter from the fascial edge. If the fascial closure is under excessive tension, that closure can be reinforced with either absorbable or nonabsorbable mesh. The former is preferred when needed to reinforce the abdominal wall in the presence of infection as the risk of a foreign induced infection will be lower than with nonabsorbable mesh

exposed bowel is covered with towels moistened by sterile saline or povidone-iodine solution. If accomplished without difficulty, eviscerated organs should be cautiously replaced back into the abdomen. The protective towels can be secured using a sterile plastic drape and reinforced with an abdominal binder. Broad-spectrum antibiotics are administered, and steps are taken to correct fluid and electrolyte abnormalities. Sedatives and analgesics can reduce intraperitoneal pressure. Intraoperatively, all layers of the wound are inspected for infection, and devitalized abdominal wall tissue is sharply debrided. The bowel and mesentery are inspected for injury, viability, hemostasis, and obstruction, and the peritoneal contents are copiously irrigated. Bowel resection is generally not necessary, but it may be required if obstruction or ischemia is present.

Vaginal Evisceration

Protrusion of viscera through the vagina has been reported in association with surgery, enterocele, trauma, Valsalva maneuver, coitus, radiation, and foreign bodies. Small bowel and mesentery are most commonly involved, but evisceration may also include large bowel and omentum. Approximately two-thirds of reported cases have occurred in patients with a history of prior surgery for pelvic relaxation or in the setting of symptomatic enterocele. Prior hysterectomy is a factor in only half of reported cases. This distressing situation tends to occur outside hospital setting and bacterial contamination is inevitable. Severe abdominal pain may indicate mesenteric compromise. Surgical preparation is similar to that for an abdominal evisceration, but in contrast, it is probably best to resist preoperative attempts at replacing the bowel transvaginally. Surgical management should be via exploratory laparotomy. During exploration, the eviscerated contents are replaced into the peritoneal cavity with a combination of gentle traction from above and guidance from below. Copious intraperitoneal irrigation and broad-spectrum antibiotics are used. Careful inspection of the bowel and mesentery are necessary to identify and repair injuries and to ensure viability. Severely damaged or obstructed bowel requires resection.

Short Bowel Syndrome

Short bowel syndrome results from loss of significant bowel length or inadequate function of normal length bowel. The net result is insufficient nutrient absorption necessary to meet the body's metabolic requirements.

Causes include extensive surgical resection, regional enteritis (Crohn's disease), and radiation injury. In women, the average length of small bowel is approximately 600 cm (range 350–700 cm). In general, 50% of the small bowel can be resected without long-term impairment of nutritional status, as long as there is normal function in the remainder of the bowel. Severe nutritional deficiencies will likely result with loss of two-thirds to three-fourths of the small intestine. Malabsorption manifest as diarrhea, dehydration, weight loss, metabolic derangement, protein and nutrient deficiencies, and anemia (iron, folate, and B_{12} deficiencies). After undergoing an intestinal resection, the remaining small bowel has adaptation capacity that begins a few weeks postoperatively and maximizes by approximately 24 months.

Compensatory adaptation is via mucosal hypertrophy with increased villus height and crypt depth. Eventually, surface area and transit time are also increased through gradual dilation and lengthening of the bowel. Enteral feeding is an important stimulus for intestinal adaptation, and use of the gut for nutrition is encouraged whenever possible. Medical management of short bowel syndrome depends on the locations of abnormalities and the severity of resultant problems. Dehydration, electrolyte abnormalities, and specific nutrient deficiencies are corrected as needed. Therapy includes histamine (H_2) blockers to reduce gastric secretions and antimotility agents, which improve absorption via increased transit time and reduced diarrhea. Broad-spectrum antibiotics may be beneficial in patients with enteric bacterial overgrowth and translocation.

Surgical therapy for short bowel syndrome begins with pre-emptive planning. A concerted effort is made to preserve as much small bowel and colon as possible at the time of any surgical resection. Whenever reasonable, therapeutic surgical procedures should be delayed until after the period of intestinal adaptation. Operative maneuvers designed to increase transit time and absorption includes stricturoplasty, tapering, serosal patching, and interposing of a colonic segment or antiperistaltic small bowel segment. Additional long-term sequelae of short bowel syndrome include gallstones in 50% of patients. Accordingly, some surgeons advocate prophylactic cholecystectomy.

Hernias

Ventral or incisional hernias occur subsequent to 1% of gynecologic surgeries. Abdominal viscera are encased by a peritoneum-lined hernia sac, which protrudes through a fascial defect. The overlying skin and subcutaneous tissue remain intact. Patients tend to describe an insidious onset of abdominal fullness or pressure and often notice a focal area of distention. Symptoms generally worsen with prolonged standing and physical activity, and lessens at rest. Hernias that reduce spontaneously and those easily reduced manually can be managed without surgery. Any suspicion of bowel obstruction, incarceration, strangulation, or necrosis requires immediate surgical evaluation. The surgical objectives are to isolate and resect the hernia sac, reduce the sac contents, lyse pertinent adhesions, and inspect the viscera to ensure GI integrity. Resection may be necessary to alleviate intestinal obstruction or remove severely damaged bowel. Before closure, steps are taken to acquire hemostasis, control infection, excise pre-existing scar tissue, and mobilize the abdominal wall to enable a tension-free fascial approximation.

General Principles

Numerous variations exist on bowel resection and anastomotic techniques. Discussed in this text are some of the more commonly used methods, instruments, and materials. This review is by no means exhaustive given the vast array of reported options on this theme. Strict adherence to the fundamental principles of anastomosis is more important to successful healing than are the specific techniques or materials used (Box 1). Broad categories for consideration include whether to use open or closed technique and whether to use hand-sewn or staple closure. Anastomotic communication can be established via an end-to-end, side-to-side, or end-to-side alignment. Hand-sewn closure may be effectively accomplished using one or two layers of absorbable or permanent suture via continuous or interrupted methods. Additionally, specific suturing techniques (i.e. Lembert, Connell) can be selected. Staple anastomoses have largely replaced hand-sewn techniques. Technical ease and equivalent to superior results are among the potential advantages of stapling methods (Box 2). An overview of selected surgical procedures in this chapter includes hand-sewn and staple techniques, with a focus on modern surgical stapling. A more expansive discussion of hand-sewn maneuvers is found in the seventh edition of TeLinde's Operative Gynecology.

Familiarity with open and closed anastomotic techniques provides the surgeon with a choice of repairs and facilitates intraoperative decision making. Open techniques (bowel lumens exposed) have gradually replaced closed techniques (lumens occluded) in most circumstances. Morbidity associated with open techniques is acceptably low. The extent of intraperitoneal spill can generally be controlled with aggressive preoperative bowel preparation and atraumatic bowel clamps. Closed techniques are potentially advantageous in reducing complications from unprepped bowel or reanastomosis involving the colon.

Angiogenesis at the anastomotic margins begins within the first 72 hours of surgery if not impeded by

Box 1 General principles of intestinal anastomosis

Intestinal anastomosis should:

- Be tension free
- Avoid intraperitoneal spill of gastrointestinal (GI) content
- Incorporate healthy tissue in the proximal and distal segments
- Preserve adequate lumen
- Be hemostatic and watertight or airtight
- Be completed under optimal surgical exposure
- Preserve maximum amount of normal bowel
- Invert the tissue edges
- Incorporate the submucosa, which is the strongest layer
- Include bowel segments of the same diameter
- Be performed in an infection free tissue bed
- Not be done with an uncorrected obstruction or fistula

Box 2 Staple techniques

Advantages

- Better blood flow and oxygen delivery across the anastomotic line
- Less operative time required
- Uniform staple placement is an inherent design of surgical staplers
- Less luminal narrowing
- Technically easier to learn and perform in most cases

Disadvantages

- Greater expense with stapling instruments
- Everted tissue edges using some techniques
- Dependence on equipment that could malfunction
- Staple lines may be less resistant to tension injury
- Technically difficult to align the surgical staplers in some anatomic locations
- Not be done with an uncorrected obstruction or fistula

infection or inflammation. The most important strength layer of the bowel wall is the submucosa, which must be incorporated into any anastomosis. Collagen is believed to be the single most important contributor to submucosal strength. The maximum anastomotic bursting pressure reflects the pressure required to disrupt an anastomosis and has been used experimentally to assess the strength of healing. The bursting pressure of an anastomosis increases rapidly during the early postoperative period. Sixty percent of the surrounding bowel wall strength is reached by postoperative day 3–4, and pressure tolerated by the anastomotic site approximates 100% of that tolerated by intact bowel wall by postoperative day 7. The ideal suture material should provide maximum strength during the lag phase of wound healing with minimal tissue reaction and inflammation. Although the perfect suture material is yet to be identified, modern monofilament and coated braided sutures represent progress towards this goal.

Double-layer intestinal closures have long been touted as more secure than single-layer closures. The traditional anastomosis includes a running inner layer of 3-0 chromic cat gut (absorbable) and an interrupted outer layer of 3-0 silk (nonabsorbable). Extensive clinical evidence, however, suggests single-layer closure to be equivalent and may offer some advantages over double layer anastomosis. Comparative animal studies have demonstrated more rapid vascularization and mucosal healing, and greater early anastomotic strength associated with single-layer repair. Double-layer closures, along with traditional sutures such as cat gut and silk, are associated with greater inflammation, reduced microneoangiogenesis, and less blood flow across the anastomosis. A single-layer reapproximation generally causes less narrowing of the intestinal lumen and can be accomplished in less time. When done properly, all hand-sewn techniques result in an inverted suture line.

Either continuous or interrupted closures can be used for intestinal anastomosis. Continuous technique is rapid and has the potential advantage of a more even tension distribution along the suture line. In comparison of running versus interrupted closure, animal studies have also shown reduced tissue oxygen tension, impaired collagen synthesis, and increased anastomotic complications using running closure. To date, however, randomized clinical trials are lacking, and retrospective studies show no consistent benefit of one technique over the other. Clinical and subclinical anastomotic leak rates, associated morbidity, and length of hospitalization are generally equivalent, even for high-risk patients (e.g. patients with prior radiation therapy, malnutrition, carcinomatosis).

SURGERY ON THE SMALL INTESTINE

Blood Supply to the Small Intestine

The small bowel receives its arterial blood supply from the superior mesenteric artery (SMA), which arises from the ventral surface of the abdominal aorta. In addition to the small bowel, the SMA also gives rise to the middle and right colic arteries, which supply those regions of the colon. The most proximal small bowel is supported by the common inferior pancreaticoduodenal artery from the SMA. Arising from the left side of the SMA is a series of jejunal and ileal arteries that branch to form anastomotic arcades. Primary arcades terminate directly into the small bowel via vasa recta or extend to form secondary, tertiary, and quaternary arcades that eventually give rise to terminal vasa recta. Avascular spaces between the vasa recta are known as windows of Deaver. In general, up to 8 cm of small intestine can remain viable distal to the closest vasa recta because of intramural vascular communications.

The ileocolic artery arises from the right side of the SMA and traverses the base of the mesentery to form a loop anastomosis with the SMA in the region of the terminal ileum. This loop encircles an area devoid of vessels known as the avascular space of Treves. The arterial blood supply to the distal ileum is considered tenuous due to a decreased number of vasa recta from only primary vascular arcades. Because of the uncertain vascular status in this area, it is recommended that 10 cm of terminal ileum also be removed during cecal resection to improve the anastomotic blood supply.

Small Bowel Resection

It is important to resect only the length of bowel necessary to adequately address the disease process, thereby sparing as much normal intestine as possible. For benign disease, bowel transection sites are located just proximal and distal to the abnormal segment. Moist laparotomy pads are positioned to isolate the surgical field from the remaining peritoneal contents. At the proposed transection sites, blunt dissection is used to make a small opening through the avascular mesenteric window adjacent to the bowel wall. The staple cartridge half of the gastrointestinal anastomotic (GIA) stapler is passed through the proximal mesenteric defect, perpendicular to the axis of the bowel. The anvil half is placed across the bowel and aligned with the cartridge. This effectively occludes the bowel as the GIA stapler is closed. Proper positioning is confirmed, and the stapler is fired by steady forward motion on the pusher-bar knife assembly. Upon release of the assembly and opening of the GIA handles, two double-staggered staple lines are noted with the intervening bowel transected. The same steps are carried out at the distal site for transection.

For benign disease, the mesenteric resection can be carried out in close proximity to the bowel, with no need to remove an intervening wedge. The objective is to preserve as much intact mesenteric blood supply as possible. The peritoneum overlying the mesentery is opened with cautery. Visual inspection and transillumination help to identify mesenteric vessels, which are clamped, cut, and suture-ligated using 2-0 silk ligatures. Division of the mesentery completes the resection. In preparation for anastomosis, tissue attachments are cleared 5 mm from both stapled bowel edges to avoid incorporation of mesenteric fat.

Staple Anastomosis

Staple end-to-end anastomosis (EEA) in the small bowel is rarely used because of excess narrowing of the lumen. More favorable are the staple side-to-side anastomotic techniques that are functionally likened to an EEA.

Staple end-to-end techniques are more aptly used for anastomosing two segments of large bowel following transverse colectomy or rectosigmoid resection.

The side-to-side, functional end-to-end staple techniques have gained wide acceptance because of the technical ease, availability of reliable instruments, and capacity to join bowel lumens of different diameters. Following resection, the occluded bowel ends are juxtaposed with the antimesenteric edges aligned in parallel along a distance of approximately 8 cm. This alignment is secured by a seromuscular 3-0 silk suture placed at the proximal end. Mayo scissors are used to excise a full-thickness oblique segment from the antimesenteric corner of each staple-occluded bowel segment. The anvil half of the GIA stapler and the cartridge half are inserted into each enterotomy. The stapler is secured into position by closing the lock lever such that the antimesenteric borders are aligned. Proper positioning is confirmed and the instrument is fired by sliding the pusher-bar knife assembly forward, and then returning it to the neutral position. This maneuver delivers two double-staggered staple rows and cuts the intervening bowel walls. The GIA instrument is disengaged and removed.

The resultant enteroenterostomy is inspected to ensure patency, viability, and hemostasis.

The open bowel edges are grasped with Allis clamps, and a linear thoracoabdominal (TA) stapler is placed across the common lumen, ensuring that full-thickness bowel wall is circumferentially elevated above the staple line. After releasing the safety, the TA stapler is fired via steady closing grip on the handles. Excess tissue above the edge of the stapler is excised, and the instrument is released. Luminal capacity is evaluated by transmural palpation between the thumb and index finger, moving in a circular motion to outline the two layers of bowel wall (in contrast to the four palpable layers proximal to the common lumen). Oversewing the staple line is unnecessary unless there is concern regarding the anastomotic integrity.

An open variation of this technique is such that after resection, the ends of the in situ bowel are not occluded. Atraumatic bowel clamps, protective moist laparotomy pads, irrigation, and povidone-iodine-soaked gauze reduce enteric contamination.

The antimesenteric borders are aligned and secured as described above. The anvil half of the GIA stapler is introduced through one open bowel lumen, and the cartridge half is introduced through the other. The GIA stapler is locked and fired along the antimesenteric borders, and the TA stapler is used to close the resultant common enterotomy. These staple techniques are also ideal for joining bowel segments of discordant diameters (i.e. ileocolonic anastomosis). The ileum and colon are aligned and secured in parallel along their antimesenteric borders. An enterotomy and colotomy are made through which the anvil and cartridge halves of the GIA stapler are placed to initiate the anastomosis as described earlier. Proper alignment minimizes the residual large bowel segment that extends beyond the anastomosis, which is at risk for nonfunction and progressive symptomatic dilation (blind loop syndrome).

Side-to-side Staple Anastomosis

Side-to-side techniques are less commonly used than they once were and have largely been replaced by end-to-end or functional end-to-end anastomoses. Nevertheless, side-to-side techniques are an effective means of reanastomosis, and they can be used to bypass an obstructed intestinal segment. Either hand-sewn or staple closure may be used. The antimesenteric borders are aligned, and the bowel segments are overlapped along 8 cm and secured into position such that the stapled bowel edges are at opposite ends of this alignment. Subsequent steps taken for the staple method are as previously described.

End-to-end Hand-sewn Double-layer Anastomosis

In performing an EEA, it is desirable to have adequate and equivalent lumens in both the proximal and distal segments. The diameter of any lumen can be increased by transecting the bowel obliquely or via linear incision along the antimesenteric border (Cheatle slit). Noncrushing linen shod or rubber shod intestinal clamps are placed across the proximal and distal bowel to decrease intestinal spill. The bowel segments and mesenteries are aligned and secured by 3-0 silk seromuscular sutures placed midway between the mesenteric and antimesenteric borders. The traditional two-layer anastomosis includes a running inner layer of 3-0 chromic catgut and an outer layer of interrupted 3-0 silk sutures.

The inner layer is closed first, starting on the mesenteric (posterior) bowel edges and continuing the closure around to incorporate the antimesenteric (anterior) edges. This is best accomplished with a double-arm needle, sewing in both directions. Suturing begins on the mucosal side, passing from in-to-out and then out-to-in, bringing the inverted bowel edges together. Full-thickness tissue bites are initiated approximately 3 mm from the edge and advanced approximately 3 mm between throws. After circumferential closure, the knot is tied toward the lumen and the bowel is rotated 180° to expose the posterior wall. Rotation is facilitated by passing one stay suture through the mesenteric defect, with sustained counterclockwise rotational traction on both stay sutures. Interrupted seromuscular 3-0 silk sutures are placed to complete the mesenteric (posterior) outer layer. The bowel is rotated back 180° into its normal anatomic position, and the anterior outer layer is lastly closed with interrupted silk Lembert sutures. If the bowel cannot be rotated, the mesenteric (posterior) outer segment must be sewn first.

Side-to-side Hand-sewn Anastomosis

For hand-sewn technique, 5 cm length parallel linear enterotomies are made along the antimesenteric borders of each bowel segment. Elevation of the anterior bowel wall with GI forceps, during either sharp or cautery incision, will reduce the likelihood of posterior wall injury. A row of interrupted 3-0 silk sutures are placed in Lembert fashion to join the posterior outer edges of the enterotomies. A running absorbable 3-0 suture is then used on the posterior inner layer sewing toward the surgeon and continuing around to the anterior edges of the enterotomies. A second posterior inner layer suture or a double-arm suture is continued away from the surgeon around the far end of the enterotomies. Suturing is continued along the anterior inner layer using the continuous over-and-over or Connell suture. The two suture ends are tied together across the anastomosis. The final anterior outer layer is placed using interrupted seromuscular sutures of 3-0 silk in Lembert fashion. Stay sutures are secured or removed, and the anastomosis is checked for integrity.

As a modification to the aforementioned procedure, the initial posterior layer of interrupted 3-0 silk Lembert sutures are placed before performing the enterotomies. Silk sutures are placed such that the knots are secured on the outside. Parallel enterotomies are made approximately 4 mm above and below the edges of the suture line. The remaining steps in the anastomosis are completed as described previously.

SURGERY ON THE LARGE INTESTINE

Blood Supply to the Large Intestine

The SMA arises from the abdominal aorta and gives rise to the ileocolic, right colic, and middle colic arteries, which supply the right and transverse portions of the colon. The inferior mesenteric artery (IMA) also arises from the abdominal aorta and gives off the left colic and sigmoid branches, which supply the descending and sigmoid colon. Each of these major vessels divide into numerous smaller branches, forming an anastomotic arcade that communicates from the cecum to the rectum via the marginal artery of Drummond. The marginal artery gives off numerous terminal vasa recta that directly supply the colon. Arterial perfusion is thus preserved to any segment of the colon as long as the marginal artery is not disrupted.

The marginal artery, however, is absent at the hepatic or splenic flexure in 1–2% of the population. This anatomic inconsistency most often affects the left side, such that colon resection in this area should include removal of the splenic flexure. Again noted is the tenuous ileocolic blood supply, such that if the cecum is resected, 10 cm of terminal ileum should also be removed. The rectum derives its oxygenation from the IMA via the superior rectal artery and from the hypogastric artery via the middle and inferior rectal arteries. An elaborate anastomotic lattice with other pelvic vessels encircles the rectum and anus.

Large Bowel Resection

The principles important in large bowel resection and anastomosis are essentially the same as those described previously for the small bowel. Segmental colon resection in gynecologic surgery is most commonly necessary because of malignancy or radiation injury. The gynecologic surgeon may also encounter benign conditions that require resection, such as severe endometriosis, diverticular disease, extensive adhesions, or nonreparable colonic injury. Large bowel resection for benign gynecologic conditions does not require segmental wedge resection of the mesentery. The integrity of the marginal artery is protected when the mesentery is transected close to the bowel wall through the vasa recta.

Mobilization of the Colon

The majority of large bowel resections require some degree of mobilization to ensure a tension-free anastomosis. The general objectives of colon mobilization are to gain retroperitoneal access and transect avascular attachments from the splenic and/or hepatic flexures. If needed, additional mobility is acquired via transecting the gastrocolic ligament. This also provides entry into the lesser omental sac, which facilitates resection of the gastrocolic ligament and infracolic omentum if necessary. Mobilization can be carried out before or after the segmental colon resection, depending on the clinical situation.

To free the right colon, retroperitoneal dissection is initiated at the base of the cecum and continued lateral and parallel to the ascending colon along the white line of Toldt. This is aided by medial traction on the ascending colon. The hepatocystocolic ligament is transected as dissection is carried into Morison's pouch and along the proximal transverse colon. Mobilization of the left colon is initiated at the most distal site of retroperitonealized sigmoid colon, which is usually located at the pelvic brim. With medial retraction on the bowel, a peritoneal incision is made lateral and parallel to the descending colon. Dissection is continued around the splenic flexure as the lienocolic and phrenicocolic ligaments are transected. Excessive traction is avoided to prevent splenic capsule injury. The left lateral portion of the gastrocolic ligament is divided to access the lesser omental sac. This ligament can be completely transected along the transverse colon by dividing the omental vessels. If necessary, division of the gastrocolic ligament is accomplished along the greater curvature of the stomach by dividing the gastroepiploic and short gastric vessels.

End-to-end Staple Anastomosis

Transverse colon resection is used as an illustrative example of this technique. After completing the resection and mobilization of the left and right colon, the proximal and distal bowel edges are brought into close opposition. Their mesenteries are aligned, and seromuscular 3-0 silk sutures are placed, dividing the bowel circumference into equal one-third segments. The mesenteric (posterior) segment of the anastomosis is completed first. Bowel rotation of 180° is facilitated by counterclockwise passage of one stay suture through the mesenteric defect, with continued counterclockwise rotational traction on the adjacent stay suture. Allis clamps are used to lift both full-thickness bowel walls into the noncutting TA stapler. The stapler is positioned such that the staple line extends just beyond the lateral edge of both stay sutures. Steady closing grip secures the device into position. After confirming proper placement, the safety latch is released, and firm closure of the handles fires the staple line. Excess tissue is sharply excised, and the stapler is released.

The bowel is rotated back 180° to its normal anatomic alignment. The two remaining equilateral segments are stapled from the serosal side in similar fashion. Alternatively, if the bowel is not easily rotated, the mesenteric (posterior) segment can be stapled first from the mucosal side. The remaining segments are closed from the serosal side as described earlier. Slight overlap of adjoining staple lines ensures complete closure without hindering anastomotic healing. Adequacy of the lumen, integrity of repair, and hemostasis are confirmed before closing the mesenteric defect.

Sigmoid Resection

The appropriate site for sigmoid transection is identified proximal to the area of diseased bowel. A small mesenteric opening is made adjacent to the colon, through which the GIA cartridge is introduced. The GIA anvil is placed across the bowel, and the stapler is secured and fired, resulting in a transected sigmoid with occluded proximal and distal segments. Moist laparotomy towels are used to pack the proximal segment above the surgical field. The mesenteric peritoneum is opened adjacent to the bowel, and the incision is continued parallel to the sigmoid as the mesentery transitions from a medial to a posterior insertion. Mesenteric vessels are clamped, cut, and secured with 2-0 silk ligatures. The rectovaginal space is opened between the uterosacral ligaments with cautery and sharp dissection. Blunt retroperitoneal dissection between the medial ureter and lateral hypogastric vessels exposes the perirectal space. Entry into the retrorectal space is aided by lifting the transected sigmoid. Retrorectal dissection is carried out to release the rectum from its attachments along the sacrum. Care is taken to avoid laceration of the presacral veins. The uterosacral ligaments are transected to gain exposure toward the distal rectum as the ureters are retracted laterally with a handheld malleable retractor. The rectal stalks are secured by dividing and ligating the posterior portion of the cardinal ligaments.

The extent of required dissection depends on the location and severity of disease. For nonmalignant pathology, dissection below the pelvic peritoneal reflection and levator ani is rarely necessary and may actually disrupt the blood supply. When normal rectum has been isolated below the diseased segment, the sigmoid resection can be finished. Pericolonic tissue attachments are cleared to expose smooth bowel wall. The TA stapler is guided across the rectum, ensuring the staple line incorporates only the rectum. The stapler is locked into position, checked for proper alignment, and fired by firm closure of the handles. Occluding clamps are placed across the bowel just above the staple line, and sharp dissection is used to transect the rectum and complete the resection.

Rectosigmoid End-to-end Staple Anastomosis

Before anastomosis, the descending colon is laid in the pelvis to ensure the colon and rectum can be approximated without tension. Redundant laxity of the colon should be observed. Any resistance or tension indicates the need for additional mobilization. The descending colonic lumen is occluded via an atraumatic clamp and the staple line is sharply excised. The appropriate diameter EEA stapler is selected based on the largest EEA sizer that can be placed into the lumen without undue stretch on the bowel wall. One milligram (one ampule) of IV glucagon causes relaxation of the muscularis and allows more accurate sizing.

Various designs of the EEA stapler exist, but generally the proximal portion consists of an anvil with a spike. An auto pursestring or hand-sewn pursestring is placed circumferentially around the open end of the descending colon. The anvil is positioned within the lumen, and the pursestring is secured around the base of the spike, the tip of which is directed towards the rectal stump. The anus is digitally dilated, and the lubricated shaft of the EEA stapler is introduced transanally. The shaft is visually and manually guided to the apex of the rectal stump. Clockwise rotation of the central wing nut advances the sharp trocar to pierce the apex of the rectal stump. The trocar is removed, leaving the hollow center shaft of the EEA in place through the rectum. The anvil spike from the descending colon is guided into the hollow center shaft of the rectal stump until it locks into place. The central wing nut is further rotated clockwise until the indicator line is readily visible in the indicator window. This rotation draws the rectum and sigmoid colon into direct opposition. Normal anatomic alignment of the mesentery is confirmed. The safety is released, and steady, firm closure of the handles fires the instrument. The handles are released, and the central wing nut is rotated counterclockwise two complete turns. A gentle rocking motion back and forth frees the instrument tip from the anastomosis, as the EEA shaft is slowly withdrawn from the rectum.

The anastomotic integrity is confirmed through a series of checks. First, the staple line is visually and manually inspected.

Second, the EEA instrument is inspected for two complete 360° tissue rings. This confirms circumferential stapling and resection of both the colonic and rectal segments. Third, the pelvis is filled with sterile crystalloid, and a rigid sigmoidoscope is used to insufflate the bowel. Manual occlusion of the proximal sigmoid ensures adequate testing pressure across the anastomosis. The anastomosis is observed while underwater, looking for air bubbles that would indicate an anastomotic leak. Rigid sigmoidoscopy also allows direct internal inspection of the staple line, if necessary.

If any of these methods suggest an incomplete anastomosis, the area in question is reinforced with interrupted 3-0 silk sutures, and the integrity is retested. Care is taken to avoid vascular compromise as the mesenteric defect is closed with interrupted sutures.

Postanastomotic morbidity and symptoms are largely related to the amount of residual rectum at the time of repair. Patients with a high colorectal anastomosis (11 cm or more above the anal verge) have relatively low morbidity and excellent functional results. Those who have undergone a low anastomosis (between 7 cm and 11 cm) have intermediate levels of morbidity, but generally have satisfactory functional results after several months of physiologic adaptation. In contrast, patients with a very low colorectal anastomosis (less than 7 cm from the anal verge) are at highest risk for complications, including anastomotic leak. These patients are also more likely to have chronic symptoms of GI frequency, urgency, and incontinence. The sigmoid J-pouch for rectosigmoid anastomosis provides a reservoir that may decrease the frequency of stools and reduce the incidence of incontinence.

Accordingly, the J-pouch is considered if resection leaves less than 7 cm of rectum and if the colon is redundant enough to allow tension-free pouch construction. Postoperatively, some patients have a sense of incomplete evacuation and require suppositories or enemas.

Anastomotic leak is more common in colorectal anastomoses than in colon-to-colon anastomoses, in part because the rectum has no serosa. In ovarian cancer surgery, the estimated incidence of clinically significant anastomotic leak is 3–5%, but a wide range of this occurrence is reported in the literature. Traditionally, temporary diverting colostomies have been used to protect distal colonic anastomoses. Clinical studies do not support the notion that routine protective colostomies reduce the risk of anastomotic breakdown. However, diversion of the fecal contents may reduce the severity of infectious complications if a leak occurs. Selective colonic diversion may be of benefit in cases of very low rectal anastomosis, prior radiation, unprepared bowel, and abscess or hematoma in the perianastomotic region.

End-to-side Staple Anastomosis

End-to-side anastomotic techniques are advantageous for intestinal closure when the anorectal region is not readily accessible (e.g. supine position) or not necessary to complete the closure (e.g. ileocolonic or high rectosigmoid anastomosis). A high rectosigmoid repair is used for illustrative purposes. Following sigmoid resection, a small colotomy is made 3–4 cm from the end of the descending colon. The EEA instrument is introduced through the open lumen, and the hollow center shaft is advanced through the colostomy. The instrument is positioned such that the tip of the EEA rests perpendicular to bowel wall. A pursestring suture is used to secure the anvil spike within the rectal lumen. The end of the rectum is brought into close proximity with the side of the descending colon as the anvil spike is secured into the EEA hollow center shaft. Clockwise rotation of the central wing nut brings the bowel edges into direct opposition. Rotation is continued until adequate closure is confirmed via the indicator window. The stapler is fired by closing the instrument grips. Counterclockwise rotation of the wing nut, followed by a subtle back and forth rocking motion, frees the instrument from the staple line. The open end of the descending colon is repaired using the TA stapler as previously described, and the integrity of the anastomosis is assessed.

End-to-end Hand-sewn Single-layer Colon Anastomosis

Before the common availability of surgical staplers, intestinal anastomoses were accomplished using hand-sewn techniques. Suture is still preferred over staple repair by some surgeons. Anastomosis can be accomplished using a single layer of delayed absorbable monofilament suture (small or large intestine) or nonabsorbable suture for large bowel (i.e. 4-0 polypropylene). The continuous closure has been proven efficacious in colon-to-colon repair and is used for this illustration. The bowel segments and mesenteric edges are aligned and secured with stay sutures. Suturing begins on the mesenteric (posterior) mucosal edges and is facilitated by a double-arm needle. The running stitch is carried out such that the needle enters near the transected mucosal edge and passes obliquely through the bowel wall to exit the serosa approximately 5 mm from the edge. The needle is passed through the adjoining segment in the same oblique fashion. Sequential tissue bites are placed 2–3 mm apart. This effectively inverts the bowel wall as the running suture is secured. Bidirectional suturing is continued around the corners onto the antimesenteric (anterior) surfaces, which are closed from the serosal side. The Gambee's single-layer technique is an equally effective method that results in end-to-end opposition of bowel edges without puckering the mucosa.

The interrupted single-layer anastomosis has generally been done as a closed technique designed to minimize intraoperative spill of enteric content. This closed technique is infrequently used today, but still plays a role in selected cases of unprepared bowel, especially those involving the colon. A pair of noncrushing clamps is placed across the lumen at both the proximal and distal sites for resection. The bowel is sharply transected between these paired clamps, and the mesenteric resection is completed as previously described. All bowel lumens remain occluded by a surgical clamp. The cut edges are held in close proximity with their respective mesenteries aligned. Interrupted 3-0 silk Lembert sutures are passed full thickness through the bowel wall, being placed approximately 3 mm apart until they encompass the entire circumference. Some surgeons prefer to exclude the mucosa, because this adds no strength and may contribute to local tissue ischemia. Gentle traction and countertraction are applied along the untied sutures to guide the opposing bowel edges together. As the clamps are slowly removed, the sutures are tied. Patency of the lumen is assessed, and any insecure anastomotic areas are reinforced with additional sutures.

COLOSTOMY

A colostomy should include tension-free bowel with noncompromised blood supply. The colon remains viable only about 2 cm beyond the closest intact vasa recta. The abdominal wall aperture must be generous enough to allow easy passage of the bowel with its intact mesentery, because even mild constriction may result in venous congestion, tissue edema, and necrosis. In gynecologic surgery, temporary colonic diversion may be necessary because of severe radiation injury (proctosigmoiditis), distal obstruction, perforation, or fistula. Permanent colostomy may be required if the rectum has been completely resected or is unacceptable for anastomosis. A diverting colostomy can also provide emergent decompression in the setting of complete large bowel obstruction at risk for perforation.

Perioperative Considerations

Preoperative consultation with an enterostomal therapist is very important in the perioperative planning and care. Counseling sessions, reading materials, support groups, and contact with other ostomy patients provide educational and emotional benefit. In nonemergent cases, the stoma appliance can be worn preoperatively to determine appropriate positioning and clarify postoperative expectations. The stoma should be located in an area that is easily seen and reached by the patient. The tentative stoma site is marked preoperatively with indelible ink. As a general guide, a line is drawn connecting the anterior-superior iliac spine to the umbilicus, and the colostomy is exteriorized through the rectus muscles at some point along this line. Placement is avoided within skin folds, surgical scars, and the umbilicus because the appliance will not seal securely with these skin irregularities.

Postoperatively, the enterostomal therapist can assist in teaching the patient independent ostomy care. Daily inspection is important to ensure tissue viability, adequate function, and nonretraction of the stoma. If tissue viability is in question, closer investigation under bright light is warranted. Insertion of a glass test tube or syringe with penlight transillumination allows for an easy bedside inspection of the internal bowel wall. If tissue viability remains uncertain, an anoscope or sigmoidoscope can be used. Focal ischemia is suggested if the mucosa is grey or dusky in appearance. Tissue necrosis distal to the skin edge may be safely observed and re-evaluated after tissue sloughing and re-epithelialization have occurred. Surgical correction is generally unnecessary in this setting. Deeper and more extensive necrosis indicates compromised blood flow and the need for colostomy revision. Excessive retraction, stricture, or peristomal herniation may also require surgical correction.

Some patients with an end sigmoid or descending colostomy prefer irrigation management over a collection appliance. Motivation, capacity for self-care, and relatively normal preoperative bowel function are requisite. Irrigation is started early in the postoperative period and is continued on a daily basis thereafter. The eventual goal is fecal continence between irrigations. Irrigation can also help reduce stoma odor and flatus, which can be further suppressed with a charcoal-based stoma cap. Some patients will develop predictable evacuation patterns such that irrigation is eventually not required. Others will be satisfied with the security of a continuous appliance.

End Colostomy Technique (Figs 11 to 21)

Efforts are made to create the stoma at the site marked on the abdominal wall preoperatively. The bowel selected for use should be adequately mobilized so the distal end can be brought beyond the abdominal wall by several centimeters. To fashion the abdominal wall aperture, a 3 cm diameter circle is drawn on the skin at the marked site. Symmetry is aided by a circular guide such as the flat, round end of a 60 cc syringe plunger. Dissection is carried through the skin and subcutaneous tissue to the level of the rectus fascia. A core of subcutaneous adipose tissue is not necessarily removed. Cruciate incisions are made in the anterior rectus sheath, with each incision being approximately 4 cm in length. The rectus muscle fibers are bluntly separated until the posterior rectus sheath and peritoneum are reached, through which similar cruciate incisions are made. When separating the rectus abdominus muscle, care is taken to avoid injury of the

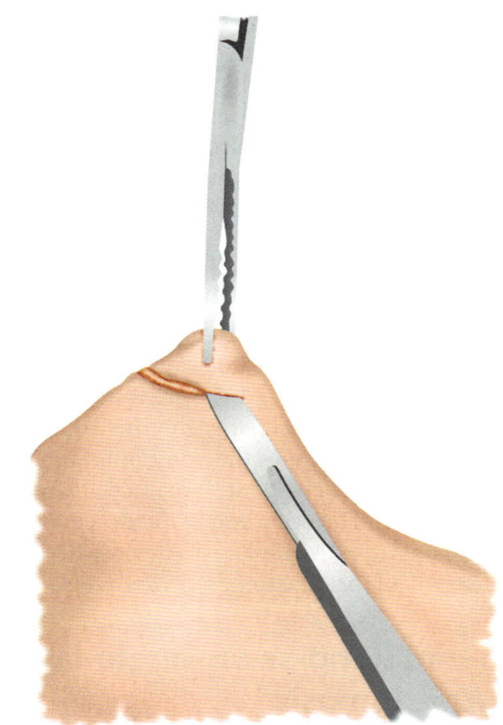

Fig. 11: The site selected for the colostomy is grasped with a Kocher clamp and excised, leaving a circular skin defect with a diameter of 3 cm

inferior epigastric vessels. All layers of the abdominal aperture are manually dilated and should easily admit three fingers without stricture.

A Babcock clamp is inserted through the aperture to grasp the colon for exteriorization. The bowel is brought through the abdominal wall, such that the occluded end rests easily above the skin surface without tension. Large epiploic appendices can be removed with electrocautery if needed to ease exteriorization. Tissue viability is assessed to ensure noncompromised blood flow. Interrupted

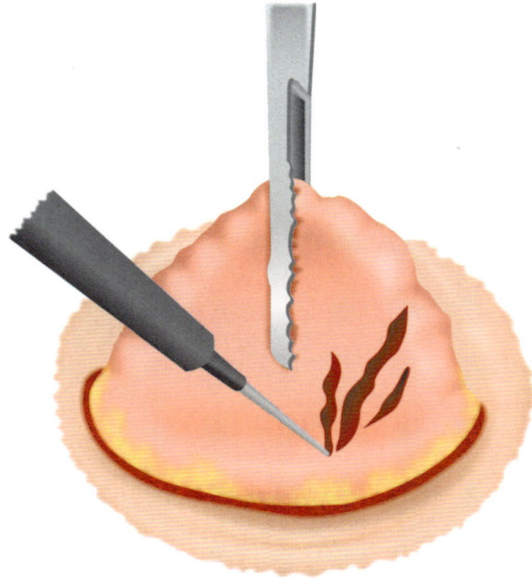

Fig. 12: The subcutaneous tissue is grasped with a Kocher clamp and is cored out to the level of the anterior rectus fascia using electrocautery

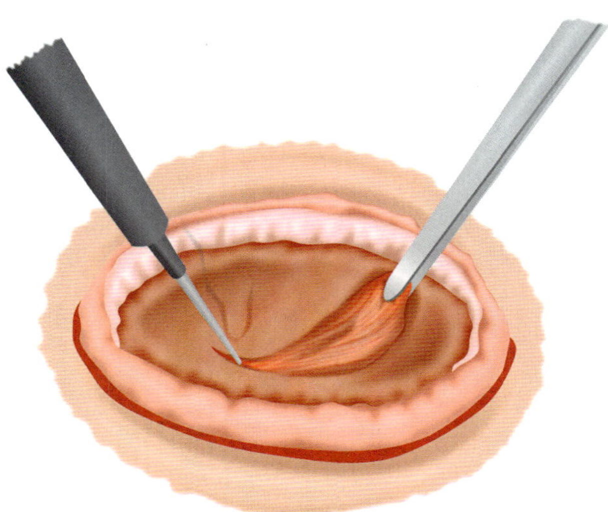

Fig. 13: The anterior rectus fascia is excised as 2–3 cm disc, exposing the rectus muscle below it

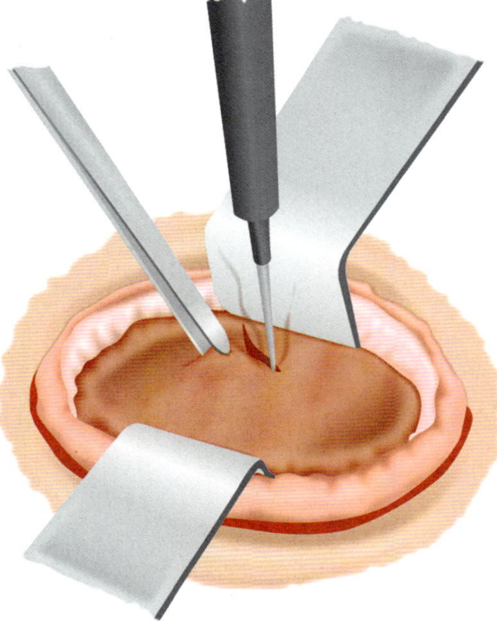

Fig. 14: The rectus muscle is separated bluntly with retractors, exposing the posterior rectus fascia, which is incised with scissors or electrocautery to provide entrance into the peritoneal cavity

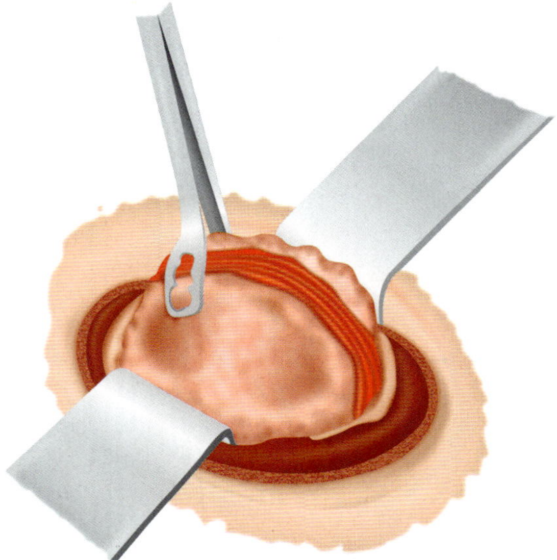

Fig. 15: The transverse colon is identified by its longitudinal taenia omental attachment and is gently pulled through the abdominal incision with a Babcock clamp

3-0 silk seromuscular sutures are fixed to the posterior and anterior rectus sheaths to secure the alignment and reduce the chance of retraction or herniation. The lateral pericolic gutter is obliterated to prevent small bowel herniation. Maturation of the stoma is deferred until after the abdomen is closed.

Any remaining surgical objectives are completed, and the peritoneal cavity is irrigated and checked for hemostasis. The intra-abdominal and extra-abdominal bowel are again inspected before closing the surgical wound. After closure, the incision is protected with collodion or sterile towels. The exteriorized colon is opened, and the cut edges are observed for bleeding to ensure viability. Excessive bowel is trimmed such that approximately 2–3 cm remain above the skin surface. If viability is questionable, the edges are trimmed further until adequate blood flow is confirmed.

The stoma is matured using interrupted delayed absorbable sutures (3-0 polyglycolic acid). Stitches are initiated at the skin surface and carried in and out through

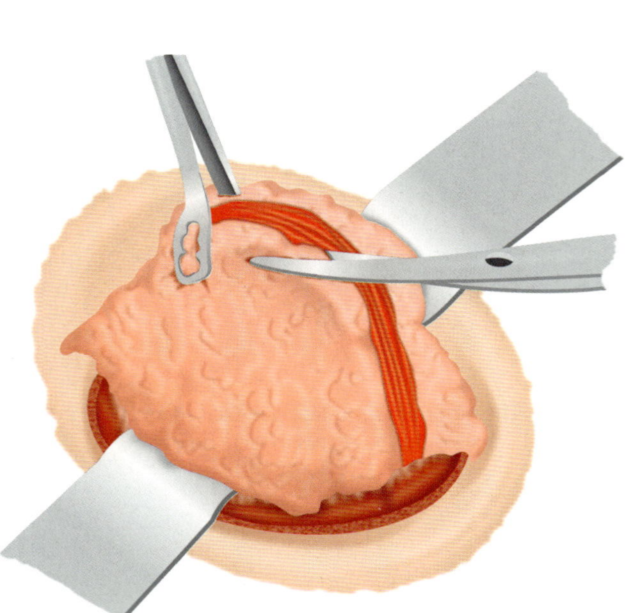

Fig. 16: The adherent omentum is dissected off the anterior aspect of the transverse colon, thereby exposing the transverse mesocolon dissection is easily accomplished without bleeding as the omental attachment to the transverse colon is avascular

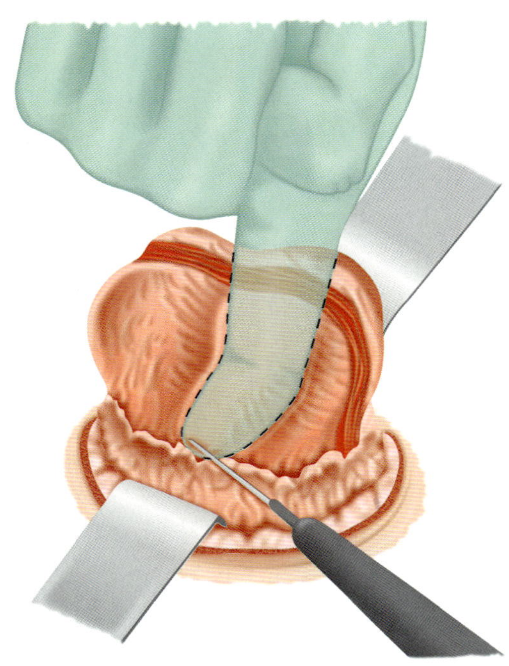

Fig. 17: Using gentle finger palpation on avascular point of attachment of the transverse colon to its mesentery is easily identified and opened

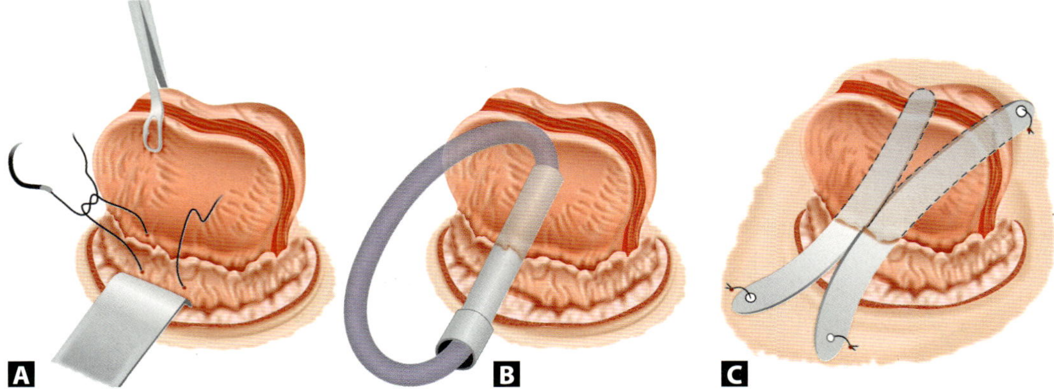

Figs 18A to C: When stomal maturation can be effected by virtue of a thorough preoperative bowel preparation, the initial step is (A) to secure the serosa and muscularis of the bowel to the incised rectus fascial edge with four to six 3-0 polyglycolic acid (PGA) sutures; (B and C) If a stoma is not to be matured at this time, a bridge is introduced through the space created on the mesenteric side of the colon

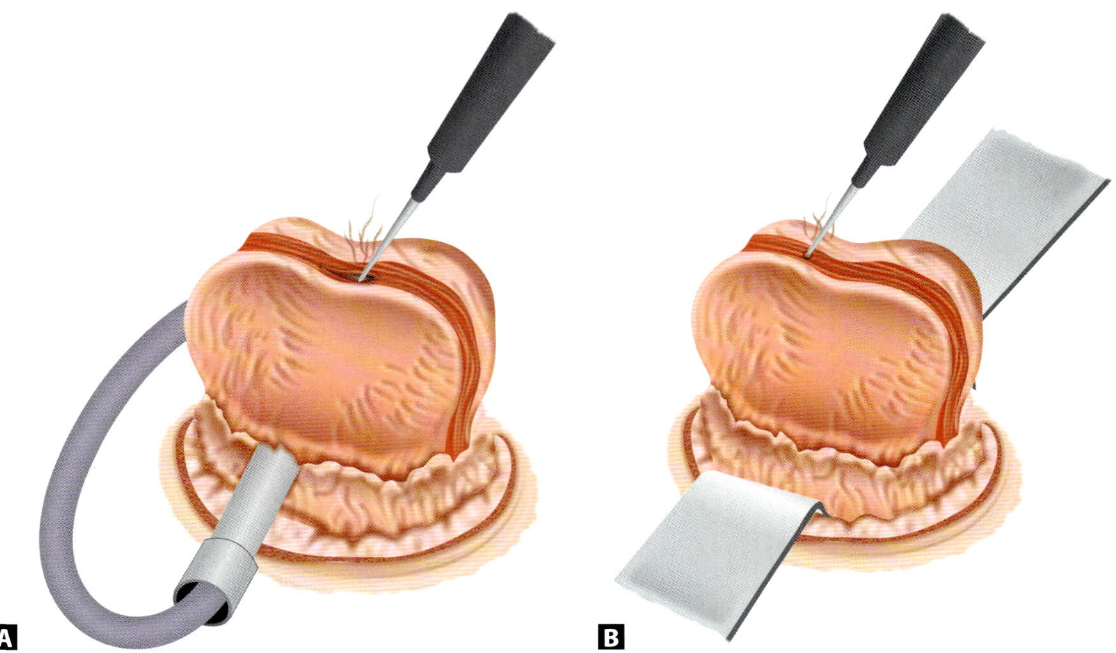

Figs 19A and B: (A) If a bridge was placed and the bowel wall left intact (Figs 18B and C), the anterior wall of the colostomy is opened with cautery at the patient's bedside the following day. The bridge is left in situ for 8 days; (B) If the stoma is to be matured during the operative procedure (Fig. 18A), the anterior wall of the colon then is opened longitudinally (preferably over a taenia) for approximately 4 cm

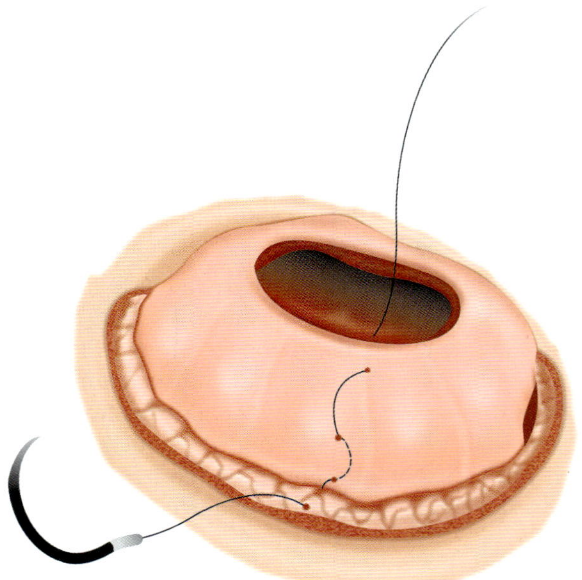

Fig. 20: Interrupted 3-0 polyglycolic acid (PGA) sutures are then placed through the full thickness of the incised colon wall, the serosa of the colon 2 cm proximal to the incised edge and then through the adjacent dermis to which it is tied

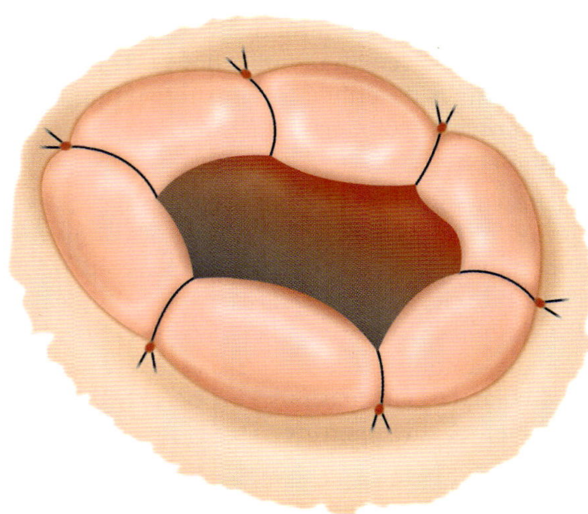

Fig. 21: Proper placement of sutures to mature the stoma will elevate the bowel wall above skin level

the seromuscular bowel wall approximately 2 cm from the distal end and then full thickness through the cut bowel edge. Sutures are placed circumferentially at about 5 mm intervals. As the sutures are tied, the everted bowel wall is folded back on itself. The result is a slightly protruding stoma that enables a better appliance fit and is less prone to retraction. In patients with a thick abdominal wall, it may not be possible to have enough viable bowel for stomal eversion. In this scenario, a stoma flush with the skin surface is matured by securing the skin to full-thickness bowel edge using interrupted sutures. The appliance is fashioned and secured intraoperatively.

Loop Transverse Colostomy

Diagrammatic representation of loop transverse colostomy shown in Figures 11 to 21.

Diverting Loop Colostomy

A loop colostomy is technically less difficult to create and reverse than an end colostomy and can often be accomplished through a single incision. This is a good technique when a temporary diverting colostomy is needed. Readily mobile transverse or sigmoid colon is preferred. As a general rule, the loop colostomy is fashioned from the most distal site along the bowel that can be effectively used. Factors to consider are that the transverse colon is generally outside of the previous surgical or radiation field and the transverse colon has a lower bacterial count than the more distal colon. Alternatively, use of the sigmoid preserves a greater length of intact bowel. The traditional loop colostomy is described for illustrative purposes and uses the transverse colon with the stoma created in the left upper quadrant.

In comparison to an end colostomy, a larger aperture is required to bring two full segments of colon through the abdominal wall. A stoma site is selected overlying the rectus muscle, which avoids skin folds, surgical scars, and the umbilicus. A transverse incision is carried down through the anterior rectus fascia. Two evenly spaced, perpendicular fascial incisions can be used to increase the diameter of this aperture. The rectus muscle fibers are bluntly separated, and the posterior rectus sheath and peritoneum are incised in a manner similar to that of the anterior fascia. The opening is manually dilated and should easily admit four fingers without stricture.

The transverse colon is identified by the presence of taenia and the omental attachment. Once isolated, the bowel is followed in a hand-over-hand fashion until the most distal yet readily mobile segment is brought through the abdominal wall. Lifting the loop is simplified by using a half-inch diameter Penrose drain passed under the intestine. A bridge device is also passed through the adjacent mesenteric window and positioned onto the skin, thereby supporting the bowel loop above the skin surface. Fascial supporting sutures are generally not necessary as the normal healing process scars the stoma into position.

Any extra length of the abdominal incision is closed. The stoma is matured by a sharp longitudinal incision through the taenia that is extended to within 1.0 cm of the skin edge at both ends. The stoma edges are everted and secured with interrupted skin to full-thickness bowel sutures using 3-0 delayed absorbable material.

The traditional Hollister bridge frequently precludes a secure appliance fit. A number of various supporting devices have been used effectively. We prefer a supporting bridge fashioned from a 20 French thoracostomy tube. A segment of about 20 cm length is cut and passed through the mesenteric window underneath the bowel. The ends are brought together over the bowel and sutured together to form a loop. This method requires no skin sutures, does not interfere with application of the collecting bag, and permits secure adherence between the stoma wafer and skin. After adequate healing (10–14 days), the bridge is easily removed by cutting the suture to open the loop and withdraw the tube.

Variations of the loop colostomy include the double-barrel colostomy in which the bowel is transected and both stomas are matured. An end colostomy with mucous fistula is used in the setting of distal obstruction, because the decompression provided by the mucous fistula avoids a closed loop obstruction. When the mucous fistula is placed immediately adjacent to the end colostomy, it is known as an end loop or terminal loop colostomy.

CHAPTER

46

Gynecologic Cancer Surgery

SPS Kochar

INTRODUCTION

The management of most gynecologic cancers involve multimodal therapy. Although some early gynecologic cancers can be eradicated by surgery alone and chemotherapy as a single modality can often cure gestational trophoblastic neoplasms, the optimal treatment of gynecologic malignancies require surgery combined with chemotherapy and/or radiation.

The major goal of this chapter is to give an appreciation and understanding of the surgical principles of the subspecialty of gynecologic oncology. Mastering the skills of surgery involves a thorough understanding of proper technique. There should be sufficient case load to insure adequate practice of the technical art of the specialty. The surgeon should also keep abreast of new suture materials, instruments and technical developments.

ANATOMY

A detailed knowledge of anatomy of the pelvis and abdomen is essential for a surgeon to perform gynecologic cancer surgery. No amount of surgical skill or knowledge can compensate for this lack of knowledge.

Lymphatic Drainage

Lymphatic drainage from the cervix follows the uterine arteries and cardinal ligaments to the pelvic nodes that include the external iliac, internal iliac and obturator nodes. From these pelvic nodes, the drainage proceeds superiorly through the common iliac nodes to the para-aortic nodes.

Lymphatic drainage from the uterine corpus and the ovaries follows one of three routes: (a) along the uterine arteries to the pelvic nodes, (b) in channels following the round ligaments to the inguinal nodes, (c) along the ovarian lymphatics directly up to the para-aortic nodes.

The para-aortic lymph nodes are part of the lumbar lymph node group. There are three subgroups: (a) preaortic, (b) retroaortic, and (c) lateral aortic (right and left). The preaortic group drains the abdominal part of the gastrointestinal tract down to the mid-rectum, whereas, the retroaortic group has no special area of drainage. The lateral group receives the lymphatic drainage from the iliac lymph nodes, ovaries and other pelvic viscera (apart from the alimentary tract), and therefore, it is this group of nodes that is sampled in the surgical staging of gynecologic malignancies.

Patient Positioning

Patient positioning for radical gynecologic oncology procedures is often critical in improving exposure. For women undergoing radical hysterectomy, the patient can be placed in "jackknife" position. The exaggerated lithotomy position is often used for improved access to the upper anterior vagina, for repair of vesicovaginal fistula, Shauta's radical vaginal hysterectomy or anterior exenteration.

SURGICAL MANAGEMENT OF CANCER CERVIX

Werthiem first described the radical hysterectomy in the year 1902. The classical Werthiem hysterectomy consists of wide resection of the parametrium, dissection of the terminal ureter from the "web" (vesicouterine ligament), wide resection of the uterosacral ligaments, and removal of the upper 3–4 cm of the vagina and paravaginal tissues, along with a thorough pelvic lymphadenectomy. Joe V Meigs made the radical hysterectomy popular in 1994.

The operative procedure popularized by Meigs included meticulous pelvic lymphadenectomy. Lymphadenectomy is now an established part of the operative procedure for any patient with disease greater than stage I. Series of cases have been reported where a radical vaginal operation has been combined with a retroperitoneal lymphadenectomy, and the results reported by Mitra, Navratil and Kastner, and McCall are good. The survival rate in patients with negative nodes is usually in the range of 90% or more.

Patients with positive pelvic nodes usually receive postoperative whole pelvis irradiation, although scientific evidence that this improves outcome, is lacking. Pelvic radiotherapy appears to effectively reduce the relapse risk when surgical margins are close or positive. The expected frequency of lymph node positivity encountered at surgery is apparently reduced by the use of preoperative external pelvic radiotherapy. These and other observations have led many to continue to recommend postoperative radiotherapy in patients with multiple positive pelvic nodes, following surgical therapy.

Types of Radical Hysterectomy

Rutledge and colleagues devised a system of rating radicality of hysterectomy used in treating women with cervical cancer at MD Anderson Hospital, which is as shown in Table 1.

Pelvic Lymphadenectomy

The lymphatic drainage of the pelvis is retroperitoneal and follows the course of the blood supply. Along the iliac vessels, dissection of the lymphatic tissue begins in the region of the bifurcation of the common iliac artery and extends upward to the bifurcation of the aorta. The ureter is easily identified at the level of pelvic brim as it enters the pelvis anterior to and at the level of bifurcation of common iliac artery. When the presacral area in the angle of the bifurcation of the aorta is being dissected, care must be taken to avoid bleeding from the middle sacral vessels and from the proximal part of the left common iliac vein, which courses through the retroperitoneal space. If the vessels are traumatized, bleeding can usually be controlled with positive pressure and small vascular clips. The lymphatic tissue along the common iliac vessels is removed by sharp dissection with the points of the Metzenbaum scissors upward, taking care to avoid the ureter. The ureter should be reflected medially during the dissection of the common iliac vessels and left attached to the parietal peritoneum in order to maintain its blood supply. The dissection is continued along the lower 2–3 cm of the aorta and vena cava, and the lymphatic tissue is clamped and excised.

The common and external iliac trunks should be rotated medially and laterally with a vein retractor during the dissection to disclose the posterior lymphatic chain behind the vessels along the psoas muscle. The genitofemoral nerve, seen lateral to the external iliac vessels, should be preserved; damage to this peripheral nerve will produce postoperative discomfort in the groin and medial aspect of the thigh. The external iliac vessels are carefully dissected to the point where they pass beneath the inguinal ligament. The external iliac vessels are reflected medially, and the areolar tissue directly beneath the vessels is freed from the lateral pelvic wall. When the obturator space has been opened, the adjacent tissue should be cleaned from the external iliac vessels. Then the artery and vein are gently retracted laterally with a vein retractor to clearly expose the obturator fossa. Lymphatic and areolar tissue should be dissected from the obturator space to the region of the pelvic floor, avoiding trauma to the obturator nerve and vessels. Damage to the obturator nerve can produce motor impairment to the adductor muscles of the thigh, and also cause sensory loss along the medial aspect of the thigh. The dissection should remove all the nodes below the bifurcation of the iliac vessels, including the hypogastric nodes and the nodes in the obturator fossa.

Table 1: Types of radical hysterectomy

Class	Description	Indication
I	Extrafascial hysterectomy; pubocervical ligament is excised, allowing lateral deflection of the ureter	CIN, early stromal invasion
II	Removal of the medial half of the cardinal and uterosacral ligaments; upper third of the vagina removed	Microcarcinoma post-irradiation
III	Removal of the entire cardinal and uterosacral ligaments; upper third of the vagina removed	Stage Ib and IIa lesions
IV	Removal of all periureteral tissue, superior vesical artery, and three-fourth of the vagina	Anteriorly occurring central recurrences where preservation of the bladder is still possible
V	Removal of portions of the distal ureter and bladder	Central recurrent cancer involving portions of the distal ureter or bladder

Abbreviation: CIN, cervical intraepithelial neoplasia

Table 2: International Federation of Gynecology and Obstetrics (FIGO) staging of endometrial carcinoma (1988)

Stage	
Ia G1,2,3	Tumor limited to endometrium
Ib G1,2,3	Invasion of less than half of the myometrium
Ic G1,2,3	Invasion of more than half of the myometrium
IIa G1,2,3	Endocervical glandular involvement only
IIb G1,2,3	Cervical stromal invasion
IIIa G1,2,3	Tumor invades serosa and/or adnexa and/or positive peritoneal cytology
IIIb G1,2,3	Vaginal metastases
IIIc G1,2,3	Metastases to pelvic or para-aortic lymph nodes
IVa G1,2,3	Tumor invasion of bladder or bowel mucosa
IVb	Distant metastases, including intra-abdominal or inguinal lymph node

Surgery for Carcinoma Endometrium

The primary treatment is total abdominal hysterectomy with bilateral salpingo-oophorectomy and selective pelvic lymph node sampling. In addition, peritoneal fluid is taken for cytology. Exploration of the abdominal cavity is done for any abdominal disease. Surgicopathological staging is done after receipt of histopathology report (Table 2).

HISTOPATHOLOGY: DEGREE OF DIFFERENTIATION

Cases of carcinoma of the corpus should be grouped according to the degree of differentiation of the adenocarcinoma as follows:

- G1: 5% or less of a non-squamous or non-morular solid growth pattern
- G2: 6–50% of a non-squamous or non-morular solid growth pattern
- G3: More than 50% of a non-squamous or non-morular solid growth pattern.

The data from the surgicopathological studies correlating multiple prognostic factors suggest criteria that could be used to allow adjuvant therapy to be planned selectively. It is recommended that except patients of stage Ia G1/G2 and stage Ib G1/G2 disease, all other patients should be offered postoperative radiotherapy as an adjuvant therapy.

A considerable data has been collected to evaluate vaginal recurrence and survival rate with surgery alone or combined with therapy, when preoperative application of radiotherapy and surgery were used. The authors believed that preoperative radiotherapy did not appear to be of benefit in the management of patients with endometrial carcinoma. The Gynecologic Oncology Group (GOG) is currently evaluating surgery plus radiotherapy versus surgery alone in moderate-risk patients. The GOG surgical-pathological study suggests that when disease is limited to the uterus, except for those with grade 3 tumors and greater than one-third myometrial invasion, radiation therapy did not offer statistically significant benefit versus surgery alone.

When disease is present in the pelvic or periaortic nodes, postoperative radiation therapy to these areas can be reasonably effective, because 40% of patients with nodal disease were tumor-free at the time of analysis.

The hysterectomy should be extrafascial and removal of the upper vagina does not appear to decrease vault recurrences. Peritoneal cytologic specimens should be obtained immediately after opening of the peritoneal cavity. If ascites is present, appropriate samples of fluid should be sent for cytologic evaluation. When lymphadenectomy is done, the retroperitoneal spaces in the pelvis are opened in routine fashion. The vessels are outlined and the lymph node bearing tissue along the external iliacs from the bifurcation to the inguinal ligament is removed. The obturator fossa anterior to the obturator nerve is cleaned of nerve tissue. Lymph nodes along the common iliacs are also removed. Retracting the small intestine into the upper abdomen and incising the peritoneum over the upper common iliac artery and lower aorta, approaches the periaortic nodes. The main vessels are outlined and the ureter is retracted laterally. The tissue overlying the vena cava and the aorta is removed en bloc, beginning at the bifurcation of the aorta and extending caudad. The upper limit of the dissection is usually the second and third portion of the duodenum as it crosses the main vessels retroperitoneally.

Patients with stage II carcinoma of the endometrium, because of extension of disease into the ectocervix, will have a greater propensity for lymph node metastasis. Primary surgery in the form of radical hysterectomy and pelvic lymphadenectomy has been the acceptable therapy in the past, but it appears that simple hysterectomy, bilateral salpingo-oophorectomy, and pelvic and para-aortic lymphadenectomy would be adequate surgery. Postoperative radiation therapy can be planned.

Treatment of stage III and stage IV disease must be individualized; however, in most cases, hormone treatment or chemotherapy, or both, must be used in addition to surgery and radiotherapy.

The recommended interval from hysterectomy to radiation, varies from immediate to 6 weeks or more. Newer forms of intracavitary radiation techniques including afterloading techniques and radium substitutes (e.g. cesium-137 and cobalt-60) have been used. Vaginal ovoids are applied to give 60–70 gray (Gy) surface dose. If deep myometrial invasion is present without extrauterine spread, 40–45 Gy external radiation to the whole pelvis is given over 4–5 weeks. The fields should cover the upper one-third to one-half of the vagina. Vaginal radium is probably unnecessary in this circumstance. When lymph node metastases have been identified, external radiation should be given to the appropriate fields. If only pelvic nodes are involved, 50 Gy over 5–6 weeks to the pelvic area can be given. If para-aortic nodes are involved, radiation to this area to the level of T-12 should be added in a dosage of 40–45 Gy. When higher doses are given to the para-aortic area, complications mainly referable to the small bowel are appreciable.

SURGICAL TREATMENT OF MALIGNANT OVARIAN NEOPLASMS

The most common epithelial cancers of the ovary are histologically categorized as serous, mucinous, endometroid and clear cell types. One theory of ovarian cancer growth suggests that the disease initially grows locally, invading the capsule and mesovarium, then invades adjacent organs by contiguous growth and lymphatic spread. When the malignant neoplasm reaches the external surface of the capsule, cells may exfoliate into the peritoneal cavity where they are free to circulate and later implant. Local and regional lymphatic metastasis may involve the uterus, fallopian tubes, and pelvic lymph nodes. Involvement of the periaortic lymph nodes by way of the infundibulopelvic ligament is also common. Probably, the variable influencing the prognosis most in each case of ovarian cancer is the stage or extent of disease. Survival depends on the stage of the lesion, the grade of differentiation of the lesion, the gross finding at surgery, the amount of residual disease after surgery and the additional treatment after surgery.

The best therapy for stage I lesions is total abdominal hysterectomy and bilateral salpingo-oophorectomy with careful surgical staging. Omentectomy is essential, as it may harbor microscopic disease in patients with apparent stage I disease. Recent evidence suggests that pelvic and periaortic nodes may be involved 10–20% of the time in apparent stage I disease, and the value of lymphadenectomy as a diagnostic and therapeutic procedure is under study. Postoperative chemotherapy is not recommended for stage Ia, grade 1 lesions. For all other cases of stage I disease, postoperative chemotherapy is recommended. Six cycles of combination chemotherapy (paclitaxel and carboplatin) are given at 3-weekly intervals. In a young woman with stage Ia disease, who is desirous of further childbearing, unilateral salpingo-oophorectomy may be associated with minimal increased risk of recurrence, provided a careful staging procedure is performed and due consideration is given to the grade of the disease.

In stage II disease, the treatment plan is to follow surgery with chemotherapy, usually a platinum based combination chemotherapy, and then to consider a second-look procedure if the patient is free of disease at completion of therapy. Omentectomy serves a valuable diagnostic tool.

In stage III disease, every effort should be made to remove the uterus with both adnexa. In addition, every effort should be made short of major bowel surgery to remove the bulk of the tumor, including the large omental cakes. Survival rate in patients with stage III disease is related to the residual tumor after surgery, such that patients with minimal residual tumor appear to have better prognosis with adjuvant therapy. The duration of multiple-agent therapy is usually 6–12 cycles. If the patient survived this period and has no clinical evidence of disease, a second-look procedure was often considered in the past. Today, it is not advocated, based on the fact that although a second-look laparotomy is diagnostic at the time, it has not had an impact on survival. In the presence of gross ascites and if the disease is considered inoperable, there is a role of giving neoadjuvant chemotherapy (3–4 cycles) to reduce the bulk of disease. This is followed by interval cytoreductive surgery. This is followed by three more cycles of adjuvant chemotherapy. Reported evidence suggests that even in optimal group (residual disease no greater than 2 cm in diameter at any site), the survival and response rate with chemotherapy are equivalent to those with abdominal and pelvic irradiation. The long-term morbidity of radiation therapy is much greater and this factor has considerably influenced postoperative therapy in favor of multiple-agent chemotherapy.

The ideal management of stage IV disease is to give neoadjuvant chemotherapy (3–4 cycles) to reduce the bulk of disease and then perform surgery. This is followed by adjuvant chemotherapy. The overall survival is poorer for this group of patients than for those assigned to other stages.

SURGICAL MANAGEMENT OF CARCINOMA VULVA

Stanley Way reported an improved survival rate in carcinoma of the vulva by use of an en bloc dissection of radical vulvectomy plus inguinal and pelvic lymphadenectomy, this has become the mainstay of treatment in vulvar cancer. With this therapy, the corrected 5 year survival rate for stage I and stage II disease has been reported as 90%. Most surgeons now limit the initial procedure to radical vulvectomy and bilateral inguinal lymphadenectomy and do not proceed with pelvic node dissection, unless metastases are demonstrated in the inguinal node area. If the presence of tumor is documented in the inguinal nodes, a pelvic lymphadenectomy is an option for therapy on the involved side only. The GOG recommends pelvic lymph node irradiation for patients with positive inguinal nodes, instead of performing pelvic lymphadenectomy.

Adjuvant radiotherapy is offered to those patients with deep stromal invasion and positive lymph nodes. The National Cancer Data Base (NCDB) noted that radiation therapy had no impact on patients with positive nodes. Those with one positive node had a 68% 5 year survival if no radiation was given compared with 46% if radiation was given. This showed that radiotherapy did not provide any survival advantage. The adjuvant therapy is given in the dose of 5,000–5,500 cGy to the inguinal nodes, with a midplane pelvic dose of 4,500–5,000 centi gray (cGy). Preoperative doses of 4,500–5,000 cGy to either groin or vulvar areas produce a hazardous situation for any subsequent surgical approach.

Complications of Radical Vulvectomy and Bilateral Inguinal Lymphadenectomy

In the early series of Stanley Way, operative mortality approached 20%. In the last 2 decades, this has been reduced to 1–2%. The complication encountered most frequently is wound breakdown, which occurs in well above 50% of patients in most series. This is usually limited to skin loss at the margin of the groin incision. Removing lesser amounts of skin and decreasing the undermining of the skin flaps have reduced the incidence of wound breakdown. Suction drainage has also added to this decreasing morbidity. Careful debridement and vigorous care to keep the wounds clean and dry almost always result in adequate healing.

Lymphedema of the lower extremities occurs, especially in patients who have had inguinal and deep pelvic node dissection. Established lymphedema can be kept under control in many patients with routine use of pneumatic hose devices that have become widely available. The development of lymphocyst in the groin area is an infrequent occurrence, and it usually resolves spontaneously.

These patients sometime report symptoms related to stress incontinence and the development of cystocele or rectocele.

Surgery for Cancer Vagina

Cases of carcinoma of vagina reported in the literature have been primarily treated by radiotherapy. In a meta-analysis of 4,885 cases, 26% were in situ carcinomas and all were treated by surgery. Patients with invasive carcinoma were treated with radiotherapy (74%), surgery (32%), and chemotherapy (12%). Surgery was used most often for stage I disease.

Treatment is tailored to the stage and extent of the disease. Large tumors are treated initially with external irradiation to shrink the disease, so that local radiation therapy will be more effective. Cancers of the upper portion of the vagina in patients with intact uteri are treated with techniques similar to those used for carcinoma of the cervix. External irradiation in a dose of 4,000–5,000 cGy is given initially, followed by vaginal ovoids and an intrauterine tandem application to deliver 6,000 cGy in 72 hours or 8,000 cGy in two applications of 48 hours, each separated by 2 weeks. For patients who have lesions involving the upper-half of the vagina, especially the upper-third, after hysterectomy, serious consideration should be given to an "open implant".

In general, the radiation therapy plan must reflect consideration of the depth of invasion of the lesion. For early lesions, particularly in the upper vagina, radical surgery may be preferred in many patients.

The proximity of relatively radiosensitive normal tissues, such as the bladder and the rectum, provides a real challenge to the radiotherapist, especially in dealing with tumors of the lower-third of the vagina. The incidence of complications after radiation therapy is relatively low. Serious complications occur in about 10% of patients and consist of rectal stenosis, rectovaginal fistulas and severe rectal bleeding requiring diversion. As many as 35% of patients experience cystitis or proctitis during or shortly after therapy, but symptoms usually resolve spontaneously.

Although, there have been few recent publications on the role of chemotherapy on vulvar carcinoma, the data that have been cited for carcinoma of the vagina are virtually non existent. The neoadjuvant regimens that have been used for vulvar cancer might theoretically be as effective. The active agents used are bleomycin, cisplatin, 5-fluorouracil (5-FU), methotrexate and mitomycin C as single agents or as combination therapy.

PELVIC EXENTERATION

Although pelvic exenteration has been used for various pelvic malignancies, its greatest and most important role is in the treatment of advanced or recurrent carcinoma of the cervix. Total exenteration with removal of the pelvic viscera, including the bladder and rectosigmoid, is the procedure of choice for carcinoma of the cervix recurrent or persistent within the pelvis after irradiation. In very selected cases, the procedure may be limited to anterior exenteration with removal of the bladder and preservation of rectosigmoid or posterior exenteration with removal of the rectosigmoid and preservation of the bladder.

One of the greatest technical advances in the evolution of pelvic exenteration is the intestinal conduit for diversion of the urinary stream. Bricker popularized the use of an ileal segment conduit for urinary diversion. Another significant advancement in surgical technique for these patients is the use of the intestinal stapling device.

Only a few patients with recurrent cancer of the cervix are suitable for this operation. Metastases outside the pelvis, whether manifested preoperatively or discovered at laparotomy is an absolute contraindication to pelvic exenteration. The triad of unilateral leg edema, sciatic pain and ureteral obstruction is pathognomonic of unresectable disease in the pelvis. A small central lesion with freely mobile parametria, reliably demonstrates resectability; however, immobility can be caused by radiation fibrosis or pelvic inflammatory disease.

Evaluation studies before surgery include chest film, computed tomography (CT) scan of the abdomen and pelvis with intravenous contrast, creatinine clearance, liver function tests, and the assessment of the patient's hemostatic mechanism.

At laparotomy, the entire abdomen and pelvis are explored for evidence of metastatic and intraperitoneal cancer. The liver should be carefully inspected visually and by palpation. The lymph nodes surrounding the lower aorta are first to be sampled if the exploration of the abdomen has revealed no evidence of disease. If the lower aorta findings are negative, a bilateral pelvic lymphadenectomy is performed. Immediate frozen section analysis of the pelvic wall nodes is necessary to determine whether the resection should continue.

Most of the morbidity and mortality directly related to exenteration occur within the first 18 months following the procedure. The commonest occurring complications are pulmonary embolism, pulmonary edema, myocardial infarction, cerebrovascular accidents, sepsis, small bowel obstruction, urinary obstruction and infection. The morbidity and mortality from radical surgery can be minimized by careful selection of the patients.

The 5-year cumulative survival rate after pelvic exenteration varies in the literature from 20% to 62%. In general, however, both morbidity and mortality and the 5-year survival have improved steadily over the last 2 decades.

LAPAROSCOPIC SURGERY IN ONCOLOGY

Several groups have demonstrated that laparoscopic gynecological oncologic procedures can be performed safely. Laparoscopic procedures that are reliable and safe when performed correctly appear potentially dangerous when the guidelines are not followed. A learning curve is necessary to develop the applications of laparoscopic surgery in oncology. Some situations are specific to laparoscopic surgery, such as increased intra-abdominal pressure and use of carbon dioxide (CO_2). This could be considered an advantage to control the intraoperative bleeding, but as a disadvantage when considering the possible dissemination and growth of malignant cells.

Laparoscopic Lymphadenectomy

Several studies have demonstrated that laparoscopic lymphadenectomy will become the standard for surgical staging in cervical or endometrial cancer. Different steps of lymphadenectomy include identification of the bifurcation of the common iliac artery and the proximal end of the obturator nerve, which is more easily identified when dissecting the external iliac vessels from the lateral pelvic wall. Para-aortic surgery usually consists of three steps: right side lymphadenectomy, left side dissection and dissection of the nodes above the inferior mesenteric artery.

Laparoscopic Radical Hysterectomy

Laparoscopic assisted radical vaginal hysterectomy (LARVH) requires in-depth knowledge of laparoscopic surgery and rigorous training in gynecologic oncology. Laparoscopic excision is easier because of the improved vision and exposure of the pelvic spaces. The first part consists of exhaustive exploration of the abdominal and pelvic anatomy with special attention to the location and boundaries of the bladder, the position of the pelvic ureters, colon, rectum and major blood vessels. Inspection of the peritoneal surface including liver, spleen, subdiaphragmatic surface is done for any evidence of disease. Bilateral pelvic lymphadenectomy is done using bipolar coagulation forceps and scissors. The extent of lymph node dissection is same as described in Wertheim's hysterectomy.

The round ligaments must be coagulated with bipolar forceps and sectioned as lateral as possible. The anterior broad ligament is opened downward and toward the bladder. Teasing the anterior peritoneum of the broad ligament with the grasping forceps, the utero-vesical junction is identified, grasped and elevated with forceps while it is cut with scissors, laser or cautery. The bladder is pushed down after coagulating the bladder pillars. The uterine artery is sutured at the origin and cut. The paravesical and pararectal spaces are identified and dissected. The cardinal ligament dissection should be done for deroofing of the ureter from the ureteric tunnel. The upper limit is the uterine artery and the posterior surface is identified while dissecting the pararectal fossa. The anterior surface can be identified in the paravesical fossa. The bladder is pushed down for obtaining adequate vaginal cuff. The rectum is pushed posteriorly using hydro-dissection. To cut the vaginal cuff, the uterine manipulator is most important for providing a satisfactory view of the area to be sectioned. After vaginal extraction of the uterus, the vagina can be repaired by suturing vaginally or through the laparoscope.

Management of Adnexal Masses

Laparoscopy should only be used for non-suspicious masses, as the technique requires the cyst to be punctured in most of the cases. However with laparotomy, the surgical rupture or puncture of a low malignant potential tumor has no influence on the prognosis, provided the tumor is removed immediately in the same surgical procedure. When the tumor is not removed immediately, laparoscopic puncture or biopsy may worsen the prognosis of a malignant ovarian tumor. Careful selection of patients is critical for the appropriate use of laparoscope for removal of adnexal masses. Laparoscopy should be used cautiously in the presence of any mass with clinical or ultrasonographic characteristics suggestive of malignancy. It is contraindicated for management of an adnexal mass in the presence of an elevated serum CA-125 value in a postmenopausal woman. The presence of irregular borders, palpitations, solitary thick septa, ascites, or matted bowel on ultrasonography should raise concern about the possibility of malignancy. CA-125 has been studied to determine its value in preoperative differentiation of benign and malignant pelvic masses. In patients younger than 50 years, an elevated CA-125 level is associated with a malignant mass lesser than 25% of the time, whereas in patients older than 50 years, it is associated with a malignant mass greater than 80% of the time. CA-125 values in excess of 300 U/mL are usually associated with malignancy even in patients younger than 50 years.

All patients scheduled for operative laparoscopy should also consent to possible laparotomy; the surgeon should be prepared to proceed with staging laparotomy without delay, if malignant disease is discovered. Cell washings are obtained from the pelvis and upper abdomen and saved for proper staging if a malignant neoplasm is found. Any suspicious area or lesion should be sampled and sent for frozen section analysis. If obvious carcinoma or ascites is found or the result of frozen section is positive, the surgeon should proceed with immediate staging laparotomy through a midline incision. Nezhat and colleagues reported their experience with 1,209 patients with adnexal masses who were managed laparoscopically. Of 1,011 cases with surgical management, ovarian cancer was discovered intraoperatively in four. This study suggests that experienced surgeons using intraoperative histology sampling may safely evaluate adnexal masses laparoscopically.

Second-look Laparoscopy

Laparoscopy appears as effective as laparotomy for second-look operations after treatment of ovarian cancer. Due to the high-risk of bowel adhesions to the anterior abdominal wall, the insertion of the primary trocar may induce bowel injuries. Bowel preparation is similar to that used for colon surgery. The first step of second-look laparoscopy is aspiration of peritoneal fluid in the posterior cul-de-sac for cytology or peritoneal washings, if necessary. The whole abdominal pelvic cavity must be explored after complete adhesiolysis to provide access to the entire pelvis and to any other abdominal area involved in the initial laparotomy, including the paracolic gutters, the diaphragm and all of the peritoneum. Any abnormal or suspicious area should be biopsied. Multiple biopsies of normal areas should be routinely performed, using 5 mm grasping forceps and laparoscopic scissors to excise a large peritoneal area.

The second-look surgery does not affect survival. In patients with advanced disease, as many as 50% with negative results of second-look operations after combination chemotherapy have experienced subsequent recurrence of their disease. Today, the second-look surgery is used infrequently, unless the patient is enrolled in a protocol.

Restaging of Ovarian Cancer

If an ovarian cancer has been treated by adnexectomy or by inadequate procedures such as puncture, biopsy or partial resection, a restaging procedure should be performed as soon as possible. The restaging of early ovarian cancer appears to be one of the most attractive indications of laparoscopy in gynecological oncology.

Endometrial Carcinoma

Surgical staging and treatment of endometrial cancer can be achieved with laparoscopy. As patients with endometrial cancer tend to be older and uterine trauma should be minimized, laparoscopic hysterectomy can be proposed in cancer cases only once sufficient experience has been gained. Peritoneal fluid is obtained for cytology as a staging procedure. After hysterectomy with bilateral salpingo-oophorectomy, pelvic lymph node sampling is done. The dissection of the para-aortic nodes is only performed in patients who have grade 3 tumors or pelvic lymph node metastases in frozen sections. The main disadvantage of the laparoscopic approach is the difficulties in obese patients and the contraindications for surgery in older patients. Laparoscopy also appears to be the best choice for endometrial cancer when a restaging procedure is decided for a patient whose cancer was diagnosed postoperatively, when examining the hysterectomy specimen.

Postoperative Complications of Radical Surgery

a. *Vesicovaginal fistula:* The posterior bladder wall may be lacerated or torn during the extensive dissection of the bladder base from the cervix and upper vagina. Suturing the bladder peritoneum to the margins of the anterior vaginal wall protects the bladder and the terminal ureters from secondary infection and subsequent fistula formation. If the patient has received irradiation treatment before surgery, bladder ischemia and vesicovaginal fistula formation may occur.
b. *Neurogenic bladder dysfunction:* Both sympathetic and parasympathetic nerve fibers are contained in the pelvic nerve plexus, and interruption of these nerve fibers produces postoperative bladder dysfunction. Prolonged postoperative bladder drainage facilitates revascularization. Adequate bladder retraining and the use of smooth-muscle relaxants can help patients control bladder symptoms. Continuous bladder catheterization should be done postoperatively for atleast 7 days and on removal of the catheter, the residual urine should be less than 75 mL.
c. *Ureterovaginal fistula:* Devascularization and ischemic necroses of the wall of the terminal ureter have proven to be the more severe complications of the radical Wertheim's procedure. The incidence of ureteric fistulas is less than 2%.
d. *Pelvic lymphocyst:* The accumulation of lymph within the pelvis from retrograde lymphatic drainage was previously noted to be a common complication. It occurred in 12–24% of cases. Prolonged drainage of the obturator space using closed suction drains (Romovac) and meticulous ligation of the pelvic lymphatics, has reduced the lymphocyst to a rare event in modern day practice. The drains should be removed only after the drainage is less than 20 mL/24 hours.
e. *Pelvic cellulitis:* Adequate vaginal and abdominal drainage of the operative site has greatly diminished the incidence of pelvic cellulitis, following radical pelvic surgery. The current practice is to begin broad-spectrum antibiotic coverage for both aerobic and anaerobic organisms immediately before surgery, and to maintain treatment for 72 hours, following surgery.
f. *Venous thrombosis:* The patient who undergoes radical pelvic surgery has a higher risk of developing venous thrombosis of the lower extremity than patients who have other kind of gynecologic surgery. Postoperative alteration of blood coagulation, trauma to the vein wall and venous stasis are commonly associated with radical pelvic surgery. Heparin, in a dose of 5,000 units, given subcutaneously three times daily, beginning 2 hours before surgery and every 8 hours thereafter for 5 days, has reduced the incidence of thrombosis from 24.6% to 7.7%. The incidence has also been found to be reduced by the intraoperative and postoperative use of pneumatic calf compression
g. *Pulmonary embolism:* Approximately 3–5% of patients with occult venous thrombosis of the lower extremities will develop a pulmonary embolus. As soon as the venous thrombosis is verified, full anticoagulation therapy can be started to prevent pulmonary embolism.
h. *Intraoperative bleeding:* Most problems with bleeding during radical surgery occur with the dissection of the cardinal ligament and the hypogastric vessels. When venous bleeding does occur, the laceration site may be difficult to identify. Compressing the pelvic floor veins with either a sponge stick or an abdominal pack for no less than 7 minutes can stop bleeding from an indefinite source. Dissection should not proceed until full control of the bleeding has been established. Vascular clips and microfibrillar bovine collagen are very helpful in controlling small areas of venous oozing. More extensive damage to the wall of the external iliac or hypogastric vein must be repaired by first placing vascular clamps above and below the area of injury and then suturing the defect.

BIBLIOGRAPHY

1. Artman LE, Hoskins WJ, Bibro MC, et al. Radical hysterectomy and pelvic lymphadenectomy for stage IB carcinoma of the cervix: 21 years experience. Gynecol Oncol. 1987;28:8-13.
2. Ball HG, Berman ML. Management of primary vaginal carcinoma. Gynecol Oncol 1982;14:154-63.
3. Barakat RR, Benjamin I. Surgery for malignant gynecologic disease. Curr Opin Obstet Gynecol. 1993;5:311-7.
4. Behbakht K, Yordan EL, Casey C, et al. Prognostic indicators of survival in advanced endometrial cancer. Gynecol Oncol. 1994;55:363-7.
5. Bloss JD, Berman ML, Mukhererjee J, et al. Bulky stage IB cervical cancer managed by primary radical hysterectomy followed by tailored radiotherapy. Gynecol Oncol. 1992;47:21-7.

6. Burchsbaum HJ, Brady MF, Delgado G, et al. Surgical staging of carcinoma of the ovaries. Surg Gynecol Obstet. 1989;169:226-32.
7. Burghardt E, Girardi F, Lahousen M, et al. Patterns of pelvic and para-aortic lymph node involvement in ovarian cancer. Gynecol Oncol. 1991;40:103-6.
8. Burghardt E, Pickel H, Lahousen M, et al. Pelvic lymphadenectomy in operative treatment of ovarian cancer. Am J Obstet Gynecol. 1986;155:315-9.
9. Burke TW. Changing surgical approaches to vulva cancer. Curr Opin Obstet Gynecol. 1992;4:86-90.
10. Canis M, Botchorishvili R, Kouyaté S, et al. Surgical management of adnexal tumours. Ann Chir. 1998;52:234-48.
11. Cavanagh D, Fiorica JV, Hoffman MS, et al. Invasive carcinoma of the vulva: Changing trends in surgical management. Am J Obstet Gynecol, 1990;163:1007-15.
12. Chi DS, Welshinger M, Venkatraman ES, et al. The role of surgical cytoreduction in stage IV endometrial carcinoma. Gynecol Oncol. 1997;67:56.
13. Copeland LJ. Second-look laparotomy for ovarian carcinoma. Clin Obstet Gynecol. 1985;28:816-23.
14. DiSaia PJ. Surgical aspects of cervical carcinoma. Cancer. 1981;48:548-59.
15. Gallup DG, Talledo OE, Shah KJ, et al. Invasive Squamous cell carcinoma of the vagina: A 14 year study. Obstet Gynecol. 1987;69:782-5.
16. Guidozzi F, Ball JH. Extensive primary cytoreductive surgery for advanced epithelial ovarian cancer. Gynecol Oncol. 1994;53:326-30.
17. Helin HL, Kirkinen P. Laparoscopic ultrasonography during conservative ovarian surgery. Surg Endosc. 2000; 14:161-3.
18. Homesley HD. Lymph node findings and outcome in squamous cell carcinoma of the vulva. Cancer. 1994;74:2399-402.
19. Jakobsen A, Bichel P, Ahrons S, et al. Is radical hysterectomy always necessary in early cervical cancer? Gynecol Oncol. 1990;39:80-1.
20. Magrina JF, Gonzalez-Bosquet J, Weaver AL, et al. Primary cell cancer of the vulva: Radical versus modified radical vulvar surgery. Gynecol Oncol. 1998;71:116-21.
21. Monson RR, MacMahon B, Austin JH. Postoperative irradiation and carcinoma endometrium. Cancer. 1973;31:630-2.
22. Morley GW. Cancer of the vulva: A review. Cancer. 1981;48:597.
23. Nezhat CR. Operative gynaecologic laparoscopy. New York: McGraw Hill; 1995.
24. Reuben SC, Young J, Mikuta JJ. Squamous carcinoma of the vagina: Treatment, complications, and long-term follow-up. Gynecol Oncol. 1985;20:346-53.
25. Sagae S, Kudo R. Surgery for germ cell tumours. Smin Surg Oncol. 2000;19:76-81.
26. Seracchioli R, Venturoli S, Colombo FM, et al. Fertility and tumour recurrence rate after conservative laparoscopic management of young women with early-stage borderline ovarian tumour. Fertil Steril. 2001;76:999-1004.
27. Sutton GP. The significance of positive peritoneal cytology in endometrial cancer. Oncology. 1990;4:21-6.
28. Trimble EL, Kosary C, Park RC. Lymph node sampling and survival in endometial cancer. Gynecol Oncol. 1998;71:340-3.
29. Vaudoyer F, Golfier F, Raudrant D. Operative technique for assumed benign ovarian cysts. J Gynecol Obstet Biol Reprod. 2001;1:68-77.
30. Zanetta G, Chiari S, Rota S, et al. Conservative surgery for stage-I ovarian carcinoma in women of childbearing age. Br J Obstet Gynecol. 1997;164:1030-5.

CHAPTER

47

Surgery for Ovarian Cancer

SPS Kochar

47.1 STAGING LAPAROTOMY FOR CANCER OVARY

SPS Kochar

INTRODUCTION

Eighty percent of patients with cancer ovary present in stage III disease at the time of diagnosis. The insidious onset of ovarian cancer needs no elaboration. A high index of suspicion is warranted in all women between the ages of 40 years and 69 years who have persistent gastrointestinal symptoms that cannot be diagnosed. It is only when the patient has gross enlargement of the abdomen marking the occurrence of ascites and extension of the neoplastic process to the abdominal cavity that she receives appropriate diagnostic evaluation. As enlargement occurs, there is progressive compression of the surrounding pelvic structures, producing vague abdominal discomfort, dyspepsia, urinary frequency and "pelvic pressure".

The ovarian neoplasms grow quickly and painlessly. Any persistent ovarian enlargement should be an immediate indication for laparotomy. The size of the tumor does not indicate the severity of the disease. Some of the largest tumors are benign histologically. At the time of surgery, it may be difficult to discriminate the malignant potential of a particular ovarian neoplasm.

Immunologic diagnosis of subclinical ovarian cancer by means of identification of specific tumor-associated antigens in the serum has yet to materialize. Several tumor-associated antigens, including the CA-125, have been identified and purified. Their detection within the serum in the presence of minimal neoplastic tissue has not been possible. It has been suggested that every woman should have a periodic pelvic examination, pelvic ultrasound examination and CA-125 test to make sure she does not harbor an occult ovarian cancer. There are no reliable data that shows screening for ovarian cancer is effective in improving length and quality of life in women with ovarian cancer. If a woman is undergoing pelvic surgery, removal of the ovaries at that time would almost fully eliminate her risk of ovarian cancer. If the woman is premenopausal, discussion of estrogen replacement therapy is important before the removal of the ovaries, because if estrogen replacement therapy is not used, the risk of premature menopause and the potential risk for cardiovascular disease and osteoporosis may outweigh the risk of ovarian conservation and the potential for ovarian cancer.

DIAGNOSIS AND STAGING

Pelvic examination remains the most practical means of detecting early disease. Routine pelvic examinations detect only 1 ovarian cancer in 10,000 asymptomatic women. Pain is usually a late complication; it is seen with early disease only in association with torsion, rupture, or infection. Any palpable ovary in postmenopausal women should be further investigated by transvaginal ultrasonography, color Doppler, laparoscopy or laparotomy. Routine laboratory tests are not of great value in the diagnosis of ovarian tumor. Pelvic ultrasound may reveal solid or cystic mass, intracystic papillations and metastatic disease. Intravenous pyelography is helpful in ruling out disease in adjacent pelvic structures. A barium enema is advisable for patients with lower intestinal symptoms. Computed tomography (CT) scan with contrast enhancement may be helpful in identifying the extent of clinical disease. Laparotomy is the ultimate test as to the nature of the disorder. Paracentesis for the purpose of obtaining a cell block and cytologic smear of the peritoneal fluid appears unnecessary and is occasionally dangerous. Regardless of whether the fluid contains neoplastic cells, laparotomy is still necessary to define the extent of the malignant process. In addition, up to 50% of ascitic fluid samples from patients with true ovarian malignant neoplasms will be negative for malignant cells on cell block analysis. Recently, interest has been generated in giving neoadjuvant chemotherapy to those patients where the disease appears clinically irrespectable, and this is followed by interval cytoreductive surgery.

Steps of Staging Laparotomy

The staging of the ovarian cancer is surgical and is based on the operative findings at the commencement of the procedure. A longitudinal midline incision is recommended to facilitate removal of the neoplasm and to permit adequate visualization of the entire abdominal cavity, including the under surface of the diaphragm. Ovarian cancer is classically a serosal spreading disease, and thus all peritoneal surfaces must be thoroughly inspected (Table 1). Although lymphatic spread to retroperitoneal nodes is common, the disease most often spreads intraperitoneally; free-floating cells shed from the primary tumor are capable of implanting on any peritoneal surface. Any peritoneal fluid found should be aspirated and submitted for cytologic examination. In the absence of peritoneal fluid, four washings should be taken by lavage of the peritoneal surfaces: the undersurface of the diaphragm, lateral to the ascending and descending colon and the pelvic peritoneal surfaces. These specimens are obtained by lavaging these areas with 50–75 mL of saline solution and retrieving the fluid for cell block analysis. Care should be taken to visualize and palpate all peritoneal surfaces, particularly the under surface of the diaphragm, the surface of the liver, the lateral abdominal gutters, and the small and large bowel mesentery (Box 1). The omentum should be scrutinized and any suspicious areas removed by excision or biopsy. If the disease is apparently limited to the pelvis, it is judicious to excise the most dependent (infracolic) of the omentum. Microscopic disease is often present in the omentum but not obvious grossly. If the disease is limited to the pelvis, great care should be taken to avoid rupture of the neoplasm during its removal. All roughened or suspicious surfaces in the peritoneal cavity should be removed as biopsy specimens. Proper staging is the key to an accurate prognosis (Table 2).

In stage III disease, every effort should be made to remove the uterus with both adnexa (Fig. 1). In addition, every effort should be made short of major bowel surgery to remove the bulk of the tumor, including the large omental cakes. Survival rate in patients with stage III disease is related to the residual tumor after surgery, such that patients with minimal residual tumor appear to have better prognosis with adjuvant therapy.

Table 1: Surgical findings

Finding	Benign	Malignant
Surface papilla	Rare	Very common
Intracystic papilla	Uncommon	Very common
Solid areas	Rare	Very common
Bilaterality	Rare	Common
Adhesions	Uncommon	Common
Ascites (100 mL)	Rare	Common
Necrosis	Rare	Common
Peritoneal implants	Rare	Common
Capsule intact	Common	Infrequent
Totally cystic	Common	Rare

Box 1 Surgical therapy in ovarian cancer

Peritoneal cytologic examination

- Determination of extent of disease
  - Pelvis
  - Peritoneal surfaces
  - Diaphragms
  - Omentum
  - Lymph nodes
- Removal of all tumor possible (total abdominal hysterectomy and bilateral salpingo-oophorectomy) plus node sampling and omentectomy

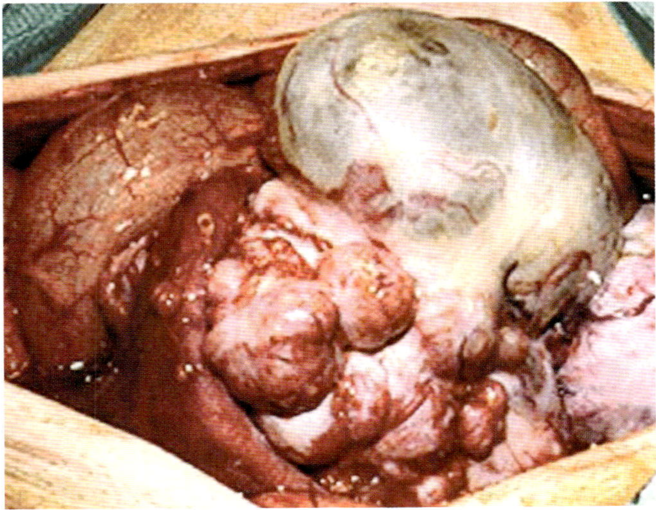

Fig. 1: Multiloculated ovarian cancer, stage III at laparotomy

Table 2: International Federation of Gynecology and Obstetrics (FIGO) staging of carcinoma ovary

Stage	Description
Stage I	Growth limited to the ovaries
Stage Ia	Growth limited to one ovary; no ascites present containing malignant cells; no tumor on the external surface; capsule intact
Stage Ib	Growth limited to both ovaries; no ascites present containing malignant cells; no tumor on the external surface; capsule intact
Stage Ic	Tumor stage Ia or stage Ib but with tumor on the surface of one or both the ovaries; or with capsule ruptured; or with ascites present containing malignant cells or with positive peritoneal washings
Stage II	Growth involving one or both ovaries with pelvic extension
Stage IIa	Extension and/or metastases to the uterus and/or tubes
Stage IIb	Extension to other pelvic tissues
Stage IIc	Tumor stage IIa or IIb but with tumor on the surface of one or both ovaries; or with capsule(s) ruptured; or with ascites present containing malignant cells or with positive peritoneal washings
Stage III	Tumor involving one or both ovaries with peritoneal implants outside the pelvis and/or positive retroperitoneal or inguinal nodes; superficial liver metastasis equals stage III; tumor is limited to the true pelvis but with histologically verified malignant extension to small bowel or omentum
Stage IIIa	Tumor grossly limited to the true pelvis with negative nodes with histologically confirmed microscopic seeding of abdominal peritoneal surfaces
Stage IIIb	Tumor of one or both ovaries; histologically confirmed implants of abdominal peritoneal surfaces, none exceeding 2 cm in diameter; nodes negative
Stage IIIc	Abdominal implants 2 cm in diameter and/or positive retroperitoneal or inguinal lymph nodes
Stage IV	Growth involving one or both ovaries with distant metastasis; if pleural effusion is present, there must be positive cytologic test results to allot a case to stage IV; parenchymal liver metastasis equals stage IV

Maximal Surgical Effort

The percentage of patients with advanced ovarian cancer who can effectively undergo cytoreductive surgery seems to range from 43–87%. It is judicious to excise as much tumor as possible when disseminated disease is encountered at the time of primary operation for ovarian cancer. The most important prognostic factors are histologic grade of the tumor and the size of the largest residual mass after primary surgery. The so-called debulking procedure has gained considerable attention in the management of ovarian cancer. The concept is to diminish the residual tumor burden to a point at which adjuvant therapy will be optimally effective. Removal of large ovarian masses and omental involvement often reduces the tumor burden by 80–90%.

Optimal cytoreduction is achieved when the largest size of residual tumor after primary surgery is less than 2 cm at any site. Gynecologic Oncology Group (GOG) study has demonstrated that optimal cytoreduction resulted in a significant survival benefit. But all residual diameters greater than 2 cm had equivalent survivals. Therefore, unless the mass can be cytoreduced to less than 2 cm, residual diameter did not influence survival. The effect of maximal cytoreductive surgery can be seen in the percentage of negative second-look procedures. A routine pelvic and periaortic lymphadenectomy should be done if the patients tumor can be optimally debulked. Benefits of lymphadenectomy in patients with bulk residual disease remain questionable.

Second-look Surgery

In ovarian cancer, the second-look operation may have following indications:

1. For restaging in a patient who probably has localized disease but who has not had an optimal staging procedure as described previously.
2. For evaluation of the effect of chemotherapy in patients receiving both standard and investigational regimens.
3. For evaluation of patients who are clinically free of disease after receiving what is considered a sufficient course of chemotherapy and are then eligible for assessment as to possible "cure" and discontinuation of therapy.

Second-look procedures begun with a laparoscopic examination to rule out widespread disease. If this lesser procedure reveals diffuse miliary studding, a laparotomy is not necessary. On the other hand, a negative laparoscopic result is not sufficient evidence for classifying the patient as without evidence of disease and a laparotomy must be performed. At the time of laparotomy, a detailed exploration of the abdominal cavity must be done in a manner similar to the initial staging procedures. If focal residual disease is encountered, it is surgically resected and the area is marked with metal clips for possible regional radiation therapy. Careful inspection of the entire abdominal cavity, including the undersurface of the diaphragm, the root of the mesentery, and all parietal and visceral peritoneal surfaces must be carried out with liberal use of biopsy from suspicious areas.

The second-look laparotomy does not affect survival. In patients with advanced disease, as many as 50% with negative results of second-look operations after combination chemotherapy have experienced subsequent recurrence of their disease. Today, the second-look laparotomy is used infrequently unless the patient is enrolled in a protocol.

BIBLIOGRAPHY

1. Barakat RR, Benjamin I. Surgery for malignant gynecologic disease. Curr Opin Obstet Gynecol. 1993;5(3):311-7.
2. Burchsbaum HJ, Brady MF, Delgado G, et al. Surgical staging of carcinoma of the ovaries. Surg Gynecol Obstet. 1989;169(3):226-32.
3. Burghardt E, Girardi F, Lahousen M, et al. Patterns of pelvic and para-aortic lymph node involvement in ovarian cancer. Gynecol Oncol. 1991;40(2):103-6.
4. Burghardt E, Pickel H, Lahousen M, et al. Pelvic lymphadenectomy in operative treatment of ovarian cancer. Am J Obstet Gynecol. 1986;155(2):315-9.
5. Copeland LJ. Second-look laparotomy for ovarian carcinoma. Clin Obstet Gynecol. 1985;28:816.
6. Eisenkop SM, Friedman RL, Wang HJ. Complete cytoreductive surgery is feasible and maximizes survival in patients with advanced ovarian cancer. Gynecol Oncol. 1998;69(2);103-8.
7. Guidozzi F, Ball JH. Extensive primary cytoreductive surgery for advanced epithelial ovarian cancer. Gynecol Oncol. 1994;53(3):326-30.
8. van Houwelingen JC, ten Bokkel Huinink WW, van der Burg ME et al. Predictability of the survival of patients with advanced ovarian cancer. J Clin Oncol. 1989;7(6):769-73.

47.2 PERI- AND PARA-AORTIC LYMPHADENECTOMY

SPS Kochar

INTRODUCTION

Retroperitoneal lymph node dissection (RPLND) has been shown to improve 5-year progression-free survival for patients with optimally debulked advanced ovarian carcinoma. It has also been shown to help prolong survival for patients with chemorefractory ovarian immature teratoma. Furthermore, RPLND is an important aspect of postchemotherapy debulking surgery for nonseminomatous germ cell tumors, which is the male counterpart of the ovarian immature teratoma. Therefore, the ability to perform an extensive RPLND is an important skill in the surgical armamentarium of the gynecologic oncologist. This chapter will focus on the performance of an aortic RPLND.

INDICATIONS FOR PARA-AORTIC NODE DISSECTION

Despite awareness of the potential for retroperitoneal spread of ovarian cancer, mandatory nodal dissection in cases of advanced ovarian cancer is not routinely performed and the prognostic benefit remains contested. Surgical studies have confirmed that the retroperitoneal lymph nodes contain disease in up to 50–70% of patients with advanced ovarian cancer.

Despite ovarian cancer being primarily an intraperitoneal disease, some believe that ignoring retroperitoneal spread may reduce the likelihood of attaining remission with first-line therapy and increase the rate of early relapse. They argue that the para-aortic lymph nodes may harbor occult tumor and act as sanctuary sites, preventing the effect of systemic therapy from reaching them. Some retrospective studies have shown benefit for performing lymphadenectomy in patients with advanced ovarian cancer.

Although removal of isolated enlarged retroperitoneal nodes is a mandatory process of the debulking procedure, the role of elective, systematic para-aortic lymphadenectomy in patients with no palpable enlargement of the retroperitoneal structures is unclear. Until definitive data exist, it does not seem logical to inflict the potential morbidity of para-aortic lymph node dissection on a patient with palpably normal retroperitoneal nodes in an attempt to by chance detect microscopic tumor deposits.

The status of the para-aortic nodes in surgical staging of cancer cervix is the most significant prognostic factor in survival.

ANATOMY

The anatomy of para-aortic lymph nodes has been well described by Fowler and Johnson (1996). The para-aortic lymph nodes are part of the lumbar lymph node group. There are three subgroups: (1) preaortic, (2) retroaortic and (3) lateral aortic (right and left). The preaortic group drains the abdominal part of the gastrointestinal tract down to the mid-rectum, whereas the retroaortic group has no special area of drainage. The lateral group receives the lymphatic drainage from the iliac lymph nodes, ovaries and other pelvic viscera (apart from the alimentary tract), and therefore, it is this group of nodes that is sampled in the surgical staging of gynecologic malignancies.

There are typically 15–20 lateral aortic nodes per side. They are located adjacent to the aorta, anterior to the lumbar spine, extending bilaterally to the medial margins of the psoas major muscles and up to the diaphragmatic crura. The lateral nodes usually dissected in gynecologic oncology span the region from the aortic bifurcation up to either the inferior mesenteric artery (IMA) or the renal veins. The first major blood vessel encountered during a caudad to cephalad para-aortic node dissection is the IMA. The IMA originates from the anterior surface of the aorta, approximately 3–4 cm above the aortic bifurcation. Next, the right and left ovarian arteries arise from their respective sides of the aorta about 5–6 cm above the bifurcation.

The right ovarian vein inserts into the right side of the inferior vena cava (IVC) approximately 1 cm below the right renal vein; however, it may insert into the right renal vein. The left ovarian vein does not insert directly into the IVC but rather follows a path close to the left ureter, inserting into the left renal vein lateral to the left border of the aorta. Three to four pairs of lumbar arteries and veins arise from the posterior surfaces of the aorta and IVC, respectively.

STEPS

An incision is made in the peritoneum overlying the right common iliac artery. The incision is carried up over the

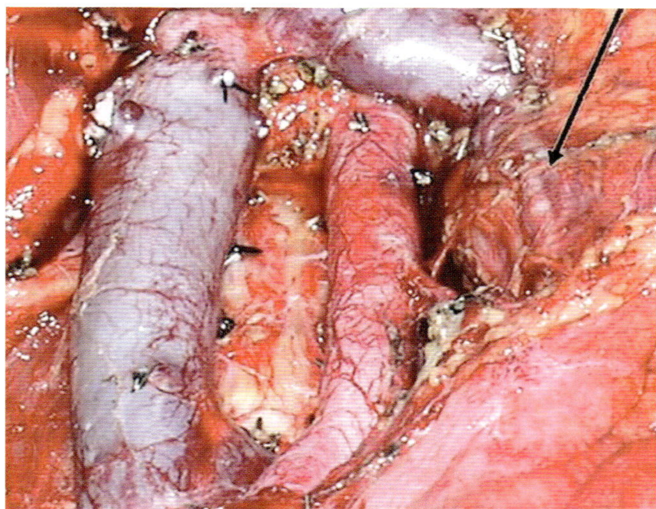

Fig. 1: Aorta and inferior vena cava denuded after completion of para-aortic lymphadenectomy

aorta to the level of the duodenum. Using blunt dissection, the ureter and the ovarian vessels are identified and mobilized laterally. In order to dissect the nodes above the IMA, the posterior peritoneum is incised from the area medial to the inferior mesenteric vein to the ileocecal region and up along the white line of Toldt. The root of the mesentery is then mobilized using sharp and blunt dissection. The small bowel contents and right colon are then moved out of the field. The fibroadipose tissue between the undersurface of the duodenum and pancreas as well as the anterior surface of the renal vein are then doubly clamped and divided in order to provide adequate exposure to the retroperitoneum. Hemoclips can be used to obtain hemostasis as needed.

A self-retaining Goligher retractor is then placed and the small bowel contents are packed away with moist laparotomy sponges. Care must be taken to prevent undue traction to the pancreas and undersurface of the duodenum. The right and left ureters are then identified and encircled with vessel loops and retracted laterally. The dissection then proceeds in a caudad-to-cephalad direction. A plane is created between the IVC and the lymphatic pedicle. The majority of the right para-aortic nodes overlie the IVC and they are generally easily dissected off the vessel. However, there is a fairly constant small vein within the lymphatics anterior to the IVC that inserts just above its bifurcation. If care is not taken to identify and ligate this so called "fellow's" vein early in dissection, it can easily be torn, with resultant heavy bleeding.

Using the "split and roll technique," all tissues within the bilateral template are removed. The vena cava is gently rolled medially and laterally. The lumbar veins are then doubly ligated and transected. Ligation of the lumbar veins allows for safe dissection behind the IVC and complete removal of the pericaval and retrocaval nodes. The split along the anterior surface of the aorta is then performed and the lumbar arteries are doubly ligated, then transected. Ligation of the lumbar arteries allows safe dissection behind the aorta and complete removal of the periaortic and retroaortic nodes (Fig. 1). Attempts should be made to preserve the IMA. The posterior limit of the dissection is the anterior spinous ligament.

COMPLICATIONS

The main complication of para-aortic lymphadenectomy is perioperative hemorrhage. The rate of this complication can be reduced by observing proper surgical techniques. Any injury to a vessel should be tackled immediately using vascular clamps and suturing with size 3-0 Mersilk sutures. Coagulation of bleeding vessels may be done using electrosurgical cautery or an argon beam coagulator. The other major complications are lymphocyst formation and deep vein thrombosis.

BIBLIOGRAPHY

1. Donohue JP. Metastatic pathways of nonseminomatous germ cell tumors. Semin Urol. 1984;2(4):217-29.
2. Fowler JM, Johnson PR. Transperitoneal para-aortic lymphadenectomy. Oper Tech Gynecolog Surg. 1996;1:8-12.
3. Panici PB, Maggioni A, Hacker N, et al. Systematic aortic and pelvic lymphadenectomy versus resection of bulky nodes only in optimally debulked advanced ovarian cancer: a randomized clinical trial. J Natl Cancer Inst. 2005;97:560-6.
4. Rezk Y, Sheinfeld J, Chi DS. Prolonged survival following salvage surgery for chemorefractory ovarian immature teratoma: a case report and review of the literature. Gynecol Oncol. 2005;96:883-7.

CHAPTER

48

Omentectomy, J Flap, TRAM Flap

Sandeep Agarwal

INTRODUCTION

Omentectomy is an integral part of many gynecological surgical procedures. Omentum has been described as a policeman of the abdomen and has an inherent property of containing and confining any aberration inside the peritoneal cavity, be it infection, inflammation hemorrhage, intestinal leaks. Hence, any shed out cells in the peritoneal cavity can theoretically be trapped by the omentum, hence, it becomes best practice to include omentum along with the excised specimen.

Omentectomy can be:

1. Partial omentectomy
2. Total omentectomy.

Partial Omentectomy

It includes excision of the part of omentum and is usually indicated in ovarian cancers, such as with:

- Small unilateral ovarian mass
- No free fluid in the abdominal cavity
- No peritoneal/serosal seedlings
- No obvious lymph node enlargement
- Clean under surfaces of diaphragm/liver surfaces.

In other malignancies also, if omentum is found adhered to a tumor (i.e. uterine mass), it is better to include a part of adhered omentum in the specimen rather than making any attempt to separate such adhesions.

Partial omentectomy usually entails excision of the infracolic part of the omentum, which is divided between the clamps and ligated.

Total Omentectomy

This includes removal of complete omentum, and is a part of surgical resection for most of the ovarian cancers, but can also be considered in other malignancies. Ovarian malignancy is peculiar as there is distinct place of debulking surgery even in advanced disease which is the case in other malignancies, such as of uterus or cervix.

Operative Technique (Figs 1 to 3)

- A liberal midline incision extending well both above and below the umbilicus is usually taken, giving good exposure up to both flexures

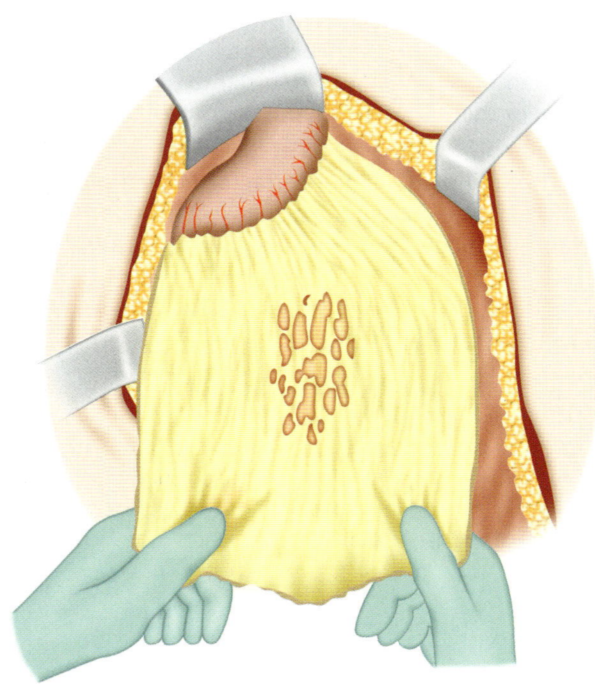

Fig. 1: The omentum is fanned-out and its attachment to the transverse colon is identified

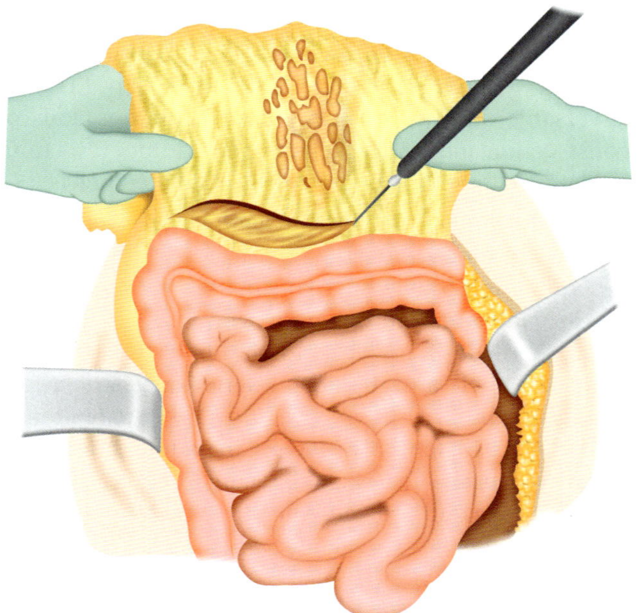

Fig. 2: An avascular plane between the transverse colon and the omentum is opened with electrocautery. Only the posterior leaf of the omentum should be incised

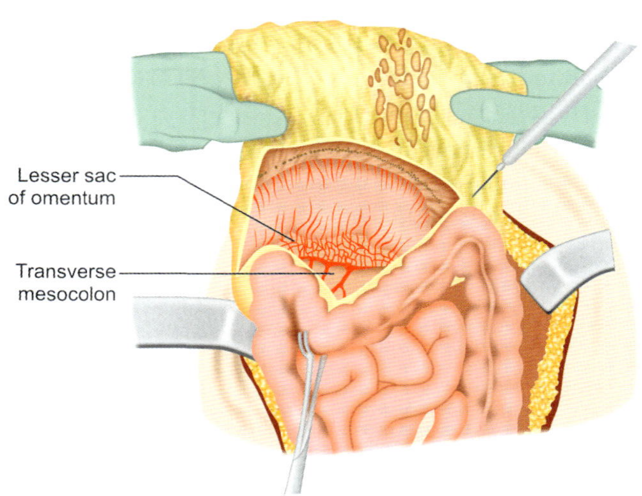

Fig. 3: An avascular plane between the omentum and underlying mesocolon is developed to the level of the lesser sac, which is anterior to the stomach wall

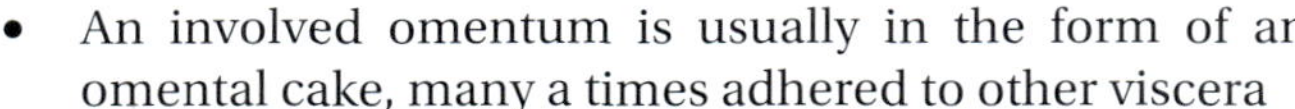

- An involved omentum is usually in the form of an omental cake, many a times adhered to other viscera
- This is best separated by finger fracture technique
- Once omentum is dissected up to transverse colon, it is lifted by an assistant with both the hands, and it is separated from transverse colon by sharp dissection, ligating vessels coming in the way till the greater curvature of stomach is reached
- The arch formed by the right and the left gastro-epiploic arteries is visualized and preserved, and branches coming toward omentum are divided and ligated moving toward the splenic flexure. Few short gastric vessels are also encountered, which are also ligated and divided, finally separating the omentum completely from the splenic flexure
- The procedure is similarly continued on the right side up to hepatic flexure finally, separating the omentum in toto as one piece
- A thorough check for hemostasis is essential, although a drain is not required.

Advantages of Omentectomy

It not only acts as a therapeutic procedure where there is involvement of omentum, but also serves as staging procedure where no obvious involvement of omentum is seen, but the most important place of omentectomy still remains in ovarian malignancies where omentum has consistently born a decent load of the disease, and role of debulking surgery is well established.

Omental "J" Flap

Omentum qualifies as an ideal interposition flap because of its rich blood supply and lymphatic drainage. Additionally, in nearly one-third cases, it can be brought to pelvis without any tension. However, in two-third cases it requires mobilization which can be done either on the left or the right gastro-epiploic vessels, allowing sufficient length, right is however preferred because of better blood supply.

An interposition flap is used in reconstructions as it increases success rate by (1) increasing neovascularity, (2) facilitating granulation formation, (3) providing cover/barrier layer as in vesicovaginal fistula (VVF) repair.

Operative Technique

Omentum is separated from the transverse colon and ligation and division of short gastric vessels further permits the mobilization of omentum from left to right, based on right gastro-epiploic artery. Absorbable suture material is used to avoid non-absorbable suture materials coming in contact of organs like urinary bladder.

The commonest application of this flap is in VVF repair where the flap is left interposed between the closed bladder and vaginal layers, anchored with the help of 3-0 vicryl sutures.

The disadvantage of this flap is that the omentum may not be available sometime or it might be diseased, an ineligible for utilization.

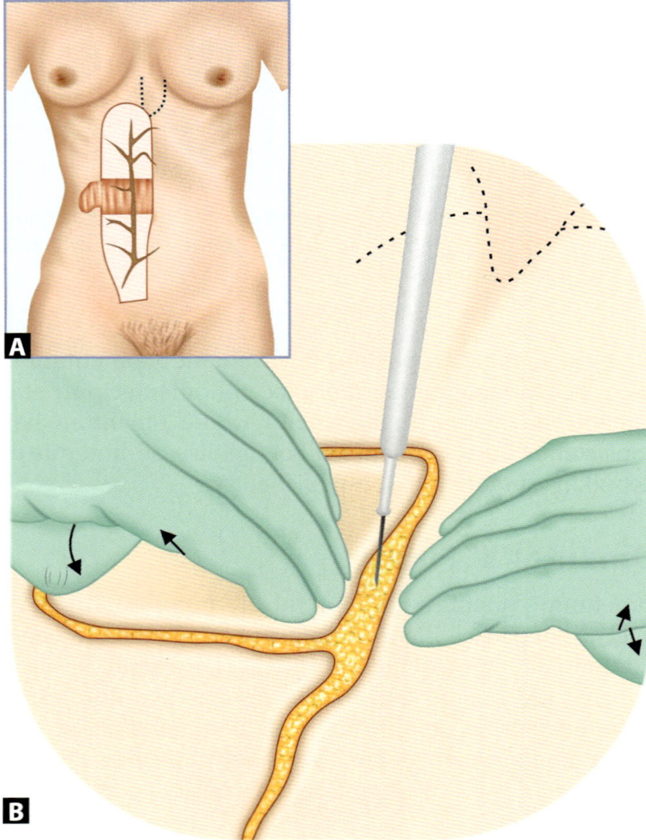

Figs 4A and B: (A) A marking pen is used to outline a 9×12 cm flap perpendicular to and extending from the midline. A skin incision is made over the outline of the flap. Typically a midline incision will include the medial border of the TRAM flap; (B) In gentle traction on the flap, the incision is carried through the cutaneous tissue to the underlying anterior rectus fascia. Care must be taken throughout the operation to avoid trauma to flap and its underlying blood supply

TRAM Flap

Reconstruction after major oncological resections is a challenge. Transverse rectus abdominis flap (TRAM) is a versatile flap which meets most of the demands of reconstruction, following extensive pelvic tumor resection, especially in the setting of previously irradiated pelvis.

The TRAM flap provides a very large skin paddle which can result in very large skin defects of perineum. It can also be used bilaterally. For the pelvic exenteration, the skin paddle can be de-epithelized and the bulk can be utilized. It has very rich blood supply based on the dominant pedicle and the deep inferior epigastric artery and vein. The bulk of the flap gives ideal tissue to obliterate the dead space in pelvis. The large skin paddle can be used to provide surface for vaginal reconstruction, perineal defect coverage and provides versatility for all patterns of reconstruction.

Operative Technique (Figs 4 to 14)

The skin island needed is marked according to the length of pedicle required and the lie of the flap along the epigastric

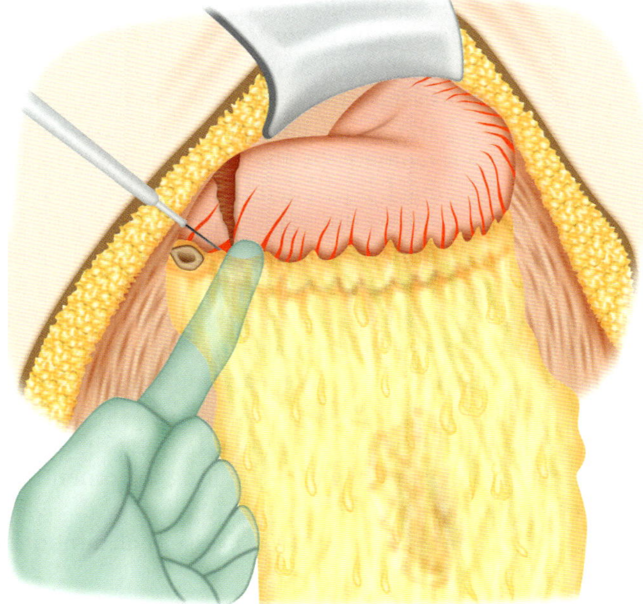

Fig. 5: The gastroepiploic and short gastric vessels are isolated by electrocautery

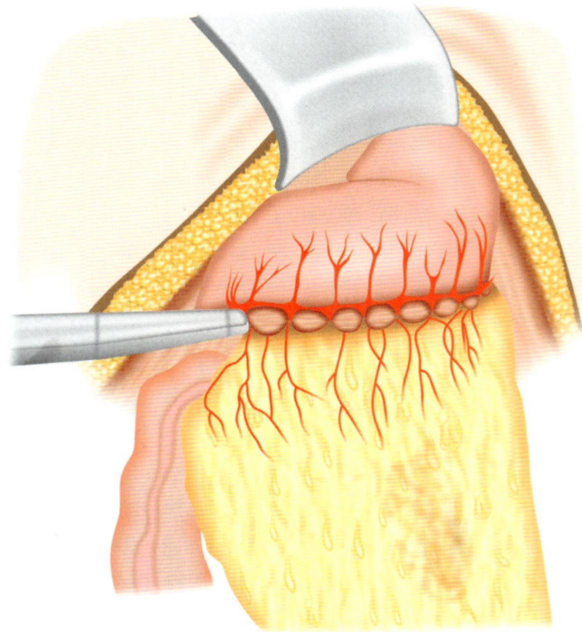

Fig. 6: The gastroepiploic and short gastric vessels are ligated with silk of absorbable ligatures or are stapled with a linear dissecting stapler

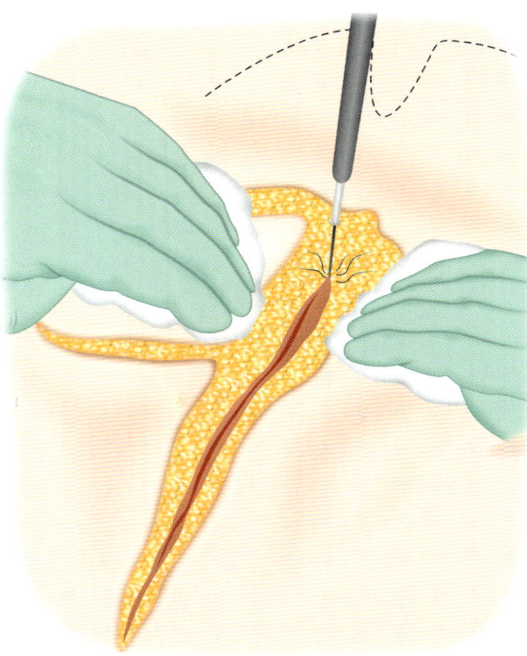

Fig. 7: The anterior rectus fascia is incised, exposing the underlying rectus abdominis muscle along the full length of the midline incision

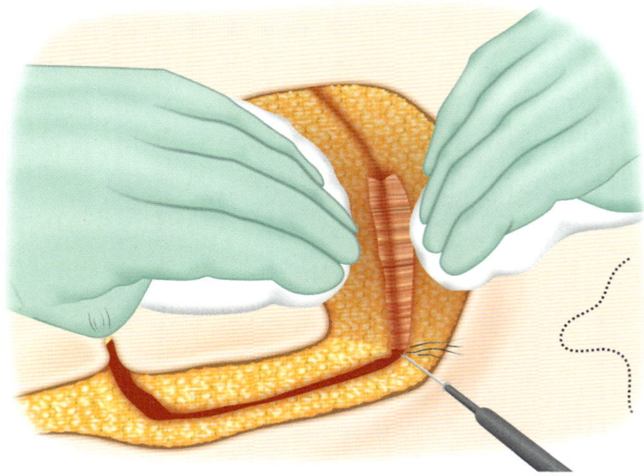

Fig. 8: The rectus abdominis muscle is transected only at the superior border of the flap (Fig. 7). The epigastric vessels located beneath the muscle must be ligated above the superior margin of the flap to protect its blood supply

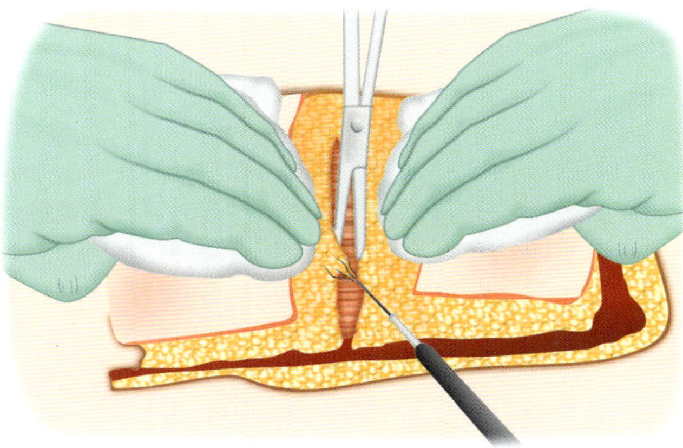

Fig. 9: The anterior rectus fascia is incised at the inferior border of the flap perpendicular to the midline. The rectus muscle is left intact

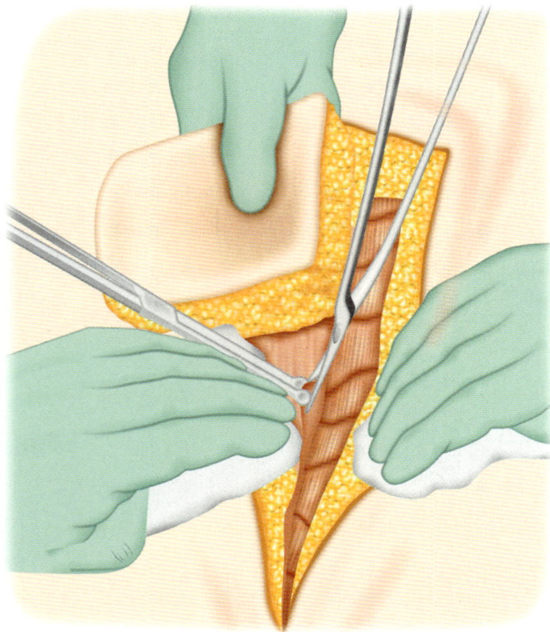

Fig. 10: If the transverse rectus abdominis flap is to be used for pelvic floor reconstruction and to form neovagina, the peritoneum of the midline incision and which underlines the myocutaneous flap is incised. The TRAM flap and the contiguous ipsilateral rectus muscle caudad to it are meticulously dissected away from the overlying anterior rectus fascia and the underlying posterior rectus sheath. Great care must be taken to avoid injury to the epigastric vessels

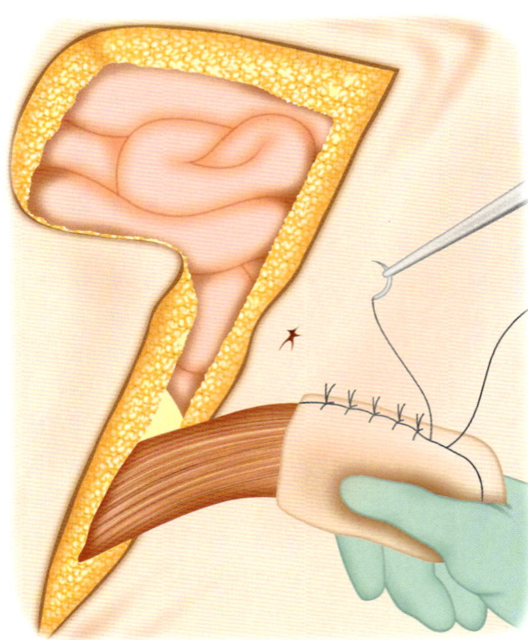

Fig. 11: When used for vaginal reconstruction, the flap is folded approximizing skin-to-skin to create a tube, the distal end of which will remain open. An interrupted 2-0 polyglycolide suture is used to fashion the new vagina. The outer portion of the tube will consist of pelvic peritoneum that envelops the rectus muscle, subcutaneous tissue and skin

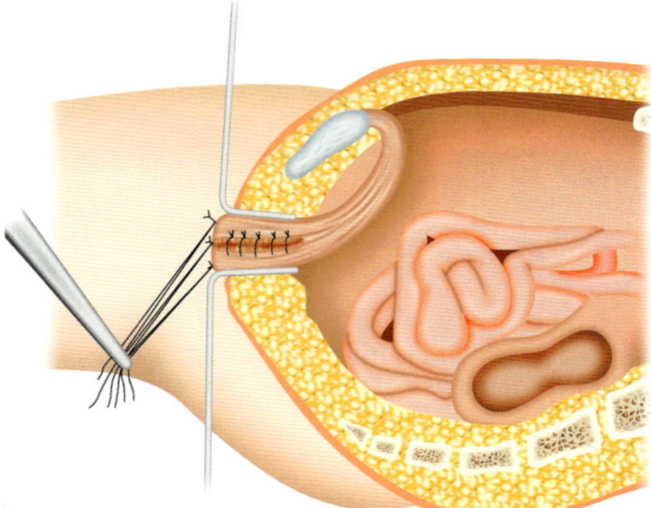

Fig. 12: The myocutaneous flap is rotated down into the pelvis and care taken to avoid torsion of its blood supply. The distal portion of the flap is tagged with several sutures to facilitate downward traction

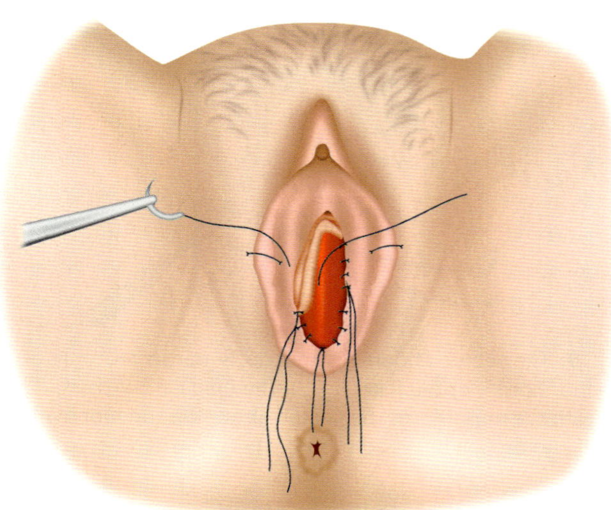

Fig. 13: The distal end of the vaginal tube is sutured to the skin of the vulva and perineum with interrupted 2-0 or 3-0 polyglycolide sutures

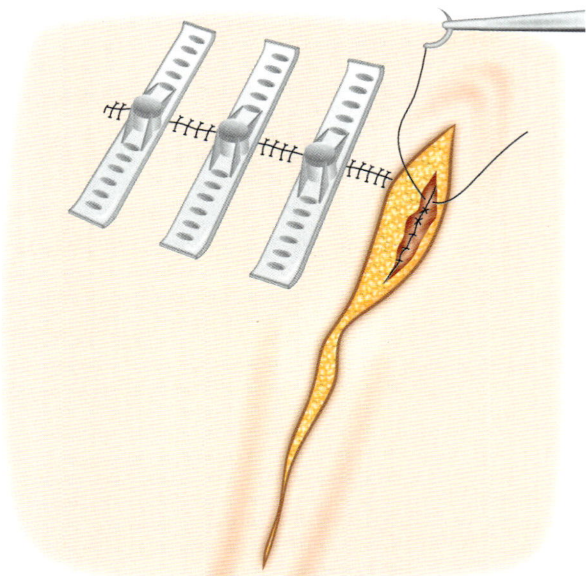

Fig. 14: Closure of the lateral abdominal wall defect from which the flap was harvested should be done with interrupted #0 or #1 permanent sutures. The skin is closed with staples (Fig. 12). When needed, nylon retention sutures or wound reinforcement with mesh should be considered

region using the superior subcostal musculocutaneous perforators of the upper abdominal wall. The area of skin overlying the rectus abdominis muscle, extending from below the costal margin to below the umbilicus for a length of 20–25 cm, is very well perfused area of skin.

After defining the skin island and dissecting it, further dissection continues caudally. Rectus muscle is detached from superior attachment to lower costal margin, and superior epigastric artery and vein divided and ligated. Rectus muscle is lifted along the flap, leaving behind the posterior rectus sheath. The anterior rectus sheath becomes narrower on the flap as it is lifted up, as a result, the lateral and medial margins of anterior rectus sheath can be closed primarily.

De-epithelization is done, so that large perineal defects can be covered.

Uses

- Defects after pelvic exenteration
- Post-irradiation pelvic defects
- Large perineal defects.

CHAPTER

49

Role of Colposcopy in Gynecology

Reshma Rafi, Sarita Bhalerao, Usha Saraiya

INTRODUCTION

Cytology and Colposcopy are two techniques which are used in the early detection of cervical cancer.

Colposcopy originated in Hamburg, Germany. Hans Hinselman, a gynecologist believed that cervical cancer must originate as a small "dot" invisible to the naked eye. He devised a series of magnifying lens which would make the dot visible and thus originated the clinical investigation called colposcopy. It remained in German speaking world for a long time. The Second World War was a great setback to its development. However, when cytology screening programs were taken up all over the world in 1950s and 1960s many cases with abnormal cytology were detected and all these cases had to be further investigated by colposcopy. Hence, 1970s saw the "renaissance" of colposcopy and its popularity increased. This was further aided by improved instrumentation and technology in all parts of the world.

Colposcopy is being widely used in western countries for precise diagnosis and management of preclinical lesions of cervix. However, it has not made an impact in developing countries like India for many reasons. The most important reason being the cost and the lack of easy availability of the equipment and lack of trained personnel in this field.

This instrument is of vital importance to those who are actively involved in early diagnosis and management of cervical cancer. Although it is possible to treat cases of early cervical neoplasia with cytomorphic, histological and clinical data, occasionally cases are over or undertreated and follow-up involves greater risks if colposcopy is not available.

Introduction of colposcopy in the evaluation of cervical lesions by clinical, cytological and histological assessment is rewarded by a higher pick-up rate and more accurate diagnosis. Being a clinical diagnostic method, the clinician can study the minute changes occurring in the cervical mucosa over a period of time. Colposcopy affords diagnostic, therapeutic and prognostic information.

NATURAL HISTORY OF CERVICAL CANCER

It has now been proved beyond doubt that invasive cervical cancer is the end result of a process of carcinogenesis which starts at its earliest stage with inflammatory reaction. When a carcinogen attacks a group of cells, they react by a process of inflammatory change. If the carcinogen keeps on acting, the cells undergo a series of changes of mild, moderate and severe dysplasia, then on to carcinoma-in-situ (CIS) and finally invasive cancer (Flow chart 1).

Up to moderate dysplasia, the lesions are reversible. But beyond that the changes are irreversible.

Flow chart 1: Natural history of cervical cancer

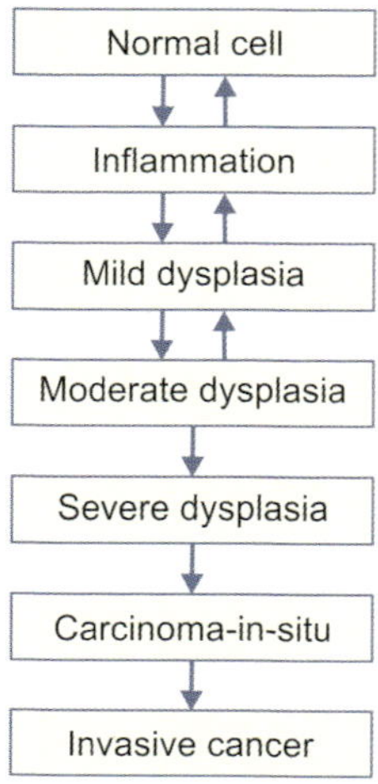

The carcinogen involved in cervical cancer is now identified as human papillomavirus (HPV). HPV 16 and 18 are oncogenic and have been proved to have a role in causation of cervical cancer.

ROLE OF HPV IN THE CAUSATION OF CERVICAL CANCER

The story of HPV is only 35 years old when Zur Hausen in 1970s proved that HPV was the causative agent of cervical cancer.

Cervical biopsies for carcinoma are positive for HPV in 99.7% of cases, supporting the fact that it is a causal and necessary factor for development of cervical cancer (Fig. 1).

Types of HPV
- HPV 6: Predilection for vulva
- HPV 16: Predilection for cervix
- HPV 16/18: Rapid progression to neoplasia
- HPV 6/11: May remain subclinical

PREVALENCE

HPV types 16, 18, 45, 31 are most important of the high-risk or the oncogenic types all over the world, according to a pooled analysis by Munoz et al. HPV 16 and 18 are the earliest most common types of HPV seen in cervical cancer across all regions and together cause nearly 71% of all cervical cancers and a vaccine that protects against both these strains has the potential to prevent this cancer.

It is a sexually transmitted virus and therefore anyone who has a normal sex life is at risk of exposure to high-risk HPV types.

Cervical cancer is the first solid tumor associated with virus infection.

In India, the incidence of cancer cervix continues to be high. Various cancer registries indicate that it is about 20–40 per 100,000 women. The tragedy is more because all cases are detected very late, in stage III and IV where treatment gives poor results. Therefore, attempts have to be made to detect it at an earlier stage.

This is possible if cytology and colposcopy are routinely used in our practice.

CYTOLOGY

Smear taking is very simple. After introducing a speculum, a smear is taken from the squamocolumnar junction with an Ayre's spatula or a cotton swab. It is smeared on a clean glass slide which is immediately dipped into a fixative consisting of equal parts of ether and 95% alcohol.

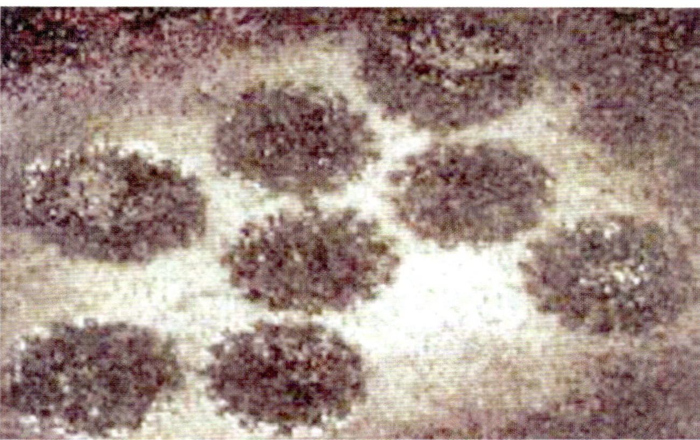

Fig. 1: Microphotograph showing highly magnified image of human papillomavirus (HPV)

This jar is taken to the laboratory where it is stained by Papanicolaou stain and then mounted in Canada balsam and covered with a cover slip.

The slide is then studied under a binocular research microscope. The report will indicate whether the cells seen are normal, atypical, precancerous or frankly malignant.

All women who have an abnormal smear on cytology have to be evaluated further by colposcopy.

COLPOSCOPIC EVALUATION

The cervix is exposed by a bivalve speculum and the colposcope is focused on it. The cervix may be cleaned with a swab soaked in normal saline.

The following factors are assessed:
- Color, tone, and opacity of the mucosa
- Surface contour
- Transformation zone or the squamocolumnar junction. It must be seen clearly as most cancers originate here (Figs 2 to 4)
- Presence or absence of abnormal vessels on the surface
- *Acetic acid application:* The cervix is painted with 3% acetic acid and then studied again. If any white patches appear now, they are called acetowhite areas and signify a thickening of the epithelium. There is a possibility of HPV infection or an early dysplasia.
- *Schiller iodine test:* This is done by painting the cervix with aqueous solution of iodine. The normal epithelium is rich in glycogen and therefore takes up a dark brown stain with iodine. Rapidly proliferating cells utilize all the glycogen and hence are deficient in glycogen. They remain unstained. Hence, iodine negative areas are considered abnormal.

The colposcopic findings are classified according to colposcopic terminology accepted at 2nd World Congress for Cervical Pathology and Colposcopy in 1975 and are modified from time to time.

The current classification was described by Walker et al. in 2003 (Box 1). Various colposcopic pictures depicting normal transformation zone to infective, epithelial changes are depicted in Figures 2 to 9.

Box 1 International terminology of colposcopy (updated January 2003)

- Normal colposcopic findings
  - Original squamous epithelium
  - Columnar epithelium
  - Transformation zone
- Abnormal colposcopic findings
  - Flat acetowhite epithelium
  - Dense acetowhite epithelium*
  - Fine mosaic—Coarse mosaic*
  - Fine punctation—Coarse punctation*
  - Iodine partial positivity—Iodine negativity*
  - Atypical vessels*
- Colposcopic features suggestive of invasive cancer
- Unsatisfactory colposcopy
  - Squamocolumnar junction not visible
  - Severe inflammation, severe atrophy, trauma
  - Cervix not visible
- Miscellaneous findings
  - Condylomata
  - Keratosis
  - Erosion
  - Inflammation
  - Atrophy
  - Deciduosis—Pregnancy
  - Polyps

*Major changes

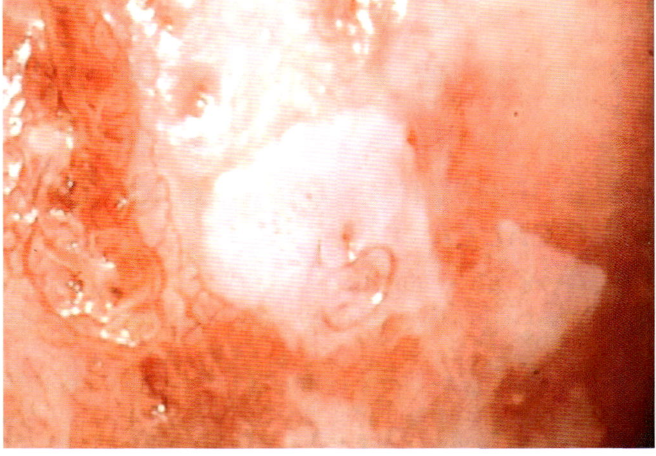

Fig. 3: Atypical metaplastic epithelium. Abnormal transformation zone

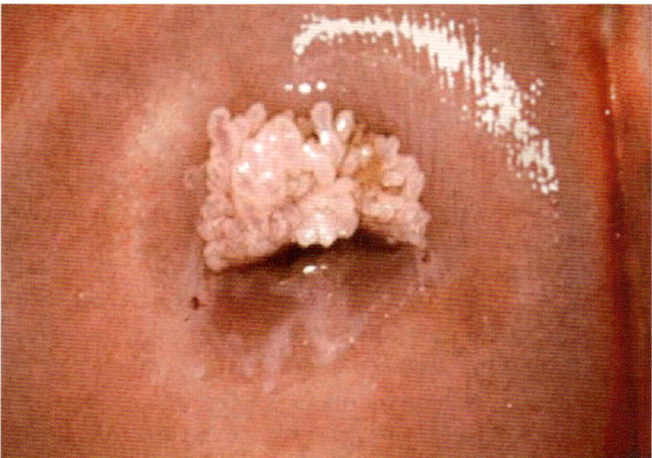

Fig. 4: Condyloma

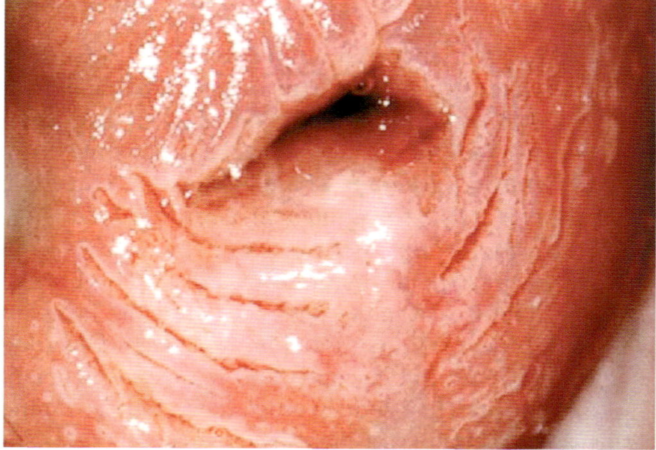

Fig. 2: Mature typical metaplastic epithelium. Normal transformation zone

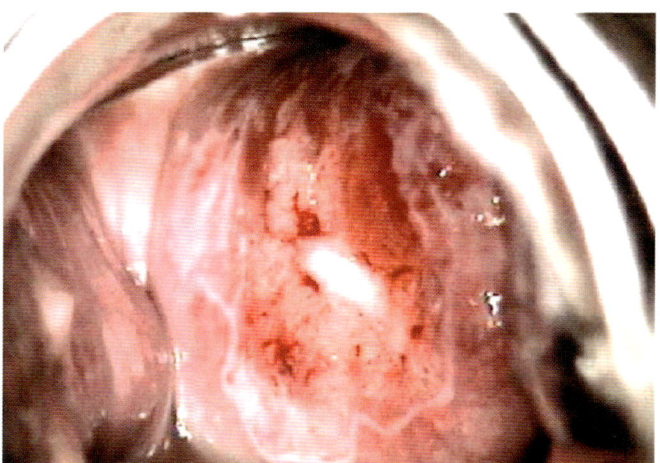

Fig. 5: Transformation zone

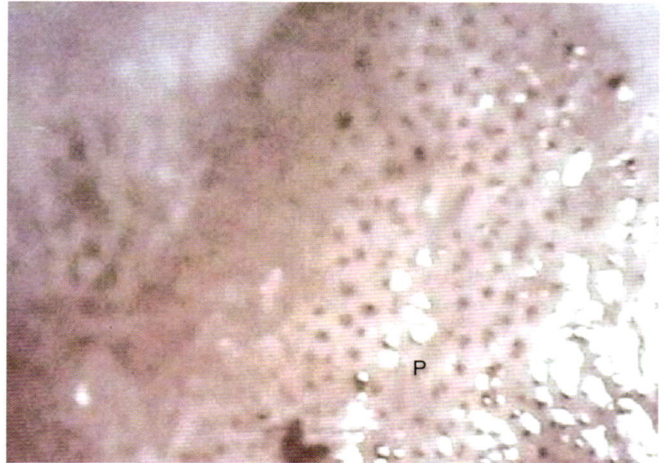

Fig. 6: Trichomoniasis

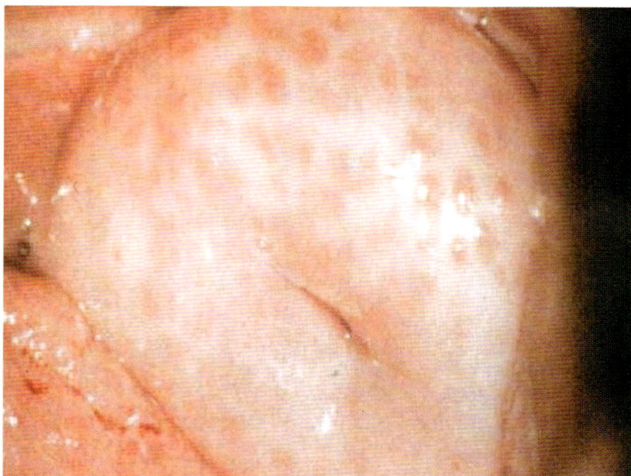

Fig. 7: Punctations

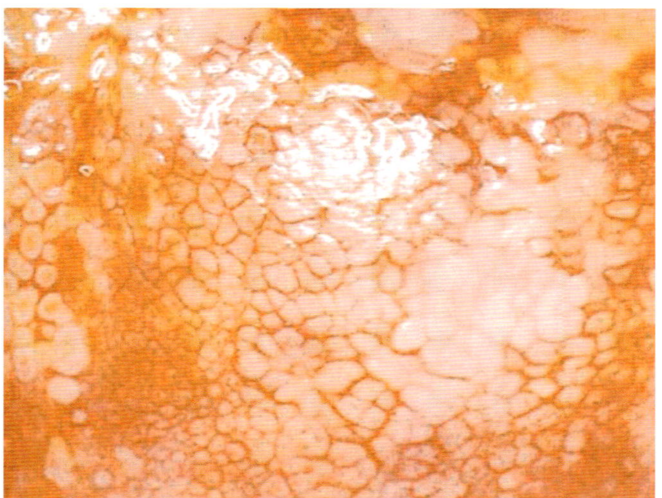

Fig. 8: Mosaic

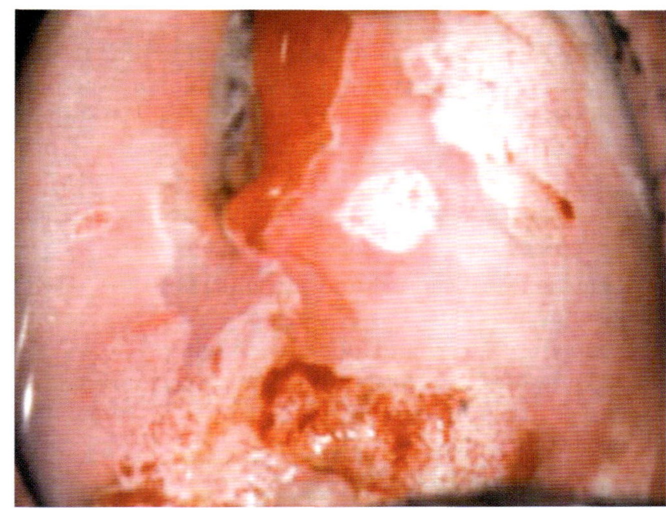

Fig. 9: Human papillomavirus (HPV) infection

MANAGEMENT OF WOMEN WITH ABNORMAL CYTOLOGY

All cases must be carefully re-examined and if possible colposcopy performed to detect the size and site of the lesion. Schiller iodine test alone is useful if colposcope is not available.

The management will depend on:

- Degree of dysplasia
- Extent of dysplasia, small or large lesion
- Age of the patient
- Desire for childbearing function
- Desire for menstrual function
- Risk factor present in the index case.

In principle, all cases of mild and moderate dysplasia should be carefully treated conservatively and followed up as regression is likely to occur.

Local destruction of a small lesion is possible by:

- Electrocautery which burns the epithelium
- Cryocautery which freezes it
- Carbon dioxide laser which destroys by evaporation.

Those who progresses further or those who are diagnosed as severe dysplasia or CIS should be treated by excisional method at the first instance.

Histopathological correlation is a must and should be done in all cases.

Excisional methods are:

- Cone biopsy which maybe diagnostic and therapeutic (Fig. 10).

This can be performed by cold knife or by carbon dioxide laser.

If the excisional biopsy has been adequate and there is no residual lesion left, the patient may be kept on

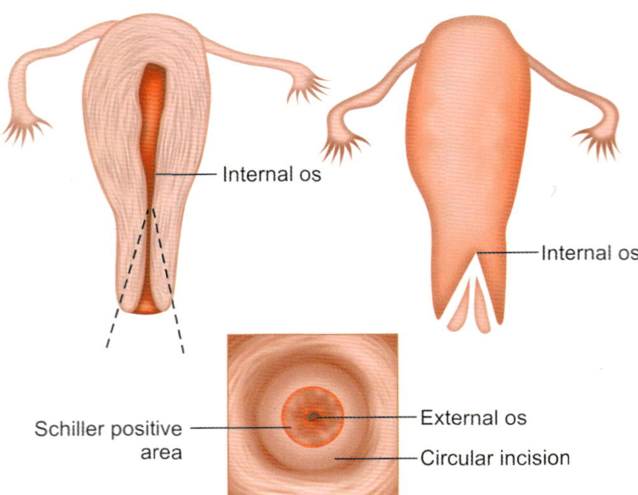

Fig. 10: Diagnostic cervical conization

follow-up. Eventually she can be considered for hysterectomy as lifelong follow-up is not possible for everyone. This hysterectomy is a simple one and not radical surgery needed for invasive cancer. Hence, it can be easily performed in any setting giving a very low morbidity rate.

The Flow chart 2 may be followed as practical application of these principles of management.

The main indications and advantages of the use of colposcopy are as follows:

- Follow-up of mild and moderate dysplasia
- To know the extent of abnormal area in severe dysplasia and CIS as a preoperative assessment. To know how big a cone to take
- When micro or early invasive cancer is diagnosed on cytology. Even though no lesion is diagnosed on naked eye inspection of cervix, it is usually obvious on colposcopy
- Follow-up of treated cases cancer of cervix to know early recurrence
- When dysplasia is treated conservatively with cryo- or CO_2 laser therapy, follow-up by colposcopy is must.

This service must be centralized in all big cities initially and with easy referral available. Training facilities have to be provided so that services can spread to many centers.

NEWER DEVELOPMENTS IN COLPOSCOPY

Since the original design of instrument in 1927, a series of changes and innovations have taken place making the colposcope more user-friendly and patient-friendly.

- *Video colposcopy:* It is no longer necessary to peer down the eye piece and try to focus. A three chip charge-coupled device (CCD) video camera is built in and a high resolution image is available on a TV monitor. This cuts down the time required for examining each patient and provides documentation. It also facilitates teaching and training of a large group. For conducting workshops it is almost a necessity. It also creates the possibility of video conferencing
- *Cervicoscope:* It is a camera attachment which takes kodachrome slides of the appearance of the cervix. This was designed by Adolf Stafl. The slides can then be reviewed by an expert Colposcopist and evaluated

Flow chart 2: Management of abnormal cytology

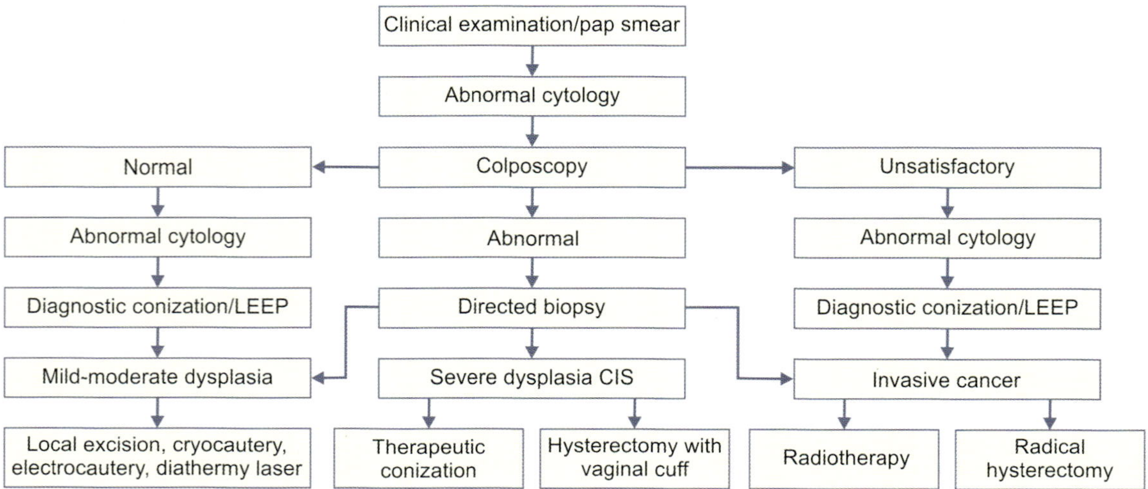

Abbreviations: LEEP, loop electrosurgical excision procedure; CIS, carcinoma in situ

along with the cytology report. The cervicoscope is a small instrument which is portable and can be handled by paramedical staff. Hence, it is very suitable for developing countries where cancer detection camps are carried out in remote areas. It also provides good documentation. Currently a digital camera can be used on the cervicoscope and images recorded on a computer

- *Chromo-colposcopy:* It was devised by Gilardi et al. in Italy. It involves the painting of the cervix with certain vital dyes and evaluating the color changes in the epithelium by Colposcopy. Traditional colposcopy gives bichromatic images both with acetic and Lugol's iodine. Chromo-colposcopy gives polychromatic images with color pattern corresponding to specific histopathology. It is a new research perspective and a new frontier for a colposcopist. Usually green indicates a metaplastic change, whereas yellow and dark brown indicate a malignant process
- *Operating colposcope with CO_2 laser:* If the laser equipment is attached to the colposcope, it can serve as a diagnostic and therapeutic tool. After evaluation of the lesion, under colposcopic control the abnormal epithelium may be treated by Laser or a small cone taken by a laser knife. This leads to less number of visits and being an OPD procedures, can be done at same sitting.

CONCLUSION

Cytology and colposcopy should be included in routine Gynecology so as to detect cervical cancer in its early stage. This will go a long way in bringing down the morbidity and mortality associated with the disease.

These techniques are simple, inexpensive and suitable for use in India. Mass screening of all women in the age of 25–55 years should be our ultimate aim. Periodic screening every 2–3 years is necessary to detect new cases. The need for periodic gynecological checkup must be stressed to all women, especially those above the age of 40 years. Facilities must be developed for the treatment of early lesions. These include cryosurgery and CO_2 laser.

BIBLIOGRAPHY

1. Burghardt E. Colposcopy Cervical Pathology. New York: Thieme Medical Publishers; 1984.
2. Coloured Atlas of Cytology and Colposcopy. In: Miniello G, Saraiya U (Eds). New Delhi: CBS publication; 1998
3. Lulla M, Saraiya U. Colposcopic and cytologic evaluation of cervical lesions. Ind J Cancer. 1983;20:156-60.
4. Saraiya U. Lasers in Gynaecological malignancies. Bio Med. 1998;5(6):14.
5. Stafl A, Wilkinson EJ, Mattingly R. Laser treatment of cervical and vaginal neoplasia. Am J Obstet Gynaecol. 1977;128:128-36.
6. Walker P, Dexeus S, De Palo, et al. International terminology of colposcopy: an updated report from the International Federation for Cervical Pathology and Colposcopy. Obstet Gynecol. 2003;101:175-7.

CHAPTER

50

Overview of Assisted Reproductive Technologies Procedures

Monesh Shah, Jaideep Malhotra

INTRODUCTION

Since time immemorial, there has been a compelling urge and necessity to propagate one's own species. Reproduction is a basic fundamental right irrespective of caste, creed, religion, race, social, economic, educational status.

Failure to conceive after attempting to do so after one or more years is termed infertility. Most infertile couples experience deep despair and despondency due to lot of social pressures coupled with physical, mental and financial stress involved in attempts to find a solution. Before the era of assisted reproductive technologies (ART), treatment options were limited in terms of techniques, medications, skills, efficacy and were associated with very low success rates in relation to the etiologic factors.

The field of ART has progressed rapidly over the past 3 decades to an extent that 80–90% of couples can be expected to have a healthy child. Louise Brown, the world's first in vitro fertilization-embryo transfer (IVF-ET) baby, was born on 25th July, 1978; this was a landmark heralding the revolutionary future of the treatment of human infertility. Indeed we are indebted to Patrick Steptoe and Robert Edwards for this marvelous breakthrough (Fig. 1).

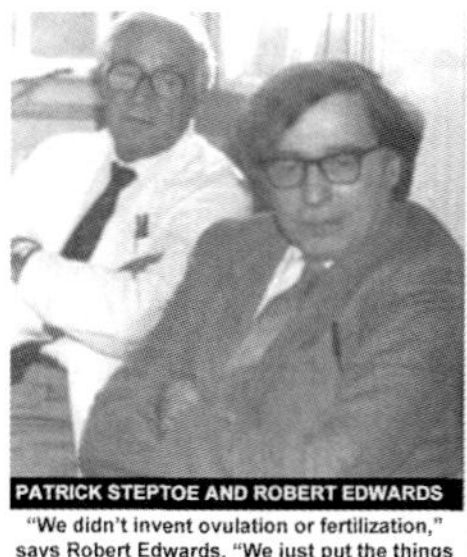

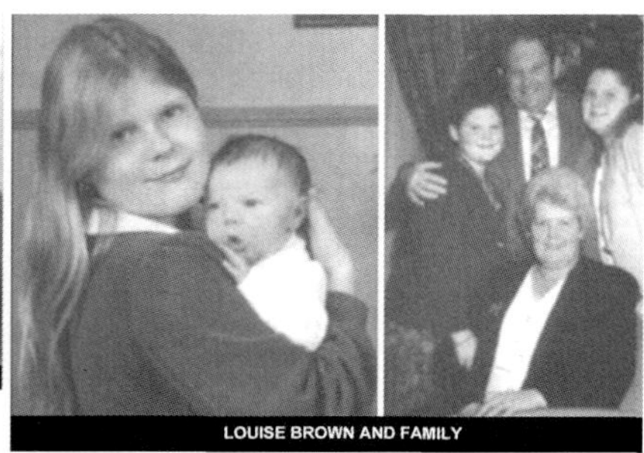

Fig. 1: First IVF baby Louise Brown and family and pioneer—in vitro fertilization team

More than two million babies have been born to date with the application of ART in almost all forms of infertility.

HISTORY

Several milestones followed the birth of Louise Brown in 1978. IVF babies were born in several parts of the world. Oocyte retrieval was done laparoscopically for nearly a decade until first sonography guided oocyte aspiration was reported in 1981 by Lenz et al. With the advent of vaginal transducers, the transvesical transabdominal oocyte pickup was replaced by transvaginal oocyte retrieval.

Gamete intrafallopian transfer (GIFT) was reported by Asch et al. This was followed by zygote intrafallopian transfer (ZIFT) in 1986. In 1992 another path breaking technique was reported by the group from Brussels, namely intracytoplasmic sperm injection (ICSI). Subsequently, pregnancies were reported with the use of testicular or epididymal sperm and even spermatids. ET graduated from the four cell stage to 6–8 cell stage and eventually progressed to the blastocyst stage transfer with increasing advances in the production of culture media and the introduction of sequential media which could sustain human life in vitro for 5–6 days.

Natural cycle treatments gave way to stimulated cycles with the advent and widespread use of gonadotropins. Urinary derived products are today available in highly purified form and recombinant technology has led to the availability of recombinant follicle stimulating hormone (FSH), lutenizing hormone (LH) and human chorionic gonadotropin (hCG). The use of gonadotropin releasing hormone (GnRH) analogs for hormone suppression during a stimulated cycle was another major event which resulted in the establishment of the long protocol as a benchmark protocol. Further research led to the development of the GnRH antagonists which are currently being used in an endeavor to minimize the cost and duration of therapy.

Methods of avoiding excessive, costly and cumbersome ovarian stimulation have resulted in in vitro maturation of oocytes (IVM) obtained from antral follicles and this approach promises to minimize disadvantages of controlled ovarian hyperstimulation.

Pregnancy following human embryo freezing was announced in 1983 by Trounson et al. Later on, human oocytes could be successfully cryopreserved. Cryopreservation techniques applied to sperms, oocytes and embryos have been streamlined to yield better success rates. Alternative methods such as vitrification of oocytes and embryos have emerged as an alternative to slow freezing methods.

Identifying a healthy genetically normal embryo for transfer has led to the development and application of preimplantation genetic diagnosis and blastomere biopsy.

Laser has also found its utility in the application of several techniques of ART including assisted hatching. Barriers of advanced maternal age and declining fertility have been broken with oocyte donation; also surrogacy has come into vogue for cases with uterine problems and medical contraindications to pregnancy.

ASSESSMENT OF OVARIAN RESERVE

Patient response to treatment is directly linked to subsequent chance of conception. Hence, prediction of ovarian reserve assumes importance as a predictor of the response to stimulation as well as the subsequent chance of pregnancy. Women with low ovarian reserve are more prone to abortions and have a higher incidence of birth defects.

- Maternal age is by far one of the most important indicators of reproductive potential with increasing age, especially after 35 years, and more so after 37 years signaling a lower chance of pregnancy irrespective of the treatment technique. The quantity and quality of oocytes determine the reproductive potential and both decline with advancing age. Also risks of abnormal progeny increases with increasing maternal age along with pregnancy related complications. Occasionally a young woman may have a low ovarian reserve but oocyte quality may not be compromised and hence she may have a better chance of pregnancy
- Day 3 FSH levels were shown to correlate with ovarian response and pregnancy outcome in IVF cycles by Muasher and Oehninger. High basal FSH levels correlate with a higher cycle cancellation rate and also denote lower chances of pregnancy. FSH levels may show intercycle variation in women with borderline ovarian reserve ranging from normal to high levels, however, finding a single raised FSH level also carries the same importance and the maximal FSH reading is the best predictor of ovarian reserve. Usually a cut off value of 10 mIU/mL is considered. In general, basal FSH correlates more with ovarian response to stimulation, the number of follicles obtained, number of oocytes retrieved and cycle cancellation rates rather than with distal events of implantation and pregnancy where maternal age assumes greater significance
- *Basal antral count on sonography evaluation:* Noting the number of antral follicles on days 3–4 of a cycle is also a reliable indicator of the response to be expected from that ovary. Fewer follicles indicate a loss of ovarian reserve and higher cycle cancellation. Antral follicle count is a better predictor compared to the ovarian volume. A multivariate analysis found antral follicle count to be a single best predictor of ovarian response
- Day 3 estradiol (E2) levels more than 80 pg/mL are thought to be an adverse signal. However, young women may exhibit both high as well as low E2 levels. High E2 may denote low ovarian reserve in women with a hurried follicular phase or may represent a high reserve in women with polycystic ovary syndrome (PCOS). Interpretation is more accurate if combined with FSH levels
- Clomiphene challenge test was first described by Navot et al. A day 3 FSH level is done and clomiphene citrate 100 mg given from days 5–9. Day 10 FSH is estimated and if it is raised more than 10–12 it indicates a low reserve
- *Day 3 Inhibin levels:* A low inhibin level is associated with high FSH levels and vice versa. This test is expensive and not routinely available.

OVARIAN STIMULATION

The oocyte that ultimately resulted in the world's first IVF conception was retrieved from a natural cycle. It was soon discovered that this method had a low efficiency and success rates as everything depended on retrieving a solitary mature oocyte. The natural cycle was also susceptible to untimely hormonal changes which would affect the oocyte quality. When clomiphene and gonadotropins were used in combination retrieval of several oocytes resulted with concomitant improved pregnancy rates. Efforts to obtain many oocytes from hormonally controlled cycles led to the further development and widespread usage of gonadotropins and later on GnRH analogs and GnRH antagonists.

Clomiphene

Clomiphene alone is rarely used in ART cycles, mainly due to the low level of response obtained. Advantages of cost and simplicity are offset by a major disadvantage of the occurrence of premature LH surges in up to 20–30% of cycles. Minimal stimulation protocols generally combine clomiphene along with small doses of gonadotropins.

Gonadotropins

These are very potent stimulators of the ovary. When started in the early follicular phase, they help in recruiting a large cohort of follicles and sustain their growth resulting in multiple follicles and subsequent retrieval of a large number of oocytes. However, the disadvantage of premature LH surge with subsequent premature luteinization of the growing cohort and subsequent low pregnancy rates remains a major disadvantage when used alone.

Gonadotropins currently available are of three types:

1. *Urinary:* These are derived from pooled urine samples of postmenopausal women and may have impurities and undesirable proteins; generally a combination of FSH and LH 75/150 IU is available.
2. *Urinary highly purified:* Here impurity levels are lower and selectively FSH alone is also available as 75/150 IU injections which can be administered subcutaneously in view of high purity levels.
3. *Recombinant:* These are genetically derived and offer advantages:
   - Highly pure with negligible contamination
   - Consistency of preparation: No batch to batch variation
   - No dependence on availability as in urinary gonadotrophins.

Currently two preparations are available: Gonal F (Serono) and Recagon (Organon). Recombinant FSH, LH (Leuvaris) and hCG (Ovidrel) are available.

Conceptually, recombinant preparations are better than urinary products with advantages of better follicular dynamics, better oocyte competence, shorter treatment duration with lower threshold and total dosage, clinical pregnancy rates appear to be higher though some have reported no significant differences as compared to urinary products. High cost is a factor to be considered.

In polycystic ovary syndrome (PCOS) patients, FSH alone is usually better suited for ovarian stimulation as compared to combined FSH due to the following reasons:

- Deficient FSH activation is important in the pathophysiology of PCOS
  - Follicle stimulating hormone prevents increased follicular apoptosis in hyperandrogenic ovaries
  - Lutenizing hormone action can increase undesirable androgen production
- Granulosa cells lack LH receptors at the start of the cycle.

The stimulation protocols in PCOS are individualized in order to obtain optimal response at a low risk of ovarian hyperstimulation syndrome (OHSS). Protocols used include:

- *Chronic low dose step-up protocol*
  75 IU FSH daily for 5–7 days increase by 37.5/75 IU if follicles less than 10 mm, every 5 days
- *Step-down protocol*
  Initial 150–225 IU/day FSH
  Later decrease to 75/37.5 IU/day once follicles are greater than or equal to 10 mm
- *Sequential protocol*
  Initial step-up followed by step-down once follicle greater than or equal to 14 mm.

GnRH Analogs (Agonists)

These are obtained by minor modifications of the GnRH molecule which result in significant prolongation of the half life. When used initially, there is a GnRH like action resulting in release of FSH and LH from the pituitary, however, continuous use results in suppression of the pituitary with downregulation. This dual action has been utilized in various protocols.

Ultra Short Protocol

The GnRH analog is given on day 2, 3 and 4 of the cycle, and the gonadotropins are started on the day following the first GnRH analog dose. This minimizes the use of gonadotropins by utilizing the initial flare-up effect of the analog. However, later on downregulatory effect can be lost as the effect wanes away, especially with longer duration of gonadotropin stimulation.

Short Protocol

Here the analog is started from day 2 of cycle and continued up to the day of hCG. Again the initial flare up is used to recruit a cohort of follicles and subsequent gonadotropin requirements may be reduced.

Long Protocol

This is the most commonly used protocol. It offers advantages of better cycle control and also facilitates scheduling of patients. In PCOS it helps in reducing the tonic LH elevation and helps in obtaining uniform follicular growth. The analog is started either in the mid-luteal phase on day 21 or on day 2 in the follicular phase. The late luteal start is preferred though there is potential risk of pregnancy; however, studies have shown no deleterious effects. A follicular start can also rescue the corpus luteum and lead to unwanted cysts. All active cysts need to be aspirated prior to starting gonadotropins.

Various molecules are available including leuprolide, triptorelin, buserelin, nafarelin.

GnRH Antagonists

These are GnRH molecules with amino-acid modifications which compete and block the GnRH receptors resulting in a decrease of FSH and more notably LH from the pituitary. In the follicular phase, they prevent or interrupt the LH surge. Two molecules cetrotide (Serono) and ganirelix (Organon) have been studied and are in clinical use today.

Two different protocols have been tried:

1. Single 3 mg dose in late follicular phase (Days 10–12).
2. Daily injections of 0.25 mg from day 7 of stimulation or from the time the leading follicle reaches 14 mm. The antagonist suppresses both FSH and LH within a few hours; there is also a concomitant reduction in estradiol. This is, however, not thought to be detrimental to subsequent implantation and embryo growth. The advantages of the antagonist protocol include:
   - Shorter cycle duration
   - Fewer injections
   - Lower gonadotropin requirement—reduction in cost
   - Lower risks of OHSS.

A few studies indicate slightly lower pregnancy rates in the antagonist cycles. This needs to be further evaluated in the light of paucity of data, lack of standardization and initial errors due to learning curve in the application of protocols. The best way to use antagonists needs further evaluation.

MAIN TREATMENT MODALITIES

Besides intrauterine insemination (IUI), which is the simplest and most basic treatment involving semen processing and deposition of sperms into the uterine cavity in a natural or stimulated cycle, the currently widely practiced treatment modalities are IVF-ET and ICSI. Despite several individual center variations in the practice of these treatments, the basic protocols are identical and involve gamete handling (both oocytes as well as sperms) in vitro. IVF relies on natural oocyte fertilization by a motile sperm and is thus suited for cases with normal seminal parameters. Presence of other female factors such as advanced age and other considerations may however lead to ICSI as the procedure of choice despite normal semen characteristics. Micromanipulation is more invasive and involves manual gamete fusion by direct injection of the sperm into the oocyte cytoplasm. Since ICSI is able to achieve fertilization and embryo development in the presence of considerable sperm hypofunction, there are natural concerns regarding the future progeny and their genetic status and fertility potential. Though fertilization and embryo numbers are higher with ICSI, there is no significant difference in the pregnancy rates between IVF and ICSI in cases with normal semen characteristics. There is no evidence favoring replacement of all IVF cases by ICSI.

In Vitro Fertilization and Embryo Transfer

In vitro fertilization-embryo transfer was initially considered a treatment of choice for tubal factor infertility. Thus cases of tubal disease, occlusion, adhesions or surgery were considered as other treatments could not offer comparable success. Subsequently, IVF indications expanded to include PCOS wherein better follicular growth and fertilization rates were obtained. Today the indications cover unexplained infertility, advancing maternal age, repeated trials of conservative treatments, ovarian failure and antisperm antibodies. IVF offers a possibility of diagnosis of gamete dysfunction. With the advent of ICSI, indications have expanded to encompass almost all cases of male infertility.

Ovarian Stimulation–Oocyte Retrieval

A couple is recruited into the IVF-ET program after proper selection and investigations. An appropriate ovarian stimulation protocol is selected and follicular growth is observed with serial sonography. Hormone tests (FSH, LH, E2, progesterone) are selectively done as per the clinical situation and when three or more follicles attain a size of 17 mm or more, hCG is administered in the dose of 5,000–10,000 IU. The oocyte retrieval is carried out 36 hours later. The hCG injection is a crucial component that initiates the changes required to prepare the oocyte to resume meiosis from the diplotene stage of prophase I in which the oocyte has been arrested. The aim is to obtain oocytes in metaphase II after the polar body has been expelled. Oocytes are ready for fertilization at this stage and earlier stage oocytes need to undergo maturation before they can be fertilized. A delay in oocyte retrieval more than 36 hours may result in ovulation and subsequent loss of oocytes in the peritoneal cavity. Very often, aspirating the periovarian fluid in the pouch of Douglas yields oocytes.

Oocyte Screening

On aspirating the follicles, the follicular fluid contents are emptied into petri dishes and screened for the presence of oocyte-cumulus-complexes (OCC). These are then transferred into flushing medium which is usually 4-(-2-hydroxyethyl)-1-piperazine ethane sulfonic acid (HEPES) buffered so that pH changes are minimal as this procedure is done under the laminar airflow system on a 37°C heated table top outside the carbon dioxide (CO_2) incubator. The OCC are rinsed with flushing medium and transferred into IVF culture medium in 4-well dishes which are placed in the CO_2 incubator for incubation for 2–6 hours.

Sperm Preparation (Fig. 2)

Semen sample is processed by layering or swimup or density gradient techniques so that a final motile sperm suspension is obtained for insemination. Sperm assessment is done by Makler chamber.

Oocyte Insemination

This is generally done after 2–6 hours of oocyte retrieval. About 5,000–100,000 sperms are gently released around the OCC in the 4-well dish and the dishes are returned to the incubator.

Fertilization Check-Day 1

Sixteen to eighteen hours post insemination, fertilization can be noted by the appearance of the second polar body and the presence of two pronuclei (PN) with aligned nucleolar bodies—the 2 PN stage. Anomalies of fertilization like 3 PN, single PN are apparent at this stage. This stage requires dissection of the cumulus cells away from the oocyte, which is usually done with the help of flexible micropipettes of 140–170 μ diameter. At this stage further incubation can be done in microdroplets of culture medium placed in single well dishes overlayed with paraffin oil. Usually zygotes are incubated in groups of two or three in each microdroplet of 40–50 μL microl. Release of paracrine factors by embryos aid in growth. This requires small volumes of culture medium which is provided by the microdroplet. Oil overlay acts as a physical barrier between the medium and the surrounding air. It reduces evaporative loss and slows the rate of gas diffusion thus buffering the medium from rapid temperature, pH and osmolality changes, especially outside the CO_2 incubator (Figs 3 to 7).

Cleavage-Day 2

Twenty six hours after insemination, cleavage begins and a two cell stage can be observed with two equal sized cells. After 44–48 hours, the four cell stage is visualized. Embryos are graded based on the number, size, shape of the blastomeres and the degree of fragmentation. Embryos can be transferred at this stage or incubated further and transferred at the 6–8 cell stage on day 3 or 4. Further incubation requires a change in the culture medium and growth can be observed until the blastocyst stage when transfer can be done. There are several advantages of transferring blastocysts as follows:

- More physiological: synchronization between the embryo and the uterus
- True assessment of embryo viability post genome activation
- Avoids exposure to a hyperstimulated setting
- Time available for diagnosis, if embryo biopsy done
- Reduced uterine contractions on day 5
- Reduced possibility of cryodamage
- Reduced pregnancy loss
- Applications in genetic diagnosis
- Assessment of development and viability.

Not all embryos may grow until the blastocyst stage and some patients may not have any ET.

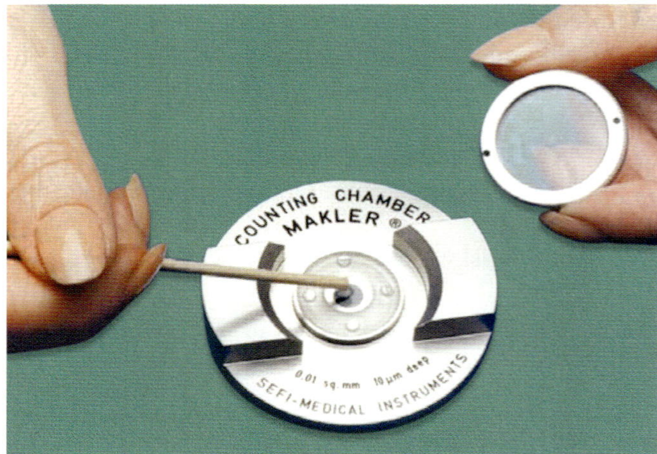

Fig. 2: Makler chamber

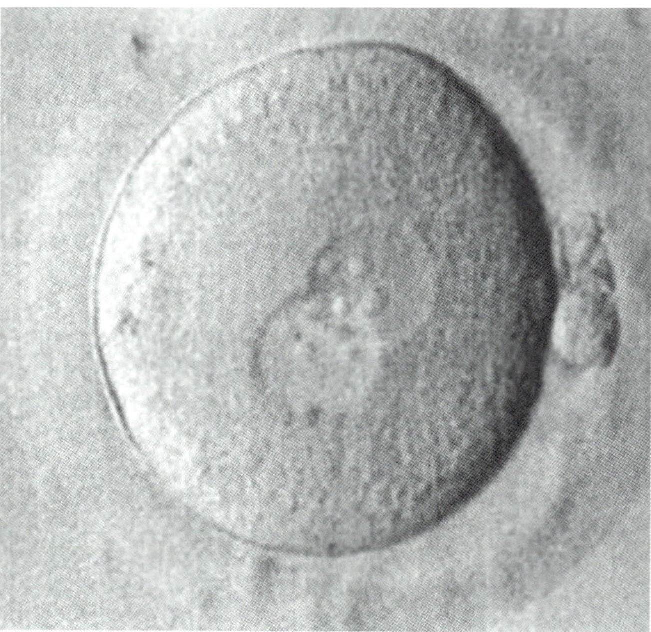

Fig. 3: Two pronuclei stage of zygote

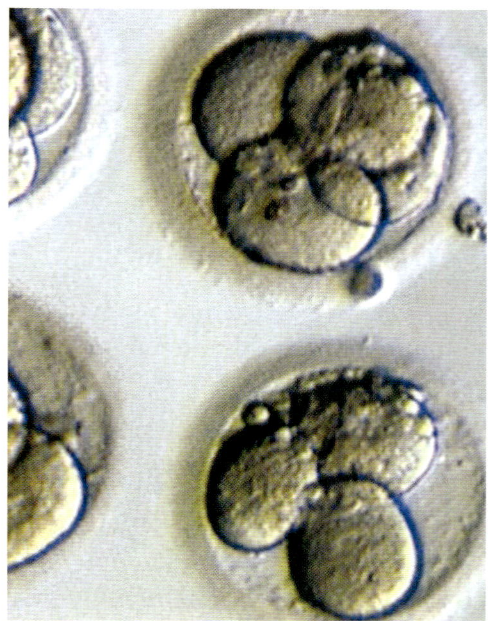

Fig. 4: Four cell embryo

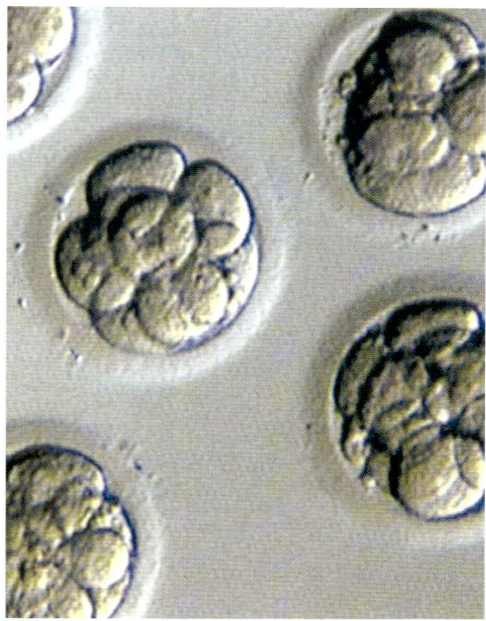

Fig. 5: Eight cell embryo

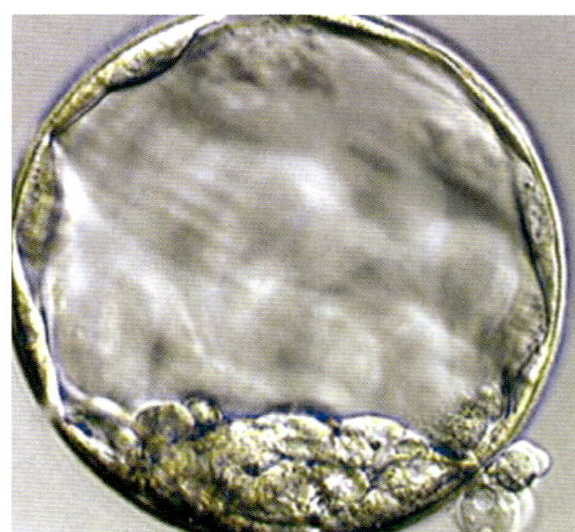

Fig. 6: Blastocyst showing blastocele

Intracytoplasmic Sperm Injection

Male infertility treatment has been revolutionized with the advent of micromanipulation. Till then recourse to medication, operative procedures like varicocele ligation, vaso-epididymal anastomosis, etc., and of course IUI, IVF-ET with pooling of semen samples was the only alternative available. This, however, could not yield desired results, especially in cases with severe oligoasthenoteratospermia. Azoospermic cases with sperm production could not benefit. IVF also could not offer a solution in cases with failed fertilization. ICSI was first reported in 1992 by the group from Brussels.

The evolution of ICSI can be traced to attempts at gamete manipulation. Partial zona dissection (PZD) was first tried out to enhance probability of sperm penetration. This was followed by subzonal insemination (SUZI) wherein sperms were injected into the perivitelline space with a micropipette. Subsequently, ICSI was tried wherein a single sperm was directly injected into the ooplasm resulting in a healthy livebirth. ICSI proved to be superior to SUZI.

Indications

- *Male subfertility:* Oligospermia, asthenospermia, teratospermia
- *Azoospermia*: Obstructive/nonobstructive techniques (Fig. 8) such as percutaneous epididymal sperm aspiration (PESA), microsurgical epididymal sperm aspiration (MESA), testicular sperm extraction (TESE) and testicular sperm aspiration (TESA) used to obtain sperms from the testes or epididymis
- *Ejaculatory dysfunction:* Retrograde ejaculation, anejaculation
- Poor post thaw sperm sample
- Poor semen sample on day of oocyte retrieval
- Fertilization failure in IVF cycles
- Unexplained infertility
- High antisperm antibodies
- IVM cycle.

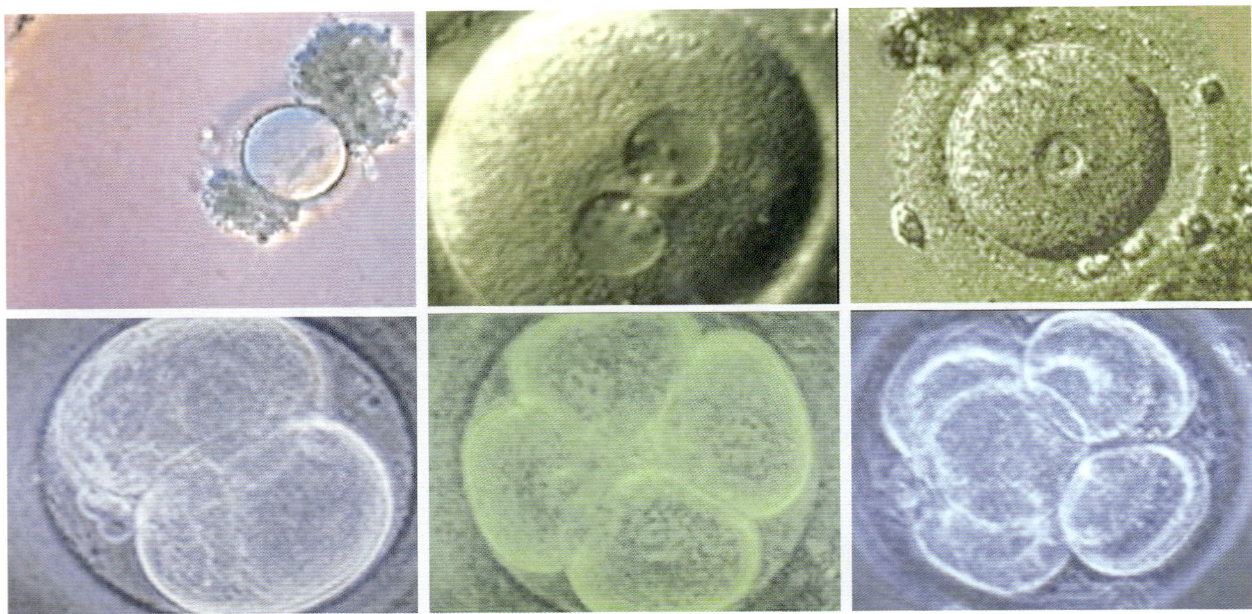

Fig. 7: Process and stages of embryo development

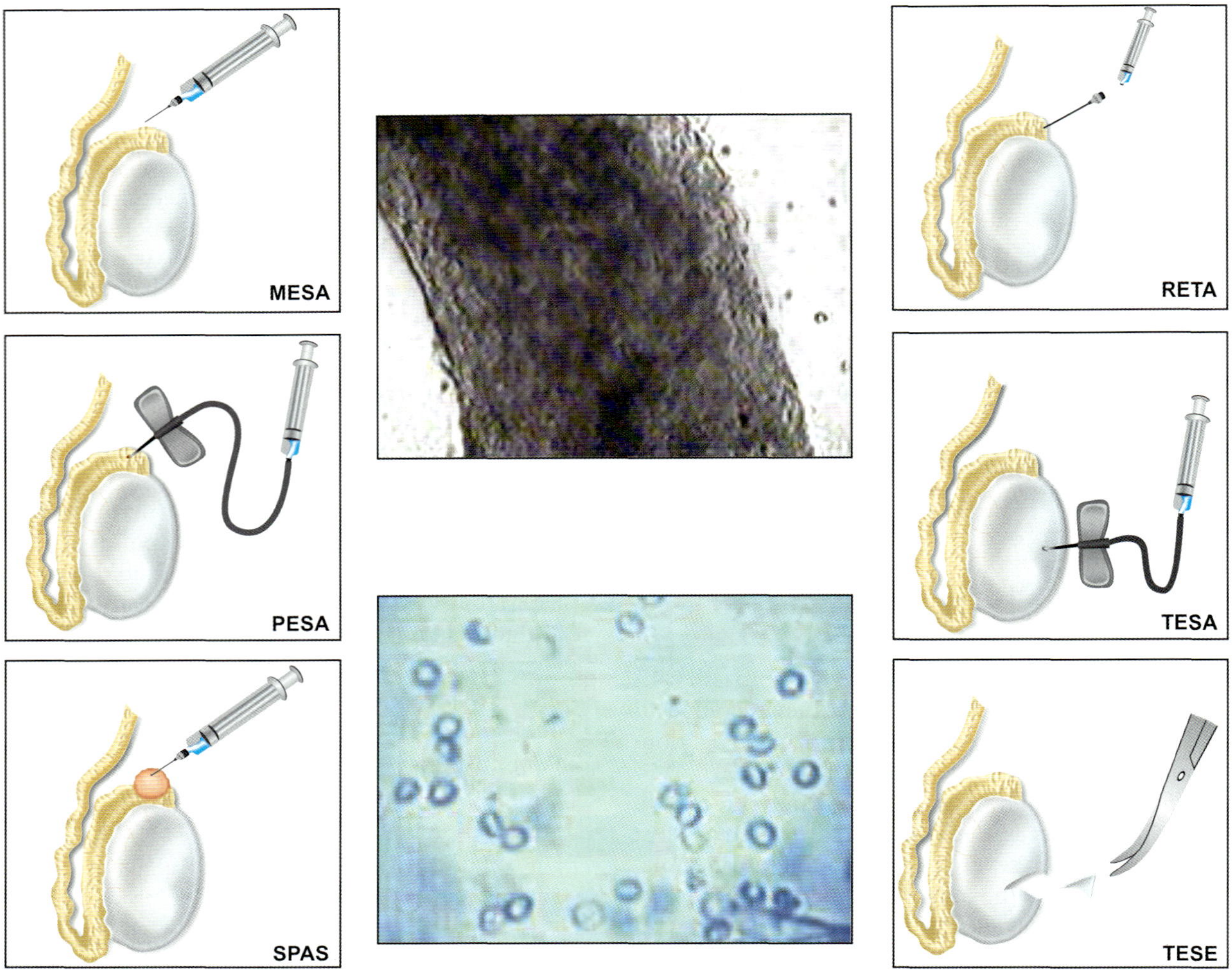

Fig. 8: Various sperm retrieval techniques

Injection of immotile sperms lowers the fertilization rate. Other factors such as sperm count, morphology (except globozoospermia) and high antisperm antibodies do not affect success rates.

Important laboratory steps which affect the success rates include:

- Concentration and duration of exposure to hyaluronidase for oocyte denudation
- Time of denudation after oocyte retrieval
- Selection of proper sperm-motile
- Position of polar body while injecting
- Aspiration of ooplasm before injection.

An appropriate stimulation protocol (long agonist or antagonist) is used and oocytes are retrieved 36 hours after hCG injection as in IVF cycle. After a short incubation of the OCC, denudation of oocytes in hyaluronidase along with mechanical aspiration is carried out and metaphase II/metaphase I/germinal vesicle oocytes are differentiated. Only metaphase II oocytes are ready for injection. Some metaphase I oocytes may undergo in vitro maturation after incubation and can be injected later; these have lower fertilization rates but similar embryos. Denuded oocytes are incubated till injection.

Sperm preparation is carried out using various techniques depending on the source:

- Ejaculated sperm are prepared by either washing and centrifuging with medium or by density gradient method
- MESA samples are collected and pooled and later centrifuged in density gradient media
- Testicular sperm are obtained by testicular aspiration or from microbiopsy and the tissue is teased under a microscope to identify sperms. The tissue is then centrifuged with medium and sperms are obtained.

Sperms are placed in a central polyvinylpyrrolidone (PVP) droplet placed in a petri dish. PVP helps in reducing sperm motility, facilitates better fluid control in the micro manipulators as well as prevents sperm from sticking to the surfaces.

The micromanipulator has a high magnification inverted microscope (Fig. 9) along with a central heated stage for maintaining temperature at 37°C in order to prevent damage to the meiotic spindle. The oocytes are placed in droplets around the central sperm containing PVP droplet under oil overlay. The micromanipulator has holding and injection pipettes which are either air or oil filled. Fine 3D movements are made through micrometers. The oocyte is held in position by gentle suction through a holding pipette (Fig. 10). The sperm injection pipette is filled with PVP and a single motile sperm is selected. This is then immobilized by gently rubbing the pipette against the base of the dish resulting in breakage of the tail. This step is important as the break in the sperm plasma membrane is important for release of sperm factors into the ooplasm resulting in oocyte activation. The immobilized sperm is then aspirated into the pipette, the oocyte held with its polar body in 6 o'clock position in order to minimize damage to the spindle body. The oolemma is pierced and ooplasm slightly aspirated into the pipette followed by injection of sperm into the ooplasm (Figs 11 and 12). The injected oocytes are rinsed and placed in culture medium droplets under oil in 5% CO_2 at 37°C in the incubator. Fertilization can be checked by observing two pronuclei and two polar bodies 16–18 hours after the injection. 1PN or 3 PN stage indicates abnormal fertilization. Generally 9% oocytes are damaged during the procedure and fertilization rates are in the range of 57–67%. Ninety percent of the fertilized

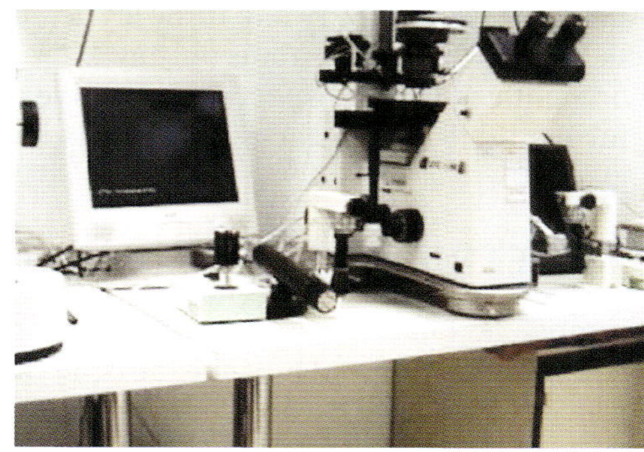

Fig. 9: ICSI setup with inverse microscope

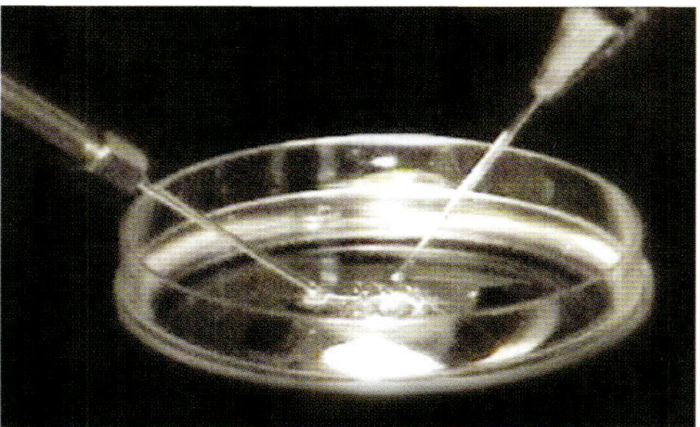

Fig. 10: Oocyte transferred in a petri dish

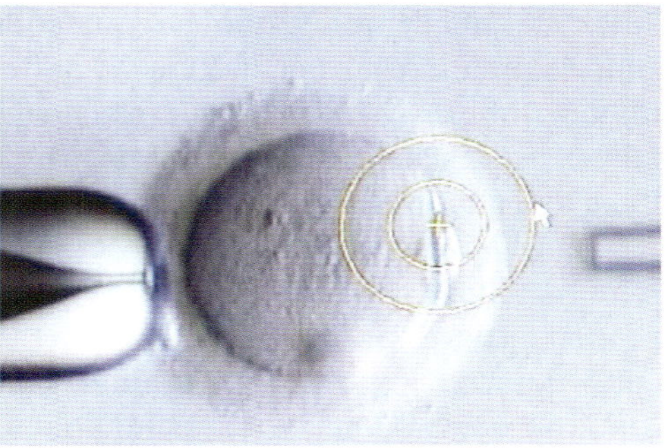

Fig. 11: Ovum being held just prior to intracytoplasmic sperm injection

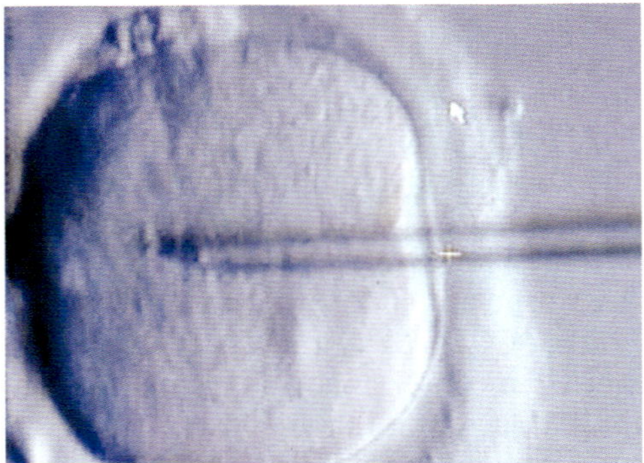

Fig. 12: Intracytoplasmic sperm injection

oocytes cleave to form embryos which reach four cell stage after 44–48 hours. Generally, two to three grade I embryos are selected for ET, which is done on day 2 or day 3 at four cell or eight cell stage, respectively. Embryos may be cultured further up to the blastocyst stage and transferred.

OOCYTE RETRIEVAL

Initial attempts at oocyte retrieval were performed at laparotomy. This was followed by a decade of laparoscopic oocyte retrieval which indeed was an integral part of several thousand IVF cycles performed in the 80s. With the advent of ovulation monitoring by sonography it was realized that oocytes could be retrieved easily by sonography guided ovarian puncture. The disadvantages of laparoscopy, namely risks of anesthesia and surgery, high costs and patient morbidity paved the way for universal sonography guided oocyte retrieval which was first performed by Lenz et al. This was done transabdominally and transvesically. Later on, vaginal transducers arrived on the scene and transvaginal oocyte retrieval became established as a simple, easy and convenient procedure which could be carried out as an outpatient procedure under sedation and local anesthesia. However, many centers use short general anesthesia and the patient frequently is discharged within a few hours of the procedure. A long vaginal transducer of 3–5 MHz frequency to ensure adequate depth of visualization is preferred. A needle biopsy guide is used along with the probe. A 17–18 gauge sharp echo tip needle is generally used. Follicle aspiration sets with needle, teflon tubing and adaptors are readily available. These are tested for mouse embryo toxicity. Suction is generated by a suction pump in the range of 90–120 mm Hg in order to ensure proper retrieval of the cumulus oocyte complex without any trauma. Some centers routinely flush the follicles until an oocyte is retrieved using double lumen aspiration needles. In a randomized study Tan et al reported no benefits of flushing. Most centers which do not practice flushing report more than 70% retrieval rates.

Complications

Though a simple procedure complications can arise during and after oocyte retrieval. The most common is vaginal bleeding at the puncture sites. Occasionaly, a large vaginal vessel may be lacerated. Bleeding generally stops with pressure, rarely a vaginal suture is required. Intra-abdominal bleeding following injury to iliac or ovarian vessels may occur and manifests as hemorrhagic shock.

Retroperitoneal bleeding can occur which may not be detectable until much later. Pelvic infection can also complicate with formation of tubo-ovarian abscess. Cases with endometriotic cysts, hydrosalpinges, and previous pelvic infections are more susceptible. A single intraoperative dose of antibiotic is given at the time of oocyte retrieval in many centers. Bowel injury and bladder injury can also occur if proper visualization before puncture is not done. Rare complications include adnexal torsion, rupture of endometriomas and even vertebral osteomyelitis.

Procedure

The patient is placed in a lithotomy position and a short general anesthesia is administered. The vagina is irrigated with normal saline and vigorously rinsed. The needle set is then connected to a tube containing some flushing medium and to the suction pump. The ovary is fixed between the probe and pelvic wall. The follicle is visualized in its maximal diameter and the needle is inserted through the needle guide into the follicle with a short jab. Suction is started and the follicle is seen to collapse completely. At the same time follicular fluid is seen in the tubing as well as the collection tube confirming aspiration. The needle is then advanced into the adjacent follicle and the procedure repeated until all follicles are completely aspirated in both ovaries (Fig. 13).

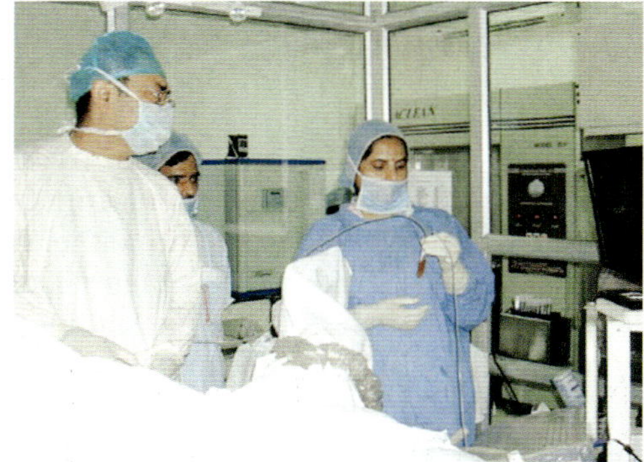

Fig. 13: Ovum pickup aspiration, in progress

EMBRYO TRANSFER (FIG. 14)

This is an important step in the entire treatment which can indeed limit the success rate of the cycle. All efforts prior to this step can go in vain if embryos are not carefully and properly transferred into the uterus. Some studies have demonstrated significant differences in pregnancy rates depending on the individual performing the ET. Whilst standardization of the procedure may eliminate this variability. Routinely, transcervical deposition of embryos is done which is essentially a blind method based on clinical feel. Thus absolute confirmation of embryo placement in the uterus is lacking. Several factors affect ET:

- *Cervical mucus:* This may plug the catheter tip leading to retention of the embryos or damage or improper placement of the embryos. Further, embryos may get stuck to the mucus and get dragged out along with the catheter. Mucus pushed into the uterus may interfere with implantation as well as may lead to contamination
- Failed negotiation of the cervical canal. Commonly acute flexion and version of the uterus hinders the passage of the catheter, which if soft, may undergo unnoticed coiling or kinking within the cervical canal
- Irritation of the uterus and initiation of uterine contractions can lead to embryo expulsion in up to 15% of cases. Higher rates of expulsion and lower pregnancy rates were noted with increasing frequency of uterine contractions.

Several methods have been demonstrated to improve the success rates after ET:

- *Dummy transfer:* This is a mock transfer done prior to the actual transfer in the same or previous cycle. This helps in noting the length and direction of the uterus as well as ease of negotiation

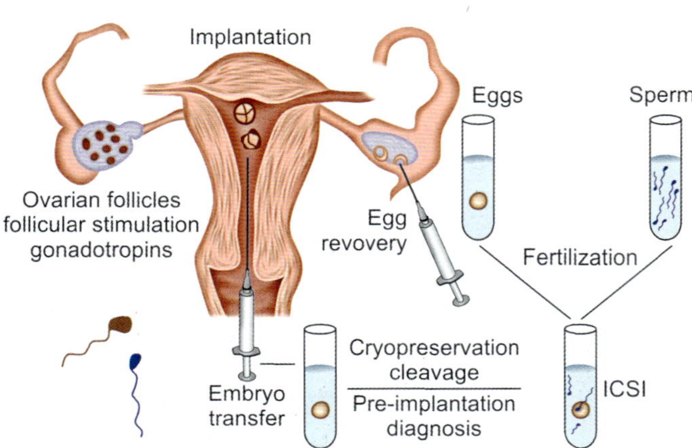

Fig. 14: Implantation

- *Ultrasonography (USG) guided transfer:* Abdominal probe placed above a filled bladder during the actual procedure helps in visualization of the passage of the catheter into the uterus and confirming the release of medium or air bubbles at the time of injection. Also, USG evaluation of the direction and length of the uterus helps
- *Avoiding initiation of uterine contractions:* Avoiding touching the fundus helps in preventing the initiation of uterine contractions. A midfundal deposition 0.5–1 cm below the fundus is ideal
- Using a soft malleable catheter to avoid trauma, as far as possible, is recommended
- As far as possible, the cervix must not be held with any instrument in order to avoid irritation to the uterus
- Blood or mucus at the catheter tip is associated with increased embryo retention in the catheter
- Cervical infection at the time of transfer also reduces the pregnancy rates
- Use of nonsteroidal antiinflammatory drug (NSAID), prostaglandin inhibitors, sedation at the time of transfer is practiced in some centers
- Loading of the embryos into the catheter should be done carefully with a small volume of 30–40 µL containing the embryos. Injection of large volumes of culture medium results in flushing of embryos into the tubes or back through the cervical canal. An ectopic pregnancy rate of nearly 5% has been reported in IVF cycles.

LUTEAL PHASE SUPPORT

Progesterone is commonly used to support the luteal phase in most ART cycles. Downregulation protocols result in low output of hormones from the corpora lutea due to suppression of FSH and LH. Also during oocyte retrieval a lot of cumulus cells and granulosa cells are sucked out leading to concerns about the adequacy of the luteal phase.

Clinical pregnancy rates were shown to improve significantly with luteal supplementation with hCG or progesterone. Various formulations of progesterone have been used.

1. Intramuscular progesterone injections 50–100 mg daily are administered up to the day of beta hCG estimation and continued thereafter if pregnancy ensues. Disadvantages are pain, discomfort and occasional pruritic rashes. The oily vehicle base is responsible for the pain and formation of nodules at the site of injection.
2. Oral or preferably vaginal micronized progesterone 200 mg three times a day can be used alternatively.
3. Vaginal progesterone cream in prefilled tube (Crinone-Serono) is also available and can be used twice daily.

4. Dydrogesterone oral tablets 10 mg twice daily can also be added.
5. Some centers also favor addition of estradiol valerate in doses of 2–4 mg daily.
6. Low dose aspirin 75 mg/day, multivitamin tablets-folate, antioxidants are also recommended in addition by some centers.

Supplementation is continued up to the day of beta hCG estimation and thereafter for 11–12 weeks, if conception occurs.

LABORATORY ASPECTS (FIGS 15 TO 19)

Equipment

Any ART setup warrants use of proper equipment placed appropriately in a proper environment. Periodic checks of equipment function and calibration, disinfection of the laboratory, standardization of protocols, monitoring the air quality and periodic assessment of the results are an integral part of any ART setup. Quality assurance and quality control is essential for obtaining standardized results on a consistent basis. Since a single variable is capable of effecting adverse outcome, stringent laboratory monitoring is vital. Some of the basic equipment includes:

- CO_2 incubator
- Laminar airflow
- Micromanipulator
- *Microscopes:* Stereo zoom microscope, binocular microscope, inverted microscope
- Centrifuge
- Heating blocks
- Standard incubator
- Refrigerator

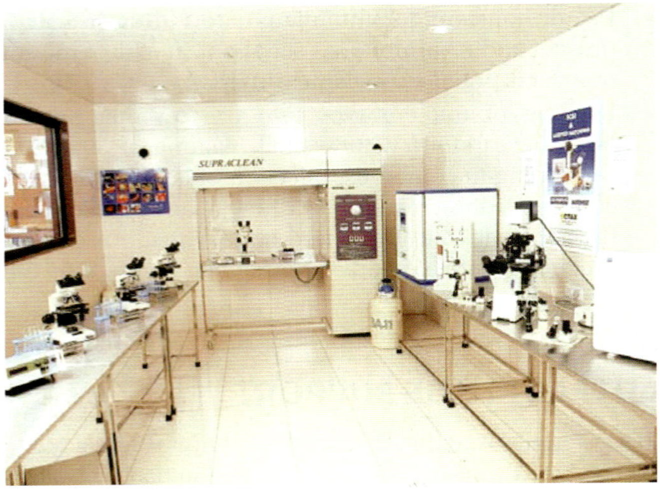

Fig. 15: An overview of ART laboratory

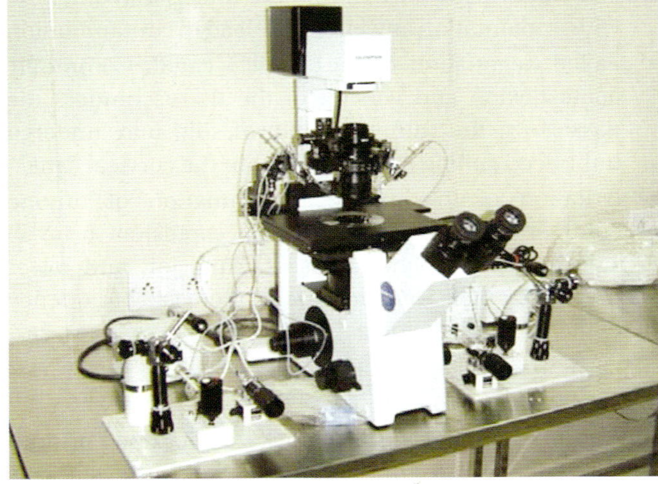

Fig. 16: Micromanipulator, complete assembly

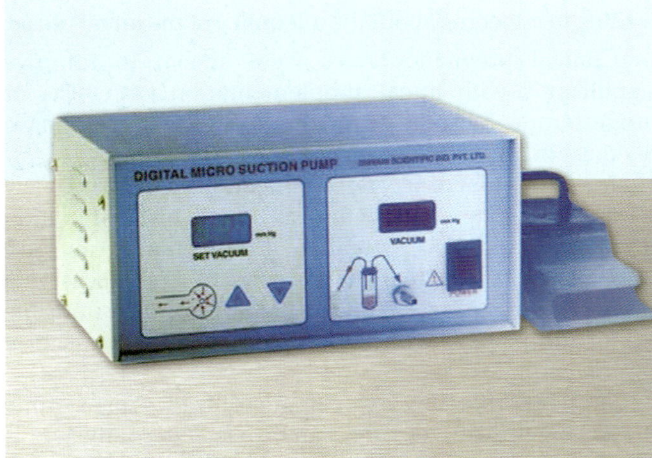

Fig. 17: Ovum pickup suction pump

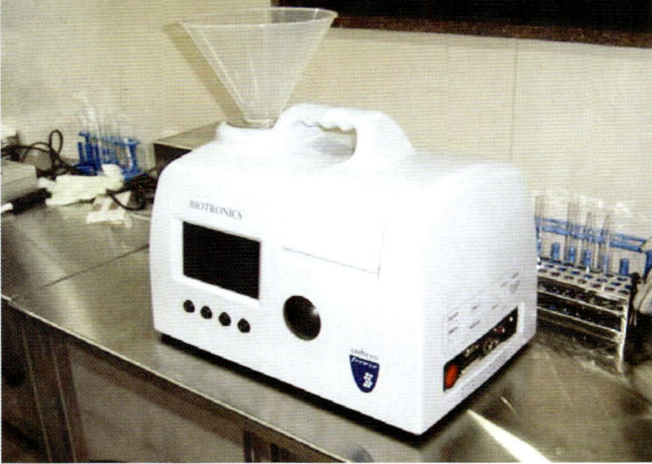

Fig. 18: Biological freezer, an instrument for cryopreservation

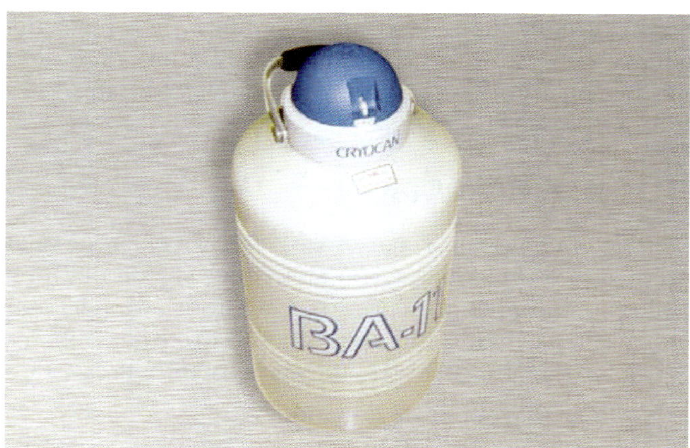

Fig. 19: Liquid nitrogen cryocan

- Liquid nitrogen canisters
- Sperm counting chamber.

Laboratory disposables: These include petri dishes, single well dishes, four well dishes, conical round bottom tubes, pipettes, oocyte pickup single/double lumen needles, ET sets, flexipets, inspection and handling sets, micropipettes amongst others.

Media and Environment

Various readymade media are available for use in ART including simple, complex, sequential media. In general, gametes must be shifted to fresh media within 48 hours. All media need to be properly equilibrated as per their composition. Proper maintenance of temperature at 37°C and a pH of 7.2–7.4 are vital. Also, media have a shelf life and need to be used within this period. Opening a media bottle several times over a long period is not recommended as this alters the composition of the medium. Various antibiotics are often added to the media in order to help avoid infection.

Common media constituents include glucose and aminoacids. These are as per the requirements of the gametes and the growing embryo. As the embryo progresses from two cell to four cell to morula to blastocyst stage, its requirements change, necessitating the use of media of different constitution. Thus sequential media cater to these requirements and assist the growing embryos in fulfilling its needs. Media available include those used for flushing, oocyte handling for a limited time, culture media for incubation within the incubator, sperm preparation media, extended culture media for growth up to blastocyst stage, special ET media, various other preparations including paraffin oil, hyaluronidase, PVP.

Embryo Culture

Maintaining a near physiologic environment in vitro is vital for the growth of embryos. Advances in the development of embryo culture systems including media, equipment and techniques have improved embryo viability significantly resulting in better pregnancy and live birth rates.

Media are vital ingredients as the gametes or embryos develop within them. Media may be of different types such as simple salt solutions with added nutrients or complex fortified media, simple optimized media or sequential media. Media use is governed by the requirements of the growing embryo and changing needs from pronucleate to cleavage stage to blastocyst stage. The chances of culture media induced trauma/damage to the embryo should be minimal. Birth defects attributable to improper media composition have been described.

Generally media are composed of the following:

- *Water:* Highly purified and endotoxin free water is a must for any medium as 99% of the medium contains water
- *Ions:* Extracellular ionic compositions alter intracellular ions and hence affect the growth. Proper concentrations of sodium (Na), chlorine (Cl), potassium (K), phosphate, calcium, magnesium is important for maintaining viability. Osmolarity also has to be maintained in the range of 275–295 mOsmol/L
- *Carbohydrates:* Differential needs of the embryo mandates the use of different carbohydrates at various growth stages. The zygote and cleavage cell embryo needs pyruvate and lactate as the major energy metabolite in contrast to glucose which is needed by the morula and blastocyst.

Proteins

Proteins, including amino acids, affect the growth of the developing embryo significantly as these are readily used for development. Also addition of amino acids results in a greater capacity to withstand stress. Nonessential amino acids and glutamine are useful as energy substrates besides helping in maintenance of pH and osmosis. There is a differential need for amino acids pre- and postcompaction and the sequential media are designed to provide this switch. Glutamine significantly affects the development of the embryo.

Ammonium accumulation as a result of amino acid metabolism adversely affects growth, hence storage of amino acid containing media at 37°C should be avoided and renewal of culture medium within 48 hours is mandatory. Increasing concentration of ammonia in the culture medium has been shown to have a negative impact on human blastocyst development.

Ethylenediaminetetraacetic acid (EDTA) is a chelator of heavy ion and addition of EDTA in the early stages enhances embryo development while it is detrimental at later stages, including post compaction.

Antibiotics such as penicillin, gentamicin, streptomycin are generally added to minimize chances of infection.

Human serum albumin (HSA) is added to alter the solvent properties of the medium. It also negates the effect of toxins. Synthetic serum substitute containing 84% HSA and 16% alpha and beta globulins is also available as an alternative. Recombinant albumin with advantages of elimination of risks of blood products and batch variability has also been found to be equally effective.

Buffers

For 6 hours post fertilization, oocytes and embryos are more susceptible to pH related damage as they lack the necessary systems to buffer the acidic/alkaline pH. To a certain extent cumulus cells help in the buffering mechanism. Various buffers have been used to protect gametes and embryos from rapid pH changes.

- Commonly a CO_2-bicarbonate buffer system is used to maintain a pH of 7.2–7.4. Most media available contain bicarbonate hence a CO_2 incubator is required with a CO_2 concentration of 5–6% in order to maintain the pH. It is important to check the calibration of the incubator with fyrite fluid or high accuracy CO_2 infrared sensors, periodically

  The main disadvantage of this system is a rapid change in pH on exposure to air
- Alternatively phosphate based buffers are available but are toxic to embryos in vitro and have limited buffering capacity in cryopreservation
- 4-(-2-hydroxyethyl)-1-piperazine ethane sulfonic acid based systems are commonly used along with some bicarbonate for gamete handling during oocyte pickup in order to maintain pH when the incubator cannot be used
- 3-(N-morpholino) propane sulfonic acid (MOPS) is another buffer recently being used with an advantage of less temperature sensitivity as compared to HEPES.

Oxygen

It has been found that lower oxygen (O_2) concentration promotes growth as compared to 20% O_2 saturation.

Temperature

Maintaining the culture medium at 37°C at all times is vital as fluctuations in temperature result in damage to the meiotic spindle. Ambient light of high intensity is damaging and low illumination is preferable while handling gametes and embryos.

Air

It is important to have pure air in the laboratory. Presence of volatile organic compounds (VOCs) and chemical airborne contaminants (CACs) significantly affects the culture process. Use of special air filtration units and positive pressure systems improves the success rates.

OOCYTE DONATION

Women of menopausal age, those with poor egg reserve or premature ovarian failure can also conceive and deliver a child with this method of using oocytes from a young donor and fertilizing them with husband's sperms to get embryos which are then transferred to the uterus of the wife.

Indications for oocyte donation:

- Premature ovarian failure congenital-gonadal dysgenesis, Turner's syndrome, post surgery infections, severe endometriosis, chemotherapy, irradiation
- Advanced maternal age—beyond 37 years
- Poor ovarian reserve
- Repeated failed IVF/ICSI cycles
- Prevention of passage of inheritable genetic disorders.

Oocyte donation using in vitro techniques was first described by Trounson in 1983. Donor screening with proper medical, surgical, family, genetic history as well as tests for infections, HIV, Hepatitis B, C need to be done. Matching of donor and recipient characteristics is preferable.

Donors undergo stimulation as in any other ART cycle. However, in vitro maturation (IVM) may be offered as an option to reluctant donors with advantages of minimal or no stimulation, fewer hospital visits and less monitoring.

Cycle synchronization between the donor and recipient is essential as oocyte retrieval and subsequent ET has to be done at an appropriate stage of endometrial development in the recipient. Generally, oral contraceptive pills along with GnRH analogs (long protocol) facilitate synchronizing both cycles. In cases of amenorrheic recipients, there is no need to use the agonists. Estradiol valerate 2 mg 2–3 times a day is generally used for a minimum of 8–10 days for endometrial growth. Sonography monitoring is done to confirm endometrial thickness greater than or equal to 7 mm. Estradiol may be continued for 4–5 weeks, if required prior to ET. In cases where the uterus is hypoplastic, several estradiol cycles with cyclical progesterone withdrawal are administered before the recipient is enrolled for ET in order to stimulate uterine and endometrial growth. Once the oocyte retrieval is scheduled for the donor, the recipient is started on progesterone a day before or on the day of oocyte retrieval. The estradiol dose may be increased to 2 mg four times a day along with daily progesterone injection 100 mg/day until the ET and up to the beta hCG estimation day. Post conception, both estradiol and progesterone are continued up to 12 weeks of gestation.

SURROGACY

Women with severe defects or damage to the uterus cannot conceive. However, they can have their biological child by undergoing ovarian stimulation, harvesting their eggs, fertilizing them with their husband's sperms and transferring the resulting embryos into another woman's uterus. This person carries the pregnancy till term and delivers a child biologically belonging to the infertile couple. The child is then legally adopted by the couple as their heir. Indications for surrogacy are:

- Uterine anomalies—severe congenital hypoplasia, rudimentary uterus
- Uterine damage—severe Asherman's syndrome post infections, post trauma
- Medical conditions precluding pregnancy.

Medicolegal and social issues need to be resolved before surrogacy is considered. Maternal child bonding may complicate the outcome. The surrogate mother is medically evaluated and undergoes the same preparatory procedures as in oocyte donation as a recipient of ET.

CRYOPRESERVATION

Cryopreservation aims at preserving living cells at subzero temperatures for extended periods of time with complete recovery of cellular function after thawing. Sperms, oocytes, zygotes, embryos as well as blastocysts have been frozen successfully. Currently either slow freezing or rapid vitrification methods are being used.

Cells undergo a lot of chemical, physical and thermal stress during freezing as well as thawing and depending on the cell type different methods are used so that there is minimal damage to cellular function. Cooling results in intracellular ice formation which is detrimental to cellular function. Special molecules called as cryoprotectants are used to facilitate the journey of the cell from 37°C to -196°C where they eventually remain in liquid nitrogen until thawing. Osmotic fluxes and changes in solute concentrations need to be minimized. Cryoprotectants can be intracellular permeating type or extracellular nonpermeating. Glycerol, propanediol, dimethylsulphoxide (DMSO) permeate into the cell across the cell membrane and replace intracellular water, whereas sucrose is extracellular cryoprotectants which increases the osmotic pressure around the cell. Gradually, these molecules help in achieving cell shrinkage with equilibrium maintained across the cell membrane. Cryoprotectant is cell-specific with cell membrane permeability and cellular water content being important determinants.

Human sperms were one of the first to be successfully cryopreserved and thawed semen was found to be capable of fertilization and induction of embryonic development. Sperms can be frozen by the ultra-rapid method. Generally after processing the semen, the sperm wash solution is diluted with the freezing medium containing glycerol in the ratio 1:1. It is cooled up to 2°C by placing it above liquid N_2 for 25 minutes and then plunged into liquid N_2. For oocytes or embryos, initially DMSO was used, but due to its disadvantages propanediol is preferred as the cryoprotectant. Blastocysts are frozen using serial concentrations of glycerol.

Vitrification is a process wherein there is rapid cooling of cells in the presence of high concentrations of cryoprotectants resulting in solidification without intracellular ice formation. The liquid cellular state is converted into a solidified state with the same molecular and ionic distribution and behaves like a viscous super cooled liquid. The cells are dehydrated by exposure to a high concentration of cryoprotectant and plunged directly into liquid N_2. Ethylene glycol is commonly used due to its rapid diffusion and equilibration properties. Oocytes, zygotes, embryos and blastocysts have been vitrified.

Results of cryopreservation vary and are generally lower than fresh cycle rates. Besides procedural damage, the initial cell quality influences future post thaw function.

IN VITRO MATURATION

Stimulating the ovaries in order to obtain several oocytes has its own disadvantages and risks. These include daily injections, long duration of treatment, necessity of monitoring with repeated sonography, blood hormonal tests besides risks of OHSS and long term associations with malignancy. PCOS patients especially are at a high risk of OHSS due to recruitment and growth of several follicles. In vitro maturation was initially proposed in this group of patients with a high basal antral count as an alternative method of obtaining oocytes without stimulating the ovaries. Earlier, Cha et al. had reported IVM of oocytes collected during gynecologic surgery, fertilization and transfer to a case of premature ovarian failure with healthy livebirths. The basic principle is to retrieve oocytes at an early stage without stimulating the ovary, maturing these in vitro, fertilizing them with IVF/ICSI and transferring the resulting embryos into the uterus. It has been demonstrated that OCC can be made to mature in vitro. In fact, cumulus cells are thought to modulate and mediate a number of beneficial cellular functions beneficial to the oocyte. They may have autocrine and paracrine effects. The culture medium is generally supplemented with small amounts of FSH, LH. Estradiol and proteins have also been added to the medium in order to mimic in vivo conditions.

With the rising success rates of IVM, its application has been extended to various other conditions besides PCOS.

High responders with exaggerated responses to small amount of gonadotropins, poor responders who need very large doses of gonadotropins and still have very few follicles, oocyte donors can avoid the long, multiple injection schedules. Recently partial gonadal dysgenesis (PGD) has also been combined with IVM resulting in a healthy livebirth. Malignancy patients requiring chemotherapy can also undergo IVM with shorter treatment duration and avoidance of hormonal stimulation.

Technique

Baseline scans are done on days 3–5 and repeated at day 7–10. hCG is administered and oocyte retrieval scheduled 36 hours later. hCG priming has been reported to increase the rates of in vitro maturation of oocytes. Oocyte retrieval is done using a low suction pressure up to 50 mm Hg. Follicular fluid is collected in 0.9% normal saline and heparin. Follicular flushing, curettage of the follicular wall and several punctures may be required in order to obtain to cumulus-oocyte complexes. The oocytes are incubated for 24–48 hours and denuded. Metaphase II oocytes are identified and either cryopreserved or subjected to ICSI. Embryos thus formed are either transferred or cryopreserved.

PARTIAL GONADAL DYSGENESIS (FIG. 20)

Initially an experimental genetic screening tool for human embryos, now it is well established clinically and used in several thousand cycles worldwide. It is used for the diagnosis of single gene defects as well as chromosomal disorders, e.g. aneuploidy, translocations. Genetically normal embryos are identified and selectively transferred thereby preventing transmission of genetic disorders.

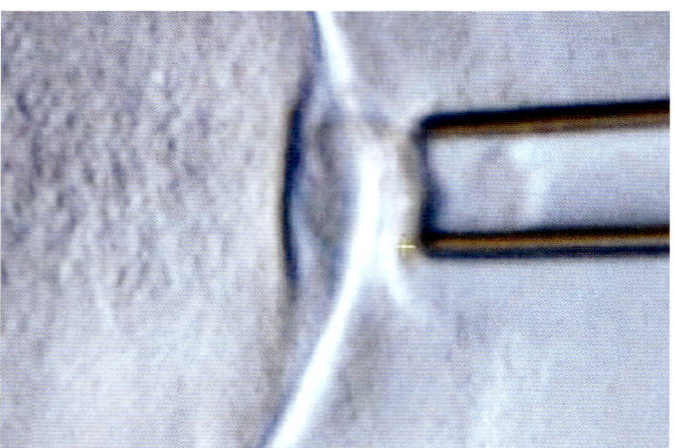

Fig. 20: Blastocyst material being picked up of prenatal genetic diagnostic screening

Polar bodies, blastomeres or blastocyst trophectoderm cells can be analyzed. The cells to be biopsied are obtained by partial zona dissection (PZD) done through chemical, mechanical or laser methods.

Either pre- or postfertilization polar body may be biopsied. The advantages include extraembryonic handling as well as time duration available between biopsy and subsequent ET. However, information about sex of the embryo and the paternal genome is not available. Also fragmentation and incomplete biopsy hinders the diagnosis.

Embryos are usually biopsied at the 6–8 cell stage on day 3 where 1–2 blastomeres are selectively obtained. The disadvantages are reduction of implantation rates if the embryo is damaged; also time between biopsy and transfer is limited, hence rapid diagnosis is essential. Further the trophectoderm may be at variance with the inner cell mass.

Various autosomal conditions like cystic fibrosis, histiocytosis as well as X-linked fragile X syndrome can be diagnosed on PGD.

Polymerase chain reaction (PCR) is the most commonly used technique with its quick and highly sensitive diagnosis. Multiplex PCR and real time PCR are also being used. Contamination from cumulus cells may cause an erroneous diagnosis, also DNA amplification failure can occur.

Fluorescence in situ hybridization (FISH) is commonly used for the diagnosis of chromosomal disorders with 9–10 chromosomes being currently studied as well as for translocations. Thus fluorescent DNA probes for sex chromosomes as well as chromosomes 13, 14, 15, 16, 18, 21, 22 are available.

Target population includes high maternal age, cases of recurrent abortions, repeated IVF cycle failures, genetically abnormal couples with translocations, inversions.

Partial gonadal dysgenesis is a safe and effective means of identifying genetically abnormal embryos with pregnancy and implantation rates comparable to conventional IVF cycles. With further advances, the scope of PGD will widen to encompass more and more genetic disorders.

LASER ASSISTED HATCHING

Lasers are widely used in medicine. Applications of laser in ART have evolved in recent years and apart from use in research, clinical use is growing as technology and instrumentation are simplifying laser availability and practical utility.

Lasers may be of contact type or non-contact type. In the latter, laser energy at the focal point is absorbed by the tissue water and macromolecules resulting in disruption of the matrix and ablation. The diode non-contact infrared lasers appear to be most appropriate for zona-cutting applications. Indium-gallium-arsenic phosphorus laser is popular with a wavelength of 1.48 μ being rapid, safe and effective.

The zona pellucida, post sperm entry, undergoes a series of mechanical and chemical changes in order to prevent polyspermy and protect the developing embryo. In some cases the zona becomes extremely hard and impairs embryo hatching. A mean zona thickness of 18 μ or more is considered significant. Lysine is important and deficiencies in action or function are important for failure to hatch. This deficiency could arise as a result of in vitro culture conditions. Zona thinning or drilling have shown improvement in implantation rates in selected cases wherein it optimizes the implantation window and promotes earlier implantation.

Indications of laser-assisted hatching (LAH) are:

- Thick zona pellucida
- Elderly patient
- Elevated basal FSH
- Failed implantation cycles
- Poor responders
- Unexplained infertility
- Slow cleaving fragmented embryos
- Very few embryos
- IVM cycles.

Laser can also be used during ICSI for sperm injection where it prevents excessive cell deformation during injection or for carrying out biopsy procedures for PGD. Zona thinning is advantageous with no loss of blastomeres or exposure to contamination with bacteria or white blood cell (WBC) or toxins as compared to zona drilling.

Generally, assisted hatching is done on day 3 at 6–8 cell stage. It can be done at the blastocyst stage also. A laser mounted micromanipulator is used. The embryo is held at one end and single or multiple small 30–40 μ holes are drilled by the laser. A large hole can result in loss of blastomeres and can increase the fragility of the embryo as well as increase its susceptibility to bacterial contamination or immune cell invasion.

COMPLICATIONS OF ART

Multiple Gestation

There has been a dramatic rise in the incidence of multiple gestation largely due to the practice of ART. The rate has nearly doubled in the last few years with 90% of the contribution coming from ART techniques and the rest from rising maternal age in the developed world. Multiple gestations has implications for the mother, risks for the children as well as financial and other concerns for the family and health providers. The practice of transferring large number of embryos is largely responsible for this outcome. Triplet gestations and higher warrant embryo reduction procedures to ensure fetal survival. Indeed current practice of ART is focused on reduction in multiple gestations by various techniques including blastocyst transfer and limitation of the number of embryos transferred. The long-term sequelae of premature births and high-order births and the costs of managing these prove to be an enormous burden and drain on the health system.

Pregnancy Complications

ART pregnancies are at increased risk of preterm delivery, intrauterine growth restriction (IUGR), low birth weight, perinatal mortality and neonatal intensive care unit (NICU) admissions. Pregnancy-induced hypertension (PIH), abruptio placentae, gestational diabetes complicate pregnancies more often and cesarean section rates are very high.

Congenital Anomalies

There is an increased risk of malformations in IVF/ICSI children and though the rise is modest, large studies are needed to address this issue. Anomalies of the genitourinary system in particular are increased in ICSI children. Part of the risk is inherent with its basis traceable to the genetic abnormalities linked to infertility and advanced maternal and paternal age. The genetic abnormalities associated with male infertility are now well known and transmission of DNA defects of sperms into the progeny is not unexpected. However, issues of in vitro culture conditions, culture media, blastomere biopsy procedures as well as drug induced abnormalities are a matter of concern.

Concerns regarding fertility of the children born as a result of IVF/ICSI need to be addressed.

In a meta-analysis Hansen et al. noted an increased risk of anomalies (odds ratio 2) compared to the natural conceptions after correcting for various parameters. However, ethnicity and duration of infertility were not factored in. In a multicentric cohort study, Bonduelle et al. noted an odds ratio for major malformations of 2.77 for ICSI children and 1.8 for IVF as compared to the natural conceptions. There were no differences in developmental milestones in IVF/ICSI children as compared to natural conception children in studies by Sutcliffe. One of the largest studies evaluating child and family outcome, an international collaborative study of ICSI: Child and Family Outcomes (ICSI-CFO) study noted no effect of conception status on neurodevelopment but highlighted increased usage and requirements of health resources by ICSI/IVF children as compared to natural conceptions.

The risks of childhood malignancy are not found to be increased in ART children.

There seems to be an association between ART and some genomic imprintable disorders like Beckwith Weideman syndrome. This has been associated with a loss of methylation at a maternal allele site. Whether this is due to inherent susceptibility of genome alterations in infertility or induced due to in vitro culture conditions need to be evaluated further.

With increasing children being born after ART these would constitute a significant proportion of the population in times to come. It is imperative to simultaneously follow up ART children diligently and thoroughly so as to detect significant markers of deviations from normalcy.

Ovarian Stimulation and Cancer

Studies by Rossing et al. indicated a higher risk of ovarian cancer associated with clomiphene citrate use for more than 1 year. A large study by Venn et al. showed no significant increase in the risk of ovarian and breast cancer in women treated with gonadotropins. Large studies are needed to evaluate the risks of prolonged usage of ovary stimulating agents and current recommendations are to use these for as short duration as possible in the smallest effective dose.

OVARIAN HYPERSTIMULATION SYNDROME

One of the most dreaded complication of ART is ovarian hyperstimulation syndrome (OHSS) which may be seen in various forms in up to 30% of all cases. Severe manifestations are associated with considerable morbidity and occasionally even mortality. Generally OHSS is classified as:

- *Mild:* Ovaries enlarged up to 5 cm with abdominal distention
- *Moderate:* Ovaries enlarged up to 12 cm with ascites, gastrointestinal symptoms of nausea, vomiting, diarrhea, abdominal pain and weight gain
- *Severe:* Ovaries enlarged more than 12 cm, massive ascites, pleural effusions, hemoconcentration, oliguria, electrolyte imbalance, disseminated intravascular coagulopathy (DIC).

It is an iatrogenic condition related to natural or exogenous hCG administration (presence of massive numbers of luteinized follicular cells).

Women at highest risk are young, thin PCOS with typical necklace sign. Very high levels of E2 s > 4000 pg/mL/1700 pg/mL in IUI cycles, more than 20 follicles or more than 6 follicles in IUI cycles, luteal phase support with hCG, conception in the treatment cycle and the long GnRH agonist protocol all increase the risk of developing OHSS.

Pathologically there is ovarian enlargement with hyperproduction of ovarian hormones and vasoactive substances resulting in a hyperpermeability state with fluid shift to extravascular spaces with hemoconcentration, renal impairment and thromboembolic phenomena. The exact mechanism is not clearly known but is thought to be related to hCG stimulated ovarian overproduction of vasoactive endothelial growth factor (VEGF) associated with angiotensin II and interleukins.

Precautions can be taken to avoid development of severe OHSS by various means:

- Low dose cautious FSH use
- Proper, continuous monitoring of follicular growth, E2 levels
- Coasting of FSH, withholding FSH and hCG doses until E2 levels reduce
- Reducing the dose of hCG to 5000 IU; replacement of hCG with GnRH agonist for ovulation induction in antagonist cycles is being studied
- Usage of GnRH antagonists/insulin sensitizers
- Thorough follicular aspiration
- 20% albumin has been administered at the time of oocyte retrieval with contrasting results
- Cryopreservation of embryos and ET in a later cycle to prevent conception in the treatment cycle
- Avoiding hCG for luteal phase support
- Finally withholding hCG and canceling the cycle.

Treatment of mild and moderate OHSS is conservative with bed rest, symptomatic treatment with antiemetics, anti-inflammatory, anticolic agents, administering intravenous fluids to replenish extracellular losses.

Severe OHSS mandates hospitalization and may even require intensive care unit (ICU) management. Principles of management are:

A. *Monitor:* Fluid intake/urine output/hematocrit/abdominal girth/electrolytes/renal function/coagulation system/liver function
B. *Replace:* Crystalloids—glucose saline vigorously colloids—20% HSA/fresh frozen plasma
C. *Aspirate:* Ascitic tap is a very simple therapeutic procedure
D. Operate only if hemoperitoneum/torsion of ovaries/life-threatening OHSS mandating medical termination of pregnancy (MTP).

JUSTIFICATION OF ART

A 20–40% success rate with ART should be compared with more traditional and conventional therapies. The latter is obviously first choice when indicated. Thus proper couple evaluation, diagnosis and counseling are vital before embarking on any treatment. The costs, risks and success rates of ART have to be clearly outlined and simpler treatments should judiciously be attempted if applicable. At the same time delaying or avoiding ART when there are clear indications is definitely not advisable considering the success rates per attempt of treatment and the potential of obtaining results in often extremely difficult cases. With ART becoming more and more invasive at the cellular level, continuous monitoring systems that identify and procrastinate potential hazards are mandated. A 25% pregnancy loss rate and 30–40% multiple gestation rate needs to be addressed. With time ART children would comprise increasing segments of the population and it is wise to check whether the future progeny is compromised in any way. Studies have indicated that ART children often require more health resources as compared to naturally conceived children. This liability needs to be quantified. The practice of ART itself is technology intensive and demands skilled manpower with deployment of quality assurance and quality control practices to sustain results.

All said and done, fertility treatment without ART today seems to be reminiscent of an era that belongs to history.

BIBLIOGRAPHY

1. Ao A, Jin S, Rao D, et al. First successful pregnancy outcome after preimplantation genetic diagnosis for aneuploidy screening in embryos generated from natural-cycle in vitro fertilization combined with an in vitro maturation procedure. Fertil Steril. 2006;85:1510.
2. Asch RH, Ellsworth LR, Balmaceda JP, et al. Birth following gamete intrafallopian transfer. Lancet. 1985;2:163.
3. Bancsi LF, Broekmans FJ, Eijlmans MJ, et al. Predictors of poor ovarian response in in vitro fertilization; a prospective study comparing basal markers of ovarian reserve. Fertil Steril. 2002;77:328-36.
4. Bavister BD, Kinsley DL, Lane M, et al. Recombinant human albumin supports hamster in vitro fertilization. Human Reprod. 2003;18:113-6.
5. Bernard A, Fuller BJ. Cryopreservation of human oocytes; a review of current problems and perspectives. Human Reprod Update. 1996;2:193-207.
6. Bonduelle M, Camus M, De Vos A, et al. Seven years of intracytoplasmic sperm injection and followup of 1987 subsequent children. Human Reprod. 1999;14:1243-64.
7. Bonduelle M, Wennerholm UB, Loft A, et al. A multi-centre cohort study of the physical health of 5-year-old children conceived after intracytoplasmic sperm injection, in vitro fertilization and natural conception. Human Reprod. 2005;20(2):413-9.
8. Cahill DJ, Fountain SA, Fox R, et al. Outcome of inadvertent administration of a gonadotropin-releasing hormone agonist (buserelin) in early pregnancy. Human Reprod. 1994;9:1243-6.
9. Cha KY, Koo JJ, Ko J, et al. Pregnancy after in vitro fertilization of human follicular oocytes collected from nonstimulated cycles, their culture in vitro and their transfer in a donor oocyte program. Fertil Steril. 1991;55:109-13.
10. Chen C. Pregnancy after human oocyte cryopreservation. Lancet. 1986;1:884-6.
11. Chian RC, Buckett WM, Tulandi T, et al. Prospective randomized study of human chorionic gonadotropin priming before immature oocyte retrieval from unstimulated women with polycystic ovarian syndrome. Human Reprod. 2000;15:165-70.
12. Cohen J, Elsner C, Kort H, et al. Impairment of the hatching process following IVF in the human and improvement of implantation by assisted hatching using micro manipulation. Human Reprod. 1999;5:7-13.
13. Cohen J, Malter H, Wright G, et al. Partial zona dissection of human oocytes when failure of zona pellucida penetration is anticipated. Human Reprod. 1989;4(4):435-42.
14. Devreker F, Winston RM, Hardy K. Glutamine improves human pre-implantation development in vitro. Fertil Steril. 1998;69: 293-9.
15. Devroey P, Braeckmans P, Smitz J, et al. Pregnancy after translaparoscopic zygote intrafallopian transfer in a patient with sperm antibodies. Lancet. 1986;1:1329.
16. El-Danasouri I, Selman H. Successful pregnancies and deliveries after a simple vitrification protocol for day 3 human embryos. Fertil Steril. 2001;76:400-2.
17. ESHRE PGD Consortium Steering Committee. ESHRE Preimplantation Genetic Diagnosis Consortium: data collection III (May 2001). Hum Reprod. 2002;17(1):233-46.
18. Fanchin R, Ayoubi JM, Righini C, et al. Uterine contractility decreases at the time of blastocyst transfers. Human Reprod. 2001;16:1115-9.
19. Fanchin R, Righini C, Olivennes F, et al. Uterine contractions at the time of embryo transfer alter pregnancy rates after in vitro fertilization. Human Reprod. 1998;13:1968-74.
20. Friedler S, Giudice LC, Lamb EJ. Cryopreservation of embryos and ova. Fertil Steril. 1988;49:743-64.
21. Gardner DK, Lane M. Culture and selection of viable blastocycts: a feasible proposition for human IVF? Human Reproduction Update. 1997;3:367.
22. Germond M, Nocera D, Senn A, et al. Microdissection of mouse and human zona pellucida using a 1.48- microns diode laser beam: efficacy and safety of the procedure. Fertil Steril. 1995;64:604-11.
23. Hackeloer BJ, Fleming R, Robinson HP, et al. Correlation of ultrasonic and endocrinologic assessment of human follicular development. Am J Obstet Gynecol. 1979;135:122-8.

24. Handyside AH, Kontogianni EH, Hardy K, et al. Pregnancies from biopsied human pre-implantation embryos sexed by Y-specific DNA amplification. Nature. 1990;344:768-70.
25. Hansen M, Kurinczuk JJ, Bower C, et al. The risk of major birth defects after intracytoplasmic sperm injection and in vitro fertilization. N Engl J Med. 2002;346(10):725-30.
26. Hoffman GE, Khoury J, Thie J. Recurrent pregnancy loss and diminished ovarian reserve. Fertil Steril. 2000;74(6):1192-5.
27. Karande VC, Morris R, Chapman C, et al. Impact of the 'Physician Factor' on pregnancy rates in a large assisted reproductive technology program: do too many cooks spoil the broth? Fertil Steril. 1999;71:1001-9.
28. Lane M, Schoolcraft WB, Gardner DK. Vitrification of mouse and human blastocysts using a novel cryo-loop container-less technique. Fertil Steril. 1999;72:1073.
29. Laws-King A, Trounson A, Sathananthan H, et al. Fertilization of human oocytes by microinjection of a single spermatozoon under the zona pellucida. Fertil Steril. 1987;48(4):637-42.
30. Lenz S, Lauritsen JG, KJellow M. Collection of human oocytes for in vitro fertilization by ultrasonically guided puncture. Lancet. 1981;1:1163-4.
31. Liu H-C, Cohen J, Alikani J, et al. Assisted hatching facilitates earlier implantation. Fertil Steril. 1993;60:871-5.
32. McClure N, Healy DL, Rogers PAW, et al. Vascular endothelial growth factor as capillary permeability agent in ovarian hyperstimulation syndrome. Lancet. 1994;344:235-6.
33. Muasher SJ, Oehninger S. The value of basal and/or stimulated gonadotropin levels in prediction of stimulation response and in vitro fertilization outcome. Fertil Steril. 1988;50(2):298-307.
34. Munne S, Lee A, Rosenwaks Z, et al. Diagnosis of major chromosome aneuploidies in human preimplantation embryos. Human Reprod. 1993;8:2185-91.
35. Nabi A, Awonuga H, Birch H, et al. Multiple attempts at embryo transfer: does this affect in vitro fertilization treatment outcome? Human Reprod. 1997;12:1188-90.
36. Nagy ZP, Liu J, Joris H, et al. The influence of the site of sperm deposition and mode of oolemma breakage at intracytoplasmic sperm injection on fertilization and embryo development rates. Human Reprod. 1995;10(12):3171-7.
37. Navot D, Rosenwaks Z, Margalioth EJ. Prognostic assessment of female fecundity. Lancet. 1987;2(8560):645-7.
38. Olivennes F, Cunha-Filho JS, Fanchin R, et al. The use of GnRH antagonists in ovarian stimulation. Human Reprod Update. 2002;8:279-90.
39. Pal L, Witt BR. Maximal historical FSH is a better predictor of cycle outcome than the baseline FSH for the IVF cycle. Fertil Steril. 2002;78:S135.
40. Palermo G, Joris H, Devroey P, et al. Pregnancies after intracytoplasmic injection of single spermatozoon into an oocyte. Lancet. 1992;340:17-8.
41. Palermo G, Joris H, Devroey P, et al. Pregnancies after intracytoplasmic injection of single spermatozoon into an oocyte. Lancet. 1992;340(8810):17-8.
42. Pensis M, Loumaye E, Psalti I. Screening of conditions for rapid freezing of human oocytes: preliminary study toward their cryopreservation. Fertil Steril. 1989;52:787-94.
43. Poindexter AN, Thompson DJ, Gibbons WE, et al. Residual embryos in failed embryo transfer. Fertil Steril. 1986;46:262-7.
44. Ponjaert-Kristoffersen I, Bonduelle M, et al. International collaborative study of intracytoplasmic sperm injection-conceived, in vitro fertilization-conceived and naturally-conceived 5-year-old child outcomes: cognitive and motor assessments. Pediatrics. 2005;115:283-9.
45. Ranieri DM, Quinn F, Makhlouf A, et al. Simultaneous evaluation of basal follicle-stimulating hormone and 17b-estradiol response to gonadotropin-releasing analogue stimulation: an improved predictor of ovarian reserve. Fertil Steril. 1998;70(2):227-33.
46. Reissmann T, Felberbaum R, Diedrich K, et al. Development and applications of luteinizing hormone- releasing antagonists in the treatment of infertility: an overview. Human Reprod. 1995;10:1974-81.
47. Rossing MA, Daling JR, Weiss NS, et al. Ovarian tumors in a cohort of infertile women. N Engl J Med. 1994;331:771-6.
48. Shaker AG, Zosmer A, Dean N, et al. Comparison of intravenous albumin and transfer of fresh embryos with cryopreservation of all embryos dfor subsequent transfer in prevention of ovarian hyperstimulation syndrome. Fertil Steril. 1996;65;992-6.
49. Soliman S, Daya S, Collins J, et al. The role of luteal phase support in infertility treatment: a metaanalysis of randomized trials. Fertil Steril. 1994;61:1068-76.
50. Steptoe PC, Edwards RG. Birth after the reimplantation of a human embryo. Lancet. 1978;2:366.
51. Sutcliffe AG, Peters CJ, Bowdin S, et al. Assisted reproductive therapies and imprinting disorders – a preliminary British survey. Hum Reprod. 2006;21:1009-11.
52. Sutcliffe AG, Taylor B, Saunders K, et al. Outcome in the second year of life after in vitro fertilization by intra-cytoplasmic sperm injection: a UK case-control study. Lancet. 2001;357(9274): 2080-4.
53. Tan SL, Waterson J, Wren M, et al. A prospective randomized study comparing aspiration only with aspiration and flushing for transvaginal ultrasound-directed oocyte recovery. Fertil Steril. 1992;58:356-60.
54. Trounson A, Leeton J, Besanko M. et al. Pregnancy established in an infertile patient after transfer of a donated embryo fertilized in vitro. Br Med J. 1983;286:835-8.
55. Trounson A, Mohr L. Human pregnancy following cryopreservation, thawing and transfer of an eight cell embryo. Nature 1983;305:707-9.
56. Trounson A, Wood C, Kausche A. In vitro maturation and fertilization and the developmental competence of oocytes recovered from untreated polycystic ovarian patients. Fertil Steril. 1994;62:353-62.
57. Ubancsek J, Witthaus E. Midluteal buserelin is superior to early follicular phase buserelin in combined gonadotropin-releasing hormone analog and gonadotropin stimulation in in vitro fertilization. Fertil Steril. 1996;65:966-71.
58. Van Steirteghem AC, Liu J, Joris H, et al. Higher success rate by intracytoplasmic sperm injection than by subzonal insemination: report of a second series of 300 consecutive treatment cycles. Human Reprod. 1993;8(7):1055-60.

59. Van Weering HG, Schats R, McDonnell J, et al. On going pregnancy rates in in vitro fertilization are not dependent on the physician performing the embryo transfer. Fertil Steril. 2005;83:316-20.

60. Veeck LL, Bodines R, Clarke RN, et al. High pregnancy rates can be achieved after freezing and thawing human blastocysts. Fertil Steril. 2004;82:1418-27.

61. Venn A, Watson L, Lumley J, et al. Breast and ovarian cancer incidence after infertility and in vitro fertilization. Lancet. 1995; 346:995-1000.

62. Virant-Klun I, Tomazevic T, Vrtacnik-Bokal E, et al. Increased ammonium in culture medium reduces the development of human embryos to the blastocyst stage. Fertil Steril. 2006;85:526-8.

CHAPTER

51

Male Infertility Surgery

Kishore M Nadkarni

INTRODUCTION

Male factor sterility is on the rise and sperm counts are dropping. Assisted reproductive technology promised new hope to infertile couples since 1978 when the world's first in vitro fertilization-embryo transfer (IVF-ET) baby was born in the United Kingdom. However, IVF-ET failed to treat severe male sterility factor, as atleast 60,000–75,000 motile sperms (post wash) were needed per oocyte to achieve IVF. The borderline cases, thus encountered embarrassing fertilization failures.

The arrival of intracytoplasmic sperm injection (ICSI) in 1992 marked a major breakthrough in the approach to male infertility. The extended indications of ICSI included azoospermia—where even spermatids, immature spermatozoa and non-motile spermatozoa could achieve fertilizations and subsequent pregnancies.

Globozoospermia, teratozoospermia, necrozoospermia, all came within the realm of ICSI.

A sizable number of patients with oligospermia, continue to get pregnant through superovulation with intrauterine insemination (IUI) of washed sperms. In these patients, no effort should be spared to increase the total motile count (TMC), so that pregnancies can be achieved through superovulation with IUI — which is more economical to the patient than entering an expensive ICSI program. Surgery still has a role in these cases.

Surgical Treatment of Infertility

Surgical treatment of male infertility can be classified as under:

- Surgery for varicocele
- Surgery for reproductive tract obstruction (RTO)
- Testicular biopsy
- Sperm retrieval techniques
- Surgery for erectile and ejaculatory dysfunction.

SURGERY FOR VARICOCELE

Varicocele is the elongation, tortuosity and pathological dilatation of the veins of the pampaniform plexus, and for long has been identified as one of the causes of male subfertility. It is frequently bilateral and long-standing varicoceles, may also cause testicular atrophy. Varicocele is more common on the left side. There are conflicting reports on the association of varicocele and infertility. Peng et al. postulated the cofactor theory in which varicocele can cause subfertility in association with a cofactor like nicotine, in which case both factors need treatment. Varicocele usually results in oligoasthenoteratozoospermia (OATS) in which, all the three parameters of sperms, viz. count, motility and morphology are affected. Total azoospermia is rare in varicocele and when present may be associated with some testicular factor. Result after varicocele ligation in such cases is poor.

Indication for varicocele surgery is a classical OATS with subfertility. Some centers advocate varicocele surgery even for patients with azoospermia with varicocele. Rarely surgery needs to be performed for pain in large adolescent varicocele.

Preferred Anesthesia

General anesthesia (GA)/spinal anesthesia.

Surgical Procedures for Varicocele Ligation

- Surgical ligation
- Laparoscopic ligation
- Microsurgical ligation
- Percutaneous occlusion of the internal spermatic vein.

Scrotal Approach

The operation is obsolete today. The veins in the pampiniform plexus are individually ligated through an

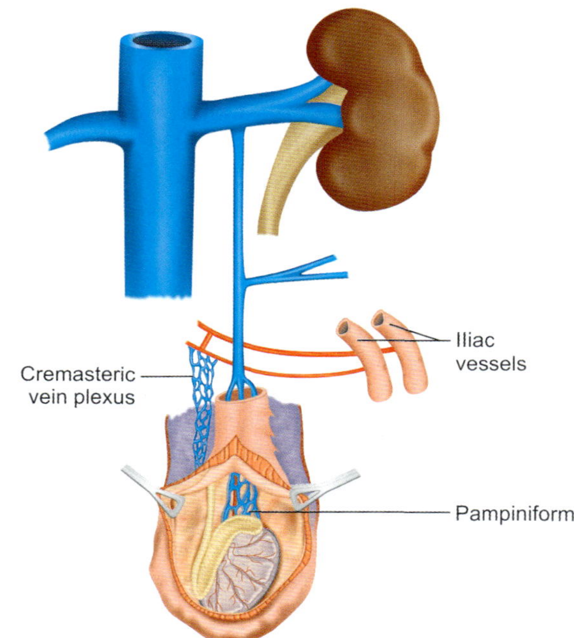

Fig. 1: Diagrammatic anatomical representation of cremasteric vein plexus

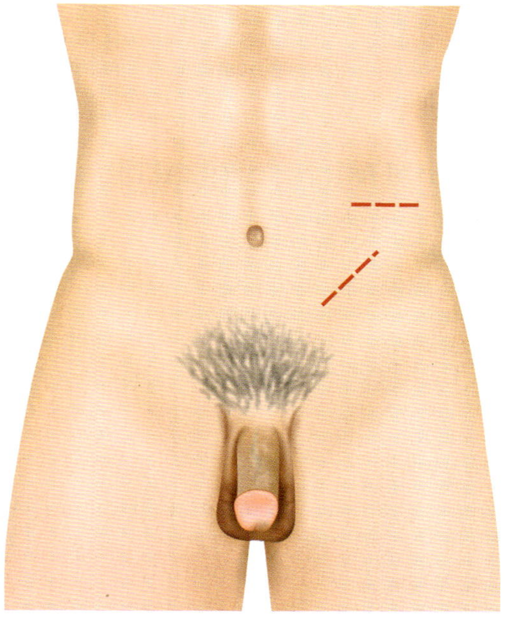

Fig. 2: Incision of varicocele surgery of cremasteric vein

incision on the scrotum. However, because the veins are too many, too close and thin, the chances of hematoma formation and the chances of damage to the spermatic artery with resulting testicular damage are very high, and hence, this approach has been abandoned.

Inguinal Approach

In this approach, the veins of the pampiniform plexus are ligated within the inguinal canal. A 3 cm incision is taken at the level of the mid-inguinal point. The external oblique aponeurosis is cut. The cord is identified and elevated out of the way. The thin layer of fascia on the cord is cut and the veins carefully dissected out of the cord. They are then cut and ligated. Care is taken to protect the artery, which lies posteriorly. Some people prefer to cut and ligate a single vein at the internal ring or just behind it.

Suprainguinal Approach (High Ligation)

A transverse lower abdominal incision is made just above the anterior super iliac spine. Layers cut include deep fascia and external oblique, internal oblique and transverses aponeurosis is split to expose the peritoneum. The peritoneum is retracted to expose the internal spermatic vein on its under surface. The vein, usually single, is identified, isolated, ligated and cut. In the modified Palomo's operation, about 2–3 cm of the vein is excised and the two ends approximated. This helps to hitch the sagging pampiniform plexus. This is the most popular method next to microsurgical varicocelectomy, which today is the gold standard.

Advantages

- Less chances of damage to the spermatic artery, which is some distance away
- Vein is dilated, turgid (2–3 mm), single and can be easily isolated
- Even damage to the spermatic artery at this level causes little testicular dysfunction. Because of extensive anastomosis between the spermatic and the cremasteric arterial systems (Fig. 1)
- There is a tributary which anastomosis with the superficial, circumflexiliac and epigastric and pudendal, and thus, with the caval system. Ligation below this tributary prevents return of varicocele (Fig. 2).

Disadvantage

Disadvantage is that the varicocele involving the cremasteric venous system cannot be ligated or even inspected in this approach.

Laparoscopic Ligation

Laparoscopic ligation is gaining popularity with more and more urosurgeons having laparoscopic set up and expertise. The vein is identified laparoscopically at the deep inguinal ring and obliterated by bipolar diathermy or clips.

Advantages

Advantages include less morbidity, early discharge from the hospital and total safety.

Disadvantages

Disadvantages are requirement of set up and expertise, inability to deal with the cremasteric veins and chances of injury to vas deferens.

Subinguinal Microsurgical Ligation

Microsurgical varicocele ligation involves ligation of each dilated vein in the spermatic cord and is carried out through a 2 cm incision just between the external ring and the base of the scrotum. A window is made and each individual vessel is ligated or coagulated. The artery is identified and protected. This is currently the gold standard operation for varicocele.

Advantage

Advantage is that the accurate individual ligation is possible and recurrence is rare, and this operation is associated with a higher pregnancy rate.

Disadvantages

Disadvantages are that it requires microsurgical expertise; microscope and lymphatics can be mistaken for veins hence, chances of hydrocele are more likely and it is possible that if the level changes, the same vein will be encountered twice or thrice.

Percutaneous Approach

Percutaneous approach to the internal spermatic vein is either through jugular or right femoral vein via inferior vena cava. Using a standard Seldinger's needle, a catheter is introduced under radiological guidance. Small substances may be injected to plug the spermatic vein such as steel coils, dacron plugs, silicon miniballoons or fibrin plugs sclerosants such as sodium morrhuate and sodium tetradecyl sulfate or phenol may also be used.

Complications of Varicocele Surgery

Complications of varicocele surgery include testicular hematoma, atrophy following damage to spermatic artery, damage to vas deferens, hydrocele formation and of course, recurrence.

SURGERY FOR MALE REPRODUCTIVE TRACT OBSTRUCTION

Obstructive azoospermia may be due to obstruction at different levels of the male reproductive tract and may be congenital or acquired as a result of trauma or infections. It must be noted that surgical reconstruction of RTO is gradually being replaced by sperm retrieval techniques with more and more patients opting for retrieval rather than reconstruction. The reasons for above may be:

- Reconstruction operation requires microsurgical expertise and results are proportional to individual skills
- The amount of motile sperms in the ejaculate may be so low after the reconstruction that ICSI will still be the assisted reproductive technology (ART) method of choice, in which case retrieval is a better option
- There is a phenomenon of inverted motility seen in the patients with long standing RTO, which prevents effective impregnation by the sperms in IUI and IVF
- There is a real chance of late treatment failures, following surgical reconstruction, hence even in patients undergoing successful operations are advised to freeze sperms for future use
- Surgery on the male reproductive tract entails high risk of antisperm antibody formation (70%), which can impair sperm motility and function.

Preferred Anesthesia

General anesthesia/spinal/regional block.

Common Operations for Male Reproductive Tract Obstruction

- Epididymovasostomy (fistula method)
- Single tubal anastomosis vaso-epididymal (VE)
- Epididymo-epididymostomy
- Vasovasostomy
- Transurethral treatment of ejaculatory duct obstruction.

All the above operation require microsurgical expertise, advanced microinstruments, surgical skills, good eye to hand coordination, suturing with vicryl/monocryl/nylon or prolene 9–10 and considerable operative time. Chances of success are variable depending on the surgical skill, but results in terms of good semen are rarely above 50% and pregnancy rates are even lower in the best of hands.

All the operations are diagrammatically represented with brief descriptions.

- Epididymovasostomy (Fig. 3)—done for vaso-epididymal obstruction as diagnosed by slightly enlarged testis with turgid epididymis (Bayle's sign), normal follicle stimulating hormone (FSH) and azoospermia. Originally performed by Edward Martin from Philadelphia. Objective of the fistula method is to create a fistula between the cut vas deferens on one side and multiple loops of epididymis on the other side. This may be end (vas deferens) to side (epididymis) or side (vas deferens) to side (epididymis)
- Vaso-epididymal single tubule anastomosis (Fig. 4)—(A) end to end (B) side to side

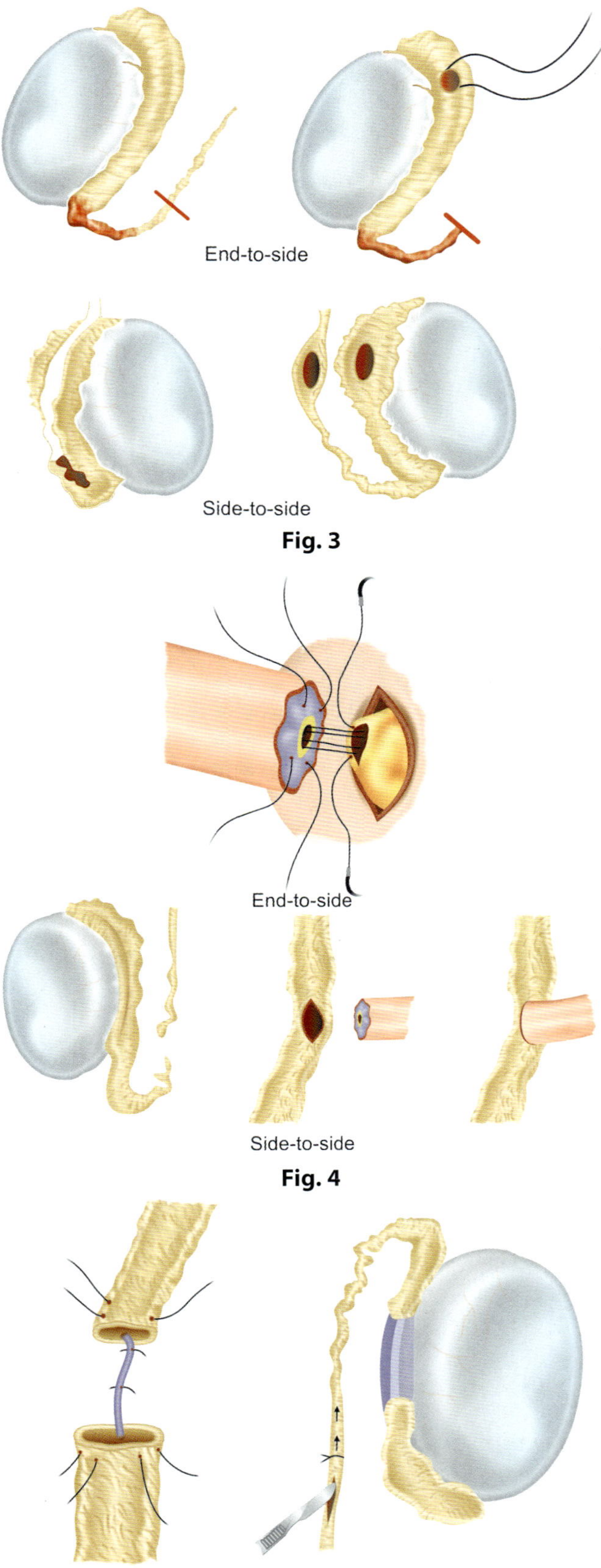

Figs 3 to 5: Common surgical approaches for reconstruction of vas deferens

Vasography is necessary to demonstrate patency of the distal vas deferens. It is also necessary to demonstrate live spermatozoa on the epididymal side in all cases of obstruction, different techniques of anastomosis have been described

- Epididymo-epididymostomy (Fig. 5) is a fine end-to-end anastomosis and is technically quite difficult
- Vasovasostomy (Fig. 6) is a simpler end-to-end anastomosis, which can be also done with an operating loop
- Transurethral treatment (Fig. 7) of ejaculatory duct obstruction can be done under vision using a cysto-resectoscope.

TESTICULAR BIOPSY

This is the age-old diagnostic method to determine the cause of azoospermics or oligospermics and is still performed today. Testicular pathology may be focal or diffuse, and hence multiple biopsies are necessary.

Open Method

Open testicular biopsy is usually performed under local anesthesia (LA). The layers of the scrotum are divided through a small incision until the tunica vaginalis is opened and the tunica albugenia exposed. As soon as this is cut, the testicular tissue pouts out, which is excised and sent for histopathological examination. The closure is done in layers.

Closed Method

Other closed methods of examining testicular tissue are:

- Fine needle aspiration cytology (FNAC) using a fine 26–28 bore needle
- Wide bore 15–18 number needle biopsy.

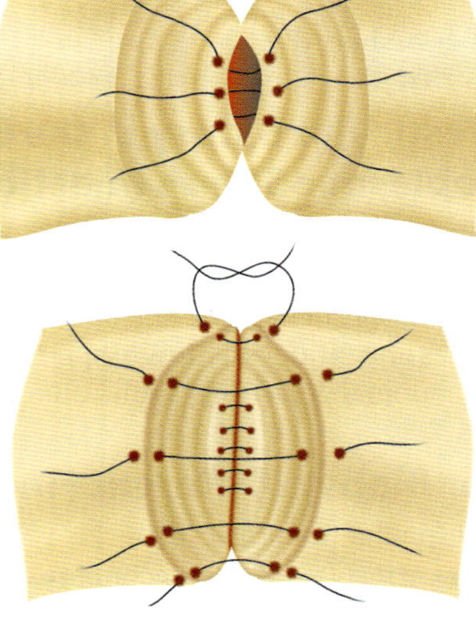

Fig. 6: Vasovasostomy

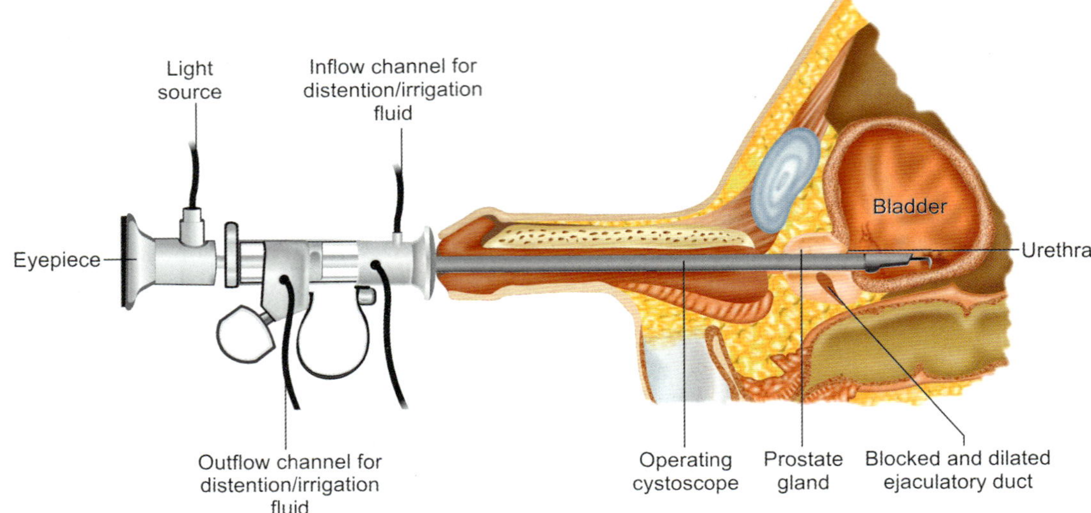

Fig. 7: Transurethral approach

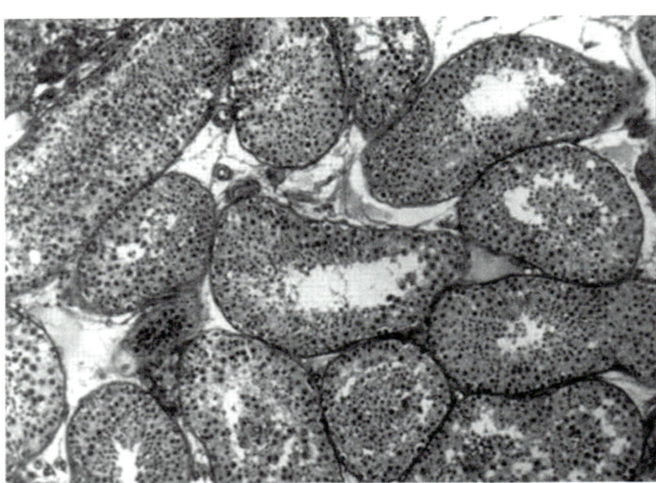

Fig. 8: Normal testicular tissue

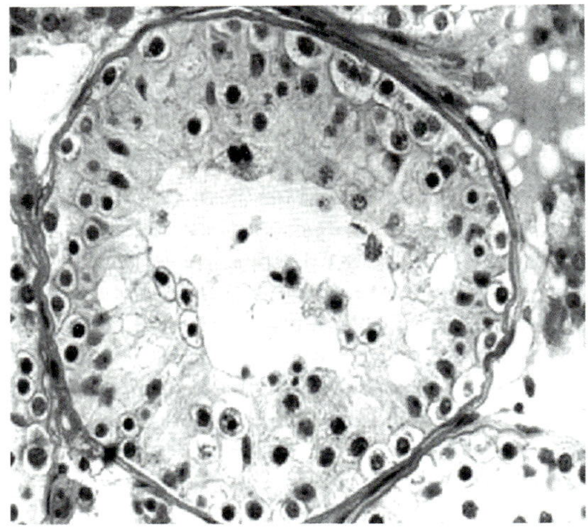

Fig. 9: Maturation arrest (usually at secondary spermatocyte stage)

Preferred Anesthesia

Local anesthesia/short GA.

Role of Testicular Biopsy in the Era of Intracytoplasmic Sperm Injection

Nowadays, testicular biopsy is almost forbidden, since it has no therapeutic value. Every attempt at testicular biopsy causes tissue damage, hematoma and fibrosis with scarring and jeopardizes any future attempts of sperm retrieval and should be abandoned. It has diagnostic value only.

Testicular Biopsy (Different Findings)

- Normal testicular tissue (Fig. 8)
- Maturation arrest (usually at secondary spermatocave stage) (Fig. 9)
- Germinal aplasia (sertoli II syndrome) (Fig. 10)

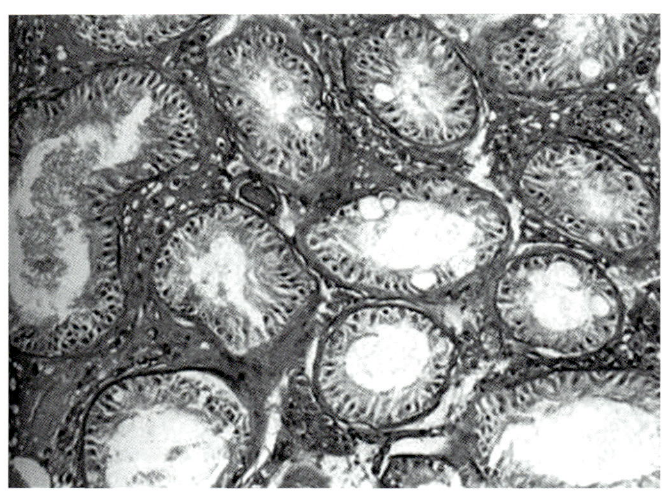

Fig. 10: Germinal aplasia

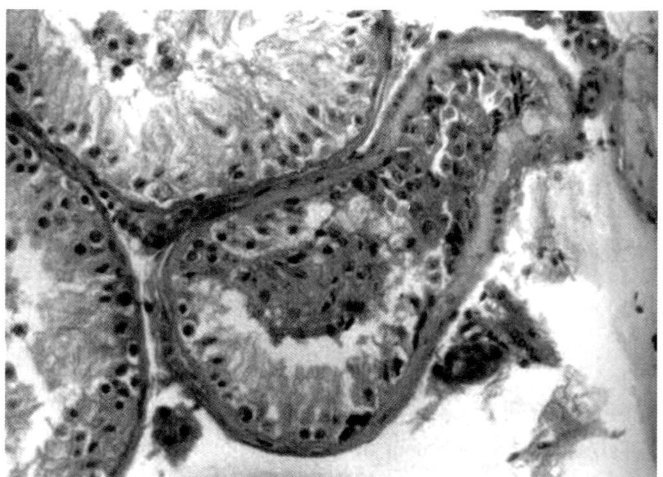

Fig. 11: Tubal atrophy

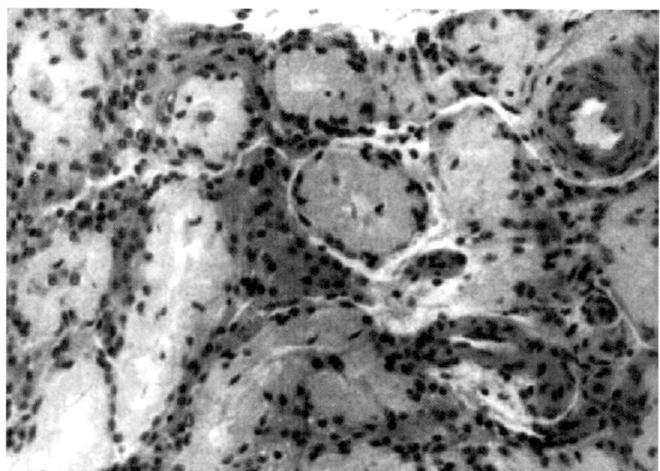

Fig. 12: Diffuse tubal atrophy

- Tubular atrophy-focal or diffuse, in which thickening of the tubular basement membrane and hylanization of tubules may be seen (Figs 11 and 12).

SPERM RETRIEVAL TECHNIQUES

Introduction

Intracytoplasmic sperm injection has changed or revolutionized the treatment of male infertility, particularly severe oligospermia and azoospermia where IVF fails to achieve fertilization.

Sperm retrieval techniques are important because they offer the only chance to patients having nil sperms to conceive their own genetic child. That is the real joy of ICSI and only by doing more such difficult cases successfully, ICSI will achieve its potential.

Indications for Sperm Retrieval Techniques

- Obstructive azoospermics
- Unreconstructable RTO or failed RTO
- Reconstructable RTO requesting retrieval instead of surgical repair.

Preferred Anesthesia

Local Anesthesia/Short GA

Relative contraindications

- Genetic mutation
- HIV (human immunodeficiency virus)
- Hepatitis
- Maternal age greater than 42 years.

Goals of Sperm Retrieval Procedures

- Obtain the best quality sperm possible
- Retrieve an adequate number of sperms both for immediate use and for cryopreservation
- Minimize damage to the reproductive tract so as not to jeopardize future attempts at sperm retrieval reconstruction.

Sperm Retrieval Indications (Etiological)

Epididymal Sperms (Obstructive Lesions)

- Congenital absence of vasovasostomy and failed reversal of vasectomy, failed vasoepididymostomy
- Vas deferens blockage following genital infections, ejaculatory duct obstruction
- Vas deferens blockage in Kartagener's syndrome
- Young's syndrome.

Testicular Sperms (Nonobstructive Lesions)

- Anejaculation
- Impotence (also, epididymal sperms)
- Non obstructive oligoasthenoteratozoospermia
- Incomplete maturation arrest
- Partial germ cell aplasia
- Undescended testis
- Klinefelter's syndrome
- Damaged testis after torsion/trauma.

Sperm Retrieval Techniques (Table 1)

Table 1: Sperm retrieval techniques

	Epididymal	Testicular
Percutaneous	PESA	TESA
	PESE	FNAC (TEFNA)
		Percutaneous biopsy
Open biopsy	MESA	TESE

Abbreviations: PESA, percutaneous epididymal sperm aspiration; TESA, testicular epididymal sperm aspiration; PESE, percutaneous biopsy; FNAC, fine needle aspirate cytology; TEFNA, testicular fine needle aspiration; MESA, microepididymal sperm aspiration; TESE, testicular sperm extraction

Other Procedures

Vas deferens sperm aspiration, spermatocele aspiration.

Microepididymal Sperm Aspiration

The first pregnancy was reported by Tembler Smith in 1985 when retrieved sperms were used for IVF. An incisions 1–2 cm is made at the base of the scrotum. Layers cut to expose epididymis and testis. The covering of the epididymis is incised using an operating loop or microscope to expose the tubules. A very small incision is made on one of the tubules using a microscalpel. A tiny needle or a hollow glass rod is passed in to the tubule under magnification and contents aspirated (Figs 13 to 15).

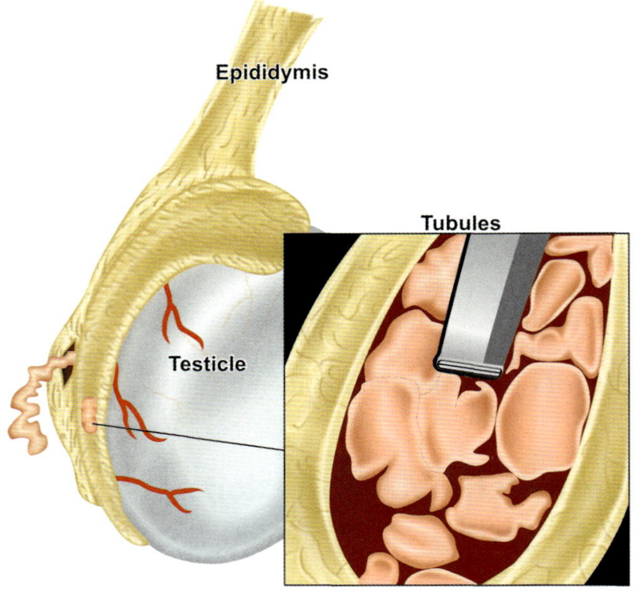

Fig. 13: Testicular anatomy

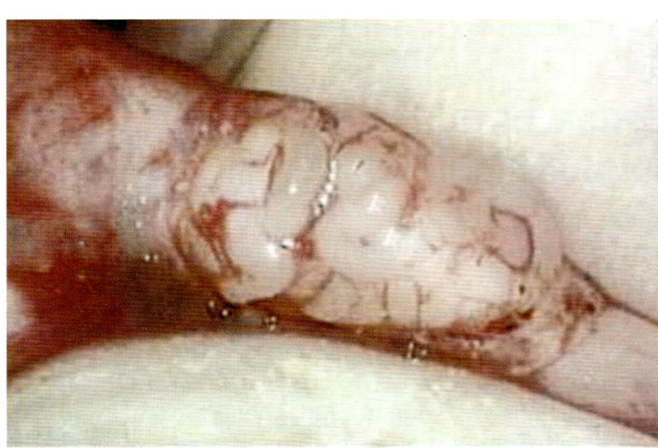

Fig. 14: Testicular tubules

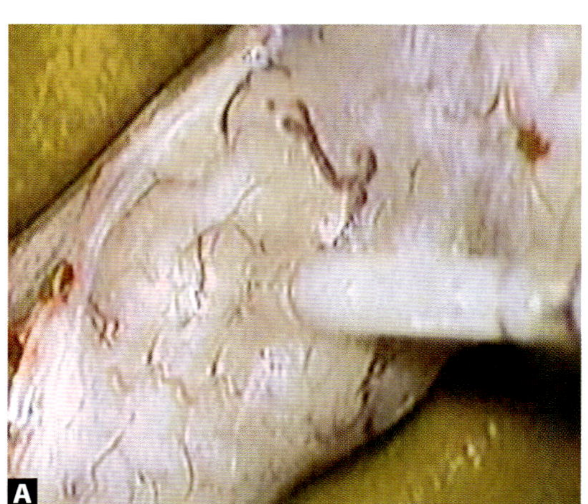

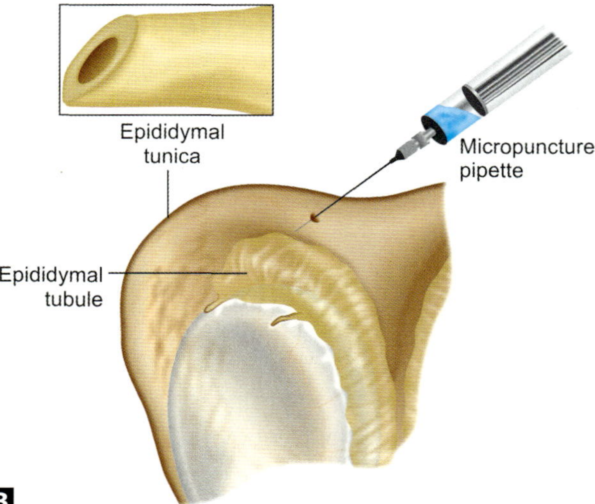

Figs 15A and B: Technique of microepididymal sperm aspiration

Advantages of MESA

- Reduced blood contamination
- Large number of sperms retrieved, can be used in many cycles
- Excellent results with cryopreservation
- Reduced risk of hematoma
- Best clinical pregnancy rates.

Disadvantages

- Requires microsurgical expertise
- Increased cost
- GA
- Postoperative discomfort
- Repeat operations are difficult because of the fibrosis and adhesions.

Percutaneous Epididymal Sperm Aspiration

Percutaneous epididymal sperm aspiration is done under LA, using number 26 scalp vein set or insulin syringe. No incision is needed (Figs 16A and B).

Advantages

- No microsurgical expertise required
- LA
- Few instruments
- Fast and repeatable
- Minimal postoperative discomfort.

Disadvantages

- Few sperms retrieved
- Risk of hematoma
- Blood contamination
- Damage to adjacent tissue.

Testicular Sperm Extraction

Testicular sperm extraction consists of doing an open testicular biopsy and then processing the tissue samples to extract spermatozoa or spermatids for ICSI (Figs 17 and 18). Pieces of tissue are kept in dishes containing culture medium at 37°C. Spermatozoa can be liberated from the tubules using mechanical methods, such as gentle grinding of tissue, crushing between glass slides, fine chopping and grating with scalpel or scissors or sharp needles, or chemical methods, such as using enzymes to digest connective tissue and red blood cells (RBCs).

Advantages

- No microsurgical expertise required
- Short local or GA
- Few instruments
- Fast and repeatable.

Disadvantages

- Few sperms retrieved
- Risk of testicular atrophy.

Percutaneous Biopsy

Percutaneous biopsy or PESE can be done in different ways, using needle and precision forceps to pull out tiny tubules directly out of the skin.

Advantages

- It is an easy procedure
- Done under LA
- Few instruments
- Fast and repeatable
- Can be done in different quadrants
- Minimal postoperative discomfort.

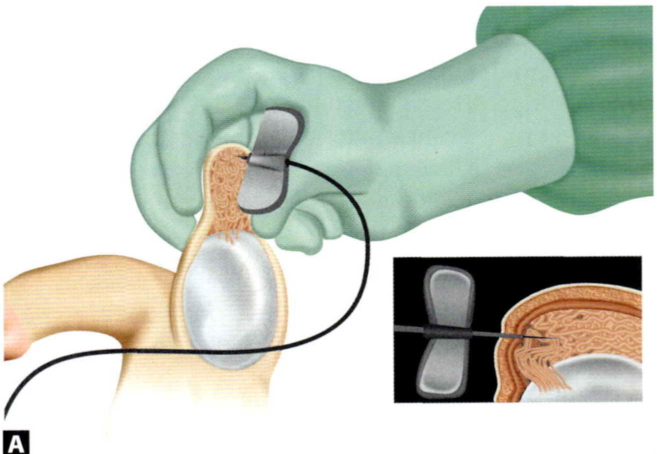

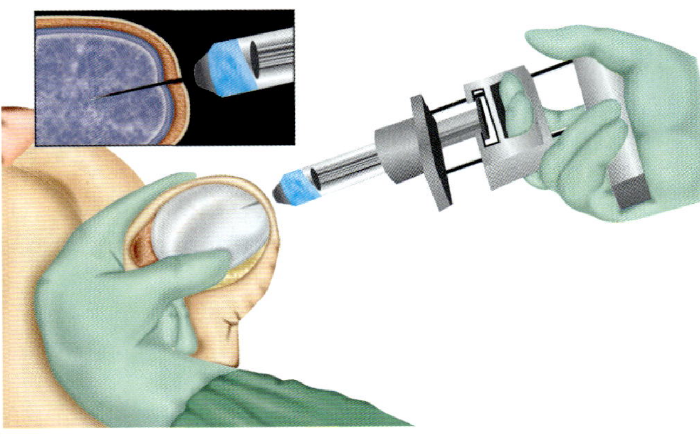

Fig. 17: Technique of percutaneous epididymal sperm aspiration

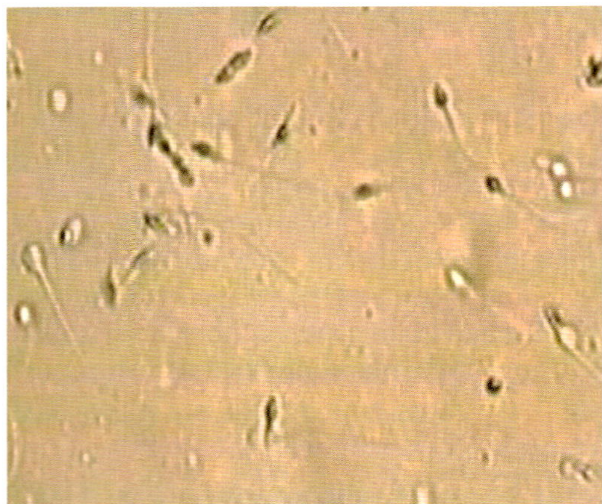

Fig. 17: Spermatids aspirated

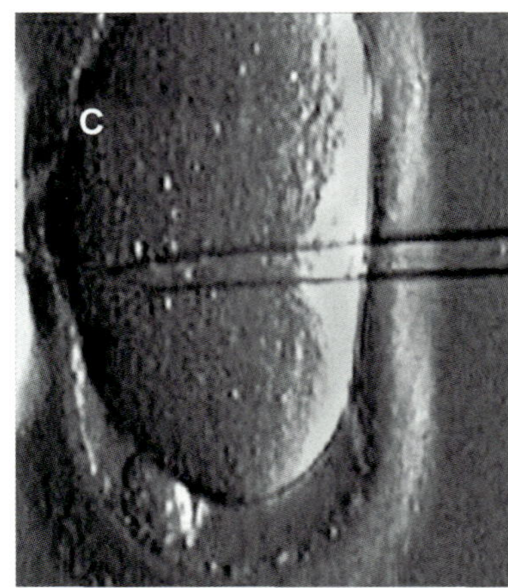

Fig. 18: Microphotograph of intracytoplasmic sperm injection

Disadvantages

- Few sperms retrieved
- Risk of testicular atrophy
- Risk of hematoma
- Blood contamination.

The ideal method of sperm retrieved is debatable. The optimal method should allow retrieval of adequate amounts of good quality semen for immediate use and future. Cryopreservation should be safe, efficient, and reliable.

Some Facts Regarding Sperm Retrieval Technique

- In 50% of azoospermic men, viable sperm could be extracted from testicular biopsies
- Apparent absence of sperm in a diagnostic open biopsy cannot be assumed to indicate that no sperm will be obtained during ICSI
- Small foci of mature (complete) spermatogenesis are present even in badly damaged testis.

SURGERY FOR ERECTILE AND EJACULATORY DYSFUNCTION

Ejaculatory Dysfunction

Ejaculatory dysfunction can be treated with a vibrator (vibroejaculation) or electroejaculator. Complex operations have been described in the region of bladder neck for retrograde ejaculation, which are rarely done in the modern days; instead, sperms are retrieved from urine in the bladder in cases of retrograde ejaculation.

Erectile Dysfunction

Erectile dysfunction is treated by psychosexual counseling, visual aids, sildenafil (viagra), mechanical devices, intracavarnosal injection of papaverine with largactil or alprostadil (PGE1) and topical agents (PGE1) applied intraurethrally. For patients who do not respond to the above, penile prosthesis may be inserted into the erectile tissue or the corpora cavernosa, which may be semirigid and malleable or inflatable.

Complex microvascular procedures have also been described for patients with impotence due to reduced arterial or venous leakage from erectile tissue.

CONCLUSION

Although ICSI has assumed center stage and is the main line therapy for male factor infertility with low sperm counts, surgical treatment still has a role to play because it offers a multiple event impact as compared to a single event impact in case of ICSI in determining the cost effectiveness of the therapy. Hence good surgical treatment can help reduce the cost per pregnancy because ART treatment (ICSI) is still out of reach for most patients.

BIBLIOGRAPHY

1. Carlsen E, Givercman A, Keiding N, et al. Evidence for decreasing quality of semen during past 50 years. British Med J. 1992;305:609-13.
2. Ferguson JM, Gillespie LN, Chalmers N, et al. Percutaneous varicocele embolization in the treatment of infertility. Br J Radiol. 1995;68:700-3.
3. Foresta C, Ruzza G, Rizzoti A, et al. Varicocele and infertility. Preoperative prognostic elements. J Androl. 1984;5:135-7.
4. Ivanissavich O. Left varicocele due to reflux. Experience with 4709 operative cases in 42 years. J Int Coll Surg. 1960;34:1287-90.
5. Jequier AM. Vasectomy related infertility, a major and costly medical problem. Hum Reprod. 1995;13:1757-9.
6. Kruger TF, Acosta AA, Simons KF, et al. Predicting value of abnormal sperm morphology factor in in vitro fertilization. Fertil Steril. 1988;49:112-7.
7. Liu J, Nagy Z, Jovis H, et al. Successful fertilization and establishment of pregnancies after ICSI in patients with Globozoospermia. Hum Reprod. 1995;10:626-9.
8. Londin K, Sjogven A, Nilsson L, et al. Fertilization and pregnancy after ICSI of acrosomeless spermatozoa: Fertil Steril. 1994;62:1266-7.
9. Martin E, Carnett JB, Levy JV, et al. The surgical treatment of sterility due to obstruction at the epididymis together with the study of the morphology of the human sperm. Univ Pa Med Bull. 1902;15(1):2-15.
10. Mehta RH, Anandkumar JC. Declining semen quality in Bangloreans: A preliminary report. Corr Sci. 1997;72:621.
11. Meniru GI, Gorgy A, Batha S, et al. Studies of percutaneous Epididymal sperm aspiration (PESA) and intracytoplasmic sperm injection. Hum Reprod Update. 1998;4:57-71.
12. Meniru GI, Gorgy A, Podsiadly BT, et al. Results of percutaneous epididymal sperm aspiration and intracytoplasmic sperm injection into major groups of patients with obstructive azoospermia. Hum Reprod. 1997;12:2443-6.
13. Nagy ZP, Verheyen G, Tournaye H, et al. An improved treatment procedure for testicular biopsy specimens offers more efficient sperm recovery: Case series. Fertil Steril. 1997;68:376-9.
14. Nieschlag E, Hertle L, Fischedick A, et al. Treatment of Varicocele counselling is as effective as occlusion of the vena spermatica. Hum Reprod. 1995;10:347-53.
15. Nilsson S, Edvinson, A, Nilsson B. Improvement of semen and pregnancy rate after ligation and division of internal spermatic vein; fact or fiction? Br J Urol. 1979;51:591-6.
16. Oehninger S, Acosta AA, Kruger TF, et al. Failure of fertilization in in vitro fertilization: The "occult" male factor. J In Vitro Fert Embryo Transf. 1988;5:181-7.
17. Palermo G, Jorish H, Devroey P, et al. Pregnancies after intracytoplasmic injection of a single spermatozoon into an oocyte. Lancet. 1992;340:17-8.
18. Palermo GD, Coben J, Alikani M, et al. Intracytoplasmic sperm injection—a novel treatment for all forms of male infertility. Fertil Steril. 1995;63:1231-40.
19. Palomo A. Radical care due to varicocele by a new technique: Preliminary report. J Urol. 1960;61:604-7.
20. Peng BC, Tomashevsky P, Nagler HM. The co-factor effect: Varicocele and infertility. Fertil Steril. 1995;54:145-8.
21. Silber SJ. Intracytoplasmic sperm injection today: A personal review. In:Devroey P, Tavalatzise BC, van Steirtghem AC (Eds). Current theory and practice of ICSI.; 1998. p. 208-58.
22. Silber SJ. Microsurgery for vasectomy reversal and vasoepididymostomy. Urology. 1984;23:505-24.
23. Tan SM, Ng FC, Ravintharan T, et al. Laparoscopic varicocelectomy: Technique and results. Br J Urol. 1995;75:523-8.
24. Temple-Smith PD, Southwick GJ, Yates CA, et al. Human pregnancy by in vitro fertilization (IVF) using sperm aspirated from the epididymis. J I n Vitro Fert Embryo Transf. 1985;2: 119-22.
25. Tesarik J. Fertilization of oocytes after injecting spermatozoa, spermatids and spermatocytes. Rev Reprod. 1996;1:149-52.
26. Tulloch WS. Varicocele in Subfertility: Results of treatment. BMJ. 1995;2:536.
27. Van Voorhis B, J sparks, Allen BD, et al. Cost effectiveness of infertility treatments: A cohort study. Fertil Steril. 1957;67:830-6.
28. Verheyan G, De Croo I, Tournaye H, et al. Comparison of four mechanical methods to retrieve spermatozoa from testicular tissue. Hum Reprod. 1995;10:2956-9.
29. Wagenknecht LV. Obstruction in the male reproductive tract. In: Bain J, Schill WB, Scjwarsteom L (Eds). Treatment of Male Infertility. Berlin: Springer; 1982. p. 221-48.
30. Winfield HN, Donovan JF. Laparoscopic varicocelectomy. Semin Urol. 1992;10:152-60.
31. Yates CA, Trounson AO, Dektreser DM. Male factor infertility and invitro fertilization, 4th International Congress in Andrology Florence, Italy 14-18. Abstract. 1989;263.

CHAPTER

52

Male Sterilization—Vasectomy

KM Nadkarni, Arun Tiwari

INTRODUCTION

With increasing awareness, information and education, male partner involvement in family planning and welfare is on the rise. Today, couples are able to discuss the family planning options amongst themselves and with their doctor and make a logical decision about the method of contraception, both temporary and permanent.

Apart from condoms and spermicidal gels, with no reliable male contraceptive pill available, vasectomy remains one of the safest and the most effective permanent contraceptive method available and is a popular male option. As compared to tubal ligation done in females, vasectomy is easier, safer, does not require opening of the abdominal cavity, quicker and can be done as an outpatient office procedure under local anesthesia. Contraception is effective, reliable and reversible. In spite of all the advantages, it is less commonly performed than tubal ligation in most countries.

Population reports (2003) have found that apart from India and China, less than 1% of women in the developing countries rely on male sterilization as a contraceptive method. In India, the figure is 2%, Nepal 6% and China 8%. Male sterilization is a major family planning method (more than 40%) in the developed countries like the United Kingdom (UK), the United States of America (USA), Canada, Australia, and New Zealand. The reason for the lower incidence in the developing countries could be gender bias, male dominance myths and misconceptions.

Vasectomy is still shrouded with fear and ignorance and many associate this procedure with loss of virility.

With the improvements and evolution in techniques such as NSV (no scalpel vasectomy), vasectomy has surpassed tubal ligation in some provinces of China.

Also, vasectomy reversal has better success rates than before. Technical success, as evidenced by live spermatozoa in the ejaculate, is achieved in more than 95% of the patients operated by trained urosurgeons. Studies suggesting increased incidence of prostatic cancer and also increased levels of antisperm antibodies have been discounted.

All these factors have led to an increase in acceptance of vasectomy as a choice of voluntary permanent sterilization (Figs 1A to H).

Indications

Vasectomy is indicated as a permanent sterilization method in couples or individual male who desires no further children. The concerned individual must be in a fit mental state and able to understand the consequences of his decision.

ELIGIBILITY CRITERIA (WHO-IPPF)

Contraindications

No permanent contraindication (irrespective of age and number of children).

Delay (Until Condition is Successfully Treated or No Longer Exists)

- Infection of operative area or acute systemic infections
- Signs and symptoms of sexually transmitted diseases (STD)
- Filariasis— elephantiasis
- Intrascrotal mass.

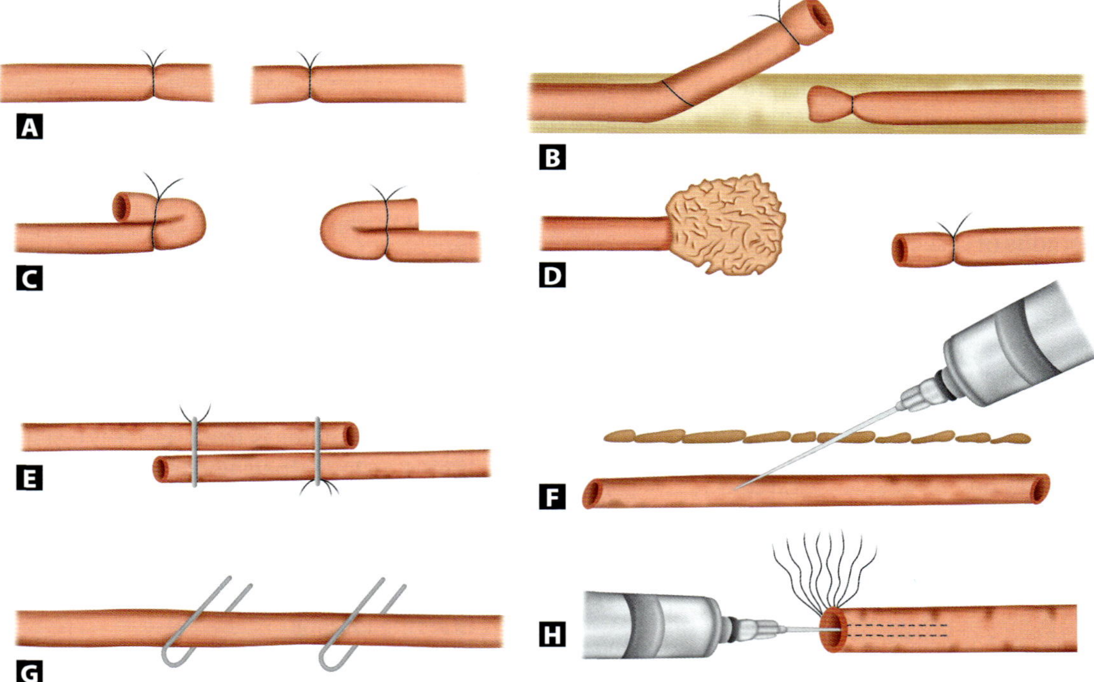

Figs 1A to H: Different methods of vas deferens occlusion

Special precautions to be done in a facility well-equipped to handle complications:

- Previous scrotal injury
- Large varicocele
- Large hydrocele
- Previous surgery for cryptorchidism
- Inguinal hernias
- Coagulation disorders.

Counseling and Preoperative Information

Males should be encouraged to undergo vasectomy as a permanent family planning procedure, particularly if the female partner is debilitated, anemic, suffering from any systemic disease, heart diseases or intra-abdominal adhesions and previous pelvic operations.

The Following Information Must be Given to the Patient

- Vasectomy is a permanent male contraception method
- It is done by a short simple office procedure under local anesthesia and does not require admission
- It does not mean castration
- It has no effect on masculinity, sexual activity, semen volume or general health
- Millions of men have undergone this safe procedure in the last 50 years
- Sterility does not occur immediately—hence other contraceptions like condom must be used until ejaculate becomes sperm-free
- There is a failure rate of 0.5%
- Reversal is possible with 70% success rate in good hands
- There is a 2% wound infection and hematoma rate
- There is no long-term effect such as testicular or prostatic cancer.

Vasectomy Procedure

- Complete preoperative counseling of patient
- Perfect choice of technique and surgery without complications at a suitable center by a trained surgeon
- Confirmation of success by semen examination showing sperm ejaculate after 12 weeks or 16–20 ejaculates.

Selection of Cases

Detailed history taking followed by local examination should be done. Local infection, scrotal problems, scrotal filariasis, hernia, hydrocele should be looked for. Psychiatric problem must be noted. Anemia, diabetes, blood pressure, recent cardiac disease should be detected. Every attempt should be made to make vasectomy safe and avoid mortality, morbidity, and subsequent discredit to the family planning program.

Techniques of Vasectomy

Anesthesia: Local anesthesia using up to 10 mL, 2% lidocaine is injected using 24 gauge needle in the 2 cm area of the incision under the median raphe; 2–3 mL of lidocaine is also injected alongside the vas deferens (into the vas deferens sheath). Occasionally, general anesthesia (GA) may be used in extremely sensitive patients. There are two methods of vasectomy

1. Conventional vasectomy (CV)
2. No-scalpel vasectomy (NSV).

Conventional Vasectomy

Steps

- A 1 cm incision is made in the skin in the median raphe at the upper end
- The vas deferens is rolled between the thumb and two fingers in the cord and palpated and brought under the skin incision
- The vas deferens is grasped with the Allis forceps. A longitudinal incision is made on the vas deferens sheath and vas deferens is pulled, dissected, exposed and held between the Allis forceps or towel clamp and brought out
- A segment of vas deferens is cut (0.5 cm) and both the ends tied. Various ligature methods are described. Hemoclips may be used or cauterization of the cut ends done. Fascial interposition (FI) may be done to prevent the cut ends from approximating. The distance between the two cut ends must be at least 2–4 cm. Too tight ligatures must be avoided as there may be chances of cut through
- Hemostasis is done, procedure repeated on the other vas deferens and skin closure done (Figs 2A to D)

No-scalpel Vasectomy

Steps

- The vas deferens is fixed under the skin at the median raphe, using a specially designed ring forceps. It holds the vas deferens extracutaneously without injuring it
- A dissecting forceps with a sharp pointed tip, similar to a curved mosquito forceps, is used to puncture the skin directly overlying the vas deferens contained in the ring forceps
- The puncture hole is enlarged to twice the diameter of the vas deferens

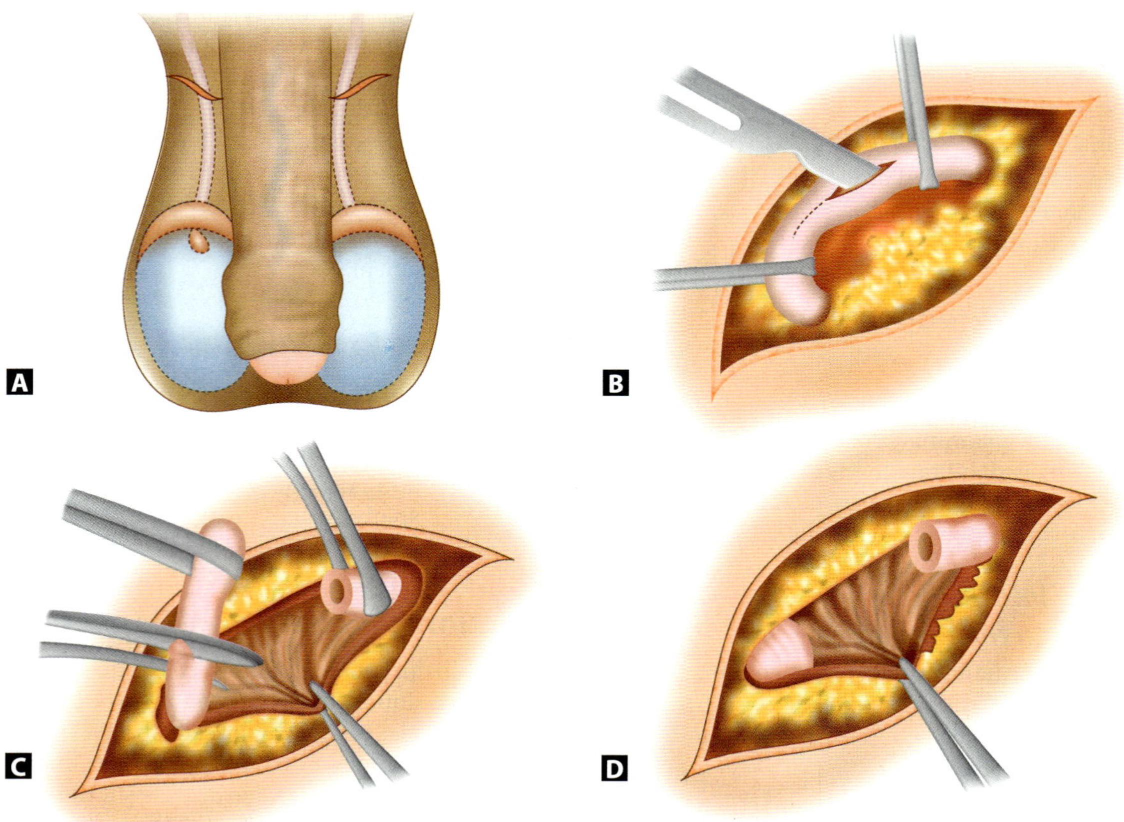

Figs 2A to D: Steps of conventional vasectomy; (A) incisions on the skin; (B) the sheath of the vas deferens is cut open; (C) a portion of the vas deferens is removed; (D) the vas deferens is ligated at the cut ends

- The next step involves a delicate but firm grasping of the vas deferens with the puncturing instrument and deliberately rotating the vas deferens in a clockwise manner to make it bare and deliver it out of the puncture wound. (This is the hallmark of the NSV)
- Subsequent handling of the vas deferens is similar to the CV
- At the end of the procedure, a tiny puncture hole results, which does not require closure
- The net result is a no-incision, no-stitch vasectomy with minimal dissection using only three instruments (vas deferens fixation forceps, vas deferens dissection forceps and a scissor) as compared to nearly 14 instruments required in CV (Fig. 3).

The NSV is being implemented in India to help male sterilization, and thus, promotes male participation in the family welfare program. Insuring availability of this new technique in the peripheral rural areas will help increase the acceptance of male sterilization in the country. The project is being funded by the United Nations Family Planning Association (UNFPA). The government of India will contribute toward providing centers for training and making available necessary infrastructure at the training sites.

Advantages of NSV over CV

- It takes less time (about 10 minutes)
- Causes faster recovery
- Less painful
- Less chances of bleeding and hematoma formation
- Only three instruments required
- No stitch required.

However, some training and special instruments are needed.

Complications include pain, swelling, discomfort, bleeding and hematoma formation. Infections may occur, sperm granuloma may result in a palpable lump. Antisperm antibodies have been demonstrated in 40–60% of men undergoing vasectomy. Failure of vasectomy may occur in 0.1–1.2% of the cases. A small percentage of people (< 10%) have chronic testicular pain after vasectomy.

Postoperatively: About 15–20 ejaculates contain sperms and 2–3 months are required to become sperm-free, during which time alternative contraceptive methods must be used.

RECENT ADVANCES

The two main components of vasectomy are isolation of the vas deferens from the scrotum and subsequent vas deferens occlusion. However, more than 30 different combinations of vas deferens occlusion have been described. Poor quality studies, heterogeneous study designs and conflicting results have made it difficult to determine which are the most effective techniques. The most common technique, especially in low resource settings is suture ligation with excision of a small segment of vas deferens. Recent evidence from Asia suggests that 95% of all vasectomies in India are done using ligation and excision. In contrast, data available indicates that only 18% of the vasectomies in the USA are done using this technique. Although vasectomy has traditionally been thought to have overall failure rates of 1–3%, recent research indicates higher failure rates for ligation and excision. A meeting

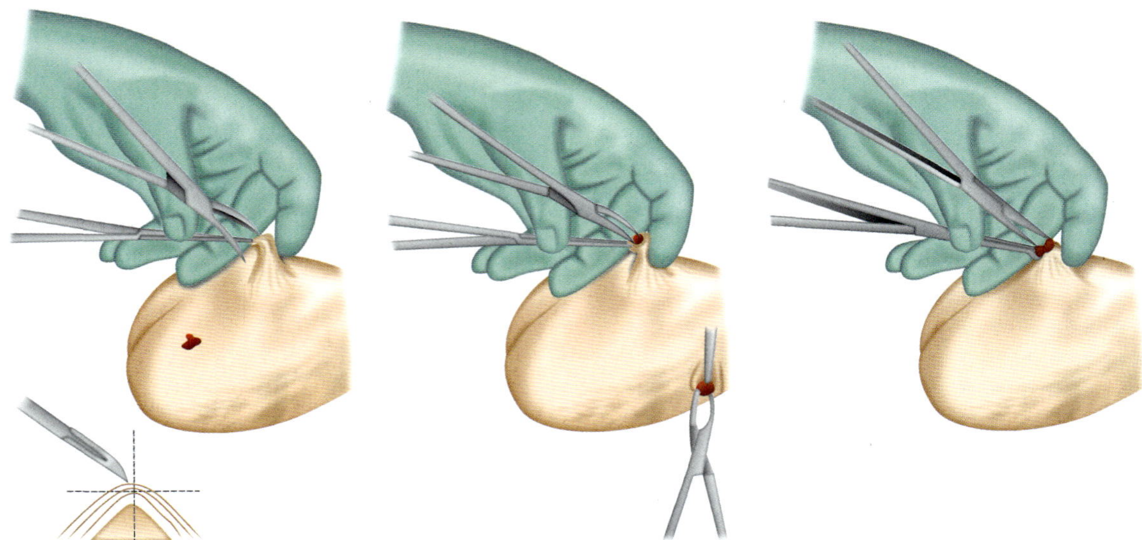

Fig. 3: Steps of no-scalpel vasectomy

of vasectomy experts held in December, 2003 came to the following conclusions:

- Ligation and excision of a small segment of the vas deferens lumen is also more effective than ligation and excision alone
- Recent evidence indicates that cautery plus FI is more effective than ligation and excision and FI, but is technically challenging.

Fascial Interposition

This is a new technique in which the sheath covering the vas deferens is pulled over one severed end and the sheath is closed to create a natural tissue barrier (Figs 1A and B). The testicular end of the vas deferens lies within the sheath and the prostatic end lies outside. Many practitioners prefer it the other way round.

REVIEW OF LITERATURE

(Author's conclusions after extensive Medline, Embase review, text books and book chapters evaluation):

1. *Vasectomy surgical techniques:* Current evidence supports no-scalpel vasectomy as the safest surgical approach to isolate the vas deferens when performing a vasectomy. Adding FI increases effectiveness beyond ligation and excision alone. Occlusion effectiveness appears to be further improved by combining FI with cautery.
2. *Scalpel versus no-scalpel vasectomy:* The no-scalpel approach to the vas deferens resulted in less bleeding, hematoma, pain and infection, as well as shorter operative time than the traditional incision technique. Although, no difference in effectiveness was found between the two approaches, the sample sizes might have been too small to detect the differences. Additional well conducted randomized trials are needed to draw any meaningful conclusions.

CONCLUSION

- Vasectomy is a simple method of permanent sterilization in males and is gradually gaining more acceptance
  - NSV is the new method promoted by the Family Planning Association of India (FPAI)—it is quicker, safer and an office procedure which can be done under LA. However, it requires a trained surgeon
- Failure rates are directly related to the experience of the operating surgeon
- Ligation, excision of a segment and vas deferens occlusion with cautery seems to be the best combination
- Fascial interposition is a new technique which reduces failures
- Making vasectomy absolutely safe with minimum complication and failure rate will boost the family planning program.

BIBLIOGRAPHY

1. Barone M, Nazerali H, Cortes M, et al. A prospective study of time and number of ejaculations to azoospermia after vasectomy by ligation and excision. J Urol. 2003;170:892-6.
2. Cook LA, Pun A, van Vliet H, et al. Christchurch School of Medicine, Public Health and General Practice, Christchurch, New Zealand. lynley.cook@xtra.co.nz
3. Haws JM, Morgan GT, Pollack AE, et al. Clinical aspects of vasectomies performed in the United States in 1995. Urology. 1998;52: 685-91.
4. IPPF Medical Bulletin London, August, 1999;33.
5. Kerry Wright Aradhya, senior science writer, Kim Best, senior science editor and David C Sokal, associate medical director.
6. Labrecque M, Dufresne C, Barone MA, et al. Clinical and Evaluative Research Unit Saint-Francois D'Assise Hospital, Centre hospitalier universitaire de Quebec, Quebec City, Canada GIL 3L5. michel.labrecque@mfa.ulaval.ca
7. Labrecque M, Dufresne C, Barone MA, et al. Vasectomy surgical techniques: A systematic review. BMC Med. 2004;2:21.
8. Labrecque M. Review of other evidence (abstract). In: Expert consultation on vasectomy: An interagency workshop organized by Family Health International, Engender Health and the ACQUIRE Project, Washington DC, Dec 3-5, 2003. Durham: Family Health International; 2004.
9. Li SQ, Goldstein M. Zhu J, et al. The no-scalpel vasectomy. J Urol. 1991;145:341-4.
10. Liskin L, Pile JM, Quillin WF. Vasectomy-safe and simple Popul Rep D. 1983;4:61-100.
11. Nazerali H, Thapa S, Hays M, et al. Vasectomy effectiveness in Nepal: A retrospective study. Contraception. 2003;67:397-401.
12. PCC. Camp SD (Ed). A guide to Methods of Birth Control. Washington: PCC; 1991.
13. Pollack A. Prevalence of occlusion techniques, vasectomy follow-up protocols and compliance with follow-up (abstract). In: Sokal DC (Ed). Proceedings of an expert consultation on vasectomy effectiveness co-sponsored by Family Health International and Engender Health, Apr 18-19, 2001, Durham, NC. Durham Family Health International; 2001.

14. Population Reports. New survey findings, Series M-17, Baltimore: Johns Hopkins Bloomberg School Of Public Health, Sept-Oct 2003.
15. Population Reports. Vasectomy: New Opportunities, Series D-5, Baltimore: Johns Hopkins University, March 1992.
16. Schmidt SS. Vasectomy. Urol Clin North Am. 1987;14:149-54.
17. Trussell J, Kowal D. The essentials of contraception: Efficacy, safety, and personal considerations. In: Hatcher RA, Trussel J, Stewart F (Eds). Contraceptive Technology, 17th Edition. New York: Irvington Publishers; 1998. p. 211-47.
18. Vessey H, Lawless M,Yates D. Lancet. 1982;1:841.
19. Wang D. Contraceptive failure in China. Contraception. 2002;66:173-8.

CHAPTER 53

Making of a Surgeon (A Practical Life and Guidance for Neosurgeons)

Randhir Puri

INTRODUCTION

"Accidents are the result of human error. Eternal vigilance is the price of safety."

"Learning is a continuous life-long process."

—**Anonymous**

Skills such as surgery are learned in life's workshop, while working in wards, operation theaters and working up patients. It is truly a life-long ergonomic art form which refines itself as one progresses in profession. Wards, operating theaters, general practice, and community clinics provide a context for active learning.

Surgery, as a speciality, has three phases, i.e. (a) deliberate learning of each step of surgical operation, (b) doing mental training and analysis of procedure and technique, and (c) doing the surgery with directions to assistants with smooth flow and coordination of the team. To be accurate, one needs to have deliberate, assiduous practice and speed, ease of operating, resulting as products of accuracy and safety.

Medical training, which includes four and half years of medical school, one year of internship, plus three or more years of residency, stands apart from ordinary human experience in much the same way that war lies outside the normal realm. Medical training like combat, involves extraordinary encounters and practices. Three factors in particular help explain why surgical training differs so much from ordinary life. First, the intensity of emotion, workload, responsibility and knowledge required is beyond the average. Very few people have to remember as many facts, work as many hours, read and absorb as many pages, interact with as many emotionally charged doctors-in-training. Second, the stakes involved in medicine are extraordinarily high. Life itself is the currency of medicine, much as it is in war.

Mistakes by physicians/surgeons are costly in terms of suffering and death. Finally, very few other human activities involve such immersion in death. One needs to only see a first-year anatomy class dissecting cadavers to appreciate how early the death immersion process begins.

She won't die. People don't die in childbirth nowadays.. .. Yes, but what if she should die?

—**Hemingway in "Farewell to Arms"**

There are some skills that trainees are expected to learn by "osmosis" while on placement and under the guidance of seniors doctors. These skills are never officially taught or examined in medical college. They are, however, a fundamental part of being a safe, good and efficient doctor.

Probably, the single most important skill a junior should acquire from day one is the ability to know when they are out of their depth and not be afraid or embarrassed to call a more senior colleague. This skill, if learned early, will save lives.

THE OPERATING THEATER

Dos

- Introduce yourself to nursing and anesthetic staff
- Engage in conversation with your colleagues
- Ask sensible questions, particularly if you do not understand something; this is the only way to learn. If you feel the timing is not appropriate, then wait until after the operation and then ask (I often do this—it shows maturity and an understanding that the surgeon is concentrating)
- Offer to make coffee/tea for your seniors after a long operation (they will be as tired as you). It shows respect for your seniors
- Ask to perform part of an operation if you think you are able or ask to be shown how to perform it so that you know it for the next time
- Ask to be taught how to write an operation note.

Don'ts

- Engage in conversation during emergencies
- Being rude to nursing staff. If you do, it will be your funeral!
- Sulk if you are not allowed to do something. Your seniors are not out to get you and there will be a good reason that you may not understand. You are within your rights to ask for an explanation after the operation. This is actually a good way to improve your surgical understanding as long as you take the correct approach
- Ever walk into theater without cover over shoes or theater clothing on. This contaminates theater floor and means that the nursing, paramedical staff will have to clean it again. Making nurses do more work than necessary is a bad move
- Ever eat or drink in theater
- Ever touch instruments on the scrub trolley without the express permission of the scrub nurse
- Ever place your gloved hands into a wound without the express permission of the surgeon
- Turn your head away from the surgical field to sneeze. The purpose of a mask is to prevent droplets from your mouth from being projected forward. There are gaps at the side of the mask to let these particles out. If you turn your head to sneeze, you will fire your germs straight into the wound. If you have to sneeze, then simply lean back but face forward.

PROFESSIONAL DEVELOPMENT

Professional development is at the cornerstone of maintaining excellence in medical and surgical practice. Although medical education plays a significant role in a physician's ongoing education, professional development encompasses a more holistic approach to learning. Professional development supports a wide range of areas including clinical education, practice management, ethical decision-making, evidence-based care and managed care principles. Unlike traditional learning, professional development facilitates a variety of learning formats, such as small groups and self-directed learning, and focuses on outcomes related to good practice.

Nurses

Nurses can be a tricky bunch, having spent years on the wards, gaining experience only to belittled by arrogant newly qualified doctors. You will see colleagues trying this approach and notice that it does not work, and furthermore, that they will quickly gain a reputation around the hospital. No one will explain when you are in medical school that qualified nurses are valuable assets. They can be your best ally or worst enemy depending on how you treat them. Most often they have been working in a particular specialty (for example maternity, laparoscopic gynecology, oncology, etc.) for many years and, while set in their ways, have a vast knowledge of the usual treatment practices that you will need for managing your patients successfully.

Nurses can be your best friend and your worst enemy, often within minutes of each other if you say the wrong thing at the wrong time. Historically, doctors have always thought themselves more hard done-by than any other medical professionals and as a response to this have always seen themselves as superior to nursing staff, both in their educational/intellectual level or in status. Nowadays, more than ever before, nurses and doctors need to work side by side as equals in the workplace, although ultimately, the overall responsibility and duty of care of the patient rests with the doctor.

Skill Acquisition

Sheer volume of exposure, rather than specifically designed curricula, is the hallmark of current surgical training. Virtual reality simulators in west are taking over training from earlier method of attachment to one senior doctor. These new training techniques are based on established theories of the ways in which motor skills are acquired and expertize is developed. Fitts and Posner's three-stage theory of motor skill acquisition is widely accepted in both the motor skills literature and the surgical literature. In the cognitive stage, the learner intellectualizes the task; performance is erratic, and the procedure is carried out in distinct steps. For example, with a surgical skill as simple as tying a knot, in the cognitive stage, the learner must understand the mechanics of the skill—how to hold the tie, how to place the throws, and how to move the hands. With practice and feedback, the learner reaches the integrative stage, in which knowledge is translated into appropriate motor behavior. The learner is still thinking about how to move the hands and hold the tie but is able to execute the task more fluidly, with fewer interruptions. In the autonomous stage, practice gradually results in smooth performance. The learner no longer needs to think about how to execute this particular task and can concentrate on other aspects of the procedure.

This model has obvious implications for surgical training. The earlier stages of teaching technical skills should take place outside the operating room; practice is the rule until automaticity in basic skills is achieved. This mastery of basic skills allows trainees to focus on more complex issues, both technical and non-technical in the operating room. To return to the example of knot tying, the learner who still has to think about how to tie a square knot is much less likely to pick up on other teaching that transpires in the operating room than is the learner who has mastered this simple skill.

Ericsson has helped to elucidate the acquisition of expertize. Expert performance represents the highest level of skill acquisition and the final result of a gradual improvement in performance through extended experience in a given domain. According to Ericsson, most professionals reach a stable, average level of performance and maintain this status for the rest of their career. In surgery, "experts" have been defined by Ericsson as experienced surgeons with consistently better outcomes than non-experts. An extensive literature on the relationship of operative volume to clinical outcomes supports the hypothesis that practice is an important determinant of outcome; the literature also provides support for Ericsson's contention that many professionals probably do not attain true expertize. However, volume alone does not account for the skill level among practitioners, since variations in performance have been shown among surgeons with high and very high volumes. Deliberate practice is a critical process for the development of mastery or expertize. Ericsson argues that the number of hours spent in deliberate practice, rather than just hours spent in surgery, is an important determinant of the level of expertize.

Deliberate Practice

Deliberate practice calls for the individual to focus on a defined task, typically identified by a teacher to improve particular aspects of performance; it involves repeated practice along with coaching and immediate feedback on performance. The attained level of expertize has been shown to be closely related to time devoted to deliberate practice in the performance of expert musicians, chess players and athletes. In the current model of surgical training, based primarily on apprenticeship, the opportunities for deliberate practice are rare. Operations are complex and it is difficult to focus on one small component of the procedure.

Virtual Reality/Simulation (Fig. 1)

Virtual reality has the potential to enhance surgical team training as well as technical skills training. In aviation, teamwork training with simulation has been instrumental in reducing errors. The importance of teamwork in preventing medical errors is well recognized and simulator-based team training has been advocated as a possible preventive approach. Early research results have been promising. Simulator-based trauma-team training has been associated with enhanced performance. Task completion and simulated survival rates have improved after emergency-team training on a simulator. Simulator-based training for crisis management in anesthesia, both for individuals and for teams, has been shown to be effective, and simulated operating room environments are being assessed for training in both technical skills and teamwork.

In summary, the report card on simulation, while not definitively positive, does suggest that it is an important addition to the training arena. The effectiveness of simulation training has been demonstrated primarily for lower-level learners, with a positive effect demonstrated for both laparoscopic and open procedures. Results to date have not been validated in large-scale studies, however, an additional research demonstrating the generalized ability of findings across institutions is required. Additional research on simulation training for more senior learners and for surgeons in practice is needed. Further, work is also needed to address important motor-learning issues, such as whether it is preferable to practice whole operation or to practice segments of operation and then build the whole from the segments, what practice schedules are optimal, and how to optimize the transfer of skills to the operating room.

As computing power expands and the cost of simulation equipment falls, it is likely that most, if not all, surgical training programs will be devoting substantial curricular time to simulator-based training. Increasing evidence of the efficacy of ex vivo training, coupled with social pressure will probably mean that future residents will need to demonstrate proficiency in basic techniques before being allowed to operate on patients.

With these and other changes in the wind, surgical educators will need to incorporate meaningful assessment into residency programs, using rigorous, reliable and regular means of assessment for all relevant surgical skills. Tools with the requisite levels of reliability and validity for summative assessment include the objective structured assessment of technical skill (OSATS) and McGill inanimate system for training and evaluation of laparoscopic skills (MISTELS) programs. For example, the MISTELS program might be used to assess a resident's performance of basic laparoscopic skills. A requisite level of performance would be required before the resident would be allowed to perform a laparoscopic hysterectomy. Similarly, OSATS stations could be used for open surgery. Residents would thus be trained in the laboratory until preset criteria is met and would only then be allowed to participate in the graduated performance of procedures in patients. Competence-based advancement, rather than time served, would become standard in surgical training.

One of the challenges of a competence-based system of education and assessment that has received little attention is how to establish pass or fail standards for the performance of technical skills. This is a major deficit in

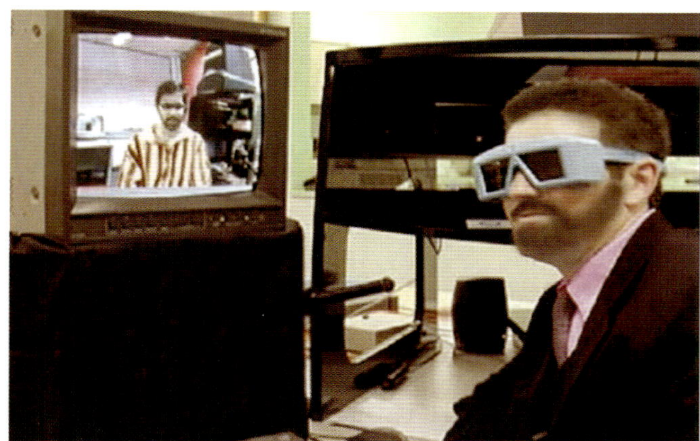

Fig. 1: Virtual reality system

the assessment literature that will require attention if a criterion-based system is implemented or if certification of technical ability is required before licensure. Given the advances in technology and the accruing evidence of their effectiveness, now is the time to take stock of the changes we can and must make to improve the assessment and training of surgeons in the future. It is proposed that in the next 10–15 years practicing surgeons will be selected, trained, credentialed, remediated and recredentialed using computerized virtual reality simulation devices. Surgeons in the future will rehearse operations on palpable holograms that were derived from patient-specific data before they actually perform the procedures on those patients the following day. Endoscopic phantoms, holographic patient simulators, and virtual surgical laboratories will revolutionize the way surgical students, interns, and residents learn and refine their techniques.

The neo-surgeons of future, thus will be products of computer trained, ergonomically skilled individuals with accuracy, speed and safety as their forte of profession.

"Cultivate the society of the young, they remain interested and never stop learning" (Cicero).

BIBLIOGRAPHY

1. Carter BN. The fruition of Halsted's concept of surgical training. Surgery. 1952;32:518-27.
2. Haluck RS, Krummel TM. Computers and virtual reality for surgical education in the 21st century. Arch Surg. 2000;135: 786-92.
3. Heppell J, Beauchamp G, Chollet A. Ten-year experience with a basic technical skills and perioperative management workshop for first-year residents. Can J Surg. 1995;38: 27-37.
4. Hutchison C, Hamstra S, Leadbetter W. The University of Toronto Surgical Skills Centre opens. Focus Surg Educ. 1998;16:22-4.
5. Leach DC. A model for GME: Shifting from process to outcomes — a progress report from the Accreditation Council for Graduate Medical Education. Med Educ. 2004;38:12-4.
6. Scallon SE, Fairholm DJ, Cochrane DD, et al. Evaluation of the operating room as a surgical teaching venue. Can J Surg. 1992;35:173-6.

CHAPTER

54 Gynecological Surgery Instruments

Sushma Gupta

INTRODUCTION

Instruments in gynecological surgery (Figs 1 to 37) are both general and specific to gynecologic surgery. Many new modification and variations in the instruments have come up but a surgeon should insist on a broad range of high quality functioning equipment that do not continually irritate by failing to work, whether it is a simple pair of scissors or the most sophisticated minimal access equipment.

In virtually all modern operating theater, instruments and drapes are prepacked and sterilized in "sets" for individual or generic procedures in a central sterile supply department. This has major advantage in terms of high standards of sterilization over selecting instruments for a specific procedure and sterilizing them immediately prior to an operation.

A wide range of prepacked and sterile disposable instruments of amazing complexity have been introduced in recent times, including much of the equipment used in minimal access surgery.

Besides the "set" and presterilized instruments, from time to time an immediate sterilizing facility is required so that in many operating theaters on the spot sterilization is available for a number of specialized pieces of equipment.

The instruments can generally be divided into:

- General operating set
- Minor procedure set
- Special instruments and laparoscopy instruments.

The general operating set commonly consists of:

- Sponge holding forceps
- Towel clips
- Bard Parker knife handle
- Hane's toothed dissecting forceps
- Non-toothed dissecting forceps
- Scissors, Mayo's dissecting
- Scissors, straight
- Lloyd Davis needle holder
- A set of Grey Turner artery forceps straight and curved
- A set of Allis forceps
- Kocher's clamps—straight and curved
- Vulsellum
- Retractors—Doyens and Langerhans'
- Babcock's forceps
- Needle holders.

Minor Procedure Set (Box 1)

One set, of cervical dilators: (i) Hagers (ii) Hawkin ambler

Some of the instruments mentioned warrant special comments.

Scissors

Often marketed as Mayo scissors, they are heavy but have a sureness about them, which allows accurate gentle

Box 1 Minor procedure set

- Sponge holder
- Blunt and sharp curette
- Sims vaginal speculum
- Needle holder
- Anterior vaginal wall
- Artery forceps
- Vulsellum
- Scissors 6"
- Simpson's uterine sound
- Bladder sound

dissection, particularly of the "separate and cut" type. The ends of the scissors are relatively blunt and will do little damage when separating tissue, while the blades are powerful enough to cut when coupled with long levers of the handles. This latter characteristic is especially important in oncosurgery work when operating on tissues previously treated with radiotherapy.

A lighter scissor with the same qualities, e.g. Monaghan's dissecting scissors is also useful.

Artery Forceps

The forceps included in the set are almost all straight. Meig's right angle forceps are of great value in dealing with vessels deep in the pelvis. They are long and allow suture to be placed around either the points or the heel of the forceps.

Tissue Clamps

On many occasions in gynecological surgery, it is necessary to clamp discrete blocks of tissues firmly and then suture the block to occlude the vessels contained with it. It is important that these clamps are strong, that the jaws oppose accurately and that tissue does not slide out from between the jaws. Many different varieties have been designed but the Kocher's clamps are the most widely used. As a general principle, the designs with longitudinal ridges have an advantage over those with transverse. In addition, a simple tooth interdigitating with a double tooth at the tips of the jaws assist correct apposition. The clamps can be straight or angled.

Uterine Sound

Designed by Simpson, they are 12" long and marked in inches. They have blunt bounded tip. The uterine end is curved and angulated. They are used to determine:

- Length of uterus and direction of uterus
- To diagnose and differentiate a polyp lying in cervix
- Locating misplaced intrauterine device (IUD)
- Correction of mobile retroversion of uterus.

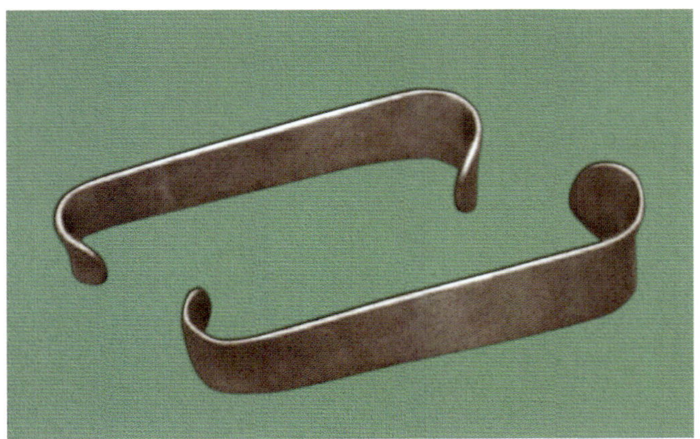

Fig. 1: Abdominal wall retractors

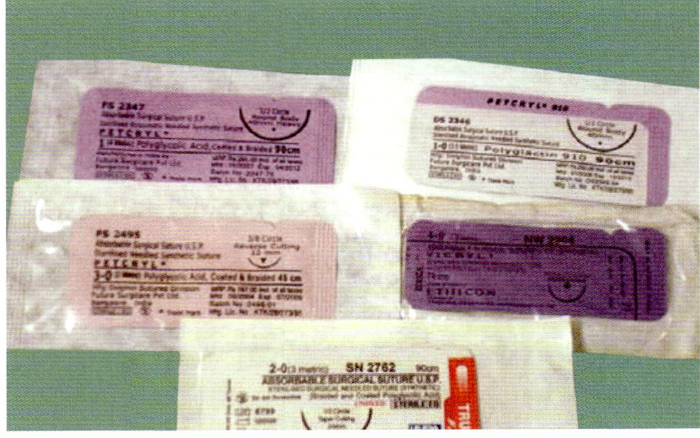

Fig. 2: Absorbable synthetic suture

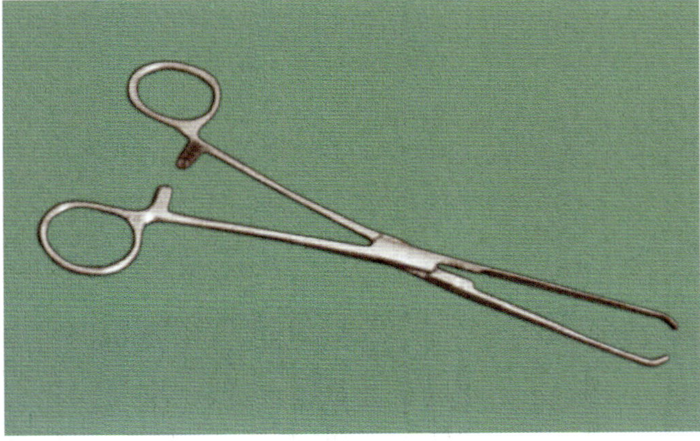

Fig. 3: Allis clamp

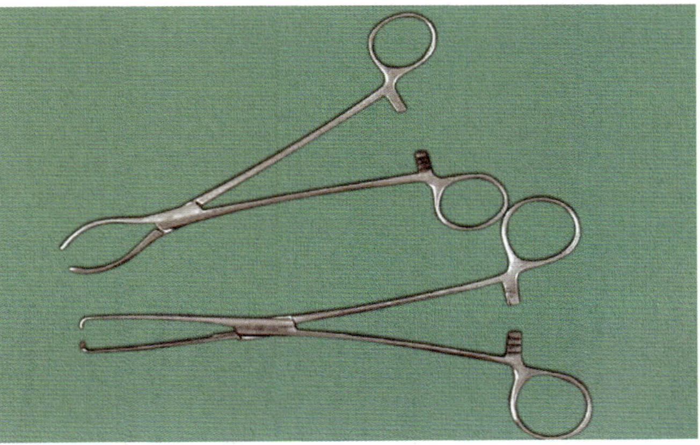

Fig. 4: Allis forceps

Blunt and Sharp Curette

Designed by Blake, one end of instrument is blunt and other end is sharp. It is used in dilation and curettage (D&C), dilation and evacuation (D&E), infertility and dysfunctional uterine bleeding (DUB).

Sims double bladed posterior vaginal speculum designed by Marion Sims, the blades are of unequal breadth. It may be single bladed also.

It is used to visualize the cervix and inspect the lesion of cervix and anterior vaginal wall. It is also used for practically all vaginal operations, e.g. D&C, D&E, vaginal hysterectomies, etc.

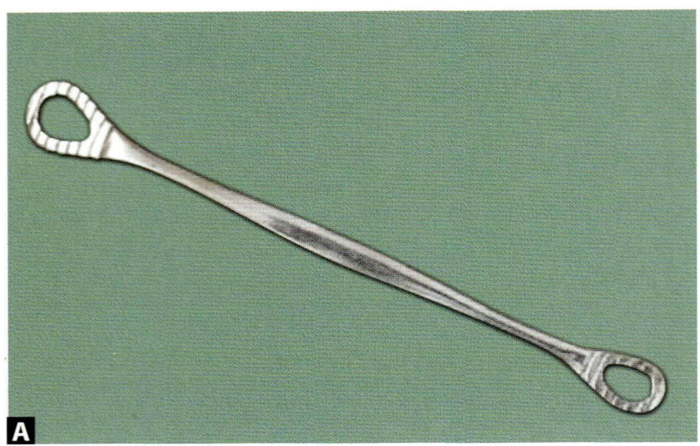

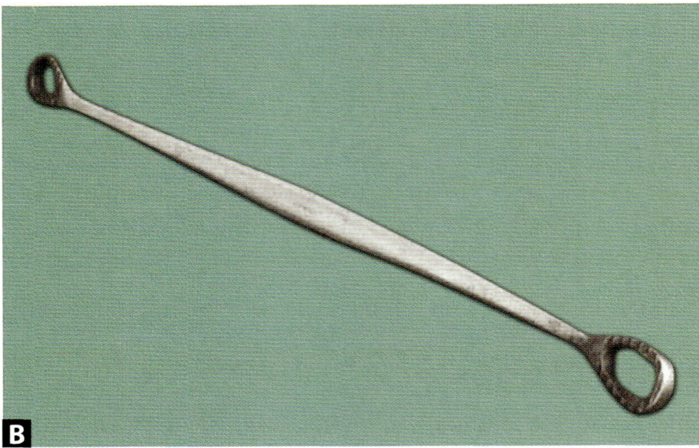

Figs 5A and B: Anterior vaginal wall retractor

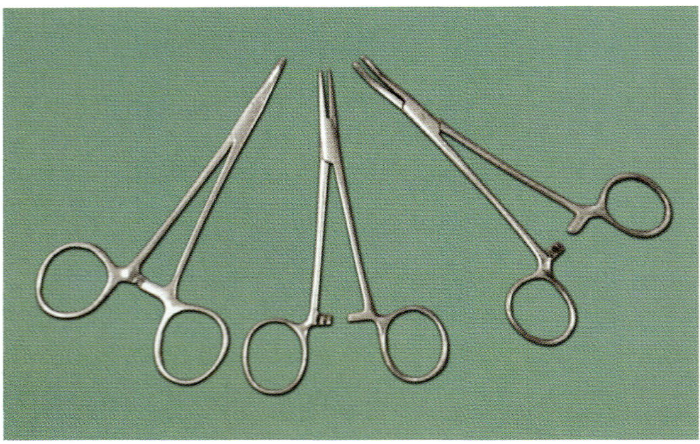

Fig. 6: Artery forceps

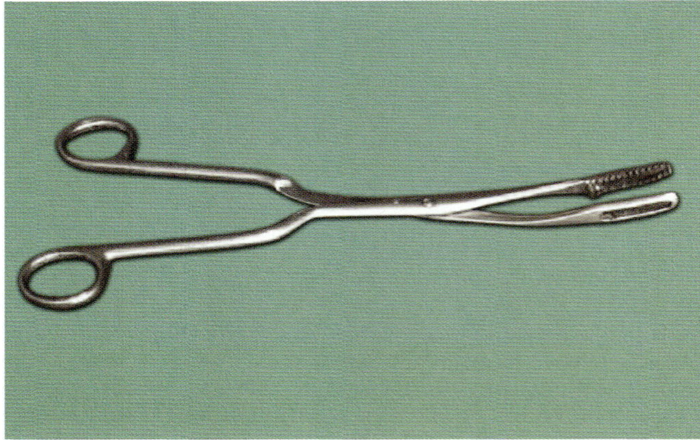

Fig. 7: Aspirotomy forceps

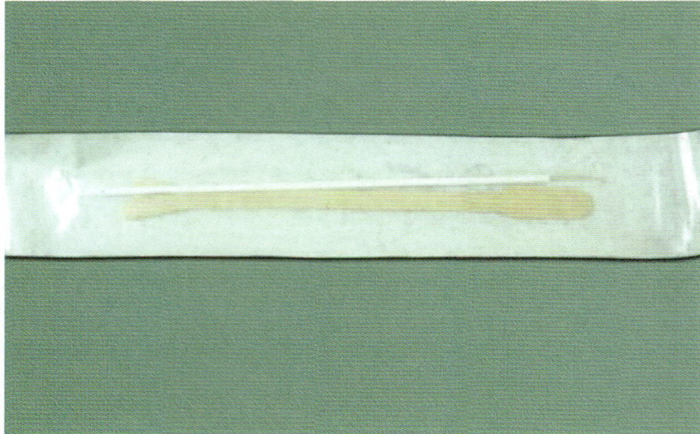

Fig. 8: Ayre's spatulate set

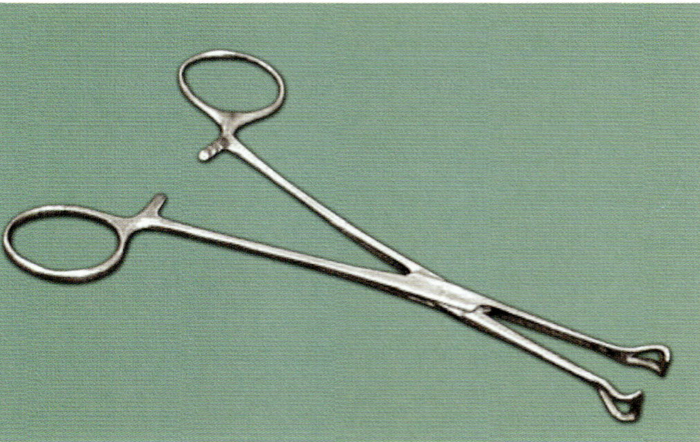

Fig. 9: Babcock

Cusco's Bivalve Self-retaining Vaginal Speculum

The valves are to retract the anterior and posterior vaginal wall to have a good look at the cervix. It is used to:

- Visualize the cervix and vaginal fornices
- Collect vaginal pool materials and scrapings for cytologic study
- Perform minor operations on the cervix.

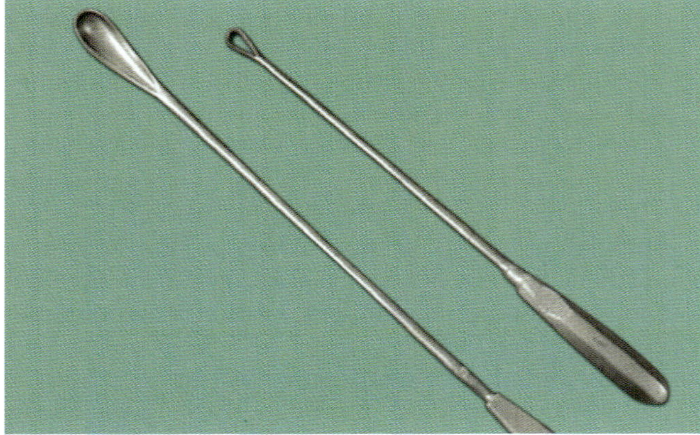

Fig. 10: Big curette

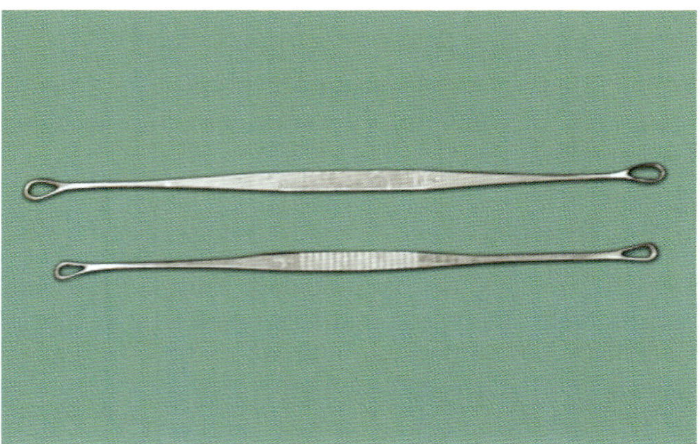

Fig. 11: Blunt and sharp curette

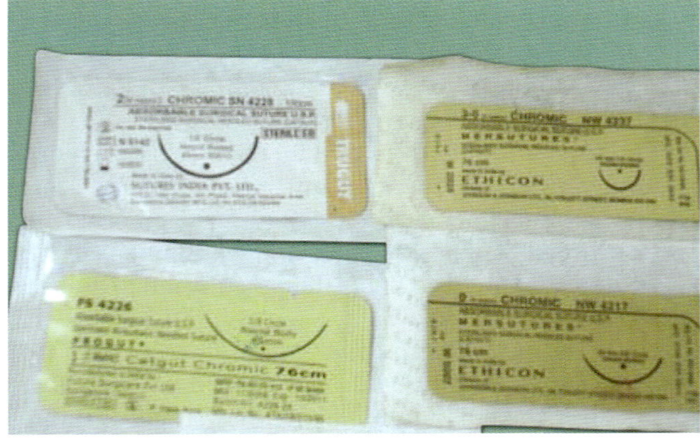

Fig. 12: Catgut sutures

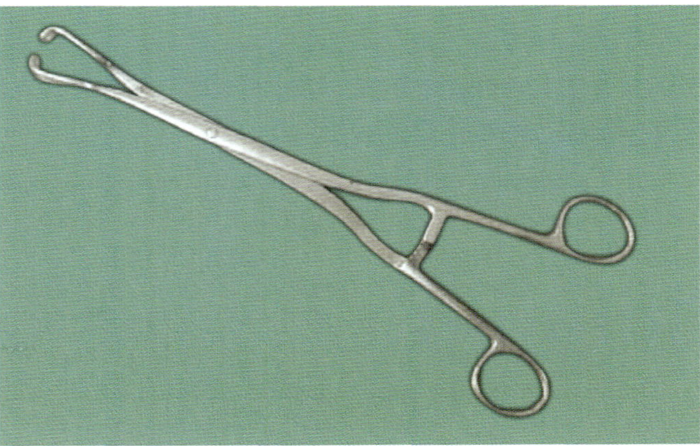

Fig. 13: Cat's paw

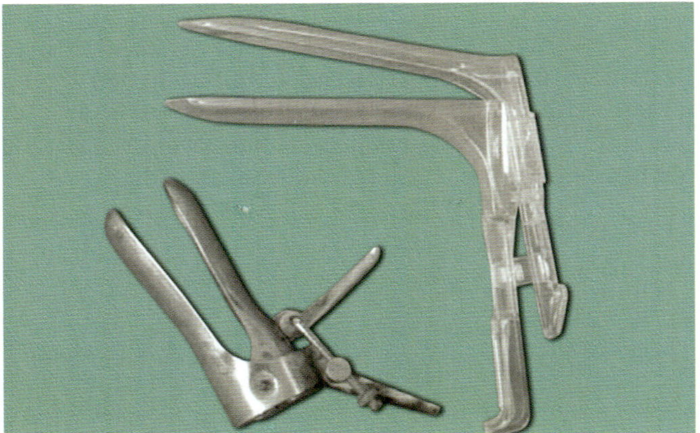

Fig. 14: Cusco's speculum

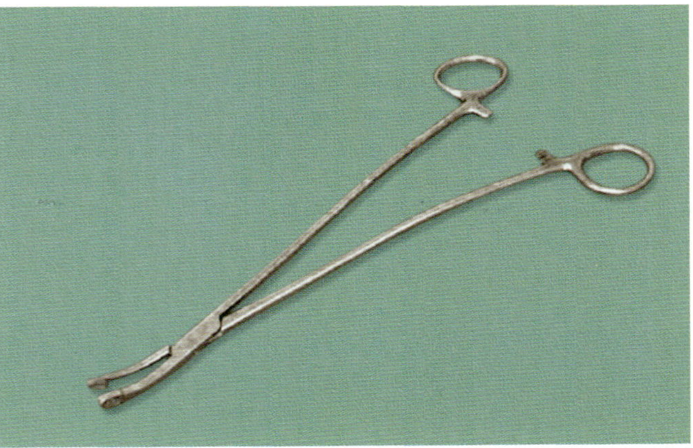

Fig. 15: Cervical punch biopsy forceps

Anterior Vaginal Wall Retractor

This instrument has loop shaped ends with transverse serrations on the loops. The loops are set at angle to the shaft. It is used along with Sims' speculum to retract the sagging vaginal wall to have a good exposure of the cervix.

Cervical Dilators

Many types are available, e.g. Hegar's, Das's, Hawkin-Ambler's, etc. They are used to dilate the cervix before D&C, D&E, pyometra, hematometra, intracavitatory radiation X-ray therapy (RXT), etc.

Vulsellum

Designed by Teals, this instrument is 8" long and is usually curved. It has sharp teeth at the end, which interlock and give a firm grip. If only 2 × 1 interlock is present, it is known as tenaculum. It is used:

- To grasp the anterior/posterior lip of cervix. To make the cervix steady during cervical operations
- To remove polyps
- To hold the fundus during abdominal hysterectomy.

Specific Instruments Used Only for Gynecological Operations

The use of general instruments is known to all, so only, a special mention for the specific instruments used for a particular gynecologic operation are being given:

1. *Boney's myomectomy clamp*: It is used to control hemorrhage during myomectomy. A piece of rubber tubing is fixed over each blade. The clamp grasps the body of uterus just above internal os of the cervix, and includes uterine vessels and both round ligaments.
2. *Myoma screw (Doyen's)*: It is used to fix the myoma after the capsule is cut opened to give traction while myoma is enucleated out of its bed. To give traction in a big uterus requiring hysterectomy.
3. *Malleable probes*: It is used in tubal recanalizations.
4. *Rubin's insufflation* cannula for tubal testing. With better diagnostic technique available, it is not much in use now.
5. *Karman's syringe* or menstrual regulation syringe, which has a capacity of 50 mL. Usually used for endometrial aspiration, especially when patient has missed her periods.
6. *Leech Wilkinson cannula*: It is used for chromopertubation during laparoscopy and hysterosalpingography.
7. *Vaginal dilators*: They are made of glass, vulcanite, plastic or steel. They are tubular in shape with one end rounded and a depression on the other end to accommodate the urethra. Available in six sizes. They are used to dilate the vagina in cases of (a) vaginismus, (b) vaginal atresia due to burn/injuries/ operations, (c) artificial vagina created in cases of congenital absence.
8. *Endometrial biopsy curette:* The name implies its use. There are slender tubular blunt-ended instruments slightly curved at the tips. There is a notch with a cutting edge near the tip. It is used to take endometrial biopsy. Endometrial sample is taken from six different areas of uterus.
9. *Ovum holding forceps:* Designed by Haywood Smiths, used during medical terminations of pregnancies and other abortions to remove retained products of conception or placenta. The blades of the instrument have spoon shaped blunt fenestrated ends. Anything held in the blades is firmly caught but not nipped at its base. It has no catch.
10. *Ayre's spatula* for taking cervical samples for Pap smear in suspected cases of cervical cancers.
11. *Cervical punch biopsy forceps* for taking cervical biopsy from any suspicious area on the cervix in cases of cervical malignancies. Designed by Gelhorns, this instrument is 22.5 cm long and has punch shaped ends inside the cup. On one fair is a tiny pin to hold the specimen punched out.
12. *Hysteroscope, laparoscope* and other endoscopy instruments are now being widely used in gynecologic practice. The era of minimal invasive surgery requires surgeon to have special training in handling and using these instruments.
13. *Microsurgery instruments* also require special training and care.

To conclude, instruments should be handled with care. Proper sterilization has to be done. Many newer and better modifications are coming up as evolution is the way of life but basic principles of usage remain as of before.

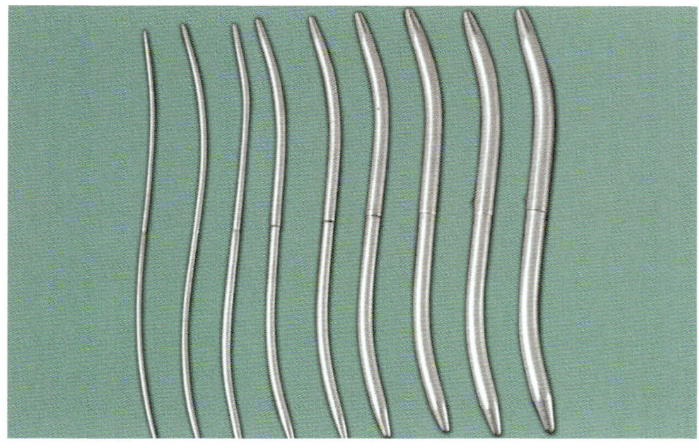

Fig. 16: Dilator set

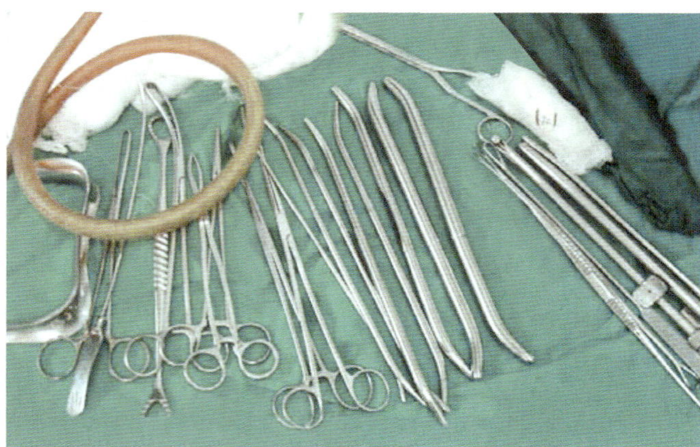

Fig. 17: Table set of instruments for D&E

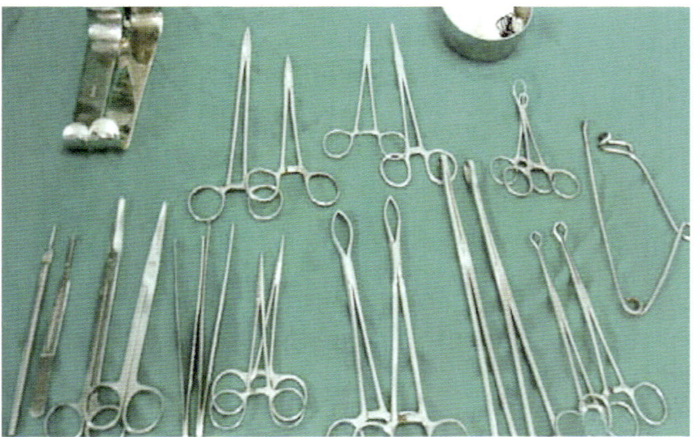

Fig. 18: Table set of instruments for tubectomy

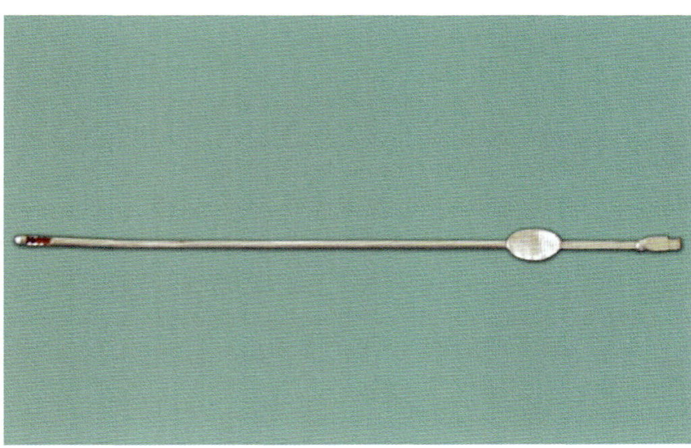

Fig. 19: Endometrial biopsy curette

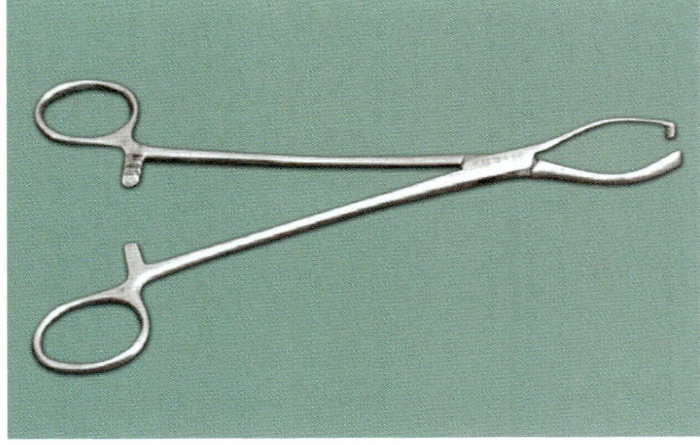

Fig. 20: Large single toothed Allis tissue holding forceps

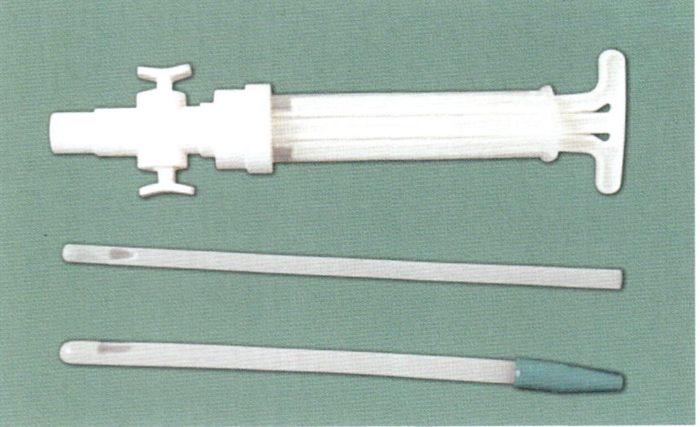

Fig. 21: Manual vacuum aspirator (MVA) set and cannulas

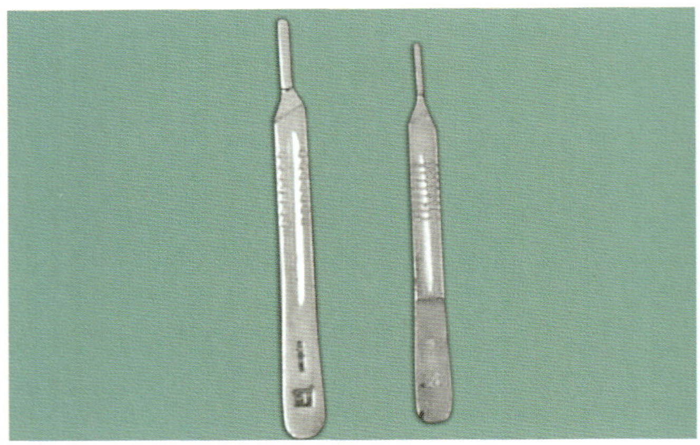

Fig. 22: Bard parker knife holder

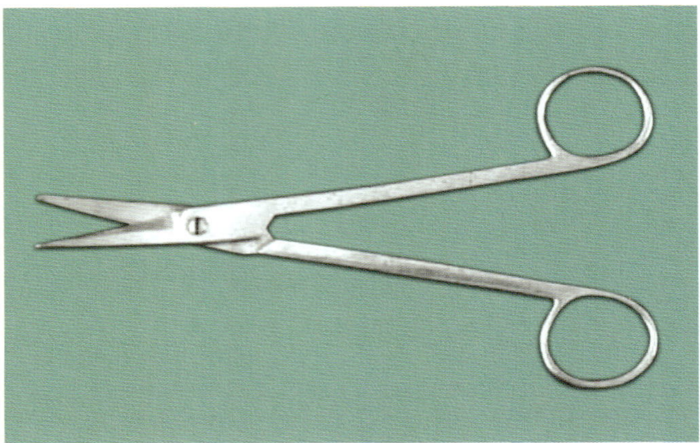

Fig. 23: Mayo scissors

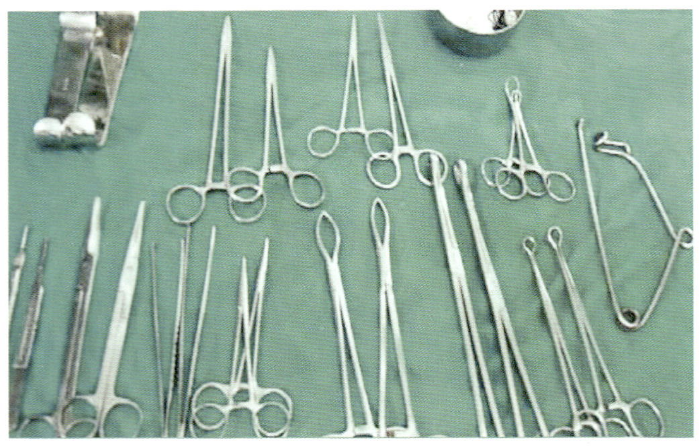

Fig. 24: Minor abdominal set

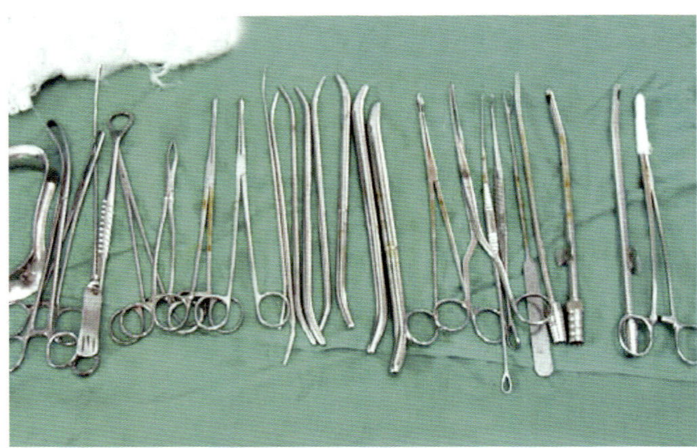

Fig. 25: Minor vaginal set

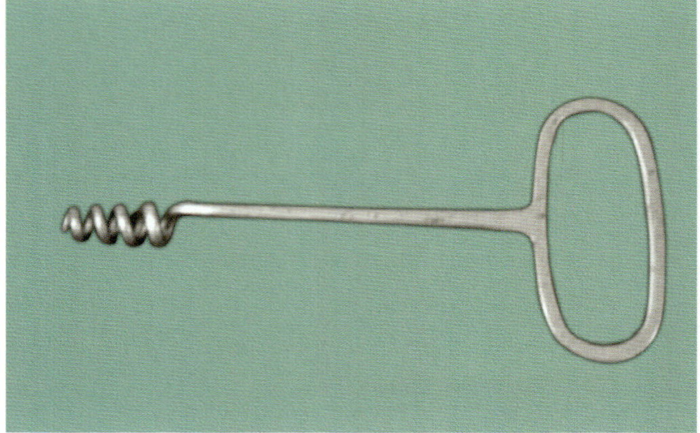

Fig. 26: Myoma screw

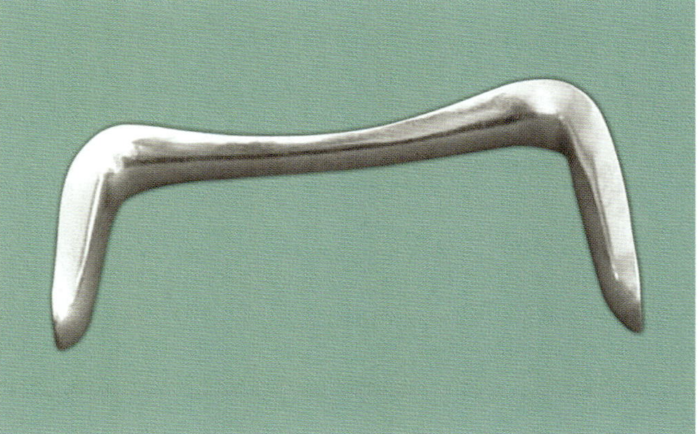

Fig. 27: Sims speculum

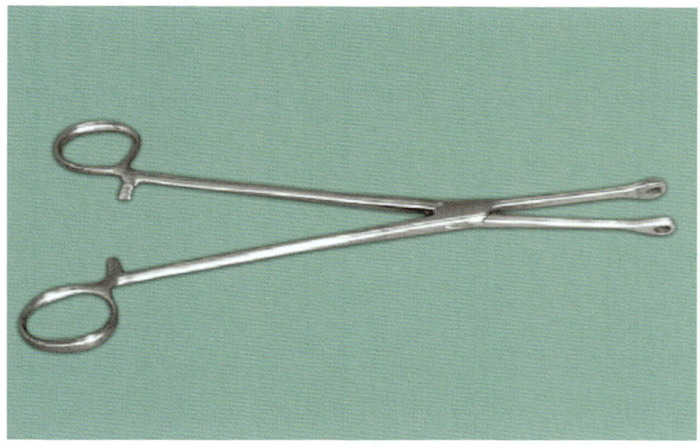

Fig. 28: Sponge holding forceps

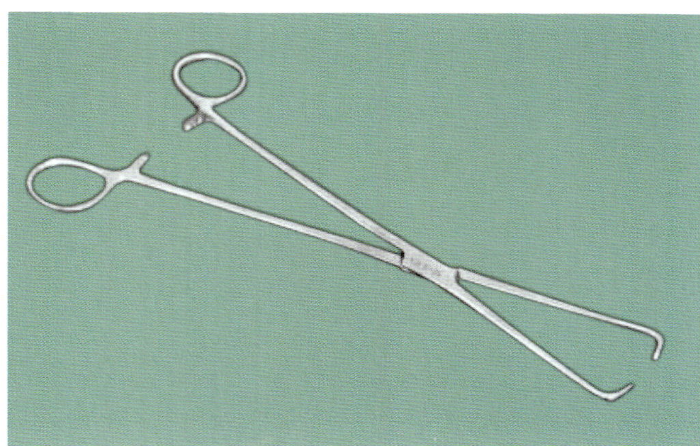

Fig. 29: Tenaculum single toothed

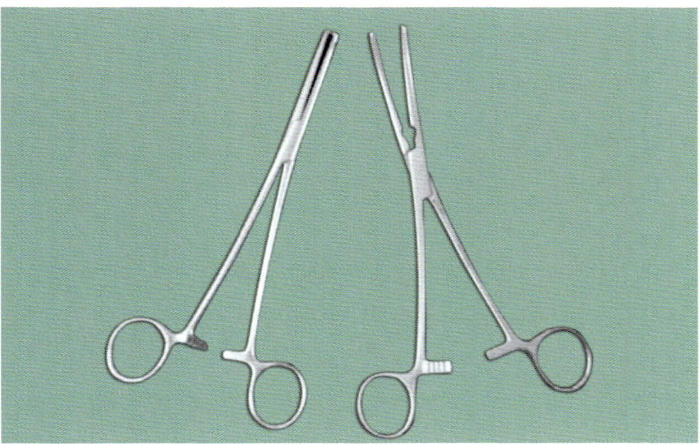

Fig. 30: Tissue clamps

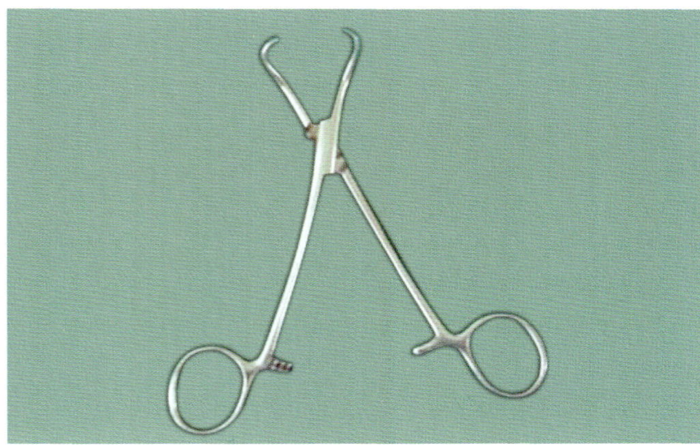

Fig. 31: Towel clip

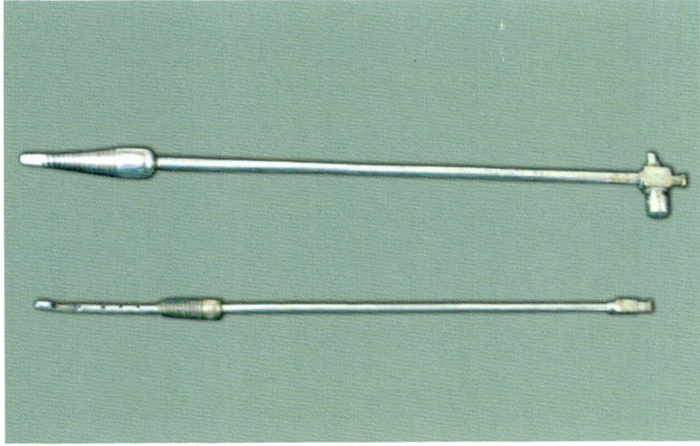

Fig. 32: Tubal patency testing cannulas

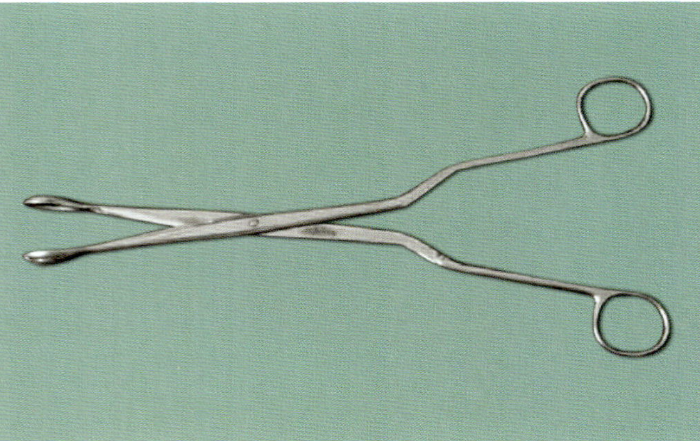

Fig. 33: Ovum forceps

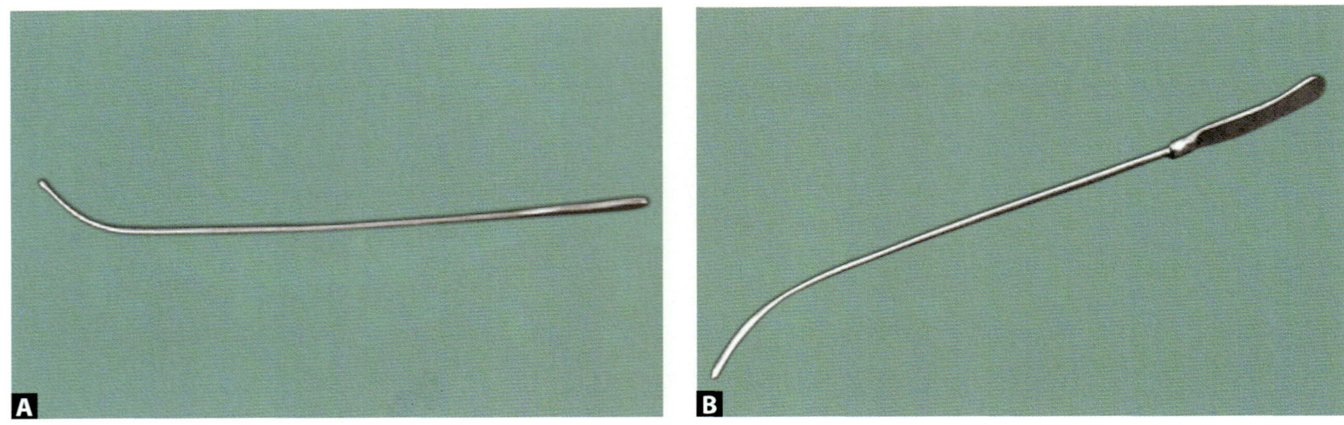

Figs 34A and B: Uterine sound

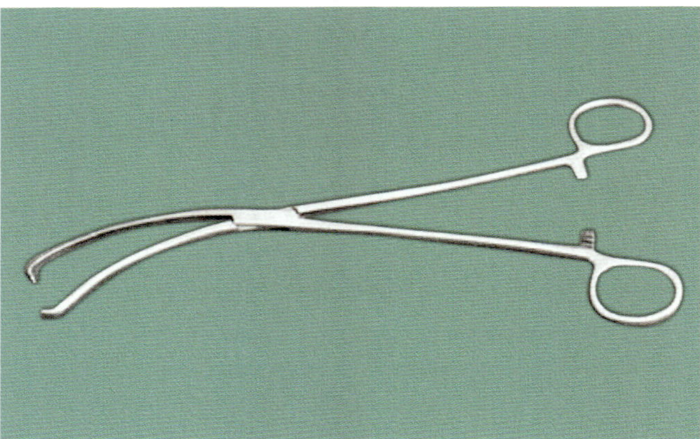

Fig. 35: Vulsellum

Section 4

Recent Advances

Section Outline

CHAPTER

55

Applications of Laser in Gynecology

Narendra Malhotra, Parul Mittal, Jaideep Malhotra

APPLICATIONS OF LASER IN GYNECOLOGY

The term laser means Light Amplification by Stimulated Emission of Radiation. Any surgical procedure which requires cutting, coagulating or removing tissues can be effectively achieved by laser. Laser surgery vaporizes tissues layer by layer without touching them, with minimal thermal damage and good clinical results.

Lasers Used in Surgeries

Various types of lasers which are used for surgery are:

- Carbon dioxide (CO_2): 1,064 nm
- Erbium: 2,940 nm
- Diode: 810 nm
- Alexandrite: 755 nm
- Ruby long pulse: 694 nm
- Neodymium-doped yttrium aluminum garnet (Nd:YAG): 1,064 nm.

LASER SURGERY FOR CERVIX

Vaporization Conization

Cervical conization is defined as removal of a volume of tissue from the central longitudinal axis of the cervix which includes the external os and some length of endocervical canal.

Requirements

Requirements for vaporization conization are:

- Lesion should be completely visualized
- Transformation zone should be completely seen
- Adenocarcinoma of endocervical canal should be ruled out
- Cervical intraepithelial neoplasia (CIN) should be confirmed.

Procedure

Vaporization conization using CO_2 laser through the colposcope can be performed in office, clinic or operating room. General anesthesia is usually not required. The margins of the transformation zone is outlined by vaporization crater using short bursts of laser energy. The craters are then connected and the cervix is divided into four quadrants and then the tissues are vaporized quadrant by quadrant to a depth of 7 mm.

Excision Laser Conization of the Cervix

This procedure produces a conization biopsy specimen which is adequate for pathologic examination and also if possible to excise the disease.

Indications for laser excisional conization are:

- Lesion extends into the canal and cannot be entirely seen
- The entire transformation zone cannot be visualized
- Abnormal cytology in absence of positive colposcopy
- Positive endocervical curettage
- Invasive cancer which cannot be ruled out by biopsy.

This procedure can be performed on an outpatient basis or under general anesthesia. After applying 4% acetic acid, borders of the lesion are noted and a cone-shaped excision is achieved. Advantages are that there is less bleeding than with scalpel, less tissue damage than with electric cautery, more precision than cryocautery and more procedures can be performed by using combination of vaporization and excision.

LASER SURGERY OF THE VULVA

Unlike cervical vaporization, depth of vaporization on vulva cannot be measured. Vulvar laser surgery is done with the aid of the colposcope.

Condyloma Accuminata

Human papillomavirus involves the epidermis and superficial portions of skin appendages. Each condyloma is identified and laser beam directed on the target. Laser vaporizes the condylomata rapidly with the beam.

Vulvar Intraepithelial Neoplasia

Local or general anesthesia can be used for vulvar laser surgery. In multiple lesions or large areas of involvement, general anesthesia is practical. Vulva is recolposcoped, 4% acetic acid is applied and affected area marked, and epidermis and superficial dermis are ablated with usual spot size of 2–3 mm and power setting of 15–50 W.

LASER SURGERY OF THE VAGINA

Vaginal intraepithelial neoplasia (VAIN) and associated—human papillomavirus (HPV) infections are difficult to treat because vagina has a large surface area which is difficult to visualize colposcopically, there are many rugae and folds in vagina, fornices may be hidden by cervix and angle of vaginal axis makes treatment by beam difficult. Most patients with VAIN require general anesthesia for the procedure. A spot size of 2 mm and power settings of 15–30 W are used, and large areas are subdivided for more accurate ablation. Often the tops of rugae are removed and troughs and valleys in between contain dysplastic epithelium which has to be overcome by proper use of speculum.

INTRA-ABDOMINAL LASER SURGERY

This is a good alternative to knife and electrosurgical instruments for surgeries. It has several advantages like precision, limited adjacent tissue damage, rapid healing, minimal scarring and ability to treat areas of difficult access.

Gynecologic Laser Laparoscopy

- *Carbon dioxide adhesiolysis:* Laser beam is delivered within the hollow ancillary probe to the pelvic adhesion. The distal end probe acts as a backstop and limits the vaporization to the tissue within the window of the probe. Advanced endometriotic adhesions can be treated with laser, omental adhesions to anterior abdominal wall are also handled rapidly and efficiently with laser. Flimsy adhesions can be vaporized and divided with low power density. Thick adhesions between tube and ovary may be lased with intermediate power density
- *Laser surgery of the Fallopian tube:* Patients with pain associated with tubal disease or patients who do not choose assisted reproductive technique (ART) can select laser tubal surgery. The tube is opened using Bruhat's procedure in which using laser three or four radial incisions are made in a closed tube with a small spot size laser beam followed by flowering of the tube using 3–5 mm spot size
- *Laser myomectomy:* Pedunculated leiomyoma can be easily removed by laser but deeply embedded intramural myomas are difficult to remove.

  During laparoscopic myomectomy, laser is used to coagulate vessels on the surface of the leiomyoma and then the base is approached to coagulate and cut the vessels. CO_2, potassium titanyl phosphate (KTP), argon and yttrium-aluminium garnet (YAG) lasers have been used during myomectomy
- *Laser surgery for endometriosis:* CO_2 or fiberoptic laser can effectively vaporize, coagulate or excuse small implants of mild to moderate endometriosis. Even the dense adhesions associated with advanced endometriosis can also be treated
- *Salphingo-oophorectomy and laparoscopically-assisted vaginal hysterectomy:* Laser energy in these operations is used mainly for dividing large pedicles which have been sutured or bipolar coagulated, dividing the peritoneum over bladder, mobilizing the bladder off the cervix and ablating endometrial implants.

Hysteroscopic Laser Surgery

Nd:YAG Laser

YAG represents an ideal laser for endometrial ablation because of its ability to penetrate tissues. It is used to effectively coagulate the endometrium and inner layers of myometrium. Advantage of hysteroscopic laser surgery is that normal saline distending medium avoids the dangers associated with vascular absorption of nonionic solutions used in electrosurgery.

Other hysteroscopic surgeries using laser include metroplasty, division of uterine septa, destruction of intrauterine synechiae and excision of submucous leiomyoma. In ovarian endometriosis, damage to the deeper stroma of the ovarian cortex can be minimized using a passed laser delivery.

Uterosacral Ligament Surgery

Carbon dioxide laser division of uterosacral ligament provided good success rates in cases of severe dysmenorrhea. The division of the uterosacral ligament is planned close to its insertion into the uterus.

Tubal Pregnancy

Ampullary ectopic pregnancies which are usually intramural are perfect for a laser incision. Laser is used for linear salpingostomy.

Isthmic tubal pregnancy usually requires partial salpingectomy in which excision of the segment is performed by coagulating on either side of the ectopic pregnancy and then excision with laser or laparoscopic scissors.

CHAPTER

56

Robotic Surgery

Narendra Malhotra, Parul Mittal, Richa Saxena

INTRODUCTION

Da Vinci® Surgical System

The da Vinci® Surgical system is a robotic surgical system made by the American company, Intuitive Surgical. Approved by the Food and Drug Administration (FDA) in 2000, it has been designed to facilitate complex surgery using a minimally invasive approach, and is controlled by a surgeon from a console.

The system is commonly being used for performing various gynecologic surgical procedures. According to the manufacturer, the da Vinci® system is called "da Vinci" in part "because Leonardo da Vinci invented the first robot", according to Italian academician Mario Taddei. Da Vinci also used anatomical accuracy and three-dimensional (3D) details in his work.

Da Vinci® robots operate in hospitals worldwide, with an estimated 200,000 surgeries conducted in 2012, most commonly for hysterectomies and prostate removals. By January 2013, more than 2,000 units had been sold worldwide. The "Si" version of the system costs on an average slightly under US $2 million, in addition to several hundred thousand dollars of annual maintenance fees.

FDA Approval

Food and Drug Administration cleared the da Vinci® Surgical system in 2000 for adult and pediatric use in urologic surgical procedures, general laparoscopic surgical procedures, gynecologic laparoscopic surgical procedures, general noncardiovascular thoracoscopic surgical procedures and thoracoscopically assisted cardiotomy procedures. The FDA also cleared the da Vinci® system to be employed with adjunctive mediastinotomy to perform coronary anastomosis during cardiac revascularization.

FEATURES OF ROBOTIC SURGERY (FIG. 1)

High-definition 3D Vision

The da Vinci® Si system offer surgeons autonomous camera control for a stable, immersive, highly magnified 3D high-definition (HD) view of the surgical field.

Precise, Collision-free Movements

Surgeon's hand movements are scaled, filtered and seamlessly translated to the instrument tips for precise instrument control. A large, open working space provides unrestricted range of motion without instrument crowding.

Ergonomic Comfort

The surgeon's console features multiple ergonomic adjustments for increased comfort and reduced fatigue during surgical procedures.

Intuitive Motion

Advanced system software correlates the surgeon's hand movements to the instrument tips, restoring intuitive control to what would otherwise be cross-handed surgery.

OVERVIEW

The da Vinci® system consists of a surgeon's console that is typically in the same room as the patient, and a patient side cart with four interactive robotic arms controlled from the console. Three of the arms are for tools that hold objects, and can also act as scalpels scissors, bovies, or unipolar or bipolar electrocautery instruments. The fourth arm

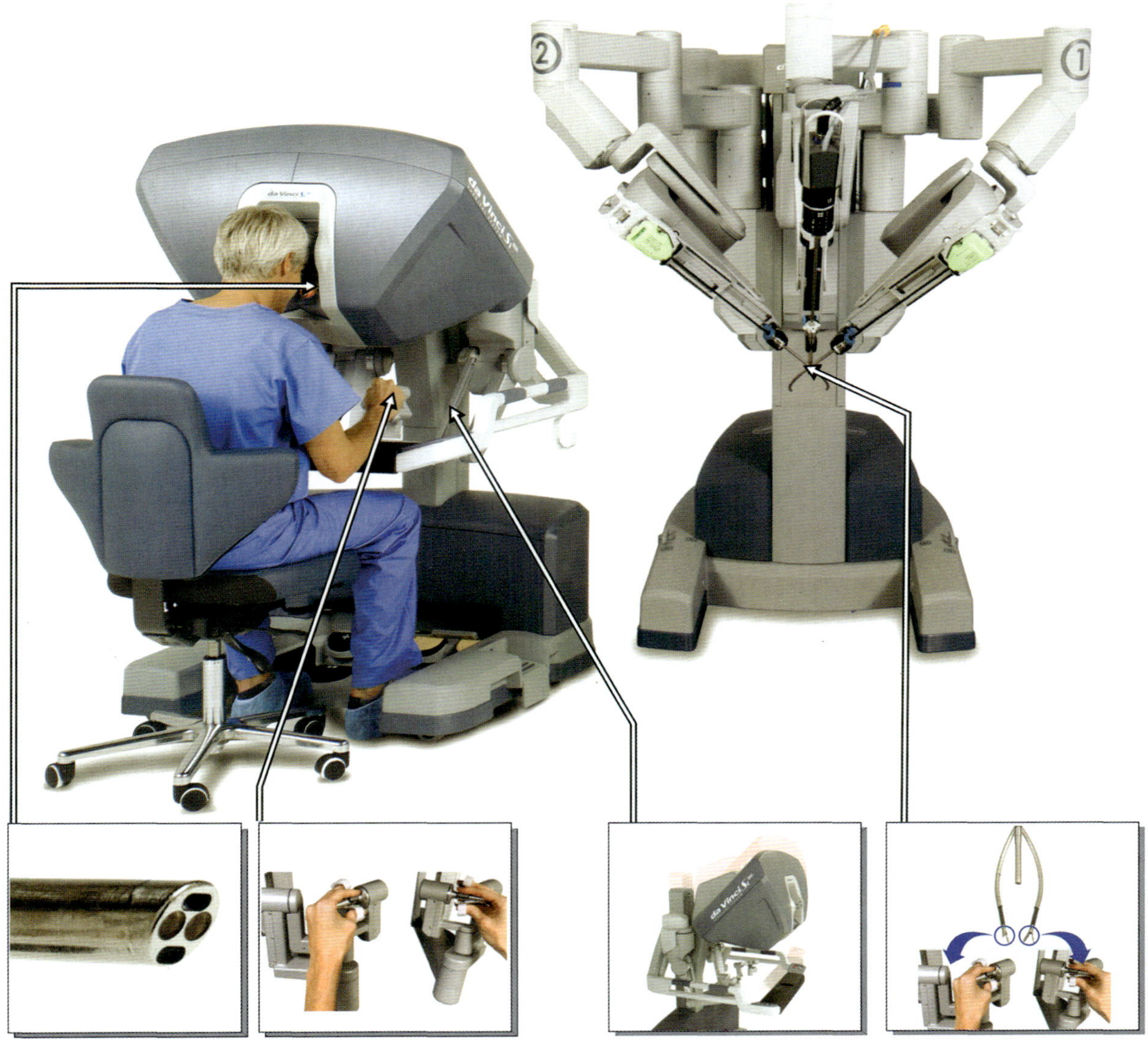

Fig. 1: Robotic surgery system

carries an endoscopic camera with two lenses that gives the surgeon full stereoscopic vision from the console. The surgeon sits at the console and looks through two eye holes at the 3D images of the procedure, while maneuvering the arms with two foot pedals and two hand controllers. This system scales, filters and translates the surgeon's hand movements into more precise micromovements of the instruments, which operates through small incisions in the body (Fig. 2).

To perform a surgical procedure, the surgeon must first use the system's weight to judge how hard it should work. Then he/she uses the console's master controls to maneuver the patient side cart's three or four robotic arms (depending on the model). The instrument's jointed wrist design exceeds the natural range of motion of the human hand; motion scaling and tremor reduction further interpret and refine the surgeon's hand movements. The da Vinci® system always requires a human operator, and incorporates multiple redundant safety features designed to minimize opportunities for human error when compared with traditional approaches.

The da Vinci® system has been designed to improve upon conventional laparoscopy, in which the surgeon operates while standing, using hand-held, long-shafted instruments, which have no wrist. With conventional laparoscopy, the surgeon must look up and away from the instruments, to a nearby two-dimensional (2D) video monitor to see an image of the target anatomy. The surgeon must also rely on his/her patient-side assistant to position the camera correctly. In contrast, the da Vinci® system's ergonomic design allows the surgeon to operate from a seated position at the console, with eyes and

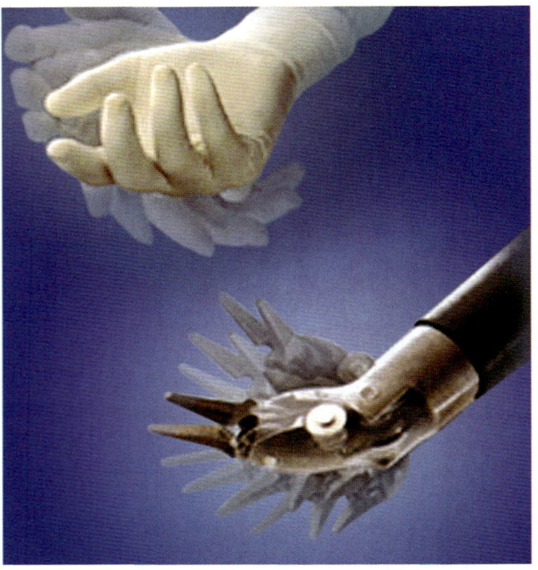

Fig. 2: Comparison of hand movements with that of da Vinci® robot
(***Source***: © 2013 Intuitive Surgical Inc.)

hands positioned in line with the instruments. To move the instruments or to reposition the camera, the surgeon simply moves his/her hands.

By providing surgeons with superior visualization, enhanced dexterity, greater precision and ergonomic comfort, the da Vinci® Surgical system makes it possible for more surgeons to perform minimally invasive procedures involving complex dissection or reconstruction. For the patient, a da Vinci® procedure can offer all the potential benefits of a minimally invasive procedure, including less pain, less blood loss and less need for blood transfusions. Moreover, the da Vinci® system can enable a shorter hospital stay, a quicker recovery and faster return to normal daily activities.

Set Up of the Operating Room

Figure 3 illustrates set up in an operating room utilizing the da Vinci® robotic equipment. The robotic surgeon operates from the remote master console and uses a

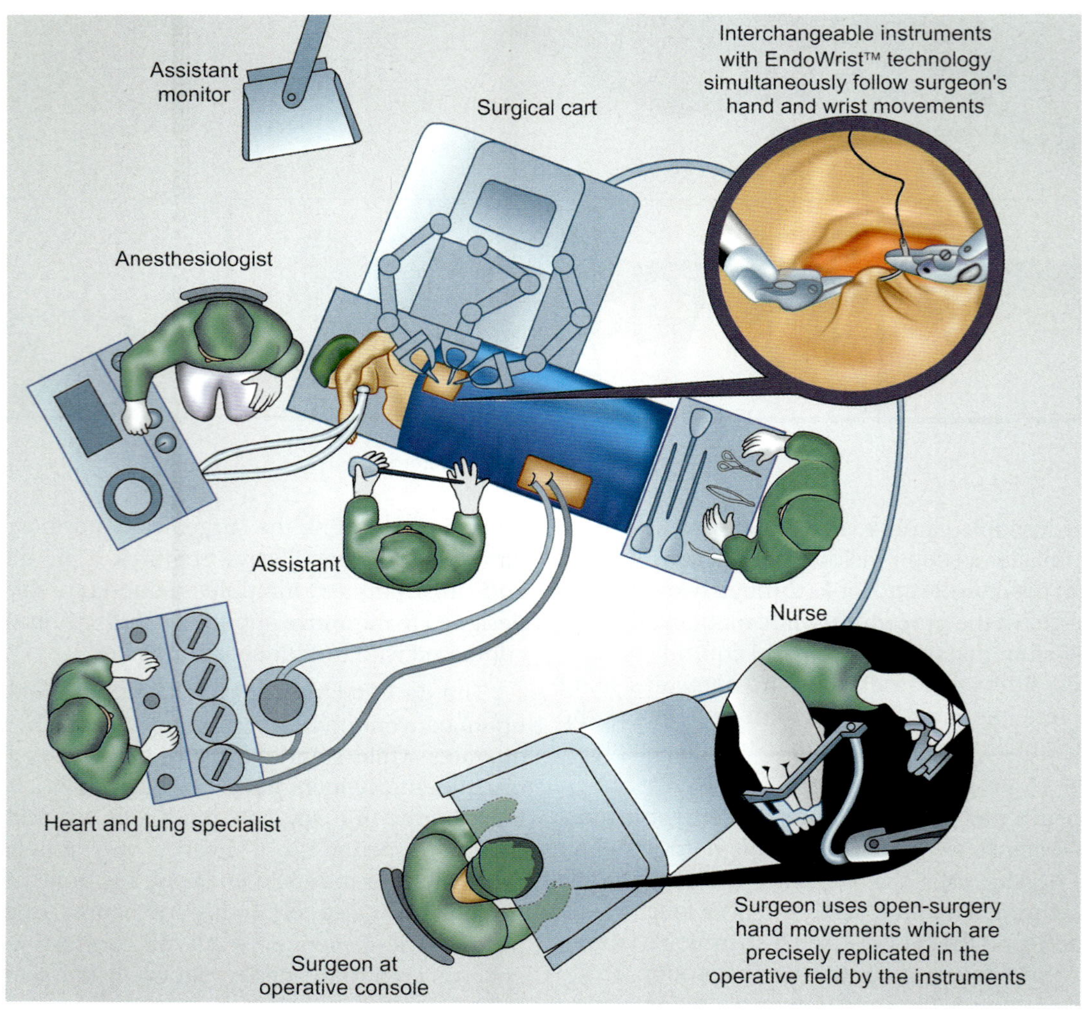

Fig. 3: Set up of the operating room
(***Source***: © 2013 Intuitive Surgical Inc.)

combination of hand controls and foot pedals. The patient-side cart is positioned in between the patient's legs, and the robotic arms are attached to stainless steel robotic trocars through a process termed as docking. One of the foot pedal (being managed by the surgeon) controls the movement of camera; another one may control the focus; another pedal helps in providing a range of motions to the robotic equipment, whereas yet another one controls both monopolar and bipolar energy sources. The hand controls of the surgeon sitting on the side console help in the movement of the camera as well as the various robotic instruments. There are about three operative robotic arms. Despite all of these advancements, a bedside assistant is still required.

ADVANTAGES OF ROBOTIC SURGERY

Advantages of Robotic Surgery for the Surgeon

The da Vinci® surgical system has the potential to change surgical procedure in three basic ways:

- *Make existing minimally invasive surgery (MIS) operations easier*: Surgical procedures routinely performed today using MIS techniques will be performed more quickly and easily
- *Making difficult MIS operations routine*: Surgical procedures that today are performed only rarely using MIS techniques are expected to be performed routinely and with confidence using the da Vinci® Surgical system. Some procedures have been adapted for port-based techniques but are extremely difficult and are currently performed by a limited number of highly skilled surgeons
- *Making new surgical procedures possible*: A number of surgeries that could not be performed in a minimal invasive manner can be performed today using the robotic system.

Advantages of Robotic Surgery for the Patient

Possible benefits of robotic surgery in comparison to open surgery include the following:

- *Minimal Scarring*: Robotic surgery is a type of minimally invasive procedure, in which several small incisions (0.25–0.75 inch) are made along the abdomen, and the surgical equipment are inserted through these incisions. In traditional abdominal surgery, a 7–8 inches long vertical or horizontal incision is usually made over the anterior abdominal wall (Fig. 4). Nowadays, an umbilical incision for minimally invasive surgery is commonly preferred. Transumbilical entry with da Vinci® single-site enables a virtually scarless surgery, providing patients one of the most cosmetically appealing results of any available surgical approach (Fig. 5).
- *Minimal Pain:* The da Vinci® System's remote center technology is designed to limit cannula movement at the patient's abdominal wall, minimizing potential port-site trauma and postoperative pain
- Reduced blood loss
- Low conversion rate to open surgery
- Low rate of complications
- Short duration of hospital stay
- Small incisions resulting in minimal scarring
- Shorter hospital stay
- Reduced requirement for narcotic pain medicine.

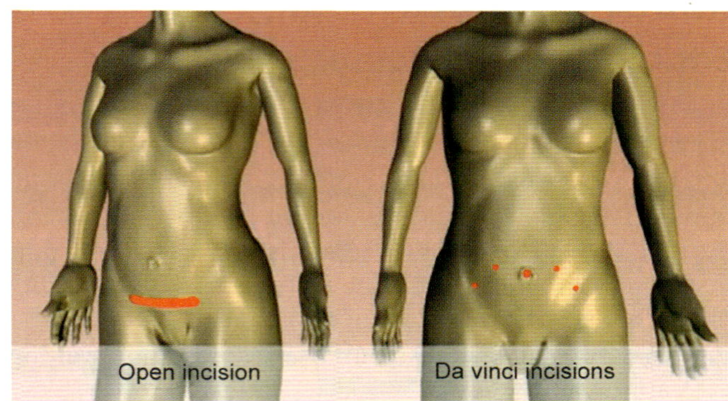

Fig. 4: Incision given in traditional open surgery compared to the minimal small incisions given in the robotic surgery

(***Source:*** © 2013 Intuitive Surgical Inc.)

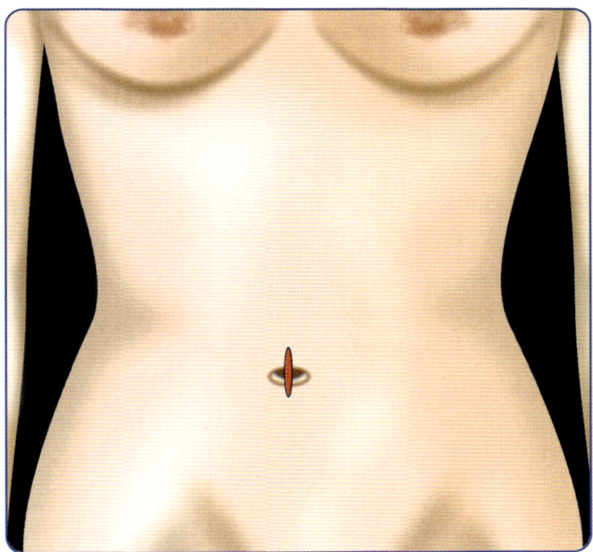

Fig. 5: Improved cosmesis due to transumbilical entry with da Vinci® single-site incision

(***Source:*** © 2013 Intuitive Surgical Inc.)

RISKS OF ROBOTIC SURGERY

Though the overall rate of complications with robotic surgery is quite low, some possible risks of robotic surgery in comparison to open surgery include the following:

- Bladder injury
- Abscess formation
- Urinary tract injury
- Bowel obstruction
- *Risks related to MIS*: These may include complications such as multiple incisions, conversion to another surgical technique and incisional hernia, pulmonary embolism, etc.

INNOVATIONS USED IN ROBOTIC SURGERY

EndoWrist® One Vessel Sealer

The EndoWrist® one vessel sealer is a fully wristed instrument, enabling an optimized approach for sealing and cutting of vessels up to 7 mm in diameter and tissue bundles. Available exclusively for the da Vinci® Si system, the EndoWrist® one vessel sealer is a single use 8 mm instrument, providing a pristine sealing surface and cutting blade for effective performance in each procedure. The EndoWrist® Stapler 45 System, however, is still awaiting FDA approval.

Features of EndoWrist® One Vessel Sealer (Fig. 6)

Uncompromised access and control: Fully wristed articulation allows surgeons to approach anatomy at optimal angles for effective sealing performance with hallmark da Vinci® precision, dexterity and control.

Optimal flexibility and efficiency: Independent seal/cut functions along with transection boundary indicator, facilitates efficient seal with confident transection, plus affords surgeons flexibility to assess the seal prior to cut.

Exceptional seal quality: The 16 mm length sealing surface and consistent computer-controlled closing pressures insure excellent tissue sealing.

Remarkable versatility: Dual-hinged, thermally isolated jaws with 40° opening angle and unique tip profile offer efficient dissection.

Proven sealing technology: The vessel sealer and stapler vision cart upgrade include the ERBE VIO 300 D especially configured for the da Vinci® system. Its optimized algorithm offers reliable sealing and minimal thermal spread.

Unparalleled ease of use: Real-time system self-checks and onscreen feedback keeps the surgeon informed.

EndoWrist® One Suction/Irrigator for Da Vinci® Myomectomy

Potential Benefits (Table 1)

The EndoWrist® one suction/irrigator (Fig. 7) offers surgeons precise control of a fully articulated suction/irrigation instrument during the various steps of myomectomy (Figs 8A and B). Use of this instrument also provides console surgeons with the following benefits:

- Greater surgeon autonomy
- Management of fluids for optimal visualization of the surgical field during enucleation
- Access to difficult-to-reach anatomy, such as myomas in posterior locations
- Ability to maintain a clear surgical field, enabling surgeon to quickly identify bleeding vessels for managing hemostasis.

Fluorescence Imaging

Firefly fluorescence imaging for da Vinci® system allows for the identification of real-time anatomy using near-infrared guidance.

Features

- Provides real-time near-infrared guidance through visualization of injectable fluorescence dye (Figs 9A and B)
- Interface allows efficient toggling between normal illumination and fluorescence imaging modes
- Incorporates illuminator utilized light emitting diode technology.

Potential Benefits

- Enables enhanced visualization capabilities for:
  - Vessel identification
  - Soft tissue perfusion
- Allows real-time identification of anatomy in fluorescence imaging mode from the Si surgeon console, in 3-dimensional, high-definition quality
- Minimizes downtime, operating expense associated with lamp replacement.

INDICATIONS FOR USE OF ROBOTIC SURGERY IN GYNECOLOGY

- Endometriosis resection
- Myomectomy

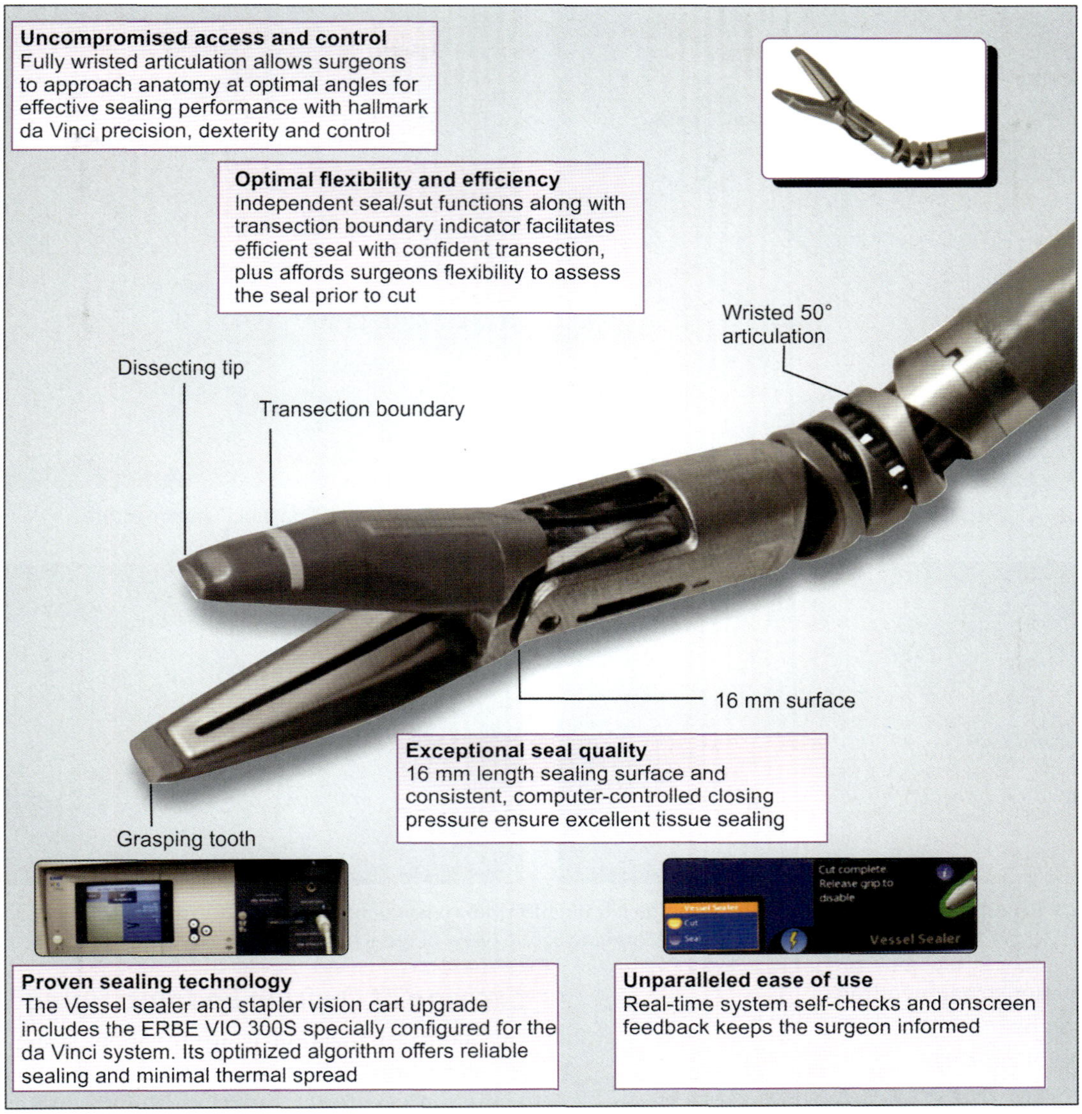

Uncompromised access and control
Fully wristed articulation allows surgeons to approach anatomy at optimal angles for effective sealing performance with hallmark da Vinci precision, dexterity and control
Optimal flexibility and efficiency
Independent seal/sut functions along with transection boundary indicator facilitates efficient seal with confident transection, plus affords surgeons flexibility to assess the seal prior to cut
Wristed 50° articulation
Dissecting tip
Transection boundary
16 mm surface
Exceptional seal quality
16 mm length sealing surface and consistent, computer-controlled closing pressure ensure excellent tissue sealing
Grasping tooth
Cut complete
Release grip to disable
Vessel Sealer
Proven sealing technology
The Vessel sealer and stapler vision cart upgrade includes the ERBE VIO 300S specially configured for the da Vinci system. Its optimized algorithm offers reliable sealing and minimal thermal spread
Unparalleled ease of use
Real-time system self-checks and onscreen feedback keeps the surgeon informed

Fig. 6: Features of the EndoWrist® one vessel sealer

Table 1: Potential benefits of EndoWrist® one suction/irrigator

Procedure step	Uses of suction/irrigator
Enucleation	• Help visualize tissue layers
Closure of deep layers	• Keep surgical site clear of blood to maintain good visualization • Achieve adequate hemostasis before moving to serosal layer closure
Closure of serosal layer	• Optimize visualization by controlling bleeding
Site clean up	• Clean anatomy with suction and irrigation after morcellation

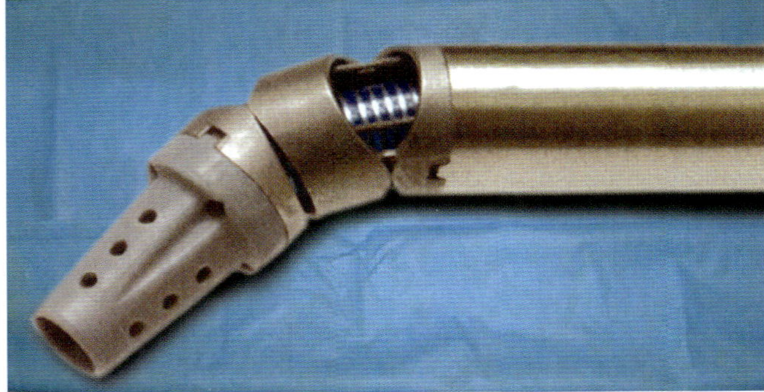

Fig. 7: EndoWrist® one suction/irrigator for da Vinci® myomectomy

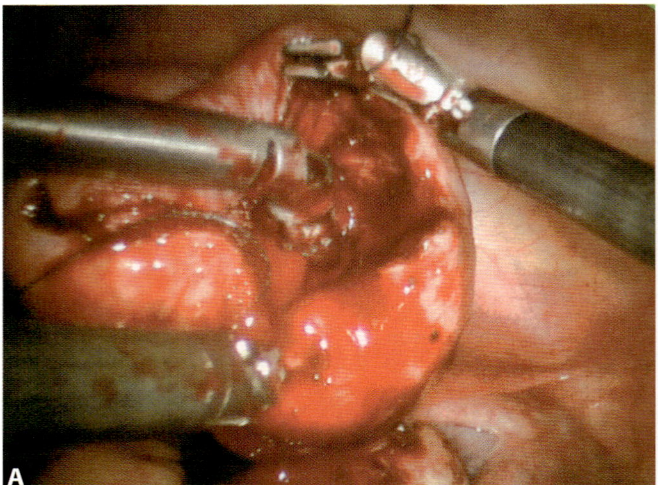
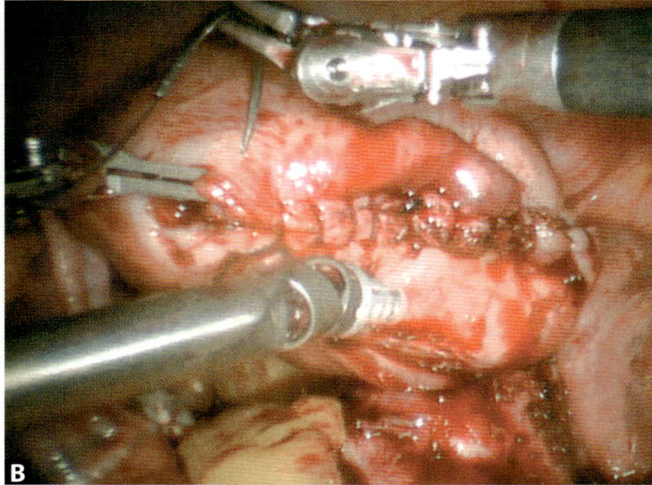

Figs 8A and B: Using EndoWrist® one suction/irrigator at the time of da Vinci® myomectomy

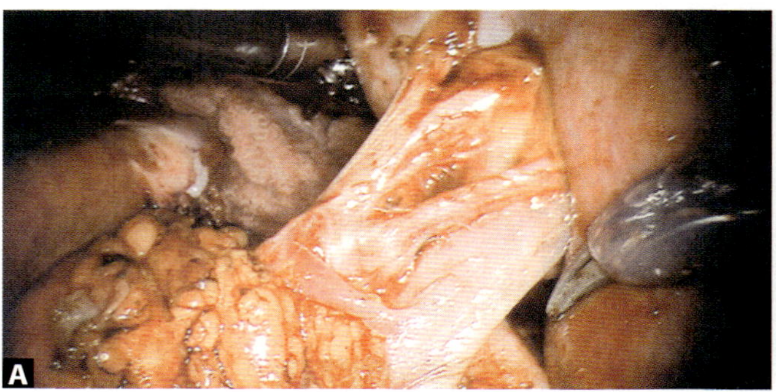
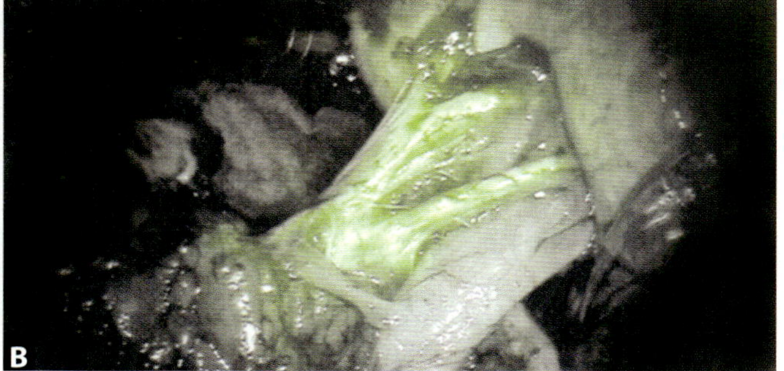

Figs 9A and B: (A) Normal 3D high-definition illumination view (view of renal hilum); (B) Vessel identification in fluorescence imaging mode (view of renal hilum)

- Excessive menstrual bleeding
- Pelvic prolapse
- Treatment of cancer
- Hysterectomy.

ENDOMETRIOSIS

Endometriotic Resection Using the Robotic System

There are four ways in which da Vinci® technology facilitates precise endometriosis resection.

Adhesiolysis

Three-dimensional HD vision provides improved visualization of tissue planes, making it easy to restore normal anatomy while avoiding injury to ureters, vasculature and other structures. In addition, hot shear (monopolar curved scissors) offers two modes for meticulous freeing of adhesions throughout the pelvic cavity (Fig. 10).

Excision of Ovarian Endometrioma

Excellent visualization using the robotic system allows easy identification of the ovary/endometrioma wall, helping to avoid damage to the ovary and to preserve functionality. The PK® dissecting forceps and long-tip forceps can be used together to provide traction/retraction for effective removal of the endometrioma (Fig. 11).

Ureterolysis

EndoWrist® instruments facilitate careful ureterolysis, even when the ureters are hidden by scar tissue and nodular disease. Wristed instrumentation also enables precise resection of lesions that have deeply infiltrated structures such as bowel and ureters. Complete autonomy can be achieved utilizing the third instrument arm to assist in tissue manipulation or retraction (Fig. 12).

Resection of Rectovaginal Nodules

Unparalleled visualization of the posterior cul-de-sac, combined with fully articulating instrumentation, enables the surgeon to identify and resect lesions and

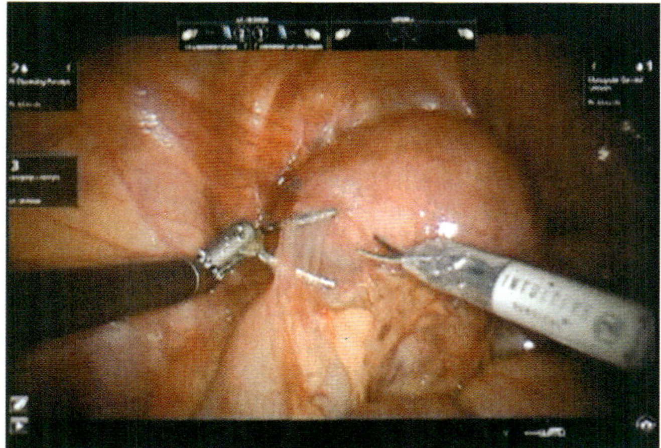

Fig. 10: Adhesiolysis

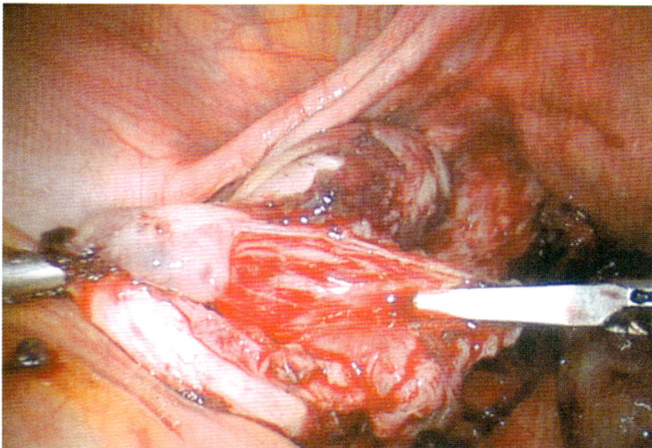

Fig. 11: Excision of ovarian endometrioma

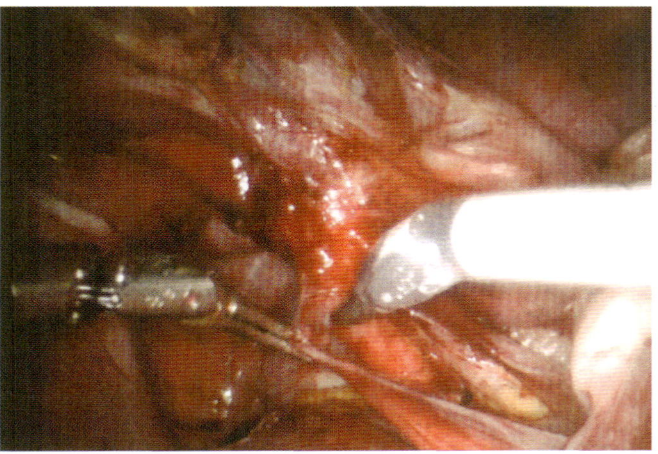

Fig. 12: Ureterolysis

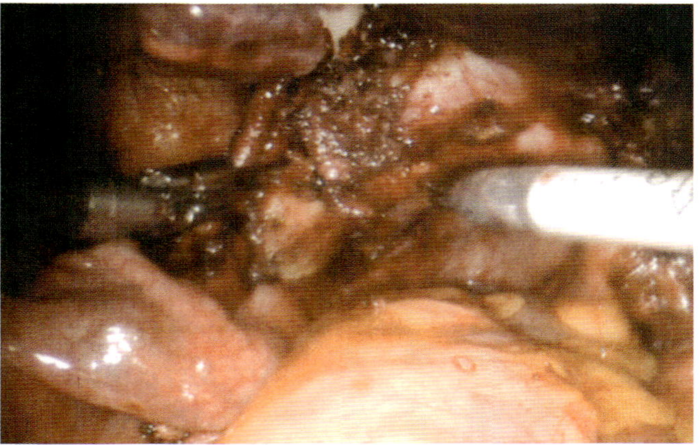

Fig. 13: Resection of rectovaginal nodules

nodules throughout the pelvic cavity. The EndoWrist® instrumentation also facilitates easy and efficient access to intraperitoneal and retroperitoneal anatomy for excision of all nodules (Fig. 13).

Surgeon Benefits

Da Vinci® surgical system enables a reproducible surgical approach for complex, diffuse or deep infiltrating endometriosis with superior visualization for complete resection of endometriotic lesion. The visualization, depth perception, dexterity and control provided by da Vinci® system offers potential for:

- D high-definition visualization of endometriotic lesions
- Ability to completely resect lesions, regardless of their location in the pelvic cavity
- Ability to precisely resect stage IV disease, including deeply infiltrating endometriosis
- Extension of a minimally invasive approach to advanced or extremely extensive cases
- Control of the camera and all three operative arms provide ultimate accuracy in maintaining surgical autonomy, accuracy and efficiency.

MYOMECTOMY

Surgeon Benefits

Robotic surgery enables gynecologists to perform uterine preserving myomectomies in a minimally invasive manner, with surgical precision and confidence in the ability to do a multilayer closure. The precision, dexterity and control provided by da Vinci® system offer potential for:

- Minimally invasive access to the myoma, potentially minimizing complications associated with a large abdominal incision
- Precise dissection of myomas using EndoWrist® instrumentation
- Precise suturing of the uterine defect for a durable, multilayer closure

- Extending a minimally invasive approach to more complex types of myomas—larger, more numerous and less accessible
- 3D vision, improved ergonomics, wide range of movements, absence of the fulcrum effect and improved instrument dexterity to eliminate most of the limitations of traditional laparoscopy.

Potential Patient Benefits

Possible benefits of robotic myomectomy in comparison to traditional laparoscopic surgery include the following:

- Minimally invasive removal of heavier, more numerous and more difficult to access fibroids
- Fever complications during surgery.

Potential Patient Risks

Possible risks of robotic myomectomy include the following:

- Weakening of the uterus during labor
- Preterm birth
- Tears or perforations in the uterine wall.

In addition to the above risks, there are risks related to MIS, such as pulmonary embolism, etc.

Myomectomy Using the Robotic System

The steps of robotic myomectomy have been illustrated in Figures 14A to F. There are four ways in which da Vinci® technology facilitates a precise myomectomy.

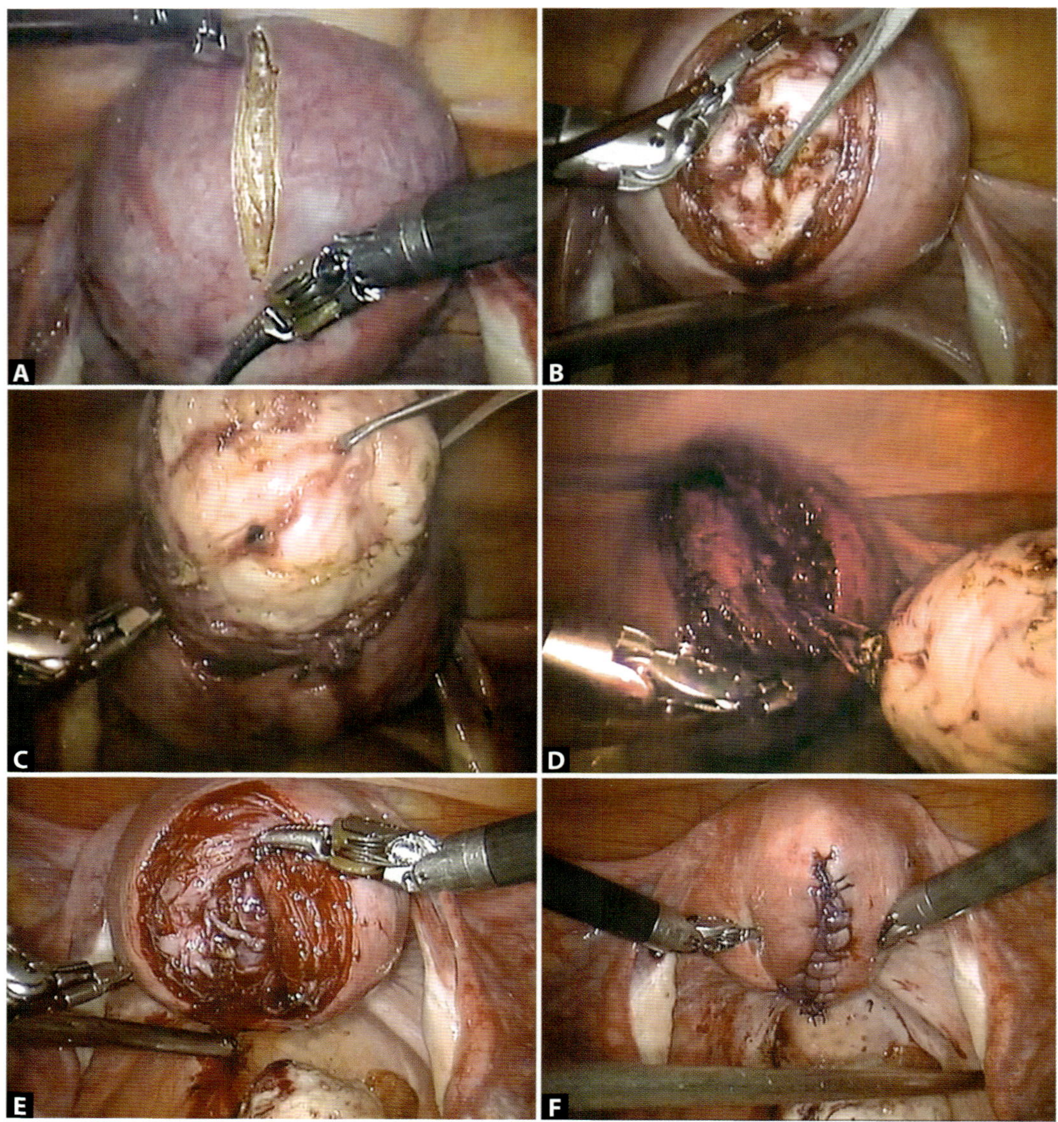

Figs 14A to F: Robotic myomectomy. (A) Using the robotic harmonic shears, a hysterotomy is made over the myoma; (B and C) Shelling out of myoma; (D) Myoma has been completely removed from the myoma bed; (E) A multilayer closure is performed employing sutures and suturing techniques that are identical to those of an open myomectomy; (F) Suturing of the uterine surface is complete

Hysterotomy

The permanent cautery hook allows the surgeon to make a horizontal or vertical incision over the uterine surface, based upon the location of the pathology, while avoiding excessive divots or tunneling within the myometrium surrounding the myoma. The PK® dissecting forceps help retract the incised myometrium and provide improved coagulation with minimal thermal spread to facilitate deliberate perpendicular cuts down to the myoma capsule.

Multilayered Suture Closure of Defect—Deep Layers

The suture cut needle driver securely holds CT-2 needles as they pass through the myometrial layers while providing integrated cutting following knot tying for improved operative efficiency. The EndoWrist® large needle driver allows for interrupted figure-of-eight or running sutures to be thrown and tied intracorporeally for a deep multilayer closure. The unsurpassed visualization of the camera allows for accurate placement of imbricated stitches in additional layers and superior ability to reconstruct the uterine defect.

Enucleation

Consistent, careful counter traction can be attained by utilizing the EndoWrist® tenaculum forceps while avoiding entrance into the endometrial cavity or premature avulsion of the myoma. The PK® dissecting forceps facilitate development of the correct dissection plane surrounding the myoma, while also providing more site-specific counter traction, facilitating a more precise dissection and enucleation of the fibroid. The hot shears is used to peel the myoma free of all attachments. Coagulation with the PK® dissecting forceps should be prudently used to pre-emptively deal with vascular attachments.

Multilayered Suture Closure of Defect—Superficial Layer

All EndoWrist® needle drivers are fully wristed, enabling quick and efficient knot typing. The long tip forcep is used to perform a running baseball stitch with an SH needle, in order to close any dead space and avoid serosal pull-through. The suture cut needle driver is used to manipulate the tissue for needle bite placement and to cut the suture upon completion of stitching for added surgical autonomy and operative efficiency.

CRITICISM AND CONTROVERSIES

The term "robotic surgery" which is commonly used to refer to this technology can give the impression that da Vinci® system is used for performing the surgeries in an autonomous manner. In contrast, the current da Vinci® surgical system does not function on its own because it has not been designed as an autonomous system. It lacks a decision-making software and relies on a human operator for all its input. Moreover, all operative steps are performed through remote human-computer interaction. The current system has been deliberately constructed in a manner so as to effortlessly duplicate the movement of the surgeon's hands with the help of the tips of microinstruments. The instrument cannot make decisions without receiving the surgeon's direct input.

Critics of robotic surgery emphasize that the technique of robotic surgery is difficult for users to learn and that this technique is not likely to be more effective than traditional laparoscopic surgery. The available evidence presents with conflicting views related to the efficacy and various side-effects related to the use of robotic equipment while performing various surgeries. Presently, there is inadequate data related to the safety of this system and the likelihood of causing injuries to the patients due to electrical currents released from the various surgical tips used by the system. As of 2013, the FDA is inquiring problems related to the use of da Vinci® robot, including fatalities that have occurred during surgeries using this device. A number of lawsuits related to the injuries and problems caused by this system are also in progress.

Also, da Vinci® system uses the software manufactured by the proprietor, which cannot be modified by surgeon. This therefore, severely limits the surgeon's ability to change the operation system. Furthermore, the cost involved in the installation and establishment of this system is quite high and may be beyond the reach of many institutions. There have also been much criticism and debate related to the procedure for obtaining the FDA approval of this system and provision of adequate training before using this system.

BIBLIOGRAPHY

1. Barakat EE, Bedaiwy MA, Zimberg S, et al. Robotic-assisted, laparoscopic, and abdominal myomectomy: A comparison of surgical outcomes. Obstet Gynecol. 2011;117(2 Pt 1):256-65.
2. Boggess JF. Robotic surgery in gynecologic oncology: Evolution of a new surgical paradigm. J Rob Surg. 2007;1:31-3.
3. Da Vinci surgery (2013). da Vinci®. Changing the Experience of Surgery. [online] Available from http://www.davincisurgery.com/ [Accessed December, 2013].
4. Intutive Surgical®. (2013). Da Vinci surgery. [online] Available from http://www.intuitivesurgical.com/company/clinical evidence/ [Accessed December, 2013].
5. Talamini MA, Chapman S, Horgan S, et al. Academic Robotics Group. A prospective analysis of 211 robotic-assisted surgical procedures. Surg Endosc. 2003;17(10):1521-4.

SHIRODKAR'S EXTENDED MANCHESTER REPAIR : A CONSERVATIVE VAGINAL SURGICAL PROCEDURE FOR GENITAL PROLAPSE REVISITED

Dr Suman P Sardesai, Dr Roohi Shaikh
Department of Obstetrics and Gynecology
Dr VM Govt. Medical College, Solapur, Maharashtra, India

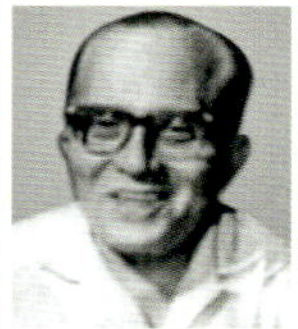

Fothergills Manchester, repair a time honored technique for young prolapse had various shortcomings. So Dr Shirodkar in 1946 came up with the Novel approach of utilizing uterosacral ligament for the repair of prolapse without amputation of cervix and concomitant enterocele repair which give a good success rate

Prerequisites for the operation:

1. Young women <35 years with II or III degree uterovaginal prolapse
2. Interested in child-bearing or preserving menstruation
3. No cervical elongation
4. Good uterosacral ligament strength

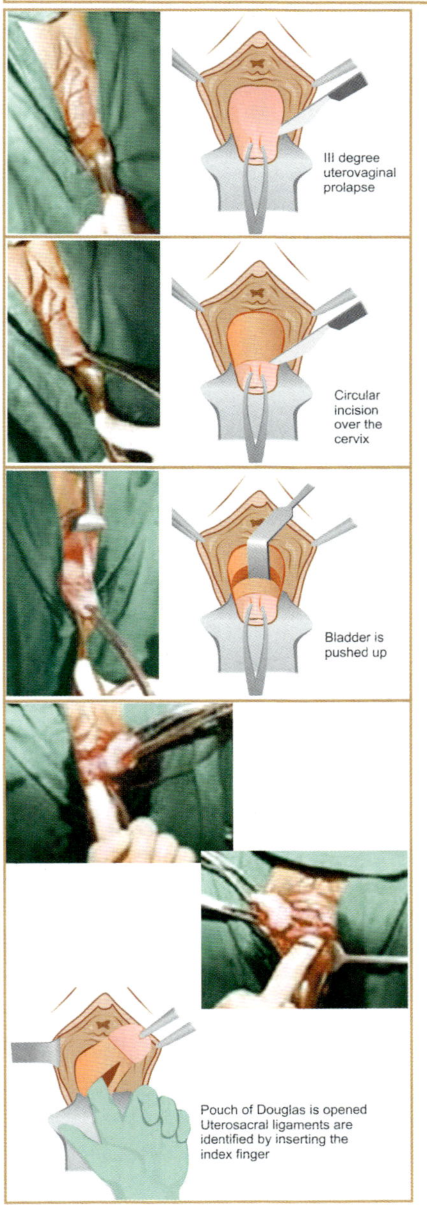

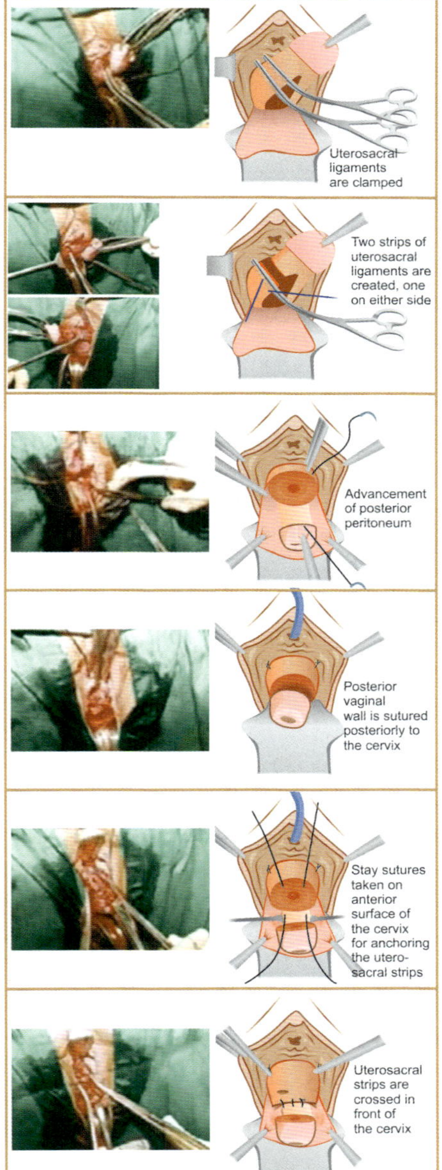

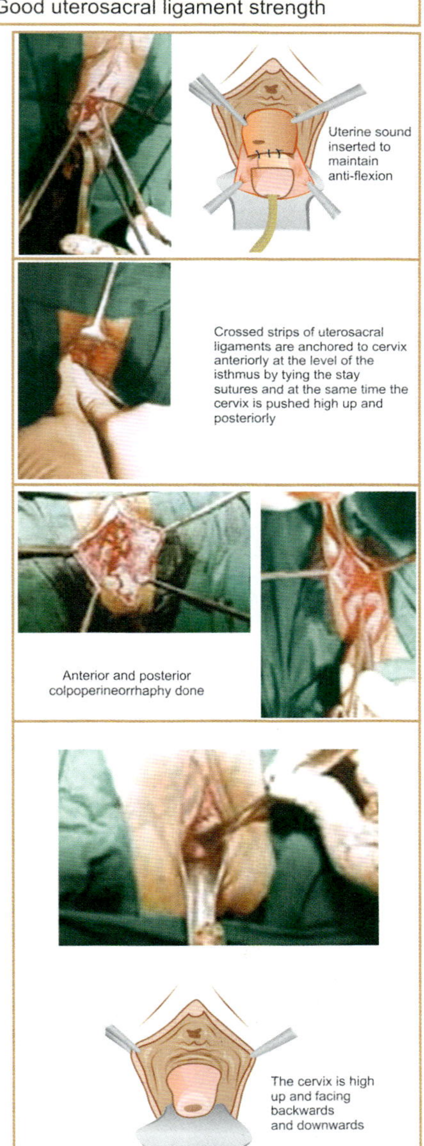

ABDOMINAL SLING OPERATIONS FOR GENITAL PROLAPSE : INDIA'S CONTRIBUTION

Dr Suman P Sardesai, Dr Rajeev Dabde, Dr Umesh Kulkarni, Dr Shweta Mittal
Department of Obstetrics and Gynecology
Dr VM Govt. Medical College, Solapur, Maharashtra, India

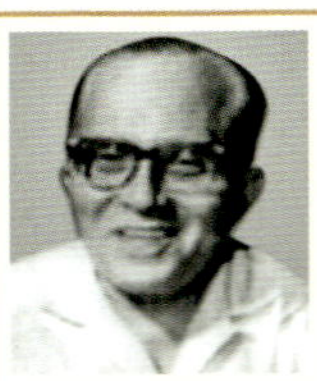

Dr VN Shirodkar

Dr Shirodkar's Bilateral Sling (1946)

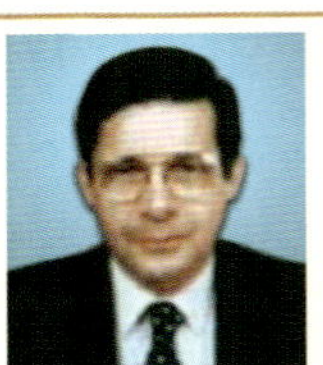

Dr RP Soonawaala

Dr Soonawaala's Unilateral Sling (1985)

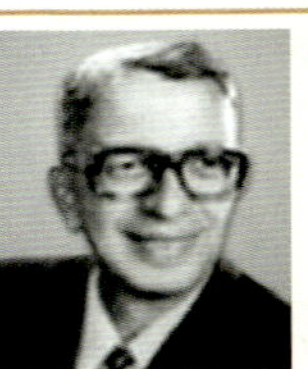

Dr BN Purandare

Dr Purandare's Cervicopexy (1956)

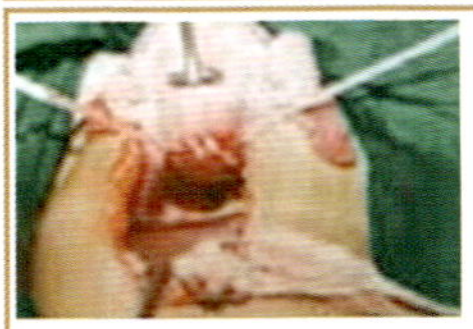
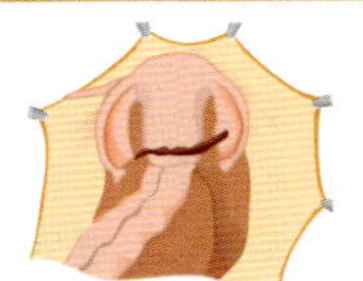

Fixatation of merselene tape on posterior aspect of cervix just above the insertion of uterosacral ligaments

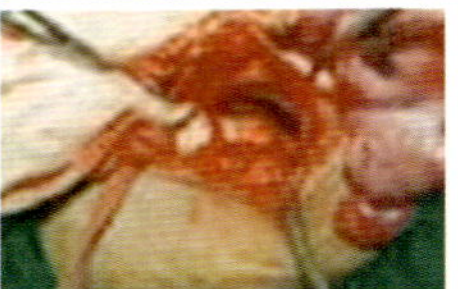
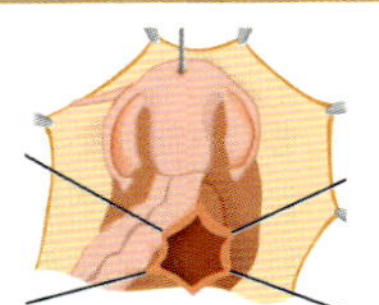

Exposer of anterior longitudinal ligament over 5th lumbar vertebra

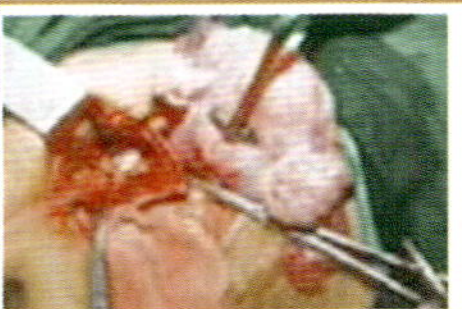
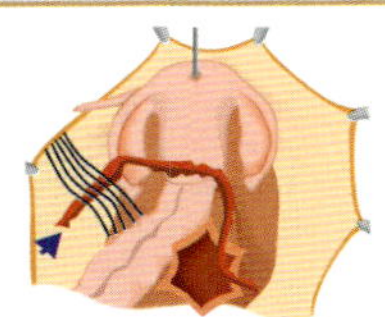

On left side merselene tape is brought out through two leaves of broad ligament and than passed through psoas loop

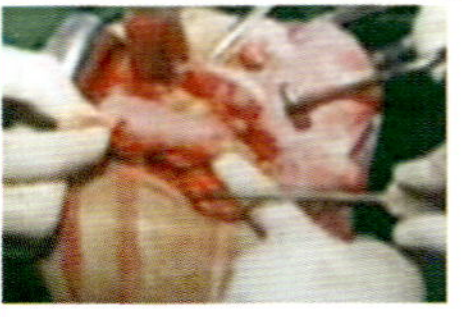
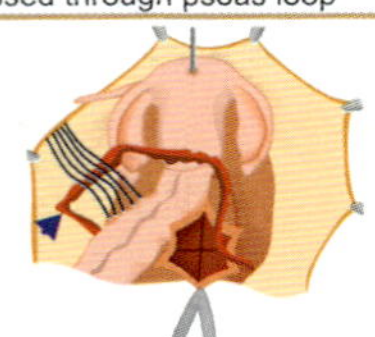

Shirodkar's needle passed beneath the pelvic colon retroperitoneally from 5th lumbar vertebra up to psoas loop

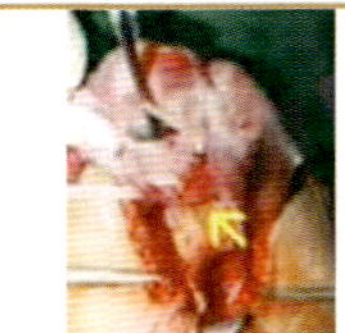
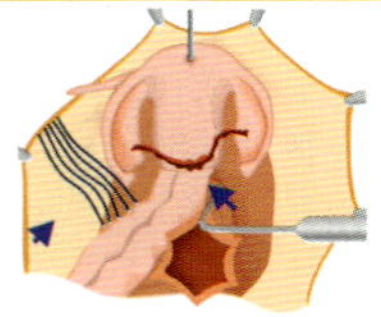

On the right side needle is passed retroperitoneally to bring the merselene tape over the 5th lumbar vertebra

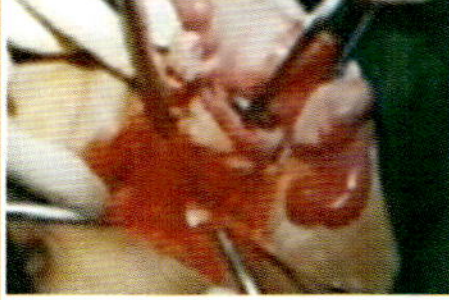
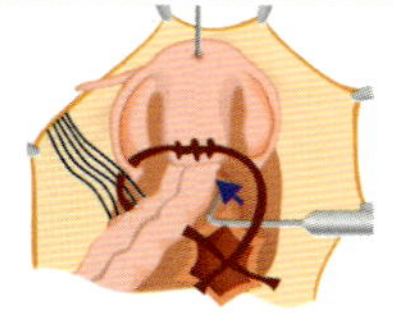

Both the ands of merselene tape fixed through the anterior longitudinal ligament in crosswise manner

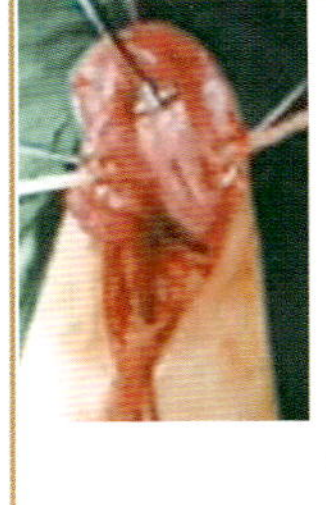
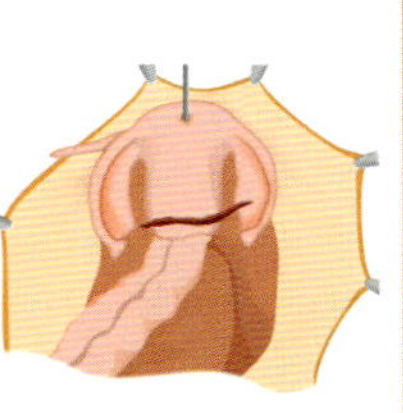

Fixation of merselene tape on posterior aspect of cervix just above the insertion of uterosacral ligaments

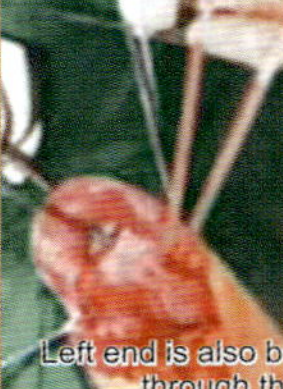
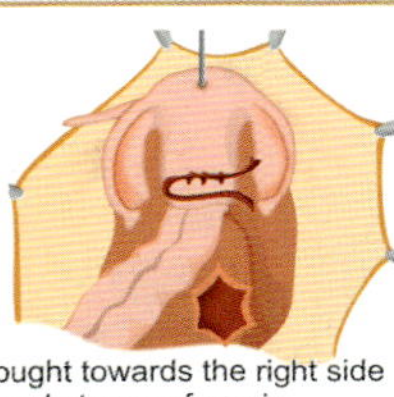

Left end is also brought towards the right side through the substance of cervix

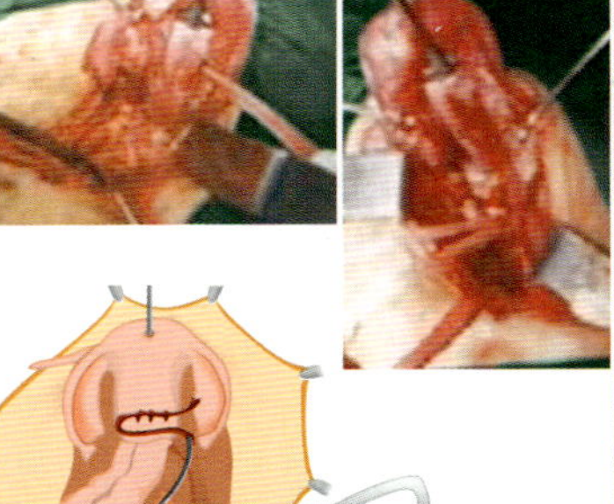

Both the ends of merselene tape brought out on right side retroperitoneally

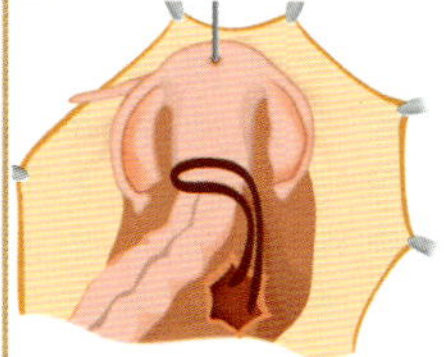

Both the ends fixed to anterior longitudinal ligament over 5th lumbar vertebra after positioning the uterus

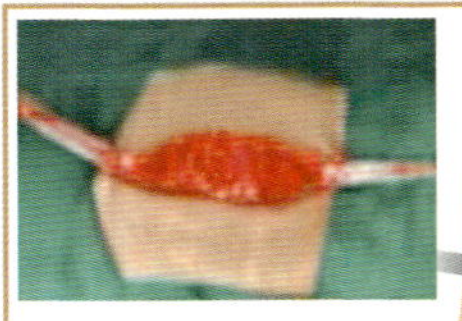

Strips of anterior rectus sheath prepared on other side at the level of anteroposterior iliac spine

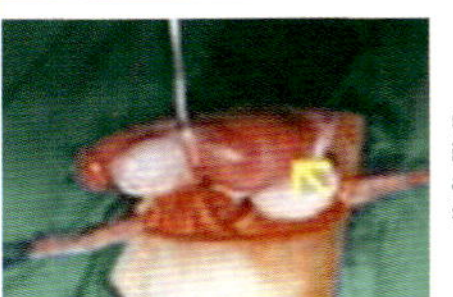

Uterus delivered through the insertion and two strips or anterior rectus sheath are seen

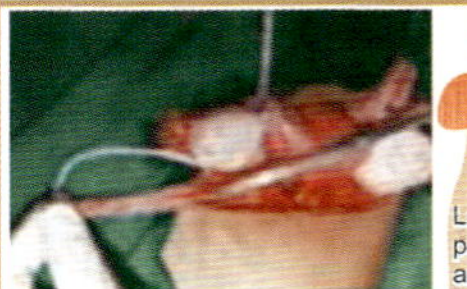
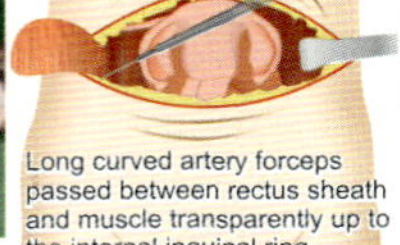

Long curved artery forceps passed between rectus sheath and muscle transparently up to the internal inguinal ring

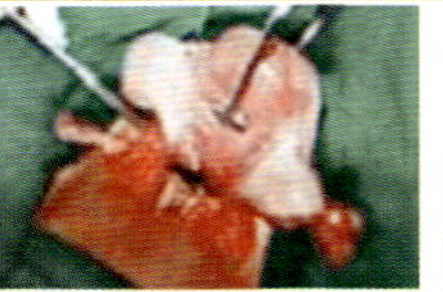
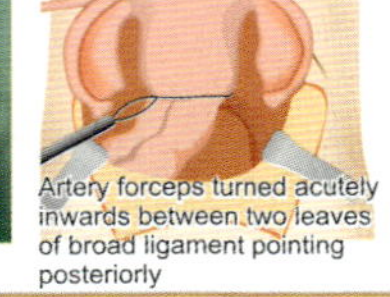

Artery forceps turned acutely inwards between two leaves of broad ligament pointing posteriorly

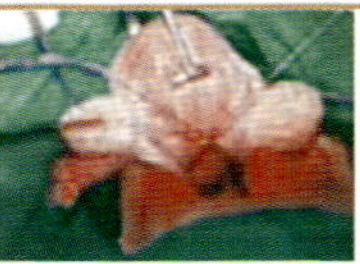

The same step is repeated on the right sides

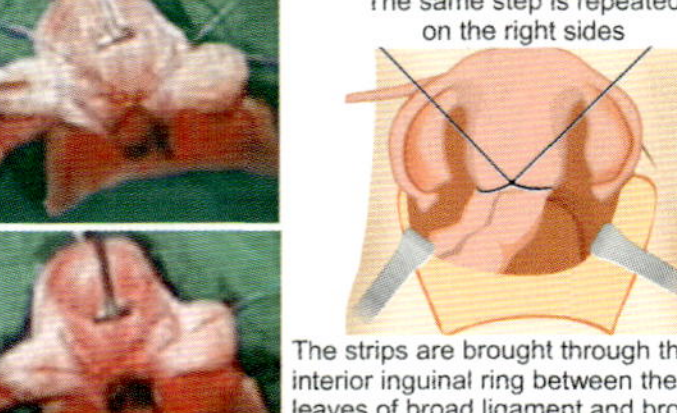

The strips are brought through the interior inguinal ring between the two leaves of broad ligament and brought out near the insertion of uterosacral ligament

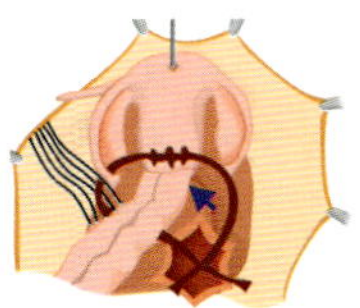

Shirodkar and Soonawaala's static siling

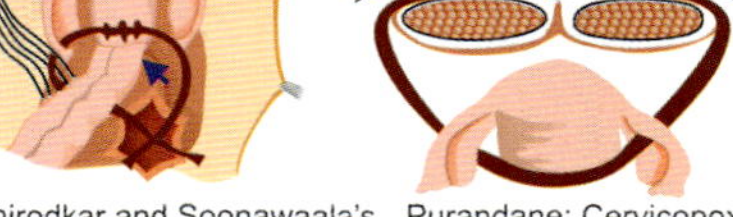

Purandane: Cervicopoxy is a Dynamic sling

Appendix 'A'

Gynecologist and Consent

By **Dr Devendra Gupta**
MS {Gen.Surg.}, PhD {Law}
Consultant General Surgeon and Medici Legal Advisor, Agra

One of the most basis of human right is freedom from physical interference, thus a woman of sufficient maturity and mental capacity can choose whether or not to submit to physical examination. Now consent to examination to obtain (except in case of emergency) may lead to recovery of damages in a civil action or even to criminal proceeding for indirect assault.
Consent may either be:

Implied Consent

This exists where no actual word of consent is spoken, but the behavior of the patient is such that it is obvious, consent is being given. Much of the medical practice depends upon this. The very fact that a patient comes to a doctor, implies that the patient is seeking medical assistance. However such implied consent only goes as far as the preliminary matters related to ordinary clinical examination consisting of inspection, palpation and auscultation. Any more complicated procedures such as vaginal or rectal examination needs more definite consent than the implication of a patient presenting himself or herself before the doctor.

Express Consent

This is where a patient responds to a direct request for consent to any particular procedure {examination or instrumentation}. Express consent should be obtained in writing. Where any surgical operation or any major diagnostic procedure is to be performed. Where patient can not write, his/her thumbprint should be taken. Written consent should refer only to one specific procedure and this should be after some explanation of what it entails. Consent obtain by deception is invalid. Example: If a doctor plays down the risk of some major surgical procedure, giving the impression that it is some trivial operation, then the patient may legitimately claim later that her consent was not for such a major procedure. Exception to this is emergency situation. Naturally, in an emergency, any operation must be carried out necessary to save the patient's life; courts will and uphold any reasonable medical descision. Where mentally defective patients and children are concerned, then consent is a matter for those persons incharge of them. The age of consent for medical treatment is not officially laid down, but eighteen years would appear to be the acceptable threshold. Below this age, young people are in the care of their guardians or parents, so for medical treatment or any operation, then it is the parents or guardians who normally give such consent.

Informed Consent

The concept of informed consent has come in force in recent years and many civil actions have been brought by patients who alleged that they did not understand the nature of the medical procedure to which they gave consent. To avoid this, all substantial risk, both of surgical operation, diagnostic procedures and drug therapy must be explained to the patient and her attendants, in comprehensive non-medical terms, every effort being made to ensure that the patient truly understands what is being said. The doctor is also entitled-indeed obliged, to modify his explanation in relation to the psychological state of the patient, in order to avoid causing any harm.

Example: The vasectomy of husband failed and his wife become pregnant and later gave birth to a child. The surgeon was held liable for not informing the patient about reversibility and compensation was awarded for upbringing of the child.

Exceeding Consent

In exceptional cases, during treatment or operation, doctor may cross the limit of the consent to save the life of the patient and the same is applicable to emergency cases. In this regard Section 92 of Indian Penal Code provides:

Section 92 {IPC}: Act done in good faith for benefit of a person without consent

Nothing is an offence by reason of any harm which it may cause to a person for whose benefit it is done in good faith, even without the person's consent, if the circumstances are such that it is impossible for that person to signify consent, or if that person is incapable of giving consent, and has no guardian or other person in lawful charge of him from whom it is possible to obtain consent in time for the thing to be done with benefit.

Thus, doctor may go beyond the consent {exceeding the previously given} in emergency and to save the life of a patient but here the burden of proof lies with the doctor to extablish validity of those circumstances.

In conclusion, it is observe that gynecologist either male or female in present sciences of CPA, informed consent from patients would be a forethought prior to taking up examination, procedures or surgeries.

Appendix 'B'

Operative Notes and Postoperative Instructions for Common Gynecological and Obstetrical Operations, Procedures

(By **Dr Sanjay Gupte**)

Section - I

Section - II

Section - III

Section - IV

SECTION-I

MTP

Preoperative Orders:

- NBM for 6 hrs.
- Consent (Form C & FOGSI Form)
- Record of preoperative all investigation reports.
- Anesthesia fitness.
- Doctor's Opinion Form 1

Operative Notes:

MTP done under GA/LA on ....at........................

LMP : ....
Indication : ....
Surgeon : ....
Anesthesia : ....

Steps:

- Patient was anesthesia.
- Lithotomy position was given.
- Painting and draping was done.
- Findings confirmed under anesthesia. Uterus................wks sized Fx clear.
- Cervix dilated up to No......................Hegar dilator.
- Suction cannula No....................inserted and products evacuated.
- Check curettage done.
- Products visualized at the end of the procedure.
- Uterus well contracted.
- Patient withstood the surgery well, Pulse......................BP.......................PV bleeding minimal at the end of the procedure.
- Entry of information in Form II.

Postoperative Orders:

- Nil By mouth for 2 hours.
- Half hourly pulse/BP/resp for first two hours.
- Sterile pads, watch for bleeding P/V
- If Rh negative Inj. Anti-D
- Antibiotics given/not given
- Counseling for contraception.
- Patient discharged from hospital at..............
- Patient's condition at discharge pulse.......................BP..........................

Postoperative Instructions for Patient:

- You will be called for follow up after 5-7 days and also after 1 month. Please make sure that you come.
- You can have full diet after going home.
- As you have been given anesthesia avoid going home on two wheeler, especially if you are feeling giddy or weak at the time of discharge.

- Take your medicines regularly.
- Do not worry about occasional vomiting, pain, bleeding from vagina.
- If vomiting, pain, PV bleeding is excessive or if there is fever, report immediately.
- Abstain from sex till next menses.
- You may get your next menses after 1 month to 6 weeks
- Rarely any MTP procedure can fail, hence, it is important to come for follow up after 1 month.
- Ask all your queries, medical (e.g. About the procedure itself) or non-medical (e.g. Bill, Discharge) well in advance.

Note: Medical method of MTP also comes under the preview of MTP Act

D & C

Preoperative Orders:

- Nil By Mouth for 6 hours.
- Consent.
- Record of all preoperative investigation reports.
- Anesthesia fitness.

Operative Notes:

D and C done under GA/LA on.............at...............

LMP : ....
Indication : ....
Surgeon : ....
Anesthesiologist : ....

Steps:

- Patient was anesthetized
- Lithotomy position was given.
- Painting and draping was done.
- Findings confirmed under anesthesia Uterus............wkshape.............fx................cervix..........................
- Cervix dilated up to no.............Hegar dilator.
- Curettage done using a sharp curett. Endometrium............... Scanty/Moderate/excessive.
- Specimen sent for HPE.
- Patient withstood the procedure well Pulse............BP.................PV bleeding minimal at the end of the procedure.

Postoperative Orders:

- Nil by mouth for 2 hours.
- Half hourly pulse/ BP / resp for 1st 2 hours.
- Sterile pads.
- Antibiotics given/not given.
- Patient discharged from hospital at...................
- Condition at discharge: Pulse........ BP..............

Postoperative Instructions for Patient:

- You will be called for follow up after 5-7 days and also after 1 month. Please bring your HPE report.
- You can have full diet after going home.
- As you have been given anesthesia avoid going home on two wheeler, especially if you are feeling giddy or weak at the time of discharge.
- Take your medicines regularly.
- Do not worry about occasional vomiting, pain, bleeding from vagina.
- If vomiting, pain, bleeding from vagina is excessive or if there is fever, report immediately.
- You may get your next menses after 1 month to 6 weeks.
- Ask all your queries, medical (e.g. About the procedure itself) or non-medical (e.g.Bill,Discharge) well in advance.

CERVICAL CAUTERY/BIOPSY

Preoperative orders:

- NBM for 6 hours.
- Consent.
- Record of all preoperative investigation reports.
- Anesthesia fitness.
- PAP Report/Colposcopy report

Operative Notes:

Cautery/Biopsy done under GA/LA on.......... at ....

LMP : ....
Indication : ....
Surgeon : ....
Anesthesiologist : ....

Steps:

- Patient was anesthetized
- Lithotomy..............................position was given.
- Painting and drapping done.
- Findings confirmed under anesthesia. Uterine size.....................wks. Shape...................cervix....................
- Biopsy taken from .... area.
- Visual lesion/acetowhite areas/colposcopy guided areas
- Cauterization done by electrocautery/cryocautery.
- Biopsy material sent for HPE.
- Colposcopy done/not done
- Pap smear taken/not taken

Postoperative orders:

- NBM................... 2 hours.
- Half hourly Pulse / BP / Resp for first 2 hours.
- Sterile Pads
- Watch for bleeding per vaginum
- Antibiotics
- Patient discharged from hospital at....................

Postoperative Instructions:

- You will be called for follow up after 5 days and again after 1 month. Please make sure that you come.
- You can have full diet after going home.
- As you have been given anesthesia avoid going home on two wheeler, especially if you are feeling giddy or weak at the time of discharge.
- Take your medicines regularly.
- Do not worry about occasional vomiting, pain, bleeding from vagina.
- If there is excessive pain, vomiting or foul smelling discharge or heavy bleeding report immediately.
- Abstain from sex till further instructions.
- Please ask all your queries, medical (e.g. About the procedure itself) or nonmedical (e.g Bill, Discharge) well in advance.

POST-IUCD INSTRUCTIONS

- This IUCD is valid for .... years.
- Please take all prescribed medicines.
- Your first followup will be after one week and on 5-10 days of your next menses.
- Next followup will be every 3 monthly for first 6 months (Post menstrually)
- Next followup will be 6 monthly for 3 years (Post menstrually)
- It is advisable to check your IUCD thread. It can be palpated by your finger.
- If any problem like heavy bleeding or abdominal pain or fever are encountered or thread is not palpable, you should come for check up as early as possible.
- IUCD can rarely fail, hence if you miss a period report for check up.

STERILIZATION/ABDOMINAL TUBAL LIGATION/TUBECTOMY

Preoperative Orders:

- Nil by mouth for 6 hours.
- Consent.
- Approved Consent Form duly signed by the patient is a must because it is the proof of coverage of the patient under F P Insurance Scheme
- Record of all preoperative investigation reports.
- Anesthesia fitness.

Operative Notes:

Bilateral tubectomy done on..........at........... under SA/GA/EA

Indication : ....
Method : ....
Surgeon : ....
Anesthesiologist : ....

Steps:

- Patient in supine position.
- Painting and draping done.
- Incision taken 2 cm below the fundus (In case of interval sterilization a suprapubic incision is taken)

- Abdomen opened in layers.
- Both tubes identified, tubes held with Babcock's forceps.
- Tube traced up to fimbrial end.
- Tube ligated with No. 1 chromic catgut at the junction of medial 1/3 and lateral 2/3 and cut (Modified Pomeroy's method)
- Same Procedure repeated on the other side.
- Hemostasis achieved. Correct count of swabs and instruments obtained.
- Abdomen closed in layers. Peritoneum sutured/ with .... , Rectus sheath with ...., Skin with ....
- Patient withstood the procedure well. GC fair pulse..............BP................. PV bleeding minimal.

Post Sterilization Instructions for Patients

- Follow up after 5-7 days for removal of skin stitches and thereafter as advised.
- Maintain personal hygiene and do not soil the dressing.
- Can use Indian toilets.
- Do not massage your abdomen.
- Regular exercise as per instructions after 4 weeks.
- Can move about in home. Avoid travelling for 1 month.
- Avoid eating outside food.
- Take your medicines regularly.
- Can eat less spicy, less chilly, Non vegetarian and fruits, however, consult doctor for proper dietary advice.
- Inform if you have excessive pain, bleeding, fever, bloating of abdomen or discharge from the wound.
- No additional external applications required for the wound.
- Ask all your queries, medical (e.g. About the procedure itself) or nonmedical (e.g. Bill, Discharge) well in advance.
- Rarely sterilization operation can fail, hence, it is important to follow up in case period is missed in future.
- In case of failure MTP can be done especially up to 1st 3 months easily, hence, it is important to report early.
- *Note:* Empanelment of doctor/health center is now compulsory
- The FP Insurance Scheme is applicable only if doctor/health center is empanelled (Registration with appropriate authority)

LAPAROSCOPIC STERILIZATION

Preoperative Orders:

- Nil by mouth for 6 hours.
- Consent.
- Record of preoperative investigation reports.
- Anesthesia fitness.

Operative Notes:

MTP/ Interval laparoscopic tubal ligation done on..................at...................... under GA/SA/EA

Surgeon : ....
Anesthesiologist : ....
LMP : ....

Steps :

- Patient was anesthetized
- Patient in .... position.
- Painting and draping done.
- Findings confirmed under anesthesia. Uterus.................. Wks sized .... shape,Fx........................... Cx.........................
- MTP/D and C done/not done.
- Uterine manipulator introduced/not introduced.
- Intra/Supra/Infra umbilical incision taken for the veress needle.
- Veress needle introduced and intraperitoneal position of the needle confirmed.
- Insufflation done with pressure................../CO2/Air.
- Veress needle removed and trocar cannula introduced.
- Trocar removed and Laparoscope introduced.
- Abdominal cavity inspected for pathology/injury.
- Both tubes visualized and traced up to the fimbrial end.
- Second puncture introduced/ not introduced.
- Silastic band applicator/cautery forceps/ clip applicator introduced.
- Both tubes occluded by silastic band/cautery/clips.
- Hemostasis and proper application of bands/clips confirmed.
- Insufflated gas removed completely.
- Scope and applicator removed.
- Ports closed with ....
- Dressing done
- Patient withstood the surgery well, GC was fair pulse............ BP....................

Postoperative Instructions Following Laparoscopic Sterilization

- You will be called for follow up after 3 days. Make sure that you come.
- You can have full diet after going home.
- As you have been given anesthesia avoid going home on two wheeler, especially if you are feeling giddy or weak at the time of discharge.
- Take your medicines regularly.
- Do not worry about occasional vomiting, pain, bleeding from vagina.
- If vomiting, pain, PV bleeding is excessive or if there is bloating or abdomen excessive oozing from operation site, report immediately.
- You may get your menses after 1 month to 6 weeks.
- Maintain personal hygiene and do not soil the dressing.
- Ask your queries, medical (e.g. About the procedure itself) or nonmedical (e.g.Bill, Discharge) well in advance.
- Rarely tubectomy operation can fail, so it is important to report it you miss your period in future.
- In case of failure MTP can be done especially) up to first 3 months easily, hence, it is important to report early.

DIAGNOSTIC LAPAROSCOPY+ HYSTEROSCOPY

Preoperative Orders:

- Nill by mouth for 6 hours.
- Consent.
- Record of all preop investigation reports.
- Anesthesia fitness.

Operative Notes:

Diagnostic laparoscopy done on .... at .... under GA/SA/EA

LMP : ....
Indication : ....
Surgeon : ....
Anesthesiologist : ....

Steps:

- Patient was anesthetized (after confirming that she has visited the toilet and passed urine before coming to the OT)
- Patient in .... postion .
- Painting and draping done.
- Findings confirmed under anesthesia Uterus size................shape, Fx.................. Cx.............................
- Hysteroscopy done
- Uterine manipulator introduced/ not introduced.
- Intra/Supra/Infra umbilical incision taken for the veress needle.
- Veress needle introduced and intraperitoneal position of the needle confirmed.
- Insufflation done with .... CO2/Air (Pressure)
- Veress needle removed and trocar cannula introduced.
- Trocar removed and Scope introduced.
- Second puncture introduced / not introduced.
- Abdominal cavity inspected for pathology/ injury.

(SPACE FOR DIAGRAM AND FINDINGS AND COMMENTS)

- Chromopertubation done spill present/not present.
- Additional surgery performed............. details.................
- Hemostasis confirmed.
- Insufflated Gas removed completely.
- Scope removed.
- Ports Closed with
- Dressing done.
- Specimen send for HPE.
- Patient withstood the surgery well. GC was fair Pulse..................... BP........................
Postoperative instructions for patients : Followup after 5 days.

POSTOPERATIVE INSTRUCTIONS FOR DIAGNOSTIC LAPAROSCOPY AND HYSTEROSCOPY

- You will be called for follow up after 3 days. Please make sure that you come.
- You can have full diet after going home.
- As you have been given anesthesia avoid going home on two wheeler, expecially if you are feeling giddy or weak at the time of discharge.
- Take your medicines regularly.
- Do not worry about occasional vomiting , pain PV bleeding.
- If vomiting, pain, PV bleeding is excessive or if there is fever report immediately. Report if there is oozing from opereation site, or bloating of abdomen.

- Abstain from sex till next menses.
- You may get your next menses after 1 month to 6 weeks.
- Maintain personal hygiene and don't soil the dressing.
- Your operative findings will be discussed with you on .... at ....
- Please ask all your queries, medical (e.g. About procedure itself) or nonmedical (e.g. Bill, Discharge) well in advance.

VAGINAL DELIVERY NOTES

Labor analgesia given/ not given. Method................

A full term/premature/IUGR, male/ female baby of .... kg weight, delivered by vertex/breech on .... at .... with/without forceps/ ventouse applied for .... (indication)

Episiotomy sutured with .... in layers.

Baby cried / didn't cry immediately after birth. Apgar at 1 min .... 5 min.......................

Placenta and membranes expelled completely. Placental wt................ inj. Ergometrine/ Prostaglandin/ oxytocin given uterus well retracted.

Blood loss...................... PPH Yes/No. If PPH Present .... cause .... Treatment......................

Patient withstood the process of delivery well. GC pulse .... BP.................. one hourly for 2 hours

POST-DELIVERY INSTRUCTIONS TO PATIENT

- You will be called for follow up after 7 days. Make sure that you come.
- Take all the medicines that are prescribed. Don't take any other medicines without consultation.
- Episiotomy care: The cut taken during the delivery of the baby is called episiotomy. It should be washed and Kept clean after passing urine and motion every time. If absorbable sutures are used, removal is not necessary.
- Maintain personal hygiene. Take laxative if a pass hard stools.
- Nipple: It is essential to keep them clean. Dry them with cotton and clean after every feed with hind milk.
- Avoid engorgement of breast.
- You will have PV discharge for 6 weeks which is normal.
- If pain, bleeding is excessive or if there is fever please inform.
- Abstinence for 6 weeks. Later contraceptives should be used.
- IUCD can be introduced within 3 months of delivery or after menses whichever is earlier.
- Return of normal menses varies with every individual, i.e. From 1½ months to 1½ years.
- Normal routine light work can be done up to 6 weeks.
- Can eat less spicy, less chilly, veg, non-veg, and fruits.
- Please make all your queries, medical (e. g. about the procedure itself) or non medical (e.g. Bill, Discharge) well in advance.

LSCS

Preoperative Orders:

- Nil by mouth for 6 hours (in case of elective LSCS)
- Consent should include indication of LSCS and should be understood by patient

- Preoperative Investigations
  haemoglobin
  Urine
  Blood grouping and Rh typing.
- Blood for grouping and cross-matching (if facilities available)
- Record of all investigations done in the antenatal period.
- Anesthesia fitness.

Operative Notes

Procedure : Emergency/ Elective LSCS done under GA/SA/EA on .... at.........................
Indication :

Steps:

- Patient anesthetized supine position and painting draping done.
- Bladder
- Catherized
- Under all aseptic precautions abdomen opened by .... incision.
- LUS identified, UV fold opened, and bladder pushed down.
- LUS opened transversely, liquor clear/meconium stained/reduced/adequate/absent.
- A full term/premature/IUGR, male/female baby of .... kg wt delivered by vertex/breech on.............. at....................with/without forceps.
- Baby cried/did not cry immediately after birth. Apgar at 1 min.................3 min.................5 min.................
- Placenta and membranes expelled out completely. Placental weight.....................
- Uterus well retracted.
- LUS stitched in single/double layer using...................
- Bilateral tubal ligation not done/done by ....method using .... suture material.
- Complete hemostasis confirmed.
- Mop and instrument and needle count checked and found to be correct.
- Abdomen closed in layers. Peritoneum with .... Rectus sheath with ....Skin with ....
- PPH Present/not present.
- Post op vaginal cleaning done with povidone-iodine.
- Urine output................ Appearance......................
- Baby Attended by.....................
  Full term/Preterm/IUGR
  Male/Female,wt..................
  on..................at....................
  Injections given.........................
- Incidental intra-abdominal findings....................... Additional findings e.g. cord round neck knot in cord amt. of liquor type of placenta any other relevant findings.
- Patient with stood the surgery well. General condition was fair.
  Pulse................BP.................PA....................PV....................Urine output................ (1 hourly for 2 hours)

Special Post op instruction (1) Encourage breastfeeding (2) Watch for bleeding per vaginum and vitals (3) BP monitoring specially in patients with PIH (4) Input-Output charting (5) Uterus well contracted

ABDOMINAL HYSTERECTOMY

Preop Orders:

- Nil by mouth for 6 hrs.
- Shaving/Enema (optional)

- Informed Consent
- Indication
- Blood for grouping and cross-matching
- Record of all-investigation done.
- Anesthesia fitness.

Operative Notes:

TAH with/without BSO done under GA/SA/EA on .... at.......................

Indication : ....
Surgeons : ....
Anesthesiologist : ....

Steps:

- Patient anesthetized.
- Patient in-supine position.
- Bladder catheterized under all aseptic precautions.
- Painting and draping done.
- Findings confirmed under anesthesia.
- Under all aseptic precautions abdomen opened in layers.
- Preoperative findings were noted as ....
- Round ligament clamped cut and ligated with .... (sature material)
- Anterior pouch opened and bladder dissected down.
- Infundibulopelvic ligament clamed, cut and ligated with..................... (If ovary is to be conserved the clamp is placed on the medial side of the tube and ovary)
- Uterine vessels on both sides clamped, cut and ligated with ....
- Uterosacrals on both the sides damped, cut and ligated with ....
- Vagina opened, specimen separated and vagina closed with..................
- Hemostasis confirmed.
- Sponge, instrument and needle count confirmed and found to be correct.
- Abdomen closed in layers. Peritoneum with .... Rectus sheath with ...., Skin with........................
- Postoperatively urine output .... appearance........................
- Patient withstood the procedure well. GC was fair, Pulse .... BP .... PA .... PV..................... urine output ....
- Average blood loss was ....
- Additional findings if any specify
  Adhesions-Intestinal/omental.
  Bladder dissection difficulties.
  Abnormal anatomical findings if any.

VAGINAL HYSTERECTOMY

Preoperative Orders:

- Nil by mouth for 6 hours.
- Shaving/Enema (optional)
- Informed consent

- Blood for grouping and cross-matching
- Record of all investigations done.
- Anesthesia fitness.

Operative Notes:

Vaginal Hysterectomy with USO or BSO with/without Ant colporrhaphy/Post colpoperineorrhaphy done under GA/SA/EA...........on...........at

Indication : ....
Surgeons : ....
Anesthesiologists : ....

Steps:

- Patient was anesthetized.
- Patient in lithotomy position.
- Painting and draping was done.
- Bladder catheterized under all aseptic precautions.
- Findings confirmed under anesthesia.
- Anterior and Posterior pouches opened taking care not to injure bladder and rectum.
- Mackenrodts ligament/uterines/Broad ligament and TO ligaments clamped, cut and ligated with .... in succession.
- Overies visualized.................... appearance................ removed/not removed.
- Hemostasis confirmed.
- Peritonization done/ not done.
- A repair and P repair done / not done.
- Vault suspension done.
- Sponge, instrument and needle count confirmed and found to be correct.
- Vaginal pack kept/not kept.
- Postoperative Urine output..................appearance....................
- Patient withstood the procedure well. GC was fair Pulse .... BP .... PA .... PV.......................
- Average blood loss.
- Additional findings if any
- Adhesions-Intestinal/omental.
- Bladder dissection difficulties.
- Abnormal anatomical findings if any.

Salient point in post op orders: Removal of pack if kept.

Watch for vitals, Input-output charting

POSTOPERATIVE INSTRUCTIONS OF MAJOR PROCEDURES

- Follow up after 5-7 days and thereafter as advised.
- Maintain personal hygiene and dont't soil the dressing (if any)
- Can use Indian toilet,
- Do not massage your abdomen.
- Do your exercise regularly as per instructions after 4 weeks.
- Avoid lifting heavy things for next 4 weeks.

- Avoid travelling but can move about at home normally.
- Avoid eating outside food.
- Take your medicines regularly.
- Can eat less spicy, less chilly,veg; nonveg and fruits, however, consult the doctor for proper dietary advice.
- Inform if you have excessive pain, bleeding, fever,vomiting,bloating of abdomen or discharge through the wound, uncontrolled passage of urine.
- No additional external application of any kind is required for the wound.
- Abstinence till further advice.
- Ask all your queries, medical (e.g. About the procedure itself) or non medical (e.g. Bill, Discharge) well in advance.

Postoperative Orders :

- Head low given/not given
- NBM till further orders
- Strict I/O chart
- TPR/BP chart
- W/F abdominal distention
- I/V fluids as per requirement
- I/V antibiotics/analgesics
- Inform pulse/BP/Urine output
- Inform abdominal distention

POSTMORTEM

The Following points should be used while

Communicating with the Aggrieved Relatives

- Postmortem is a scientific process of studying the internal parts of the body to evalute the time and cause of death. This helps in arriving at correct diagnosis and in Medicolegal cases it helps in proving or disproving negligence.
- Postmortem does not amount to unnecessary mutilation of the body. The performing doctor never treats the body with disrespect and always takes care not to unsult the religious feelings of the diseased or the relatives.
- We all understand the feelings of the relatives and as doctors we never would want to add further stress to their grief. But there are situations during which the law of the land forces us to send the body for postmortem.
- If the present situation demands that PM be done, then refusing to allow the body to be shifted for PM is not in the best interest of all the involved parties. Such an act can be illegal and punishable by law.
- So we request you to co-operate with us to shift the body with dignity and respect and allow the law enforcing authorities to give justice to the deceased.

Special Notes:

1. Postmortem is mandatory in the following situations:
    - Table Death
    - Suicidal Death
    - Homicidal Death
    - Death within 24 hrs of admission if the case was undermined
    - MLC PM can be asked by the doctor for which relatives consent is not required
    - Whenever MLC PM is indicated refusal by patient's relative cannot be an excuse.

ANTENATAL CHECK LIST

Pt Name

Blood Group

Allergies

ANTENATAL CHECK LIST

Bld Invest	1st trimester	2nd trimester	3rd trimester
USG	11 to 13 weeks	20 to 22 weeks	
InjTT			
Registration	Place of Delievery		
	Lactation Advise		
	Exercise Chart		
	Charges		
	Blood Arrangement		
	Communicate risk		
Special Invest for: Associated Medical Problem			
Prev Surg	Minor/Major/Gyn	Complications	
Prev Anes	SA/EA/GA/LA	Complications	
Labor	Relative Attendance		
Instructions	Blood Donors		
	Complications		
	Risk Factors	Infertility	Short height
		BOH	Obesity
		Prev LSCS	CPD
		IUGR	Surgery
		Incomp Os	Elderly
		Hydramnios	Prev abortion
		Rh Factor	Postdatism
		PIH	Prev Bid Tr
		Threatened abortion	Hepatitis
		Prematurity	Thyroid
		DM	Oligohydramnios
		H/vPPH	Anemia
		APH/PP	

ANTENATAL INVESTIGATIONS

Name :		Bld Group :	Allergy		
Date	1	2	3	4	5
Laboratory					
Hb					
Hemogram					
Urine : A					
: S					
: Micro					
BSL : F					
: PP					
VDRL HIV			HbsAg		
OGCT TSH			Triple Test		

IF Rh Negative

Husb Bld Gp	ICT

IF DM

Glyco Hb	1	2		
BSL : F	1	2	3	4
: PP	1	2	3	4

If Thyroid Problem

FT3	1	2	3
FT 14	1	2	3
TSH	1	2	3

Special tests as per indications

SECTION-II

TIPS ON PNDT ACT

PREVENTION IS BETTER THAN CURE
IGNORANCE OF LAW IS NO EXCUSE

Why Prevention is Necessary?

Offences and Penalties

Prohibition of advertisement relating to preconception and prenatal determination of sex

Owner of the place or any employee (Permanent or honorary)

- For first contravention—imprisonment up to 3 years and with fine which may extend to 10,000 rupees
- For subsequent Contravention—imprisonment up to 5 years and with fine which may extend up to Rs 50,000
- The name of the Registered Medical practitioner shall be reported by the AA to the State Medical Council concerned for taking necessary actions.
- Suspension of registration—if the charges are framed by the court and till case is disposed off.
- Removal of the name from the register of the council
  - For Five Years — for the first conviction
  - Permanently — for subsequent offence

Contravention of any provisions or any rules for which no penalty has been 1
Elsewhere provided in this act punishment is imprisonment up to 3 months or fine up to Rs. 1000/- or both.
Continuing contravention additional Rs five hundred for every day during which such
Contravention continues after conviction for the first such contravention

Every offence under this Act shall be

Cognizable non-bailable non-compoundable

Cognizance of offences

- Only Metropolitan Magistrate or Judicial Magistrate of the first class
- Only on a complaint by
  - The AA Concerned or authorized officer
  - A Person who has given at least 15 days notice to the AA of alleged offence and of his intention to make a complaint to the court.

Registration of the center is mandatory as

- Genetic counseling center
- Genetic laboratory
- Genetic clinic
- Ultrasonography center
- Imaging science center

-No center can function without registration

Registration of center

- Application to appropriate authority
- Form A in duplicate— Properly filled
- Mention procedure for which approval is asked for i.e.
  - Ultrasound
  - Chorion biopsy
  - Amniocentesis
  - Cordocentesis
  - Foetoscopy
  - Fetal biopsy
- List of employees with address and registration number—employee includes visiting doctors also.

- Prescribed documents of
  - Degree certificate
  - Experience certificate
  - Registration certificate
  - Undertaking on stamp paper of Rs 50.00

Undertaking

Center do not/shall not conduct any technique, test or procedure for preconceptions sex selection and/or prenatal sex determination

- Details of Sonography Machine
  - Make
  - Manufacturer
  - Model
  - Portability
- Prescribed fees by DD drawn in favor of AA on any scheduled bank

  Rs 3000.00
  - Genetic counseling center
  - Genetic laboratory
  - Genetic Clinic

  Rs. 4000.00
  - Combination
  - Organization
  - Institution

Certificate of Registration

- Form B in duplicate provided by Appropriate Authority in duplicate
- One copy is to be displayed at a conspicuous place at the place of business
- Non transferable
- Both copies of registration shall be surrendered to Appropriate Aurthority in case of
  - Change of ownership
  - Change of manangement
  - Ceasing to function
- New owner/manager will have to apply afresh for registration

Rejection of Application

- Form C
- Within 90 days—for the reasons recorded in writing by Appropriate Authority
- Re-submission within 90 days
- Within 90 days—no new fees
- Any subsequent application shall be accompanied with the prescribed fees
- Application fees is nonrefundable
- Fees collected shall be utilized by appropriate authority in activities connected with implementation of provisions of the act.

Validity of Registration— Five years from date of issue

Renewal of Registration

- Form A in duplicate to appropriate authority
- Thirty days before the date of expiry of certificate of registration
- Will be given in Form B
- For five years from date of expiry
- Application may be rejected for reasons
- Will be communicated in Form C giving reasons in writing
- Fees payable—one half of the fee paid for authorization
- Surrender immediately both copies of earlier certificate of registration to AA in case of
  - Renewal of registration
  - Rejection of renewal

Deemed Renewal

In event of failure of the appropriate authority to renew the certificate of registration or to communicate within a period of 90 days from the date of receipt of application for renewal of registration, the certificate of registration shall be deemed to have been renewed

Display at conspicuous place-3 feet × 2 feet board (blue background and white text)
Name of the hospital/nursing home ______________________________
Address ______________________________
Antenatal sex determination is punishable offence.
Sex determination is not done here.

Maintenance and Preservation of Records

- Register containing - Serial No., Name, Age, and Address of patient, Name of husband/father, Date of counseling, Procedure and test, Parity, Indication of procedure and Name of the person performing procedure (To be preserved for two years and kept ready for inspection whenever demanded by AA)

What to Preserve

Form of consent	Laboratory results	Microscopic pictures
Sonographic plates	Slides	Recommendation chits/letters

Prescribed Forms—to be filled and signed properly
Form D : Genetic Counseling Center
Form E : Genetic Laboratory
Form F : Genetic Clinic/Ultrasonography center/ Imaging science center Form G: Invasive procedure

- Duly signed by patient
- Risk should be explained in language in which patient understands
- You can send specimen to registered genetic laboratory only
- Genetic laboratory can receive specimen from registered center only
- It shall no: be necessary for genetic laboratory to obtain a fresh consent.

Any deficiency or inaccuracy found in record shall amount to contravention of provisions

Of Act unless contrary is proved by person conducting antenatal ultrasonography.
Form H : Appropriate authority shall maintain a permanent record of

- Applications for grant of renewal of certificate of registration.
- Letter of intimation of every change of employee, place, machine, etc.
- Address and equipment installed.

Prescribed Form of Declaration of Pregnant Woman

- I Mrs .... declare that by undergoing ultrasonography/ image scanning, etc. I do not want to know the sex of my fetus.

Date: Signature/thumb impression of pregnant woman

Place:

Prescribed Forms declaration of doctor/person conducting ultrasonography/imaging scanning

- I, Dr... declare that while conducting ultrasonography/image scanning on Ms...................................., I have neither detected nor disclosed the sex of her fetus to any body in any manner.

Date:

Place: Signature

(Declaration below each and every report of antenatal sonography is mandatory)

Written consent of pregnant woman is mandatory, if you do ultrasound examination or invasive procedures irrespective of gestational age.

- Form should be filled up in triplicate
- One Form is to be given to the patient
- One is to be kept for office record
- One is to be sent to the appropriate authority every month before 5th of next month

Period of Preservation

- For two years from the date of completion of date of counseling, prenatal diagnostic procedure or prenatal diagnostic test.
- In event of any legal proceeding till the final disposal of legal proceeding or for two years whichever is later.

Record on Computer or other Electronic Equipment

Printed copy of records shall be taken and preserved after authentication by a person responsible for such records

Intimation of Change within Thirty Days of

– Employee – Place – Address – Equipment installed

Registration of USG machine—Detail of machine

– Make – Model – Manufacturer – Immovable/portable

Sale of machine—to registered center only

One can not buy, install or use USG machine for antenatal sonography unless center and machine are registered

Non use of machine—Intimate appropriate authority

- Due to Repair, Permanent non use or Buy back to company
- Surrender certificate of registration to Appropriate Authority

Bare act on demand for persual—Copy both in English and local language (with latest amendments) shall be available to patient and their relatives and each and every visitor.

Remedies—when?

– Notice issued – Machine seized – Registration suspended/cancelled

Doctor's Reaction to the Notice

– Hide – Ignore – Panic – Influence – Advice

What happens next—Exploitation by

– Patient/relatives – Politician – Police – Pleader – Press

– Panchayat (So called social group) – Protection groups (NGOs)

What to do on Receiving Notice

- Do not panic
- Do not ignore
- Discuss with friends/seniors—medical opinion
- Advocate-legal opinion
- Take Medicolegal opinion
- Reply within 30 days or in a stipulated time given in notice
- Reply on letter pad
- Reply to the point—No unnecessary writing
- No admissions
- Attach documents with your reply

Search and Seizures

- Appropriate Authority or person designated by appropriate authority suo moto or on complaint may visit center for
  - Inspection
  - Search
  - Seizure
- Cooperate with them—not your enemy
- Answer their questions patiently

Appeal Within 30 Days

On satisfaction of the sufficient cause of delay the appropriate authority may condone the dalay. Appeal shall be made to the

- Sub district appropriate authority
- District appropriate authority if order is passed by Sub District AA
- State appropriate authority/UTAA if order is passed by District AA
- State Government if order is passed by state AA
- Central appropriate authority
- Central Government if order is passed by central AA
  Each appeal shall be disposed of within sixty days of its receipt.

Judicial Remedies

- Judicial Magistrate first class
- Metropolitan Magistrate
- Sessions Court
- High Court
- Supreme Court

Code of Conduct

1. Do not conduct or associate with sex detection and disclosure
2. Do not employ unqualified person
3. Don't refer for sex determination
4. Do not do procedure at unregistered place
5. Ensure no violation of rules

6. Help law enforcing agency to book violators
7. Display name and designation prominently on the dress worn
8. Write name and designation in full under signature
9. Do not conduct female feticide
10. No professional misconduct

FORM A

[See Rules 4(1) and 8(i)]

(To be submitted in duplicate with supporting documents as enclosures)

FORM OF APPLICATION FOR REGISTRATION OR RENEWAL OF REGISTRATION OF A GENETIC COUNSELING CENTER/GENETIC LABORATORY/GENETIC CLINIC/ ULTRASOUND CLINIC/IMAGING CENTER

1. Name of the applicant________________________________
   (Indicate name of the organization sought to be registered)
2. Address of the applicant________________________________
3. Type of facility to be registered____________________________
   (Please specify whether the application is for registration of a Genetic Counseling Center/Genetic Laboratory/ Genetic Clinic/Ultrasound Clinic/Imaging Center or any combination of these)
4. Full name and address/addresses of Genetic Counseling Center/Genetic Laboratory/Genetic Clinic/Ultrasound Clinic/Imaging Center with Telephone/Fax number(s) Telegraphic/Telex/E-mail address(s).
5. Type of ownership of Organization(individual ownership/partnership/company/cooperative/any other to be specified). In case type of organization is other than individual ownership, furnish copy of articles of association and names and addresses of other persons responsible for management, as enclosure.
6. Type of Institution (Govt. Hospital/Municipal Hospital/Public Hospital/Private Hospital/Private Nursing Home/ Private Clinic/Private Laboratory/any other to be stated.)
7. Specific prenatal diagnostic procedures/tests for which approval is sought
   (a) Invasive (i) amniocentesis/chorionic villi aspiration/chromosomal/biochemical/molecular studies
   (b) Non-Invasive Ultrasonography
   Leave blank if registration is sought for Genetic Counselling Center only.
8. Equipment available with the make and model of each equipment (List to be attached on a separate sheet).
9. (a) Facilities available in the Counselling Center.
   (b) Whether facilities are or would be available in the Laboratory/Clinic for the following tests:
      i. Ultrasound
      ii. Amniocentesis
      iii. Chorionic villi aspiration
      iv. Fetoscopy
      v. Fetal biopsy
      vi. Cordocentesis
   Whether facilities are available in the Laboratory/Clinic for the following:
   i. Chromosomal studies
   ii. Biochemical studies
   iii. Molecular studies
   iv. Preimplantation genetic diagnosis
10. Names, qualifications, experience, and registration number of employees (may be furnished as an enclosure).

11. State whether the Genetic Counseling Center/Genetic Laboratory/Genetic Clinic/Ultrasound Clinic/imaging center qualifies for registration in terms of requirements laid down in Rule 3.
12. For renewal applications only:
    (a) Registration No.
    (b) Date of issue and date of expiry of existing certificate of registration.
13. List of Enclosures:
    (Please attach a list of enclosures supporting documents attached to this application.)

Date:

Place: (..)

Name, designation and signature of the person authorized to sign on behalf of the organization to be resistered.

DECLARATION

I, Shri/Smt/Kum./Dr. .... son/daughter/wife of .... aged .... years resident of .... working as (indicate designation) .... in (indicate name of the organization to be registered) .... hereby declare that I have read and understood the Prenatal Diagnostic

Techniques (Regulation and Prevention of Misuse) Act,1994 (57 of 1994) and the prenatal Diagnostic Techniques (Regulation and prevention of Misuse) Rules,1996,

I also undertake to explain the said Act and Rules to all employees of the Genetic Counseling Center/Genetic Laoratory/Genetic Clinic/ultrasound clinic/imaging center in respect of which registration is sought and to ensure that Act and Rules are fully compiled with.

Date:

Place: (..)

Name, designation and signature of the person authorized to sign on behalf of the organization to be registered
[SEAL OF THE ORGANIZATION SOUGHT TO BE REGISTERED]

ACKNOWLEDGMENT

The application in Form A in duplicate for grant*/renewal of registration of Genetic Counseling Center*/Genetic Laboratory*/Genetic Clinic*/Ultrasound Clinic*/Imaging Center* by .... (Name and address of applicant) has been received by the Appropriate Authority .... on (date).

The list of enclosures attached to the application in Form A has been verified with the enclosures submitted and found to be correct.

Or

*On verification it is found that the following documents mentioned in the list of enclosures are not actually enclosed. This acknowledgment does not confer any rights on the applicant for grant or renewal of registration.

Date: (..)

Place:
SEAL

Signature and Designation of Appropriate Authority or authorized person in the office of the Appropriate Authority.

Strike out whichever is not applicable or not necessary. All enclosures are to be authenticated by signature of the applicant.

FORM B

[See Rules 6(2), 6(5) and 8(2)]
CERTIFICATE OF REGISTRATION
(To be issued in duplicate)

1. In exercise of the powers conferred under Section 19 (1) of the prenatal Diagnostic Techniques (Regulation and Prevention of Misuse) Act,1994 (57 of 1994), the Appropriate Authority hereby grants registration to the Genetic Counseling Center*/Genetic Laboratory/Genetic Clinic/Ultrasound Clinic/Imaging Center named below for purposes of carrying out Genetic Counseling/Prenatal Diagnostic Procedures*/Prenatal Diagnostic Tests/ ultrasonography under the aforesaid Act for a period of five years ending on
2. This registation is granted subject to the aforesaid Act and Rules thereunder and any contravention thereof shall result in suspension or cancellation of this certificate of Registration before the expiry of the said period of five years apart from prosecution.
   A. Name and address of the Genetic Counseling Center*/Genetic Laboratory*/Genetic Clinic/Ultrasound Clinic/ Imaging Center*
   B. Prenatal diagnostic procedures* approved for (Genetic clinic)

      Non-Invasive
      i. Ultrasound

      Invasive
      ii. Amniocentesis
      iii. Chorionic villi biopsy
      iv. Fetoscopy
      v. Fetal skin or organ biopsy
      vi. Cordocentesis
      vii. Any other (specify)
   C. Prenatal diagnostic tests* approved (for Genetic laboratory)
      i. Chromosomal studies
      ii. Biochemical studies
      iii. Molecular studies
   D. Any other purpose (please specify)
3. Model and make of equipment being used (any change is to be intimated to the Appropriate Authority under Rule 13).
4. Registration No. allotted
5. Period of validity of earlier Certificate of Registration.
   (For renewal Certificate of Registration only) From.........To...........

Signature, name and designation of
the Appropriate Authority
SEAL

Date:
Place:

DISPLAY ONE COPY OF THIS CERTIFICATE AT A CONSPICUOUS PLACE AT THE PLACE OF BUSINESS

FORM C

[See Rules 6(3) 6(5) and 8(3)]
FORM FOR REJECTION OF APPLICATION FOR GRANT/RENEWAL OF REGISTRATION

In exercise of the powers conferred under Section 19(2) of the prenatal Diagnostic Techniques (Regulation and Prevention of Misuse) Act,1994, the Appropriate Authority hereby rejects the application for grant*/renewal of registration of the undermentioned Genetic Counseling Center*/Genetic Laboratory*/Genetic Clinic*/Ultrasound Clinic*/Imaging Center*

1. Name and address of the Genetic Counseling Center*/Genetic Laboratory*/Genetic Clinic*/Ultrasound Clinic*/ Imaging Center
2. Reasons for rejection of application for grant/renewal of registration: (..)

Date: Signature, name and designation of the Appropriate Authority with SEAL of Office

Place:

*Strike out whichever is not applicable or necessary.

FORM D

[See Rule 9(2)]
FORM FOR MAINTENANCE OF RECORDS BY THE GENETIC COUNSELING CENTER

1. Name and address of Genetic Counseling center.
2. Registration No
3. Patient's name
4. Age
5. Husband's/Father's name
6. Full address with Tel.No, if any
7. Referred by (Full name and address of Doctor(s) with registration No.(s) (Referral note to be preserved carefully with case papers)
8. Last menstrual period/weeks of pregnancy
9. History of genetic/medical disease in the family (specify)
   Basis of diagnosis:
   (a) Clinical
   (b) Biochemical
   (c) Cytogenetic
   (d) Other (e.g. radiological, ultrasonography)
10. Indication for prenatal diagnosis
    A. Previous child/children with:
       i. Chromosomal disorders
       ii. Metabolic disorders
       iii. Congenital anomaly
       iv. Mental retardation
       v. Hemoglobinopathy
       vi. Sex linked disorders
       vii. Single gene disorder
       viii. Any other (specify)

B. Advanced maternal age (35 years or above)
C. Mother/Father/sibling having genetic disease (specify)
D. Others (specify)

11. Procedure advised
    i. Ultrasound
    ii. Amniocentesis
    iii. Chorionic villi biopsy
    iv. Fetoscopy
    v. Fetal skin or organ biopsy
    vi. Cordocentesis
    vii. Any other (specify)
12. Laboratory tests to be carried out
    i. Chromosomal studies
    ii. Biochemical studies
    iii. Molecular studies
    iv. Preimplantation genetic diagnosis
13. Result of diagnosis If abnormal give details. Normal/Abnormal
14. Was MTP advised?
15. Name and address of Genetic Clinic* to which patient is referred
16. Dates of commencement and completion of genetic counseling

Place:

Date:

Name, Signature and Registration No. of the Medical Genesticist/Gynecologist/Pediatrician administering Genetic Counseling.

FORM E

[See Rule 9(3)]

FORM FOR MAINTENANCE OF RECORDS BY GENETIC LABORATORY

1. Name and address of Genetic Laboratory
2. Registation Number
3. Patient's name
4. Age
5. Husband's/Father's name
6. Full address with Tel.No, if any
7. Referred by/sample sent of (full name and address of Genetic Clinic) (Referral note to be preserved carefully with case papers)
8. Type of sample: Maternal blood/Chorionic villus sample/amniotic fluid/Fetal blood or other fetal tissue (specify)
9. Specify indication for prenatal diagnosis
   A. Previous child/children with
      i. Chromosomal disorders
      ii. Metabolic disorders
      iii. Malformation(s)
      iv. Mental retardation
      v. Hereditary hemolytic anemia
      vi. Sex linked disorder
      vii. Single gene disorder
      viii. Any other (specify)

B. Advanced maternal age (35 years or above)
C. Mother/father/sibling having genetic disease (specify)
D. Other (specify)

10. Laboratory tests carried out (give details)
    i. Chromosomal studies
    ii. Biochemical studies
    iii. Molecular studies
    iv. Preimplantation genetic diagnosis
11. Result of diagnosis If abnormal give details. Normal/Abnormal
12. Date(s) on which tests carried out.
    The results of the prenatal diagnostic tests were conveyed to..............on...................

Place: Name, Signature and Registration No. of the
Date: Medical Geneticist/Director of the Institute

FORM F

[See provision to Section 4(3), Rule 9(4) and Rule 10 (1A)]

FORM FOR MAINTENANCE OF RECORD IN RESPECT OF PREGNANT WOMAN BY GENETIC CLINIC/ULTRASOUND CLINIC/IMAGING CENTER

1. Name and address of the Genetic Clinic/Ultrasound Clinic/Imaging Center.
2. Registration No.
3. Patient's name and her age
4. Number of children with sex of each child
5. Husband's/Father's name
6. Full address with Tel.No.,if any
7. Referred by (full name and address of Doctor(s)/Genetic Counseling Center(Referral note to be preserved carefully with case papers)/self referral
8. Last menstrual period/weeks of pregnancy
9. History of genetic/medical disease in the family (specify)
   Basis of diagnosis:
   (a) Clinical
   (b) Biochemical
   (c) Cytogenetic
   (d) Other(e.g.radiological,ultrasonography, etc. specify)
10. Indication for prenatal diagnosis
    A. Previous child/children with:
        i. Chromosomal disorders
        ii. Metabolic disorders
        iii. Congenital anomaly
        iv. Mental retardation
        v. Hemoglobinopathy
        vi. Sex linked disorders
        vii. Single gene disorder
        viii. Any other (specify)
    B. Advanced maternal age (35 years)
    C. Mother/father/sibling has genetic disease (specify)
    D. Other (specify)

11. Procedures carried out (with name and registration No. of Gynecologist/Radiologist/Registered Medical Practitioner) who performed it.

    Non-Invasive

    i. Ultrasound (specify purpose for which ultrasound is to be done during pregnancy (List of indications for ultrasonography of pregnant women are given in the note below.)

    Invasive

    ii. Amniocentesis
    iii. Chorionic villi aspiration
    iv. Fetal biopsy
    v. Cordocentesis
    vi. Any other (specify)
12. Any complication of procedure-please specify
13. Laboratory tests recommended 3[3]
    i. Chromosomal studies
    ii. Biochemical studies
    iii. Molecular studies
    iv. Preimplantation genetic diagnosis
14. Result of
    a. Prenatal diagnostic procedure (given details)
    b. Ultrasonography Normal/Abnormal
       (specify abnormality detected, if any)
15. Date(s) on which procedures carried out.
16. Date on which consent obtained. (In case of invasive)
17. The result of prenatal diagnostic procedure were conveyed to on
18. Was MTP advised/conducted?
19. Date on which MTP carried out.

Date: Name, Signature and Registration number of the Gynecologist/Radiologist/Director of the Clinic

Place:

DECLARATION OF PREGNANT WOMAN

I, Ms...........................(name of the pregnant woman) declare that by undergoing ultrasonography/image scanning, etc. I do not want to know the sex of my fetus.

Date: Signature/Thump impression of pregnant woman

Place:

DECLARATION OF DOCTOR/PERSON CONDUCTING ULTRASONOGRAPHY/IMAGE SCANNING

I, ... (name of the person conducting ultrasonography/image scanning) declare that while conducting ultrasonography/image scanning on Ms..............(name of the pregnant woman), I have neither detected nor disclosed the sex of her fetus to any body in any manner.

Place: Name and signature of the person conducting ultrasonography/image scanning/Director or owner of genetic clinic/ultrasound clinic/imaging center.

Date:

IMPORTANT NOTE

i. Ultrasound is not indicated/advised performed to determine the sex of fetus except for diagnosis of sex-linked diseases such as Duchenne Muscular Dystrophy, Hemophilia A and B, etc.

ii. During pregnancy ultrasonography should only be performed when indicated. The following is the representative list of indications for ultrasound during pregnancy.

1. To diagnose intrauterine and/or ectopic pregnancy and confirm viability.
2. Estimation of gestational age (dating)
3. Detection of number of fetuses and their chorionicity.
4. Suspected pregnancy with IUCD in situ or suspected pregnancy following contraceptive failure/MTP failure.
5. Vaginal bleeding/leaking.
6. Follow-up of cases of abortion
7. Assessment of cervical canal and diameter of internal os.
8. Discrepancy between uterine size and period of amenorrhea.
9. Any suspected adnexal or uterine pathology/abnormality
10. Detection of chromosomal abnormalities, fetal structural defects and other abnormalities and their follow up.
11. To evaluate fetal presentation and position
12. Assessment of liquor amnii.
13. Preterm labor/preterm premature rupture of membranes.
14. Evaluation of placental position, thickness, grading and abnormalities (placenta previa, retroplacental hemorrhage, abnormal adherence, etc.)
15. Evaluation of umbilical cord—presentation,insertion, nuchal encirclement, number of vessels and presence of true knot.
16. Evaluation of previous cesarean section scars.
17. Evaluation of fetal growth parameters, fetal weight and fetal well being.
18. Color flow mapping and duplex Doppler studies.
19. Ultrasound guided procedures such as medical termination of pregnancy, external cephalic version, etc. and their follow-up.
20. Adjunct to diagnostic and therapeutic invasive interventions such as chorionic villus sampling (CVS) amniocentesis, fetal blood sampling, fetal skin biopsy, amnio-infusion, intrauterine infusion, placement of shunts, etc.
21. Observation of intra-partum events.
22. Medical/surgical conditions complicating pregnancy.
23. Research/scientific studies in recognized institutions.

Person conducting ultrasonography on a pregnant woman shall keep complete record thereof in the clinic/center in Form-F and any deficiency or Inaccuracy found therein shall amount to contravention of provisions of Section 5 or Section 6 of the Act, unless contrary is proved by the person conducting such ultrasonography.

FORM G

[See Rule 10]
FORM OF CONSENT
(For invasive techniques)

I,............... wife/daughter of .... Age .... years residing at .... hereby state that I have been explained fully the probable side effects and after effects of the prenatal diagnostic procedures.

I wish to undergo the preimplantation/prenatal diagnostic technique/test/procedures in my own interest to find out the possibility of any abnormality (i.e. disease/deformity/disorder) in the child I am carrying.

I undertake not to terminate the pregnancy if the prenatal procedure Technique/test conducted shows the absence of disease/deformity/disorder.

I understand that the sex of the fetus will not be disclosed to me.

I understand that breach of this undertaking will make me liable to penalty as prescribed in the Prenatal Diagnostic Techniques (Regulation and Prevention of Misuse) Act 1994 (57 of 1994) and rules framed thereunder.

Date: Signature of the pregnant woman

Place:

I have explained the contents of the above to the patient and her companion (Name .... Address .... Relationship ....) in a language she/they understand.

Date: Name, Signature and/Registration number of Gynecologist/Medical Geneticist/Radiologist/Pediatrician/Director of the Clinic/Center/Laboratory

Place: Name, Address and Registration number of Genetic Clinic/Institute

SEAL

FORM H

[See Rule 9(5)]

Form for maintenance of permanent record of applications for grant/rejection of registration under the prenatal diagnostic techniques (Regulation and Prevention of Misuse Act, 1994.

1. Sr.No.
2. File number of Appropriate Authority.
3. Date of receipt of application for grant of registration.
4. Name, Address, Phone/Fax etc. of Applicant:
5. Name and address(es) of Genetic Counseling Center*/Genetic Laboratory*/Genetic Clinic*/Ultrasound Clinic/Imaging Center*
6. Date of consideration by Advisory Committee and recommendation of Advisory Committee, in summary.
7. Outcome of application (state granted/rejected and date of issue of orders—record date of issue of order in Form B or Form C).
8. Registration number allotted and date of expiry of registration.
9. Renewals (date of renewal and renewed up to)
10. File number in which renewals dealt.
11. Additional information, if any.

Name, Designation and Signature of Appropriate Authority

GUIDANCE FOR APPROPRIATE AUTHORITY

a. Form H is a permanent record to be maintained as a register, in the custody of the Appropriate Authority.
b. *Means strike out whichever is not applicable.
c. On renewal, the Registration Number of the Genetic Counseling Center/Genetic Laboratory/Genetic Clinic/ultrasoundClinic/Imaging Center will not change. A fresh registration Number will be allotted in the event of change of ownership or management.
d. Registration number shall not be allotted twice.
e. Each Genetic Counseling Center/Genetic Laboratory/Genetic Clinic/Ultrasound Clinic/Imaging Center may be allotted a folio consisting of two pages of the Register for recording Form H.

f. The space provided for 'additional information' may be used for recording suspension, cancellations, rejection of application for renewal, change of ownership/management, outcome of any legal proceedings, etc.
g. Every folio (i.e. 2 pages) of the Register shall be authenticated by signature of the Appropriate Authority with date, and every subsequent entry shall also be similarly authenticated.

Format of Form for Submission of monthly report to the Appropriate Authority. Do not forget to take a copy of acknowledgment duly signed by Appropriate Authority. Preserve it in your records

Registration No............

To,
The Appropriate Authority and CDHO.

Date:

Sub: Submission of Forms-F for Sonography of Patients.

Respected Sir,

In the month of .... I have done................................ no. of Sonographies in connection of PNDT Act. I herewith submitting.............. number of Form-F

Please accept it and do needful.

Truly Yours

(Name of the Doctor)

Seal of Hospital

Registration No. ....

Date:

To,
The Appropriate Authority and CDHO.

Sub: Submission of Forms-F for Sonography of Patients.

Respected Sir,

In the month of .... I have done.......................... no. of Sonographies in connection of PNDT Act. I herewith submitting.......... number of Form-F.

Please accept it and do needful

Truly Yours

(Name of the Doctor)

Seal of Hospital

TIPS ON MTP ACT

MTPs can only be conducted in places that have been approved under the Act.

1. Application for approval of a place should be made in Form-A and must be addressed to the CDMO of the District.
2. The committee after recommendation of CDMO approve the place and grant a certificate of approval in Form-B
3. Certificate of approval-Form-B is to be conspicuously displayed at the approved place.

4. Cooperate during monitoring or inspection with the Authorities.
5. Requirements for obtaining MTPR 1. Indications 2. Woman's consent and 3. RMP(s) opinion.
6. Record Keeping: Records have to be maintained for all MTP procedures conducted by the unit.
   1. Form-I- To record the opinion of the RMP conducting the MTP procedure.
   2. Form-C- To record consent of the woman undergoing the MTP procedure. Consent of only the woman has to be obtained prior to conducting the MTP procedure. Spousal consent is not required. However in case of minor and mentally ill women, the consent of the guardian will have to be obtained.
   3. Form-III-Is The Admission register for recording details of the MTPs conducted. Such register is to be kept for a period of five years from the year it relates to . The entries in the admission register are to be made serially, with a fresh serial no. to be started at the commencement of a new year from 1st January. Serial number of a particular year will be distinguished from the serial number of other years by mentioning the year against the serial number. Admission register is a secret document and the information contained therein is to be strictly confidential. It is to be kept in the custody of the head of the hospital or the owner of the Approved place and is not open to inspection except under some special circumstances, such as:
      a. Woman applying for a certificate for obtaining leave.
      b. Under authority of Law.

      No entries pertaining to the name of the pregnant woman can be made in Case-sheets, Operation theater register, Follow-up card or any other document or register other than the Admission Register and all such references to the pregnant woman in such places other than the Admission Register is to be made by the Serial number assigned to the woman, and not by her name, in the Admission Register.
   4. Form-II- All forms are to be kept in the custody of the owner of the unit and a monthly statement of all the MTP cases have to be sent to the CDMO in Form-II

Custody of Forms: Procedure to be followed

The following documents are to be kept in a sealed envelope within three hours of doing MTP by the RMP who perform the MTP and Kept in safe custody till the envelope is sent to the head of the hospital or the owner of the approved place or the CDMO of the state:

1. Consent given by a pregnant woman for the MTP, i.e Form-C
2. Certified opinion of the RMP(s) i.e Form-I and
   - Intimation of the MTP-(every month)
   - Envelope should be marked "SECRET" should contain serial number assigned to the pregnant woman in the Admission Register Name of the RMP(s) by whom pregnancy was terminated.

Envelope Specimen
to be sealed.

SECRET

Serial No........................
Name of the RMP

Reporting and Record Maintenance in Situation of Emergencies

The address of the Approved place or hospital and Date of termination of the pregnancy. Strict confidentiality has to be maintained for all records maintained under this Law.

In the case of an MTP performed under Section 5 of the Act, i.e, those necessary immediately to save the life of the woman, the columns pertaining to

1. The hospital or the approved place and
2. The serial number assigned to the pregnant woman, is to be left blank in Form I

In such a case, the following details should be noted on the envelope marked "SECRET"

1. The name and address of the RMP by whom the MTP was carried out, and
2. Date on which it was carried out.

If pregnancy is not terminated in an approved place or hospital, every envelope should be sent by registered post to the CDMO of the state on the same day on which the pregnancy was terminated or on the next working day following day on which the pregnancy was terminated.

FORM A

[See sub-Rule(2) of Rule(5)

Form of application for the approval of a place under clause(b) of Section 4

Category of approved place:

A. Pregnancy can be terminated up to 12 weeks

B. Pregnancy can be terminated up to 20 weeks

   1. Name of the place (in capital letters)
   2. Address in full
   3. Non-Government/Private/Nursing Home/Other Institutions
   4. State, if the following facilities are available at the place

Category A

i. Gynecological examination/labor table,
ii. Resuscitation equipment
iii. Sterilization equipment
iv. Facilities for treatment of shock, including emergency drugs
v. Facilities for transportation, if required.

Category B

i. Gynecological examination/labor table.
ii. An operation table and Instruments for performing abdominal or gynecological surgery.
iii. Drugs and parental fluid in sufficient supply for emergency cases.
iv. Anesthetic equipment, resuscitation equipment and sterilization equipment.

Place:

Date: Signature of the owner of the place

FORM B

(See sub-Rule (6) of Rule 5)

Certificate of approval

The place described below is hereby approved for the purpose of the Medical Termination of Pregnancy Act, 1971 (34 of 1971)

As read within up to................................. Weeks.
Name of the place
Address and other descriptions
Name of the owner place:
Date:

To the government of the ....

FORM C

(See Rule 8)

I .... daughter/wife of .... aged about .... years at present residing at.........................(here state the permanent address) do hereby give my consent to the termination of my pregnancy at

(State the name of place where the pregnancy is to be terminated)

Place:

Date: Signature

(To be filled in by guardian where the woman is a mentally ill person or minor)

I.. son/daughter/wife of .... aged about..............................years at present residing at..............(here state the permanent address) ....do hereby give my consent to the termination of the pregnancy of my ward who is a minor/lunatic at (state the name of place where the pregnancy is to be terminated) ....(place of termination of my pregnancy)

Place:

Date: Signature

FORM I

[See Regulation 3]

I................. (Name and qualifications of the Registered Medical practitioner in block letters) .... (Full address of the Registered Medical practitioner)

I .... (Name and qualifications of the Registered Medical practitioner in block letters).....................(Full address of the Registered Medical practitioner)... hereby certify that* I/We am/are of opinion, formed in good faith, that it is necessary to terminate the pregnancy of ....(Full name of pregnant woman in block letters)........................... resident of............................(Full address of pregnant woman in block letters)...................... for the reasons given below**

*I/We hereby give intimation that *I/We terminated the pregnancy of the woman referred to above who bears the serial no. in the Admission Register of the hospital/approved place.

Place: Signature of the Registered Medical Practitioner

Date:

Strike out whichever is not applicable

** of the reasons specified items(i) to (v) write the one which is appropriate

i. in order to save the life of the pregnant woman
ii. in order to prevent grave injury to the physical and mental health of the pregnant woman
iii. in view of the substantial risk that if the child was born it would suffer from such physical or mental abnormalities as to be seriously handicapped
iv. as the pregnancy is alleged by pregnant woman to have been caused by rape.
v. as the pregnancy has occurred as result of failure of any contraceptive device or methods used by married woman or her husband for the purpose of limiting the number of children

Note: Account may be taken of the pregnant woman's actual or reasonably foreseeable environment in determining whether the continuance of her pregnancy would involve a grave injury to her physical or mental health

Place: Signature of the Registered Medical Practitioner

Date:

FORM II

(See Regulation 4(5)

1. Name of the state
2. Name of the Hospital/approved place
3. Duration of pregnancy (give total no.only)
   a. Up to 12 weeks
   b. Between 12 and 20 weeks
4. Religion of woman
   a. Hindu
   b. Muslim
   c. Christian
   d. Others
   e. Total
5. Termination with acceptance of contraception
   a. Sterilization
   b. IUD
6. Reasons for termination:
   (give total number under each subhead)
   a. Danger to life of the pregnant woman
   b. Grave injury to the physical health of the pregnant woman
   c. Grave injury to the mental health of the pregnant woman
   d. Pregnancy caused by rape.
   e. Substantial risk that if the child was born, it would suffer from such physical or mental abnormalities as to be seriously handicapped
   f. Failure of any contraceptive device or method.

Signature of the Officer Incharge with Date

FORM III

[See Regulation 5]

ADMISSION REGISTER

(To be destroyed on the expiry of five years from the date of the last entry in the Register).

1	2	3	4	5	6	7
S.No. Admission	Date of	Name of the patient	Wife/ Daughter of	Age	Religion	Address

8	9	10	11	12	13	14
Duration of Pregnancy	Reasons on which Pregnancy is terminated	Date of termination of Pregnancy	Date of discharge of patient	Result and Remarks	Name of RMP(s) by whom the opinion	Name of RMP(s) by whom Pregnancies terminated

OFFENCES AND PENALTIES MTP

The MTP a recognizes offences committed by the RMPs or any other persons conducting MTPS without following the provisions of the Law.

However, it must be noted that there is no liability on RMPS if it is shown that the MTP was conducted in good faith. The conduct of MTPS in places that are, not registered are penalized under this Act.

A woman does not attract any penalties for a breach of the provisions of this Act. However, she may be prosecuted under the provisions of the IPC if she does not fulfill the conditions of this Act.

Nature of offence	*Person liable*	*Penalty imposed*
Termination of pregnancy by any person other than an RMP	Non-RMR who terminates the pregnancy	Imprisonment for a term not less than 2 years which may extend to 7 years
Termination of pregnancy by any person in any other place other than an approved place	RMP or non-RMR whoever terminates the pregnancy owner of such an unapproved place	Imprisonment for a term not less than 2 years which may extend 10 years
Contravention of requirement of record-keeping	RMP	Fine which may extend to Rs 1000

AN OVERVIEW

MTP ACT: An Overview

1. Who can apply for MTP Registration?
   a. Anybody who is an owner of the MTP center can apply for the MTP Registration
   b. The person should be responsible for the administration and supervision of the MTP center
   c. It is not necessary for the person to be a doctor.
2. Who can provide the sevices in registered MTP centers?
   Doctors who are willing to provide their services to the MTP center must be registered under the State Medical Council and having the experience as follows:
   a. Six months of house surgery in Gynecology and obstetrics
      OR
   b. Experience at any hospital for a period of not less than one year in the practice of Gynecology and Obstetrics
      OR
   c. Having assisted a registered medical practitioner in the performance of 25 cases of MTP in a good hospital or an approved training institute
3. Instruments and equipment required for an MTP Center
   1. Operation theater
   2. Operation table
   3. Equipment for resuscitation and anesthesia
      a. Oxygen cylinder
      b. Bellows for oxygen supply
   4. Vacuum aspiration
   5. Parenteral fluids
   6. Sterilization equipment
   7. Autoclave.
4. To whom and in what circumstances can the MTP Register be divulged.
   MTP register is a secret document. This can only be divulged in following circumstances:
   a. If it is asked by the Chief Surgeon
   b. If it is asked by a Magistrate of the First Class in the case of an investigation into an offence.

   c. If it is asked by the District Judge
   d. On the application of an employed woman whose pregnancy has been terminated, to grant a certificate for the purpose of enabling her to obtain leave from her employer.
5. How to maintain the MTP register.
   a. At every abortion center there should be a Govt. approved MTP register as mentioned in Form III.
   b. This register will start at the beginning of every New Year with a new serial number, e.g. 5th case 1972 or 5th case of 1973 will be numbered as 5/1972 or 5/1973.
6. Period of record keeping of the MTP register.
   a. The MTP register has to be maintained for minimum 5 years after the last entry made.
   b. Other important documents regarding the MTP Register are to be maintained for 3 years.
7. To whom and when a report on the MTP Register is sent.
   A report on the MTP Register should be sent to the District Surgeon at the end of every month.
8. Conditions regarding preservation of MTP Registration Certificate.
   The MTP Registration Certificate should be prominently displayed in the center.
9. Precautions that should be taken if there is change in place of MTP center.
   If the place of MTP center is changed it should be registered afresh at the new address.
10. Essential and complementary services at the MTP center
    A. Manpower for essential services
       1. Trained doctors
       2. Trained anesthetist
    B. Essential equipment for MTP Center
       1. Anesthesia equipment
       2. Oxygen cylinder.
       3. Equipment and instruments for pelvic and abdominal surgery
    C. Routine medicines required in the center
       1. Injection Atropine
       2. IV Glucose
       3. Ringer's Lacate Solutions
       4. Injection Lignocaine
       5. Amoxycillin
       6. Paracetamol
       7. Injectable Prostaglandins
       8. Injection Promethazine
          Additional drugs for second trimester:
       9. Ethacridine lactate
       10. Methergin.
    D. Emergency medicines required for the MTP Center
       1. Injection Adrenaline
       2. Injection Hydrocorcisone
       3. Injection Dopamine
       4. Injection Frusemide
       5. Injection Oxytocin
    E. Essential facilities at MTP Center
       1. Generator
       2. Fire extinguisher.
    F. Complementary facilities
       1. Trained lab technician
       2. Trained nurses and *ayas*.

3. Medical social worker and staff
4. Availability of information
5. Telephone facility
6. Ambulance
7. Food.

MISCONCEPTIONS ABOUT MTP REGISTRATION AND THEIR EXPLANATIONS

Misconception	*Explanation*
If the MTP Center is registered, it is mandatory to perform free MTP.	There is no legal binding of performing free MTP if the center is registered.
Government officials ask for the record of past 15 MTP procedures performed by the center if you apply to government register the center.	From legal point of view it is not correct to perform MTP prior to registration of the center and officials should not ask for past record.
Qualified obstetricians need not register their center/ hospital.	Legally even qualified obstetricians need to register their center/hospital.
If a family planning center is registered there is no need to register as MTP center	MTP Center registration and family planning center registration are two separate procedures. It is essential to register MTP center separately
It is not necessary to register the centre if the number of MTP procedures conducted is not very high	MTP Center needs to be registered irrespective of the number of MTP procedures being performed.
Private medical centers are not allowed to provide MTP facility	After MTP registration the private center is allowed to carry out MTP procedures.
If MTP is performed by induction method or medical methods no registration is required.	Centers which perform any type of MTP need registration.
Qualified obstetrician (MD Obs Gyn or DGO) needs to attach certificate of experience to carry out MTP along with the center registration application.	Qualified Obstetrician (MD Obs Gyn or DGO) need not attach experience certificate along with center registration application.

THE REGISTRATION OF BIRTH AND DEATHS ACT

1. Persons required to register births and deaths-(1) It shall be the duty of the persons specified below to give or cause to be given, either orally or in writing, according to the best of their knowledge and belief, within such time as may be prescribed, information to the Registrar of the several particulars required to be entered in the forms prescribed by the State Government under sub-Section (1) of Section 16
   a. In respect of births and deaths in a house, whether residential or non-residential, not being any place referred to in clauses (b) to (e), the head of the house or, in case more than one household live in the house, the head of the household, the head being the person, who is so recognized by the house or the household, and if he is not present in the house at any time during the period within which the birth or death has to be reported, the nearest relative of the head present in the house, and in the absence of any such person, the oldest adult male person present therein during the said period;
   b. In respect of births and deaths in a hospital, health center, maternity or nursing home or other like institution, the medical officer in charge or any person authorized by him in this behalf;
   c. In respect of births and deaths in a jail, the jailor in charge;
   d. In respect of births and deaths in hostel, *dharmasala*, boarding-house, lodging-house, tavern, barrack, toddy shop or place of public resort the person in charge thereof;

e. In respect of any new-born child or dead body found deserted in a public place, the head-man or other corresponding officer of the village in the case of a village and the officer in charge of the local police station elsewhere:
   Provided that any person who finds such child or dead body, or in whose charge such child or dead body may be placed, shall notify such fact to the headman or officer aforesaid;
f. In any other place, such person as may be prescribed.

2. Not with standing anything contained in sub-Section (1), the State Government, having regard to the conditions obtaining in a registration division, may be order require that for such period as may be specified in the order, any person specified by the State Government by designation in this behalf, shall give or cause to be given information regarding births and deaths in a house referred to in clause (a) of sub-Section (1) instead of the persons specified in that clause.

Duty of certain persons to notify births and deaths and to certify cause of death:

1. It shall be the duty of
   i. The midwife or any other medical or health attendant at a birth or death, the keeper or the owner of a place set apart for the disposal of dead bodies or any person required by a local authority to be present at such place, or
   ii. Any other person whom the State Government may specify in this behalf by his designation, to notify every birth or deaths or both at which he or she attended or was present, or which occurred in such areas as may be prescribed, to the Registrar within such time and in such manner as may be prescribed.
2. In any area, the State Government, having regard to the facilities available therein in this behalf, may require that a certificate as to the cause of death shall be obtained by the Registrar from such person and in such form as may be prescribed.
3. Where the State Government has required under sub-Section (2) that a certificate as to the cause of deaths shall be obtained, in the event of the death of any person, who, during his last illness, was attended by a medical practitioner, the medical practitioner shall, after the death of that person, forthwith, issue without charging any fee, to the person required under this Act to give information concerning the death, a certificate in the prescribed form stating to the best of his knowledge and belief the cause of death; and the certificate shall be received and delivered by such person to the Registrar at the time of giving information concerning the death as required by this Act. Sec 11.

Informant to sign the register- Every person who has orally given to the Registrar any information required under this Act shall write in the register maintained in this behalf, his name description and place of abode, and, if he cannot write, shall put his thumb mark in the register against his name, description and place of abode, the pariculars being in such a case entered by the Registrar, Sec 12.

Extracts of registration entries to be given to informant- The Registrar shall, as soon as the registration of a birth or death has been completed, give, free of charge, to the person who gives information under Section 8 or Section 9 an extract of the prescribed particulars under his hand from the register relating to such birth or death, Sec13.

Delayed registration of births and deaths:

1. Any birth or death of which information is given to the Registrar after the expiry of the period specified, therefore, but within thirty days of its occurrence, shall be registered on payment of such late fee as may be prescribed.
2. Any birth or death of which delayed information is given to the Registrar after thirty days but within one year of its occurrence shall be registered only with the written permission of the prescribed authority and on payment of the prescribed fee and the production of an affidavit made before a notary public or nay other officer authorized in this behalf by the State Government.
3. Any birth or death, which has not been registered within one year of its occurrence, shall be registered only on an order made by a Magistrate of the first class or a Presidency Magistrate after verifying the correctness of the birth or death and on payment of the prescribed fee.

4. The provisions of this section shall be without prejudice to any action that may be taken against a person for failure on his part to register any birth or death within the time specified, therefore, and any such birth or death may be registered during the pendency of any such action. Section 14

Registration of name of child—Where the birth of any child has been registered without a name, the parent or guardian of such child shall within the prescribed period give information regarding the name of the child to the registrar either orally or in writing and thereupon the Registrar shall enter such name in the register and initial and date the entry. Section 15

Correction or cancellation of entry in the register of births and deaths—If it is proved to the satisfaction of the Registrar that any entry of a birth or death in any register kept by him under this Act is erroneous in form or substance, or has been fraudulently or improperly made, he may, subject to such rules as may be made by the State Government with respect to the conditions on which and the circumstances in which such entries may be corrected or cancelled, correct the error or cancel the entry by suitable entry in the margin, without any alteration of the original entry, and shall sign the marginal entry and add thereto the date of the correction or cancellation.

Penalties

1. Any person who:
   a. Fails without reasonable cause to give any information which it is his duty to give under any of the provisions of Sections 8 and 9; or
   b. Give or causes to be given, for the purpose of being inserted in any register of births and deaths, any information which he knows or believes to be false regarding any of the particulars required to be known and registered; or
   c. Refuses to write his name-description and place of abode or to put his thumb mark in the register as required by Section-11, shall be punishable with fine which may extend to fifty rupees.
2. Any Registrar or Sub-Registrar who neglects or refuses, without reasonable cause, to register any birth or deaths occurring in his jurisdiction or to submit any returns as required by sub-Section (1) of Section 19 shall be punishable with fine which may extend to fifty rupees.
3. Any medical practitioner who neglects or refuses to issue a certificate under sub-Section (3) of Section 10 and any person who neglects or refuses to deliver such certificate shall be punishable with fine, which may extend to fifty rupees.
4. Any person who, without reasonable cause, contravenes any provision of this Act for the contravention of which no penalty is provided for in this section shall be punishable with fine, which may extend to ten rupees.
5. Notwithstanding anyting contained in the Code of Criminal Procedure, 1898(5 of 1898), an offence under this section shall be tried summarily by a Magistrate.

TIPS OF BIOMEDICAL WASTE ACT

Mandatory Things in the Hospital Premises

1. Needle destroyer
2. Syringe destroyer
3. Three colored bags or Two combined color bags
4. Sodium hypochlorite solution
5. Segregation training of staff by the service provider.

Advices

1. Registration under Biomedical Waste Act is mandatory
2. Send report to SPCB every year before 31st January
3. Renewal of SPCB certificate every three years.
4. Display of SPCB certificate–Not mandatory.
5. Display of service certificate–Not mandatory.
6. Preserve the bills and receipts of payment of every month of service provider.
7. Make a habit to give a certificate if you are handing over a missed fetus.

Fee Structure

Bedless Hospital - Rs 1000/-
Up to 50 Beds Hospital - Rs 2000/-

Note Addresses of Authorities

1. Regional Office : State Pollution Control Board (As per area)
2. Head Office : As per the area

Duty of Occupier

It shall be the duty of every occupier of an institution generating bio-medical waste, which includes a hospital nursing home, clinic, dispensary, veterinary institutions, and animal house, pathological laboratory, blood bank by whatever name called to take all steps to ensure that such waste is handled without any adverse effect to human health and the environment.

Authorization

a. Every occupier of an institution generating, collecting, receiving, storing, transporting, treating disposing and/or handling biomedical waste in any other manner, except such occupier of clinic, dispensaries, pathological laboratories, blood banks providing treatment/service to less than 1000 (one thousand) patients per month, shall make an application in Form I to the prescribed authority for grant of authorization.
b. Every operator of a Biomedical waste facility shall make an application in Form I to the prescribed authority for grant of authorization.
c. Every application in Form I for grant of authorization shall be accompanied by a fee as may be prescribed by the Government of the State of Union Territory.

Annual Report

Every occupier/operator submit an annual report to the prescribed authority in Form II by 31 January every year, to include information about the categories and quantities of biomedical wates handled during the preceding year. The prescribed authority shall send this information in a compiled form to the Central Pollution Control Board by 31 March every year.

Maintenance of Records

a. Every authorized person shall maintain records related to the generation, collection, reception, storage, transportation, treatment, disposal and/or any form of handling of biomedical waste in accordance with these rules and any guidelines issued.
b. All records shall be subjected to inspection and verification by the prescribed authority at any time.

Accident Reporting

When any accidents occur at any institution or facility or any other site where biomedical waste is handled or during transportation of such waste, the authorized person shall report the accident in Form III to the prescribed authority forth with.

ENVIRONMENT (PROTECTION) ACT 1986

SCHEDULE-I

(See Rule 5)

CATEGORIES OF BIOMEDICAL WASTE

1 (Waste Category No.) *1*	*Waste Category (Type)* *2*	*3 (Treatment and Disposal option 4)* *3*
Category No.1	Human Anatomical waste (human tissues, organs, body part)	incineration@/deep burial
Category No.2	Animal Waste (Animal tissues, organs, body parts carcasses bleeding parts, fluid, blood and experimental animals used in research waste generated by veterinary hospitals colleges, discharge from hospitals animal houses)	incineration@/deep burial
Category No.3	Microbiology and Biotechnology Waste (Waste from laboratory cultures, Stock or local specimens of micro-organisms live or attenuated vaccines, human and animal cell culture used in research and infectious agents from research and industrial laboratories, wastes from production of biological, toxins, dishes and devices used for transfer of cultures)	local autoclaving/microwaving incineration@
Category No.4	Waste sharps (needles, syringes, scalpels, blades, glass, etc. that may cause punctuator and cut. This includes both used and unused sharps)	disinfection (chemical treatment @@/auto autoclaving/ microwaving and mutilation/shredding##
Category No. 5	Discarded Medicines and Cytotoxic drugs (wastes comprising or outdated, contaminated and discarded medicines	Incineration@/destruction and drugs disposal in secured land-fills
Category No. 6	(Soiled) Waste (Items contaminated with blood, and body fluid's including cotton, dressings, soiled plaster casts, lines, bedding, other material contaminated with blood)	Incineration@/auto autoclaving/ microwaving
Category No. 7	Solid Waste (waste generated from disposable items other than the wate sharps such as tubings, catheters, intravenous sets, etc.)	disinfection by chemical treatment @@ autoclaving/microwaving and mutilation/shredding##
Category No. 8	Liquid Waste (waste generated from laboratory and washing cleaning housekeeping and disinfection activities	disinfection by chemical treatment @@ and discharge into drains.
Category No. 9	Incineration Ash (ash from incineration of any bio-medical waste)	disposal in municipal landfill
Category No. 10	Chemical Waste (chemical used in production of biologicals, chemicals used in disinfection, as insecticides, etc.)	chemical treatment @@ and discharge into drains for liquids and secured landfill for solids

1. Subs, for "option" by S.O.545(E) dated 2nd June. 2000 (w.e.f. 2nd June, 2000)
2. Added by ibid.
3. Subs by ibid.
4. *Options given above are based on available technologies, Occupies/Operator wishing to use other state-of-the-art technologies shall approach the Central Pollution Control Board to get the Standards laid down to enable the prescribed authority to consider grant of authorization.

@@ Chemicals treatment using at least 1 percent hypochlorite solution or any other equivalent chemical reagent. It must be ensured that chemical treatment ensures disinfection.

Multilation/shredding must be such so as to prevent unauthorised re-use.

@ There will be no chemical pre-treatment before incineration. Chlorinated plastics shall not be incinerated. Deep burial shall be an option available only in towns with population less than five lakhs and in rural areas

SCHEDULE-II

(See Rule 6)

COLOR CODING AND TYPE OF CONTAINER FOR DISPOSAL OF BIOMEDICAL WASTES

Color Coding	Type of container	Waste category	Treatment options as per Sch.1
Yellow	Plastic bag	Cat.1.Cat. 2, and Cat. 3, Cat.6	Incineration/deep burial
Red	Disinfected container/ Plastic bag	Cat.3, Cat.6, Cat.7.	Autoclaving/Microwaving. Chemical Treatment
Blue/White translucent	Plastic bag/puncture proof container	Cat.4.Cat.7	Autoclaving/Microwaving Chemical Treatment and destruction/shredding
Black	Plastic bag	Cat.5 and Cat.9 and Cat.10 (solid)	Disposal in secured landfill

Notes:
1. Color coding of waste categories with multiple treatment options as defined in Sch-1, shall be selected depending on treatment option chosen. Which shall be as specified in Sch-I
2. Waste collection bags for types needing incineration shall not be made of chlorinated plastics
3. Categories No. 8 to 10 (liquid) do not require containers/bags.
4. Categories No.3 if disinfected Ideally need not be put in containers/bags.

AN APPLICATION FORM UNDER RULES 8 OF THE BIOMEDICAL WASTE (REGULATION AND CONTROL) RULES, 2000

FORM-I

(See Rule 8)

APPLICATION FOR AUTHORIZATION

(To be submitted in duplicate)

Rs. 50/-

To,
The Member Secretary
State Pollution Control Board

1. Particulars of Applicant : ....
   i. Name of the applicant : ....
   (In block letters and in full)

ii. Name of the Institution : ....
Address ....
Tele. No/Fax No./Telex No. : ....
iii. Type of Institution : ....
iv. No. of bed : ....

2. Activity for which Authorization is sought : ....
   i. Generation : ....
   ii. Collection : ....
   iii. Reception : ....
   iv. Storage : ....
   v. Transportation : ....
   vi. Treatment : ....
   vii. Disposal : ....
   viii. Any other form of Handling : ....
3. Please state whether applying for fresh authorization or for renewal (In case of renewal previous authorization No. and date) : ....
4. i. Address of the institution handling biomedical wastes : ....
   ii. Address of the place of the treatment facility : ....
   iii. Address of the place of disposal of the wastes : ....
5. i. Mode of transportation (in any) of biomedical wastes : ....
   ii. Mode(s) of treatment (categorywise) : ....
6. Brief description of method of treatment and disposal (Attach details) : ....
7. i. Category (See Schedule-I) of waste to be handled : ....
   ii. Quantity of waste (Categorywise) to be handled per month : ....
8. Declaration

I do hereby declare that the statements made and information given above are true to the best of my knowledge and belief and that I have not concealed any information.

I do also hereby undertake to provide any further information sought by the prescribed authority in relation to these rules and to fulfill any conditions stipulated by the prescribed authority.

Date: Signature of the Applicant

Place: Designation of the Applicant

BIOMEDICAL WASTE (MANAGEMENT AND HANDLING RULES,1998)

FORM II

(See Rule 10)

Annual report

(To be submitted to the prescribed authority by 31st January every year)

1. Particulars of applicant.
   Person in charge of Hospital:
   Name and address of the Hospital:
2. Categories of waste generated and quantity on a monthly average basis:
   As per Annexure-I
3. Brief details of the treatment facility
   1. Name of the Operator:
   2. Name and address of facility:
      Tel. No:
4. Categorywise Quantity of Waste treated: As per Annexure-II
5. Modo of treatment with details:
   Incineration — Incinerator: 200 kg/hour, Two chamber, Scrubber stack
   Autoclaving — Autoclave: 600 liter, Two Programmer Automatic
   Shredding — Shredder: 75 k/hour with Automatic Dejamming Mechanism
6. Any other information:
   Method of segregation: Different colored Non-Chlorinated Polyethylene Bags. Method of collection and storage: As per norms, we have closed area for storage. Treatment and Disposal facilities: as per local contract (Incineration, Autoclaving, Shredding, landfilling)
7. Certified that the above report is for the period from 01/01/0 to 31/12/0

Date: Signature:

Place: Designation:

ANNEXURE-I

Categories of waste generated and quantity on a monthly average basis:

S. No.	*Category of waste treated*	*Description of the waste as per category*	*Quantity(In kg)*
1.	1.	Human Anatomical waste	
2.	2.	Animal waste	
3.	3.	Microbiology and Bio-technology waste	
4.	4.	Sharp waste	
5.	5.	Discarded Medicines and Cytotoxic drugs	
6.	6.	Solid waste cottons, Dressings Materials, etc.	
7.	7.	Solid waste catheters, tubing	
8.	8.	Liquid waste	
9.	9.	Incineration	
10.	10.	Ash Chemical Waste	

ANNEXURE-II

Categorywise Quantity of Waste treated: For the year 200...

Month	Incin.Category 1,2,3,5, and 6 Quantity (kg)	Autoclaving/ Shredding category 3,4,6, and 7 Quantity (kg)	Month	Incin.Category 1,2,3,5, and 6 Quantity (kg)	Autoclaving/ Shredding Category 3,4,6, and 7 Quantity (kg)
January			July		
February			August		
March			September		
April			October		
May			November		
June			December		

FORM-III

V (See Rule 12)

Accident reporting

1. Date and time of accident:
2. Sequence of events leading to accident:
3. The waste involved in accident:
4. Assessment of the effect of the accidents on human health and the environment:
5. Emergency measures taken:
6. Steps taken to alleviate the effects of the accidents:
7. Steps taken to prevent the recurrence of such an accident:

Date: Signature

Place: Designation

AUTHORIZATON FEES

S. No.	*Particulars*	*Rate of fees Rs.*
A	Hospital and nursing home	
	a. with 500 beds and above	05,000/-
	b. with 200 beds and above, but less than...500 beds	04,000/-
	c. with 50 beds and above, but less than...200 beds	03,000/-
	d. with less than 50 beds.	02,000/-
B.	Every occupier of an institution generating, collecting, receiving, storing, transporting, treating, disposing and/or hurdling biomedical waste in any other manner, including clinics,dispensaries, pathological laboratories, blood banks, veterinary institution animal house, by whatever name called, but not included in A above	01,000/-
C.	Every institution and operator connected with Management and Handling of Bio-Medical waste...	
	i. The operations having an incinerator with capacity up to 50 kg per hour	10,000/-
	ii. Waste operations having an incinerator with capacity of more than 50 kg per hour	20,000/-
	iii. Operators having facilities other than incinerator	01,000/-

TIPS OF BOMBAY NURSING HOMES REGISTRATION ACT

- Form 2'C' is now a days demanded by insurance companies for claim.
- Keep ready xerox copies of 2 'C' Form.
- Although not mandatory but one should display 2 'C' Form in OPD
- Place to be registered in Health Department (Local)
- Fee Structure

  1 to 5 beds Rs. 500/- per annum

  6 to 10 beds Rs. 1000/- per annum

  >10 beds Rs. 1500/- per annum
- Registration is done maximum for five years. Yearly registration is also available.
- Financial year under BNHR Act is 1st April to 31 st March.
- Display OPD Charges and emergency charges in OPD.

Documents required for BNH Registration

1. Degree Certificate
2. Medical Council Registration
3. Bio-medical Registration
4. Shop Establishment Registration
5. Last year's Municipal Tax Bill with Receipts
6. Electric Bill/Telephone Bill Any One
7. BU permission copy
8. Partnership Deed copy In case of Partnership
9. Article of Memorandum in Ltd.and Pvt Ltd hospital
10. Visiting card
11. Letter pad
12. Service certificate of agency

FORM 'B'

Sr.No. Rs. 50/-

Application for Registration Renewal of Registration under Section 5 of the Bombay Nursing Homes Registration Act, 1949

(See Rules 4 and 6)

The replies to be written in the column

1. Full name of the applicant*.
2. *Full residential address of the applicant

   Telephone No.
3. Technical Qualifications, if any, of the applicant
4. Nationality of the applicant
5. Situation of the registered or principal office of the company, Society, Association or other body corporate
6. Name and other particulars of the nursing home in respect of which the registration is applied for
7. Place where the nursing home is situated

   Telephone No.
8. Brief description of the construction size and equipment of the nursing home or any premises used in connection therewith.
9. Whether the nursing home or any premises used in connection therewith are used or are to be used for purpose other than that of carrying on a nursing home.
10. a. Number of beds for maternity patients,

    b. Number of beds for other patients.
11. Names, ages, and qualifications of the members of the nursing staff in the nursing home.
12. Place where the nursing staff is accommodated

13. Name, ages, and qualifications of the resident of visiting physicians or surgeons in the nursing home.
14. a. Whether the nursing home is under the supervision of a qualified nurse and, if so, his on her name, age and qualifications.
    b. Proportion of the qualified and unqualified nurses on the nursing staff.
15. a. Whether the nursing home is under the supervision of a qualified nurse or midwife and, if so, his name, age and qualifications.
    b. Whether any medical practitioner or unqualified midwife is employed for nursing any patient in the nursing home.
16. Whether any person of alien nationality is employed in the nursing home and, if so, his name and other particulars.
17. Fees charges to patients
18. Whether the applicant is interested in any other nursing home or business and, if so, the place where such nursing home is situated or where such businesses is conducted
19. *No. and date of expiry of the certificate of registration.

I solemnly declare the above statements are true to the best of my knowledge and belief.

Date: Signature of the applicant

In case the applicant is made on behalf of a company society, Association or other body corporate the name and residential address of the person In charge of the management of such company society, Association of body corporate should be given.

This Item is applicable only when the application is made on behalf of company Association or other body corporate.

The queries made in this item should be answered/only when the Nursing home is a non-maternity or mixed home (i.e home having maternity and non-maternity words.). In the case of mixed home the queries should be answered with reference.

The queries made in this should be answered only when the nursing home is a meternity or mixed home (i.e home having maternity and non-maternity words). In the case of a mixed home the queries should be answered with reference the maternity word.

Following Documents should be attached with the Form

1. Registration Certificate of Medical Council.
2. Degree Certificate.
3. Evidence for place of Nursing Home.
   i.e. Electrictiy Bill, Tax Bill, Building used Permission, Telephone Bill.

MUNICIPAL CORPORATION

Certificate of Registration Under Section 5 of the Bombay Nursing Homes Registration Act 1949 (See Rule 5)

This is to certify that Shri/Shrimati .... has been registered under the Bombay Nursing Homes Registration Act 1949 in respect of .... (here insert the name of the Nursing Home) situated at .... City and has been authorized to carry on the said Nursing Home.
Registration No:
Date of Registration:
Date of Issue of the certificate:
This certificate of registration shaft be valid up to ....

FORM 'C'

Medical Officer of Health
Municipal Corporation

BOMBAY SHOPS AND ESTABLISHMENT ACT

- It is a District and corporation Act.
- It is not applied to the hospitals without bed.
- It is applied only to the hospitals containing bed(s) and providing 24 hours services. So, Radiologists, Pathologists, etc. who do not provide their services for 24 hours are exempted from this Act.
- It is applied in all the corporation and certain districts.
- Previously MBBS Doctors were also registered under this Act but, now a days authority does not give registration to MBBS Doctors under this Act. Old registered MBBS doctors may continue as such.
- List of documents required at the time of registration/renewal of the licence.
  - Municipal Tax Bill of Hospital/Residence/Shop
  - In case of rented shop rent deed or rent contract
  - In case of rented house rent deed or rent contract
  - Electric bill xerox copy
  - Telephone bill xerox copy
  - Two passport size photographs
  - Doctor's degree certificate
  - If partnership firm then partnership deed and Article of memorandum
  - Authority Letter
  - Visiting Card
  - Letter pad
- Certificate of Registration is to be displayed at the premises of the hospital.
- A Name plate bearing the name of the owner of the hospital is also to be displayed.
- Form 'A' -For new registration
- Form 'D' - For renewal of registration
- Form 'E' - For any changes in address, partnership, etc.

SECTION-III

HOSPITAL DOCUMENTS–MODEL FORMS

CONSENT-FORM

Patient's Information	*Relative's Information*
Name:	Name:
Sex: Age: Yr.	Sex: Age: Yr:
Registration No:	Address:
Diagnosis:	
Operation's Title:	Relationship with the patient:

I.................................... the undersigned GIVE CONSENT for

☐ MY OWN/☐ AFOREMENTIONED PATIENT'S above mentioned operation and /or medication/investigation/anesthesia/therapy/procedure, etc.

1. The necessity of this medication/investigation/anesthesia/operation/therapy/procedure, the ill-effects if this is not performed, hazards and complications in the therapeutic modalities other than operation, have been explained to me by Dr. ....
2. I have been explained clearly that any medication/investigation/operation/therapy is not totally safe and that such procedure or anesthesia can be a risk to life of an otherwise healthy person also.
3. Doctors have explained to me that excessive bleeding, infection, cardiac arrest, pulmonary embolism and complications like this can arise suddenly and unexpectedly while undergoing medication/investigation/operation/therapy/procedure or anesthesia.
4. I give consent for any change in the anesthesia or operative procedure as well as for removal of any organ as deemed necessary by the Doctors at the time of medication/investigation/operation/therapy/procedure.
5. I have been made aware that after the above operation/medication/investigation/therapy/procedure and anesthesia instead of desired benefit, some complication may arise e.g. .... and I believe that to avoid such complications, if any, appropriate care shall be taken by

Dr (Surgeon) ____

Dr (Anesthetist) ____

or any other doctors suggested by them. ☐ have read the above writing. ☐ The above writing has been read out to me. I have understood the aforesaid and I am giving my consent willingly.

Witness	*Witness*	*Patient/Relative*
Sign: Name: Address: Age: Yrs. Date Date	Sign: Name: Address: Age: Yrs. Date Date	Sign and/or LHTI Time Date

NAME AND ADDRESS OF THE HOSPITAL/NURSING HOME WITH 2 'C' FORM REGISTRATION NO.

Proforma of Medical Certificate

Patient - ______________________

Age - ______________________

Diagnosis - ______________________

Date of admission - ______________________

Date of operation - ______________________

Date of discharge - ______________________

Operative details - ______________________

Advice - ______________________

Patient's signature and/or thumb impression
Date:
Place:

Doctor's signature and stamp with registration no.
Date:
Place:

NAME AND ADDRESS OF THE HOSPITAL/NURSING HOME

Sterilization and IUCD Register

S. No.	*Name and Address with prominent and marks*	*Details of couple*	*Husband*	*Wife*	*Patient's History*	*STERILIZATION No*	*IUCD Insertion No*
		Age	Yrs	Yrs	Total pregnancies	Abdominal/	LMR
		Education			Living M..... F.......	Laparoscopic	
		Occupation			Abortions	Vasectomy	Date of Insertion
		Mthly Income			Age of last issue	Date of op.	of IUCD
	Urban/Rural *Religion-	Caste			Years M...... F.......	Type of Ane. G/S/L/E	

OPD Case Register

Date:........../............/ As per IT Rule: Appendix-IV, Form No. 3C [see Rule 6F (3)]

S. No.	*Name*	*Reg./Case Paper No.*	*Professional Services rendered*	*Fees Received Rs.*	*Date of Receipt*	*Remarks if Any*
1.						
2.						
3.						
4.						
5.						

Indoor Case Register

Reg. No. Sr.	*Date and Time of Admission*	*Date and Time of Discharge*	*Name of the Patient and Address*	*Sex Age*	*Diagnosis*	*Nature of Professional Services rendered*	*Bill No. and Date*	*Receipt No. and Date*	*Remarks/ Any Comments*
	A.M/R.M	A.M/R.M		M/F					

Operation Theater Register

Sr. No.	Date	Indoor/ OPD Reg. No.	Name of the patient	Type of Anesthesia	Provisional Diagnosis	Procedure done	Operating Surgeon	Anesthesia tist	Names Assisting Doctor/s	Assisting Nurse/s	Remarks
			Male/Female Age: Yrs.		GA/SA/LA/EA Dur.of Surge am/pm to am/pm.			Material for HPE-Yes/No			

NAME AND ADDRESS OF THE HOSPITAL/NURSING HOME

This type of details of vaccination with dates put in front of all vaccines shall be provided to all the delievered patients at the time of discharge

Name .... scheduled dates of vaccination

Vaccination Profile

At Birth	-BCG	______
At 1st Month	-OPV+Hepatitis-B	______
At 2nd Month	-OPV+Hepatitis-B+DPT+HIB	______
At 3rd Month	-OPV+DPT+HIB	______
At 4th Month	-OPV+DPT+HIB	______
At 5th Month	-OPV+HIB	______
At 6th Month	-Hepatitis-B	______
At 9th Month	-Measles	______
At 15th Month	-MMR	______
At 18th Month	-OPV+DPT+HIB	______
At 5 Yrs	-OPV+DT	______

Special Vaccines

HEPATITIS-A	-At 1 Yr.	______
	-At 1 1/2 Yr.	______
CHICKENPOX	-At 1 Yr.	______

INDOOR CASE PAPER

- Majority complaints are filed by the indoor patients.
- Majority doctors do not keep it properly.

MODEL INDOOR CASE

Name : .... O.RD. No. : ....

Age/Sex : .... Occupation : .... Indoor No. : ....

Address : ....

DOA : ....

DOO : ....

DOD : ....

Provisional diagnosis:...

Final diagnosis:..

i. History :...

a. Complaint ....

b. Past history ....

c. Personal history ....

d. Family history ....

ii. Examination: ....

a. General ....

b. Local ....

c. Systemic ....

iii. Investigations: ....

a. Pathological ....

b. Radiological ....

c. Other ....

iv. Indoor Treatment: ....

Date/Time	Findings	Treatment

v. Operative Note:

vi. Note on Discharge

DISCHARGE CARD

- It is good documentary evidence.
- Mention condition of the patient at that time.
- You may not give indoor case papers but you have to give this to all the patients.

Discharge Card

Indoor No: .... OPD No. : ....

Name : ....

Address:...

DOA: .... DOO: .... DOD: ....

....

Investigations: Reports:

....

Operative Note:

....

Advice: Diagnosis:

....

Condition on discharge:

....

Follow-up dates:

Signature
Dr ABC
'X' Nursing

Note: All the reports, treatment given and date of follow-up.

CERTIFICATE

- Only RMP can give it.
- A Patient has all the right to ask for a genuine medical certificate related to his illness.
- A reasonable charge may be taken.

Dr. ABC
Reg. No
Address
Regn. No. of 2 'C' Form

Model Certificate

No.: .... Date: ....

1. This is to certify that Mr/Mrs/Miss .... is /was under my treatment for since
2. He/She has been advised complete rest/light work from.. to ....
3. In continuation of the previous certificate No.: .... dated:.................................. given by me/by Dr XYZ, he/she is further advised rest till ....
4. He/She is examined by me today and is found fit for duty from...
5. Identification Mark :...

Signature/thumb impression of patient.

Signature of Doctor (Rubber stamp)

DEATH CERTIFICATE

- It is misnomer, more accurately it is the Cause of Death Certificate.
- You are bound to issue it if the patient is under your treatment.

A Model Death Certificate

(Medical Certificate of Cause of Death)

1. Name of the deceased:..
2. Address ....
3. Date/time of death:..
4. Sex: .... 5. Marital Status :................................ 6. Occupation: ....
7. Date of birth: .... 8. Age: ....
9. a. Cause of death : ....
   b. Immediate cause : ....
   c. Other significant conditions : ....
10. How did injury occur: ....
    Accident/suicide/homicide.
11. If deceased was a female:
    Was the death associated with pregnancy? Yes/No.
    If yes, was there a delivery? Yes/No.
    If yes, has it taken place within 42 days of delivery?

Name of Doctor:
Reg. No.

Rubber Stamp

Signature and Address of Doctor

GENERAL CONSENT FORM

(To be modified as per the procedure)

I .... Case Paper No .... Register No .... in .... hospital give consent for my own/relative medication/ investigation/anesthesia/operation/therapy/procedure.

1. The necessity of this medication/investigation/anesthesia/operation/therapy/procedure, the ill-effects if this is not performed; hazards and complications in the therapeutic modalities other than operation have been explained to me by Dr...
2. I have been explained clearly that any medication/investigation/operation/therapy is not totally safe and that such procedure or anesthesia can be a risk of life of an otherwise healthy person also.
3. Doctors have explained to me that excessive bleeding, infection, cardiac arrest, pulmonary embolism and complications like this can arise suddenly and unexpectedly while undergoing medication/investigation/operation/ therapy/precedure or anesthesia.
4. I give consent for any change in the anesthesia or operative procedure as well as for removal of any organ as deemed necessary by the doctors at the time of medication/investigation/operation/therapy/procedure.
5. I am aware that after medication/investigation/operation/therapy/procedure and anesthesia instead of desired benefits some complications, e.g.

   ....

   ....

   and I believe that to avoid such complication appropriate care shall be taken by

   Dr (Surgeon)..

   Dr (Anesthetist)..

   Or any other doctors appointed by them.

   I have understood the aforesaid and I willingly give my consent.

Signature:
Witness: Date:
Time:

CERTIFICATION OF CAUSE OF DEATH

Registration of Births and Deaths Act (RBD), 1969 provides for certification by a medical practitioner who has attended the deceased during the latter's last illness.

A cause of death is a desease, abnormality, injury or poisoning that contributed directly or indirectly to death. A death often results from a combined effect of two or more conditions. These conditions may be completely unrelated, arising independently of each other; or they may be causally related to each other, that is, one condition may lead to another, which in turn leads to a third condition and so on. Where there is a sequence, the underlying cause,i.e the disease or injury which initiated the sequence of events will get selected for the purpose of tabulation.

The underlying cause of death is:

a. The disease or injury which initiated the train of events leading directly to death, or
b. The circumstances of the accident or violence which produced the fatal injury.

All these morbid conditions or injuries consequent to the underlying cause relating to death are termed as antecedent and immediate cause.

Physician's Responsibility

1. To complete the medical part of the certificate regarding all diseases, morbid conditions or injuries either resulted in or contributed to death.
2. Indicate specifically all the several conditions and the chain of events if a sequence can be identified.
3. Put any other condition contributing to death separately if not directly forming part of the fatal sequence.
4. The various particulars, other than those of the medical part on cause of death, are also required for reporting the death by the hospital to the registration authority in the prescribed format.
5. The detachable portion of the form containing only the fact of death without disclosing the cause of death may either be signed by the certifier or the medical officer of the hospital, and handed over to the relatives of the deceased.
6. The form of medical certificate of cause of death is to be sent to the local registrar of Births and Deaths along with the death report in the prescribed format within the prescribed time limit.
7. The certificate should be filled by the attending physician or a physician having personal knowledge of the case history.
8. The names of the disease should be written in full and legible to avoid the risk of their being misread.
9. He should avoid indefinite or inadequate terms.

INCORRECT FILLING AND THE CORRECT FILLING OF THE MEDICAL PART OF THE CERTIFICATE

		Incorrect Certificate	*Correct Certificate*
1.	Part I	a. Diabetes b. Gangrene Foot c. Carcinoma pancreas and chronic bronchitis	a. Gangrene Foot b. Diabetes c. Carcinoma Pancreas
	Part II	....	Chronic Bronchitis
2.	Part I	a. Polycystic kidney b. Renal failure and hypertension c. Ischemic heart disease	a. Renal failure(b) b. Hypertension c. Polycystic kidney
	Part II	....	Ischemic Heart Disease
3.	Part I	a. Intestinal obstruction b. Femoral hernia c.	a. Femoral Hernia with obstruction b. .... c. ....
	Part II		
4.	Part I	a. Retention of urine with hypertrophy of prostate with uremia b. Cataract c. Ischemic heart disease	a. Uremia b. Retention of urine c. Hypertrophy of prostate
	Part II	....	Cataract, Ischemic heart disease.
5.	Part I	a. Primary Bronchogenic Carcinoma of Rt.Lung b. Emaciation c. Metastasis of lymph nodes to liver	a. Emaciation b. Metastasis to lymph nodes and liver c. Bronchogenic carcinoma of rt. lung
	Part II	....	....

DAMA

- It must be remembered that a patient cannot be kept in the hospital against his will, it is illegal.
- A doctor may obtain his signature in following form and if he does not sign then do not insist but put appropriate remark in the form.

Date: Dr ABC
Time: XYZ Nursing Home

Discharge Against Medical Advice

Patients Name: ....

No.: .... Age : .... Sex : ....

Address : ....

This is to certify that I am leaving this hospital at my own request, at my own risk and on my own responsibility and against the advice of the medical staff.

Witness: Signature

- Remember, that it itself shows that the patient is not satisfied with you
- Keep the records of such a patient.

DEATH OF A PATIENT ON OPERATION TABLE

Whenever one hears news about death of a patient on the operation table while the surgery was being performed our immediate reaction points towards negligence on the part of the team of doctors in the operation room. This is more so in Gynecological and obstetric patients because these patients are young and healthy and most of them do not have any major medical problem. A successful out come is, therefore, taken for granted by the relatives of the patient. They are shocked while facing this unexpected event.There is disbelief about the incidence, a feeling of helplessness and a strong sense of suspicion about whatever happened within the four walls of the operation theater. What follows, therefore, is a knee jerk reaction which on several occasions can lead to mob violence especially if the diseased is related to a socially impotant personality.

This article is an attempt to get an insight of the situation which leads to death of a patient on table and its aftermath. Idea is to learn our lesson so that the involved doctors, hospital staff, and the relative can conduct themselves well while facing such a mishap with dignity and respect towards each other and also to the dead person.

Why does such suspicion occur?

- Relatives feel that in this era of technical advances made in the field of medicine, mishaps can never occur during surgery.
- Doctors don't counsel the patient and the relatives about their condition, the complications expected during any surgery because of surgery of anesthesia.
- Relatives are often not satisfied with the explanation given by the doctors after the mishap and feel that lots of facts are hidden. They feel cheated if the communication after the mishap is not transparent and with empathy.
- Relatives are further hurt if the hospital staff ask for payment of bills incurred after they have lost their patient.
- Relatives get carried away by adverse remarks about the case by hospital staff, other doctors or any one else who may not be present in the theater.

Are Doctors always responsible for the event?

- In spite of all the advances that have occurred in the field of medicine in terms of drugs and equipment certain conditions is still out side the control of any doctor. We have yet to achieve a zero percent mortality rate (Percentage of chances of death) for any surgery. Some of the conditions which deserve mention are as follows:
- Embolism–In this condition a clot develops within the circulatory system and if it get dislodged and blocks the blood vessels supplying blood to vital organs like brain and heart, there can be a sudden collapse and death.
- Anaphylaxis to any drug during surgery can be fatal
- Certain conditions are specific to the disease process
- Fat embolism is common in certain orthopedic patients
- Obstetric patients can suffer from various complications of child birth which are unforeseen and can cause fatality suddenly
- Some patients can be "high risk" cases for anesthesia due to cardiorespiratory problems. The level of such risk is mentioned in ASA grading, grade 4 being the highest risk patient. If surgery has to be done in spite of anesthesia risk, patient is prone to complications due to anesthesia. Such calculated risks are needed to be taken various situations of emergency.

Can Doctors be occasionally responsible for such deaths?

- If the operation theater is not equipped enough to manage the kind of case that was undertaken. E.g. oxygen cylinders, anesthesia equipment, etc.
- A rule of locality is employed while deciding the minimum requirement of an operation theater. An operation theater in a remote village is not expected to be as equipped as an operation theater of a hospital in metropolitan cities. But doctors in village are also expected to use their good sense in selecting patients.
- Not keeping blood ready for surgery which is likely to bleed. Here again rule of locality is employed to give benefit of doubt to palces where blood bank facilities are not available.
- Knowingly taking up a high risk case in a set up not equipped enough to manage such a risky patient
- Not following standard protocols of preoperative, operative and postoperative management which is accepted by a body of doctors of similar qualifications
- Any other situation in which it is proved that doctors failed in his duty to give a standard of care towards his patient during the conduct of the case.

What the Doctors should expect from the relatives in such a situation?

- Communicate with the doctor and get satisfied about the reasons leading to such a death. Don't try to get information from the staff nurses and other staff member of the hospital. They will not be able to give a true picture of the situation in the operation theater.
- Don't bother the doctor with barrage of questions asked again and again. In stead let the senior most and understanding relative talk to the doctor and give the information to all other relatives.
- Don't prevent the doctor from doing a post mortem. We are all legally bound in a situation of a table death to avoid resisting postmortem. It is in the interest of all of us because,
- It tells us about the cause of death
- It clears out doubt about the role of doctor in the mishap. Negligence of the doctor can be diagnosed from post mortem report
- Don't prevent to smooth conduct of police panchanama. All the documentation is to collect evidence which can prove or disprove the negligence of the doctors involved
- Under no circumstance should you allow anti-social elements or aggressive relatives or friends or acquaintances known to you to create mob violence in the hospital. This is not only unethical but is also illegal and can attract arrest on criminal charges

- Pay the bill in full and take a receipt of the same because it is a good evidence of treatment being taken and paid for by the patient.

Remember that courts have time and again agreed that doctors are not always expected to create miracles and just because in a particular case mishap occurred, it doesn't always mean that doctor was negligent. If the doctor has taken reasonable care and followed all standard accepted treatment protocols then he can not be considered to have done negligence. Always give due consideration to the fact that doctors in our country often have to perform in trying situations due to non-affordability of the patients, non availability of blood and proper transport facility. And to top it all the menace of spurious drugs keeps a hanging sword on the top of both the doctors and the patients.

IDEAL ANTENATAL CASE SHEET

OPD Reg No. : .... IPD No. : .... Dt. of First visit: ....

Name : .... Age : .... yrs. Education : ....

Address : .... Occupation : .... Contact No. : ....

Husband's Name : .... Age : .... yrs. Education : ....

Occupation : .... Family I/c Rs. .... /mth. Age at Marriage .... yrs.

Consanguinous/Non-Consanguinous................................ Menarche .... yrs. PMH.......................

LMP ☐☐ ☐☐ ☐☐ **EDD** ☐☐ ☐☐ ☐☐

Obstetric History

G ☐ P ☐ A ☐ L ☐

Sr No.	Type of delivery/ abortion	L or D	Sex	Age yrs.	Birth BW(kg)	Complication's in pregnancy or labor or Peurperium	Indication for Intervention	Child Health
1								
2								
3								
4								
5								

If LSCS	Indication :	
	SA	Complications: ....
Elective/Emergency	GA/EA	Baby Outcome: ....

Past History

☐ Heart Disease ☐ Hypertension ☐ Diabetes ☐ Renal Disease ☐ Jaundice
☐ Operations ☐ Tuberculosis ☐ Blood Transfusion ☐ Bronchial Asthma ☐ Thyroid Dysfunction
☐ PIH ☐ Allergy ☐ Epilepsy ☐ Fever with erruptions ☐ Drugs

Family History

☐ Multifetal Pregnancy ☐ Hypertension ☐ Diabetes ☐ Anomalies

Dietary Recall

☐ Adequate ☐ Not adequate

I-Examination (Gest.Age-wks.)

Height .... cm. Weight .... kg. Pallor .... Pulse .... /min BP ..../
.... mm of Hg Thyroid .... Breast .... CVS .... RS ....
Varicose veins .... P/A .... Obst/E: Height of uterus .... wks .... cm
Abd Girth : .... cm. Pres : .... Pos : ....
FHS......................... /min other : .... Int/E:P/Sp : .... P/V : ....

Investigations

Blood Group : ABO: ☐ Rh ☐ Husb:Blood Group: ABO: ☐ Rh ☐

Date	Lab	Hb	Urine	BSL	ICT

GTT: ....
HIV: .... VDRL .... HBsAg: ....
TORCHT: ....
TFT: ....
Karyotype: ....
Pap smear: ....
PIH Profile: ....
Anemia Profile: ....

LMP: ....

Date	Complaints	WKS			WT	P	BP	OE	PP	POS	ENG	FHS	Treatment
		Date	USG	Fundus									

Date	Wks	Cx	Pelvimetry	inj. TT (dt.)	Special tests for Fetal Welbeing:

Sonography

1st Trimester:

Date	Dr.	Uterus	GS	FP	CRL	FCA	Ov.	Int OS	NT	Others	Impression

2nd/3rd Trimester:

Date	Dr.	Gestational Age					Placenta		FCA	Abn.	AF	Int OS	FW	Comments
		BPD	FL	HC	AC	Wks	Loc	Mat						

HIGH RISK FACTORS :
....

LIST OF MEDICAL RECORDS

List of Records

1. Case Papers
2. Prescriptions
3. Investigation and Reports
4. USG Reports
5. HPE Reports
6. Consent Forms
7. Anesthesia Forms
8. Operation Notes
9. Referral Notes
10. Discharge summary
11. Certificates.

Registers

A. OPD Register
B. Indoor Register
C. Operation Theater Register
D. Delivery Register
E. Birth and Death Register
F. Lab Register
G. Radiology including Imaging Register
H. Nurses GOB Register
I. M L C Register
J. M T P Register
K. Family Planning Device Register
L. Fumigation Register
M. Autoclave Register
N. Equipment Receipts.

SECTION-IV

PREOPERATIVE QUESTIONNAIRE

Date: ....

Name: .... Age: .... Sex: M/F

Address:...

This questionnaire is designed to assist the anesthesiologist who will be taking care of you during operation

	No	Yes
Have you had any previous operations?		
If yes, was there any problem in relation to anesthesia?		
Have you ever been admitted to hospital?		
Do you suffer from heart disease?		
Do you suffer from high blood pressure?		
Do you get breathless/chest pain on mild exercise or at night?		
Do you have asthma or bronchitis?		
Do you have diabetes?		
Do you have epilepsy/fits?		
Have you ever had liver disease/jaundice?		
Have you ever suffered from tuberculosis?		
Do you have tendency to:bruise easily/bleed excessively following minor injury?		
Have you recently suffered from cough, fever, running nose/sore throat?		
Do you smoke?		
Do you drink alcohol habitually?		
Do you have any loose/false teeth?		
Do you were contact lenses?		
Are you taking any medications?		
Do you suffer from backache?		
For women: are you pregnant?		

If answer to any of the above questions is yes, please bring the relevant papers at the time of surgery. Any other information you would like to give:

Signature of patient/parent/guardian

PREOPERATIVE INVESTIGATIONS

Based on the Age of the Patient

Age (Years)	*Hb*	*Urine*	*PT PTTK*	*Platelet BT*	*Elect Great*	*BUN Creat*	*BSL*	*LFT*	*CXR*	*ECG*
<40	•	•								
40-49	•	•								•
50-64	•	•							•	•
65-74	•	•					•	•	•	•
>75	•	•					•	•	•	•

Based on Pre Existing Medical Condition

Preoperative Disease	*PT PTTK*	*Platelet BT*	*Elect*	*BUN Creat*	*BSL*	*LFT*	*CXR*	*ECC*
Cardiovascular				•			•	•
Pulmonary							•	•
Hepatic	•					•		
Renal disease			•	•				
Diabetes			•	•	•			•
CNS			•	•	•			•
Malignancy								
Bleeding disorder	•	•						

Based on Preoperative Drug Therapy

Preoperative Drug therapy	*PT PTTK*	*Platelet BT*	*Elect*	*BUN Creat*	*BSL*	*LFT*	*CXR*	*ECC*
Diuretics			•	•				
Digoxin			•	•				•
Steroid			•		•			
Anticoagulants	•							
Smoking>20 pack year							•	•
Alcohol>80 gm/day						•		•

PREOPERATIVE INSTRUCTIONS FOR THE PATIENT

Mr./Mrs...Date:

Before coming to the hospital for any operation it is necessary to follow these instructions religiously for your own safety.

Do not take any solid foods from am/pm.on

Do not take any liquids from am/pm.on

Remove all the ornaments and jewellery before coming to the hospital

Remove nail paint, lip stick or any cosmetics before coming to the hospital

On the day prior to operation take all the medicines as advised by the doctor.

Avoid drinking alcohol, smoking or eating tobacco at least 24 hours prior to operation

Bring one responsible relative with you, who would stay with you during the operative and post-operative period

Remove the wrist watch, contact lenses, removable dentures before coming to the operation theater. Before coming to the operation theater wear loose cotton gown and avoid tight and synthetic clothes. For 24 hours after the operation avoid cooking, driving vehicle and handling machinery.

If you have not been able to follow a particular instruction for some reason; or if there is any change in your health condition, please inform the operating surgeon or the anesthetist.

Minimum Intraoperative Monitoring

Minor surgeries:	Pulse Blood Pressure Respiration Colour of nails/tongue
Major surgeries:	As above+ Urine output Temperature Pulse oximetry Electrocardiogram
If available:	End-tidal carbon dioxide monitor Peripheral nerve stimulator Central venous pressure Direct arterial pressure Blood gas analysis.

LIST OF ESSENTIAL EMERGENCY DRUGS

Medicine	*Trade name*	*Qty*	*Exp*
Adrenaline			
Aminophylline			
Atropine			
Calcium gluconate			
Deriphylline			
Dexamethasone			
Dextrose 25 percent			
Diazepam			
Dobutamine			
Dopamine			
Frusemide			
Glyceryl trinitrate (Tab/Inj)./ Patch)			
Hydrocortisone sodium succinate			
Kesol			
Mannitol			
Mephentermine			
Metoclopramide			
Nifedipine			
Pheniramine maleate			
Polygelatin or other plasma expanders			
Promethazine			
Sodium bicarbonate			
Suxamethonium			
Thiopentone sodium			
Verapamil			
Xylocaine			

LIST OF ADDITIONAL DRUGS FOR OPERATION THEATER

Medicine	*Qty*	*Exp. Date*
Adrenaline	10	
Aminophylline	5	
Antibiotics		
Atropine	5	
Calcium gluconate	5	
Chlorpheniramine maleate	5	
Deriphylline	5	
Dexamethasone	5	
Dextrose 25 percent	5	
Distilled water/Normal saline Ampoules	50	
Chloramphenicol Aplicap	10	
Dopamine	5	
Frusemide	10	
Glyco pyrolate	10	
Heparin/Logiparin	1	
Hydrocortisone sodium	5	
Kesol	5	
Mannitol	2	
Mephentermine	5	
Metoclopramide	10	
Midazolam	2 vial	
NSAID Inj.Diclofenac/Piroxicam	5	
Ondansetron	5	
Paracetamol	1vial	
Pentazocine	10	
Phenytoin sodium	5	
Polygelatin	2	
Prochlorperazine	5	
Promethazine	5	
Ranitidine	5	
Sodium bicarbonate	10	
Tramadol hydrochloride	10	
Xylocaine without preservative(Xylocard)	1	
Xylocaine with Adrenaline	5	
Xylocaine without Adrenaline.	5	
Xylocaine	4 percent	
Lignocaine 10 percent spray	1	
Cardarone	1	
Nicoran	1	
Betaloc	1	

LIST OF "ANESTHETIC DRUGS" GA/REGIONAL

Drug	*Qty.*
Bupivacaine (for spinal)	5 amp
Bupivacaine	3 vial
Ketamine	2 vial
Neostigmine	20 amp
Pancuronium or Atracurium or Vecuronium	5 amp
Suxame honium	3 vial
Thiopentone sodium	5 vial
Xylocaine 5 percent	5 amp

SPECIAL DRUGS FOR OBSTETRIC OPERATION THEATER

Drug	*Brand*	*Qty.*
Carboprost	Prostodin	2
Methylergometrine	Methergine	5
Oxytocin	Pitocin	15
Hyoscine hydrobromide	Buscopan	5
Magnesium sulphate	Magsulf	10

CHECK LIST OF PREOPERATIVE PREPARATION

Patient Preparation

Match the name of the patient with surgery to be done and confirm the side

Confirm: NBM status
Consent is taken
Allergies if any
Notes and investigation reports are entered on the case paper.
Blood has been sent for grouping and cross-matching if indicated.
Presence of responsible relative.
Language of communication
Enema, shaving, etc. if indicated.
Remove jewellery, nail polish, contact lenses, and dentures.

Theater Preparation

Confirm: Date of fumigation.
Drums are autoclaved and ready as per schedule.
All the disposables are ready (as per requirement of the case.)

1. Syringes 2 cc, 5 cc, 10 cc, 20 cc
2. Needles: 24,25,26,20,18
3. Scalp vein-20,21,22,24
4. Intracath No 24,22,20,18,16.
5. Three way/Bivalve.
6. IV sets, Blood set, Microdrip set.
7. IV bottles: RL, DNS,D5,D10,NS, dextrose 25 percent, Hemaccel or Hestar, etc.

8. Spinal needles (23,25,26,27,29)
9. Epidural catheter and set.16,18
10. Cavafix
11. Urethral catheters, urine bags.
12. Ryle's tube
13. Drain:Corrugated, Suction drain.
14. Gel foam
15. Cloves, caps, drapes, growns, etc.
16. Anesthesia equipment to be checked with availability of oxygen, suction, alternative light source.

ANESTHESIA RECORD

Name : .... Sex:M/F Age: .... Yrs: ....
Date : .... Reg. No: ....Wt: ....Kgs
Surgeon : Dr. .... Anesthetist: Dr. ....
Operation : ....

Preoperative Assessment

H/O Previous Anesthesia:
H/O Past Medical Problems:
H/O Allergy:
H/O Smoking/Alcohol/Tobacco chewing
Drug history:
O/E: Pulse: BP.:
Airway: MP Teeth: TM Dist:
Resp. syst.:
CVS :
Exercise Tolerance:

Premedication:

NBM*
Ranitidine/Omeprazole: mg.}Orally with sip of water
Metoclopramide/Ondansetron: mg.}2 hrs before Operation, (at)
Atropine/Glycopyrolate: mg.IM half an hour before sending to OT.
Steam Inhalation:
Nebulization with saline/salbutamol

Investigations:

Hb: WBC: Platelets: 10/lit
Urine: BSL:
Urea: Creatinine:
Electrolyte:Na: sec K: INR:
Coagulation:PT:
X-ray Chest:
ECG:
Others:

ANESTHESIA NOTES

Details:

Induction: Inhalational/IV
General/Spinal/Epidural/Local/Stand-by
Regional:Aseptic Technique
ASA Score

Maintenance: Airway ETT No.Spot.Resp/IPPV with O2+N2O+

Position: Sitting/Lateral

Space: L1/2, L2/3, L3/4, L4/5
LM No. Betadine and Spirit for Preparation

mis Percent Lignocaine for LA Needle: No: G.Spinal/Tuohy

Reversal: Neostigmine mg; Epi.Space cm.
Atrop/Clycop mg; cath in space cm.

Drugs:

Time																											
O2																											
N2O																											
Fluids																											
Chart																											
Code																											
Pulse																											
BP																											
^																											
V																											

Position: Approx Blood Loss:

Postoperative Progress:

Patient:awake/obeying commands pules: BP: SaO2%

Postoperative Instruction:

Inform SOS{Contact No.}

POSTOPERATIVE INSTRUCTIONS DURING RECOVERY

NBM for Hours
Position: head low/head up/propped up/lateral (as applicable)
O2 by mask (If required)
Watch for response to verbal commands.
Watch for vomiting:Oral suction if required
Monitoring: TPR/BPI/O chart Sao2, ECG if required
IV fluids: as required
Analgesics: as required Antiemetics:as required Antibiotics: as required Physiotherapy:(if applicable)
Inform SOS.
Tel numbers of:
Surgeon:
Anesthetist:
Hospital owner:

CHART FOR DISPLAY

Cardiac Arrest Management Protocol

CARDIAC ARREST

Basic Life Support
Open Airway
Check Breathing
Assess Circulation
Chest compression 100/min
Ventilation

Advanced Life Support
Precordial Thump
Attach Monitor/Defibrillator

Ventricular Fibrillation or Ventricular Tachycardia

Defibrillate × 3 (1st series 200 200 360 j Subse. series 360 360 360j

CPR (1 min) Chest Compression (100/min) Ventilation 15:2

Assess Rhythm Non VFA/T Asystole/Electro-Mechanical dissociation(Check pulse)

CPR (3 min) Chest Compression (100/min Ventilation 15:2

During CPR

1. Correct Reversible Causes

Hypoxia Hypovolemia Hypothermia Hupo/hyperkalemia and Metabolic disorders	Tension Pneumothorax Tamponade Toxic Disorders Thromboembolic and Mechanical obstruction

2. If not done already check electrode paddle position and contact Attempt and verify-Airway and Oxygen and venous access Give adrenaline (1 mg) every 3 min (1ml of 1 in 1000 solution)

3. Consider Antiarrhythmic drugs-Lignocaine,Bretylium Atropine 3 mg iv once only/Pacing if there is P wave activity Buffers-50 ml of NaHCO3 (8.4%) only when pH<7.0 and BE>-10 mmol/lit

Ref.: Guidelines published by the European Resuscitation Council (1998) and the resuscitation council (UK)

ALGORITHMS

Bradycardia Algorithm

Bradycardia
Heart rate <60 bpm and inadequate for clinical condition

↓

- Maintain patent airway; assist breathing as needed
- Give Oxygen
- Monitor ECG (identify mythm), blood pressure, oximetry
- Establish IV access

↓

Signs or symptoms of poor perfusion caused by the bradycardia?

(e.g. acute altered mental status, ongoing chest pain, hypotension or other signs of shock

Adequate perfusion → **Observe/Monitor**

Poor perfusion →

- Prepare for transcutaneous pacing; use without delay for high-degree block (type II second-degree block or third-degree AV block)
- Consider atropine 0.5 mg IV while awaiting pacer. May repeat to a total dose of 3 mg. If ineffective, begin pacing
- Consider epinephrine (2 to 10 μg/min) or dopamine (2 to 10 μg/kg per minute) infusion while awaiting pacer or if pacing ineffective

↓

- Prepare for transvenous pacing
- Treat contributing causes
- Consider expert consultation

Reminders

- If pulseless arrest develops, go to pulseless Arrest Algorithm
- Search for and treat possible contributing factors:
  - -Hypovolemia
  - -Hypoxia
  - -Hydrogen ion (acidosis)
  - -Hypo-/hyperkalemia
  - -Hypoglycemia
  - -Toxins
  - -Tamponade,cardiac
  - -Tension pneumothorax
  - -Thrombosis (coronary or pulmonary)
  - -Trauma (hypovolemia, Increased ICP)

HEALTHCARE PROVIDER ALGORITHM

(Adopted from BLS (Basic Life Support) AHA (American Heart Association))

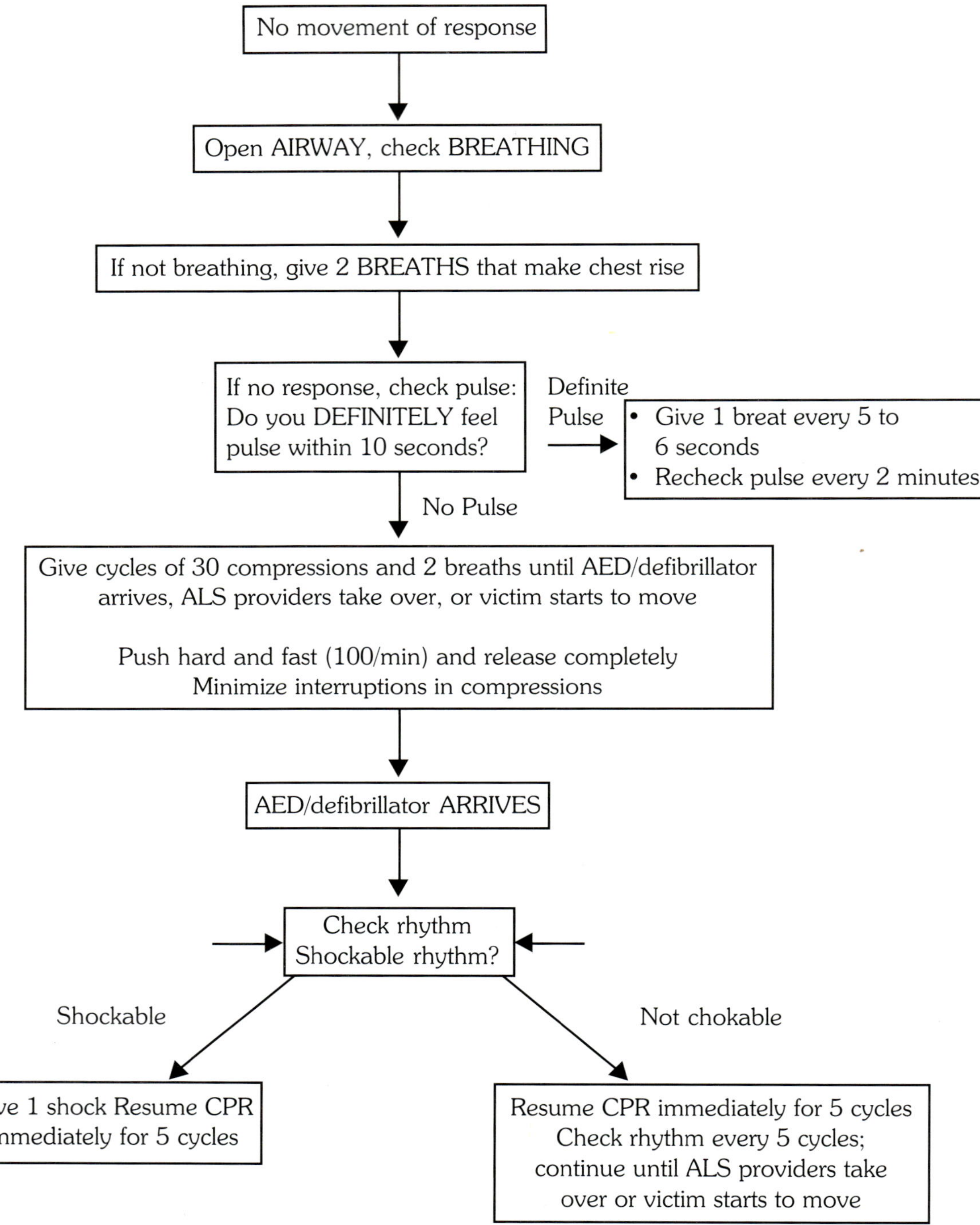

PULSELESS ARREST ALGORITHM

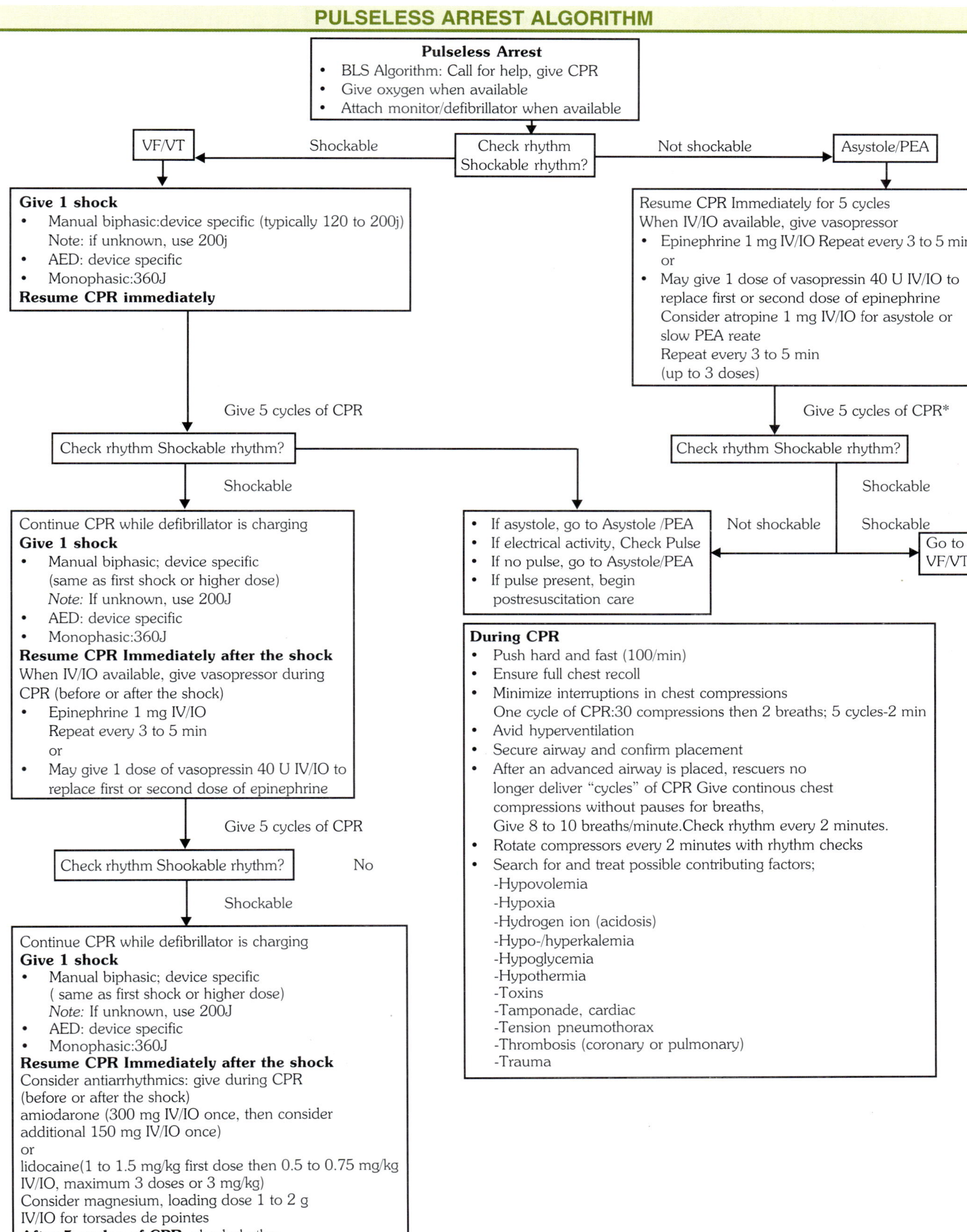

TACHYCARDIA ALGORITHM

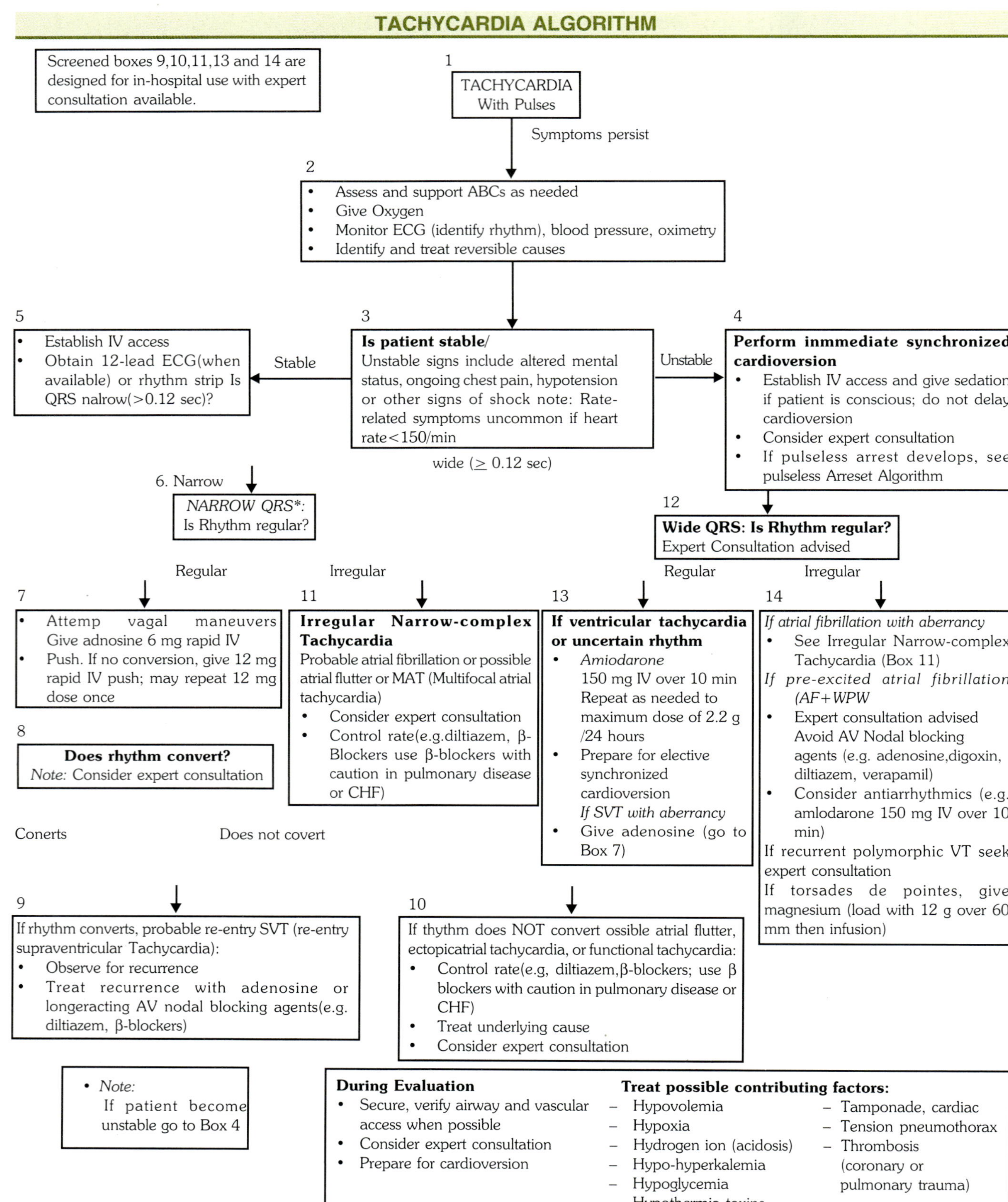

INFUSION RATES FOR SELECTED CARDIOVASCULAR MEDICATIONS

Nitroglycerin (25 mg/250 ml]= SO mg/500 ml= 100/ig/mi)

Dosage(ug/min)	*Infusion rate microdrops/min= ml/hr(60 microdrops/ml*
5	3
10	6
20	12
30	18
40	24
50	30
60	36
70	42
80	48
90	54
100	60
110	66
120	72
130	78
140	84
150	90
160	96
170	102
180	108
190	114
200	120

Lidocaine (2 gm/500 ml=4 mg/ml)

Dosage(mg/min)	*Infusion rate microdrops/min=ml/hr(60 microdrops/ml)*
1	15
2	30
3	45
4	60

Dopamine Hydrochloride (800 mg/500 ml = 1600 ug/ml

	Body weight								
Dosage	88	99	110	121	132	143	154	165	176
(ug/kg/min)	40	45	50	55	60	65	70	75	80
1.0	2	2	2	2	2	2	3	3	3
2.5	4	4	5	5	6	6	7	7	8
5.0	8	8	9	10	11	12	13	14	15
7.5	11	13	14	15	17	18	20	21	23
10.0	15	17	19	21	23	24	26	28	30
15.0	23	25	28	31	34	37	39	42	45
20.0	30	34	38	41	45	49	52	56	60
25.0	38	42	47	52	56	61	66	70	75
30.0	45	51	56	62	67	73	78	84	90

Infusion rate: microdrops/min = ml/hr (60 microdrops/ml)

Dobutamine Hydrochloride (250 mg/250 ml = 1000 ug/ml)

					Body weight				
Dosage	88	99	110	121	132	143	154	165	176
(ug/kg/min)	40	45	50	55	60	65	70	75	80
1.0	2	3	3	3	4	4	4	5	5
2.5		7	8	8	9	10	11	11	12
5.0	12	14	15	17	18	20	21	23	24
7.5	18	20	23	25	27	29	32	34	36
10.0	24	27	30	33	36	39	42	45	48
12.5	30	34	38	41	45	49	53	56	60
15.0	36	41	45	50	54	59	63	68	72
20.0	48	54	60	66	72	78	84	90	96
30.0	72	81	90	99	108	117	126	135	144
40.0	96	108	120	132	144	156	168	180	192

Infusion rate: microdrops/min= ml/hr (60 microdrops/ml)

INFUSION RATES FOR SELECTED CARDIOVASCULAR MEDICATIONS

Norepinephrine (4 mg/250 ml = 16/zg/ml)

Dosage(μg/min)	*Infusion rate microdrops/min=ml/hr(60 microdrops/ml)*	
1	4	
	1	8
4	15	
6	23	
8	30	
	10	38
	12	45
	16	60
	20	75
	24	90
	28	105

Isoproterenol (2 mg/250 ml = 8/ug/ml)

Dosage(ug/min)	*Infusion rate microdrops/min= ml/hr (60 microdrops/ml)*	
1	8	
	2	15
4	30	
6	45	
8	60	
	10	75
	12	90
	16	120
	20	150

Oxytocin Infusion Sharing Relationship Between drops/min and milliunits

Drops/min	*5 Units/500 ml (milliunits/min)*	*2.5 units/500 ml (milliunits/min)*
10	5	2.5
20	10	5
30	15.0	7.5
40	20	9.80
50	25.0	12.30
60	29.0	14.80

GUIDELINE FOR MANAGEMENT OF AN ADULT PATIENT WITH SUSPECTED ANAPHYLAXIS DURING ANESTHESIA

Initial Therapy

1. Stop administration of drug(s) likely to have caused the anaphylaxis.
2. Maintain airways: give 100 percent oxygen.
3. Lay patient flat with legs elevated
4. Give epinephrine. Intravenously in a dose of 0.1-1 mg (0.1-1.0 ml of 1:1000 solution) and it is further titrated according to the blood pressure response. Patient with cardiovascular collapse require endo-tracheal intubation, artifical ventilation with 100 percent oxygen and titration of Adrenaline drip.
5. Rapid introvenous volume replacement with 1-2 lit of colloid initially. For maintenance of blood pressure several liters of crystalloid may be necessary.

Secondary Therapy

1. Antihistamines: H1 blockers like Chlorpheniramine or Promethazine and H2 blockers like Ranitidine.
2. Corticosteroids (100-300 mg hydrocortisone iv)
3. Catecholamine infusions (starting doses: epinephrine 4-8 ug min [0.05-0.1 ug kg^{-1} min^{-1}]; norepinephrine 4-8 ug min^{-1} [0.04-0.1/ug kg^{-1} min^{-1}]; isoproterenol 0.05-0.1 ug min^{-1}]
4. Nebulization with bronchodilator like Salbutamol to treat persistent bronchospasm.
5. Once the systems start stabilizing gradual weaning off the inotropic support and ventilation support.

REQUISITES FOR INSTITUTING EPIDURAL ANALGESIA

A. Resuscotative equipment:
   1. Adequate supply of oxygen and ventimask with reservoir bag
   2. Ventilation apparatus
   3. A laryngoscope with blades 3,4,5
   4. Range of endotracheal tubes from size 6 to 8.
   5. The table should have facility for quick Trendelenburg position.
   6. Suction apparatus.
   7. Intravenous cannulae, colloids, and crystalloids.
   8. Drugs to treat hypotension and bradycardia, i.e Atropine, Ephedrine and Dopamine.

B. Regional block equipment
   1. Epidural set with needle, catheter, LOR syringe and bacterial filter (16g/18g)
   2. Drugs:
      Lignocaine 2 percent with or without Adrenaline
      Bupivacaine: 0.25 percent or 0.5 percent Normal saline ampoules
      Fentany (2 ml = 100 mcg)

C. Sterile items
   1. Sterile trolly with gowns and gloves.
   2. Sterile drapes
   3. Betadine, spirit with sponge holding forceps
   4. Syringes: 2 ml 5 ml 10 ml (2 each)
   5. Needles: No 18, No 24 (2 each)

PROTOCOL FOR INSTITUTING EPIDURAL LABOR ANALGESIA

A. Preparation

Introduction of the anesthesiologist to the patient.

The anesthesiologist should explain the procedure, the possible complications and obtain an informed consent. Check all resuscitation equipment and drugs

Take complete medical history from patient and the medical records, thorough clinical examination and examine the lab reports

Rule out contraindications for epidural injection: e.g. bleeding disorder, anticoagulant therapy.

Establish intravenous access and pre-load with appropriate quantity of crystalloid.

B. Technique

Thorough hand wash with sterile gown and gloves

Disposables are taken on sterile trolley: Epidural set, syringes 10,5,2 Needles 21,24 Antiseptic care of the back. Position is either sitting or lateral depending on the choice of the anesthesiologist. Lumbar interspace 2/3 or 3/4 is identified.

Local infiltration analgesia. Ask the patient not to move without warning and informing the anesthesiologist at every contraction.

The epidural space is identified using loss of resistance to air or saline.

Catheter is passed, the needle is removed and excess of catheter is withdrawn leaving 3-5 cm. in the epidural space. The catheter is then taped to the back of the patient.

C. Test Dose and Top-up Doses

Loading dose of 10 to 15 ml. is administered containing Bupivacaine in the range of 0.0625 percent to 0.2 percent with Fentany 2 mcg/ml

Careful monitoring of vital parameters especially blood pressure throughout the labor.

Further top-ups are given based on patient's demand or at fixed time intervals.

Maintain the lateral position so as to prevent caval compression.

Fetal heart and uterine contractions are monitored at regular intervals.

The anesthesiologist should remain available in close vicinity to handle a medical of obstetric emergency.

EPIDURAL LABOR ANALGESIA:RECORD SHEET

Name: Date:

Age yrs Parity: Primi/Multi

Obstetrician-Dr Anesthetist-Dr.

Indication-Patient's Request ☐ Obstetrician's Request ☐ Patient's Condition ☐

Induction of labor-Spontaneous Oxytocin Prostaglandin ☐

Procedure

Position-Sitting ☐ Lateral ☐ Lumbar Space-L1-2qL2-3qL3-4qL4-5

Tuohy Needle-no. 16qNo. 18 ☐ Loss of resistance to-Saline ☐ Air ☐

Epidural space cm Catheter in space cm

Drugs

Initial set-up: Bupivacaine percent Fentanyl ugm/ml

Dose- ml

Subsequent Top-ups Bupivacaine percent Fentanyl ugm/ml

Dose- ml

Problems

1. Bony Obstruction ☐
2. 1 Space Attempted ☐
3. Bloody Tap ☐
4. Dural Puncture a ☐
5. Difficulty in Threading The Catheter a ☐
6. Bloody Tap with Catheter ☐
7. Dural Tap with Catheter ☐
8. Inadequate Block ☐
9. Unilateral Block ☐
10. Others ☐

Complications

Immediate 1. Hypotension 2. Bradycardia 3. Total Spinal ltching

Late 1. PDP Headache 2. Neurological Sequelae 3. Others

Mode of delivery- 1. NVD ☐ 2. Instrumental ☐ 3. LSCS ☐

Duration of labor-hrs min

APCAR score- 0 MIN 1 MIN 5 MIN

Monitoring

Time	*Dose*	*B.P: 5 Min*	*10 Min*	*15 Min*	*Cx Dil*

Appendix 'C'

Application for Registration of Indian Nationals U/S 13(3) of the Indian Medical Council Act, 1956

(By Dr RN Goel)

1. Name of the applicant (block capital letters)
2. Father's name (block letters)
3. Date and place of birth
4. Preliminary education (full particulars of matriculation or equivalent examination passed with name of the examination body and with year of obtaining)
5. Date of passing inter science or equivalent examination with name of the university.
6. Name of the medical school/college attended with the date of joining and leaving (block capital letters)
7. Name of the medical degree/diploma obtained and univ/licensing body with the year of obtaining the qualifications.
8. a. Whether s/he has undergone practical training before or after obtaining the medical qualification required by the rules of the concerned foreign country, give details.
   b. If not, then has s/he undergone the prescribed training in and approved hospital in India, give details.
9. Was any recognized medical college/school in India attended before departure from India, outside countries (give names of period of study undergone and examination passed).
10. If the language of study in the country be other than English, please indicate if it was studied in India before departure or was studied in that country. Please indicate the time taken for that study and whether any examination was passed.
11. Do the medical examination(s) passed *ipso facto* entitle one to register in the country in which they were taken or a separate examination for registration has to be passed.
12. If s/he is registered in any foreign country? If so, give the name of the body with which registered and the number and date of registration.
13. Is he a citizen of India
    a. by birth or
    b. by domicile
    If (b) state the date of becoming Indian citizen.
14. Present address (capital letter) with pin code and phone
    Remarks of the state medical
15. Council how the information contained above has been verified as authentic.

Date: Signature of the applicant

Note: The application form should be properly and neatly filled in.

PROCEDURE FOR REGISTRATION

1. a. Attested xerox copies (two each) of the following certificates/testimonials must be attached. Degree/diploma (if the same in language other than English then an authentic translation in English)
   b. Certificate of having undergone the practical training
   c. Certificate of Indian citizenship duly attested by a 1st class magistrate or an attested xerox copy of Indian pass-port
   d. X pass/matriculation certificate.
   e. XII pass/Sr. Secondary/Intermediate/+2 marksheet along with(returnable) original documents.
   f. Two recent passport size photographs front view.
   g. Signature on two self adhesive slip provided with application.
2. The total registration fee is Rs 1500/- (Rupees one thousand five hundred only).
   However, if a candidate has obtained provisional registration in India s/he is required to pay only Rs 1000/- a bank draft for Rs.1000/- (or Rs 1500/- or Rs 500/- as applicable) drawn in favor of the secretary, medical council of India, New Delhi payable at New Delhi, must be sent along with the applicable for registration with Medical Council of India.
   In case registration is sought with a State Medical Council of India the registration fee will be as per rules of the concerned State Medical Council.
3. The certificate will be sent by Regd. Post/speed post.
4. Provisional registration certificate in original issued by State Medical Council/Medical Council of India, has to be surrendered alongwith application for permanent registration.

Procedure Regarding Registration and Related Matters

The Council issues Provisional Registration u/s 25(2) of the IMC Act, 1956 to the candidates possessing recognized medical qualifications awarded by the Indian Universities to undergo one year internship training provided the candidates submit a copy of pass certificate and NOC from the Dean of the college and the required fee for Rs. 500/- by a Bank Draft in favor of Secretary, Medical Council of India.

The Council issues Permanent Registration u/s 23 of the IMC Act, 1956 to the candidates possessing recognized medical qualifications awarded by the Indian Universities Provided the candidate surrender Provisional Registration certificate (in original), Internship completion Certificate and the required fee for Rs.1000/- by a Bank Draft in favor of Secretary, Medical Council of India.

The Council issues Conditional Provisional Registration u/s 25(1) of the IMC Act,1956 to the Candidates possessing recognized foreign medical qualification to undergo one year internship training provided the candidate submits the copy of degree, passport and 10+2 mark sheet or its equivalent (in original) with the required fee for Rs. 500/- by a Bank Draft in favor of Secretary, Medical Council of India subject to verification of degree, passport and 10+2 mark sheet or its equivalent from the authorities concerned.

If the Council receives the authenticity of the documents from the authority concerned, the Council issues Permanent Registration u/s 13(3) of the IMC Act, 1956 to the candidate possessing recognized foreign medical qualification provided the candidate surrenders the Provisional Registration Certificate and submits a copy of one year internship training certificate, with the required fee for Rs. 1000/- by a Bank Draft in favor of Secretary, Medical Council of India and the prescribed form duly filled by the Candidate.

Procedure for Getting IMR Certificate

The following are requirements for obtaining IMR Certificate:

1. A hand written/typed application addressed to the Secretary, Medical Council of India, New Delhi, requesting for getting IMR Certificate.
2. An attested Xerox copy of registration with Medical Council of India or with any State Medical Council
3. A demand draft of Rs. 100/- in favor of Secretary, Medical Council of India payable at New Delhi at any Bank.

MEDICAL COUNCIL OF INDIA
Pocket-14, Sector-8, Dwarka Phase-1
New Delhi-110075
India

Phones: 091-011-25367033, 25367035, 25367036
Fax: 25367025 Telegrams: MEDCONCIND
E-mail: mci@bol.net.in
Website: http//www.mciindia.org

APPLICATION FORM
FOR REGISTRATION OF ADDITIONAL QUALIFICATION/S
U/S 26(1) OF THE INDIAN MEDICAL COUNCIL ACT,1956

1. Name of the Doctor
2. Address as given in the Indian Medical Register
3. Present address in block capitals with pincode and phone no.
4. Permanent address in block capitals with pincode and phone no.
5. a. Primary qualification (i.e 'MBBS' or equvalent) with year of obtaining.
   b. Name and address of College/Institute attended for the same alongwith duration of course.
   c. Date of completion of internship.
   d. University awarding the qualification.
6. a. Name of the State Medical Council with which registered.
   b. Registration number (as it appears on the registration certificate).
   c. Date of registration
7. Additional qualification for which certificate is requested with documentary proof. column

Details to be furnised in the Table given as under (Please do not fill the remarks)

Qualification	*College attended*	*University*	*Date of qualification*	*Remarks R/NR etc.*

Declaration

8. I solemnly affirm and declare that the above entries made by me are correct.

Date:

Signature of the candidate

Important Instructions

The following instructions should be read carefully before filling up the forms:

- Incomplete documents will be rejected.
- The forms should be COMPLETE IN ALL THE RESPECT and SHOULD BE filled up in capital letters in candidate's own legible handwriting.
- All the documents should be signed and dated by the applicant only.
- The addresses, wherever required, should be complete in all respect.
- The date, wherever required, should be mentioned in complete i.e. year, month, and the day.
- The fee is non-refundable and is accepted by Demand Draft only in favor of Secretary, Medical Council of India payable at New Delhi.

- Public dealing will be between 3:00 and 5:00 PM only.
- No enquiry will be entertained over telephone during office hours.
- Candidates are requested to not to approach the office before 30 days of submission of the Application form alongwith other documents/receipt of the verification from the concerned issuing authorities, if any.
- The certificate will be issued only to those who possess a registrable basic medical qualification and subsequently have obtained recognized postgraduate medical qualification(s) as per the provisions of the IMC Act,1956.
- The candidates are requested to ensure that the documents be enclosed as per the order in the Checklist. All the certificates should be submitted in original alongwith 2 clear attested photocopies of each of these certificates. All papers/documents should be numbered according to the checklist.

CHECK LIST

Check List for Enclosures

1. Bank draft @ Rs. 100/- (Rupees one hundred only) for each qualificaton in favor of Secretary, Medical Council of India, New Delhi, payable at New Delhi.
2. The degrees/diplomas or provisional certificate of postgraduate qualification issued by the Principal/Dean of the college concerned, as shown in Col. '7' of the application form.
3. The degrees/diplomas or provisional certificate of postgraduate qualification issued by the Registrar of the University concerned, as shown in Col. '7' of the application form.
4. The candidate is required to send the original as well as a copy, duly attested by Magistrate/Gazetted Officer, of the originals will be returned alongwith the certificate of registration of additional qualification and the attested copies will be retained in this office.
5. Copy of permanent reigstration certificate.
6. Attested copy of the pass certificate from the college.
7. Those who are already registered with State Medical Council there is no need for re-registration with MCI.
8. Two recent passport size photographs front view and two adhesive signature slips.

MINISTRY OF HEALTH AND FAMILY WELFARE

(Department of Family Welfare)

Notification

New Delhi, the 13th June, 2003

GSR 485 (E) - In exercise of powers conferred by Section 6 of the Medical Termination of Pregnancy Act, 1971 (34 of 1971), the Central Government hereby makes the following rules, namely:

1. Short title and commencement—
    1. These rules may be called the Medical Termination of Pregnancy Rules, 2003.
    2. They shall come into force on the date of their publication in the Official Gazette.
2. Definitions: In this rules, unless the context otherwise requires,
    a. "Act" means the Medical Termination of Pregnancy Act, 1971 (34 of 1971) and the Medical Termination of Pregnancy (Amendment) Act, 2002 (64 of 2002).
    b. "Chief Medical Officer of the District" means the Chief Medical Officer of a District, by whatever name called;
    c. "Form" means a form appended to these rules.
    d. "Owner" in relation to a place means any person who is the administrative head or otherwise responsible for the working or maintenance of a hospital or place, by whatever name called, where the pregnancy may be terminated under this Act.

   e. "Committee" means a committee constituted at the district level under the proviso to clause (b) of Section 4 read Rule 3.

3. Composition and tenure of District Level Committee
   1. One member of the district level committee shall be the Gynecologist/surgeon/Anesthetist and other members from the local medical profession, nongovernmental organization, and Panchayati Raj Institution of the District. Provided that one of the members of the Committee shall be a woman.
   2. Tenure of the Committee shall be for two calendar years and the tenure of the non-government members shall not be more than two terms.
4. Experience and training under clause (d) of Section 2:
   For the purpose of clause (d) of Section (2), a registered medical practitioner shall have one or more of the following experience or training in gynecology and obstetrics, namely;
   a. In the case of a medical practitioner, who was registered in a State Medical Register immediately before the commencement of the Act, experience in the practice of gynecology and obstetrics for a period of not less than three years;
   b. In the case of a medical practitioner, who is registered in a State Medical Register:
      i. If he has completed six months of house surgery in gynecology and obstetrics; or
      ii. Unless the following facilities are provided therein, if he had experience at any hospital for a period of not less than one year in the practice of obstetrics and gynecology; or
   c. If he has assisted a registered medical practitioner in the performance of twenty-five cases of medical termination of pregnancy of which at least five have been performed independently, in a hospital established or maintained or a training institute approved for this purpose by the government.
      i. This training would enable the Registered Medical Practitioner (RMP) to do only 1st Trimester terminations (up to 12 weeks of gestation).
      ii. For terminations up to twenty weeks the experience or training as prescribed under sub rules (a), (b), and (d) shall apply.
   d. In case of a medical practitioner who has been registered in a State Medical Register and who holds a post-graduate degree or diploma in gynecology and obstetrics, the experience or training gained during the course of such degree of diploma.
5. Approval of a place
   - No palce shall be approved under clause (b) of Section 4
      i. Unless the Government is satisfied that termination of pregnancies may be done therein under safe and hygienic conditions; and
      ii. Unless the following facilities are provided therein, namely

   In case of first trimester, that is, up to 12 weeks of pregnancy: A gynecology examination/lab our table, resuscitation and sterilization equipment, drugs and parental fluid, back up facilities for treatment of shock and facilities for transportation; and

   In case of second trimester, that is, up to 20 weeks of pregnancy:
   a. An operation table and instruments for performing abdominal or gynecological surgery;
   b. Anesthetic equipment, resuscitation equipment and sterilization equipment;
   c. Drugs and parental fluids for emergency use.
6. *Form of consent:* The consent referred to in sub-Section(4) of Section 3 shall be given in Form C.

FORM B

(See sub-Rule (6) of Rule 5)

Certificate of Approval

The place described below is hereby approved for the purpose of the Medical termination of Pregnancy Act, 1971 (34 of 1971).

As read within up to .... weeks

Name of the Place

Address and other descriptions

Name of the owner

Place :

Date:

To the Government of the ....

FORM C

(See Rule 8)

I .... daughter/wife of .... aged about .... years of .... (Here state the permanent address). At Present residing at do hereby give me consent to the termination of my pregnancy .... (State the name of place where the pregnancy is to be terminated).

Place:

Date: Signature

(To be filled in by guardian where the woman is a mentally ill person or minor)

I .... son/daughter/wife of .... aged about .... years of .... at present residing at (Permanent address) .... do hereby give my consent to the termination of the pregnancy of my ward .... who is a minor/ lunatic at .... (Place of termination of my pregnancy)

Place:

Date: Signature

PREGNANCY TERMINATION ACT

FORM 'A'

(See Sub-Rule (1) of Rule 5)

Application for Registration and Grant of Certificate

I, ... a registered medical practitioner within the meaning of Section 2 (d) of the Medical Termination of Pregnancy Act, 1971 (34 of 1971), hereby apply for the registration of my name and issue of certificate to the effect that I possess the prescribed experience or training referred to in the said section. My other particulars are as follows:

1. Address:...
2. Designation:
3. Name of the State Medical Register in which registered and the registration no.
4. Qualification:

Qualification	*Year*	*University*
a. Medical degree or Equivalent qualification b. Post-graduate medical degree or diploma		

5. Experience in practice of Gynecology and Obstetrics:

6. Training in termination of pregnancy: Duration... Place of training...Certified that the particulars given above are correct to the best of my knowledge.

Place : ....
Date : ....

Signature ....

NB: For ready reference the relevant rule is reproduced below:

"5.(1) For the purpose of establishing that he possess such degree or diploma and experience or training or both in Gynecology and Obstetrics as is referred to in Rule 4. Every registered medical practitioner who intends to terminate any pregnancy in accordance with the provisions of the Act shall make an applicaton Form 'A' to the State Family Welfare Officer for the registration of his name and for the issue of a certificate to him to the effect that he possessed the said degree or diploma and the said experience or training or both."

FORM 'B'

(See sub-Rule (6) of Rule 5)

Certificate of approval

The place described below is hereby approved for the purpose of the Medical termination of Pregnancy Act, 1971 (34 of 1971).

As read within up to...................... weeks

Name of the Place

Address and other descriptions

Name of the owner

Place:
Date:

To the Government of the ....

FORM 'C'

(See Rule 8)

I, ... daughter/wife of .... aged about .... years of .... (Here state the permanent address) At present residing at .... do hereby give my consent to the termination of my pregnancy at .... (State the name of place where the pregnancy is to be terminated)

Place:

Date: Signature

(To be filled in by guardian where the woman is a mentally ill person or minor)

I, ... son/daughter/wife of .... aged about .... years of .... at present residing at (Permanent address) .... do hereby give my consent to the termination of the pregnancy of my ward .... who is a minor/ lunatic at ....

(Place of termination of my pregnancy)

Place:

Date: Signature

FORM A

[See Rules 4(1) and 8(1)]
(To be submitted in duplicate)

With supporting documents as enclosures, also in duplicate form of application for registration or renewal of registration of a genetic counselling center/genetic laboratory/genetic clinic

1. Name of the applicant (specify Shri/Smt/Km/Dr)
2. Address of the applicant
3. Type of facility to be registered
   (specify Genetic Counseling Center/Genetic Laboratory/Genetic Clinic/any combination of these)
4. Full name and address/addresses
   of Genetic Counseling Center/Genetic Laboratory/Genetic Clinic/with Telephone/Telegraphic/Telex/Fax E-mail numbers.
5. Type of ownership and organization
   (specify individual ownership/partnership/company/co-operative/any other).In case of type of organization other than individual ownership, furnish copy of articles of association and names and addresses of other persons responsible for management, as enclosure.
6. Type of Institution
   (Govt Hospital/Municipal Hospital/Public Hospital/Private Hospital/Private Nursing Home/Private Clinic/Private Laboratory/any other to be stated.)
7. Specific prenatal diagnostic procedures/tests for which approval is sought
   (for example amniocentesis, Chorionic villi aspiration/Chromosomal/biochemical/molecular studies, etc.)
   Leave blank if registration sought for Genetic Counselling Center only.
8. Equipment available with the make and model of each equipment
   List to be attached on a separate sheet.
9. a. Facilities available in the Counseling Center
      i. Ultrasound
      ii. Amniocentesis
      iii. Chorionic villi aspiration
      iv. Fetoscopy
      v. Fetal biopsy
      vi. Cordocentesis
   b. Whether facilities are available in the Laboratory/Clinic for the following tests:
      i. Chromosomal studies
      ii. Biochemical studies
      iii. Molecular studies
10. Names, qualifications, experience and registration number of employees may be furnished as an enclosure (Refer Schedules I, II or III).
11. State whether the Genetic Counseling Center/Genetic Laboratory/Genetic Clinic [1[1]] qualifies for registration in terms of minimum requirements laid down in Schedule I, II, and III and if not, reasons therefore.
12. For renewal applications only:
    a. Registration No.
    b. Date of issue and date of expiry of existing certificate of registration.
13. List of Enclosures:
    Please attach a list of enclosures giving the supporting documents enclosed to this application.

Date:
Place: Name and Signature of applicant

[1[1]] Stike out whichever is not applicable or not necessary. All enclosures are to be authenticated by signature of the applicant.

FORM F

[See Proviso to Section 4(3), Rule 9(4) and Rule 10(1A)

Form for maintenance of record in respect of pregnant woman by genetic clinic/ultrasound clinic/imaging center

1. Name and address of the Genetic Clinic/Ultrasound Clinic/Imaging Center.
2. Registration No.
3. Patient's name and her age
4. Number of children with sex of each child
5. Husband's/Father's name
6. Full address with Tel. No., if any
7. Referred by (full name and address of Doctor(s)/Genetic Counseling Center (Referral note to be preserved carefully with case papers)/self referral
8. Last menstrual period/weeks of pregnancy
9. History of genetic/medical disease in the family(specify)

   Basis of diagnosis:
   a. Clinical
   b. Bio-chemical
   c. Cytogenetic
   d. Other (e.g. radiological, ultrasonography, etc. specify)
10. Indication for Prenatal diagnosis
    A. Previous child/children with:
       i. Chromosomal disorders
       ii. Metabolic disorders
       iii. Congenital anomaly
       iv. Mental retardation
       v. Hemoglobinopathy
       vi. Sex linked disorders
       vii. Single gene disorder
       viii. Any other (specify)
    B. Advanced maternal age (35 years)
    C. Mother/father/sibling has genetic disease (specify)
    D. Other (specify)
11. Procedures carried out (with name and registration No. of Gynecologist/Radiologist/Registered Medical Practitioner) who performed it.

    Non-Invasive
    i. Ultrasound (specify purpose for which ultrasound is to done during pregnancy)
       [List of indications for ultrasonography of pregnant women are given in the note below]

    Invasive
    ii. Amniocentesis
    iii. Chorionic villi aspiration
    iv. Fetal biopsy
    v. Cordocentesis
    vi. Any other (specify)
12. Any complication of procedure—please specify

13. Laboratory tests recommended [3]
    i. Chromosomal studies
    ii. Biochemical studies
    iii. Molecular studies
    iv. Preimplantation genetic diagnosis
14. Result of
    a. Prenatal diagnostic procedure (give details)
    b. Ultrasonography Normal/Abnormal
    (specify abnormality detected, if any).
15. Date(s) on which procedures carried out.
16. Date on which consent obtained. (In case of invasive)
17. The result of prenatal diagnostic procedure were conveyed to .... on ....
18. Was MTP advised/conducted?
19. Date on which MTP carried out.
20. Declaration of doctor conducting ultrasonography

I, ... (name of the person conducting ultrasonography/image scanning) declare that while conducting ultrasonography/image scanning on Ms .... (name of the pregnant woman), I have neither detected nor disclosed the sex of her fetus to any body in any manner.

Date:
Place:

Name, Signature and Registration number
of the Gynecologist/Radiologist/Director of the Clinic

Declaration of Pregnant Woman

I, Ms .... (name of the pregnant woman) declare that by undergoing ultrasonography/image scanning, etc. I do not want to know the sex of my fetus.

Signature/Thump impression of pregnant woman

Important Note

i. Ultrasound is not indicated/advised/performed to determine the sex of fetus except for diagnosis of sex-linked disease such as Duchenne Muscular Dystrophy, Hemophilia A and B, etc.
ii. During pregnancy Ultrasonography should only be performed when indicated. The following is the representive list of indications for ultrasound during pregnancy.

1. To diagnose intrauterine and/or ectopic pregnancy and confirm viavility.
2. Estimation of gestational age (dating)
3. Detection of number of fetuses and their chorionicity.
4. Suspected pregnancy with IUCD *in situ* or suspected pregnancy following contraceptive failure/MTP failure.
5. Vaginal bleeding/leaking.
6. Follow-up of cases of abortion
7. Assessment of cervical canal and diameter of internal os.
8. Discrepancy between uterine size and period of amenorrhea.
9. Any suspected adenexal or uterine pathology/abnormality
10. Detection of chromosomal abnormalities, fetal structural defects and other abnormalities and their follow-up.
11. To evalute fetal presentation and position
12. Assessment of liquor amnii.
13. Preterm labor/preterm premature rupture of membranes.

14. Evaluation of placental position, thickness, grading and abnormalities (placenta praevia, retroplacental hemorrhage, abnormal adherence, etc.)
15. Evaluation of umbilical cord-presentation, insertion, nuchal encirclement, number of vessels and presence of true knot.
16. Evaluation of previous cesarean section scars.
17. Evaluation of fetal growth parameters, fetal weight and fetal well being.
18. Color flow mapping and duplex Doppler studies.
19. Ultrasound guided procedures such as medical termination of pregnancy, external cephalic version, etc. and their follow-up.
20. Adjunct to diagnostic and therapeutic invasive interventions such as chorionic villus sampling (CVS), amniocenteses, fetal blood sampling, fetal skin biopsy, amnio-infusion, intrauterine infusion, placement of shunts, etc.
21. Observation of intra-partum events.
22. Medical/surgical conditions complicating pregnancy.
23. Research/scientific studies in recognized institutions.

Person conducting ultrasonography on a pregnant woman shall keep complete record thereof in the clinic/center in Form-F and any deficiency or inaccuracy found therein shall amount to contravention of provisions of Section 5 or Section 6 of the Act, unless contrary is proved by the person conducting such ultrasonography.

DECLARATION

I, Sh/Smt/Kum/Dr.................................... son/daughter/wife of .... aged .... years resident of.. hereby declare that I have read and understood the Prenatal Diagnostic Techniques (Regulation and Prevention of Misuse) Act, 1994 (57 of 1994) and the Prenatal Diagnostic Techniques (Regulation and Prevention of Misuse) Rules, 1995.

I also undertake to explain the said Act and Rules to all employees of the Genetic Counseling Center/Genetic Laboratory/Genetic Clinic in respect of which registration is sought and to ensure that Act and Rules are fully compiled with

Date:
Place: Name and Signature of applicant

ACKNOWLEDGEMENT

[See Rules 4(2) and 8 (1)]

The application in Form A in duplicate for grant*/renewal* of registration of Genetic Counseling Center*/ Genetic Laboratory*/Genetic Clinic* by................................... (Name and address of applicant) has been received by the Appropriate Authority......................On (date.)

The list of enclosures attached to the application in Form A has been verified with the enclosures submitted and found to be correct.

OR

On verification it is found that the following documents mentioned in the list of enclosures are not actually enclosed.

The acknowledgement does not confer any rights on the applicant for grant or renewal of registration.

Date: Signature and Designation of Appropriate Authority, or authorized person in the office of the Appropriate Authority.

SEAL

Original
Duplicate for display

FORM B

[See Rules 6(2),6(5) and 8(2)]

CERTIFICATE OF REGISTRATION

(To be issued in duplicate)

1. In exercise of the powers conferred under Section 19 (1) of the Pre-natal Diagnostic Techniques (Regulation and Prevention of Misuse) Act, 1994 (57 of 1994), the Appropriate Authority.................................hereby grants registration to the Genetic Counseling Center*/Genetic Laboratory*/Genetic Clinic* named below for purposes of carrying out Genetic Counseling/Prenatal Diagnostic Procedures*/Prenatal Diagnostic Tests as defined in the aforesaid Act for a period of five years ending on..........................
2. This registration is granted subject to the aforesaid Act and Rules thereunder and any contravention thereof shall result in suspension or cancellation of this Certificate of Registration before the expiry of the said period of five years.
   A. Name and address of the Genetic Counseling Center*/Genetic Laboratory*/Genetic Clinic*
   B. Name of Applicant for registration.
   C. Pre-natal diagnostic procedures approved for (Genetic Clinic)
      i. Ultrasound
      ii. Amniocentesis
      iii. Chorionic villi biopsy
      iv. Fetoscopy
      v. Fetal skin or organ biopsy
      vi. Cordocentesis
         i. Any other (specify)
   D. Pre-natal diagnostic tests* approved (for genetic laboratory)
      i. Chromosomal studies
      ii. Biochemical studies
      iii. Molecular studies
3. Registration No. allotted
4. For renewed Certificate of Registration only
   Period of validity of earlier Certificate From .... To .... Or Registration.

Date:

Signature, name and designation
of the Appropriate Authority

Seal

Display one copy of this certificate at a conspicuous place at the place of business

FORM C

[See Rules 6(3), 6(5) and 8(3)]

REJECTION OF APPLICATION FOR REGISTRATION OR RENEWAL OF REGISTRATION

In exercise of the powers conferred under Section 19(2) of the Prenatal Diagnostic Techniques (Regulation and Prevention of Misuse) Act, 1994, the Appropriate Authority .... Hereby rejects the application for grant*/ renewal* of registration of the Genetic counseling center* Genetic Laboratory*/ Genetic Clinic* named below for the reasons stated.

Name and address of the Genetic Counseling Center*/Genetic Laboratory*/Genetic Clinic*

Name of Applicant who has applied for registration

Reasons for rejection of application for registration

Signature, name and designation of the Appropriate Authority

Date:

Seal

*Strike out whichever is not applicable or necessary.

FORM D

[See Rule 9(2)]

Name, address and registration no. of genetic counseling center record To be maintained by the genetic counseling center

1. Patient's name
2. Age
3. Husband's/Father's name
4. Full address with Tel. No., if any
5. Referred by (Full name and address of Doctor(s) with registration No.(s) (Referred note to be preserved carefully with case papers)
6. Last menstrual period/weeks of pregnancy
7. History of genetic/medical disease in the family (specify) Basis of diagnosis:
   a. Clinical
   b. Biochemical
   c. Cytogenetic
   d. Other (e.g. radiological)
8. Indication for prenatal diagnosis
   A. Previous child/children with:
      i. Chromosomal disorders
      ii. Metabolic disorders
      iii. Congenital anomaly
      iv. Mental retardation
      v. Hemoglobinopathy
      vi. Sex linked disorders
      vii. Any other(specify)

B. Advanced maternal age (35 years)
C. Mother/father/sibling has genetic disease (specify)
D. Others (specify)

9. Procedure advised [1[2]]
   i. Ultrasound
   ii. Amniocentesis
   iii. Chorionic villi biopsy
   iv. Fetoscopy
   v. Fetal skin or organ biopsy
   vi. Cordocentesis
   vii. Any other (specify)
10. Laboratory tests to be carried out
    i. Chromosomal studies
    ii. Biochemical studies
    iii. Molecular studies
11. Result of prenatal diagnosis
    If abnormal give details. Normal/Abnormal
12. Was MTP advised?
13. Name and address of Genetic Clinic* to which patient referred.
14. Dates of commencement and completion of genetic counseling.

Date:

Name, Signature and Registration No. of the Medical Geneticist/Gynecologist/pediatrician

[1[2]] Strike out whichever is not applicable or necessary.

FORM E

[See Rules 9(3)]

Name, address and registration no. of genetic laboratory record To be maintained by the genetic laboratory

1. Patient's name
2. Age
3. Husband's/Father's name
4. Full address with Tel.No., if any
5. Referred by/sample sent by (full name and address of Genetic Clinic) (Referral note to be preserved carefully with case papers)
6. Type of sample: Maternal blood/Chorionic villus sample/amniotic fluid/Fetal blood or other fetal tissue (specify)
7. Specify indication for prenatal diagnosis
   A. Previous child/children with:
      i. Chromosomal disorders
      ii. Metabolic disorders
      iii. Malformation(s)
      iv. Mental retardation
      v. Hereditary hemolytic anemia
      vi. Sex linked disorder
      vii. Any other(specify)

B. Advanced maternal age(-35 years)
C. Mother/father/sibling has genetic disease(specify)
D. Other(specify)

8. Laboratory tests carried out(give details)
   i. Chromosomal studies
   ii. Biochemical studies
   iii. Molecular studies
9. Result of prenatal diagnosis
   If abnormal give details. Normal/Abnormal
10. Date(s) on which tests carried out.
   The results of the Prenatal diagnostic tests were conveyed to .... on ....

Date:

Name, Signature and Registration No.
of the Medical Geneticist

FORM G

[See Rule 10]

FORM OF CONSENT

I, ... wife/daughter of .... Age .... years residing at .... hereby state that I have been explained fully the probable side effects and after effects of the prenatal diagnostic procedures. I wish to undergo the prenatal diagnostic procedures in my interest to find out the possibility of any abnormality (i.e. deformity or disorder) in the child I am carrying.

I undertake not to terminate the pregnancy if the prenatal procedure and any prenatal tests conducted show the absence of deformity or disorders. I understand that the sex of the fetus will not be disclosed to me.

I understand that breach of this undertaking will make me liable to penalty as prescribed in the Prenatal Diagnostic Techniques (Regulation and Prevention of Misuse) Act, 1994 (57 of 1994)

Date
Place

Signature

I have explained the contents of the above consent to the patient and her companion (Name .... Address .... Relationship ....) in a language she/they understand.

Name, Signature and/Registration number of Gynecologist

Date

Name, Address and Registration number of Genetic Clinic

FORM H

[See Rule 9(5)]

Permanent record of application for registration, grant of registration rejection of application for registration and renewals of registration

1. Sl.No.
2. File number of Appropriate Authority.
3. Date of receipt of application for grant of registration.
4. Name, Address, Phone/Fax, etc. of Applicant:
5. Name and address(es) of Genetic Counseling Center*/Genetic Laboratory*/Genetic Clinic*
6. Date on which case considered by Advisory Committee and recommendation of Advisory Committee. In summary.
7. Outcome of application(state granted/rejected and date of issue of orders)
8. Registration number allotted and date of expiry of registration.
9. Renewals (date of renewal and renewed up to).
10. File number in which renewals dealt.
11. Additional information, if any.

Name, Designation and Signature of
Appropriate Authority

Guidance for Appropriate Authority

a. Form H is a permanent record to be maintained as a register, in the custody of the Appropriate Authority.
b. *Means strike out whichever is not applicable.
c. Against item 7, record date of issue of order in Form B or Form C.
d. On renewal, the Registration Number of the Genetic Counseling Center/Genetic Laboratory/Genetic Clinic will not change. A fresh registration Number will be allotted in the event of change of ownership or management.
e. No Registration number shall be allotted twice.
f. Each Genetic Counseling Center/Genetic Laboratory/Genetic Clinic may be allotted a folio consisting of two facing pages of the Register for recording Form H.
g. The space provided for 'additional information' may be used for recording suspension, cancellations, rejection of application for renewal, change of ownership/management, outcome of any legal proceedings, etc.
h. Every folio (i.e. 2 pages) of the Register shall be authenticated by signature of the Appropriate Authority with date, and every subsequent entry shall also be similarly authenticated.

PNDT Act

"3. The qualifications of the employees, the requirement of equipment, etc. for a Genetic Counseling Center, Genetic Laboratory, Genetic Clinic, Ultrasound Clinic and Imaging Centre shall be as under:

1. Any person being or employing
   i. A gynecologist or a pediatrician having six months experience or four weeks training in genetic counseling or
   ii. A medical geneticists, having adequate space and educational charts/models/equipment for carrying out genetic counseling may set up a genetic counseling center and get it registered as a genetic counseling center.

2. (a) Any person having adequate space and being or employing
   i. A Medical Geneticist and
   ii. A laboratory technician, having a BSc degree in Biological Sciences or a degree or diploma in medical laboratory course with at least one year experience in conducting appropriate prenatal diagnostic techniques, tests or procedures may set up a genetic laboratory
3. 1. Any person having adequate space and being or employing
      a. Gynecologist having experience of performing at least 20 procedures in chorionic villi aspirations per vagina or per abdomen, chorionic villi biopsy, amniocentesis, cordocentesis fetoscopy, fetal skin or organ biopsy or fetal blood sampling, etc. under supervision of an experienced gynecologist in these fields, or
      b. a Sonologist, Imaging Specialist, Radiologist or Registered Medical Practitioner having post graduate degree or diploma or six months training or one year experience in sonography or image scanning, or.
      c. A medical geneticist may set up a genetic clinic/ultrasound clinic/imaging center.
   2. The Genetic Clinic/ultrasound clinic/imaging center should have or acquire such of the following equipment, as may be necessary for carrying out the tests or procedures.
      a. Equipment and accessories necessary for carrying out clinical examination by an obstetrician or gynecologist.
      b. An ultra-sonography machine including mobile ultrasound machine, imaging machine or any other equipment capable of conducting fetal ultrasonography.
      c. Appropriate catheters and equipment for carrying out chorionic villi aspirations per vagina or per abdomen.
      d. Appropriate sterile needles for amniocentesis or cordocentesis.
      e. A suitable fetoscope with appropriate accessories for fetoscopy, fetal skin or organ biopsy or fetal blood sampling shall be optional.
      f. Equipment for dry and wet sterilization.
      g. Equipment for carrying out emergency procedures such as evacuation of uterus or resuscitation in case of need.
      h. Genetic Works Station.
7. In the said rules, for Rule 5, the following rule shall be substituted, namely:
   "5. Application Fee-(1) Every application for registration under Rule 4 shall be accompanied by an application fee of:
   a. Rs. 3000.00 for Genetic Counseling Center, Genetic Laboratory, Genetic Clinic, Ultrasound Clinic or Imaging Center.
   b. Rs. 4000.00 for an institute, hospital, nursing home, or any place providing jointly the service of a Genetic Counseling Center, Genetic Laboratory and Genetic Clinic, Ultrasound Clinic or Imaging Center or any combination thereof.

Provided that if an application for registration of any Genetic Clinic/Laboratory/Center, etc. has been rejected by the Appropriate Authority, no fee shall be required to be paid on re-submission of the application by the applicant for the same body within 90 days of rejection. Provided further that any subsequent application shall be accompanied with the prescribed fee. Application fee once paid will not be refunded.

CONSENT FOR ADMISSION AND DELIVERY AND SURGERY

I undersigned, Miss/Mrs. ....
Name... (Husband's/Father's Name)........................... (Surname).................
.... completed years and residing at .... give my free consent for the operation/delivery of .... to be performed on myself by Dr. .... and MOI/c under general spinal/epidural/local anesthesia. Supplemented or combined with any other type of anesthesia as found necessary, to be administered by Dr. .... MOI/c. I also understand that procedures other than the proposed ones or in addition to them may be found necessary and/or desirable while operating of anesthetising and I consent for them if the surgeon and/or the anesthetist think them essential and beneficial to me.

I have been explained and I have understood:

1. There are unimaginary risks during anesthesia.
2. Detection of cancer after operation.
3. The patient has tendency of heart disease.
4. The patient is serious and under risk.
5. Family doctor is allowed into the operation theater with lady patients otherwise she has full faith to surgeon and staff.
6. I, ... give the authority to the surgeon to send the patient for operation/medication/nursing home.
7. Disputes subject to .... Jurisdiction only
8. Expenses of medicines after operation are additional. In serious condition relatives are free to take advice of any other doctor.
9. The necessity, nature, procedure, consequences, risks and complications of the operation.
10. The procedure of administration of anesthesia.
11. Risks and possibilities of complications to my unborn child resulting from the operation and the anesthesia.

Signature of Patient

Staff on Duty Signature of Husband/Father/Mother ....

* The same consent should be taken in local language also.

CONSENT FOR STERILIZATION

I, the undersigned Mrs... age .... year .... wife/widow of .... residing at .... (Husband's full name) and having .... male children aged .... and .... female children aged .... give my free consent for the (Other method) operation of Abdominal/Vaginal/ Laparoscopic .... Sterilization to be performed upon myself by Dr .... and MOI/c of .... under general/spinal/local anesthesia to be administered by Dr. .... and MOI/c. (Full name)

I have been explained and I have understood

i. The technique of the operation
ii. The procedure of anesthesia
iii. The consequence of the operation
iv. The risks and complications of the operation and the anesthesia including the remote possibility of the operation resulting in future pregnancy.

I also understand that the procedures other than the proposed ones in addition to them, for the operation and/or the anesthesia may be found necessary or desirable and I consent for them, if the surgeon and/or the anesthetist think them essential and beneficial to me.

I, Mr. ...., husband of the patient, concur with the above consent.
.... (Signature of witness) ....

Signed in my presence (Name and address of witness)

(Signature of Husband) Staff on Duty Date Signature (Patient)

* The same consent should be taken in local language also.

CONSENT FORM FOR MTP IN ADULT

I, undersigned, Mrs/Miss ....D/o, W/o, M/o...
(Name)..(Husband's/Father's Name)......................................(Surname).............
Aged... completed years and residing at .... admitted under IPD No. .... with OPD NO. .... request .... to terminate my pregnancy.
...................................Give my free consent for the operation/Medical Termination of my pregnancy by Dr .... and MOI/c of ...., Agra, under General/Spinal/ Local anesthesia to be administered by Dr .... MOI/c. (a) the pregnancy has occurred as a result of failure of the contraceptive technique of IUD/oral pills/condom/coitus interrupts/periodic abstinence/ tubectomy/vasectomy/.. (any other) employed by us. (b) in view of the substantial risk that if the child were born it would suffer from such physical or mental abnormalities as to be seriously handicapped. (c) as this pregnancy has resulted from my being raped. (d) in order to prevent risk of injury to my physical or mental health by reason of my actual/reasonably foreseeable environment.

I have been explained and I have understood the procedure proposed to be employed for terminating the pregnancy and for anesthetizing me along with the likely risks and complications of both these, including the remote possibility of this pregnancy continuing in spite of the procedures employed for terminating it. I also understand that procedures other than the proposed ones: or in addition to them for terminating the pregnancy and/or for anesthetizing may be found necessary or desirable and I consent for them, if the surgeon and/or the anesthetist think them essential and beneficial to me.

Signed in my presence.. Signature (Patient)
Signature of the witness (Husband)..

* The same consent should be taken in local language also.

CONSENT FOR LAPAROSCOPY

- I have been explained the risks of laparoscopy operation at each step. I have been explained of possible small risk of injury to bowel, bladder and blood vessels during verres needle insertion, trocar insertion, gas insufflation, use of cautery. I have also been explained the limitation of Endoscopy operations and a small chance of conversion to open laparotomy to complete the operation.
- I have no objections to my operation being recorded on video and shown on CCTV to doctors for learning and training purpose.

Signature of Husband   Witness   Date   Signature (Patient)

* The same consent should be taken in local language also.

OPERATION NOTES

Name.. Time ....

Surgeons 1 .... Anesthetists 1 ....

.... 2. ....

....

....

O.T. Staff 1 ....

2. ....

3. ....

4. ....

Anesthesia: ....

....

....

Operation steps:

....

....

....

....

Drugs used during operation: ....

....

....

....

Postoperative progress

Time	*Pulse*	*BP*	*IV Fluid*	*Urine output*	*Drain*	*Pt. complaint*
0 Hours						
1 Hour						
2 Hours						
3 Hours						

PREANESTHETIC ASSESSMENT SPECIAL SYSTEMIC AND CARDIO-RESP. REPORT

Name: .... Age: .... Sex: ....

Past history: CCF operation — Minor / Major

1 HD/MI	EKG	Drugs	Koch's	Hypertension
Diabetes	Icterus	Skiagram	Allergy	Palpitation/Ghabraht
Pedal edema	Bleeding	Arrhythmias	UTI	Nephropathy
COAD	Convulsions	PND	Steroids	APD/GERD

Family History

1 HD Kock's Hypertension COAD Diabetes Allergy

Personal History

Tobacco	Smoking	Personality	Dietary pattern	Drug sensitivity
Alcohol	Physical activity	Obesity	Psychosocial tension	Addition

Examination

Pulse (Radial) — R / L

Other peripheral pulses

BP (Sitting)

Heart

Lungs

Abdomen/GIT

LVE/RVF/CCF CNS

Edema
Anemia
Jaundice
Clubbing
Cyanosis

Present Complaints

Investigation profile: Hb .... Blood group .... B1 Sugar .... Routine Urine .... Others .... EKG/Dynamic Monitoring/Skiagram

Cardio-respiratory status

Goldman cardiac risk index grade

Clinical impression

Any specific drug instructions

Advice: ....

....

Note: This report may reflect personal impression of the consultant, not valid for mediolegal purposes.

Date	*Treatment*	*Treatment child*	*Temp. pulse resp.*

ANNEXURE-1

Check List to be Filled in before Sterilization Operation of A Male/Female by the Doctor Concerned

1. Whether the age of the client is within laid down norms(Male clients should be below the age of 60 years, for Female should be below the age of 45 years and above 22 years) Yes/No
2. Whether information relating to marital status, No. of living children and age of the youngest child obtained. Yes/No
3. Whether the client has been counseled regarding sterilization so as to help the clients make informed and voluntary decision. Yes/No
4. Consent form—whether the client has understood the consent for and the following relative contraindications. Yes/No
5. Whether the client has been examined for excluding medical contraindication i.e. psychiatric disorder and physical illness. The surgeon/doctor should examine for the following relative contraindications. Yes/No
   a. Psychiatric disorder
   b. Physical illness
      i. Acute febrile illness
      ii. Jaundice or other chronic liver disease
      iii. Anemia (hemoglobin less than 8 gm%)
      iv. Chronic systemic disease, including tuberculosis, bronchial asthma, blood dyscrasias, heart disease, uncontrolled diabetes, hypertension and thyrotoxicosis
      v. Malignancy
      vi. Skin conditions, including infection involving operative site
      vii. Pelvic infection, adhesions or mass
      viii. Severe nutritional deficiency, such as generalized edemas, anemia and vitamin deficiency
   a. Allergy to local anesthesia (alternative anesthesia or procedure must be provided)
   b. Gross obesity
   b. The following conditions in postpartum clients:
      i. Puerperal fever
      ii. Prolonged rupture of membranes (24 hrs)
      iii. Preeclampsia or eclampsia
      iv. Ante-partum or postpartum hemorrhage resulting in hemoglobin less than 8 gm percent
      v. Trauma to the genital tract
      vi. History of postpartum psychosis.
6. Whether assessment and screening of the client has been done as follows:
   6.1 Whether the client has been physically examined—pulse, blood pressure, respiratory rate, temperature, body weight, general condition and nutritional status, auscultation of heart, lungs, examination of abdomen, pelvic examination and other examination as indicated by the clients medical history or general physical examination. Yes/No
   6.2 Laboratory Examination: Blood test for hemoglobin, urine analysis for sugar, and albumin and other laboratory examination. Yes/No
   6.3 Final Medical Assessment of the operating Surgeons: Whether sugeon has verified fitness of the client including abdominal/pelvic examination before conducting the surgery. Yes/No
7. Whether instructions relating to prevention of infection has been followed? Yes/No
   7.1 Whether cleaning and fumigation of the OT has been done. Yes/No
   7.2 Proper arrangement for decontamination of articles after surgery is available for items that come in contact with blood or other body fluids by placing in solution of disinfectant for 10 minutes (surgical instruments gloves needles and syringes, cotton gauze, etc.) Yes/No
   7.3 Sterilization procedure of equipment/instruments required for surgery has been carried out as laid down in the guidelines. Yes/No

Signature...
Name of the Surgeon...........................
Date..

ANNEXURE-2

Application For Sterilization Operation And Consent Form

1. Name: Shri/Smt...
2. Husband's Name and Address...
3. Father's Name and Address...
4. Operation Center...

Dear Sir/Madam

Kindly make arrangements for my sterilization operation. My age is .... years and my husband/wife's age is .... years.

I am married and my husband/wife is alive. We have .... male and ....female living children. The age of my youngest living child is ....yrs. I have decided to undergo sterilization operation independently and on my own without any outside pressure, inducement or force. I am aware that other methods of contraception are available to me. I know that for all practicle purpose this operation is permanent and that after the operation will be unable to have any more children. I also know that there are still some chances of failure of the operation for which the hospital / institution and operating doctor will not be held responsible by me or my relative or any other person whomsoever. My husband / wife has not been sterilized previously. I am aware that I am undergoing operation, which carries an element of risk. I have been explained the eligibility criteria for the operation and I affirm that I am eligible to undergo operation according to criteria. I agree to undergo the operation under any type of anesthesia which the doctor thinks suitable for me. After sterilization operation if I get pregnant, then I shall report within four weeks to the doctor / hospital and will get abortion done free of cost. Under such circumstances, the State Government will pay a compensation of Rs. 5000/- to me which will be acceptable to me. I know that if I am unable to get the pregnancy aborted within four weeks of pregnancy, then I will not be entitled to claim any compensation from any court of law in this regard. I agree to come for follow-up to the center / doctor as instructed, failing which I shall be responsible for the consequences, if any.

I have read the above-mentioned facts/information* in my own language.

Religion: ....

Age: ....

Business / Occupation: ....

Signature of the acceptor/applicant

Signature of the witness

Full Name :..

Full Address :..

(only for those beneficiaries who cannot read and write)

Shri /Smt .... have been explained other methods of contraception available and the failures associated with other methods have been explained fully.

Signature of Counselors
Full Name:...............................
Full Address : ....

I Know very well Shri / Smt...................................... and the information given by me / her is correct. His / her name has been registered with health center / city center at Sal. No...............................

Signature of Promoter......................................
Full Name..
Full Address...

CERTIFICATE OF MEDICAL OFFICER

I certify that I have satisfied myself that Shri/Smt .... is within the eligible age-group and is mentally and medically fit for a sterilization operation. There is no evidence that he / she has undergone a sterilization operation previously. I have explained all clauses to the client and that this form has the authority of a legal document.

Signature of Operating Doctor
(Name and Address)

Signature of Medical Officer
(Name and Address)

DENIAL OF STERILIZATION

I Certify that Shri / Smt..is not suitable client for re-sterilization for the following reasons.

1...

2...

He/she has been provided the following alternative methods of contraception.

Signature of counsellor** or
Doctor making decision
(Name and Address)

**Counsellor can be any health personnel including doctor.

FOR OFFICIAL USE ONLY

(d) To be filled by examining doctor

Note : If the surgeon is himself health examiner, the certificate may be given by him.

Age of the client according to appearance..

Urine analysis for sugar...

Blood pressure..

Whether client has gone sterilization earlier or not...

As per examination by the doctor, the client is mentally and medically fit for sterilization operation.

I have confirmed from the client regarding his / her marital status and number of living children. I have explained pros and cons of the sterilization operation to the client and he himself is mentally ready for the operation.

Signature of the client.................................

Signature of the surgeon
(Name in capital letter)...................................
Present place of posting.................................

(E) CERTIFICATE OF THE SURGEON

I have performed sterilization operation. During the operation there was no visible signs of earlier sterilization and as per appearance he/she was within the age limit for sterilization. If it is female sterilization, the type of operation performed.

Abdominal/Vaginal/Laparoscopic/Minilap

General/Local anesthesia used.

Signature of the surgeon
(Name in capital letters).....................................
Present place posting...

Economic, social and demographic details of the client under going sterilization operation

Monthly report of the District Family Welfare Bureau should be accompanied by the following proforma:

1. Name of Client:...
2. Name of head of the family : Shri :..
3. Name of Father / Husband :......................................
4. Mohalla :.. House No.: ....
5. PHC/Urban Center :.....................
6. Ward:...
7. Religion:..
8. Caste General / SC /ST /NT / VJNT / OBC Class:..............................
9. Whether Married (Yes/No)
10. Age of Applicant (complete years....................)
11. Age of Husband / Wife (complete years...............)
12. No. of alive children
    (a) Sons.................. (b) Daughters................
    Age.......................Months............................
    Husband....................Wife............................
13. Age at Marriage.............................
14. Educational qualification
    Husband: Illiterate / Literate / Primary / Junior High School / High School / Graduate and above.
    Wife: Illiterate / Literate / Primary / Junior High School / High School / Graduate and above.
15. Difference from the last termination of pregnancy (Delivery or abortion) .... years .... and ....

Payment Particulars

Amount given to applicant Rupees................Paise...............

For...................... Sterilization

Date:..........................

Signature of applicant

Name........................

FOLLOW UP

Person concerned with the service of the applicant name .... Post...............................

Place of Appointment...

1. Promoter.........................
2. Health Worker...........................
3. Medical Officer, PHC ....
4. Surgeon.........................

If tubectomy methods adopted.

Abdominal/Vaginal/Laparoscopic/Laparotomy

Type of Anesthesia : General/Local/Spinal

Full name of the person going to give follow up ....

Present Address:...

OTHER INFORMATION

1. Whether any contraceptive method has been adopted earlier YES/NO
   if yes (1) Name of the Method .... (2) Period of the Method ....
2. Whether promoter of applicant is regional worker of family welfare program Yes/No
   If yes, whether applicant is inhabitant of the jurisdiction of that worker: Yes/No
3. Reason for the application of sterilization: Limited family/diseases/financial or other
   I certify that above mentioned particulars are correct.

Place:.......................

Signature
Full Name ....
Present Address ....

THE APPLICATION FOR THE APPROVAL OF PRIVATE MEDICAL PRACTICENER/ CLINIC/NURSING HOME/MATERNITY HOMES FOR CARRYING OUT TUBECTOMIS

1. Name of Applicant Doctor:
2. Qualification:
3. Registration No.:
4. Experience in the performance of Tubectomy Operation
5. Address in full
6. Whether has Clinic/Nursing Home/Maternity Hospital?
7. State, if the following facilities are available with him/her:
   - i. Beds for Gynecological Cases No.
   - ii. Operation table
   - iii. Shadow less lamp
   - iv. Oxygen cylinder
   - v. Apparatus for resuscitation
   - vi. Suction apparatus
   - vii. Instrument sets for carrying out tubectomies (Give name of instruments and quantity)
   - viii. Autoclave with drums
   - ix. Sterilizer for Instruments
   - x. Necessary equipment and Instruments for instiling anesthesia:
   - xi. Separate operation room
   - xii. Availability of Drugs for Pre-and Post-operative Medication as well as for Emergencies:

Place........................

Date........................

Appendix 'D'

Doctor's Liability Under Consumer Protection Act and Preventive Steps to Avoid Litigation and its Outcome with Important Dos and Don'ts

Nidhi Gupta, Anurag Gupta

INTRODUCTION

The classical concept of doctor-patient relationship born in the earlier years of family physicians has undergone a drastic change in this materialistic world where doctors are treated as service providers and patients as consumers under the Consumer Protection Act (CPA). It is unfortunate to put the medical professional service providers under the same consumer laws and courts who deal with faulty pressure cookers and substandard air conditioners (ACs).

A doctor is definitely not making pressure cookers and ACs of his patients, as the human body's complexities and response to drugs and stress are still not fully understood.

The medical professional is answerable to the patient and the law if he/she is negligent in performing his/her duty.

This chapter deals with the doctor's liability under CPA and preventive steps to avoid litigation and its outcome with important dos and don'ts for the doctors.

CONSUMER PROTECTION ACT, 1986

General

This Act is enacted to provide better protection of the interests of the consumers and for the establishment of consumer councils for settlement of consumer's disputes.

Application

It is applicable to all goods and services, unless otherwise, expressly provided by the Central Government by notification.

Consumer

Any person who buys any good or avails/hires any service against consideration, which has been paid/promised/under system of deferred payment is a consumer.

Deficiency

Any fault, imperfection, shortcoming, inadequacy in the quality, nature and performance of a service, which is required to be maintained under law or has been undertaken by the opposite party to be performed under a contract is a deficiency.

Medical Services

Services rendered by doctors and hospitals, which comes within the purview of personal service has been held by courts to be within the jurisdiction of this Act. In India, there are several kinds of medical-pathies in vogue, i.e., allopathy, homeopathy, ayurvedic, unani, acupuncture, electropathy, acupressure, naturopathy, hydrotherapy, etc., and they all provide services to the consumer and come under this Act.

Reliefs

The court may direct the complainant the following:
- To remove the defect
- To replace the goods with new goods
- To return to the complainant the price paid by him
- To pay compensation to the consumers for any loss/injury suffered by him due to negligence of the opposite party
- To remove the defects on deficiencies in the service in question
- To discontinue unfair trade practice/restrictive trade practice/not to repeat it
- Not to offer/withdraw hazardous goods for sale
- To provide for adequate cost to the parties.

Rights of Consumer as Patients

- The right to be protected against marketing of goods and services, which are hazardous to life and property
- The right to be informed about the quality, quantity, potency, purity, standards, and price of goods and services to protect against unfair trade practices
- The right to be heard and receive due consideration at appropriate forums
- The right to seek redressal against unfair trade practices
- The right to consumer education.

Consumer Agencies

For speedy, inexpensive and simple quasi-judicial machinery of redressal, agencies to adjudicate consumer complaints have been set up at the district, state and national levels.

These bodies decide disputes keeping in mind the basic principles of natural justice and have the power to grant certain reliefs as provided in the Act.

Power of Consumer Agencies

They are vested with same powers as in a civil court under the Code of Civil Procedure, 1908. The details of the agencies are given in Table 1.

Table 1: Details of the consumer forum agencies

S. No.	Details	District forum	State commission	National commission
1.	Composition	District judge as chairman and 2 other members, one of which shall be a woman	High Court judge as the chairman and 2 other members, one of which shall be a woman	Supreme Court judge as chairman and 2 other members one of which shall be a woman
2.	Jurisdiction	In district where dispute arose	In state where dispute arose	Whole of India, except Jammu and Kashmir
3.	Amount	Up to 20 lacs	Exceeds 20 lacs but less than 1 crore	> 1 crore
4.	Time limit	Within 2 years	Within 2 years	Within 2 years
5.	Appeal where time limit	State Commission, within 30 days	National Commission, within 30 days	Supreme Court, within 30 days

Who Can File a Complaint?

- Consumer (patient/purchaser)
- Registered consumer organization
- Central/State Government
- One or more consumers together
- In case of death of consumer, his legal heir or representative.

Basis of the Complaint

- Deficiency in service (treatment)
- Misrepresentation about the type, quality and standard of service
- False claim that the service/treatment is recognized by some institution or Government.

Time Limit

It specifically provides that the district forum, state commission or the national commission shall not admit a complaint unless it is filed within 2 years from the date on which the cause of action arose.

The delay maybe condoned if the complainant satisfies the forum/commission that he had sufficient cause for not filing that complaint within such period.

Procedure

Complaint can be filed on plain paper through ordinary post, or in person by the patient. It must contain details of deficiency in service with proof in four copies. It bears no court fees.

Where to File a Complaint

Complaints in which claim for compensation is up to 20 lacs is filed before district forum within whose jurisdiction the opposite party actually and voluntarily resides/carries on business has a branch office.

Complaints in which claim of compensation is more than 20 lacs but less than one crore is filed before state commission.

Complaints in which claim of compensation is more than/one crore is filed before the national commission.

Punishment for Noncompliance of Order of Forum/Commission

Noncompliance of any order of forum or commission warrants imprisonment for a term not less than 1 month, maybe extended to 3 years or with fine, which shall be not less than Rs. 2,000, but maybe extended to Rs 10,000, or both.

Frivolous/Vexatious Complaints

Section 26 of CPA clearly states that any complaints found to be frivolous or vexatious shall be dismissed. Forum/commission will apply its mind to contemplate the bonafides of allegation, to test the truth and veracity of evidence.

For such complaints, an order is also passed that the complainant shall pay to the opposite party such cost, not exceeding Rs. 10,000, as may be specified in the order.

Appeal

District Forum

Any person aggrieved by an order passed by the district forum can file an appeal to the state commission within a period of 30 days from the date of the order. Appeal can only be filed after the appellant has deposited 50% of the amount he is required to pay in terms of the order of district forum or Rs. 25,000, whichever is less.

State Commission

Appeal is filed to the national commission within 30 days from the date of the order. Appellant has to deposit 50% of the amount he is required to pay in terms of order of state commission or Rs. 35,000, whichever is less.

National Commission

Appeal can be filed to the Supreme Court within 30 days from the date of order. Appellant has to deposit 50% of the amount he is required to pay in terms of order of national commission or Rs 50,000, whichever is less.

PREVENTIVE STEPS TO AVOID LITIGATION AND ITS OUTCOME

Preventive Steps

Level I: Primary prevention/protection against complaint being filed.

Level II: Secondary prevention/protection against the defendant from being held negligent.

Level III: Tertiary prevention/protection against direct financial consequence in case compensation is awarded.

Level IV: Quartic protection/protection against professional and psychological stresses.

Level I/Primary Prevention

- Behavior
  - Commercial behavior is to be discouraged
  - Behavior of the entire team matters
  - Should be courteous and sympathetic
- Counseling
  - All queries of the patient and attendants should be patiently heard and answered in simple language
  - Details regarding the disease, risks, complication and treatment modality must be given
  - No false guarantees should be given
  - Communication between the patient and doctor must be two-way
  - Compassionate care should be provided
- Second opinion/referral
  - In case a doctor needs a second opinion or the attendants demand the same, then the doctor should accept such demands
  - Referral to a higher center with better facilities to save the life of a patient should always be sought for after explaining the attendants, the need
- Facilities/training
  - All the facilities available in the institute should be displayed
  - Prescription heads/sign boards should depict the true qualifications, designation, training experience and facilities
  - The doctor and the staff should regularly update their knowledge, skills and facilities according to the claims made by the clinic/hospital
- Medical ethics
  - Knowledge of medical ethics and laws in practice are very useful in improving practicing methods of doctors
- Grievance redressal cell
  - In very big institutions, a cell can be established to tackle a potential problem of dissatisfaction on the spot.

Level II/Secondary Prevention

The key words are:

- Exercising reasonable skill and care in diagnosis and treatment
- Proper documentation
- Legally valid consent.

Reasonable skill and care: It has three aspects:
1. Medical: Every doctor/medical establishment must exercise reasonable skill and care as expected from an average person with equivalent qualifications and experience in similar circumstances.
2. Social: Reasonable skill and care must be exhibited to the patient/attendants/relatives through expressions, actions and discussions on the part of the doctor.
3. Legal: Documentation about doctor exercising reasonable skill and care in consultation, diagnosis and treatment of the patient.

Proper documentation and record keeping: Date, time, history, positive physical findings and investigations, treatment and instructions given should be mentioned.

History of drug allergies, referrals and second opinions should also be mentioned. A note of erring patients should be made, e.g., unreliable history, refusing admission, not following instructions, etc. The prognosis should be explained to the patient/attendant in simple comprehensible language, and preferably in writing, especially in complicated and serious cases.

Preservation of record: Record of patients should be preserved for 3 years because:
- Under CPA, limitation of filing a complaint is 2 years
- Under law of tort, limitation is 3 years. Legally valid consent should be taken in all the cases as and when required.

Level III/Tertiary Prevention

Professional indemnity insurance: In India, all insurance companies are nationalized, and hence, terms and conditions are almost identical. The following points should be kept in mind while taking a policy:
- Take policy of a company where you know somebody as it will be easy dealing when actual need arises
- The insurance company takes the liability for "policy period", so pay the premium on time
- Inform the company:
  - Change of your address of clinic/hospital
  - Attachments with other hospitals
  - Specialty in which doctor is practicing
  - Receive a notice/complaint
- The company is not responsible for:
  - Unqualified employee
  - Claims arising from specific facilities like X-ray, ultrasonography (USG), etc., unless mentioned in the form
  - If doctor practices a specialty other than mentioned on the form
  - A specific contract of 100% cure or similar is made by doctor
- No liability will arise on part of the company in respect of:
  - Any criminal act/unlawful act
  - Service rendered under influence of intoxicants or narcotics
  - Claims arising from any condition directly/indirectly caused by human immunodeficiency virus (HIV)
  - Third party public liability
  - Use of drugs for weight reduction, cosmetic surgery, dental surgery, liability caused by use of radioactive substance
  - Other doctors using the nursing home under contract without knowledge of the company
- The policy is void if there is a misstatement in, or if a material fact is suppressed or omitted from the proposal.

Level IV/Defending Litigation by Forming Medical Defense Societies and Strong Peer Support

The professional, social and psychological aspects of litigations and its absence can only be fought by providing a strong peer support and by formation of medical defense organizations at the district, state and national levels to:
- Assist in such situations
- Help the doctor to collect literature on the subject of litigation from standard textbooks and judgements
- Get senior and experienced doctors to give their opinion about the merits of the case
- Take up cover of defense on behalf of the doctors against medical negligence. However, no attempt should be made in diagnosis and treatment to defend cases of gross negligence or glaring deviations from the accepted norms of code of ethics for medical professionals.

Nine Rs of Preventive Steps

1. *Rapport*: Maintain a healthy rapport and communication with the patient, attendants, fellow doctors and subordinate staff.
2. *Rationale*: The doctor must have in his mind, the provisional diagnosis and the planned treatment, and this diagnostic and therapeutic rationale must be mentioned in the medical record.
3. *Record*: It should be carefully prepared, complete, accurate, legible, germane, relevant, timely and generously informative.
4. *Remarks*: Derogatory remarks to the patient, attendants, other doctors should always be avoided. The patient's ailment should always be kept confidential.
5. *RS*: A doctor should not prescribe/administer any medication without an appropriate medical indication. He should be aware of the possible side effects and contraindications of the drugs he is using. Drug allergy histories should be documented in the records.
6. *Res ipsa loquitur* are situations when a layman could presume malpractice without the testimony of an expert witness, e.g. instruments left in the abdomen of a patient who undergoes laparotomy.
7. *Respect*: Doctor should always give due respect and show concern to a patient as an individual, as a human being and as a person. "A humanistic approach solves more problems, melts more hostilities and eliminates more law suits."
8. *Results*: The patient and family should be made aware of the possible outcome of the diagnostic and therapeutic efforts.
9. *Risks*: These should always be discussed with the patient/attendants before obtaining consent to proceed.

Physician should tell about the relevant risks involved according to the patient in question, the serious ones that may have a slight chance of occurring and the minor ones which might occur with significant frequency.

Risk Management

New mantra to avoid litigation risk management involves the development of strategies to optimize the patient's well-being and to prevent or limit health risk to the patient, as well as the legal risk to the caregiver.

It involves the following:

- *Identification of risk*: Risk can be identified by the history and examination of the patient and patients marked as "high-risk" patients
- *Risk assessment*: Assessment of individual risks must be done as:
  - Frequency of risk.
  - Cost of risk and its effect on progress of the case.
  - Under what circumstances is the likelihood of risk to increase
- *Risk management strategies*:
  - Avoidance: A doctor can stop taking care of high risk cases.
  - Prevention: Clinical practice guidelines in the form of flow charts or ready reckoners should be provided to the staff to deal with situations and these may prevent events from occurring which could lead to adverse outcomes, and thereby litigations.
  - Transfer: A "high-risk" case may be transferred to a better equipped center.
  - Reduction: A reduction in risks can be done if the doctor is aware of them, outlines a thorough investigation and takes preparatory measures to deal with them
  - Segregation: In difficult and complicated cases, consultation or second opinion should be obtained and step-by-step treatment of complications must be undertaken
- *Strategy implementation*: The implementation of strategy should take into account the awareness of current practice and of alternatives that are both practical and compatible with the objectives of care that has to be rendered
- *Evaluation of experience*: Risk management is a continuous process and a committee must be appointed to study the risk and the strategy applied, and thence evaluates the success or pitfalls of such applications.

In view of the Supreme Court affixing its seal of approval on the applicability of the CPA to the service provided by the medical profession, it has become all the more imperative for the medical professionals to exercise a greater degree of caution while undertaking diagnosis and treatment of patients. It is, therefore, felt necessary to make the doctors aware of certain precautions which ought to be taken. Such precautions have been summarized thereafter as dos and don'ts for doctors.

It is also desirable for the patients and their attendants to observe certain norms so that they benefit most out of the medical help sought, and healthy relationship with the doctor/hospital is maintained.

DOS FOR DOCTORS

- Mention your qualifications/training/experience/designation on the prescription. Qualification means recognized degrees/diplomas as regulated by the Indian Medical Degrees Act, 1916, as amended from time to time. Mention of scholarships/membership/awards, which are not qualifications, should be avoided
- Always mention date and timing of the consultation
- Mention age and sex of the patient. In a pediatric prescription, weight of the patient must also be mentioned
- Always put your hand on the part that the patient says is painful. Apply your stethoscope on him/her, even if it is for cosmetic reasons
- Listen attentively; look carefully; ask questions intelligently
- If, after completing the examination, the patient/attendant feels that something has been left out or wants something to be re-examined, oblige him
- Always face the patient. Maintain eye contact that is comfortable to the patient. Do not stare. Some patients tolerate very little eye contact. Learn to observe out from the corner of your eyes
- In case you have been distracted/inattentive during the history taking, ask the patient/attendant to start all over again. He will never mind it. As far as possible, consultations should not be interrupted for nonurgent calls
- Ask the patient to come back for review the next day in case you have examined him hurriedly, or if you are not sure about the diagnosis/treatment
- Mention "diagnosis under review" or "under evaluation" until the diagnosis is finally settled
- In complicated cases, record precisely the history of illness and substantial physical finding about the patient on your prescription
- If the patient/attending are erring on any count (history not reliable, refusing investigations, refusing admission) make a note of it or seek written refusal preferably in local language with proper witness
- Mention the condition of patient in specific/objective terms. Avoid vague/nonspecific terminology
- Record history of drug allergy
- Write names of drugs clearly. Use correct dosage (by revising knowledge periodically), and mention clearly, method and interval of administration. Here one must use local or sign language. Do not forget writing precautions like AST/per orally (PO)/intramuscular (IM)/intravenous (IV)/locally/with milk/HS/OD/BD/TDS/pc (after food)/ac (before food) etc. in local language
- If a drug is a poison (e.g. certain local applications), warn in writing
- Mention additional precautions, e.g. food, rest, avoidance of certain drugs, allergens, alcohol, smoking, etc. if indicated
- Give instructions to the patient in comprehensible terms, making sure that the patient understands both the instruction and the importance of strictly adhering to them, e.g. while prescribing a potent anti-inflammatory drug, warn that if he experiences any stomach trouble, he should stop taking the drug and consult a doctor immediately
- Mention likely side effects and action to be taken, if they occur
- Remember to advise in writing, pathological tests/radiological tests at specified intervals for certain drugs, which require such monitoring, if such drugs are prescribed. Some examples are sodium valproate, carbamazepine, methotrexate and other immunosuppressives
- Always advise the patient not to stop taking a drug suddenly, which is required to be tapered before it is stopped
- Remember major drug interactions
- Specifically mention review, or follow-up schedule
- Mention if patient(s)/attendant(s) is/are under effect of alcohol/drugs
- In case of a particular drug/equipment is not available, make a note
- Prescription with caution during pregnancy/lactation
- Adjust doses in case of a child/elderly patient and in renal or hepatic disorders
- In case of chronic ailments, mention treatment to be taken immediately in case of an emergency. For example, a patient on antiepileptic treatment should be advised to take an injection of diazepam when convulsions occur

- In case of any deviation from care, mention reasons; mention whether prognosis explained. If necessary, take signature of the patient/attendant after explaining the prognosis in written local language
- Mention where the patient should contact in case of your nonavailability/emergency
- If you are not sure what disease the patient has after a thorough work-up, get a consultation. Develop a list of physicians you trust and respect in each of the specialties. Nurture your relationship with them and consult them in difficult cases
- Whenever referring a patient, provide him with a referring note. In case of emergency/serious illness, ring up the concerned doctor in the patient's presence. Show your concern
- Always keep with you and refer to, the latest edition of the standard textbook of your branch of medicine. Always subscribe to at least one standard journal and participate in at least two updates/conferences every year
- Update your knowledge and skill from time to time. If a doctor does not keep pace with recent advances, the quality of care suffers, and does not measure up to the standards of reasonable care and skill and attitude, over a period of time. Not only do they make any attempt to update themselves, but they slip downwards also. Doctors may become incompetent due to other causes—age, mental illness, addiction to alcohol or drug abuse
- Update not only your own knowledge and skill, but also that of your staff. Update the facilities and equipment according to prevailing current standards in your area
- Preferably employ qualified assistants. If not available, impart proper training and skill at your or some appropriate center, and obtain the same
- Medication to relieve pain, especially in postoperative and cancer cases must be carried out carefully
- Always obtain a legally valid consent before undertaking a surgical/diagnostic procedure. Learn the difference between "informed persuasion" and "informed consent". The first is legally wrong. Though, at times it may be medically correct
- It is important to screen every patient for hepatitis B/HIV infection before every surgery/blood transfusion, so that false claims are not made at a later date
- In case of medically terminating pregnancy (MTP)/sterilization, always follow the guideline issued by the Government of India
- Before administering an injection/vaccination, always check:
  - Name of the injection (a wrong injection may be given through mistake or oversight)
  - Reconfirm the route of administration
  - If it is to be diluted, check the dilution factor (1:2, 1:4, etc.)
  - Rate of the administration (fast, slow, in drip, etc.)
  - Site of injection, e.g., anterolateral thigh (if age < 2 years), gluteal region, deltoid, etc.
  - That a disposable syringe and needle are used. If that is not possible, use syringe and needle after proper sterilization
  - In case the patient is agitated/not cooperating, restrain him properly with 1 or 2 assistants, or wait until he calms down. It is not unusual for the broken needle leading to a claim for compensation
  - Confirm that it has been kept at the required temperature
  - If it is required to be reconstituted, check the diluent and also whether it has got to be cooled before using, and
  - Ensure that an injection is not given intravenously, if contraindicated
- Routinely advise X-rays in injury to bones and joints, and related diseases of bones/joints
- Always rule out pregnancy before subjecting the uterus to X-rays
- Always read reports carefully, and interpret the results of tests/X-rays properly and make a note of it. In case of any doubts, recheck with the laboratory/diagnostic center
- A patient who is undergoing labor should be attended to without any lapse
- In a complex medical situation, a doctor would be expected to conduct more frequent and more extensive examinations, and would be expected in making his assessment to seek all ancillary assistance, e.g., by means of tests, etc.
- In all instances of "swab cases" and "instrument cases", the surgeon in charge is generally held directly or vicariously liable for negligence. The surgeon in charge must therefore, personally ensure that such mishaps do not occur
- The period for the responsibility of the surgeon extends to and includes the postoperative care. He must, therefore, ensure proper postoperative care to the patient
- In the case of death of the patient occurring while undergoing a surgery/diagnostic procedure, the higher hospital authorities/police authorities must be informed without loss of time. In such cases, autopsy/postmortem is mandatory

- In case the hospital/clinic claims to provide 24 hour emergency service, availability of necessary equipment in working order and competent staff within reasonable time is mandatory
- Always seek proper legal and medical advice before sending reply to the notice sent by the patient or his representative, or to the complaint referred to you from a consumer court.

DON'TS FOR DOCTORS

- Don't prescribe without examining the patient, even if he is a close friend or relative
- Never examine a female patient without the presence of female nurse/attendant, especially during genital and breast examinations
- Don't insist on the patient to tell the history of illness or be examined in presence of others. He/she has a right to privacy and confidentiality
- Do not permit considerations of religion, nationality, race, party politics or social standing to intervene between you and your patient
- It may not be reasonable for a doctor to assume what the patient is saying, is truthful, when what the patient/attendant says is clearly contradicted by the symptoms
- Don't smoke while examining a patient
- Don't examine a patient when you are sick, exhausted, or under influence of alcohol or any intoxicating substance
- Don't be overconfident. Don't look overconfident
- Don't prescribe a drug or indulge in a procedure if you cannot justify its indications
- Don't prescribe/administer a drug which is banned, e.g. analgin, oxyphenbutazone, etc.
- Don't over-prescribe too much of the drug—too large a dose for too long days
- Don't under prescribe—not prescribing the needed drug dose is too small, length of treatment is too short
- Don't prescribe multiple drugs. Such prescription, maybe due to inability to form a correct diagnosis. Possibilities of drug interactions increase with polypharmacy
- Don't write instructions on a separate slip. Don't allow substitutions
- Don't indulge in self-serving notes. A self-serving note is one in which the factual content or the general tone suggests that the writer's principal aim was to protect himself from a subsequent complaint rather than to make a genuine record
- Don't adopt experimental method in treatment. If there is some rationale, do it only after informed consent
- Don't do anything beyond your level of competence. Competence of doctors, nursing staff is defined by their qualification, training, experience and competence of a hospital/nursing home is defined by competent staff by the availability of various equipment in working order and back-up support, e.g. handling of cases of accident/emergency, severe reaction to drugs, anesthesia, etc., and availability of resuscitative equipment, etc.
- Don't give a drug parenterally if it can be given orally. There maybe some exceptions
- When you are not sure what to do, consult your senior/specialist/colleague
- Don't refuse if the patient/attendants want to leave against medical advice. It is their right. Document this properly
- Never avoid a call for help from a nurse on duty at night. In all probability a genuine emergency may be there
- Never order an investigation unless the result is likely to help you direct the treatment or make a difference in what you tell a patient
- Don't allow modern diagnostic tests to substitute your clinical judgment. At best, they can only supplement it. Always analyze the cost-benefit rationale before rushing to get these tests done. In case of a particular test has a high false-positive or false-negative results, explain this to the patient before getting it done
- Never label any condition as "functional" until it has been accurately ascertained that it is not due to any other cause
- Don't talk to an angry patient about any other subject until you understand the reason of his anger. Then take necessary time and steps to calm him down
- Never scold attendants of a seriously or terminally ill patient
- Don't challenge anybody
- Don't refuse the patient's right to know about diagnosis and treatment of his illness

- Don't withhold information, however harsh and difficult, in seriously/terminally ill patient. It must be conveyed with compassion and gradually, if time permits. The doctors, and especially their assistant, must train themselves in the art of sensitive communication. It would be wise to take into confidence the family members, close relatives and friends; this would often make the acceptance easier and quicker
- Don't tell patient/attendant bad news until you are as certain as possible on the accuracy of the finding
- Don't leave at the moment of death. There is a tendency, especially on the part of senior doctors, to go away at this time when their presence and experience are most needed
- Don't hesitate to extend your condolences and sympathies to the bereaved persons
- Don't forget to provide genetic counseling to couples and parents with known family history/children having genetic abnormalities, e.g., thalassemia, hemophilia, etc.
- Don't issue death certificates unless you have yourself verified it
- Don't divulge secrets you come to know during discharge of your professional duties unless there are exceptions as carved out in the Code of Medical Ethics. There are some exceptions to this general principal:
  - If the patient gives consent
  - When it is undesirable on medical grounds to seek patient's consent
  - The doctor's overriding duty to society
  - The information is required for legal process
  - For the purpose of medical research, after obtaining permission from competent authority
- Don't deny medical care to a patient with HIV infection/AIDS (acquired immunodeficiency syndrome). Observe all necessary precautions
- Don't inform that the person is infected with HIV unless confirmatory test results are received
- Don't issue a false medical certificate
- Don't give untrue, misleading or improper reports, documents, etc.
- Don't refuse the patient's right to examine and receive an explanation about your bill regarding the source of payment; whether or not it is reimbursed by the government or by his employer/insurance company
- Don't refuse the patient's right to know about the hospital rules and regulations
- Don't purchase costly sophisticated equipment only for the sake of prestige. It may induce you to indulge in malpractice
- Don't dump hospital garbage, including used disposables in the open. It is criminal. It should be properly incinerated/destroyed to prevent spread of disease or reuse by unscrupulous persons
- Don't refuse first-aid/medical care to accident and emergency cases, even if it is a medicolegal case. It is a primary duty of every doctor/hospital to provide treatment up to its true level of competence in such cases before referring them to a higher center, if required
- Never talk loosely with your colleagues, despite intense professional rivalry. Never criticize your colleagues. The patients/attendants may incite you to say/do something. They may seek your comments on the other doctor's treatment. There is always a polite way to set aside their comments and queries. Remember, if you had seen the case from the start, you would have done the same. If your colleague has made an error of judgment regarding diagnosis or treatment, you never know under what circumstances this happened.

CONCLUSION

Though, the inclusion of the medical profession in purview of CPA is gift from the West, the law makers of India fail to understand that the medical and healthcare system in India is different from the West, as even today, health and medical system is the responsibility of the state and not of the individual, and is further more not insurance based.

In view of the Supreme Court affixing its seal of approval on the applicability of the CPA to the service provided by the medical profession, it has become all the more imperative for the medical professionals to exercise a greater degree of caution while undertaking diagnosis and treatment of patients. It is, therefore, felt necessary to make the doctors aware of certain precautions which ought to be taken. Furthermore, the doctors must be well informed of the law regarding this, and also the latest amendments made in the legal procedures plus how to proceed in case a complaint is lodged against them.

It is also desirable for the patients and their attendants to observe certain norms so that they benefit most out of the medical help sought, and healthy relationship with the doctor/hospital is maintained.

Appendix 'E'

Instruments

S Inamdar

SIM'S SPECULUM (FIG. 1)

Material: Stainless steel

Sterilization: (i) autoclave, (ii) boiling.

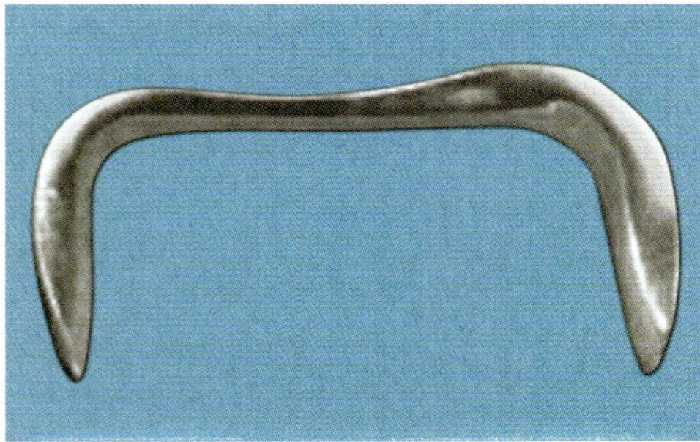

Fig. 1: Sim's speculum

Uses

- *Gynecologic*:
  - Routine gynecological examination to visualize vagina and cervix
  - To collect discharge from posterior fornix
  - Hysterosalpingography (HSG)
  - Gynecological operations.
- *Obstetric:*
  - Routine per speculum examination
  - Manual vacuum aspiration (MVA), first trimester medical termination of pregnancy (MTP)
  - Cervical cerclage
  - Diagnose and repair cervical tear.

SIM'S ANTERIOR VAGINAL WALL RETRACTOR (FIG. 2)

Material: Stainless steel

Sterilization: (i) autoclave, (ii) boiling.

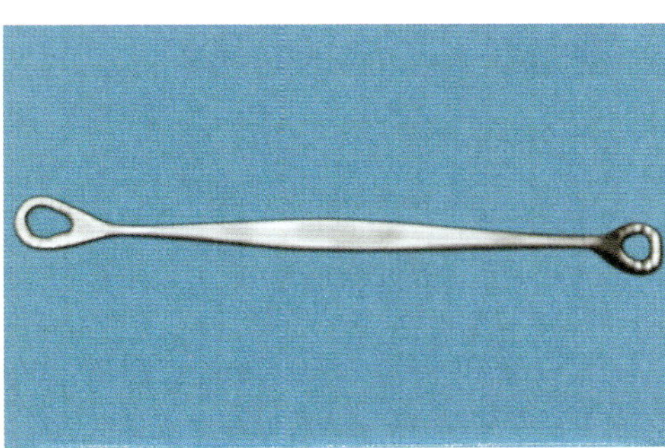

Fig. 2: Sim's anterior vaginal wall retractor

Use

Along with Sim's speculum, to visualize cervix by retracting anterior vaginal wall.

DOYEN'S RETRACTOR (FIG. 3)

Material: Stainless steel

Sterilization: Autoclaving.

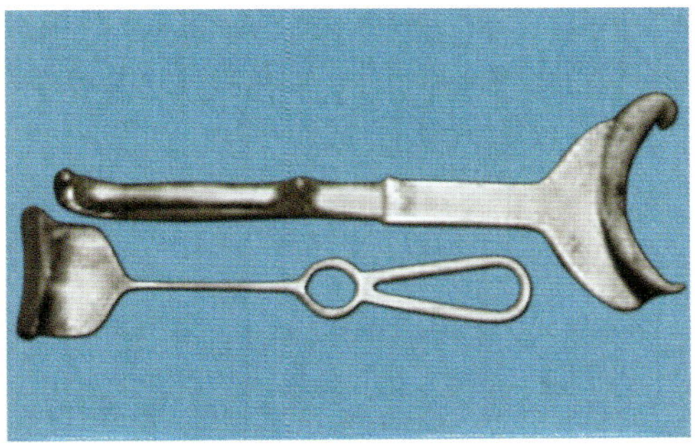

Fig. 3: Doyen's retractor

Uses

- *Gynecologic:*
  - Abdominal hysterectomy

- Wertheim's hysterectomy
- Tuboplasty
- Sling operation
- Purandare's cervicopexy
- Exploratory laparotomy for ovarian tumors
- Myomectomy.
- *Obstetric:*
  - Cesarean section
  - Cesarean hysterectomy
  - Exploratory laparotomy for ruptured tubal ectopic pregnancy.

CUSCO'S BIVALVED SELF-RETAINING VAGINAL SPECULUM (FIG. 4)

Material: Stainless steel

Sterilization: (i) autoclave, (ii) boiling.

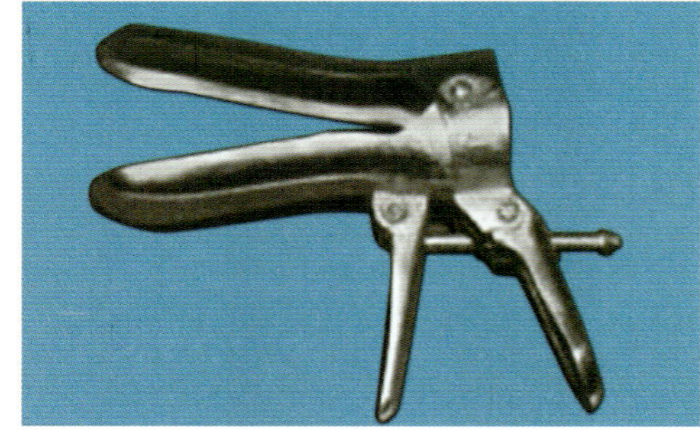

Fig. 4: Cusco's speculum

Uses

- Routine per speculum examination in gynecology
- Colposcopy
- Endometrial biopsy
- Cervical punch biopsy
- PAP smear
- Insertion and removal of intrauterine contraceptive device (IUCD)
- Intrauterine insemination.

AUVARD'S WEIGHTED SELF-RETAINING POSTERIOR VAGINAL SPECULUM (FIG. 5)

Material: Stainless steel

Sterilization: Autoclaving.

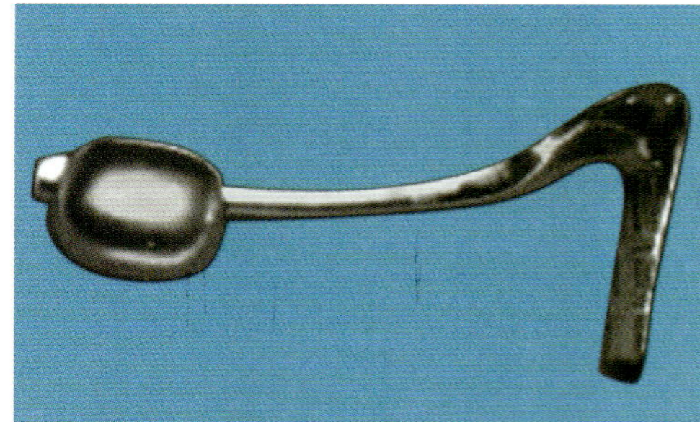

Fig. 5: Auvard's speculum

Uses

- Vaginal hysterectomy
- Anterior colporrhaphy
- Kelly's repair
- Fothergill's/modified Fothergill's repair
- Vesicovaginal fistula repair
- Schauta's hysterectomy.

SONAWALLA'S SELF-RETAINING VAGINAL SPECULUM (FIG. 6)

Material: Stainless steel

Sterilization: Autoclaving.

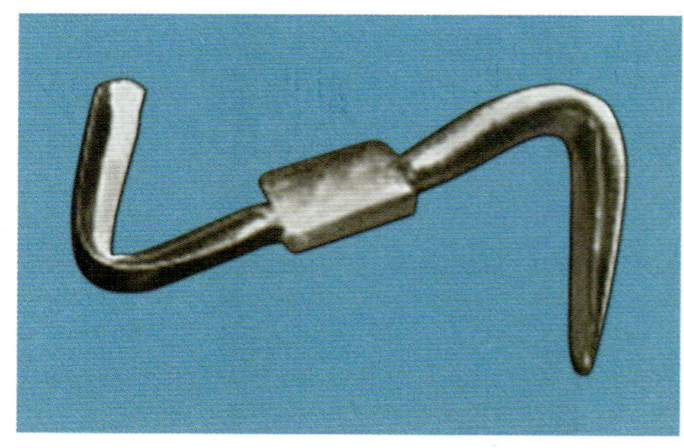

Fig. 6: Sonawalla's speculum

Uses

- Vaginal hysterectomy
- Vaginal tubal sterilization

- Vesicovaginal fistula repair
- Fothergill's repair/modified Fothergill's repair
- Schauta's radical hysterectomy.

LANDON BLADDER RETRACTOR (FIG. 7)

Material: Stainless steel

Sterilization: Autoclaving and boiling.

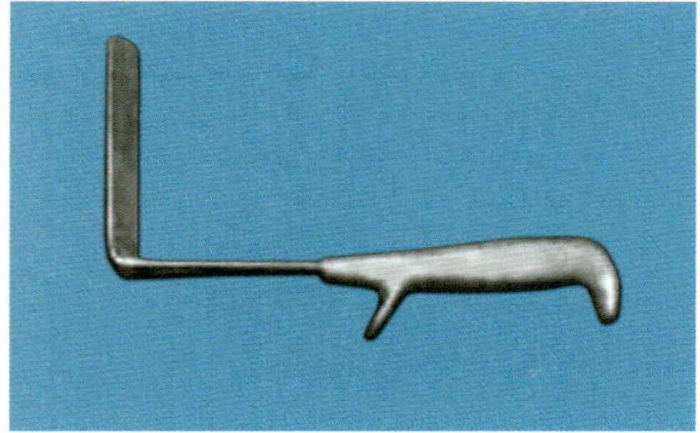

Fig. 7: Landon retractor

Uses

- To retract the bladder away from cervix and uterus during vaginal hysterectomy. It is introduced into anterior pouch after the uterovesical fold of peritoneum has been opened
- To retract lateral and anterior vaginal walls during any vaginal operation.

TONGUE DEPRESSOR (FIG. 8)

Material: Stainless steel

Sterilization: (i) autoclaving, (ii) boiling.

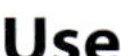

Use

To examine oral cavity

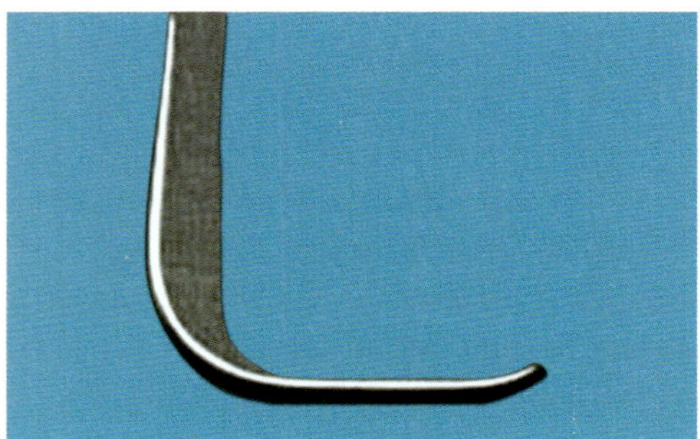

Fig. 8: Tongue depressor

RIGHT ANGLE RETRACTOR (FIG. 9)

Material: Stainless steel

Sterilization: (i) autoclaving, (ii) boiling.

Uses

- To retract abdominal wall during tubal ligation
- To retract bladder and posterior vaginal wall during hysterectomy
- To retract bladder during abdominal hysterectomy.

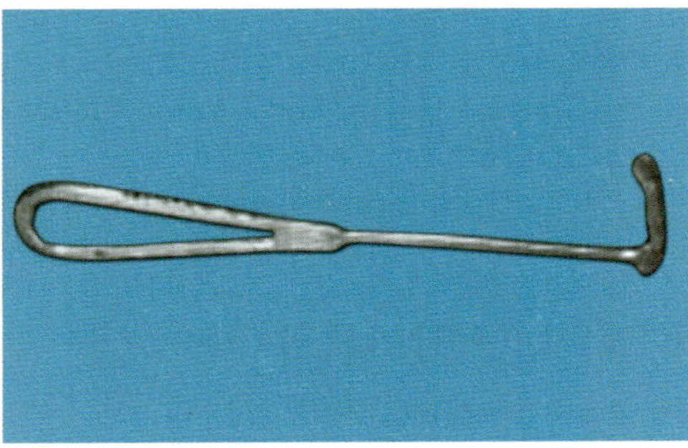

Fig. 9: Right angle retractor

FLUSHING CURETTE (FIG. 10)

Material: Stainless steel

Sterilization: (i) autoclaving, (ii) boiling.

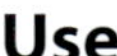

Use

Dilatation and evacuation operation.

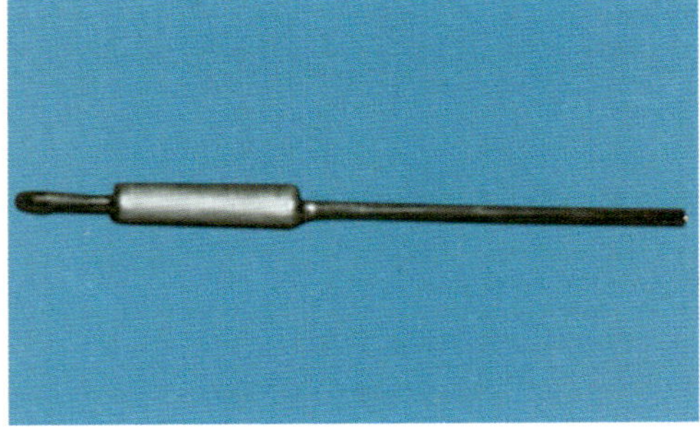

Fig. 10: Flushing curette

TOWEL CLIP (FIG. 11)

Material: Stainless steel

Sterilization: Autoclaving and boiling.

Uses

- For draping
- Can be used for hemostasis.

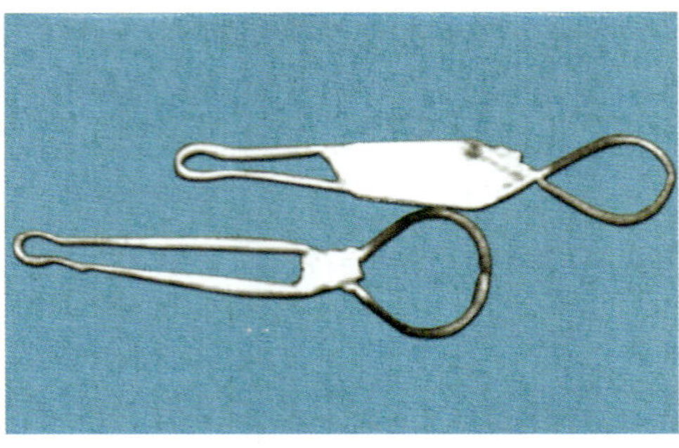

Fig. 11: Towel clip

ALLIS TISSUE HOLDING FORCEPS (FIG. 12)

Material: Stainless steel

Sterilization: (i) autoclaving, (ii) boiling.

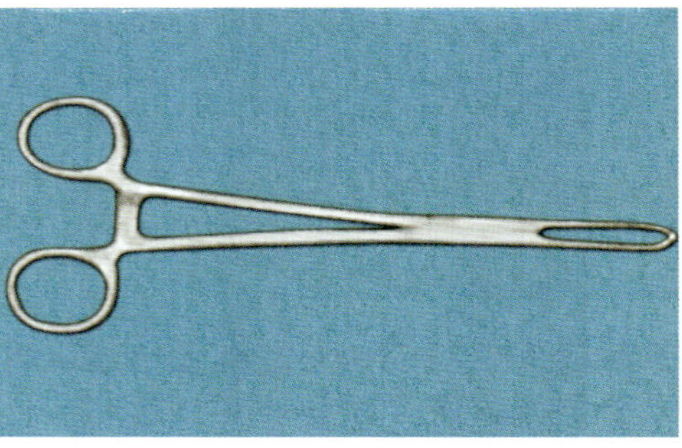

Fig. 12: Allis forceps

Uses

- *General:* To hold the rectus sheath while opening and closing abdominal wall
- *Gynecologic:* To hold the edges of vagina
  - In anterior colporrhaphy, enterocele repair, colpoperineorrhaphy
  - In vaginal hysterectomy, abdominal hysterectomy
  - Fothergill's repair
  - Repair of vesicovaginal/rectovaginal fistula
  - To hold the cervix
  - Abdominal hysterectomy
  - To hold the lips of pediatric cervix
  - To hold the uterus
  - Vaginal and abdominal hysterectomy, myomec-tomy, utriculoplasty
  - Marchetti test for detection of stress urinary incontinence.
- *Obstetric:*
  - In lower segment cesarean section (LSCS) to hold angles of uterine incision
  - For correction of acute inversion of uterus.

NEEDLE HOLDER (FIG. 13)

Material: Stainless steel

Sterilization: Autoclaving.

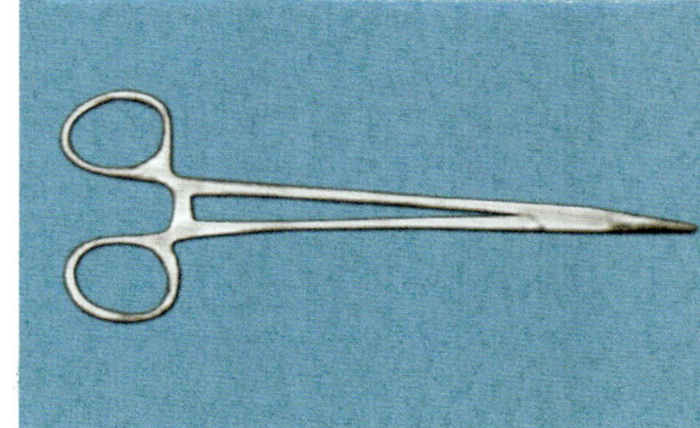

Fig. 13: Needle holder

Use

To hold needle during suturing.

ARTERY FORCEPS (FIG. 14)

Material: Stainless steel

Sterilization: Autoclaving.

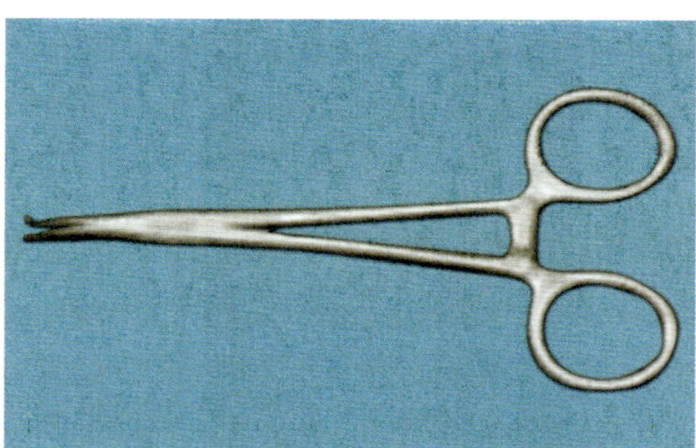

Fig. 14: Curved artery forceps

Uses

- For hemostasis
- Holding structures like peritonium, rectus sheath, vessels, muscles, etc. during any operative procedure
- For suture removal
- Can be used for clamping placenta after delivery of baby.

SPONGE HOLDING FORCEPS (FIG. 15)

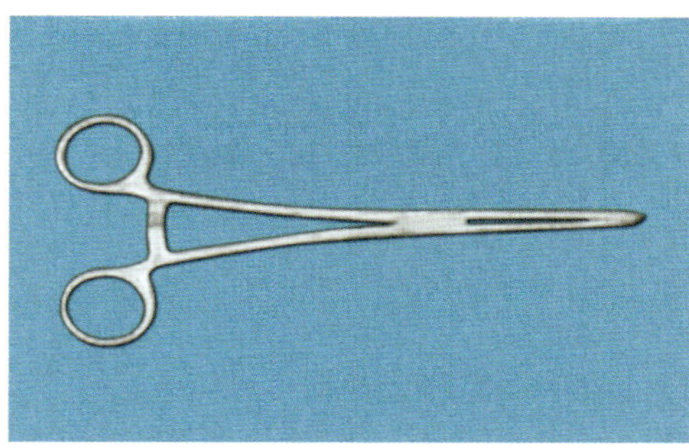

Fig. 15: Sponge holding forceps

Material: Stainless steel

Sterilization: (i) autoclaving, (ii) boiling.

Uses

- *General:*
  - Painting and preparing parts preoperatively
  - Swab out cavities like vagina, pelvic cavity
- *Gynecologic:*
  - For applying pressure over deep bleeding points during pelvic surgery
  - To check hemostasis of stumps during vaginal hysterectomy
  - For packing away omentum and intestines out of pelvis in gynecological operations
- *Obstetric:*
  - To hold lips of pregnant cervix during tightening of os
  - For diagnosis and repair of cervical tear
  - Swab out blood in uterine cavity.

KIDNEY TRAY (FIG. 16)

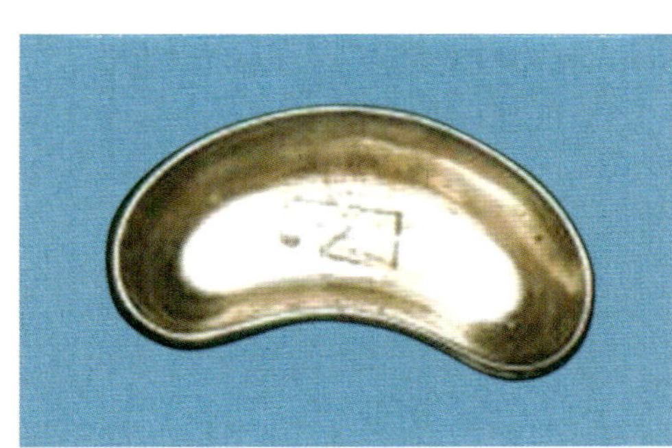

Fig. 16: Kidney tray

Material: Stainless steel

Sterilization: Autoclaving and boiling.

Uses

- To collect and hold urine
- To hold swabs for painting before any operation
- To collect placenta after delivery of baby
- To collect blood in ruptured ectopic pregnancy
- To collect vomitus.

KOCHER'S CLAMP (FIG. 17)

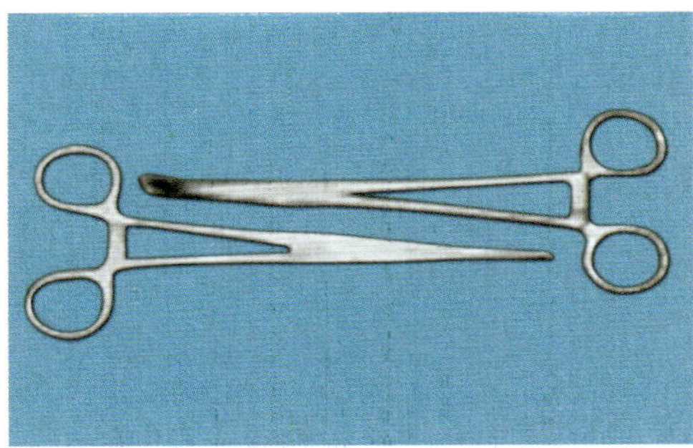

Fig. 17: Kocher's clamp

Material: Stainless steel

Sterilization: (i) autoclaving, (ii) boiling

The blades may be curved or flat or straight. One blade has a longitudinal ridge which fits in a longitudinal groove on the other blade. It has transverse serrations on its blade.

Uses

Hysterectomy: To clamp the uterosacral ligaments, uterine blood vessels and the cornual structures or the infundibulopelvic ligaments in vaginal hysterectomy.

- Oophorectomy for ovarian cysts or tumors
- Removal of pedunculated leiomyomatous polyps
- Salpingectomy for tubal ectopic gestation
- Cesarean hysterectomy
- Clamping the umbilical cord of the newborn
- Artificial low rupture of membranes
- To hold the uterus during abdominal hysterectomy.

TENACULUM (FIG. 18)

Material: Stainless steel

Sterilization: (i) autoclaving, (ii) boiling.

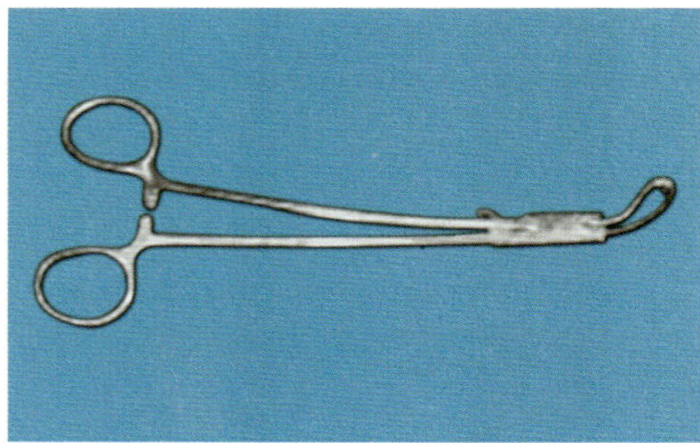

Fig. 18: Tenaculum

Uses

- To hold the lips of nulliparous cervix
- To hold cervical stump in subtotal hysterectomy.

Special use

- HSG
- Chromopertubation test
- Rubin's test.

BABCOCK FORCEPS (CURVED AND STRAIGHT) (FIG. 19)

Material: Stainless steel

Sterilization: (i) autoclaving, (ii) boiling.

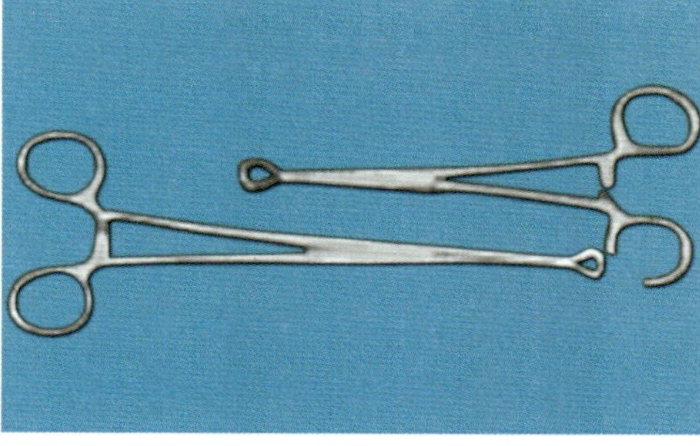

Fig. 19: Straight Babcock forceps

Uses

To hold tubular structures like:

- Fallopian tubes in tubal sterilization, ruptured tubal ectopic pregnancy
- Round ligaments
- Ureters in Wertheim's hysterectomy
- Vas in vasectomy
- Appendix and cecum in appendicectomy.

GREEN ARMYTAGE FORCEPS (FIG. 20)

Material: Stainless steel

Sterilization: (i) autoclaving, (ii) boiling.

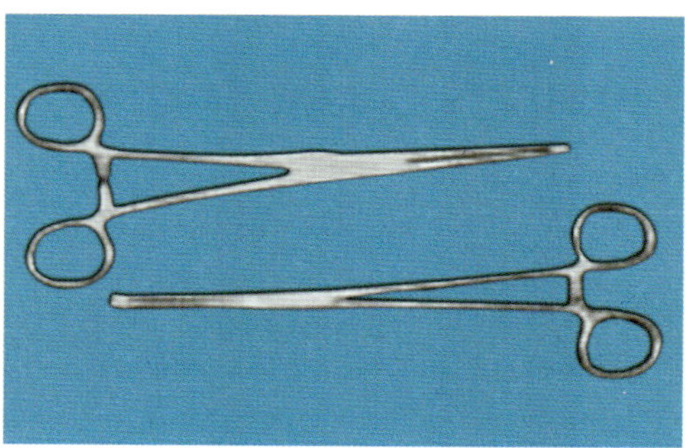

Fig. 20: Green armytage forceps

Uses

- To achieve hemostasis by compressing the bleeding uterine vessels during LSCS
- To lift uterine edges during suturing of uterus
- To trace and repair cervical tears after vaginal delivery.

BLADDER SOUND (FIG. 21)

Material: Stainless steel

Sterilization: (i) autoclaving, (ii) boiling.

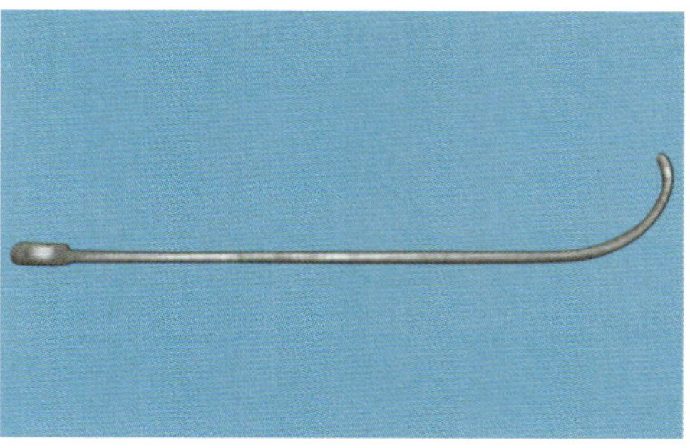

Fig. 21: Bladder sound

Uses

- To define the limits of bladder during operation
- To confirm a suspected bladder injury during vaginal hysterectomy
- To determine length and direction of vesicovaginal fistulae
- To sound a calculus or foreign body in the bladder
- To differentiate bladder or urethral diverticulum from anterior vaginal wall cyst.

LEECH WILKINSON'S CANNULA (FIG. 22)

Material: Stainless steel

Sterilization: (i) autoclaving, (ii) boiling

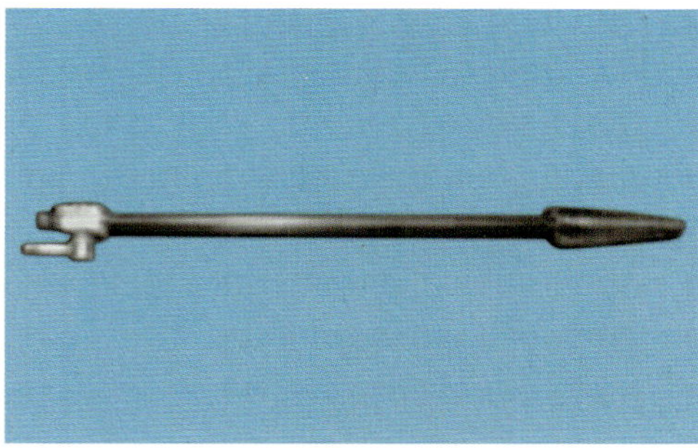

Fig. 22: Leech Wilkinson's cannula

Uses

- HSG
- Chromopertubation test in laparoscopy
- Hydrotubation.

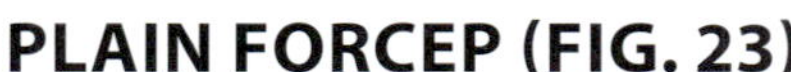

PLAIN FORCEP (FIG. 23)

Material: Stainless steel

Sterilization: Autoclaving and boiling.

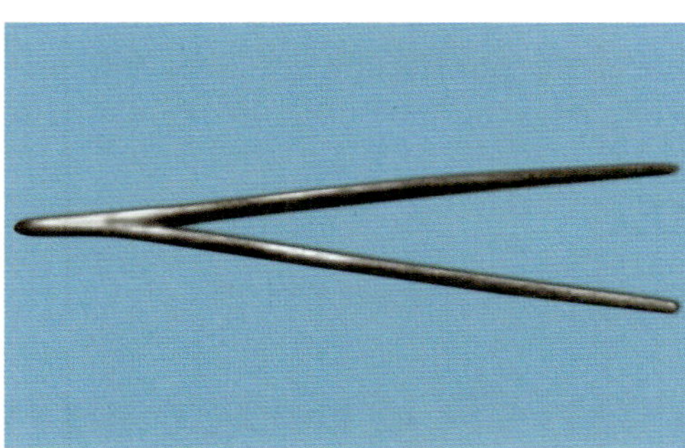

Fig. 23: Plain forcep

Uses

- To hold thin delicate structures such as peritoneum
- Muscles, vessels, thin fascia, intestinal wall, bladder wall, etc.
- During suture removal
- Packing abdominal cavity during abdominal operations.

TOOTH FORCEP (FIG. 24)

Material: Stainless steel

Sterilization: Autoclaving and boiling

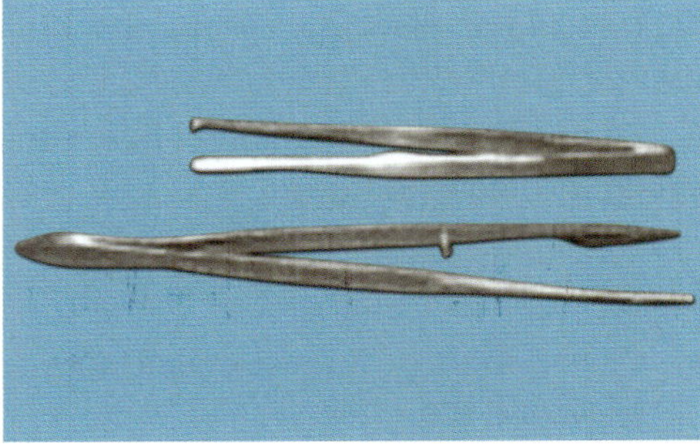

Fig. 24: Tooth forcep

Uses

- To hold tough structures like:
  - Tendon
  - Fascia
  - Skin
  - Rectus sheath
  - Uterine wall, etc.
- Can be used for hemostasis.

HEGAR'S DILATOR (FIG. 25)

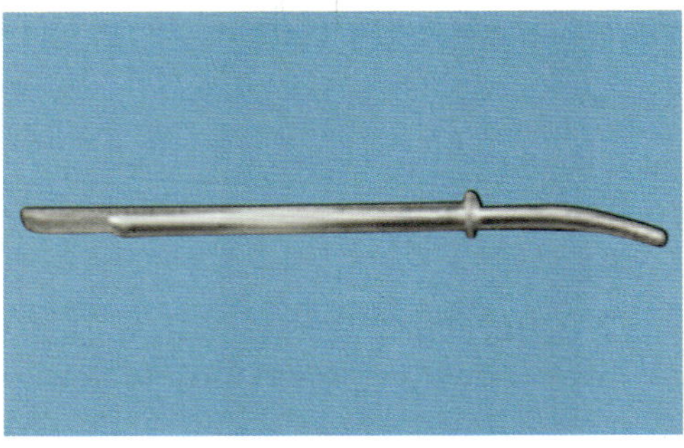

Fig. 25: Hegar's dilator

Material: Stainless steel

Sterilization: (i) autoclaving, (ii) boiling.

It is a solid rod curved near the tip and tapering towards the tip. The curve is shallow and the dilating portion is within terminal 1.5 cm of the dilator.

Uses

For the rapid dilatation in:

- Prior to endometrial curettage
- Prior to suction aspiration for first trimester MTP
- Prior to suction evacuation of mole
- Removal of endometrial polyp, placental polyp, leiomyomatous polyp
- Hysteroscopy
- Amputation of cervix, Fothergill's operation, following cervical conization
- Cervical stenosis
- Application of intrauterine radiotherapy
- Primary dysmenorrhea
- Diagnosis of incompetent os.

FENTON'S DILATOR (FIG. 26)

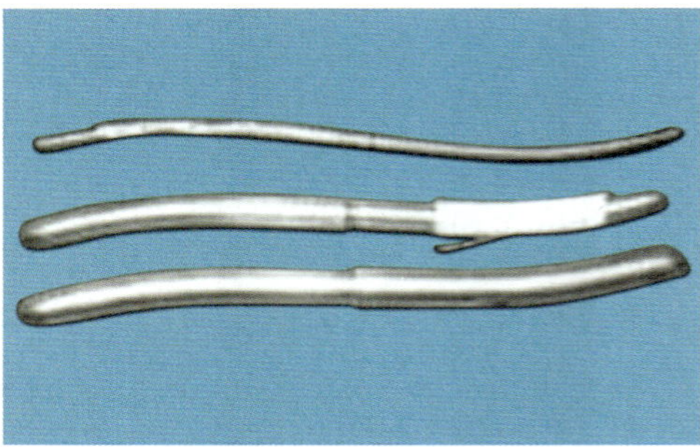

Fig. 26: Fenton's dilator

It is similar to Hegar's dilator except for two important differences—it is more tapering and hollow inside.

Use

Same as that of Hegar's dilator.

CUZZI'S PLACENTAL CURETTE (FIG. 27)

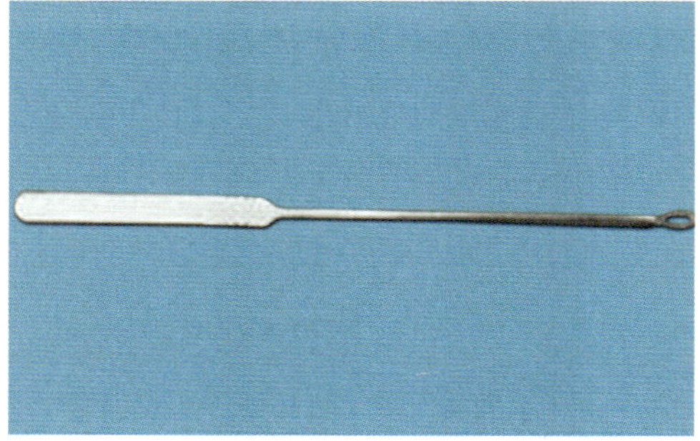

Fig. 27: Cuzzi's placental curette

Material: Stainless steel

Sterilization: (i) autoclaving, (ii) boiling.

It is a long instrument with a handle at one hand and curette at the other. The curette is spoon-shaped.

The outer surface of curette has transverse serrations and the rim of spoon is somewhat sharp.

Uses

- Check curettage for incomplete abortion and retention of the placenta in second trimester
- Retained segments or bits of placenta after delivery of a viable fetus.

UTERINE CURETTE (FIG. 28)

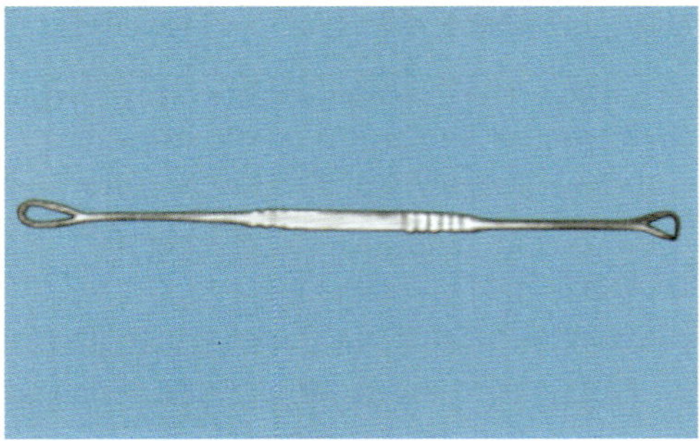

Fig. 28: Sharp and blunt curette

Uses

- Gynecological uses
  - *Diagnostic:*
    - Primary or secondary infertility for ovulation detection
    - Tuberculous endometritis
    - Abnormal uterine bleeding
    - Endometrial hyperplasia/endometrial carcinoma
    - Carcinoma cervix
    - Secondary amenorrhea
    - Postmenopausal bleeding
  - *Therapeutic:*
    - Dysfunctional uterine bleeding (DUB)
- Asherman's syndrome
- To remove embedded intrauterine device (IUD).
- *Obstetrical uses*
  - MTP, check curettage
  - Blunt curettage in abortions
  - Secondary persistent pulmonary hypertension (PPH), subinvolution.

AYRE'S WOODEN SPATULA (FIG. 29)

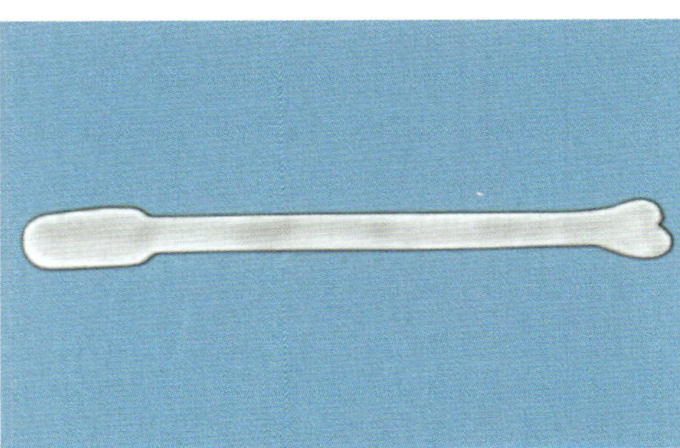

Fig. 29: Ayre's wooden spatula

Material: Wood

Sterilization: Dry heat.

Uses

- Pap smear
- To take surface biopsy in obvious cases of carcinoma cervix
- Hormonal cytology
- Cervicovaginal smear
- Buccal smear.

IUCD REMOVING HOOK (FIG. 30)

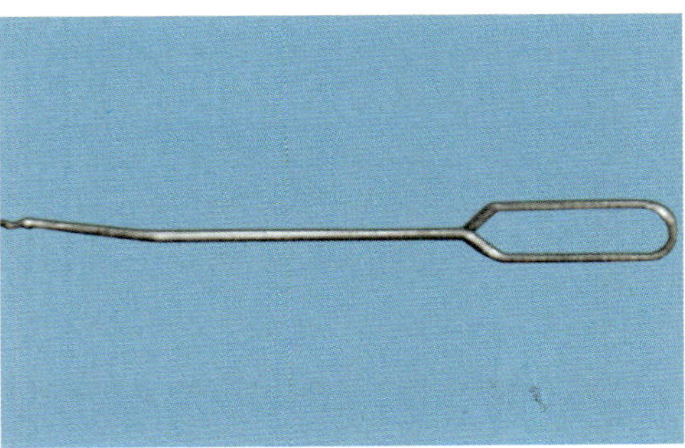

Fig. 30: IUCD removing hook

Material: Stainless steel

Sterilization: (i) autoclaving, (ii) boiling.

Uses

- Removal of an embedded IUD from the uterine cavity
- Removal of tubal prosthesis from the uterine cavity.

VACUUM EXTRACTOR (FIG. 31)

A vacuum extractor has a suction cup, a traction handle, a source of creating vacuum and a vacuum gauge to note the negative pressure created. The cup may be made up of metal or softer material like silastic.

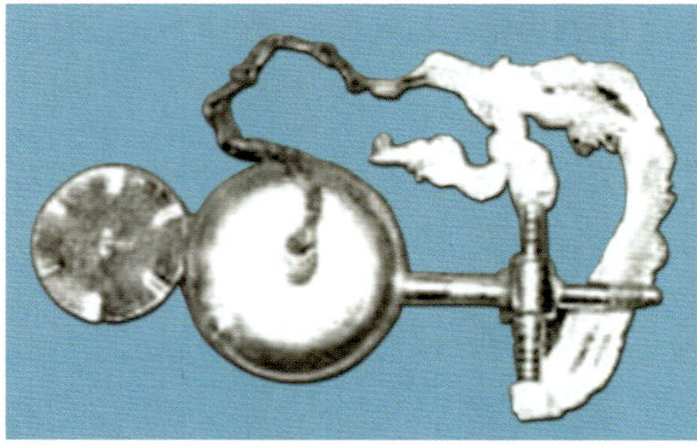

Fig. 31: Vacuum extractor

Uses

- Deep transverse arrest with adequate pelvis
- Delay in descent of high head in case of second baby of twins
- As an alternative of forceps operation
- Delay in late first stage due to uterine inertia or primary cervical dystocia
- As an adjunct to symphysiotomy.

VULSELLUM (FIG. 32)

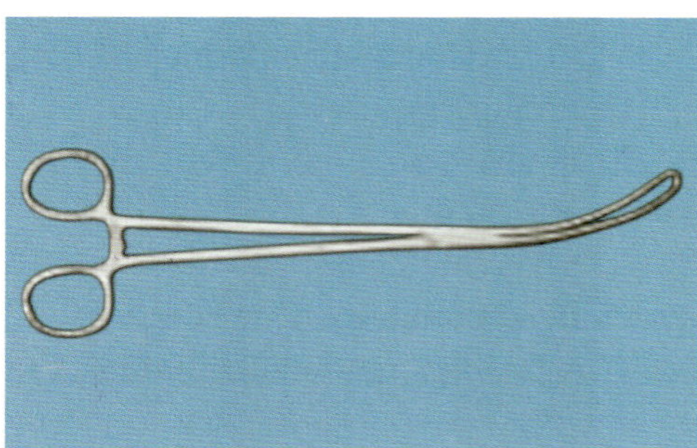

Fig. 32: Vulsellum

Material: Stainless steel

Sterilization: (i) autoclaving, (ii) boiling.

Uses

- Anterior lip held in:
  - Endometrial biopsy
  - IUCD insertion
  - Intrauterine insemination
  - Vaginal hysterectomy
  - Cauterization of cervix and cervical biopsy
- Posterior lip held in:
  - Colpopincture for suspected ruptured ectopic pregnancy
  - Culdoscopy
  - Posterior colpotomy.

HULKA'S UTERINE MANIPULATOR (FIG. 33)

Fig. 33: Hulka's uterine manipulator

Material: Stainless steel

Sterilization: (i) autoclaving, (ii) boiling.

Uses

- It is used to elevate and manipulate position of uterus for following:
  - Laparoscopic sterilization
  - Sterilization by mini laparotomy
  - Visualization of pelvic structures by laparoscopy.

VITOON'S UTERINE MANIPULATOR (FIG. 34)

Fig. 34: Vitoon's uterine manipulator

Material: Stainless steel

Sterilization: (i) autoclaving, (ii) boiling.

Uses

Same as that of Hulka's uterine manipulator.

DREW SMITH'S CATHETER (FIG. 35)

Material: Stainless steel

Sterilization: (i) autoclaving, (ii) boiling.

It is S-shaped and has a side opening to drain liquor amnii. It has a spring loaded stylet with a blunt tip.

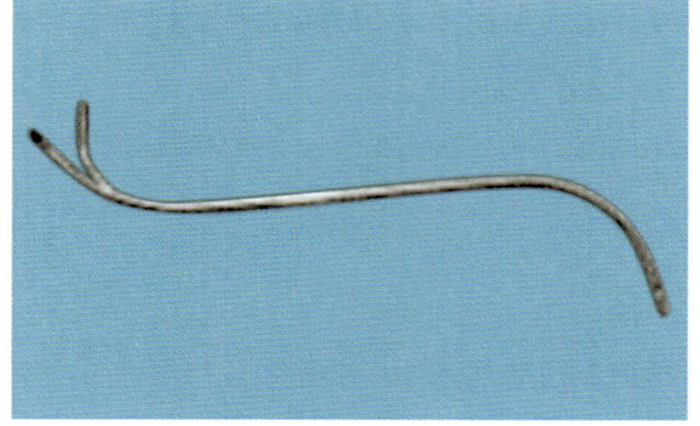

Fig. 35: Drew Smith's catheter

Uses

- High amniotomy
- To drain a hydrocephalic head through a spina bifida, in case of a breech delivered up to the head.

FLUSHING CANNULA (FIG. 36)

Material: Stainless steel

Sterilization: (i) autoclaving, (ii) boiling.

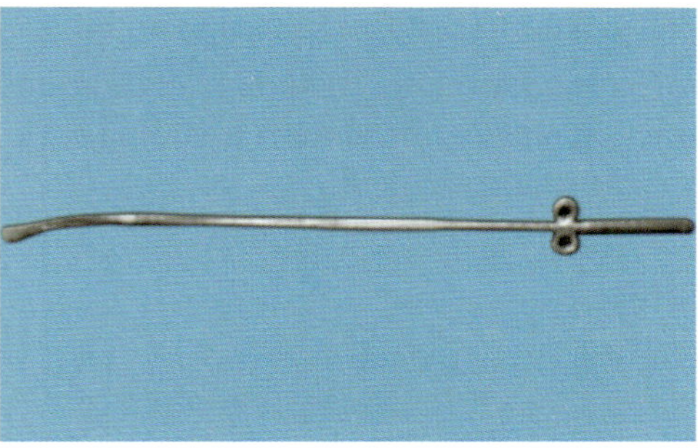

Fig. 36: Flushing cannula

Uses

Used for suction to keep the operating field dry during operation in narrow field, e.g.—

- Tuboplasty
- Repair of vesicovaginal fistula and rectovaginal fistulae.

LONG-CURVED OBSTETRICS FORCEPS (FIGS 37 AND 38)

Material: Stainless steel

Sterilization: (i) autoclaving, (ii) boiling

Measurement: Length is 37 cm; distance between the tips is 2.5 cm and widest diameter between the blades is 9 cm.

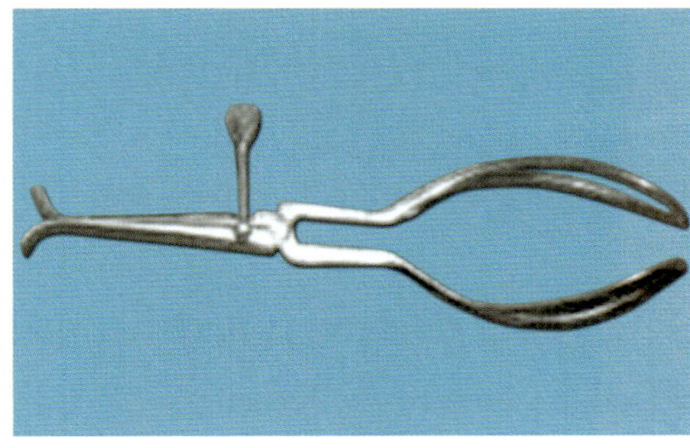

Fig. 37: Long-curved obstetrics forceps

Uses

- Delay in the second stage
- *Fetal indications*:
  - Appearance of fetal distress in the second stage when the prospect of vaginal delivery is safe
  - Cord prolapse
  - Aftercoming head of breech
  - Low-birthweight baby
  - Postmaturity
- *Maternal indications:*
  - Maternal distress
  - Preeclampsia
  - Postcesarean pregnancy
  - Heart disease.

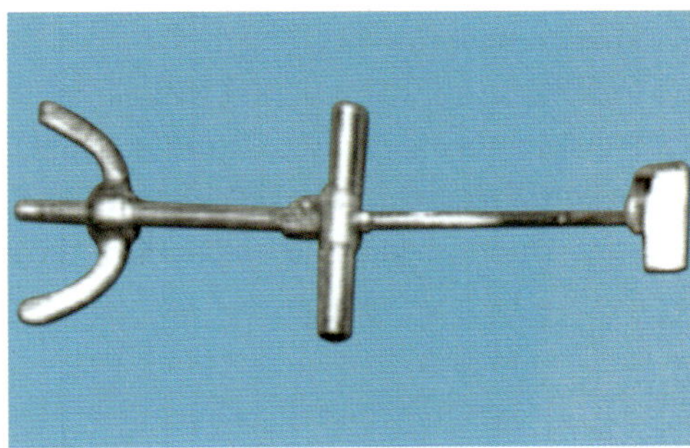

Fig. 38: Axis-traction device

WRIGLEY'S FORCEPS (FIG. 39)

Material: Stainless steel

Sterilization: (i) autoclaving (ii) boiling

Measurement: Length 27.5 cm, light construction, English lock.

Use

Used for low forceps delivery.

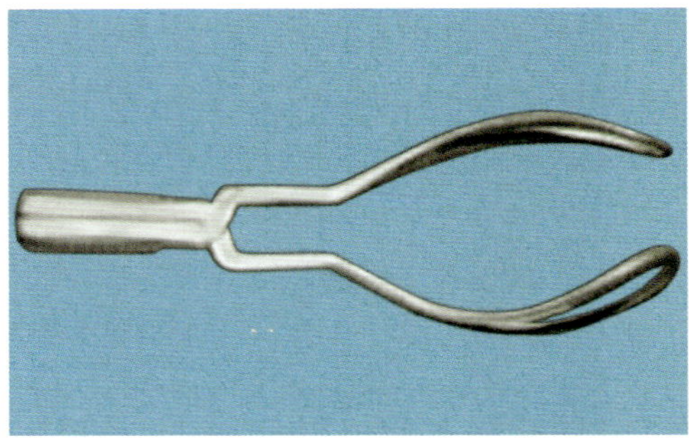

Fig. 39: Wrigley's forceps

KIELLAND'S FORCEPS (FIG. 40)

Material: Stainless steel

Sterilization: (i) autoclaving, (ii) boiling

Measurement: Length 40 cm, straight obstetric forceps without any axis traction device. It has got a sliding lock which facilitates correction of synclitism of the head.

Use

Same as other obstetric forceps.

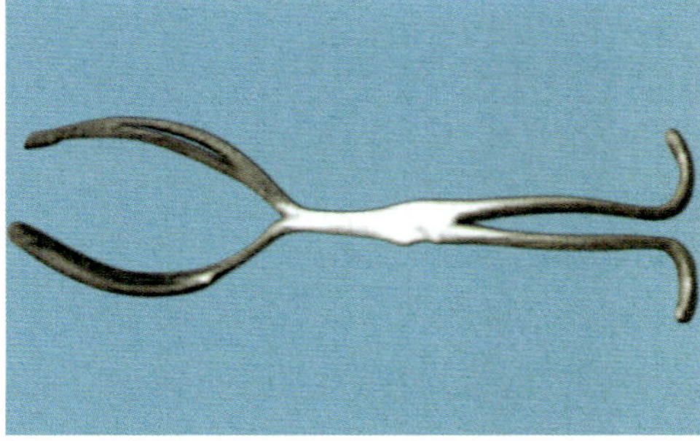

Fig. 40: Keilland's forceps

MIXTER FORCEPS (FIG. 41)

Material: Stainless steel

Sterilization: Autoclaving and boiling

Uses

- To ligate internal iliac artery
- Can be used for ligating any vessel.

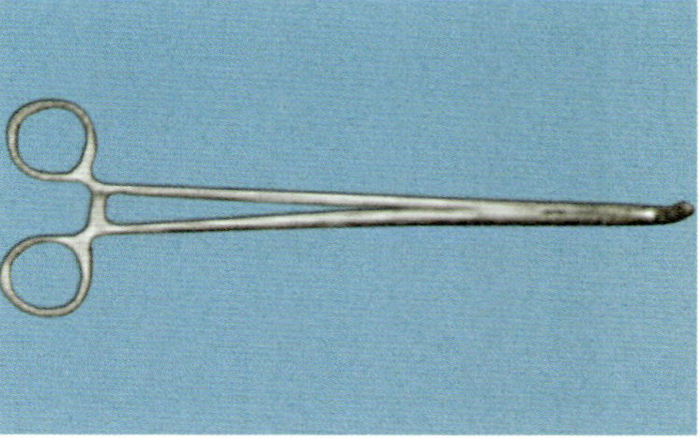

Fig. 41: Mixter forceps

SUCTION CANNULA (FIG. 42)

Material: Stainless steel, plastic

Sterilization: Autoclaving or boiling for stainless steel; gamma irradiation for plastic.

Uses

- First trimester MTP
- Inevitable abortion in first trimester
- Flexible plastic cannula for menstrual regulation
- Suction evacuation of vesicular mole
- Large suction cannula for second trimester pregnancy termination.

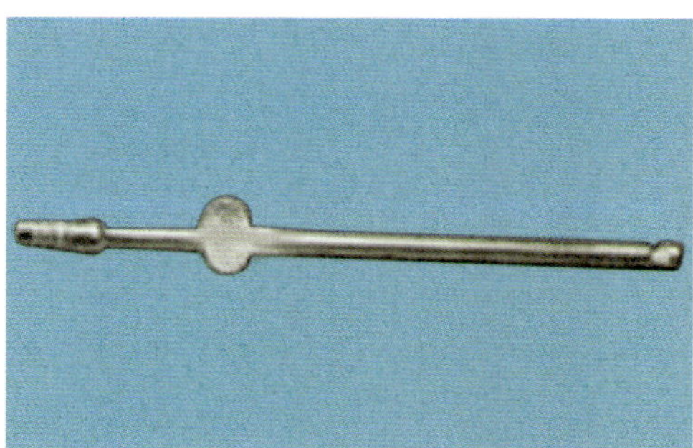

Fig. 42: Suction cannula

DOYEN'S MYOMA SCREW (FIG. 43)

Material: Stainless steel

Sterilization: (i) autoclaving, (ii) boiling.

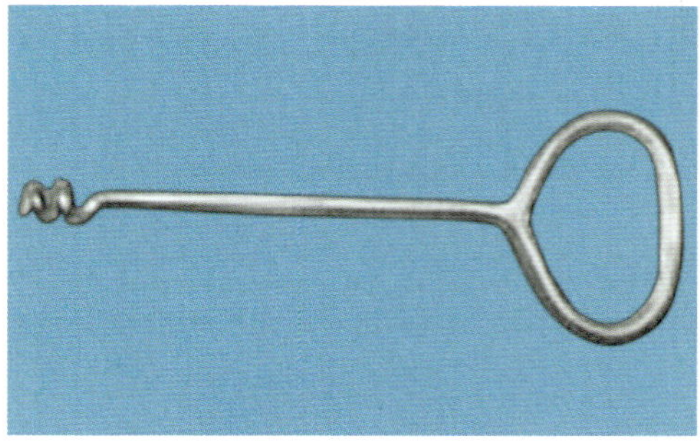

Fig. 43: Doyen's myoma screw

Use

To hold steady and apply traction on a fibroid during abdominal vaginal myomectomy.

SHIRODKAR CERVICAL CERCLAGE NEEDLE (FIG. 44)

Material: Stainless steel

Sterilization: Autoclaving

Parts: Business end—5 cm half circle needle with a blunt tip and a subterminal broad eye, short handle with serrations. Two needles—right and left sided.

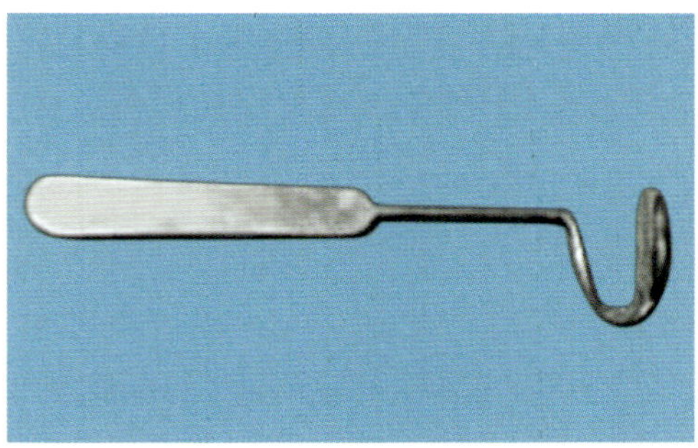

Fig. 44: Shirodkar's needle

Use

Shirodkar cervical circlage operation for treatment of incompetent os.

OLDHAM'S PERFORATOR (FIG. 45)

Material: Stainless steel

Sterilization: (i) autoclaving, (ii) boiling

The blades are as in Simpson's perforator, but have only one shoulder. There is neither any spring nor any lock.

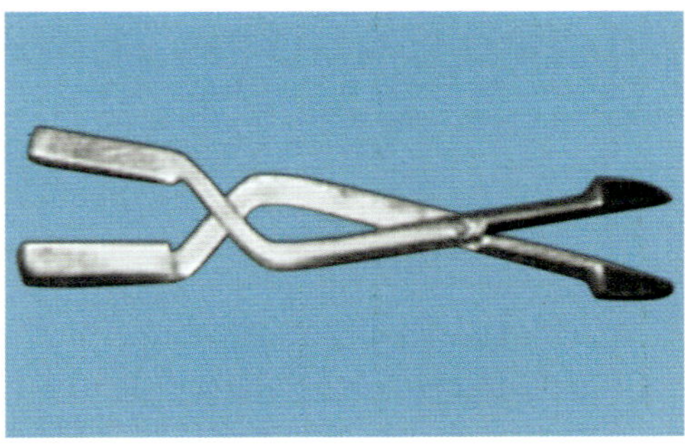

Fig. 45: Oldham's perforator

Use

- Craniotomy
  - Opening fetal thorax or abdomen for evisceration.

SIMPSON'S PERFORATOR (FIG. 46)

Material: Stainless steel

Sterilization: (i) autoclaving, (ii) boiling

Its blade has triangular tips with outer cutting edges. There are two shoulders on the blades. There is a locking system between the ends of the handles which locks the blades in closed position.

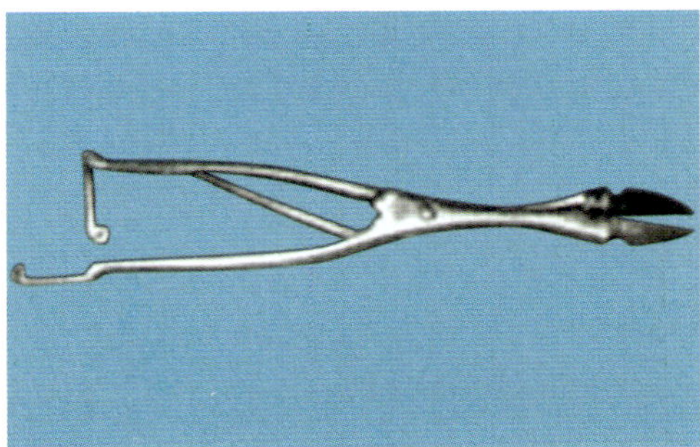

Fig. 46: Simpson's perforator

Use

Same as Oldham's perforator.

BRAUN'S CRANIOCLAST (FIG. 47)

Material: Stainless steel

Sterilization: (i) autoclaving, (ii) boiling.

Uses

- To crush the vault of skull after craniotomy
- To crush the base of skull after craniotomy
- To break up the vault of skull and remove it piecemeal
- To extract the fetal head after craniotomy and crushing.

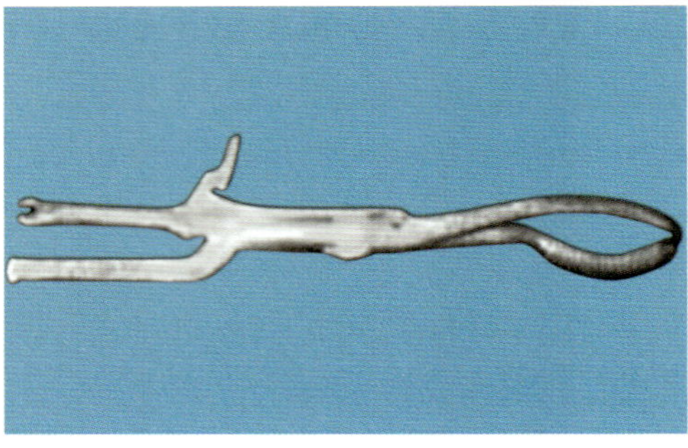

Fig. 47: Braun's cranioclast

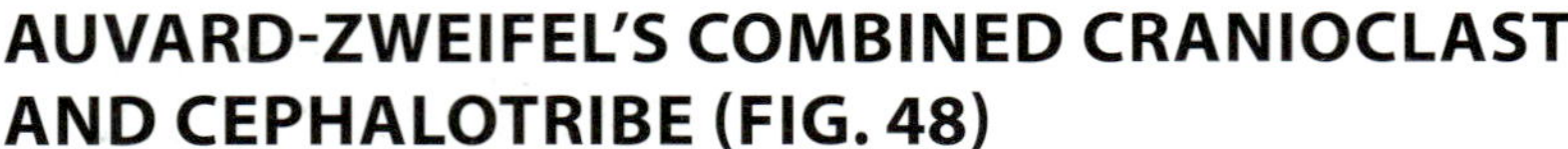

AUVARD-ZWEIFEL'S COMBINED CRANIOCLAST AND CEPHALOTRIBE (FIG. 48)

Material: Stainless steel

Sterilization: (i) autoclaving, (ii) boiling.

Uses

- To crush the vault and base of fetal skull after craniotomy
- To extract fetal head after craniotomy and crushing
- Blades 1 and 2 can be used as cranioclast.

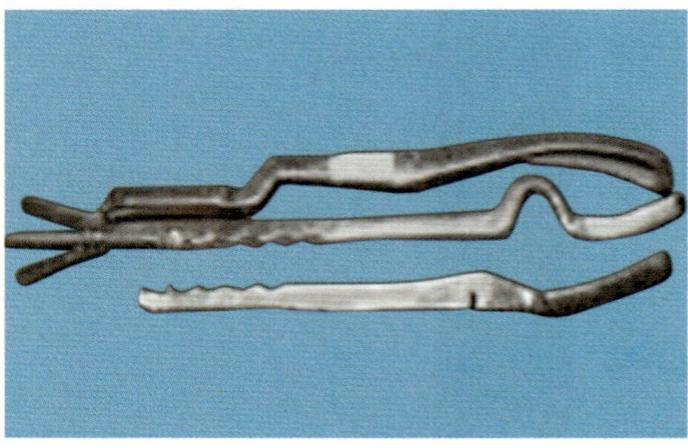

Fig. 48: Auvard-Weifel's combined cranioclast and cephalotribe

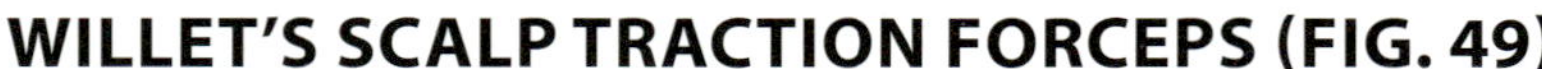

WILLET'S SCALP TRACTION FORCEPS (FIG. 49)

Material: Stainless steel

Sterilization: (i) autoclaving, (ii) boiling.

Uses

- To control bleeding due to degree 1 or 2 placenta previa
- To give traction on fetal head after craniotomy, to hasten delivery
- To give scalp traction to deliver fetal head during cesarean section
- Scalp traction to prevent recurrence of cord prolapse after replacement of the prolapsed cord above the level of fetal head.

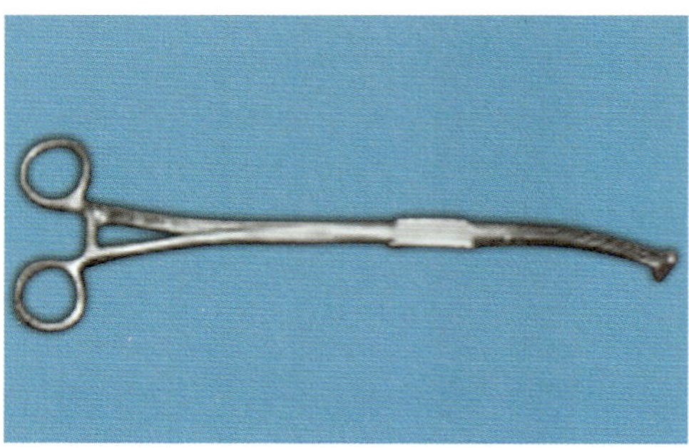

Fig. 49: Willet's scalp traction forceps

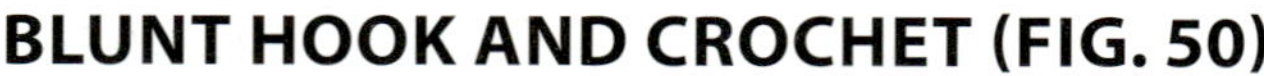

BLUNT HOOK AND CROCHET (FIG. 50)

Material: Stainless steel

Sterilization: (i) autoclaving, (ii) boiling.

Uses

- Uses for the hook:
  - To apply groin traction in case of a breech presentation
  - To pull down a fetal leg in case of a transverse lie
- Uses of the crochet:
  - To extract decapitated head
  - To aid delivery of fetal head after craniotomy.

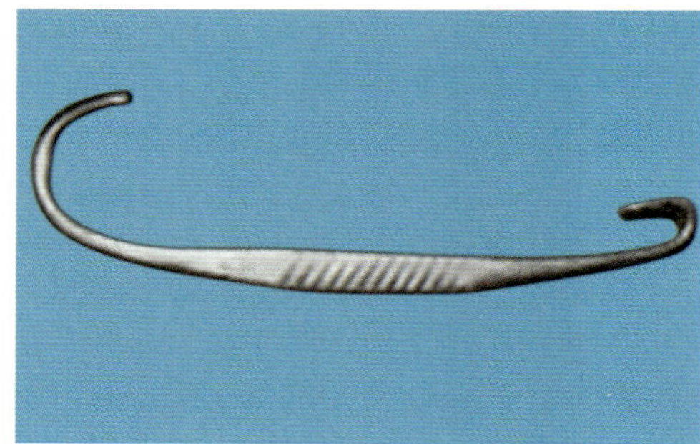

Fig. 50: Blunt hook and crochet

MARTIN'S PELVIMETER (FIG. 51)

Material: Stainless steel.

Uses

The instrument was used in past for external pelvimetry. Various diameters such as external conjugate, intercristal, intertuberous, interspinous diameters were measured in the past.

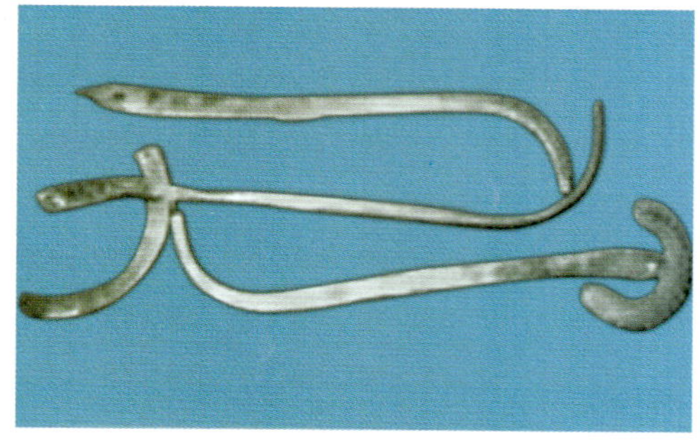

Fig. 51: Martin's pelvimeter

RUBBER RING PESSARY (FIG. 52)

Material: Rubber or polyethylene

Sterilization: Plastic pessaries available presterilized; rubber ring pessaries can be sterilized by chemical methods.

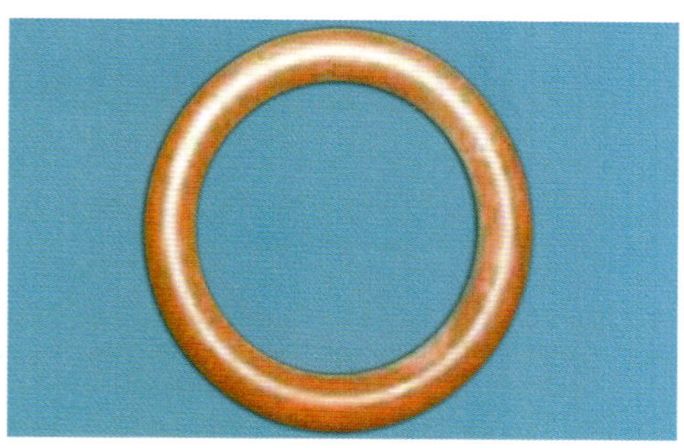

Fig. 52: Rubber ring pessary

Use

In uterocervical descent.

Indications

- Pregnancy up to 12–14 weeks
- During lactation
- When further child bearing is intended in near future
- When surgery is contraindicated in a patient
- If patient refuses operation
- As a therapeutic test to confirm whether the symptoms are due to prolapse
- To promote healing of the decubitus ulcer prior to surgery.

Action

Supports the uterus by resting on the two levator ani muscles acting as shelves.

Index

Page numbers followed by *f*, *b* and *t* indicate figure, box and table respectively.

A

B

C

D

E

F

G

I

J

K

L

M

R

T

U

V